COMBAT AND OPERATIONAL BEHAVIORAL HEALTH

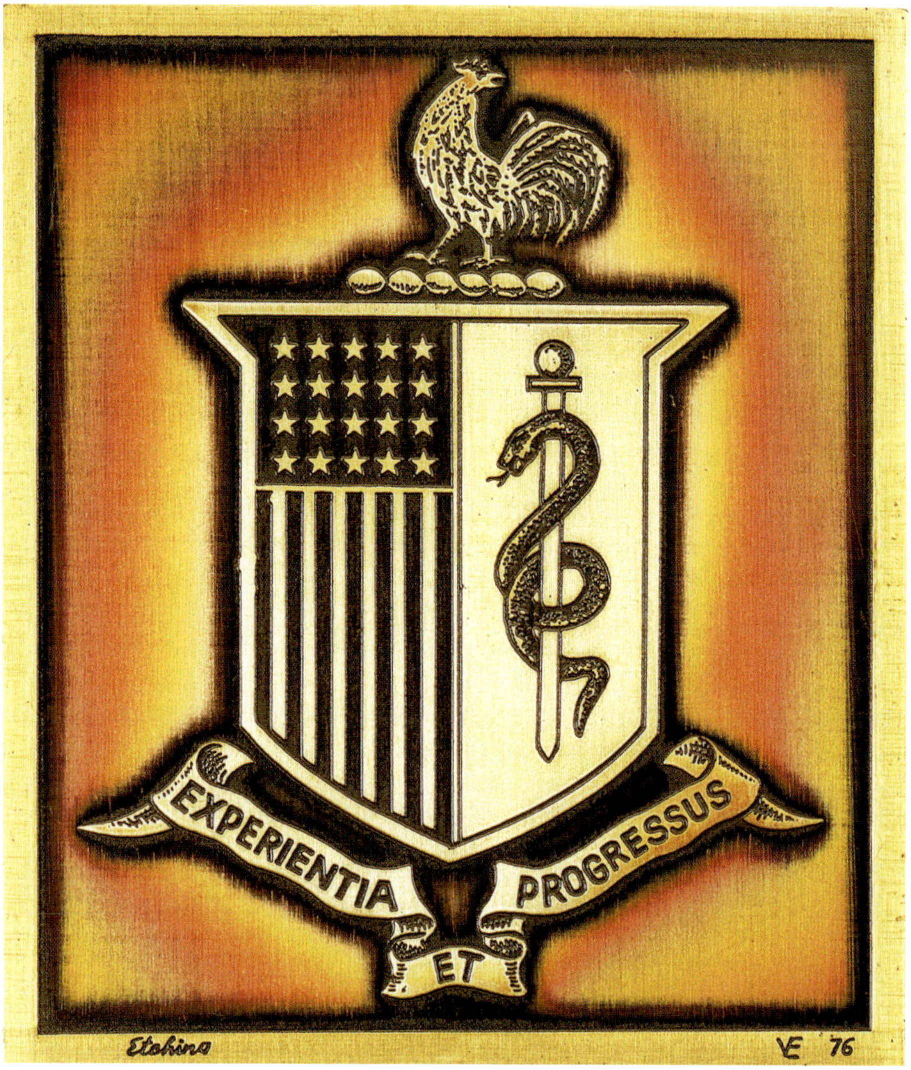

The Coat of Arms
1818
Medical Department of the Army

A 1976 etching by Vassil Ekimov of an original color print that appeared in *The Military Surgeon*, Vol XLI, No 2, 1917

This book is dedicated to the many professionals committed to diagnosing and treating combat and operational stress casualties. These include our predecessors—Doctors Frank Jones, Kenneth Artiss, and Albert Glass—as well as the many who worked on this project, and those who will no doubt labor many years from now on the next volume in this series. All of these caregivers pursue this effort not just to conserve the nation's fighting strength. They also believe, as do all military personnel, that we take care of our own—the service members who face the difficulties of combat and the families who support them.

The *TMM* Series

Published Textbooks

- Medical Consequences of Nuclear Warfare (1989)
- Conventional Warfare: Ballistic, Blast, and Burn Injuries (1991)
- Occupational Health: The Soldier and the Industrial Base (1993)
- Military Dermatology (1994)
- Military Psychiatry: Preparing in Peace for War (1994)
- Anesthesia and Perioperative Care of the Combat Casualty (1995)
- War Psychiatry (1995)
- Medical Aspects of Chemical and Biological Warfare (1997)
- Rehabilitation of the Injured Soldier, Volume 1 (1998)
- Rehabilitation of the Injured Soldier, Volume 2 (1999)
- Medical Aspects of Harsh Environments, Volume 1 (2001)
- Medical Aspects of Harsh Environments, Volume 2 (2002)
- Ophthalmic Care of the Combat Casualty (2003)
- Military Medical Ethics, Volume 1 (2003)
- Military Medical Ethics, Volume 2 (2003)
- Military Preventive Medicine, Volume 1 (2003)
- Military Preventive Medicine, Volume 2 (2005)
- Recruit Medicine (2006)
- Medical Aspects of Biological Warfare (2007)
- Medical Aspects of Chemical Warfare (2008)
- Care of the Combat Amputee (2009)
- Combat and Operational Behavioral Health (2011)

For sale by the Superintendent of Documents, U.S. Government Printing Office
Internet: bookstore.gpo.gov Phone: toll free (866) 512-1800; DC area (202) 512-1800
Fax: (202) 512-2104 Mail: Stop IDCC, Washington, DC 20402-0001

ISBN 978-0-16-088756-7

Textbooks of Military Medicine

Published by the

Office of The Surgeon General
Department of the Army, United States of America

and

US Army Medical Department Center and School
Fort Sam Houston, Texas

Editor in Chief
Martha K. Lenhart, MD, PhD
Colonel, MC, US Army
Director, Borden Institute
Assistant Professor of Surgery
F. Edward Hébert School of Medicine
Uniformed Services University of the Health Sciences

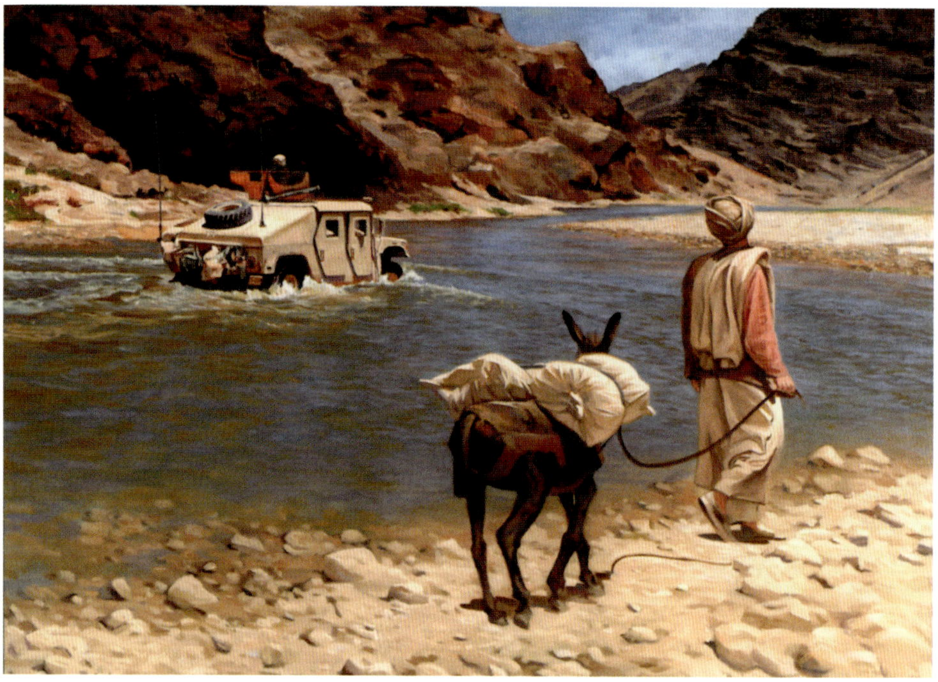

Tracking Bin Laden, by Sergeant First Class Elzie Golden, oil on canvas, 2002. First place winner of the DINFOS MILGRAPH 2002 Military Graphic Competition, fine art category.

Art: Courtesy of the Army Art Collection, US Army Center of Military History.

COMBAT AND OPERATIONAL BEHAVIORAL HEALTH

Senior Editor

ELSPETH CAMERON RITCHIE, MD, MPH
Colonel, Medical Corps, US Army (Retired)
Chief Clinical Officer, District of Columbia Department of Mental Health
Former Psychiatry Consultant to The Army Surgeon General and Director,
Behavioral Health Proponency, Office of The Surgeon General

Office of The Surgeon General
United States Army
Falls Church, Virginia

Borden Institute
Fort Detrick, Maryland

2011

Editorial Staff: Linette Sparacino
Volume Editor

Ronda Lindsay
Technical Editor

Douglas Wise
Illustrator

Joan Redding
Senior Production Editor

Bruce Maston
Illustrator

This volume was prepared for military medical educational use. The focus of the information is to foster discussion that may form the basis of doctrine and policy. The opinions or assertions contained herein are the private views of the authors and are not to be construed as official or as reflecting the views of the Department of the Army or the Department of Defense.

Dosage Selection:

The authors and publisher have made every effort to ensure the accuracy of dosages cited herein. However, it is the responsibility of every practitioner to consult appropriate information sources to ascertain correct dosages for each clinical situation, especially for new or unfamiliar drugs and procedures. The authors, editors, publisher, and the Department of Defense cannot be held responsible for any errors found in this book.

Use of Trade or Brand Names:

Use of trade or brand names in this publication is for illustrative purposes only and does not imply endorsement by the Department of Defense.

Neutral Language:

Unless this publication states otherwise, masculine nouns and pronouns do not refer exclusively to men.

Published by the Office of The Surgeon General at TMM Publications
Borden Institute
Fort Detrick, Maryland

Library of Congress Cataloging-in-Publication Data

Combat and operational behavioral health / senior editor, Elspeth Cameron Ritchie.
p. ; cm. -- (TMM series)
Includes bibliographical references and index.
1. Veterans--Mental health. 2. Post-traumatic stress disorder. 3. Combat--Psychological aspects. 4. War neuroses--Prevention. I. Ritchie, Elspeth Cameron. II. United States. Dept. of the Army. Office of the Surgeon General. III. Borden Institute (U.S.) IV. Series: Textbooks of military medicine.
[DNLM: 1. Combat Disorders--prevention & control. 2. Combat Disorders--psychology. 3. Military Personnel--psychology. 4. Military ychiatry. 5. Veterans--psychology. 6. Veterans Health. WM 184]
RC550.C653 2011
616.85'212--dc23

2011017013

PRINTED IN THE UNITED STATES OF AMERICA

18, 17, 16, 15, 14, 13, 12, 11 5 4 3 2 1

Contents

Contributors

AMY B. ADLER, PhD
Research Psychologist, US Army Research Unit—Europe, Walter Reed Army Institute of Research, CMR 442, APO AE 09042-1030

GEORGE N. APPENZELLER, MD
Lieutenant Colonel, Medical Corps, US Army; Commander, US Army Medical Activity, Alaska, 1060 Gaffney Road #7400, Fort Wainwright, Alaska 99703-7400; formerly, Deputy Commander for Clinical Services, Command Group, Winn Army Community Hospital, Fort Stewart, Georgia

BRYAN L. BACON, DO
Major, Medical Corps, US Army; Disaster Psychiatry Fellow, Department of Psychiatry, Uniformed Services University of the Health Sciences, 4301 Jones Bridge Road, Bethesda, Maryland 20814; formerly, Chief, Behavioral Health, Bavaria Medical Department, Vilseck, Germany

MONTY T. BAKER, PhD
Major, Biomedical Sciences Corps, US Air Force; Director of Clinical Research, Warrior Resiliency Program, San Antonio Military Medical Center, 2200 Bergquist Drive, Suite 1, Lackland Air Force Base, Texas 78236; formerly, Element Leader, Mental Health Clinic, 59th Military Health System, Lackland Air Force Base, Texas

MATTHEW J. BARRY, DO
Major, Medical Corps, US Army Reserve; Staff Psychiatrist, Department of Behavioral Health, Rochester Veterans Affairs Outpatient Clinic, 465 Westfall Road, Rochester, New York 14620; formerly, Major, Medical Corps, US Army; Chief of Psychiatric Service USA MEDDAC and 10th Mountain Division Psychiatrist, Fort Drum, New York

ALFONSO R. BATRES, PhD
Chief Officer and Director, Readjustment Counseling Service, Department of Veterans Affairs, 810 Vermont Avenue NW, Washington, DC 20420

TRISHA BENDER, MD
Major, Medical Corps, US Army; Division Psychiatrist, 25th Infantry Division Headquarters, Building 580, DIVSURG CELL, Schofield Barracks, Hawaii 95857-6000; formerly, Child and Adolescent Fellow, Tripler Army Medical Center, Honolulu, Hawaii

DAVID M. BENEDEK, MD
Colonel, Medical Corps, US Army; Professor and Deputy Chair, Department of Psychiatry, Uniformed Services University of the Health Sciences, 4301 Jones Bridge Road, Bethesda, Maryland 20814

RICHARD D. BERGTHOLD, PsyD
Commander, Medical Service Corps, US Navy; Chief of Staff, Wounded, Ill and Injured, Bureau of Medicine and Surgery, 2300 E Street NW, Washington, DC 20372

GRAEME C. BICKNELL, PhD, LISW
Lieutenant Colonel, Medical Service Corps, US Army; Deputy Chief, Behavioral Health Division, US Medical Command, Building 2792, Room 112, 2050 Worth Road, Fort Sam Houston, San Antonio, Texas 78234-6010

NANCY BLACK, MD
Colonel, Medical Corps, US Army; Training and Program Director, National Capital Consortium of Child and Adolescent Psychiatry Fellowships, Department of Psychiatry, Walter Reed Army Medical Center, Borden Pavilion, 6900 Georgia Avenue NW, Washington, DC 20307-5001

PAUL D. BLIESE, PhD
Colonel, Medical Service Corps, US Army; Director, Psychiatry and Neuroscience, Walter Reed Army Institute of Research, 503 Robert Grant Avenue, Silver Spring, Maryland 20910

ANDREE BOUTERIE, MD
Staff Psychiatrist, Psychiatry Consultation Liaison Service, Walter Reed Army Medical Center, 6900 Georgia Avenue NW, Washington, DC 20307-5100

WAYNE BOYD, MDiv
Colonel, Chaplain Corps, US Army; Staff Officer, Comprehensive Soldier Fitness, Headquarters, Department of the Army, Zachary Taylor Building (NC3), 2530 Crystal Drive, Room 512B, Arlington, Virginia 22202; formerly, Program Manager, Directorate of Health Promotion and Wellness, US Army Center for Health Promotion and Preventive Medicine, Aberdeen Proving Ground, Maryland

CHAD BRADFORD, MD
Commander, Medical Corps, US Navy; Division Psychiatrist, 2nd Marine Division, Division Surgeon's Office, Attn: Division Psychiatry, HQBN 2MAR DIV, Camp Lejeune, North Carolina 28547; formerly, Forensic Psychiatry Fellow, National Capital Consortium, Washington, DC

JOHN C. BRADLEY, MD
Colonel, Medical Corps, US Army; Chair, Department of Psychiatry, Borden Pavilion, Room 2022, Walter Reed Army Medical Center, 6900 Georgia Avenue NW, Washington, DC 20307; Psychiatry Consultant, North Atlantic Regional Medical Command and Vice Chair, Department of Psychiatry, Uniformed Services University of the Health Sciences, Bethesda, Maryland

JILL E. BREITBACH, PsyD
Major, Medical Service Corps, US Army; Neuropsychologist, Department of Psychology, Evans Army Community Hospital, USAMEDDAC, 1650 Cochrane Circle, Fort Carson, Colorado 80913; formerly, Group Psychologist, 1st Special Warfare Training Group, Fort Bragg, North Carolina

STEVEN BREWSTER, MD, MPH
Colonel, Medical Corps, US Army; Commander, US Army Medical Activity–Bavaria, Vilseck, Germany, Unit 28038, APO AE 09112; formerly, Director, Epidemiology and Disease Surveillance, US Army Center for Health Promotion and Preventive Medicine, Public Health Command, Aberdeen Proving Ground, Maryland

SUSAN MILLER BRIGGS, MD, MPH
Associate Professor of Surgery, Harvard Medical School, Director, International Trauma and Disaster Institute, Massachusetts General Hospital, 55 Fruit Street, White 506, Boston, Massachusetts 02114

TERESA L. BRININGER, PhD, CHT, OTR/L
Lieutenant Colonel, Medical Specialist Corps, US Army; Deputy for Rehabilitation and Reintegration, Telemedicine and Advanced Technology Research Center, Medical Research and Materiel Command, 504 Scott Street, Building 722, Room 30, Fort Detrick, Maryland 21702

MILLARD D. BROWN, MD
Major, Medical Corps, US Army; Psychiatry Residency Director, Department of Psychiatry, Tripler Army Medical Center, 1 Jarrett White Road, Honolulu, Hawaii 96859

EDWARD A. BRUSHER, LCSW, BCD
Lieutenant Colonel, Medical Service Corps, US Army; Deputy Director, Behavioral Health Proponency, Office of The Surgeon General, 5109 Leesburg Pike, Skyline 6, Suite 693, Falls Church, Virginia 22041-3258; formerly, Combat Operational Stress Control Program Manager, US Army Medical Command, Fort Sam Houston, Texas

GABRIELLE BRYEN, MSW, LCSW
Major, Medical Service Corps, US Army; Deputy Chief, Department of Social Work, Womack Army Medical Center, Stop A, Fort Bragg, North Carolina 28310; formerly, Brigade Behavioral Health Officer, 3rd Brigade Combat Team, 4th Infantry Division, Fort Carson, Colorado

JAMES P. BURNS, OTR/L, MOT
Major, Medical Specialist Corps, US Army; Occupational Therapist, Department of Orthopaedics and Rehabilitation, Building 2, Room 3J04, Walter Reed Army Medical Center, 6900 Georgia Avenue, NW, Washington, DC 20307-5001; formerly, Chief Occupational Therapist, Department of Surgery, Fort Jackson, South Carolina

DANIEL J. BUSHEME, MA, LCDC
Lieutenant Colonel, Nurse Corps, US Air Force; Chief, Mental Health Nursing, US Air Force Medical Operations Agency, 485 Quentin Roosevelt Road, Suite 400, San Antonio, Texas 78226-2017; formerly, Deputy Squadron Commander and Inpatient Mental Health Flight Commander, Travis Air Force Base, California

NORMAN M. CAMP, MD
Colonel, US Army (Retired); 3105-D Stony Point Road, Richmond, Virginia 23235; Clinical Professor of Psychiatry, Department of Psychiatry, Medical College of Virginia, Virginia Commonwealth University, Richmond, Virginia 23298

JUSTIN S. CAMPBELL, PhD
Lieutenant, Medical Service Corps, US Navy; Deployment Health Senior Analyst, Department of the Navy, Bureau of Medicine and Surgery, Deployment Health (M3C3), 2300 E Street NW, Washington, DC 20372

RONALD CAMPBELL, MD
Chief, Inpatient Psychiatry Service, Department of Behavioral Health, Landstuhl Regional Medical Center, CMR 462, APO AE 09180

RICK L. CAMPISE, PhD, ABPP
Colonel, Biomedical Sciences Corps, US Air Force; Commander, 559th Medical Group, 1920 Biggs Avenue, Lackland Air Force Base, Texas 78236; formerly, Commander, 1st Medical Operations Squadron, Langley Air Force Base, Virginia

JANIS CARLTON, MD, PhD
Commander, Medical Corps, US Navy; Department Head, Psychological Health and Traumatic Brain Injury, Building 7, Room 600, National Naval Medical Center, 8901 Wisconsin Avenue, Bethesda, Maryland 20889; formerly, Department Head, Mental Health, Naval Hospital, Camp Lejeune, North Carolina

CARL A. CASTRO, PhD
Colonel, Medical Service Corps, US Army; Director, Military Operational Medicine Research Program, US Army Medical Research and Materiel Command, 504 Scott Street, Fort Detrick, Maryland 21702-5012; formerly, Chief, Department of Military Psychiatry and Chief, Soldier and Family Readiness, Walter Reed Army Institute of Research, Silver Spring, Maryland

ASHLEY CHATIGNY, DO
Captain, Medical Corps, US Army; Fellow, Department of Child and Adolescent Psychiatry, Tripler Army Medical Center, 1 Jarrett White Road, Honolulu, Hawaii 96859-5000

RYO S. CHUN, MD
Colonel, US Army (Retired); Clinical Director, Child and Adolescent Psychiatry Service, Department of Psychiatry, Walter Reed Army Medical Center, 6900 Georgia Avenue NW, Washington, DC 20307; formerly, Chief, Child and Adolescent Psychiatry Service, Department of Psychiatry, Walter Reed Army Medical Center, Washington, DC

JEFFREY COADY, PsyD
Commander, Scientist Corps, US Public Health Service; Deputy Team Leader, US Public Health Service Disaster Mental Health Team II, Department of Health and Human Services, 233 North Michigan Avenue, Suite 600, Chicago, Illinois 60601

PAUL COLTHIRST, DDS, MS
Major, Dental Corps, US Army; Dental Public Health, Department of Leadership Development, US Army Medical Department Center and School, 2250 Stanley Road, Fort Sam Houston, Texas 78234-6100; formerly, Staff Officer, Dental Command Headquarters, Fort Sam Houston, Texas

MARC A. COOPER, MD
Chief, Community Mental Health Service, Moncrief Army Community Hospital, 4500 Stuart Street, Fort Jackson, South Carolina 29207; formerly, Major, Medical Corps, US Army; OIF 05-07 Theater Mental Health Consultant, Task Force 30th Medical Brigade, Baghdad, Iraq

ANTHONY COX, MSW
Lieutenant Colonel, Medical Service Corps, US Army; Social Work Consultant, Great Plains Regional Medical Command; Chief, Social Work, Brooke Army Medical Center, 3851 Roger Brooke Drive, Fort Sam Houston, Texas 78234

STEPHEN J. COZZA, MD
Colonel, US Army (Retired); Associate Director, Center for the Study of Traumatic Stress, and Professor, Department of Psychiatry, Uniformed Services University of the Health Sciences, 4301 Jones Bridge Road, Bethesda, Maryland 20814; formerly, Chief, Department of Psychiatry, Walter Reed Army Medical Center, Washington, DC

BRUCE E. CROW, PsyD
Colonel, Medical Service Corps, US Army; Clinical Psychology Consultant to The Surgeon General, US Army, and Director, Warrior Resiliency Program, Southern Regional Medical Command, Brooke Army Medical Center, Fort Sam Houston, Texas 78234

DEBORAH CROWLEY, MD
Captain, Medical Corps, US Army; Child Psychiatry Fellow, Department of Psychiatry, 1 Jarrett White Road, Tripler Army Medical Center, Hawaii 96859

JAMES E. CZARNIK, MD
Colonel, Medical Corps, US Army; Command Surgeon, Joint Special Operations Command, PO Box 70239, Fort Bragg, North Carolina 28307-5000; formerly, Deputy Command Surgeon, US Army Special Operations Command, Fort Bragg, North Carolina

COLIN DANIELS, MD, MBA
Lieutenant Colonel, Medical Corps, US Army; Psychiatrist, Department of Psychiatry, Madigan Army Medical Center, 9040 Fitzsimmons Drive, 7BLM, Tacoma, Washington 98431; formerly, Chief, Behavioral Health Services, 28th Combat Support Hospital, Operation Iraqi Freedom 2003

VIRGIL T. DEAL, MD
Colonel, Medical Corps, US Army; Surgeon, United States Special Operations Command, 7701 Tampa Point Boulevard, MacDill Air Force Base, Florida 33621-5323; formerly, Commander, Walter Reed Health Care System, Washington, DC

GEORGIA DELA CRUZ, DMD, MPH
Lieutenant Colonel, Dental Corps, US Army; Dental Staff Officer, Dental Corps Office, Office of The Surgeon General, US Army, 5109 Leesburg Pike, Suite 682, Falls Church, Virginia 22041; formerly, Army Dental Representative, TriService Center for Oral Health Studies, Uniformed Services University of the Health Sciences, Bethesda, Maryland

JAMES DEMER, MD
Attending Child Psychiatrist, Inpatient Child Psychiatry Service, Hutchings Psychiatric Center, 7682 Warrior's Path, Baldwinsville, New York 13027; formerly, Major, Medical Corps, US Army; Division Psychiatrist, 10th Mountain Division, Fort Drum, New York

CARROLL J. DIEBOLD, MD
Colonel, Medical Corps, US Army; Chief, Department of Psychiatry, 1 Jarrett White Road, Tripler Army Medical Center, Honolulu, Hawaii 96859

THOMAS F. DITZLER, PhD
Director of Research, Department of Psychiatry, Tripler Army Medical Center, 1 Jarrett White Road, Honolulu, Hawaii 96859

MICHAEL E. DOYLE, MD
Lieutenant Colonel, Medical Corps, US Army; Deputy Commander for Clinical Services, USAMEDDAC West Point, 900 Washington Road, West Point, New York 10996; formerly, Commander, US Army Health Clinic, Wiesbaden, Germany

GARY J. DROUILLARD, MD
Lieutenant Colonel, Medical Corps, US Army; Chief, Chemical Addiction Treatment Service, Department of Psychiatry 1 Jarrett White Road, Tripler Army Medical Center, Hawaii 96859; formerly, Chief, Consultation Liaison Psychiatry, Tripler Army Medical Center, Honolulu, Hawaii

JASON E. DUCKWORTH, DMin, MDiv
Lieutenant Colonel, Chaplain Corps, US Army; Garrison Chaplain, Religious Support Office, US Army Garrison, Heidelberg, Germany, CMR 419 Box 1876, APO AE 09102; formerly, Training Developer, Chaplain Basic Officer Leader Course, US Army Chaplain Center and School, Fort Jackson, South Carolina

MARK EARNSHAW, BA(Hons), MSc
Lieutenant Colonel, QARANC, Ministry of Defence, St Georges Court, Bloomsbury Way, London, WC1A 2SH, United Kingdom; formerly, Research Fellow, Academic Centre for Defence Mental Health, London, United Kingdom

MARY W. ERICKSON, MAOL, OTR/L
Colonel, US Army (Retired); formerly, Reintegration Branch Chief, Proponency Office for Rehabilitation and Reintegeration, The Office of The Surgeon General, US Army, 5109 Leesburg Pike, Suite 684, Falls Church, Virginia

MICHAEL E. FARAN, MD, PhD
Colonel, US Army (Retired); Director, Child, Adolescent, and Family Behavior Health Proponency, Madigan Army Medical Center, Madigan Annex Building 9913A, Ramp 2, McKinnley Road, Tacoma, Washington 98431; Director, School Based Mental Health, Child and Adolescent Psychiatry Service, Department of Psychiatry, Tripler Army Medical Center, Honolulu, Hawaii

CHARLES M. FLORA, MSW
Associate Director, Readjustment Counseling Service, Department of Veterans Affairs, 810 Vermont Avenue NW, Washington, DC 20420

ROBERT D. FORSTEN, DO
Colonel, Medical Corps, US Army; Command Psychiatrist, US Army Special Operations Command (AOMD), 2929 Desert Storm Drive (Stop A), Fort Bragg, North Carolina 28310-9110; formerly, Staff Psychiatrist, Department of Psychiatry, Walter Reed Army Medical Center, Washington, DC

KELLY FORYS, PhD
Psychologist, Department of Outpatient Behavioral Health, Landstuhl Regional Medical Center, CMR 402, Box 1045, APO AE 09180; formerly, Psychologist, US Army Center for Health Promotion and Preventive Medicine, Aberdeen Proving Ground, Maryland

PETER FREDERICH, MDiv
Lieutenant Colonel, Chaplain Corps, US Army; Family Ministries Officer, Directorate of Ministry Initiatives, US Army Chief of Chaplains Office, 1421 Jefferson Davis Highway, Suite 10600, Arlington, Virginia 22202; formerly, Director, US Army Family Life Chaplain Training Center, Fort Benning, Georgia

LOUIS M. FRENCH, PsyD
Director, Traumatic Brain Injury Service, Defense and Veterans Brain Injury Center and Department of Orthopaedics and Rehabilitation, Walter Reed Army Medical Center, 6900 Georgia Avenue NW, Washington, DC 20307; Department of Neurology, Uniformed Services University of the Health Sciences, Bethesda, Maryland

GREGORY A. GAHM, PhD
Colonel, Medical Service Corps, US Army; Chief, Department of Psychology, Madigan Army Medical Center, 9933C West Hayes Street, Fort Lewis, Washington 98431

THOMAS A. GASKIN, PhD
Commander, US Navy (Retired); Director of Combat Operational Stress Control, US Marine Corps, Manpower and Reserve Affairs, Personal and Family Readiness Division, 3280 Russell Road, Quantico, Virginia 22134; formerly, Head, Combat and Operational Stress Control Program, Headquarters, US Marine Corps, Quantico, Virginia

MARSHALL J. GOBY, PhD
Colonel, US Army (Retired); Team Leader/Supervisory Psychologist, Veterans Affairs Readjustment Counseling Service, Palm Beach Veterans Center, 2311 10th Avenue North, #13, Lake Worth, Florida 33461; formerly, Reserve Psychology Consultant, Office of The Surgeon General, US Army, Falls Church, Virginia

EILEEN U. GODINEZ, PhD
Inspector General Chief, Inspections and Outreach Branch, US European Command, CMR 480, Box 1865, APO AE 09128; formerly, Chief, Plans Analysis and Integration Office, US Army Garrison, Hawaii

GEOFFREY GRAMMER, MD
Lieutenant Colonel, Medical Corps, US Army; Chief, Inpatient Psychiatry, Department of Psychiatry, Walter Reed Army Medical Center, 6900 Georgia Avenue NW, Washington, DC 20307

SHARETTE KIRSTEN GRAY, MD
Lieutenant Colonel, Medical Corps, US Army; Chief, Hospital and Administrative Psychiatry Services, Department of Behavioral Health, Carl R. Darnell Army Medical Center, Building 36000, Darnell Loop, Fort Hood, Texas 76544; formerly, Division Psychiatrist, 4th Infantry Division, Fort Hood, Texas

NEIL GREENBERG, MD
Commander, Medical Corps, United Kingdom Armed Forces; Defence Professor of Mental Health, King's College, London, Weston Education Centre, Cutcombe Road, London SE5 9RJ; formerly, Senior Lecturer in Military Psychiatry, Academic Center for Defence Mental Health, King's College, London

THOMAS GRIEGER, MD
Captain, US Navy (Retired); Associate Professor, Department of Psychiatry, Uniformed Services University of the Health Sciences, 4301 Jones Bridge Road, Bethesda, Maryland 20814

PAUL HAMMER, MD
Captain, Medical Corps, US Navy; Director, Naval Center for Combat and Operational Stress Control, 34960 Bob Wilson Drive, Suite 400, San Diego, California 92134-6400

DARYL HAWKINS, PhD
Alcohol and Drug Control Officer, Army Substance Abuse Program, Building 6, Room 2066, Walter Reed Army Medical Center, 6900 Georgia Avenue NW, Washington, DC 20307-5001

KATHY HELMICK, MS, CNRN, CRNP
Senior Executive Director, Traumatic Brain Injury, Defense Center of Excellence for Psychological Health and Traumatic Brain Injury, 1335 East-West Highway, 9th Floor, Suite 700, Silver Spring, MD 20910; formerly, Deputy Director, Defense and Veterans Brain Injury Center, Walter Reed Army Medical Center, Washington, DC

JEFFREY V. HILL, MD
Lieutenant Colonel, Medical Corps, US Army; Chief, Child and Adolescent Psychiatry, Landstuhl Regional Medical Center, CMR 402 Box 1356, APO AE 09180; formerly, Chief, Outpatient Psychiatry, Landstuhl Regional Medical Center, Landstuhl, Germany

CHARLES W. HOGE, MD
Colonel, US Army (Retired); formerly, Director, Division of Psychiatry and Neuroscience, Walter Reed Army Institute of Research, 503 Robert Grant Avenue, Silver Spring, Maryland 20910

EDMUND G. HOWE, MD, JD
Professor of Psychiatry, Associate Professor of Medicine, and Director, Programs in Medical Ethics, Uniformed Services University of the Health Sciences, 4301 Jones Bridge Road, Bethesda, Maryland 20814; and Senior Scientist, Center for the Study of Traumatic Stress, Bethesda, Maryland; formerly, Major, Medical Corps, US Army

JAMIE HACKER HUGHES, PsychD
Head of Defence Clinical Psychology, Ministry of Defence, Joint Medical Command, Coltman House, Whittington Barracks, Lichfield, United Kingdom WS14 9PY; formerly, Senior Lecturer in Military Psychology, Academic Center for Defence Mental Health, London, United Kingdom

ROBIN A. HURLEY, MD
Associate Director, Education, WG Hefner Veterans Affairs Medical Center (Mailcode 11F), 1601 Brenner Avenue, Salisbury, North Carolina 28144; formerly, Associate Director, Mental Health, WG Hefner Veterans Affairs Medical Center, Salisbury, North Carolina

CHRISTOPHER G. IVANY, MD
Major, Medical Corps, US Army; Psychiatrist, Department of Behavioral Health, Evans Army Community Hospital, Building 7500, 1650 Cochrane Circle, Fort Carson, Colorado 80913; formerly, Division Psychiatrist, 4th Infantry Division, Fort Hood, Texas

DAVID E. JOHNSON, MD
Major, Medical Corps, US Army; Chief, Behavioral Health, Department of Psychiatry, US Army MEDDAC Bavaria, IMEU-SFT-DHR, ATTN: OMDC Schweinfurt, Unit 25850, APO AE 09033

AILEEN KIM, MD
Lieutenant Commander, Medical Corps, US Navy; Staff Psychiatrist, Department of Behavioral Health, Building 7, 3rd Floor, National Naval Medical Center, 8901 Wisconsin Avenue, Bethesda, Maryland 20889; formerly, Chief Resident, Department of Psychiatry, Naval Medical Center Portsmouth, Portsmouth, Virginia

ROBERT L. KOFFMAN, MD, MPH
Captain, Medical Corps, US Navy; Director of Deployment Health, Department of the Navy, Bureau of Medicine and Surgery, Deployment Health, 2300 E Street NW, Washington, DC, 20372

HAROLD KUDLER, MD
Associate Clinical Professor, Department of Psychiatry, Duke University Medical Center, Durham, North Carolina; Associate Director, Mental Illness Research, Education and Clinical Center, Mid-Atlantic Veterans Integrated Service Network (VISN 6), VA Medical Center, 508 Fulton Street, #166A, Durham, North Carolina 27705

R. GREGORY LANDE, DO
Chief, Psychiatry Continuity Service, Department of Psychiatry, Walter Reed Army Medical Center, 6900 Georgia Avenue NW, Building 2, Room 5343, Washington, DC 20307; Clinical Consultant, Walter Reed Army Medical Center Substance Abuse Program, Washington, DC

LISA LANDRY, PhD
Instructor/Writer, Department of Behavioral Health Sciences, Army Medical Department Center and School, 3151 Scott Road, Building 2840, Office 32, Fort Sam Houston, Texas 78234

CHRISTOPHER L. LANGE, MD
Lieutenant Colonel, Medical Corps, US Army; Program Director, National Capital Consortium Forsenic Psychiatry Fellowship Program, Department of Psychiatry, Walter Reed Army Medical Center, 6900 Georgia Avenue NW, Building 6, Room 3038, Washington, DC 20307; formerly, Staff Psychiatrist, Psychiatry Consultation Liaison Service, Walter Reed Army Medical Center, Washington, DC

JENNIFER T. LANGE, MD
Lieutenant Colonel, Medical Corps, US Army; Medical Director, Behavioral Health Clinic, Department of Psychiatry, Walter Reed Army Medical Center, 6900 Georgia Avenue NW, Washington, DC 20307-5001

DOUGLAS H. LEHMAN, MSW, LCSW
Treatment Provider, Department of Behavioral Health and Family Advocacy, Evans Army Community Hospital, 7500 Cochrane Circle, Fort Carson, Colorado 80913

LAURENT S. LEHMANN, MD
Associate Chief Consultant in Mental Health, Office of Mental Health Services, Department of Veterans Affairs, 810 Vermont Avenue NW, Room 966, Washington, DC 20420

BARBARA LEINER, MSW, LCSW-C
Psychiatric Social Worker, Department of Child Psychiatry, Walter Reed Army Medical Center, Borden Pavilion, 6900 Georgia Avenue NW, Washington, DC 20307-5001; formerly, Clinical Case Manager, Department of Child Psychiatry, Kaiser Permanente Mid-Atlantic States, Rockville, Maryland

STEVEN LINDLEY, MD, PhD
Director of Outpatient Mental Health, Department of Veterans Affairs Palo Alto Health Care System, 795 Willow Road, 116R/MHC, Menlo Park, California 94025; and, Associate Professor, Department of Psychiatry, Stanford University, Palo Alto, California

BRETT LITZ, PhD
Professor, Department of Psychiatry, Boston University School of Medicine, 77 East Concord Street, Boston, Massachusetts 02118; Associate Director, Behavioral Sciences Division, Department of Veterans Affairs National Center for Posttraumatic Stress Disorder, White River Junction, Vermont

GAIL H. MANOS, MD
Captain, Medical Corps, US Navy; Navy Psychiatry Specialty Leader and Senior Medical Officer, Director of Mental Health, Naval Medical Center Portsmouth, 620 John Paul Jones Road, Portsmouth, Virginia 23708; formerly, Psychiatry Residency Training Director, Department of Psychiatry, Naval Medical Center Portsmouth, Portsmouth, Virginia

BARBARA A. MARIN, PhD
Integrated Chief, Department of Addictions Treatment and Clinical Director, Army Substance Abuse Program, Walter Reed Army Medical Center, 6900 Georgia Avenue NW, Washington, DC 20307-5001

JEEVENDRA MARTYN, MD
Professor/Chief, Department of Anesthesiology and Critical Care, Harvard Medical School/Shriners Hospital for Children, 51 Blossom Street, Room 206, Boston, Massachusetts 02114

AMY M. MATTILA, MS, MBA
Captain, Medical Specialist Corps, US Army; Chief, Department of Occupational Therapy, Reynolds Army Community Hospital, 4301 Wilson Street, Fort Sill, Oklahoma 73503; formerly, Chief, Occupational Therapy, 254th Medical Detachment (Combat Operational Stress Control), Germany

JAMES E. McCARROLL, PhD, MPH
Colonel, US Army (Retired); Psychologist, Center for the Study of Traumatic Stress and Department of Psychiatry, Room B3068, Uniformed Services University of the Health Sciences, 4301 Jones Bridge Road, Bethesda, Maryland 20814; formerly, Psychologist, Walter Reed Army Institute of Research, Silver Spring, Maryland

KELLY R. McCARTHY, MA
Captain, Nurse Corps, US Air Force; Historian, Peterson Air Force Base, 150 Vandenberg, Suite 110S, Peterson Air Force Base, Colorado 80914; formerly, Chief, Behavioral Health Nursing Management, Life Skills Center, United States Air Force Academy, Colorado Springs, Colorado

KEVIN M. McGUINNESS, PhD
Captain, Scientist Corps, US Public Health Service; Director and Medical Psychologist, HRSA/BCRS National Health Service Corps, Ready Responder Program, Department of Health and Human Services, c/o La Clinica de Familia, 510 East Lisa Drive, Chaparral, New Mexico 88081; formerly, Senior Clinical Scientist, Health and Human Services, US Department of Justice, Bureau of Prisons, Federal Correctional Institution La Tuna, New Mexico

DENNIS McGURK, PhD
Major, Medical Service Corps, US Army; Commander, US Army Medical Research Unit—Europe, Walter Reed Army Institute of Research, CMR 442, Box 777, APO AE 09042

ROBERT C. McKENZIE, DO
Lieutenant Colonel, Medical Corps, US Army; Department of Behavioral Health, US Army Health Clinic-Vicenza, Caserma Ederle, Italy, Unit 31401, Box 13, APO AE 09042

MARGARET A. McNULTY, DrPH
Captain, US Navy (Retired); Assistant Professor, Department of Nursing, Kapiolani Community College, 4303 Diamond Head Road, Honolulu, Hawaii 96816

CORINA MILLER, MSW
Clinical Social Worker, Department of Psychiatry, Walter Reed Army Medical Center, Building 2, Office #6317, 6900 Georgia Avenue NW, Washington, DC 20307-5001; formerly, Clinical Social Worker, National Naval Medical Center, Bethesda, Maryland

CHARLES MILLIKEN, MD
Colonel, Medical Corps, US Army; Program Director, National Capital Consortium Psychosomatic Medicine/Geriatric Psychiatry Fellowship, Walter Reed Army Medical Center, 6900 Georgia Avenue NW, Washington, DC; formerly, Principal Investigator, Division of Psychiatry and Neuroscience, Walter Reed Army Institute of Research, 503 Grant Avenue, Silver Spring, Maryland

ANGELA MOBBS, PsyD
Captain, Medical Service Corps, US Army; Special Forces Assignment and Selection Psychologist, Special Warfare Center and School, Rowe Training Facility, Building T-5167, 1500 Camp Mackall Place, Marston, North Carolina 28363; formerly, Brigade Psychologist, 3rd Brigade Combat Team, 3rd Infantry Division, Fort Benning, Georgia

WALTER MORALES, MSA
Sergeant Major, US Army (Retired); Program Manager, Army Suicide Prevention Program, Army G-1, Headquarters, Department of the Army, 300 Army Pentagon, ATTN: Army G-1 (DAPE-HR), Washington, DC 20310-0300

SCOTT C. MORAN, MD
Major (P), Medical Corps, US Army; Psychiatry Residency Training Program Director, Psychiatry Consultation Liaison Service, Department of Psychiatry, Building 6, Room 2060, Walter Reed Army Medical Center, 6900 Georgia Avenue NW, Washington, DC 20307-5100

ANTHONY J. MORTON, MD
Major, Medical Corps, US Army; Medical Director, Department of Behavioral Health, Moncrief Army Community Hospital, 4500 Stuart Street, Fort Jackson, South Carolina 29207-5720; formerly, Division Psychiatrist, 1st Armored Division, Wiesbaden, Germany

WILLIAM P. NASH, MD
Captain, US Navy (Retired); Assistant Clinical Professor, Department of Psychiatry, University of California at San Diego, 6326 Timarron Cove Lane, Burke, Virginia 22015; formerly, Senior Consultant, Defense Centers of Excellence for Psychological Health and Traumatic Brain Injury, Rosslyn, Virginia

SHARON M. NEWTON, OTR/L, MHS
Lieutenant Colonel, Medical Specialist Corps, US Army; Command Inspector General, 30th Medical Command, CMR 442, APO AE 09042; formerly, Theater Consultant for Combat and Operational Stress Control, Iraq

MARVIN OLESHANSKY, MD
Colonel, US Army (Retired); Staff Psychiatrist, Psychiatric Outpatient Service, Department of Psychiatry, Tripler Army Medical Center, 1 Jarrett White Road, Honolulu, Hawaii 96822; formerly, Staff Psychiatrist, Psychiatry Consultation Liaison Service, Walter Reed Army Medical Center, 6900 Georgia Avenue NW, Washington, DC

VICTORIA W. OLSON, MBA
Executive Director, Hawai'i Army Museum Society, Post Office Box 8064, Honolulu, Hawaii 96830-0064

JESSICA PARKER, PsyD
Captain, Medical Service Corps, US Army; Chief, Warrior Restoration Center, Department of Behavioral Medicine, Winn Army Community Hospital, 541 East 9th Street, Building 359, Fort Stewart, Georgia 31314-5674; formerly, Psychology Resident, Traumatic Brain Injury, Brooke Army Medical Center, San Antonio, Texas

ROSS H. PASTEL, PhD
Lieutenant Colonel, Medical Service Corps, US Army; Chief, Division of Traumatic Brain Injury, Research Directorate, Defense Centers of Excellence for Psychological Health and Traumatic Brain Injury, 1335 East-West Highway, Suite 900, Silver Spring, Maryland 20910; formerly, Assistant Professor, Department of Medical and Clinical Psychology, Uniformed Services University of the Health Sciences, Bethesda, Maryland

SAMUEL E. PAYNE, MD
Colonel, Medical Corps, US Army; Chief, Outpatient Behavioral Health Services, Dwight D. Eisenhower Army Medical Center, Building 300, Room 13A-15, 300 South Hospital Road, Fort Gordon, Georgia 30905

MARY ANN PECHACEK, PsyD, LMFT
Psychologist and Instructor/Writer, Department of Behavioral Health Sciences, Special Subjects Branch, Army Medical Department Center and School, 3151 Scott Road, Building 2840, Office #033-B9, Fort Sam Houston, Texas 78234; formerly, Psychologist and Instructor/Writer, Soldier and Family Support Branch/Special Subjects, Fort Sam Houston, Texas

JON T. PEREZ, PhD
Captain, Scientist Corps, US Public Health Service; Team Leader, US Public Health Service Disaster Mental Health Team II, Department of Health and Human Services, Indian Health Service Headquarters, 801 Thompson Avenue, Suite 300, Rockville, Maryland 20852

ALAN L. PETERSON, PhD, ABPP
Professor, Department of Psychiatry, Mail Code 7792, University of Texas Health Science Center at San Antonio, 7703 Floyd Curl Drive, San Antonio, Texas 78229; formerly, Chair, Department of Psychology, Wilford Hall Medical Center, San Antonio, Texas

KRIS A. PETERSON, MD
Colonel, Medical Corps, US Army; Chief, Department of Psychiatry, Madigan Army Medical Center, Building 9040, Fitzsimmons Drive, Tacoma, Washington 98431; formerly, Child and Adolescent Psychiatry Consultant to The Surgeon General, US Army

SIMON PINCUS, MD
Colonel, US Army (Retired); Clinical Director, Department of Mental Health, McChord Medical Clinic, 690 Barnes Boulevard, Joint Base Lewis-McChord (McChord Field), Washington 98438; formerly, Chief, Inpatient Psychiatry, Madigan Army Medical Center, Tacoma, Washington

CHRISTINE M. PIPER, APRN, BC
Colonel, US Army (Retired); Coaching Trainer/Instructor, LivingWorks, Inc.; formerly, Chief, Soldier and Family Assistance Center, Schofield Barracks, Hawaii

JOHN RALPH, PhD
Commander, Medical Service Corps, US Navy; Director, Department of Mental Health, National Naval Medical Center, 8901 Wisconsin Avenue, Bethesda, Maryland 20889; formerly, Officer-in-Command, Presidential Support Program, Marine Barracks, Washington, DC

MARK A. REGER, PhD
Research Psychologist, Department of Psychology, Madigan Army Medical Center, 9933C West Hayes Street, Fort Lewis, Washington 98431; and Affiliate Assistant Professor, Department of Psychiatry and Behavioral Sciences, University of Washington School of Medicine, 1925 NE Pacific Street, Seattle, Washington 98195-6340

DAVID REYNOLDS, PhD
Major, Biomedical Sciences Corps, US Air Force; Mental Health Element Leader, Department of Psychology, Malcolm Grow Medical Center, 1050 West Perimeter Road, 779 MDOS/SGOH, Andrews Air Force Base, Maryland 20762; formerly, Chief, Department of Health Psychology, Landstuhl Regional Medical Center, Landstuhl, Germany

ELSPETH CAMERON RITCHIE, MD, MPH
Colonel, US Army (Retired); formerly, Psychiatry Consultant to The Surgeon General, US Army, and Director, Behavioral Health Proponency, Office of The Surgeon General, Falls Church, Virginia; currently, Chief Clinical Officer, District of Columbia Department of Mental Health, 64 New York Avenue NE, 4th Floor, Washington, DC 20002

AMANDA ROBBINS, PsyD
Captain, Medical Service Corps, US Army; Brigade Combat Team Behavioral Health Officer, 4th Brigade Combat Team, 10th Mountain Division, Fort Polk, Louisiana 71459

RENÉ J. ROBICHAUX, PhD, LCSW
Colonel, US Army (Retired); Social Work Programs Manager, Behavioral Health Division, US Army Medical Command, 2050 Worth Road, Suite 10, Fort Sam Houston, Texas 78234; formerly, Chief, Department of Social Work, Brooke Army Medical Center, Fort Sam Houston, Texas

MICHAEL RUSSELL, PhD
Lieutenant Colonel, Medical Service Corps, US Army; Army Medical Department Neuropsychology Consultant, Warrior Resiliency Program, Lincoln Center, Suite 300, 7800 Interstate 10 West, San Antonio, Texas 78230

JOSEF I. RUZEK, PhD
Director, Dissemination and Training Division, National Center for Posttraumatic Stress Disorder, Veterans Affairs Palo Alto Health Care System, 795 Willow Road, Menlo Park, California 94025

ALBERT Y. SAITO, MD
Clinical Director, Child and Adolescent Psychiatry Service, Department of Psychiatry, Tripler Army Medical Center, 1 Jarrett White Road, Honolulu, Hawaii 96859-5000; formerly, Staff Psychiatrist, Department of Child Psychiatry, Tripler Army Medical Center, Honolulu, Hawaii

BRETT J. SCHNEIDER, MD
Lieutenant Colonel, Medical Corps, US Army; Deputy Chief, Department of Psychiatry, Building 61, Child and Adolescent Psychiatry Clinic, Walter Reed Army Medical Center, 6900 Georgia Avenue NW, Washington, DC 20307

MERRITT SCHREIBER, PhD
Captain, Scientist Corps, US Public Health Service (Inactive Reserve Corps); Senior Program Manager, Center for Public Health and Disasters, University of California at Los Angeles Center for the Health Sciences, 1145 Gayley Avenue, Suite 304, Los Angeles, California 90024; and Operations Lead, USPHS Mental Health Team II

ROBERT L. SHERIDAN, MD
Associate Director, Department of Surgery, Harvard Medical School at the Massachusetts General Hospital; Assistant Chief of Staff, Shriners Burn Hospital, 51 Blossom Street, Boston, Massachusetts 02114; formerly, Lieutenant Colonel, Medical Corps, US Army; US Army Institute of Surgical Research, Brooke Army Medical Center, San Antonio, Texas

EDWARD SIMMER, MD, MPH
Captain, Medical Corps, US Navy; Executive Officer, Naval Hospital, 1 Pinckney, Beaufort, South Carolina 29902; formerly, Senior Executive Director for Psychological Health, Defense Centers of Excellence for Psychological Health and Traumatic Brain Injury, Silver Spring, Maryland

TANGENEARE WARD SINGH, MD
Major, Medical Corps, US Army; Chief, Department of Behavioral Health, Blanchfield Army Community Hospital, 650 Joel Drive, Fort Campbell, Kentucky 42223

MARSHALL SMITH, MD
Lieutenant Colonel, Medical Corps, US Army; Chief, Behavioral Health, Landstuhl Regional Medical Center, CMR 402, Box 1357, APO AE 09180; formerly, Chief, Outpatient Behavioral Health, Landstuhl Regional Medical Center, Landstuhl, Germany

STEVEN SOUTHWICK, MD
Professor, Department of Psychiatry, Yale University School of Medicine and Yale Child Study Center, 333 Cedar Street, New Haven, Connecticut 06510; Adjunct Professor, Department of Psychiatry, Mount Sinai School of Medicine, One Gustave L. Levy Place, New York, New York 10029; Deputy Director, Clinical Neurosciences Division, Department of Veterans Affairs National Center for Posttraumatic Stress Disorder, White River Junction, Vermont

JAMES J. STAUDENMEIER, MD, MPH
Colonel, Medical Corps, US Army; Consultant, Army Substance Abuse Program, Department of Psychiatry, USAMEDDAC, 11050 Mount Belvedere Boulevard, BMD (Wilcox), Fort Drum, New York 13602; formerly, Fellow in Geriatric Psychiatry, Walter Reed Army Medical Center, Washington, DC

FREDERICK J. STODDARD JR, MD
Associate Clinical Professor, Department of Psychiatry, Harvard Medical School at the Massachusetts General Hospital; and Chief of Psychiatry, Shriners Burn Hospital, 51 Blossom Street, Boston, Massachusetts 02114; formerly, Senior Surgeon, US Public Health Service

KATHERINE H. TABER, PhD
Research Health Scientist, Department of Research and Education, WG Hefner Veterans Affairs Medical Center, Mailstation 11M, 1601 Brenner Avenue, Salisbury, North Carolina 28144; formerly, Research Fellow, School of Health Information Sciences, University of Texas at Houston

ARTIN TERHAKOPIAN, MD, MPH
Major, Medical Corps, US Army; Chief, Inpatient Psychiatry, Department of Behavioral Health, William Beaumont Army Medical Center, 5005 North Piedras Street, El Paso, Texas 79920; formerly, Chief, Behavioral Health, 10th Combat Support Hospital, Baghdad, Iraq

RICHARD TOYE, PhD
Lieutenant Colonel, Medical Service Corps, US Army Reserve; Company Commander, 883rd Medical Company (Combat Stress Control), 495 Summer Street, Boston, Massachusetts 02210; formerly, Brigade Behavioral Health Consultant, 804th Medical Brigade, Fort Devens, Massachusetts

TINA TRUDEL, PhD
Site Director, Defense and Veterans Brain Injury Center at Virginia NeuroCare, 1101-B East High Street, Charlottesville, Virginia 22902; Assistant Clinical Professor of Psychiatry and Behavioral Neurobehavioral Sciences, University of Virginia Medical School, Charlottesville, Virginia 22902; formerly, Executive Director, Lakeview NeuroRehabilitation Center, Effingham Falls, New Hampshire

ROBERT J. URSANO, MD
Colonel, US Air Force (Retired); Director, Center for the Study of Traumatic Stress, and Chair, Department of Psychiatry, Room B3068, Uniformed Services University of the Health Sciences, 4301 Jones Bridge Road, Bethesda, Maryland 20814

JEFFREY L. VOYLES, MDIV
Lieutenant Colonel, Chaplain Corps, US Army; Director and Clinical Supervisor, Chaplain Family Life Training Program, Building 2606 Collins Loop, Fort Benning, Georgia 31905

HAROLD J. WAIN, PHD
Chief, Psychiatry Consultation Liaison Service, Department of Psychiatry, Building 2, Room 6238, Walter Reed Army Medical Center, 6900 Georgia Avenue NW, Washington, DC 20307-5100

WENDI M. WAITS, MD
Lieutenant Colonel, Medical Corps, US Army; Chief, Inpatient Psychiatry Service, Department of Psychiatry, Tripler Army Medical Center, 1 Jarrett White Road, Room 4B106, Honolulu, Hawaii 96859-5000; formerly, Child and Adolescent Psychiatry Fellow, Tripler Army Medical Center, Honolulu, Hawaii

DEBORAH L. WARDEN, MD
Formerly, National Director, Defense and Veterans Brain Injury Center Headquarters; Departments of Neurology and Psychiatry, Walter Reed Army Medical Center, 6900 Georgia Avenue NW, Washington, DC 20307; Departments of Neurology and Psychiatry, Walter Reed Army Medical Center, 6900 Georgia Avenue NW, Washington, DC 20307-5001

CHRISTOPHER H. WARNER, MD
Major, Medical Corps, US Army; Chief, Department of Behavioral Medicine, Winn Army Community Hospital, Building 9242, Room 20, 1083 Worcester Drive, Fort Stewart, Georgia 31324; formerly, Division Psychiatrist, 3rd Infantry Division, Fort Stewart, Georgia

TERRY C. WASHAM, MSSA, LISW
Colonel, Medical Service Corps, US Army Reserve; Military Liaison Coordinator, Office of Seamless Transition, Department of Veterans Affairs, VA Medical Center, 10000 Brecksville Road, Brecksville, Ohio 44141

PATRICIA WATSON, PHD
Assistant Professor, Dartmouth Medical School, 1 Rope Ferry Road, Hanover, New Hampshire 03755-1404; Senior Educational Specialist, Executive Division, Department of Veterans Affairs National Center for Posttraumatic Stress Disorder, White River Junction, Vermont

THOMAS C. WAYNICK, MDIV
Lieutenant Colonel, Chaplain Corps, US Army; Command Chaplain, Family, Morale, Welfare, and Recreation Command, 4700 King Street, Alexandria, Virginia 22301; formerly, Director and Clinical Supervisor, US Army Family Life Chaplain Training Program, Fort Benning, Georgia

SIMON WESSELY, MD
Department Head, Department of Psychological Medicine, King's Centre for Military Health Research, King's College, Weston Education Centre, 10 Cutcombe Road, London SE5 9RJ United Kingdom; formerly, Honorary Lecturer in Forensic Psychiatry, Institute of Psychiatry, London, United Kingdom

RICHARD J. WESTPHAL, PHD, RN
Captain, Nurse Corps, US Navy; Psychological Health Promotion Programs, Department of the Navy, Bureau of Medicine and Surgery, Deployment Health, 2300 E Street NW, Washington, DC 20372

KATHLEEN M. WRIGHT, PHD
Research Psychologist, US Army Medical Research-Europe, Walter Reed Army Institute of Research, CMR 442, Box 94, APO AE 09042; formerly, Deputy Chief, Department of Military Psychiatry, Walter Reed Army Institute of Research, Silver Spring, Maryland

JEFFREY S. YARVIS, MSW, PHD
Lieutenant Colonel, Medical Service Corps, US Army; Chief, Behavioral Health, Department of Psychiatry, Borden Pavilion, Walter Reed Army Medical Center, 6900 Georgia Avenue NW, Washington, DC 20307; formerly, Director of Social Work, Uniformed Services University of the Health Sciences, Bethesda, Maryland

TODD YOSICK, LISW
Major, Medical Service Corps, US Army; Deputy Director, Resilience and Prevention Directorate, Office of the Assistant Secretary of Defense for Health Affairs, Defense Centers of Excellence for Psychological Health and Traumatic Brain Injury, 1335 East-West Highway, Silver Spring, Maryland 20910; formerly, Chief, Battlemind Training Office/Chief, Combat and Operational Stress Control, Army Medical Department Center and School, Fort Sam Houston, Texas

Foreword

Military healthcare has the unique opportunity of truly addressing the full continuum of illness, injury, disease, and health. Just as military healthcare professionals have made significant contributions to the improvement of physical health and lessening of injury and disease over the history of the United States, we are now a leading proponent of changes in prevention, recognition, and treatment in multiple areas of behavioral health.

Essential to progress in this arena is developing awareness of behavioral health needs and educating our beneficiaries about the appropriateness of receiving care for what are often "invisible" diseases or injuries. The need for this education and developing a toolkit of successful skills, techniques, and strategies for resilience have never been more apparent than during what has become a persistent state of conflict. We are committed to leading the Nation in eliminating the stigma of behavioral health problems. Men and women within our militaries and across America must learn that it is just as acceptable and appropriate to seek behavioral healthcare as it is to seek treatment for a broken bone.

Since the publication of the two *Textbooks of Military Medicine* psychiatry volumes—*Military Psychiatry: Preparing in Peace for War* (1994) and *War Psychiatry* (1995)—we have made tremendous strides. This volume, *Combat and Operational Behavioral Health*, expands on these previous two volumes, covering the full breadth of the psychological and behavioral health continuum. Important contributions include preparation for deployment and resiliency training; the provision of services in theater; recovery after physical or emotional injury due to combat; reunion and reintegration; military children and families; operational psychiatry; and the daunting challenge to prevent suicide.

I see our effect on social attitudes toward behavioral and/or psychological health as potentially substantial. Our prospects are good for a better understanding of the neurochemistry and basic pathophysiology of many common stress-related problems, and our grasp and management of millennia-old problems of armed conflict are much improved. However, major challenges remain. One may think the diagnosis of posttraumatic stress disorder (PTSD), for example, would be straightforward. On the contrary, it varies widely among different stakeholders. The more complex issues of the etiology of PTSD and traumatic brain injury, and effective treatments for these conditions, as well as their interaction with age, gender, and other medical issues, are far more daunting.

This new textbook is an excellent resource for all healthcare professionals as they strive to provide the finest quality and most compassionate care of the men and women in uniform and their spouses, significant others, and children. Every person who is in contact with a military member struggling to cope with the emotional trauma of war, disease, or injury needs our support and best efforts.

The contributions of the exceptional civilian and military professionals in this outstanding text can raise the quality of behavioral healthcare across our land and help eliminate the stigma of requesting this care. Although we talk a lot about the reduction of stigma, to actually reduce it and improve Soldiers' willingness to seek treatment is a Herculean task. Therefore, let us all participate in this essential step forward for the health and well-being of those who have often suffered in silence and alone.

Lieutenant General Eric B. Schoomaker, MD, PhD
The Surgeon General and
Commanding General, US Army Medical Command

Washington, DC
February 2010

Preface

This book was begun in 2005 when it became apparent that an update to the previous volumes on military psychiatry—*Military Psychiatry: Preparing in Peace for War* (1994) and *War Psychiatry* (1995)—was needed. In the almost 20 years since the chapters in those two volumes were drafted, enormous changes and advancements in classification, diagnosis, and treatment of combat stress have occurred. The pace of change has accelerated with the wars in Afghanistan and Iraq. These wars have become known by many names: Operations Enduring Freedom and Iraqi Freedom, the Long War, and continuous overseas contingency operations, among others.

In the early years of the operations in Afghanistan (2001) and Iraq (2003), changes in operational tempo and resulting extended deployments were extremely taxing for military families. What was problematic in these early years (tempo and deployment) because of the change from past experience has now become problematic because it is the norm. The murders and murder/suicides at Fort Bragg, North Carolina, in 2002 highlighted the perils of soldiers' rapid return from Afghanistan battlefields to civilian life. The investigations at Fort Bragg and other installations revealed continuing problems with access to care, as well as reluctance of career-minded soldiers to seek treatment.

In response to these and other events, training and systems were put into place to prepare soldiers for "redeployment" (return to garrison). One of the earlier approaches, "Battlemind," was designed to help reintegrate service members and families. Battlemind recently evolved into the Comprehensive Soldier Fitness program, which is focused on enhancing resiliency. Despite these various new programs, many soldiers remain reluctant to seek behavioral healthcare for many reasons, perhaps the greatest of which is worry about its effects on their careers. Stigma is a persistent problem, despite numerous efforts to reduce its prevalence. Often it is the soldiers' families who try to get these service members in for treatment. To improve access to care, the Army and other services have dramatically increased their number of mental health providers, up about 70% between 2007 and 2010.

To assist this growing population of service members, the military behavioral health community has added many new systems of evaluation and care. The Post-Deployment Health Assessment (PDHA), which screens soldiers on return from theater, was implemented after the Persian Gulf War (1990–1991). However, soldiers often did not admit to symptoms after deployment because they wanted to get home as soon as possible. Beginning in 2005, the PDHA was joined by the Post-Deployment Health Re-Assessment (PDHRA), administered at 3 to 6 months after return. It was designed to connect with service members after "the honeymoon" of returning home was over.

Family programs have been expanded to help with issues that arise during both deployment and redeployment. There are specialized programs at Walter Reed Army Medical Center and other facilities for families of the wounded that attempt to prepare children to see parents missing a limb or disfigured from a blast. Another difficult area has been support to families of the deceased. US military families have not faced these numbers of service-connected fatalities since the Vietnam War. In the past, spouses and children were required to leave base housing and service-centered support systems relatively soon after their loved one's death. This policy has changed over time, with longer access to housing and healthcare afforded these families.

Traumatic brain injury (TBI) is another major concern and affects families as well as service members. The sources of these injuries are varied: blasts, gunshot wounds, accidents. TBI can present with many symptoms, some similar to posttraumatic stress disorder, including irritability, impulsiveness, and personality changes.

The rising suicide rate has been a major concern for all in the Army. The combination of unit and individual risk factors include high operations tempo, feelings of disconnectedness on return home, problems at work or home, pain and disability, alcohol, and easy access to weapons. Consistent and high-profile attempts have been made to reduce suicide with numerous training programs for service members, focusing on buddy aid and gatekeepers. However, thus far these efforts have been only partially successful. The prolonged effects of exposure to violence and death are not easy to change.

New efforts to assist service members continue. The Defense Center of Excellence was stood up in November 2007, with a focus on best practices and reducing stigma. Other programs are the Comprehensive Behavioral Health Campaign Plan, the Department of Defense–Department of Veterans Affairs Integrated Mental Health Plan, and the National Intrepid Center of Excellence.

An ongoing concern is the long-term effects of the Long War, for the next 20, 30, or 50 years. After the Vietnam War, far too many veterans ended up on the streets—unemployed, homeless, and addicted. By examining the potential causes of combat stress and emotional trauma, the various approaches to diagnosis and treatment, the roles of providers (and their own resiliency), and the many programs available to help, this volume seeks to reduce the difficulties faced by veterans as they reenter civilian life. However, success in this area will require a concerted effort by all on the home front, including the Army, other branches of the military, the Department of Veterans Affairs, other federal agencies, and state and local agencies, as well as civilian and private organizations. It is hoped that the interventions described in this volume will contribute to that effort by informing and guiding military and civilian healthcare providers, the public, and both active duty service members and veterans of these most recent conflicts.

Elspeth Cameron Ritchie, MD, MPH, Colonel, US Army (Retired)
Chief Clinical Officer, District of Columbia Department of Mental Health
Formerly, Psychiatry Consultant to The Army Surgeon General, and Director, Behavioral Health Proponency, Office of The Surgeon General

Washington, DC
December 2010

COMBAT AND OPERATIONAL BEHAVIORAL HEALTH

Section I: Setting the Stage

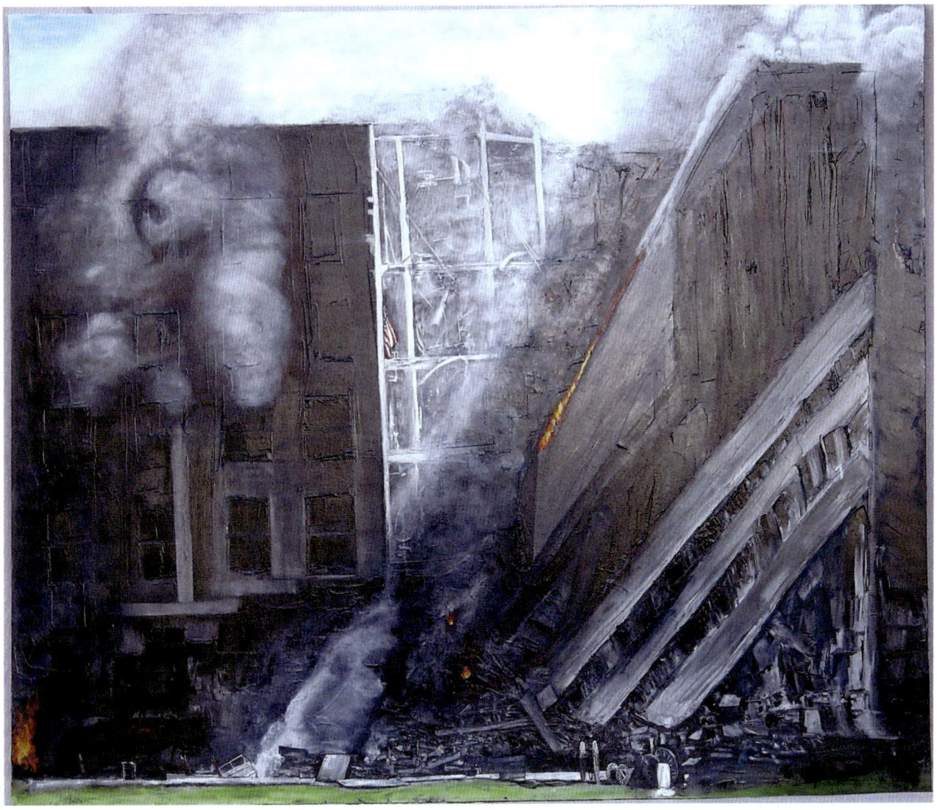

Plan Accordingly, by Gary N. "Butch" Cassidy, oil on canvas, 2002.

Art: Courtesy of the Army Art Collection, US Army Center of Military History.

Chapter 1

COMBAT AND OPERATIONAL BEHAVIORAL HEALTH: AN UPDATE TO AN OLD HISTORY

ELSPETH CAMERON RITCHIE, MD, MPH*; AND CHRISTOPHER G. IVANY, MD†

*Colonel, US Army (Retired); formerly, Psychiatry Consultant to The Surgeon General, US Army, and Director, Behavioral Health Proponency, Office of The Surgeon General, Falls Church, Virginia; currently, Chief Clinical Officer, District of Columbia Department of Mental Health, 64 New York Avenue NE, 4th Floor, Washington, DC 20002

†Major, Medical Corps, Psychiatrist, Department of Behavioral Health, Evans Army Community Hospital, Building 7500, 1650 Cochrane Circle, Fort Carson, Colorado 80913; formerly, Division Psychiatrist, 4th Infantry Division, Fort Hood, Texas

INTRODUCTION

In the years since the attacks of September 11, 2001 (also known simply as "9/11"), the United States has been at war in both Iraq and Afghanistan, and has responded to myriad natural disasters and terrorist incidents. Although all wars produce stress casualties, during and after different wars these casualties have manifested in many ways, both with physical and psychological symptoms. With the notable exceptions of the data collected by the Walter Reed Institute of Research and the Mental Health Assessment Teams (to be described later in this volume), only a few articles have begun to appear in the literature about the behavioral health lessons learned during the conflicts in Afghanistan and Iraq. A plethora of practical information is not yet in the scientific literature. This volume seeks to consolidate, in real time, the information that is emerging, both to guide current policy and practice, and for the future.

Lessons learned include areas such as: (*a*) management of behavioral health issues on the battlefront; (*b*) care of the physical and psychological needs of the wounded; (*c*) reintegration of soldiers with their families; (*d*) return of soldiers with psychological symptoms to the battlefield; (*e*) deployment of troops into humanitarian and disaster situations, such as the 2004 tsunami and Hurricane Katrina in 2005; and (*f*) the special needs of children of service members, including the families of the wounded and deceased.

The disaster literature, which draws heavily on the combat literature, tends to focus on a single traumatic event. War is related to, but different from, disasters. It may start as unexpectedly as disasters do, but then persist for years. Unlike victims of disaster, service members are generally prepared for battle. They may or may not, however, be prepared for the sights, sounds, and smells of starving populations as seen in Somalia or mass graves, such as in Bosnia.

BEHAVIORAL HEALTH CHALLENGES FOR THE US MILITARY

The military has extensive mental health capabilities. Yet these capabilities sometimes fail to meet significant needs that emerge from recent deployments. These include service members home on leave brought to a civilian emergency room by a concerned family member; demobilized National Guard and reservists who may be remote from a military treatment facility or Veterans Affairs (VA) facility; and family members distraught over the frequent deployments of their soldier kin.

A recurrent issue is that of stigma and barriers to care. Numerous programs, which will be described in this volume, exist to encourage military personnel to seek help. But there are also considerable potential consequences of seeking mental healthcare. These include: leadership ignorance of psychological issues; the requirement to report to command if a soldier enrolls in the Alcohol and Substance Abuse Program; security clearances; and other potential impacts on the soldier's career. All of these issues are currently being addressed by the leadership.

Suicides are highly publicized, but they do not necessarily represent the status of the mental health of the force. US forces are all screened, employed, and have access to free healthcare—all factors that reduce the incidence of suicide. The Army continues to strive to reduce these rates further. However, the rate of suicide in the Army has continued to rise every year since 2004. The rate has just surpassed that in the civilian world, where age- and gender-adjusted rates are about 20/100,000/year. The US Army's suicide prevention training has been revised to reflect the motivations of soldiers who kill themselves. Suicide prevention, therefore, is a topic of enormous significance to the Army.

Over the next few years, based on historical data, many service members will leave the Army or other military services. Traditionally, about 10% of former soldiers who seek care do so through the VA. At the present time (late 2009), about 40% of former soldiers who seek care are using the VA. Most of the rest obtain it through standard civilian healthcare sources. Thus it is critically important that civilian providers know about the psychological issues facing soldiers and families.

The signature weapon of today' wars, both in Iraq and Afghanistan, is the blast. The clinicians' experience of caring for victims of these weapons is the result of years of technological, medical, and psychiatric advancements. But the history of military psychiatry is replete with attempts to answer many questions similar to the ones that the US military now faces. Military psychiatrists have only intermittently succeeded in capturing those historical lessons learned for contemporary application.

Many questions remain. How can the responses of military and civilian mental health systems be optimized? What has been learned about mental health risks facing today's soldiers and their families? How can practitioners engage returning soldiers, and what are likely pitfalls they may encounter? These dilemmas apply to all services, but the Army and Marines have been most heavily involved in the ground conflict and therefore constitute the focus of the text.

HISTORY OF THE PSYCHIATRY VOLUMES OF THE TEXTBOOKS OF MILITARY MEDICINE

As the American military engaged in the armed conflicts of the 19th and 20th centuries, its mental health officers fought parallel battles treating service members' psychiatric wounds. Like battlefield commanders learning from past successes and failures, these pioneering clinicians developed potent strategies in the war against mental illness. For decades, however, despite numerous therapeutic advances, only a small number published their findings, leaving invaluable lessons vulnerable to the passage of time.

The disparate preservation and distribution of these "lessons learned" hindered future generations of mental health clinicians from acquiring crucial lessons on war psychiatry. For example, the World War II psychiatrist Frederick Hanson had to rediscover the principles of forward treatment of combat stress casualties in the midst of the North African campaign even though Thomas Salmon had established their effectiveness 25 years earlier during World War I.[1,2] Likewise, in the opening months of the Korean conflict, US Army physicians, unaware of the benefit of quickly treating combat stress cases close to their units, evacuated nearly one quarter of the fighting force as psychological casualties.[3] Fortunately, Colonel Albert Glass, well-versed in the practice of combat psychiatry in the course of his World War II tour under Hanson, sharply reduced combat stress casualties by implementing principles now known as "PIES," or proximity, immediacy, expectancy, and simplicity.

It was not until 20 years after the conclusion of World War II that the preeminent Army psychiatrists of the day, led by Colonel Glass, compiled the key behavioral health lessons of the campaign. The first volume of *Neuropsychiatry in World War II* appeared in print in 1966[4] and the second in 1973.[5] These two volumes became the foundation of modern combat psychiatry. Although valuable for their historical preservation of the failures and ultimate successes of psychiatry in World War II, the delay in publication prevented two decades of clinicians from applying their messages. In addition, the volumes could not account for the sizable cultural shifts of the 1960s, which would heavily influence the presentation of combat stress in the Vietnam War.

The Vietnam War and its social aftermath further demonstrated the effectiveness of forward treatment of combat stress and introduced new principles, such as the etiology and management of disorders of frustration and loneliness.[6,7] At the conclusion of the Vietnam era, these essential tenets, hard won through decades of painful experience, were preserved only as an oral tradition and in scattered literary sources.

Even before the end of the Vietnam War, several luminaries of the military psychiatric community realized that a comprehensively compiled, refined, and codified source of military psychiatric experience from this era was required to preserve the accumulated data and perpetuate its application in future conflicts. Lieutenant Colonel Kenneth Artiss took an interest in producing an inclusive textbook but left military service in 1964. Even before the beginning of the Vietnam War, Colonel Franklin Del Jones emerged as the lead editor of the daunting project.[8,9] Jones, one of the few career military psychiatrists who had completed a tour in Vietnam, also distinguished himself as a pragmatic clinician, expert pharmacotherapist, knowledgeable military historian, and master teacher.

Jones, a humble, soft-spoken Texan, had been mentored by Albert Glass, well-known throughout the military for his implementation of the forward treatment of combat stress casualties in Korea. Jones also shared Glass' steadfast commitment to preserve and develop the psychiatric lessons learned in past armed conflicts.[9] Throughout his Army career, Jones had held numerous prominent clinical, academic, and administrative positions such as Director of Psychiatric Education at Walter Reed Army Medical Center and the Consultant to the Surgeon General, US Army, but his greatest passion remained writing. As the leader of the textbook project, Jones invited authors from all armed services, multiple backgrounds, and various disciplines, but imbued the work with his own belief that practical experience takes precedence over speculation and theory. Jones retired from active military service in 1988 with the rank of colonel. He battled a severe autoimmune disorder, but nonetheless poured himself into the textbook project by personally authoring or coauthoring 18 of the 38 chapters, and researching and editing the remaining 20. During the first Gulf War (Operations Desert Shield and Desert Storm, 1990–1991), Jones provided bound copies of relevant draft chapters to the psychiatry consultants for the Army, Navy, and Air Force. These consultants, in turn, distributed these to psychiatrists throughout the theater of operations to enable them to use the lessons learned from previous wars in this rapidly evolving conflict. Through collaboration with the

Borden Institute, the endeavor blossomed into two volumes, one published in 1994 (*Military Psychiatry: Preparing in Peace for War*[2]) and the other in 1995 (*War Psychiatry*[10]) in the *Textbooks of Military Medicine* series. Jones died in 2005, remembered as an epic contributor in the annals of military psychiatry.

With the publication of *Military Psychiatry* and *War Psychiatry*, members of the military mental health community could for the first time quickly reference a central repository of military-specific psychiatric knowledge from Napoleonic times through the Persian Gulf War. Faculty at the Army's teaching hospitals integrated the texts into the curriculum for psychiatric residents and distributed them to psychologists, social workers, chaplains, and even to the US Army War College, which educates the Army's most promising combat arms leaders. Behavioral health clinicians based much of their intervention at the Pentagon on September 11, 2001, on the principles of forward treatment.[8,11] Perhaps most significantly, the generation of mental heath officers deployed as part of Operation Enduring Freedom (OEF) and Operation Iraqi Freedom (OIF) avoided mistakes made by their predecessors in the opening stages of previous wars. Instead, they rapidly adapted and implemented time-tested psychiatric treatment of US military fighters.

Lessons found within the volumes can guide contemporary mental health leaders as they set policies that improve on those of the past. The importance of an efficient transition of care for soldiers from active duty to the VA system is highlighted by the difficulties in the post-Vietnam era. The clinical presentation of posttraumatic stress disorder (PTSD) in OIF and OEF soldiers is presaged by Jones' description of the evolution of the syndrome from World War I through the Vietnam War. Post–World-War-II lessons depict the benefit of systematic emphasis on education and rehabilitation in recovery from PTSD. The textbooks present historical insights into many contemporary mental health issues.

Military Psychiatry and *War Psychiatry* spurred further useful debate about military and combat psychiatry. Since their publication in the mid-1990s, clinicians, researchers, and administrators have made countless advances integrating surveillance, education, treatment, and new neurobiological research, and adapting their practice to the post-9/11 world. These advances will be described further in this volume.

Today's military mission also differs greatly from that of Jones' era. Combat doctrine now emphasizes modular forces engaging in asymmetric wars involving multiple deployments, intense urban warfare, and without clearly defined front lines. An expanding body of research and clinical experience is illuminating the psychiatric impact of these new and demanding missions on service members and their families. Inspired by the Jones' texts, the military mental health community continues on a historically informed journey of debate and documentation.

SUMMARY

Although it has only been 15 years since the publication of Jones' two volumes on military psychiatry, a contemporary literary resource that encapsulates military behavioral health knowledge and experience has been overdue. Inspired by Doctors Glass, Jones, Artiss, and many others, this newest version of the behavioral health volumes of the *Textbooks of Military Medicine* provides clinicians with an indispensable weapon in the battle against the psychiatric illnesses that affect the men and women in uniform and their families.

There has been considerable discussion about the title of this book, which will be briefly summarized here. Early on, it was clear that "psychiatry" was too discipline specific. However, the question was what to replace it with. The Army has shifted from "mental health" to "behavioral health." The Department of Defense is beginning to use "psychological health." Some like the term "behavioral medicine"; other dislike the apparent emphasis on disease.

Parallel discussions ensued about whether to use the term "military" or "uniformed," as the Public Health Service plays a central role in responding to disasters. "Combat" describes the wars, but also leaves out the responses to natural disasters. Thus the title, "Combat and Operational Behavioral Health," was chosen to cast the widest net possible.

There are some caveats. Inevitably, this is not the whole story. In the 4 years it has taken to produce the book, there have been multiple new efforts. Rather than hold off publication to have time to judge their effectiveness, they are simply mentioned in the conclusion. Although there has been an effort to include as many sources and military services as possible, many practitioners are too busy during these times to write. In addition, new lessons are learned all the time. There are two first-person accounts, which are included as appendices, as they are more first-person accounts than scholarly chapters. However, their stories add to the depth of understanding of what it is like to be a practitioner in an immature and dangerous theater. There is also an account of media coverage of soldiers' behavioral health in Iraq during Operation

Iraqi Freedom 05-07, which is included as the third appendix. Finally it is hoped that this volume is a valuable addition to the literature, and a timely guide for practitioners and leaders.

REFERENCES

1. Glass AJ. Psychiatry at the division level. In: Hanson FR, ed. *Combat Psychiatry: Experiences in the North African and Mediterranean Theaters of Operation, American Ground Forces, World War II.* Bulletin of the US Army Medical Department. Washington, DC: Government Printing Office; 1949: 45–73.

2. Jones FD, Sparacino LR, Wilcox VL, Rothberg JM, eds. *Military Psychiatry: Preparing in Peace for War.* In: Zajtchuk R, Bellamy RF, eds. *The Textbooks of Military Medicine.* Washington, DC: Department of the Army, Office of The Surgeon General, Borden Institute; 1994.

3. Ritchie EC. Psychiatry in the Korean War: perils, PIES, and prisoners of war. *Mil Med.* 2002;167:898–903.

4. Anderson RS, Glass AJ, Bernucci RJ, eds. *Neuropsychiatry in World War II.* Vol I. *Zone of the Interior.* Washington, DC: Government Printing Office; 1966.

5. Anderson RS, Glass AJ, Bernucci RJ, eds. *Neuropsychiatry in World War II.* Vol II. *Overseas Theaters.* Washington, DC: Government Printing Office; 1973.

6. Jones FD. Experiences of a division psychiatrist in Vietnam. *Mil Med.* 1967;132:1003–1008.

7. Jones FD, Johnson AW. Medical and psychiatric treatment policy and practice in Vietnam. *J Soc Issues.* 1975;31:49–65.

8. Ritchie EC, Cassimatis E, Emanuel R, Milliken C, Gray SH. The contributions of Kenneth Leslie Artiss, MD. *J Am Acad Psychoanalysis Dynamic Psychiatry.* 2003;31:663–673.

9. Ivany CG, Gray SH. Franklin Delano Jones, MD, and *War Psychiatry. J Am Acad Psychoanalysis Dynamic Psychiatry.* 2007;35:1–12.

10. Jones FD, Sparacino LR, Wilcox VL, Rothberg JM, Stokes JW, eds. *War Psychiatry.* In: Zajtchuk R, Bellamy RF, eds. *Textbook of Military Medicine.* Washington, DC: Department of the Army, Office of The Surgeon General, Borden Institute; 1995.

11. Milliken CS, Leavitt WT, Murdock P, Orman DT, Ritchie EC, Hoge CW. Principles guiding implementation of the Operation Solace plan: "Pieces of PIES," therapy by walking around, and care management. *Mil Med.* 2002;167(9 suppl):48–57.

Chapter 2

US ARMY PSYCHIATRY LEGACIES OF THE VIETNAM WAR

NORMAN M. CAMP, MD*

*Colonel, US Army (Retired); 3105-D Stony Point Road, Richmond, Virginia 23235; Clinical Professor of Psychiatry, Department of Psychiatry, Medical College of Virginia, Virginia Commonwealth University, Richmond, Virginia 23298

INTRODUCTION

The US ground war in Vietnam (1965–1972) began on March 8, 1965, when over 3,500 men of the 9th Marine Expeditionary Brigade made an unopposed amphibious landing on the northern coast of the Republic of South Vietnam. This was in response to intensification in the fighting between South Vietnam—an ally of the United States—and indigenous communist forces (Viet Cong guerrillas) and those from South Vietnam's neighbor to the north, the Democratic Republic of Vietnam (North Vietnam). In early May, the first US Army troops (the 173rd Airborne Brigade) arrived in South Vietnam, landing at the mouth of the Saigon River at Vung Tau. Thus began an enormous military effort by the United States and other allies who sought to block the spread of communism in Southeast Asia.

Considering the limited resources of the enemy and the superior military might of the United States, it was anticipated that the threat could be quickly contained. Only belatedly was it discovered that the resolve of the communists had been underestimated. The war became a drawn out, mostly "low intensity," "irregular," counterinsurgency/guerrilla conflict, which was far more challenging than expected. The United States and its allies had become intractably ensnared in Vietnam's simultaneous and protracted social revolution, civil war, and nationalistic opposition to foreign domination. In time, the cost of the war far exceeded the tolerance of the American people (over 58,000 Americans died and over 300,000 were wounded) and produced great national agony and incalculable cultural aftereffects. Finally, just over 2 years after the last US military personnel were withdrawn (March 29, 1973) under a negotiated truce, North Vietnam violated the truce and overran South Vietnam, which surrendered on April 30, 1975.

The war effort also assumed a central role in a decade of social and political upheaval in the United States—a nightmare that threatened its most basic institutions, including the US military. Through the second half of the war (1969–1972), an increasing proportion of US troops in Vietnam came to question their purpose there. They expressed, in every way except for collective mutiny (including psychiatric conditions), their inability or unwillingness to accept the risks of combat, acknowledge the authority of military leaders, or tolerate the hardships of an assignment in Vietnam. This all occurred in a setting where combat objectives were still in effect, weapons were ubiquitous, violence was adaptive, and illicit drugs were effectively marketed and widely used by US troops. The attitudes of these young replacement soldiers, most of whom were draftees or reluctant volunteers, were strongly resonant with the growing opposition to the war in the United States. A radicalized, liberal, "counterculture" youth movement emerged, along with antagonism toward American institutions and, especially, military service among younger, black Americans. Facilitative, but also emblematic, this dissenting subculture especially rallied around the burgeoning drug culture of the times.

The severe breakdown in soldier morale and discipline suffered by the US Army during the drawdown years in Vietnam struck at the heart of military leadership. It also overlapped with the mission of Army psychiatry. From the outset, the organization of psychiatric services in Vietnam was especially weighted in favor of the treatment and rehabilitation of combat stress casualties. These did not materialize in the numbers envisioned, however, and instead an unprecedented flood of psychosocial casualties emerged. These consisted of disciplinary problems, racial disturbances, attacks on superiors, drug abuse, and the rising prevalence of soldiers diagnosed with character disorders, especially for those in noncombat units and with assignments relatively unrelated to combat risks.[1] Military leaders, as well as law enforcement, administrative, and medical/psychiatric elements, were all severely tested until the remaining US ground forces were withdrawn.

Following the war, the Army Medical Department did not commit to developing a historical summary of psychiatry in Vietnam or study these problems for "lessons learned." Furthermore, the Army evidently lost, abandoned, or destroyed documentation at the conclusion of hostilities that could serve as primary source material.[2] Vietnam has been referred to as America's first computerized war. Ironically, however, the Army apparently emerged from this experience with far fewer records pertaining to the provision of military psychiatric services than in earlier and less "sophisticated" times. In lieu of a more systematic approach, this chapter will draw upon the extant literature from the war to provide a composite of the stressors affecting soldiers sent to Vietnam. It will provide an overview of the emergent trends in psychiatric conditions and behavioral problems faced by Army leaders and the deployed psychiatric specialists and their mental health colleagues. It also will raise important questions that seem to linger despite the three-and-a-half decades since US troops left Vietnam—questions for which the answers may have considerable bearing for such troops in similar wars in the future.

THE INCOMPLETE HISTORY OF ARMY PSYCHIATRY IN THE VIETNAM WAR

Spanning approximately a decade, from late 1962 through early 1972, an estimated 135 psychiatrists served with the US Army in Vietnam in successive cohorts, typically for 1-year assignments.[3] Roughly one third of these psychiatrists were trained in Army residency programs; the other two thirds received their psychiatric education in civilian settings. The number of psychiatrists who served in Vietnam was considerably fewer than the more than 2,400 psychiatrists who served in World War II. However, those who served in Vietnam participated in a war that became surrounded with unparalleled social and political discord. The associated polarization and tensions of the period, especially later in the war, clearly affected attitudes within psychiatry and particularly challenged the role and ethics of psychiatry in support of the military.

A few publications summarize Army psychiatry experience in Vietnam. They primarily focus, however, on observations from the advisor period and the buildup phase of the war (1962–1969)[3–6] and fail to draw sufficient attention to the rampant psychiatric and behavioral problems that subsequently developed there. Also misleading is the commonly published Army psychiatric admission rate for the Vietnam War of 12–16/1,000 soldiers per year,[7–10] which appears quite favorable compared to Korea (28/1,000/y)[10] and World War II (28–101/1,000/y).[11] Utilizing a single outcome measure and averaging all 7 years of experience in Vietnam effectively dilutes the 4-fold increase in the last few years and minimizes both the breadth and the depth of the intersecting morale and psychiatric problems in Vietnam.

In 1975, Jones and Johnson published a preliminary overview of Army psychiatry in Vietnam when Johnson was serving as the psychiatric consultant to the Office of The Surgeon General, US Army.[7] They described common clinical entities and provided gross prevalence data, which they associated with changing theater circumstances and policy features of the war. They left greater detail and synthesis for other accounts that, regrettably, failed to materialize.

Other circumstances also help explain the absence of a more complete Vietnam military psychiatry history. Until it was forced to study heroin use among soldiers late in the war,[12–14] the Army undertook relatively little formal psychiatric field research in Vietnam after regular forces were committed in 1965. Notable exceptions are the study of physiological, psychological, and social correlates of stress by Major Peter Bourne, Medical Corps, and his colleagues from Walter Reed Army Institute of Research (WRAIR), conducted in 1965 and 1966,[15] and the surveys of illegal drug use in 1967 by RA Roffman and E Sapol,[16] and in 1969 by MD Stanton.[17] Also helpful are publications regarding the theater drug abuse epidemic derived from investigative visits to Vietnam late in the war by senior military psychiatrists—Colonel Stewart L Baker Jr, Medical Corps,[18] Colonel Harry C Holloway, Medical Corps,[19] and Norman Zinberg, MD, a civilian psychiatrist.[20]

Anecdotal accounts published by psychiatrists who served in the war are also a useful source of information.[21] Regrettably, some measure of skew is introduced because, of the 27 psychiatrists who served with the Army and who published accounts, 82% (22) were assigned there during the first half of the war (1965–1968). Also, of 46 publications from the entire group of 24 individuals, half appeared in the *US Army Vietnam Medical Journal*—a nonjuried publication that was circulated primarily in Vietnam and ceased publication in 1970. The few articles by psychiatrists who served during the drawdown phase of the war when psychiatric attrition rates were highest are primarily limited to descriptions of local patterns of drug abuse or drug treatment programs.

Besides being generally spotty, the available research and historical literature specifically lacks validation of the field psychiatric practices and results in Vietnam,[22] especially the adaptation of the classic combat psychiatry "doctrine" (informal) to the irregular, counterinsurgency war that was mostly fought in Vietnam and under increasingly controversial circumstances. This chapter will make additional references to this doctrine, but it can be summarized as the provision of brief, simple, mostly field treatments (eg, safety, rest, and physical replenishment); peer support; sedation, if necessary; and opportunities for emotional catharsis of the soldier's traumatic events—applied as close to the affected soldier's unit as practical and accompanied by expectations that the individual quickly recover, rejoin comrades, and reenter the combat situation.[23,24]

Similar uncertainties surround the use in theater of recently developed pharmacologic agents. Vietnam provided military medicine with its first set of physicians—especially psychiatrists—routinely trained in the use of neuroleptic (antipsychotic), anxiolytic (antianxiety), and tricyclic (antidepressant) medications. The discovery of these medications revolutionized the practice of psychiatry generally; they had considerable promise in the management of combat stress reactions (CSRs) and other conditions in Vietnam. Anecdotal reports indicate that they were commonly prescribed throughout the theater for a full range of symptoms related to combat stress. A limited survey in 1967 confirmed their high use by Army physicians, including psychiatrists.[25] However, there were no associated clinical or research studies, and, in the aftermath of the war, some have raised questions as to whether prescribing psychoactive medications for combat-exposed soldiers represented unethical medical practice by coercing participation among dissenting soldiers.

It is also critical to try to reconstruct the military psychiatry experience in Vietnam to consider the impact of the reversal in American approval of the war on the clinical decisions of the deployed psychiatrists. Ethical and moral reactions to a war and its politics can influence military psychiatrists regarding the diagnosis and management of their cases (eg, encourage sympathetic overdiagnosis and overevacuation—decisions proven in past wars to prolong morbidity in combat-affected soldiers).[26]

In 1982, in an attempt to fill in this missing information, WRAIR queried all veteran Army psychiatrists who could be located about their professional experiences in the war. Of the estimated 135 psychiatrists who served in Vietnam (133 were men, two were women), 115 were located. Of those, 85 (74%) responded to a structured questionnaire exploring patterns of psychiatric problems encountered, types and effectiveness of clinical approaches, and personal reactions to the associated professional challenges and dilemmas.[2,27] Selected study findings will be summarized later in this chapter.

THE WAR'S RATIONALE AND PROVOCATION

To understand how the US government could reach a point where it would expend American lives and resources to fight a counterinsurgency in Vietnam, one must remember that following the end of World War II (1945), the United States and its allies soon found themselves again in an epic struggle against the menace of totalitarianism—this time, Soviet-sponsored Marxist communism (the "Cold War"). Relations between the two ideological camps were typically strained, and a catastrophic nuclear war seemed frighteningly possible. For example, between 1950 and 1953, the United States waged a costly war in support of South Korea's defense against a communist takeover by North Korea. Even closer to home, in 1961 the United States came perilously close to nuclear war with the former Soviet Union when it was discovered that the communist regime of Fidel Castro in Cuba had permitted the Soviet placement of nuclear missiles on that Caribbean island. The growing perception among Americans was that without vigorous opposition by the United States and its allies, democracy could be obliterated by a cascade of communist revolutions (the "domino theory") throughout the developing nations of the world, such as those in Southeast Asia. Because the United States was a signatory of the 1954 Southeast Asia Treaty Organization (with France, the United Kingdom, Thailand, Pakistan, Australia, New Zealand, and the Philippines),[28] South Vietnam's struggle to defend itself against armed aggression from North Vietnam (in violation of the 1954 Geneva Agreement that brought an end to the First Indochina War)[28] presented a compelling opportunity to draw the line with respect to the perceived threat.

THE SCOPE OF AMERICA'S WAR IN VIETNAM

America's enemies in Southeast Asia were 2-fold: (1) the indigenous Viet Cong guerrilla forces who operated in South Vietnam and who used harassment, terrorism, and sabotage as tactics to destabilize the government of South Vietnam, and (2) their allies—the regular units of North Vietnamese Army, who likewise sought a takeover of South Vietnam.

The pursuit of US military objectives in Vietnam became a huge undertaking. The ground war spanned over 8 years and by the time the remaining military personnel were withdrawn in 1973, 3.4 million American military men and women had served in the theater (typically a single, 1-year assignment), as well as offshore with the US Navy and at US Air Force bases in Thailand and Guam. When it ended, more than 58,000 Americans had died (over 47,000 due to enemy action or missing in action),[29] and more than 300,000 had been wounded.

The majority of those who were sent to Vietnam served in the Army (60%–80%), thus the majority of the casualties also were from the ranks of the Army (over 30,000 killed in action [KIA] and over 200,000 wounded in action [WIA]). Roughly 20% of troops actually served in first echelon combat arms, and the remainder served in combat support and service support roles. For the most part, Reserve and National Guard units were not called up, and the US military, especially the Army, resorted to increased conscription rates to meet its needs. Although only 25% of the total American forces deployed were technically draftees (vs 66% in World War II), many more were "draft-motivated" (ie, they enlisted in anticipation of being drafted because enlisting improved their chances of obtaining a noncombat assignment[30(p32)]). The average age of the Vietnam War soldier was younger (19 years old) than those who served in World War II (26 years old). They were also better educated than their fathers' generation of soldiers.

The war in Vietnam is classified as a "limited conventional war" because there were units larger than 4,000 soldiers operating in the field. However, it became mostly a counterinsurgency war. The war in Vietnam is also referred to as "low intensity" because of the low ratio of KIA and WIA to the numbers of personnel deployed compared to previous American wars. For example, a comparison of the peak years of US Army WIA rates during Vietnam (1968 = 120/1,000 troops) and Korea (1950 = 460/1,000 troops) suggests a lower combat intensity in Vietnam.[31] This can be misleading because of the smaller proportion of combat personnel compared to those in combat support and service support positions in Vietnam (a "tooth-to-tail" ratio of 1:5) and the availability of improved medical care. According to Ronald Spector, a military historian,

> Men in "maneuver battalions," the units that actually did the fighting, continued to run about the same chance of death or injury as their older relatives who had fought in Korea or in the Pacific [in World War II]. Indeed, during the first half of 1968, the *overall* [author's italics] Vietnam casualty rate exceeded the overall rate for all theatres in World War II, while the casualty rates for Army and Marine maneuver battalions were more than four times as high.[30(p55)]

The data accumulated on the types of wounds sustained in Vietnam are also revealing of the nature of combat there. Many more American casualties were caused by small arms fire or by booby traps and mines than in previous wars, and many fewer were caused by artillery and other explosive projectile fragments.

At home, an estimated quarter of a million Americans lost an immediate family member to the war. South Vietnam's military casualties numbered 220,357, with almost a half million becoming wounded. The United States spent $189 billion prosecuting the war and supporting the South Vietnamese government. In one 12-month period alone—mid-1968 through mid-1969, the peak year of US combat activities—America and its allies had over 1.5 million military personnel deployed (543,000 Americans, 819,200 South Vietnamese, and 231,100 from South Korea, Australia, New Zealand, Thailand, and the Philippines combined); US forces staged 1,100 ground attacks of battalion size or larger (compared to only 126 by the communist forces); and there were 400,000 American air attacks that dropped 1.2 million tons of bombs, costing $14 billion.[32]

AMERICA'S TWO VIETNAM WARS: PRE-TET '68 AND POST-TET '68

The American story of the ground war in Vietnam should be considered as two Vietnam War stories—starkly different, sequential stories that pivot on the events occurring in 1968. Taken together, these two stories portray a dramatic reversal of fortune for the United States, a reversal that powerfully shaped American culture.

The Buildup Phase (1965–1967): Lyndon Johnson's War

Lyndon Johnson was sworn into his first full term as President in January 1965, riding the crest of a national political consensus and overall prosperity. It was only, in the words of *Newsweek*, that "[n]agging little war in Vietnam,"[33(p58)] that cast a shadow on his ambition to create a "Great Society" of social reforms as his legacy. Nonetheless, the administration was determined to pursue those political agendas as well as ensure that South Vietnam did not fall into the communist sphere.

Preceded by over 10 years of US financial assistance and military advisors, US military presence expanded rapidly in South Vietnam after the Marine landing in 1965. By June 1966, American troops numbered 285,000, and another 100,000 would be pouring in by the end of the year. The number of inductions into the US military in 1966 alone was almost 320,000 men, a 250% increase over the previous year.[30]

The US Army, Marine Corps, and, in the Mekong River Delta, Navy units committed in South Vietnam typically found themselves operating in a rugged, tropical environment with formidable impediments to movement over the ground, extraordinary heat and humidity, and monsoonal rains for months at a time. Furthermore, combat operations conducted 10,000 miles from the United States required a very long logistical network. These troops also operated among an indigenous population of an exotic, Asian culture who spoke an exceptionally difficult language for Americans to learn. The local Vietnamese appeared to tolerate the presence of US troops, but it was common for them to be ambivalent about the government of South Vietnam and to harbor Viet Cong guerrillas. The relationships between US forces and the South Vietnamese were generally strained; US troops regarded them warily at best.[34] US combat units sponsored public relations programs designed to "win the hearts and minds" (ie, recruit the loyalty of villagers by providing for their welfare and security), but these brought only qualified success.

The combat strategy employed by the US Army in the buildup phase in Vietnam was one of attrition (body counts and kill ratios),[35] primarily through search-and-destroy missions initiated from well-defended enclaves. Guerrilla and terrorist operations by Viet Cong forces and periodic attacks by North Vietnamese regular units were the principle tactics of the communist forces. As a consequence, military engagements more often involved clashes between highly mobile, small tactical units as opposed to battles between major military formations. Furthermore, US successes were limited because the Viet Cong guerrillas were elusive, dictated the tempo of the fighting, and too often were content to snipe, set booby traps, and stage ambushes. Their hit-and-run tactics allowed them to fade safely into the jungle or into the local populace if the fight turned against them—tactics ingrained in their culture from centuries of guerrilla warfare against foreign invaders. US forces were more likely to find themselves in conventional war engagements against regular North Vietnamese divisions in the northern provinces. However, even these main force units more often than not staged combat initiatives from behind the safety of the 17th parallel demilitarized zone that separated North Vietnam from South Vietnam, thereby eluding pursuit by US units and their allies. Consequently, most combat activity for US forces involved brief encounters between isolated, small units—a war of no fronts. A Joint Chiefs of Staff study reported that of all the US patrols conducted in 1967 and 1968, less than 1% resulted in contact with the enemy.[35] Still, when there was contact, the fighting was as bloody and intense as any that had occurred during World War II. US forces did periodically stage larger scale operations during this phase of the war, and some elements of these engagements exacted heavy tolls on the enemy.

The US military in the late 1960s enjoyed remarkable technological advantages in Vietnam. Weaponry was a prime example. Whether carried with them into the field, or employed as tactical support from air strikes or artillery, field commanders could bring to bear formidable firepower on the enemy. If the enemy began to outnumber an allied force in an engagement, close support from the air or from artillery quickly reversed the equation. Another element of US technical superiority in Vietnam was that of air mobility—the ubiquitous helicopter. This was unprecedented in US warfare and allowed reconnaissance and ordnance delivery from the air, heliborne movement of troops for tactical advantage, timely evacuation of the wounded, and frequent resupply. In fact, the first full US Army combat division to be sent to Vietnam was the 1st Cavalry Division (Airmobile).

US Army Medical and Psychiatric Support

A third element in the Vietnam theater that greatly enhanced life for the US combat soldier in Vietnam was the outstanding medical support available. From the outset of the war, the US military made every effort to ensure that troops received timely, sophisticated medical attention, including psychiatric care, despite the hostile physical environment and Vietnam's geographical remoteness. The build up of Army medical units was completed in 1968 when 11 evacuation, 5 field, and 7 surgical hospitals were in place. These facilities, plus the 6th Convalescent Center in Cam Ranh Bay, brought the total bed capacity in South Vietnam to 5,283.[31] Most importantly, the new helicopter ambulance capability also permitted rapid evacuation of the wounded to the most appropriate level of medical care. As far as physical casualties, these efforts achieved remarkable success throughout the war. Comparing the ratio of KIA to WIA across wars attests to the superiority of medical care provided in Vietnam (World War II, 1:3.1; Korea, 1:4.1; and Vietnam, 1:5.6).[31]

The Organization and Preparation of Army Psychiatrists for Vietnam

Once the mobilization was under way in 1965, Army psychiatrists and allied mental health personnel were rapidly assigned and widely distributed throughout the theater. This peaked during the 4 full-strength years (1967–1970) when approximately 23 Army psychiatrist positions per year were available. In planning to fight in Vietnam, the Army Medical Department assumed that the greatest psychological threat to the force would be the "breaking point" of soldiers exposed to sustained enemy fire (eg, "combat exhaustion"—now labeled "combat stress reaction"). In anticipating large numbers of these casualties, they not only promulgated the treatment philosophy developed and refined in World War II and Korea (doctrine described earlier),[8] they also established policies and organizational structures[36] borrowed from those earlier engagements—a system that weighted the psychiatric assets in favor of combat units, even though combat-exposed troops would represent less than 20% of the Army deployed in South Vietnam.[30] Military planners were not only confident that this system would promote the conservation of military strength, they also believed that it would reduce morbidity in affected soldiers. This system centered upon assignment of psychiatrists to either a combat unit, typically as a division psychiatrist, or to a combat service support medical unit, typically a hospital (or specialized psychiatric detachment).

Assignment as a Division Psychiatrist. Throughout the war only the combat divisions (composed of 15,000–20,000 soldiers), that is, their medical battalions, had their own, directly assigned (eg, "organic") psychiatrists (along with allied mental health personnel). The rationale was to embed mental health personnel within combat units to provide psychiatric treatment capability as far forward as could practically be accomplished.[7] It also permitted the psychiatrist to serve as a staff officer of the command of the division and thereby provide timely advice on matters affecting morale and mental health (eg, "command consultation").

Assignment as a Hospital Psychiatrist. Alternatively, psychiatrists (along with allied mental health personnel) were assigned to Army-level hospitals or to the two specialized medical/psychiatric detachments (98th and 935th) in Vietnam. They functioned more often in a clinical role, and their command authority was from higher levels of Army medical command in Vietnam (ultimately the US Army Medical Command, Vietnam, or USAMEDCOMV, as it came to be called). The first priority for these psychiatric elements was to provide inpatient treatment for referrals from the combat divisions or other primary care facilities. In the case of the specialized psychiatric detachments ("KO teams" [the "KO" arbitrarily indicated that these were hospital augmentation detachments]), they offered more extended hospitalized care (up to 30 days) as well as serving as staging centers for out-of-country evacuations for soldiers needing additional care. The mission for hospital psychiatrists and their mental health colleagues also included the provision of outpatient care (eg, the Mental Health Consultation Service) for the soldiers from nondivisional (primarily noncombat) units on a regional basis. However, because these mental health assets were not part of the command structure of these units, mental health "command consultation" was far less predictable than would be the case in the combat divisions.

One psychiatrist slot was allocated to each of the seven full combat divisions deployed in Vietnam, as well as one each to the evacuation and field hospitals. These were filled depending on anticipated need and psychiatrist availability. In addition, throughout most of the war, the two Army neuropsychiatric specialty centers were operational and each was to be staffed with three psychiatrists. Furthermore, each year of the war a senior psychiatrist was to serve in a staff position with US Army Vietnam Headquarters as the Neuropsychiatric Consultant to the Commanding General, United States Army Republic of Vietnam (CG/USARV) Surgeon. The central task of the Consultant was to direct the coordination of psychiatric facilities and program planning, which required extensive travel throughout Vietnam to visit psychiatrists and programs, to provide clinical leadership, and to serve as consultant to senior military leaders about psychiatric issues.

The training and indoctrination provided for physicians, including psychiatrists, who would be assigned in Vietnam also centered on the limits of soldiers in combat, the causes of breakdown under sustained fire (social, physical, and emotional), and the prevention or management of large numbers of combat-generated psychiatric casualties as were encountered in the wars preceding Vietnam. This was the case in the Army's two psychiatric residency-training programs (Walter Reed General Hospital, Washington, DC, and Letterman General Hospital, San Francisco, California) where the principles of prevention and treatment of combat breakdown were emphasized in the curricula. It was also the case regarding newly commissioned, civilian-trained psychiatrists who would be assigned in Vietnam. They received their primary orientation to military psychiatry at the Army's Medical Field Service School, which was located at Fort Sam Houston in San Antonio, Texas. This preparation included only a few hours of didactic instruction in military psychiatry, and this was primarily regarding the pathogenesis, symptoms, and management of combat exhaustion[37] and the organization of psychiatric services within the combat division.[38]

The Relative Infrequency of Classic Combat Exhaustion Casualties in Vietnam

In time it became evident that the large numbers of combat exhaustion casualties that were predicted and planned for in Vietnam never materialized. The only overview of the psychiatric problems in the Vietnam War, published by Jones and Johnson, did not report theater-wide incidence statistics for combat exhaustion specifically,[7] although they were apparently collected by USAMEDCOMV.[9] Although these authors attested to the fact that the incidence throughout the war was "extremely low,"[7(p53)] Jones and Johnson added some confusion by referring to all hospitalized psychiatric patients in Vietnam as "combat psychiatric casualties." They also acknowledged that disagreements as to diagnostic criteria produced major problems in collecting and comparing incidence statistics for combat exhaustion in Vietnam, or even between wars. Boman, an Australian psychiatrist, provided corroboration in his postwar analysis of military psychiatry practices in Vietnam. He illustrated significant diagnostic confusion in the literature, and he posited that US military psychiatrists systematically, if inadvertently, mislabeled combat-generated psychological problems as character disorders, resulting in inappropriate administrative or disciplinary dispositions as well as spuriously lowering apparent incidence rates.[39] Finally, the only official summary of US Army medical experience in Vietnam (covering the war up through May 1970, two thirds into the war), which was authored by Major General Spurgeon Neel, does not mention combat exhaustion or any other forms of combat-generated psychopathology.[31]

Also hampering the collection of data regarding combat exhaustion casualties in Vietnam was the fact that, by definition, it is a reversible, stress-generated, psychosomatic regression that, when treated early and effectively, typically remits within a couple of days. As a consequence, many cases would have been treated at lower echelons of medical care and thus not be included in hospitalization rates.[40,41]

Approximations of CSR incidence measures in Vietnam came in the form of comparisons of the number of hospitalized CSR cases with those for other psychiatric conditions. The overview by Colbach and Parrish of US Army mental health activities in Vietnam through the first two thirds of the war reported 7% of all psychiatric admissions were diagnosed as CSR, but unfortunately they did not include data sources.[6] A smaller window, but one with more specific data, is provided by Major Peter Bourne, Medical Corps, Chief, Neuropsychiatry, WRAIR Medical Research Team in Vietnam (1965–1966). While comparing US Army psychiatric hospitalization rates in Vietnam with those of the Army of the Republic of Vietnam during the first 6 months of 1966, Bourne found 6% of US Army psychiatric admissions were diagnosed as combat exhaustion.[9] Captain HSR Byrdy, Medical Corps, division psychiatrist (1965–1966) with the 1st Cavalry Division (Airmobile) reported a true CSR rate for his division of 1.6 / 1,000 troops per year; however, he also comments, "What gets referred [to the division psychiatrist] depends on the tactical situation of the unit [and] one is hard-pressed to know what a real incidence is."[41(p50)] Still, these figures are consistent with an unusually low incidence, at least for the first half to two thirds of the war. In addition, in a postwar survey of psychiatrists who served with the Army in Vietnam, 32% reported that they had only rare exposure to combat-induced psychiatric casualties.[27]

All this is not to say that the specialized treatment of combat exhaustion was not an important challenge in Vietnam; just that it was never at the level (numbers) that had been anticipated, and that in time it was greatly overshadowed by other unanticipated psychiatric conditions and behavior problems.

Morale in the Buildup Phase: Consensus at Home and Esprit in Vietnam

During the war's first 3 years, opposition at home was only gradually building, whereas draft call-ups quickly gathered momentum to meet the huge personnel needs in Southeast Asia. Because reserve units and the National Guard were, for all practical purposes, exempted from deployment in Vietnam throughout the war, the ground forces were composed of a mix of career soldiers, draftees, and volunteers (including many draft-motivated volunteers). Although the combat could at times be very intense during these initial years, and the cities and countryside were not secure, morale and sense of purpose remained high among the troops fighting in Vietnam. Furthermore, attrition due to psychiatric or behavioral problems was exceptionally low compared to previous conflicts. This was somewhat surprising considering the psychologically depleting nature of the remote, exotic, hostile, tropical setting and the enemy's guerrilla tactics and resolute tenacity.[42]

Throughout the war, soldiers fighting in Vietnam encountered certain novel features that distinguished the theater from those of previous wars and invariably affected morale. For example, the battlefield ecology was powerfully affected by the helicopter mobility of US ground forces; the enemy's elusiveness but lack of a capacity to deliver sustained, precision-guided indirect fire (as with artillery and combat aircraft); and, especially, the overall US strategy of fighting a war of attrition as opposed to one for territorial control. The psychosocial complexion of the "rear" was unique. US troops typically staged combat activities from geographically isolated, fixed, relatively secure enclaves that were easily resupplied by helicopter. The high ratio of combat support and service support troops to combat troops (5:1) was also unusual compared to earlier wars.

Efforts to understand soldier stress and resilience in Vietnam also have to take into account the influence of the draft (stress inducing) as well as the effect of the military's replacement policy of individualized, 1-year tours. The 1-year tour was intended to be stress reducing because these soldiers would perceive their obligation and risk as limited.[9,31] However, over time the resultant churning and ultimate depletion of experienced military personnel in the theater (including officers and noncommissioned officers [NCOs]) also had a hugely negative effect on commitment and cohesion, and consequently morale.[29,30]

Still, according to General Westmoreland, Commander, US Military Assistance Command, Vietnam (COMUSMACV), the troops operating in Vietnam during the buildup years were "the toughest, best trained, most dedicated American servicemen in history."[43(p34)] More specific to the Army in Vietnam, Retired Brigadier General SLA Marshall, combat veteran of World War I and front-line observer in World War II and Korea, commented after his extended visit in 1966:

> My overall estimate was that the morale of the troops and the level of discipline of the Army were higher than I had ever known them in any of our wars. There was no lack of will to fight and the average soldier withstood the stress of engagement better than ever before.[43(p34)]

The observations and interpretations by military sociologist Charles Moskos from his time in Vietnam as a war correspondent between 1965 and 1967 are especially useful in understanding the morale, stress, and psychosocial adaptations of the soldiers serving in those initial years. Moskos reported high morale and combat motivation despite the rigors of the counterinsurgency warfare and the extremely inhospitable setting. He believed this arose out of the linkage between the soldiers' individual self-concern (heightened because of the 1-year, individual rotation system) and devotion to the other soldiers in the immediate combat group (eg, instrumental interdependencies motivated by the functional goal of survival). He also observed their shared belief in an exaggerated masculine ethic as well as a "latent ideology" of devotion to US ideals, which stemmed from their conviction regarding the supremacy of the US way of life. Furthermore, the soldiers he studied were notably apolitical and antagonistic toward peace demonstrators ("privileged anarchists") at home.[44]

Psychiatric investigator Bourne's comments from his year in Vietnam are also illuminating. He reported that soldiers in these early years maintained a positive motivation in part through what he labeled "combat provincialism."

> They are not only unconcerned about the political and strategic aspects of the war; they are also disinterested in the outcome of any battle that is not in their own immediate vicinity. . . . [The soldier] retains certain deep allegiances and beliefs in an . . . amorphous positive entity, "Americanism," which allow him to justify his being sent to Vietnam.[9(p44)]

Bourne especially credited the fixed, 1-year tour for soldiers for the continued high morale, but he also expressed concern for its consequent disturbance to the "solidarity of the small unit"—the traditional stress protection system for combat soldiers.

Buildup Phase Psychiatric Overview

Correlating with the observations of high esprit and commitment, troop attrition due to psychiatric or behavioral dysfunction was exceptionally low as well during those first few years. The proportion of medevacs out of Vietnam for psychiatric reasons (3%–4%) compared quite favorably with that for the Korean conflict (6%) and for World War II (23%).[23] Rates for deviant behaviors for the same period were also low (eg, the annual stockade confinement rate was 1.15/1,000, compared to the expected overseas rate of 2.2).[4] Some senior Army psychiatric observers attributed this to an array of operational and preventive factors that appeared to protect the soldiers from psychiatric and behavioral difficulties: (*a*) technological superiority and the professionalism of the troops; (*b*) fixed, 1-year assignments; (*c*) high-quality leadership; and (*d*) adequate supplies, equipment, and support—especially medical support.[7,23,45,46] Others also credited the application of the aforementioned doctrine of combat psychiatry.[47,48]

Although alcohol use and abuse was predictably a common stress outlet for these soldiers,[7] military leaders and the psychiatric contingent were primarily concerned with the use of illegal drugs by troops, especially the locally grown marijuana, which was readily available and highly potent. In their survey regarding drug use patterns of 584 lower ranking enlisted soldiers departing Vietnam in 1967, Roffman and Sapol reported that of the 32% who acknowledged ever smoking marijuana, 61% began in Vietnam and one quarter were considered heavy users (greater than 20 times during their 1-year tour in Vietnam). The authors concluded that the extent of marijuana use in Vietnam was very similar to that among civilian peers.[16] Furthermore, in the opinion of Bourne, marijuana use created almost no psychiatric problems.[9] Use of opiates was also reported in Vietnam, but it was not as pure as that sold after 1970 and was not used by soldiers in sufficient numbers to constitute a serious problem for command.[17]

One psychological phenomenon that did attract a fair amount of attention from military psychiatrists was the phasic nature of moods and attitudes affecting soldiers during the course of their 12-month tour of duty in Vietnam: (*a*) "immersion shock" and fearfulness; (*b*) then mastery and reduced preoccupation with home, but with some depression, resignation, and flight into a "hedonistic psuedocommunity"; (*c*) followed by growing combat apprehension and a "short-timers syndrome."[7,49,50] The latter refers to a low-grade form of disability often exhibited in combat soldiers who were within 4 to 6 weeks of their date of expected return from overseas (DEROS). Symptoms consisted of reduced combat tolerance and efficiency; increasing fear about being killed or wounded; and sullen, irritable, or withdrawn behavior. This had also been noted among troops serving in the Korean War after fixed, individualized tours were first introduced there in mid-1951.[51]

Overall, the incidence of psychiatric and behavioral difficulties among the deployed Army troops in Vietnam in these initial years was held to levels no greater than if they were still stateside. Satisfaction was expressed that adequate psychiatric resources had been deployed from the start in contrast to previous wars.[3,8] To that effect, Bourne confidently, if prematurely, declared the end of the military-medical problem of combat psychiatric casualties: "The Vietnam experience has shown that we have now successfully identified most of the major correlates of psychiatric attrition in the combat zone."[47(p487)]

Buildup Phase Psychiatrist Reports

The morale and confidence of the deployed Army psychiatrists during these early years also appeared to be high. This is suggested both in the large numbers who were inspired to publish professional accounts and the role satisfaction that these reports reveal. Taken together, these psychiatrists reflect optimism and tout the effectiveness of the traditional doctrine of combat psychiatry in Vietnam, the utilization of newly developed pharmacologic agents (anxiolytics and neuroleptics), and the extension of principles of social psychiatry to military leaders (command consultation). Simply scanning selected titles provides an impression as to the predominant psychiatric challenges faced through these early years in the war (Exhibit 2-1).

More specific to the growing antiwar sentiment in the United States, two Army psychiatrists who served in the buildup phase and published accounts, Captain AS Blank Jr and Captain HS Bloch, commented specifically that they did not believe the growing opposition to the war was significantly affecting their patients. Blank, who served early in this phase (1965–1966), commented,

> Do the ambiguities of the war seem to be a problem for the soldiers? The answer is very simply, "No." I did not see a single patient in whom I felt that any kind of conflict about the war on any level was primary in precipitating his visits to me.[41(p58)]

Bloch, who served 2 years later (1967–1968) in the same area as Blank, asserted that in his experience, soldiers who struggled with concerns regarding the morality of the conflict typically were driven by pre-Vietnam psychological conflicts.[40] Nonetheless, considering what followed, it is apparent that time was running out on positive morale in Vietnam.

The Transition From Buildup to Drawdown (1968–1969)

1968 Surprise "Tet" Offensives and Perceptions of a Lost War

The year 1968 was the bloodiest year in Vietnam for US forces (16,592 KIA), and events both at home and in Southeast Asia served as the tipping point in US sentiment for pursuing military objectives there. During the month of May alone, 2,000 Americans were killed—the highest monthly death toll of the war.[52] June 13th marked the day that Americans had been fighting in Vietnam longer than any prior war. However, the greatest negative effect arose from the enemy's "Tet" offensives.

On the morning of January 31st, communist guerillas broke the Tet (or Lunar New Year) truce and launched coordinated attacks on cities and towns throughout South Vietnam. Although they were ultimately extremely costly to the communist forces and achieved little militarily, their political yield was enormous. Many held the US media accountable for misinterpreting these events as signaling a US defeat and provoking a reversal in public and political support for war.[53] Nonetheless, these attacks, as well as the month-long, bloody battle to retake Hue and the prolonged siege of the Marine base of Khe Sanh, created the indelible perception in the United States that the war could not be won. The enemy appeared to defy the Johnson administration's assurances of imminent defeat, and nowhere in the country seemed secure despite great expenditures of lives and money. As a consequence, calls for the war to end became urgent and trumped most other considerations.

On March 31, 1968, President Johnson announced that he would halt the bombing over North Vietnam as a prelude to peace negotiations. He also declared that he would not seek reelection in service of that end. Ten days later he announced that General Creighton Abrams would relieve General William Westmoreland, the original commander, United States Military Assistance Command, Vietnam (USMACV). Still, it wasn't until a year later, mid-1969, that the first Army units pulled out of South Vietnam. America had begun to disengage, yet the fighting continued amid tortuous peace negotiations, continued assignment

EXHIBIT 2-1

SELECTED PUBLICATIONS BY BUILDUP-PHASE ARMY PSYCHIATRISTS (INCLUDING RESEARCH REPORTS)

Year in Vietnam	No. Who Published Articles/Total No. Deployed Army Psychiatrists (as a percentage)*	Publications
1965	1/7 (14.2%)	Huffman RE. Which soldiers break down: a survey of 610 psychiatric patients in Vietnam. *Bull Menninger Clin*. 1970;34:343–351.
		Bourne PG. Urinary 17-OHCS levels in two combat situations. In: Bourne PG, ed. *The Psychology and Physiology of Stress: With Reference To Special Studies of the Viet Nam War*. New York, NY: Academic Press; 1969: 95–116. Research report.
1966	6/16 (37.5%)	Conte LR. A neuropsychiatric team in Vietnam 1966–1967: an overview. In: Parker RS, ed. *The Emotional Stress of War, Violence, and Peace*. Pittsburgh, Penn: Stanwix House; 1972: 163–168.
		Johnson AW. Psychiatric treatment in the combat situation. *US Army Vietnam Med Bull*. 1967;January/February:38–45.
		Jones FD. Experiences of a division psychiatrist in Vietnam. *Mil Med*. 1967;132:1003–1008.
		Dowling JJ. Psychological aspects of the year in Vietnam. *US Army Vietnam Med Bull*. 1967;May/June:45–48.
		Tischler GL. Patterns of psychiatric attrition and of behavior in a combat zone. In: Bourne PG, ed. *The Psychology and Physiology of Stress: With Reference to Special Studies of the Viet Nam War*. New York: Academic Press; 1969: 19–44.
		Kenny WF. Psychiatric disorders among support personnel. *US Army Vietnam Med Bull*. 1967;January/February:34–37.
1967	12/22 (54.6%)	Roffman RA, Sapol E. Marijuana in Vietnam: a survey of use among Army enlisted men in two southern corps. *Int J Addict*. 1970;5:1–42. Research report.
		Anderson JR. Psychiatric support of the 3rd and 4th Corps tactical zone. *US Army Vietnam Med Bull*. 1968;January/February:37–39.
		Baker WL. Division psychiatry in the 9th Infantry Division. *US Army Vietnam Med Bull*. 1967;November/December:5–9.
		Bloch HS. Brief sleep treatment with chlorpromazine. *Comp Psychiatry*. 1970;11:346–355.
		Bostrom JA. Management of combat reactions. *US Army Vietnam Med Bull*. 1967;July/August:6–8.
		Casper E, Janacek J, Martinelli H. Marijuana in Vietnam. *US Army Vietnam Med Bull*. 1968;September/October:60–72.
		Evans ON. Army aviation psychiatry in Vietnam. *US Army Vietnam Med Bull*. 1968;May/June:54–58.
		Fidaleo RA Marijuana: social and clinical observations. *US Army Vietnam Med Bull*. 1968;March/April:58–59.
		Gordon EL. Division psychiatry: documents of a tour. *US Army Vietnam Med Bull*. 1968;November/December:62–69.
		Motis G. Psychiatry at the battle of Dak To. *US Army Vietnam Med Bull*. 1968;March/April:57.
		Pettera RL, Johnson BM, Zimmer R. Psychiatric management of combat reactions with emphasis on a reaction unique to Vietnam. *Mil Med*. 1969;134:673–678.
		Talbott JA. The Saigon warriors during Tet. *US Army Vietnam Med Bull*. 1968;March/April:60–61.

*These numbers do not count research reports, although they are listed in the Publications column.

of replacement troops (albeit in decreasing numbers after mid-1969), and a progressively confrontational antiwar/antimilitary faction stateside. The war took on characteristics of a tedious, agonizing stalemate, and the lack of tangible measures of progress contributed to the widespread feelings of futility and frustration about the war.

Emerging Demoralization and Dissent

The contentious and protracted counterinsurgency war soon started to have corrosive effects on successive cohorts of replacements sent to fight there. Budding demoralization and dissent during these pivotal years began to reveal itself especially in racial incidents and widening drug use (particularly marijuana, but also commercially marketed stimulants and barbiturates) by soldiers. Law enforcement figures demonstrated an increase of over 260% in the number of soldiers involved with possession or use of marijuana during 1968 as compared to the previous year.[30] Also, excessive combat aggression (atrocities) seemed to become more prevalent.[54–57] According to Ronald Spector, who served as a Marine field historian in Vietnam (1968–1969),

> as the war ground on through its third and fourth year, the prestige of performing a mission well proved increasingly inadequate to men who more and more could see no larger purpose in that mission, and no end to the incessant patrols, sweeps, and ambushes which appeared to result only in more danger, discomfort, and casualties.[30(p61)]

Spector also noted that the evolving stalemate in Vietnam came to resemble the bloody trench warfare of World War I, a battle in which both sides grossly underestimated the other.[30(p314)]

Journalist Donald Kirk reported from the field in 1969 that

> [t]he attitudes of GIs [slang for "government issue"] did not turn seriously until Fall of 1968 when President Johnson stopped the bombing of North Vietnam and agreed to enter into peace talks . . . .The change in [soldier] attitudes was so sudden . . . [as compared to earlier] they by and large applauded the [antiwar] demonstrators . . . the senselessness of the struggle.[58(p61)]

Correspondent JP Sterba provides observations on the shifting demographics and particularly the attitudes of the soldiers who went to fight in Vietnam in 1969. He demonstrated how the rapidly unfolding political events in the United States caused the romance and idealism of the early war to be replaced by a "hated, dreary struggle" in which the soldier's overriding preoccupation was that of self-protection:

> These were the grunts of the class of 1968—they had come out of that America some of their commanders had seen only from the windows of the Pentagon. They were the graduates of an American nightmare in 1968 that stemmed mostly from the war they had now come to fight—the year of riots and dissention, of assassinations and Chicago, the year America's ulcer burst.[59(p447)]

Transition Phase Psychiatric Overview

The official summary of US Army medical experience in Vietnam through May 1970 made note of rising annual incidence rates for psychiatric conditions beginning in 1969 (from 13.3/1,000 for 1968, to 25.1/1,000 through first quarter of 1970). It also underscored that this increase did not covary with the dropping rates for WIA, the traditional measure of combat intensity—a correlation that had been true in previous wars.[31] The principle author of this report, Major General Spurgeon Neel, attributed this uncharacteristic rise in psychiatric disorders to dissenting soldier subgroups who were motivated by racial, political, or drug culture priorities, and to the widening use of illegal drugs by soldiers in Vietnam. However, because this review only encompassed the first two thirds of the war and was not published until 1973, after the troops were withdrawn, it failed to illuminate the fuller, more ominous picture in a timely fashion.

Published more contemporarily in 1970, the Army Psychiatry Consultant to the Surgeon General, Colonel Matthew Parrish, and the Assistant Consultant, Major Edward Colbach, both of whom had served in Vietnam, did broadcast their concern about the rise in the psychiatric casualty rate in Vietnam up through mid-1970. In their opinion this was a consequence of the increase in racial tensions and the general decrement in perception of military purpose within the soldier. They correctly predicted that the intent to disengage from Vietnam would likely produce accelerating psychiatric problems among those newly assigned there.[6] However, despite this warning, there were no structural changes in the organization of mental health assets in Vietnam nor modifications in the selection, preparation, or deployment of mental health personnel sent as replacements to the theater.

MD Stanton[17] reported sizable increases in the use of most drugs from a survey of drug use patterns among soldiers entering or departing Vietnam in late 1969, which he compared with results from the 1967 survey by Roffman and Sapol. Stanton speculated, however, that marijuana and some other drugs might actually allow certain types of individuals to function under the stresses of a combat environment and separation from home.

As far as comparisons with the US Marines fighting in Vietnam, Lieutenant Commander JA Renner Jr, a Navy psychiatrist who served in the Vietnam theater in 1969, noted a similar rise regarding disciplinary problems, including racial disturbances, attacks on superiors, drug abuse, and the number of men diagnosed with character disorders ("hidden casualties"). He expressed his concern that military psychiatrists were premature in touting the low rate for psychiatric difficulties in the war.[60] (He did not publish until 1973, after the Marines had left Vietnam.)

Transition Phase Psychiatrist Reports

Army psychiatrists serving in these years were mostly not inspired to publish accounts of their professional experience in Vietnam compared to those who served in the buildup phase. Indeed, the titles suggest increasing attention to challenges surrounding GI drug use and other morale issues and away from combat-related problems. Still, dissent within the ranks appears not to be a subject of major concern by these psychiatrists (Exhibit 2-2).

The Drawdown Phase (1969–1972): Richard Nixon's War

The second half of the war took on a starkly different character from the first half. By January 1969, when President Nixon succeeded President Johnson, the United States had been at war in Vietnam for 4 years. Nixon promised "peace with honor," negotiations with the enemy, and a gradual withdrawal of troops, while confronting extreme impatience and often violent protest in America.[61] With the change of command in Vietnam, the military strategy of attrition shifted to a defensive one that sought area security and "Vietnamization" of the fighting. Enemy offensive activity also slackened. Overall US troop strength in Vietnam peaked at 543,400 in mid-1969 and declined through the next 3 years until all combat forces were

EXHIBIT 2-2

SELECTED PUBLICATIONS BY TRANSITION-PHASE ARMY PSYCHIATRISTS (INCLUDING RESEARCH REPORTS)

Year in Vietnam	No. Who Published Articles/Total No. Deployed Army Psychiatrists (as a percentage)*	Publications
1968	3/22 (13.6%)	Colbach EM, Crowe RR. Marijuana associated psychosis in Vietnam. *Mil Med*. 1970;135:571–573.
		Colbach EM, Willson SM. The binoctal craze. *US Army Vietnam Med Bull*. 1969;March/April:40–44.
		Forest DV, Bey DR, Bourne PG. The American soldier and Vietnamese women. *Sex Behav*. 1972;2:8–15.
		Postel WB. Marijuana use in Vietnam: a preliminary report. *US Army Vietnam Med Bull*. 1968;September/October:56–59.
1969	2/22 (9.1%)	Bey DR. Change in command in combat: a locus of stress. *Am J Psychiatry*. 1972;129:698–702.
		Bey DR, Smith WE. Organizational consultant in a combat unit. *Am J Psychiatry*. 1970;128:401–406.
		Bey DR, Zecchinelli VA. Marijuana as a coping device in Vietnam. *Mil Med*. 1971;136:448–450.
		Master FD. Some clinical observations of drug abuse among GIs in Vietnam. *J Kentucky Med Assn*. 1971;69:193–195.
		Stanton MD. Drug use in Vietnam. *Arch Gen Psychiatry*. 1972;26:279–286. Research report.

*These numbers do not count research reports, although they are listed in the Publications column.

withdrawn. US operations of battalion size or larger slowly began to decline beginning in mid-1968.[62] Still, despite the reduction of combat operations and the peace negotiations, which proceeded erratically, US service personnel continued to die there (15,316 from 1969–1972).

In 1969, the US public was horrified to learn that in 1968 several hundred Vietnamese civilians of the hamlet of My Lai had been massacred by a US Army unit.[63] Although there had been previous reports of atrocities by US troops, this incident seemed to verify the public's worst fears about the war being senseless and destructive.

"America's war" had become prolonged, stalemated, and costly; the sense of national purpose and resolve was dropping fast. Furthermore, the abandonment of hopes for military victory in Vietnam had a powerfully negative effect on the country, the institution of the US Army,[64–66] and especially those whose fate it would be to serve during the drawdown in Vietnam and who would be required to fight battles of disengagement amid pressures from home to oppose the war and the military.[62] Simultaneously waging war and pursuing a peace with the enemy undermined the commitment of these soldiers compared to those deployed in the first few years of the war. This commitment was replaced with alienation, disaffection, and sagging morale. In retrospect, gradually rising rates for psychiatric conditions and behavior problems during 1968 and 1969 signaled a brewing discontent and dissent within the ground forces deployed on a massive scale.

Cultural Polarization in America and the Vietnam War

To fully understand the psychosocial forces affecting the soldiers sent to Vietnam, one must appreciate the powerful and often clashing cultural crosscurrents in the United States that surrounded them in the late 1960s and early 1970s. This history must be viewed against the backdrop not only of the nation's post–World-War-II experience and subsequent Cold War tensions between the United States and the former Soviet Union, but also of the advent of television coverage of the war, the assassination of President John Kennedy in 1963, and the coming of age of the post–World-War-II "baby boom" generation.

The years surrounding the Vietnam War (1965–1975) represented an excruciatingly volatile period in American life. Intense and often militant challenges to government institutions, especially the military and the war in Vietnam, were increasingly made by: (*a*) a progressively disapproving American public, (*b*) the rising civil rights and black pride movements, and (*c*) the emerging New Left and a dissenting youth counterculture (the "generation gap"). They, in turn, were opposed by an equally fervent and reactive conservative sector. The prolonged, costly war in Vietnam served as a rallying point, both pro and con, for their passions and ambitions. These three movements, fostered by an expanding drug culture, variously fed and were fed by a widening crisis within the military overall (unprecedented demoralization and alienation), and in Vietnam especially. As they synergistically intersected, they generated a groundswell of opposition to military service among draft-eligible men.

Public Opposition to the War and Political Activism. Over the course of the war larger and louder antiwar protest rallies, marches, and demonstrations took place in the United States, with some reaching the level of riots. The new television coverage of the war brought the costs and the political turmoil in Vietnam straight into the living rooms of US citizens and most likely accelerated the public's perception that the war's justification was questionable, despite reassurances from both the Johnson and Nixon administrations.

The steadily growing public disapproval of the war in Vietnam can be traced through a series of nationwide Gallup opinion polls conducted during the war years in which respondents were asked: "In view of the developments since we entered the fighting in Vietnam, do you think the US made a mistake sending troops to fight in Vietnam?" In 1965, only 25% thought US military involvement was a mistake (vs 60% who said "No"), but by 1971 these factions had almost completely reversed (60% saying "yes," it was a mistake, and only 30% disagreeing).[67]

Following the insertion of ground troops in March 1965, the growing personnel requirements in Vietnam resulted in dramatically accelerated draft calls. For example, total inductions in 1965 were about 120,000; those for 1966 and 1967 were two-and-a-half times the 1965 figure. As opposition to the war mounted, the draft became the epicenter of the antiwar protest until the military switched to an all-volunteer force in 1973.[30] With each passing year, as the need for more troops became evident, additional criteria for draft exemption were removed to increase the pool of eligible draftees. In 1968, in an effort to blunt the public's growing concern for unevenness and inconsistency in the Selective Service System, the draft was modified to a lottery system, based on birthdays. On December 1, 1969, the first drawing was held. Men then knew the likelihood of being drafted based on where their birthdays fell; however, for those selected and sent to Vietnam under this new, random system, their sense of injustice was compounded.[68] Ultimately 4 million young men were exempted by high lottery numbers;

more than 200,000 young men were accused of draft offenses.[68]

The Counterculture and Youth/Student Opposition to the Vietnam War. Opposition to US involvement in Vietnam began slowly in 1964 on various college campuses as part of a more general rising spirit of student activism. In addition to various liberal causes, "free speech," "free love," "peace," and "do your own thing" were also popular. The means employed to indicate opposition included political advocacy, civil disobedience, "sit-ins," "teach-ins," and generally nonviolent resistance to the status quo.

A succession of tremendous shocks ushered in a more fervent antiestablishment spirit: the assassination of President Kennedy in the autumn of 1963; the first ghetto uprisings in the summer of 1964; the escalation of the war in Vietnam beginning in 1965 and the impact of the draft; the 1968 assassinations of presidential candidate Robert Kennedy and civil rights leader Reverend Martin Luther King; and, also in 1968, the enemy's surprise Tet offensives and other seeming military setbacks in Vietnam. The result was widespread impatience with the prospects for orderly change through more peaceful, passive means, and deep cynicism and mistrust of American institutions and "anyone over 30." The "Woodstock generation," named after the huge rock festival held in upstate New York in August 1969, and it's "summer of peace and love" were quickly fading memories as the movement took on a more radical perspective and accepted a more open, and at times violent, revolutionary approach.

As one measure, surveys of student attitudes in 1969 revealed that although only 2% of college youth were highly visible activists, roughly 40% of their peers held similar views ("protest prone"), signifying a true generation gap. Among this larger group, approximately half endorsed the belief that the United States was a sick society and acknowledged a loss of faith in democratic institutions. Two thirds endorsed civil disobedience to promote their causes, especially antiwar protests and draft resistance.[69]

Emergent Black Pride Movement and Racial Tensions. In 1948, President Harry Truman put forth an executive order directing the nation's military services to eliminate all vestiges of racial segregation. Since then, many positive gains made in the status of black Americans can be directly attributed to the men and women who served in the military. However, the burgeoning civil rights movement in the 1960s heightened black soldiers' awareness of disparities (with accusations of discrimination) in positions and roles for blacks in the military, especially among the younger soldiers and particularly regarding combat exposure and risk.[62,70]

For instance, during the initial years in Vietnam, questions were raised as to whether blacks represented an unfair proportion of the combat casualties. In fact, for the period 1965 to 1966 in each of the deployed combat divisions, the proportion of deaths of African-Americans exceeded the proportion of African-American soldiers in the division. However, closer analysis revealed that, overall, blacks did not serve in Vietnam out of proportion to their numbers in the general population; and rather than racially-driven policies, various other social and cultural factors (eg, levels of education and socioeconomic status) served to select African-Americans for greater risk in Vietnam.[30] Still, beginning in 1967, the military began to reduce the numbers of black soldiers assigned to infantry, armor, and cavalry units in Vietnam, and by mid-1969 the percentage of black casualties was close to the percentage of blacks serving in Vietnam.[70]

Racial tensions in America became explosive following the assassination of Reverend Martin Luther King in April 1968. Racial protests and riots erupted at numerous US military installations worldwide, including in Vietnam. The most notorious in Vietnam was in August 1968, when black confinees seized the Long Binh stockade and held it for almost a month. These sentiments coincided with the rapid evolution of a more radical "black power" faction, which advocated a black pride revolution and rejected assimilation in American culture as a central goal for African-Americans. Career military blacks were often caught between their loyalty to the military and the attitudes of the younger, black enlisted soldiers who were restive and expected solidarity from them regarding questions of discrimination. As the war wound on, younger blacks increasingly opposed sacrifices and risks in what they perceived as a racially inspired war (eg, against other people of color).[71,72] They dismissed it as a "white man's war" and asserted their intention to return home to take up the fight against repression and racism in America.[73]

Soldier Resistance and the "GI" Underground Movement. As opposition to the war mounted, public attitudes in the United States toward returning veterans reversed from acceptance to scorn. This left those who chose, or were directed, to serve in Vietnam as replacements conflicted as to what represented patriotic, morally justifiable behavior, as well as less certain regarding the inherent risks and hardships they faced there. Johnston and Bachman[74] compared results of surveys of draft-eligible men conducted in spring 1969 and again in summer 1970, regarding their plans and attitudes toward military service. In that short span of time the majority shifted from identifying with US political and military policies in Vietnam to feeling alienated from the greater society, the government, and US involvement there.[74] The roughly 4-fold Army-wide increase in rates for absent without leave (AWOL) and desertion during the period from 1964 to 1974 provides a measure of the growing opposition to serving over the course of the war.[75]

Organized dissent within the military did not emerge until 1967 and disappeared in 1973 once combat units were out of Vietnam. It apparently was slow in its development because its inspiration required the angst of returning veterans to be combined with draftee resistance. In time, a vicious cycle developed in which returning veterans publicly repudiated their Vietnam service record, including joining war protest organizations such as Vietnam Veterans Against the War, which in turn encouraged prospective Vietnam soldiers to oppose service there. In the United States this essentially first-term enlistee and draftee antiwar resistance movement was especially promulgated through "alternative culture" GI coffee houses, underground newspapers (estimated to exist on 300 posts and bases),[51(p234)] antiwar protest petitions, and support from civilian antiwar groups.

As it turned out, most soldiers in Vietnam were not true antiwar protestors and, overall, the GI resistance movement had only limited success.[76] Still, although the antiwar movement within the Vietnam-era military failed to reach revolutionary proportions for several reasons, especially the lack of sympathetic civilians in Vietnam, its emergence was unique in US history and some believed it accelerated withdrawal from the war.[51] Others argued that it emboldened the enemy and thus dragged out the peace negotiations and prolonged the war. Nonetheless, military and government officials were quite concerned about its effects.

The Spreading Drug Culture and Its Effects on Soldiers Sent to Vietnam. The incidence of illegal drug use among teens and young adults in the United States, especially psychedelics and marijuana, rose rapidly in the 1960s in tandem with the emerging dissidence of this group. Various studies were conducted during the Vietnam era comparing drug use among soldiers with their civilian peers. For example, a nationwide study of psychoactive drug use by young men at the close of the Vietnam War indicated that the peak of the drug epidemic was 1969 to 1973, and that veterans, regardless of where they served, showed no higher rates than nonveterans.[77] Regarding measures among the military in the United States, a survey of drug use at a stateside military installation in 1970, 1971, and 1972 showed the percentage of respondents reporting premilitary drug use increased as did the amount of use and the number of current users.[78] A study of pattterns of drug use among 5,482 active duty enlisted men assigned to 56 separate Army units in the United States between January 1969 and April 1969 found one quarter of subjects acknowledged past use of marijuana, amphetamines, lysergic acid diethylamide (LSD), or heroin.[79] Two years later a similar survey of 19,948 new military inductees between January 1971 and June 1971 found that almost one third acknowledged civilian drug use.[80]

Among soldiers sent to Vietnam, Sapol and Roffman surveyed 584 enlisted soldiers departing Vietnam in 1967 (31.7% reported use of marijuana at least once) and concluded that the rates were comparable with those reported in published studies among university students.[81] In a survey of soldiers entering or departing Vietnam 2 years later, Stanton found a sizable increase in the reported use of marijuana among those leaving Vietnam (28.9% vs 50.1% respectively compared to the 1967 survey). Most of this was accounted for by the increase reported by soldiers entering Vietnam. However, Stanton did find a shift toward heavier use among his sample of departing enlisted soldiers (29.6% compared to the 7.4% from the earlier study). Nonetheless, his impression was that the rise in casual marijuana use in Vietnam mostly mirrored rising use patterns among civilian peers.[82]

Regarding heroin use, a 1972 heroin use survey comparing 1,007 noncombat Army soldiers in Vietnam simultaneously with 856 counterparts assigned to a stateside post found that 13.5% of Vietnam soldiers and 14.5% of those stateside reported previous use of heroin. The authors compared their findings with published surveys, concluding that a heroin epidemic occurred in Vietnam earlier in the 1970s, but that any conclusion that "such an epidemic '[w]as unique' . . . and 'infected' many average US soldiers appears inaccurate and misleading."[83] Taken together, these studies strongly verify that younger enlisted soldiers, not surprisingly, brought into the service and into Vietnam their drug use habits from civilian life.

Disputes About the Ethics of Combat Psychiatry

The shifting social and political zeitgeist in the latter half of the war—particularly the accelerating antiwar and antimilitary sentiment—began to affect psychiatrists and psychiatry, and provoked concerns about cooperating with the military. Debates—typically quite passionate—that questioned the ethics of psychiatrists who performed draft evaluations[84–88] or served with the military, especially in Vietnam[39,89–93] appeared in the professional literature beginning in 1970. Denunciation of military psychiatry came both from psychiatrists and other physicians who had served in Vietnam, as well as from those who had not.[26]

Mental health organizations also sought to take official positions on the war. Even if not specifically questioning the ethics of their colleagues in uniform, they nevertheless questioned the morality of the US military and government. In March 1971, 67% of members responding to a poll of the American Psychiatric Association voted that the United States should terminate all military activity in Vietnam.[94] In July 1972, the American Psychological Association joined seven other mental health associations in attacking the US role in the war. Their public statement included, "we find it morally repugnant for any government to exact such heavy costs in human suffering for the sake of abstract conceptions of national pride or honor."[95] Defense of professional support for the US forces was published by several psychiatrists, most of whom had served in Vietnam.[5,6,96–99]

Mounting Biopsychosocial Stressors in the Combat Theater Ecology

In the second half of the war, even though more troops were leaving than were sent as replacements, hostilities and dangers continued. The successive cohorts of replacement soldiers in Vietnam were deeply affected by the moral crisis at home, which included increasingly radical US politics, especially regarding the war, and a rapidly expanding drug culture. Furthermore, the annualized troop rotation schedules, rapid and wholesale transportation of soldiers and media representatives, and modern technology all promoted the accelerated infusion of a growing antiwar, antimilitary sentiment into the ranks of the military there. Unrelenting public opposition to the war may have accelerated the US pullout, but the process demoralized those who were sent there during the drawdown years. Understandably, many soldiers interpreted antiwar sentiment as criticism of them personally—not the war more generally. The uncertain combat results in the theater and vacillating—at times contradictory—government policies and military strategies regarding prosecuting the war and pursuing the peace were also demoralizing.

This demoralization and alienation of soldiers in the Vietnam theater often took the form of psychiatric and behavioral problems, especially drug abuse, racial incidents, and misconduct, and presented problems for the Army and Army psychiatrists on an unprecedented scale. These were even more of a problem among soldiers in the "rear," but even within combat units, troops covertly, and at times overtly, challenged authority (eg, combat refusal incidents, "search and avoid" missions, excess combat aggression). Matters became even more serious after a Vietnamese-based heroin market began to flourish in the spring of 1970 and large numbers of US soldiers became users. It took 9 months to institute an effective urine drug screening system that would permit the military to comprehend and react to this insidious and widespread problem of self-inflicted soldier dissent and disability. Equally disturbing to the Army in Vietnam were the incidents of soldiers attacking their superiors, typically with explosives ("fragging"—named after the fragmentation grenade). Like the widening use of heroin by soldiers, such attacks became increasingly common in the drawdown phase of the war.[62,100] Although there are no official figures, data presented by Gabriel and Savage identified a total of 1,016 incidents (for all branches) for the years 1969 through 1972 (eg, "actual assaults" combined with incidents where "intent to kill, do bodily harm, or to intimidate" was suspected).[65] Whereas assassination of officers and NCOs had been seen in earlier wars to a limited degree, typically under combat circumstances, the Vietnam theater is distinct in that not only was the prevalence of such incidents exceptionally high, but these attacks occurred more often in rear areas with the tacit approval of peers.[101]

Thus, despite the reduction in combat levels, Army leadership and the medical/psychiatric contingent in Vietnam became increasingly consumed with problems associated with the wholesale demoralization and alienation of soldiers—symptoms of a seriously compromised Army that were competing for attention with the challenge of preparing the South Vietnamese military to take over from the United States and its allies. Furthermore, by now the deployed psychiatrists were surrounded by a professional literature that was mostly critical of the military psychiatric structures and doctrine that were applied in Vietnam.[26]

An especially thorough historical series on the Vietnam War by the Boston Publishing Company included vivid descriptions of the various expressions of the contempt for the war and the South Vietnamese shared by US military forces in the last years of the war:

> The daily round of random death and incapacitation from mines and booby traps, combined with short-timers fever and skepticism about the worth of "search and clear" steadily lowered American morale.[62(p97)]

The authors give ample witness to the pervasive demoralization in the theater and the brittle nature of race relations, primarily within noncombat units. They also document the associated weakening of the military legal system. According to these authors, combat refusals, drug problems, and racial strife often proved impossible to resolve in the last years in Vietnam. While punishments tended to be increasingly lenient, commanders openly acknowledged that rather than hunt the enemy or carry out a tactical mission, they considered their primary responsibility to be to return their men safely home. "It sometimes seemed to be little more than a ragtag band of men wearing bandannas, peace symbols, and floppy bush hats, with little or no fight left in it."[43(p16)]

Similarly, Balkin's historical review of the severe breakdown in morale and effectiveness of the US military in Southeast Asia during this phase of the war provided thoroughly referenced data indicating an unprecedented increase in rates of combat refusals, combat atrocities, heroin use, assassinations (or threats) of military leaders, racial conflicts, desertion and AWOL, and the emergence of the GI antiwar movement.[51] It also underscored the corrosive effects on morale and cohesion consequent to pervasive careerism among military leaders ("ticket punching," an emphasis similarly brought to bear by Gabriel and Savage[65]).

Kirk, a journalist reporting from the last years of the war, noted that,

> [i]t is, in reality, a desultory kind of struggle, punctuated by occasional explosions and tragedy, for the last Americans in combat in Vietnam. It is a limbo between victory and defeat, a period of lull before the North Vietnamese again seriously challenge allied control over the coastal plain, as they did for the last time in the Tet, May and September offensives of 1968. For the average "grunt," or infantryman, the war is not so much a test of strength under pressure, as it often was a few years ago, as a daily hassle to avoid patrols, avoid the enemy, avoid contact—to keep out of trouble and not be the last American killed in Vietnam.[58(p65)]

More ominous is the investigative report by Linden, another journalist, about his visit in 1971. Linden covered much of the same ground as those mentioned above, but he provided case examples and other observations. These included corroboration from Captain Robert Landeen, an Army psychiatrist assigned to the 101st Airborne Division. Linden dynamically depicted the circumstances and meanings that combined to produce a class war between leaders and subordinates in Vietnam, often with fragging as its final result. He described how fraggings and other threats of violence were commonly used as a means of controlling officers and NCOs: "[fragging in Vietnam became] prevalent, passionless, and apparently unprovoked, representing the grisly game of psychological warfare that GIs use."[100(p12)]

Not surprisingly, the Army's pernicious morale and discipline problems were mirrored on a comparable scale among the Marines fighting in Vietnam. The official review of US Marine activities late in the war acknowledged rampant combat atrocities, "friendly fire" accidents, combat refusals, racial strife, drug abuse, fraggings, and dissent.[102] William Corson, a retired Marine lieutenant colonel (expert on revolution and counterinsurgency warfare, and a veteran of World War II, Korea, and Vietnam), blamed the military's demobilization problems in late Vietnam (drug use, dissent, and racial incidents) on both America's failure in Vietnam and to an "erosion of moral principle within the military."[103(p100)] He referred to the rise in fragging incidents as a new service-wide form of psychological warfare and an aspect of institutionalized mutinous behaviors (along with sabotage, evasion of leadership responsibilities, and internecine conflict). According to Corson, "[a]s with fragging, the potential for a mutinous refusal to carry out an order is so widespread [in Vietnam] that routine actions are being avoided by those in charge."[103(p99)]

Drawdown Phase Psychiatric Overview

Traditional Military Psychiatry Indices. The summary of Army neuropsychiatry in the Vietnam War provided by Jones and Johnson illustrated a dramatic rise in the standard indices of psychiatric attrition during the last few years of the war.[7] As noted previously, the inpatient hospitalization rate had hovered around 12–14/1,000 soldiers per year through the first 3 years of the war[7–9]—favorable compared to figures for Korea (73/1,000) and World War II (28–101/1,000).[11] However, the rate started to rise in 1968, doubled by April 1970, and doubled again by July 1971, reaching an annualized rate of 40/1,000. From there it dropped rapidly until the remaining troops were pulled out in March 1973, apparently primarily because the Army relaxed its medevac policies (in Vietnam only) for drug-dependent soldiers, which ordinarily would have excluded them[104] (Figure 2-1).

Especially dramatic is the skyrocketing out-of-country psychiatric evacuation rate, which had remained below 4–5/1,000 troops per year throughout the war until 1971. By July 1971, it had risen to 42.3, and by the following year, July 1972, the rate had climbed to 129.8. In other words, at that point in the war, *one out of every eight soldiers* was being medically evacuated from Vietnam for psychiatric reasons (primarily for heroin dependency).

As a corollary, the percentage of neuropsychiatric evacuations among all medevacs from Vietnam also accelerated. It had remained below 5% but rose to 30% in late 1971, and by late 1972 it was at 61%. By 1971,

EXHIBIT 2-3

SELECTED PUBLICATIONS BY DRAWDOWN-PHASE ARMY PSYCHIATRISTS (INCLUDING RESEARCH REPORTS)

Year in Vietnam	No. Who Published Articles/Total No. Deployed Army Psychiatrists (as a percentage)*	Publications
1970	2/20 (10%)	Char J. Drug abuse in Vietnam. *Am J Psychiatry*. 1972;129:463–465. Ratner RA. Drugs and despair in Vietnam. *U Chicago Magazine*. 1972;64:15–23.
1971	1/13 (7.7%)	Joseph BS. Lessons on heroin abuse from treating users in Vietnam. *Hosp Community Psychiatry*. 1974;25:742–744. Holloway HC. Epidemiology of heroin dependency among soldiers in Vietnam. *Mil Med*. 1974;139:108–113. Research report.
1972	0/1 (0.0%)	Holloway HC, Sodetz FJ, Elsmore TF, and the members of Work Unit 102. Heroin dependence and withdrawal in the military heroin user in the US Army, Vietnam. In: *Annual Progress Report, 1973*. Washington, DC: Walter Reed Army Institute of Research; 1973: 1244–1246. Research report.

*These numbers do not count research reports, although they are listed in the Publications column.

the pervasive demoralization within the larger military population in Vietnam. Although alluding to likely individual premorbidity factors in the drug-dependent soldier, Ratner credited more their universal despair, which he attributed to a combination of societal factors (eg, America's motivation for waging war in Southeast Asia represented a displacement of its internal "racial hostilities") and an "inhumane" Army. Furthermore, he acknowledged the sense of clinical impotence he shared with his colleagues ("there seems to be no place for a psychiatrist to begin") and appeared to echo the cynicism of his soldier-patients.[118]

Equally troubling is the publication of Lieutenant Commander HW Fisher, a Navy psychiatrist who served with the 1st Marine Division during the same year as Ratner, only far to the north near Da Nang. According to Fisher, of 1,000 consecutive referrals, he diagnosed 960 Marines as personality disorders, usually antisocial.[119] Furthermore, although he differs from Ratner in attributing their military dysfunction to predisposition (eg, he labels them with personality disorder diagnoses), Fisher especially faulted their officers and NCOs for encouraging indiscipline. He felt that this occurred through vacillations in enforcing regulations and argued that these problems were exacerbated by expectations that psychiatry provide medical evacuation out of Vietnam or recommend administrative separation from the service in lieu of punishment, thus serving as encouragement of the deviant Marine's rebellion.[119]

Taken together, the record from this phase suggests the morale of some of these psychiatrists suffered a serious decrement parallel to that of the typical soldier of that period. More importantly, it also indicates that the psychiatric contingent, like the military leadership in Vietnam, was wholly unprepared to contend with the extensive proportion of US troops who would in time oppose serving under the post-Tet (1968) circumstances through antimilitary behaviors and psychological disability.

POSTWAR FEATURES

Vietnam Veterans and the High Prevalence of Readjustment Problems

A comprehensive review of postdeployment adjustment and psychiatric morbidity is outside the scope of this chapter. However, the data indicate that many who served in Vietnam subsequently experienced serious and sustained readjustment problems, including frank posttraumatic stress disorder (PTSD). Some suggest that the prevalence of debilitating psychological and social problems among Vietnam veterans greatly exceeds that for earlier US wars. Additionally, when postdeployment adjustment difficulties are included with psychological problems that arose in the theater, the psychosocial cost for the Vietnam War appears unprecedented.

However, estimates as to the prevalence of sustained postwar adjustment and psychiatric problems for Vietnam veterans seem to vary as widely as the political reactions to the war itself.[22,120–125] Furthermore, comparisons of the psychosocial effect of combat service across US wars is especially difficult because measures are inconsistent. Somewhat reassuring, a 1980 Harris Poll of Vietnam veterans commissioned by the then Veterans Administration found 91% reporting they were glad they had served their country, 74% said they enjoyed their time in the service, and nearly two thirds said they would go to Vietnam again, even knowing how the war would end.[29]

Nonetheless, rising professional concern for the psychological injury of veterans secondary to service in Vietnam brought about a revolutionary change in the taxonomy of psychiatric disorders in civilian medicine. In the decade that followed the war, the *International Classification of Disease,* 9th edition, *Clinical Modification* (ICD-9-CM),[126] and the *Diagnostic and Statistical Manual of Mental Disorders,* 3rd edition (DSM-III),[127] both contained the new category "Post-Traumatic Stress Disorder or PTSD," which had been originally called "post-Vietnam syndrome." The inclusion of PTSD in DSM-III reflected the political efforts of the Vietnam veterans who were seeking greater recognition, as well as the efforts of Americans with residual antiwar sentiment and psychiatrists who believed that DSM-II had neglected the ordeal of combat veterans.[128] In that DSM-III includes combat as an etiological factor for PTSD, it suggests that overwhelming combat stress and civilian catastrophes are identical—a proposition that seems arguable.

The most definitive findings regarding PTSD prevalence and incidence following the Vietnam War come from the government-sponsored National Vietnam Veterans Readjustment Study (NVVRS). At the time of the study (mid-1980s), approximately 30% of male and 27% of female study participants had evidenced PTSD at some point since serving in Vietnam, and for many PTSD had become persistent and incapacitating (15% and 9% of study participants respectively).[129]

However, divergence from the emphasis in the original PTSD model (the traumatic event is singularly explanatory) has occurred. Over the years since the war, disputes have arisen as to the relative weight to give various etiologic influences (eg, predisposition and personality, traumatic extent of combat theater circumstance, and post-Vietnam experience). These disputes have complicated the diagnosis and treatment of PTSD and related adjustment difficulties. Many behavioral science observers have commented on the considerable potential for postwar adjustment difficulties to be powerfully affected by psychological and social dynamics that are not the direct consequence of combat zone "trauma."[39,123,130–132] According to Arthur S Blank Jr, a former Army psychiatrist who was assigned in Vietnam and who subsequently served for many years as National Director for the Department of Veterans Affairs Readjustment Counseling Centers,

> [s]ince 1973 I have treated, evaluated, supervised the treatment of, or discussed the cases of approximately 1,400 veterans of Viet Nam with PTSD and have yet to hear a single case where the veteran's symptoms were not accompanied by either (1) significant doubts or conflicts about the worthiness of the war, or (2) considerable anger about perceived lack of support for the war by the government or the nation. Furthermore, although researchers have been barred from exploring the relationship between the occurrence of PTSD and the overwhelmingly conflicted nature of the war, it is the observation of almost all clinicians who have treated substantial numbers of Viet Nam veterans with PTSD that the clinical condition is almost always accompanied by a deeply flawed sense of purpose concerning what happened in Viet Nam.[133]

Following the cessation of hostilities in Southeast Asia, the ethical challenges to military psychiatry, which were voiced during the war, shifted to retrospectively critical conclusions regarding negative long-term consequences of field psychiatric practices in Vietnam (the aforementioned doctrine). The perspective seems to be that the implementation of these practices may have been in the service of collective goals (eg, military objectives), but in the process it ignored the needs of the soldier and fostered the development of PTSD.[39,134–136] Offsetting opinion came from Blank, who noted that acute CSRs usually do not meet the criteria for PTSD and do not generally evolve into diagnosable PTSD later.[137] It also came from Jones, who argued vigorously that postwar sympathies for maligned Vietnam veterans may have led psychiatrists without military experience to misunderstand the unique aspects of a soldier's state when psychological defenses become overwhelmed in combat. As a consequence they fail to appreciate the characteristically fluid and reversible nature of the resultant acute stress disorder and the increased risk for psychiatric morbidity (including PTSD) if treatments do not promote symptom suppression and rapid return to military function and comrades.[138]

Survey of Veteran Army Psychiatrists Who Served in Vietnam

As mentioned earlier, in 1982 WRAIR queried veteran Army psychiatrists who served in Vietnam about their experiences in the war.[2,27] Of the estimated 135 who served in Vietnam, 115 were located, and of those, 74% (85) completed a structured questionnaire exploring patterns of psychiatric problems encountered, types and effectiveness of clinical approaches, and personal reactions to the associated professional challenges and dilemmas. Study respondents were evenly distributed over the years of deployment in Vietnam so that the gleaned information can be considered representative. Also, in the theater, 21% (18) served exclusively in combat units (roughly one third of the slots each year), 49% (42) served exclusively in combat service support medical units (eg, with hospitals or the psychiatric specialty teams), and 25% (21) spent some time assigned to each. The remaining four served exclusively as the theater "Neuropsychiatric Consultant" to the CG/USARV Surgeon. The following summarizes the most salient findings from the study:

- *Unprecedented levels of predeployment professional training*. The degree of formal psychiatric training shared by these psychiatrists was unprecedented in contrast to World War I and World War II, as was the proportion of deployed psychiatrists who received residency training in Army programs (one third).[139]
- *As theater problems progressively increased, predeployment military experience among replacement psychiatrists decreased.* Although the psychiatrists who served in Vietnam averaged little postprofessional training experience in the military, greater numbers of civilian-trained psychiatrists with no practical military background, as well as an increasing proportion of military-trained psychiatrists with no field experience, were sent during the second half of the war. In the first half of the war these two groups constituted only one quarter of the assigned psychiatrist strength. In the second half they represented three quarters. This decline in practical experience, which characterized successive groups of psychiatrists sent to Vietnam, was mirrored in an equally salient reduction in relevant background experience, though not rank, of the Vietnam theater Neuropsychiatric Consultant to the CG/USARV Surgeon.
- *Psychosocial disorders progressively outweighed combat-generated ones.* Regarding the distribution of patients by standard psychiatric diagnoses, these veteran psychiatrists reported over one half of their clinical efforts were devoted to personality disorders, adjustment reactions, or substance abuse syndromes. Furthermore, 32% (24) of the study participants reported that they had only rare exposure to combat-induced psychiatric casualties during their tours. Similarly, the mean percentage of clinical caseload devoted to "combat reactions" for all psychiatrists in the study was only 12.6%. These findings appear to validate that Vietnam was a "low-intensity" war,[31] at least by the measure of its potential to psychologically overwhelm soldiers committed to combat. Furthermore, the burden of treating various psychosocial problems rose dramatically as the war passed the halfway mark. In comparing ratings of 16 behavioral problems by the study participants from the first half of the war with those of the second half, the exponential rise in the heroin problem was distinguishable from the steady, although not insignificant, problems associated with the use of other drugs such as alcohol and marijuana. This finding held true when comparing psychiatrists who served only with combat units with those who served only in hospital assignments. Also, like the jump in problems associated with heroin use in the latter third of the war, the study psychiatrists overall reported a significant rise in their involvement in group racial conflicts and with individuals responsible for violent incidents.
- *Psychoactive medications were extensively prescribed, but risks and benefits were not monitored.* The descriptive and quantitative data from the 48% (41) of the study psychiatrists who acknowledged some exposure to combat reaction cases indicate that they extensively used and highly valued these medications (neuroleptics and anxiolytics) in the treatment and management of soldiers suffering from a wide variety of combat-generated symptoms. (The Army psychiatrists in Vietnam, however, had little or no way to measure the subsequent effects of such medications on the combat effectiveness, or vulnerability, of solders who were returned to duty following such treatment, or regarding their long-term effects including postwar adjustment.)

- *Many Vietnam psychiatrists still felt embittered, especially those who served in the latter half of the war.* A large proportion of the study psychiatrists emphasized, often eloquently, that they still felt quite strongly—typically negatively—about the war and their role in it. This was primarily the case among those who served in the second half of the war. These psychiatrists' responses indicate that in many respects they felt overwhelmed when trying to treat soldiers (and advise commanders) affected by a raging drug epidemic, eruptions of racial animosities, and outbreaks of violence, while using staffing and policies instead designed to manage large numbers of combat-generated casualties. Compared to their counterparts in the first half of the war, these psychiatrists tended to be more vocal, more divided (according to training differences), and, in some cases, quite defensive. The psychiatrists of this latter period also appeared more likely to perceive inequities and to be critical of their preparation and utilization by the Army.[2,27]

LINGERING QUESTIONS AND CONSIDERATIONS

This review indicates that during the drawdown years in Vietnam (1969–1973), Army psychiatrists faced a different and more challenging scenario than that encountered by those who preceded them—one that suggests a dangerous erosion of Army morale and discipline and an associated epidemic of psychiatric conditions and misconduct. It also raises important questions that might have been more easily answered at the conclusion of hostilities if a thorough and systematic study of the psychiatric and behavioral crisis there had been conducted—questions for which the answers may be critical in preparing for a similar military engagement in America's future.

Should more have been done by military and medical/psychiatric leaders to preserve the mental health, psychosocial resiliency, and, by implication, the combat readiness of the replacement soldiers sent to fight in Vietnam? Did the military leadership and the psychiatric component in Vietnam ignore the mounting evidence and warnings by senior medical and psychiatric observers[6,31] and fail to adjust psychiatric perspectives or modify the preparation, deployment, and organization of psychiatric assets in order to meet these challenges? By way of response, the following considerations are offered despite the late date and incomplete information.

The Larger Army During the War

Although the troops in Vietnam were more demonstrative, clearly the long and controversial war took a massive toll on the morale and mental health of the US Army generally.[64–66,140] The troops in Vietnam were resonant with the restive, antiestablishment sentiments of their military peers outside the theater. More specific to mental health, epidemiological data provided by Datel regarding the larger US Army indicate that by mid-1973:

- the worldwide incidence of neuropsychiatric disease among Army personnel rose to near the peak level seen during the Korean War;
- the psychosis rate for the worldwide active duty Army had never been higher;
- character and behavior disorder diagnoses also peaked; and
- the proportion of Army hospital beds in the United States occupied for all psychiatric causes was greater than it had ever been,[25] including during the so-called "psychiatric disaster period"[10] of World War II.

The Soldiers Who Served in Vietnam

The reduction in combat activities and the perception of demobilization surely explains some of the rise in psychiatric conditions and behavioral problems from 1969 on. These kinds of problems were predictable based on data from World War II and Korea, where large numbers of soldiers were stationed far from home, living in confined and isolated groups, and serving primarily in service and support roles.[141,142] Similar problems have been associated with constabulary forces and those in the process of demobilization in an overseas setting who resent being asked to sustain further sacrifices beyond the conclusion of hostilities.[104,143] Even a dramatic increase in the use of narcotics by US soldiers was seen at the close of the Korean War, which was also attributed to service in the Asian theater.[144] Should all of these problems be lumped under a concept like a collective "short-timer's syndrome" (ie, impatient to complete their assignment and return to their stateside lives)? In the case of the skyrocketing evacuation rates in Vietnam for soldiers with opium breakdown products detected in their urine, Jones referred to these casualties as "evacuation syndromes" (eg, efforts by soldiers to manipulate the system to get relief from foreign deployment and, perhaps, combat risks).[105]

However, beyond these familiar stressors, the troops in the latter part of the war in Vietnam also exhibited intense opposition to military authority—an attitude that coincided with the virulent antiwar and antimilitary feelings of those at home. Should it be concluded that the pervasive psychiatric and behavioral problems in these individuals were primarily expressions of an embittered aggregate of soldiers who resented being asked to make sacrifices to salvage America's lost cause there while surrounded by the moral outrage and blame of the US public? Some consider these soldier behaviors to have collectively represented a "macromutiny."[145] But was Vietnam so sociopolitically unique that the US experience there can be discounted as unlikely to repeat? Or does a closer look need to be taken at what happened there? What can it teach about the limitations of human nature, including among the civilian population at home, under these specific conditions of war and deployment, especially from the standpoint of the social psychology of military groups?

The Army Psychiatric Component in Vietnam

Certainly the overall record of psychiatric care provided through the course of the war in Vietnam was laudatory. But the traditional psychiatric models for the management and treatment of this avalanche of demoralization and alienation seem to have mostly been ineffective by the end of the war. It does appear that military psychiatry failed to extrapolate from drawdown and demobilization problems seen in earlier wars. A failure to anticipate the growing demoralization and dissent in Vietnam secondary to public repudiation of the war resulted in a failure to modify the system of mental health resources and the selection and preparation of replacement psychiatrists.

A Social Stress and "Disease" Model

On the other hand, perhaps these problems were insoluble on any terms pertaining to clinical psychiatry. First, the overlap between matters bearing on morale and mental health ultimately became quite entangled as the war progressed, and yet those primarily responsible for the former (military commanders) and those responsible for the latter (military mental health personnel) did not typically maintain a running dialogue, especially in instances of divergent command structures, which was most usually the case. Second, considering the exceptionally high prevalence of problems that arose among previously functional soldiers, the pathogenesis is more suggestive of a social–psychiatric disorder of the collective (eg, Goffman's pathogenic "total institution,"[146] Fleming's "sociosis,"[131] or Rose's "macromutiny"[145]), as opposed to one primarily centered on the individual soldier. In this regard, it should be noted that the psychiatric training of the times, including in the Army settings (and despite intents otherwise[23]) did not emphasize social pathology and interventions (including at the macro level) nor provide sufficient practical training.

In other words, in that these problems were epidemic in the Vietnam theater and were not, for the most part, combat-related, a social stress model seems especially warranted because these seem to represent failures of adaptation at the group level. They evidently arose from complex interactions combining personal circumstance with powerful biological (often including drug-induced), psychological, and social stressors (in Vietnam as well as from home)—stressors that became progressively onerous for sequential cohorts of replacement soldiers as the war wound to its bitter conclusion.

Veteran Postwar Adjustment Problems

As noted earlier, the important subject of the adjustment problems of veterans after the war is beyond the scope of this chapter, but it should be mentioned that the clash of values affecting soldiers in Vietnam also invariably complicated the reintegration of returning soldiers. For many, it may have contributed to chronic psychiatric conditions and serious adjustment difficulties because some symptom formation may have served to obtain, through the "sick role,"[147] an honorable adaptation to impossibly contradictory public (moral) pressures (eg, "damned for going, blamed for losing"). Furthermore, in most cases the symptoms and difficulties of these veterans remained unaddressed because of the unavailability of the PTSD diagnosis prior to 1980. Following the promulgation of the PTSD diagnosis through the publication of DSM-III, the problems and conditions of this group of veterans began to be more systematically addressed by the Department of Veterans Affairs, which began the gradual implementation of the Vet Centers—a nationwide system of community-based, war veteran counseling centers[133] (totaling 260 centers by 2009). More information on the Vet Centers is available at their Web site: http://www.vetcenter.va.gov.

Final Considerations

In his book, *Psychiatry in a Troubled World*,[148] Dr William C Menninger, the Army Surgeon General's chief psychiatrist through most of World War II, described military psychiatry as a "dirty job," one in which the psychiatrist helps a normal individual adjust to the abnormal situation of combat. He was primarily referring to the moral weight inherent in expecting soldiers to return to combat duty and additional risks following the brief, simple measures associated with the classic combat psychiatry treatment regimen (the doctrine mentioned earlier). Following military psychiatry's experience in Vietnam, it can surely be acknowledged that it is a "messy job" as well. As such, attention can be drawn to the multivariate social and environmental stressors that can also serve to corrupt soldier morale, commitment, and discipline, as well as mental health, under certain adverse combat theater circumstances, and psychiatry's limited capabilities for making this bearable for them.

SUMMARY

The commitment of US forces in Southeast Asia resulted in 7 exhausting years of combat activities. Ultimately, however, despite their material and technological inferiority, the enemy's resolve and resilience outlasted the tolerance of the US public, and US involvement ended following mounting protest in the United States, withdrawal of US military forces and civilian advisors in 1973, and, finally, the defeat and surrender of the Saigon government to North Vietnam in April 1975—little more than 2 years after the negotiated truce in January 1973. More specific to military psychiatry, these remarkable events and circumstances—and the attendant social and political convulsion in America—adversely affected the mental health and psychological resilience of a large proportion of the military service members assigned in Vietnam, and the task for military psychiatrists there broadened and became more complex.

Even if widely scattered, the various publications from psychiatrists and other professionals who served in Vietnam, visited the theater, or were in a position to review the circumstances there, do comprise a partial historical record. These reports and the WRAIR survey of veteran Army psychiatrists suggest a number of characteristics regarding the psychiatric challenge in Vietnam, some of which appear to be unique compared to the wars that preceded it. They also provoke additional important questions.

In the beginning, when US ground troops were first committed and throughout the buildup phase (1965–1967), adequate psychiatric resources were deployed with the combat forces, and psychiatric and behavioral problems were manageable. Rates of psychiatric evacuations from Vietnam were exceptionally low, as were rates for disciplinary problems. Morale and commitment of Army troops, including psychiatrists, proved to be high. Of special note is that newly developed psychoactive medications, especially neuroleptics and anxiolytics, were enthusiastically used throughout the theater by psychiatrists and other medical officers, but their use and effects were never studied.

The US public's attitude toward the war reversed dramatically following the enemy's bold surprise attacks in 1968. These events heralded the withdrawal of US forces and demobilization from the war. Despite this, there continued the assignment of replacement soldiers (in decreasing numbers), including psychiatrists; killing and wounding of more US service members; and passionate antiwar, antimilitary sentiment within US society. These years also saw the beginning of a surge in psychiatric admissions and behavioral problems throughout the Army—and especially in Vietnam.

Over time, the reality in Vietnam proved to be far different than expected. The combat exhaustion casualties that were predicted never materialized and the replacement Army psychiatrists and allied personnel who served in Vietnam from 1969 on found themselves in a radically different war (and with a radically different Army) than was faced by those who served in previous wars (with their emphasis on psychiatric attrition among soldiers worn down by sustained combat) or those who preceded them in Vietnam. Furthermore, psychiatrists with appreciably less military experience, including those in leadership positions, were sent even as the problems in the theater were multiplying. Not only were they challenged with unprecedented levels of psychiatric and behavior problems, it was unprecedented for these rates to rise while the United States was reducing its military and political presence in South Vietnam, US forces were gradually turning the fighting over to the Army of the Republic of South Vietnam, and US casualty rates were declining.

What military psychiatry ultimately encountered in large numbers were young troops with severe demoralization, a progressive reluctance to soldier, antagonism—sometimes violent—toward military authority, and a variety of psychiatric conditions and behavioral disorders. Theater psychiatric hospitalization statistics indicate a 4-fold increase compared to the early war years. Related, and even more remarkable, was the common and casual use of heroin by a large proportion of US troops, although most were not addicted. At its worst point, one out of every eight enlisted soldiers was medically evacuated from Vietnam because of narcotic use.

These accelerating psychiatric conditions and behavior problems, which coincided with America's repudiation of the war and the counterculture passions of their civilian peers, were certainly consequential to serving in the combat theater, but in most cases they had little or no direct connection to combat activity. It appears that many soldiers more or less disabled (or demobilized) themselves through mental disorders, drug use, and other symptoms and forms of misconduct.

Regarding the response of the deployed mental health elements, because the rising theater and deployment demoralization and alienation-driven problems arose far more predictably among noncombat troops, the center of effort shifted to hospital-based mental health assets and gradually overtaxed the psychiatric and related medical resources. These problems mostly failed to yield to conventional psychiatric approaches, and increasingly drastic administrative and law enforcement measures were required. The late-war psychiatrists complained about being unprepared and may have become uncertain of their goals and structures. They may have also shared, to some degree, the demoralization and antimilitary passions of the soldiers with whom they served. Combat readiness went thankfully untested by the enemy. Nonetheless, it is striking that there were no structural changes in the organization of mental health assets in Vietnam or modifications in the selection, preparation, or deployment of mental health personnel sent as replacements to the theater.

With the advantage of the relative objectivity offered by the passage of time, it can now be acknowledged that the models for understanding and anticipating casualties both from combat stress and from deployment stress are considerably more complex than was understood before—or even during—the Vietnam War. The earlier model was derived from observations of troops fighting in sustained, intense combat environments, and it primarily weighed combat stress against resiliency of the individual soldier (although the buffering effects of allegiance to combat buddies and other factors were considered to be vital). But in an extended, "low-intensity," counterinsurgency conflict the model must be broadened to also take into account other critical, compounding, and often indirect influences of the combat theater. A list centered around "soldier variables" might include the usual ones, that is, (*a*) the nature and setting of the fighting; (*b*) training and expertise; (*c*) physical condition; (*d*) background and personality; (*e*) social circumstance (within the small combat unit as well as the soldier's network of family and friends); (*f*) confidence in military leaders and equipment; and (*g*) commitment to the military goals. It might also, and surely not least, include the necessity to ensure that soldiers believe the country requires, as well as values, the inherent risks and sacrifices they undertake.

Retrospective suggestions generated out of the Vietnam War especially include the need for the military to develop a multivariate concept of combat "theater" breakdown (as opposed to combat breakdown) that considers both the symptomatic soldier and the dysfunction arising in groups of soldiers, and to employ an epidemiological approach for early recognition of deteriorating psychosocial and psychiatric circumstances. For example, in Vietnam a psychiatric field research team could have been created for the sole purpose of collecting, analyzing, and disseminating information regarding a wide array of often initially innocuous indices of flagging morale (eg, rising malaria rates among soldiers subverting malaria prophylaxis as a means of avoiding service). This information could have then served for clinicians and commanders as a timely map of the psychosocial "terrain" of stressors, morale, performance, and symptom patterns of the troops, which would have permitted the development of early intervention measures. Such an epidemiologic approach could have been combined with systematic debriefing of returning psychiatrists to redirect some of the attention of replacement psychiatrists from a combat stress model toward a social stress model of psychiatric dysfunction.

Other structural adaptations as the war in Vietnam lengthened might have included: (*a*) extending the tours of each of the theater Neuropsychiatry Consultants (as well as tours of other psychiatrists in leadership positions) to provide needed continuity; (*b*) increasing the level of seniority of the replacement military psychiatrists as the pool of experienced civilian psychiatrists unavoidably decreased; and (*c*) linking numbers of deployed psychiatrists to epidemiologically documented need, rather than to overall troop strength. Finally, a policy could have been established, presuming it met overall mobilization needs, requiring that each recently graduated psychiatrist serve some time with a stateside military unit before departing for Vietnam.

REFERENCES

1. Jones FD. Reactions to stress: combat versus combat support troops. Paper presented at: World Psychiatric Association; August 19, 1977; Honolulu, Hi.

2. Camp NM, Carney CM. US Army psychiatry in Vietnam: preliminary findings of a survey, I: background and method. *Bull Menninger Clin.* 1987;51:6–18.

3. Allerton WS. Army psychiatry in Vietnam. In: Bourne PG, ed. *The Psychology and Physiology of Stress: With Reference to Special Studies of the Viet Nam War.* New York, NY: Academic Press; 1969: 219–236.

4. Johnson AW Jr. Combat psychiatry, I: a historical review. *Med Bull U S Army Europe.* 1969;26(10):305–308.

5. Johnson AW Jr. Combat psychiatry, II: the US Army in Vietnam. *Med Bull U S Army Europe.* 1969;26(11):335–339. [Reprinted as: Psychiatry stresses activity in Vietnam. *U S Medicine.* June 1, 1970: 8–13.]

6. Colbach EM, Parrish MD. Army mental health activities in Vietnam: 1965–1970. *Bull Menninger Clin.* 1970;31:333–342.

7. Jones FD, Johnson AW Jr. Medical and psychiatric treatment policy and practice in Vietnam. *J Soc Issues.* 1975;31(4):49–65.

8. Baker SL Jr. Traumatic war disorders. In: Kaplan HI, Freedman AM, Sadock BJ, eds. *Comprehensive Textbook of Psychiatry III.* Baltimore, Md: Williams and Wilkins; 1980: Chap 25.3: 1829–1842.

9. Bourne PG. *Men, Stress, and Vietnam.* Boston, Mass: Little Brown; 1970.

10. Datel WE. *A Summary of Source Data in Military Psychiatric Epidemiology.* Alexandria, Va: Defense Documentation Center; 1976. Document AD No A 021-265.

11. Tiffany WJ Jr. The mental health of Army troops in Vietnam. *Am J Psychiatry.* 1967;123:1585–1586.

12. Holloway HC, Sodetz FJ, Elsmore TF, and the members of Work Unit 102. Heroin dependence and withdrawal in the military heroin user in the US Army, Vietnam. In: *Annual Progress Report.* Washington, DC: Walter Reed Army Institute of Research; 1973: 1244–1246.

13. Howe RC, Hegge FW, Phillips JL. Acute heroin abstinence in man, I: changes in behavior and sleep. *Drug Alcohol Dependence.* 1980;5:341–356.

14. Howe RC, Hegge FW, Phillips JL. Acute heroin abstinence in man, II: alterations in rapid eye movement (REM) sleep. *Drug Alcohol Dependence.* 1980;6:149–161.

15. Bourne PG, ed. *The Psychology and Physiology of Stress: With Reference to Special Studies of the Viet Nam War.* New York, NY: Academic Press; 1969.

16. Roffman RA, Sapol E. Marijuana in Vietnam: a survey of use among Army enlisted men in two southern corps. *Int J Addict.* 1970;5:1–42.

17. Stanton MD. Drug use in Vietnam. *Arch Gen Psychiatry.* 1972;26:279–286.

18. Baker SL. US Army heroin abuse identification program in Vietnam: implications for a methadone program. *Am J Public Health.* 1972;62:857–860.

19. Holloway HC. Epidemiology of heroin dependency among soldiers in Vietnam. *Mil Med.* 1974;139:108–113.

20. Zinberg NE. Rehabilitation of heroin users in Vietnam. *Contemp Drug Problems.* 1972;1:263–294.

21. Camp NM, Stretch RH, Marshall WC. *Stress, Strain, and Vietnam: An Annotated Bibliography of Two Decades of Psychiatric and Social Sciences Literature Reflecting the Effect of the War on the American Soldier.* Westport, Conn: Greenwood Press; 1988.

22. Pols H, Oak S. War and military mental health: the US response in the 20th century. *Am J Public Health.* 2007;97:2132–2142.

23. Tiffany WJ Jr, Allerton WS. Army psychiatry in the mid-'60s. *Am J Psychiatry*. 1967;123:810–819.

24. Jones FD. Traditional warfare combat stress casualties. In: Jones FD, Sparacino LR, Wilcox VL, Rothberg JM, Stokes JW, eds. *War Psychiatry*. In: *Textbooks of Military Medicine*. Washington, DC: Office of The Surgeon General, US Department of the Army and Borden Institute; 1995: 35–61.

25. Datel WE, Johnson AW Jr. *Psychotropic Prescription Medication in Vietnam*. Alexandria, Va: Defense Technical Information Center; 1981. Document No A097-610.

26. Camp NM. The Vietnam War and the ethics of combat psychiatry. *Am J Psychiatry*. 1993;150:1000–1010.

27. Camp NM, Carney CM. US Army psychiatry in Vietnam: preliminary findings of a survey, II: results and discussion. *Bull Menninger Clin*. 1987;51:19–37.

28. US Department of State. *Why We Fight in Viet-Nam*. Washington, DC: Office of Media Services, US Department of State; 1967. Viet-Nam Information Notes No. 6.

29. Sorley L. *A Better War: The Unexamined Victories and Final Tragedy of America's Last Years in Vietnam.* New York, NY: Harcourt Books; 1999.

30. Spector RH. *After Tet: The Bloodiest Year in Vietnam*. New York, NY: The Free Press; 1993.

31. Neel S. *Medical Support of the US Army in Vietnam, 1965–1970*. Washington, DC: Government Printing Office; 1973.

32. Doyle E, Lipsman S, and the editors of Boston Publishing Co. *The Vietnam Experience: Setting the Stage*. Boston, Mass: Boston Publishing Co; 1981.

33. Dougan C, Lipsman E, Doyle C, and the editors of Boston Publishing Co. *The Vietnam Experience: A Nation Divided*. Boston, Mass: Boston Publishing Co; 1984.

34. Doyle E, Weiss S, and the editors of Boston Publishing Co. *The Vietnam Experience: A Collision of Cultures*. Boston, Mass: Boston Publishing Co; 1984.

35. Doyle E, Lipsman S, and the editors of Boston Publishing Co. *The Vietnam Experience: America Takes over*. Boston, Mass: Boston Publishing Co; 1982.

36. US Department of the Army, Vietnam. *Medical Services: Mental Health and Neuropsychiatry*. APO San Francisco, Calif: HQ USARV; October 15, 1970. USARV Regulation No. 40-34.

37. Cooke ET. Another look at combat exhaustion. Medical Field Service School Department of Neuropsychiatry. Training document GR 51-400-320. [Distributed to the author, July, 1967.]

38. Training documents GR 51-400-960 and TABLE GR 51-400-104-105. Army Medical Field Service School. San Antonio, Tex. [Distributed to the author, July, 1967.]

39. Boman B. The Vietnam veteran ten years on. *Aust N Z J Psychiatry*. 1982;16:107–127.

40. Bloch HS. Army clinical psychiatry in the combat zone: 1967–1968. *Am J Psychiatry*. 1969;126:289–298.

41. Johnson AW Jr, Bowman JA, Byrdy HS, Blank AS Jr. Panel discussion: Army psychiatry in Vietnam. In: Jones FD, ed. *Proceedings: Social and Preventive Psychiatry Course, 1967*. Washington, DC: Government Printing Office; 1968: 41–76. [See also Alexandria, Va: Defense Documentation Center (Document ADA950-058).]

42. Moskos CC Jr. Military made scapegoat for Vietnam. In: Millett AR, ed. *A Short History of the Vietnam War*. Bloomington, Ind: Indiana University Press; 1978: 67–72.

43. Fulghum D, Maitland T, and the editors of Boston Publishing Co. *The Vietnam Experience: South Vietnam on Trial*. Boston, Mass: Boston Publishing Co; 1984.

44. Moskos CC Jr. *The American Enlisted Man: The Rank and File in Today's Military*. New York, NY: Russell Sage Foundation; 1970.

45. Edmendson SW, Platner DJ. Psychiatric referrals from Khe Sanh during siege. *U S Army Vietnam Med Bull*. 1968;July / August:67–72.

46. Glass AJ. Introduction. In: Bourne PG, ed. *The Psychology and Physiology of Stress*. New York, NY: Academic Press; 1969: xiii–xxx.

47. Bourne PG. Military psychiatry and the Vietnam experience. *Am J Psychiatry*. 1970;127(suppl):481–488.

48. Hays FW. Psychiatric aeromedical evacuation patients during the Tet I and Tet II offensives. *Am J Psychiatry*. 1970;127:503–508.

49. Tischler GL. Patterns of psychiatric attrition and of behavior in a combat zone. In: Bourne PG, ed. *The Psychology and Physiology of Stress: With Reference to Special Studies of the Viet Nam War*. New York, NY: Academic Press; 1969: 19–44.

50. Dowling JJ. Psychological aspects of the year in Vietnam. *U S Army Vietnam Med Bull*. 1967;May / June:45–48.

51. Balkind JJ. *Morale Deterioration in the United States Military During the Vietnam Period*. Ann Arbor, Mich: University Microfilms International. [Dissertations Abstracts International, 39 (1-A), 438. Order No. 78-11, 333]; 1978.

52. Dougan C, Weiss S, and the editors of Boston Publishing Co. *The Vietnam Experience: Nineteen Sixty-Eight*. Boston, Mass: Boston Publishing Co; 1983.

53. Braestrup P. *Big Story: How the American Press and Television Reported and Interpreted the Crisis of Tet 1968 in Vietnam and Washington*. Boulder, Colo: Westview Press; 1977.

54. Yager J. Personal violence in infantry combat. *Arch Gen Psychiatry*. 1975;32:257–261.

55. Schell J. *The Military Half: An Account of Destruction in Quang Ngai and Quang Tin*. New York, NY: Alfred A. Knopf; 1968.

56. Norden E. American atrocities in Vietnam. In: Falk RA, Kolko G, Lifton RJ, eds. *Crimes of War*. New York, NY: Random House; 1971: 265–284.

57. Vietnam Veterans Against the War. *The Winter Soldier Investigation: An Inquiry Into American War Crimes*. Boston, Mass: Beacon Press; 1972.

58. Kirk D. *Tell It to the Dead: Memories of a War*. Chicago, Ill: Nelson-Hall; 1975.

59. Sterba JP. Cover your ass. In: Falk RA, Kolko G, Lifton RJ, eds. *Crimes of War*. New York, NY: Random House; 1971: 445–458. [Originally printed as: Close up of the grunt: the hours of boredom, the seconds of terror. *New York Times Magazine*. February 8, 1970.]

60. Renner JA Jr. The changing patterns of psychiatric problems in Vietnam. *Comp Psychiatry*. 1973;14:169–181.

61. Mueller JE. Trends in popular support for the wars in Korea and Vietnam. *Am Political Science Rev*. 1971;65:358–375.

62. Lipsman S, Doyle E, and the editors of Boston Publishing Co. *The Vietnam Experience: Fighting For Time*. Boston, Mass: Boston Publishing Co; 1983.

63. Hersh SM. *My Lai 4: A Report on the Massacre and its Aftermath*. New York, NY: Random House; 1970.

64. Johnson H, Wilson GC. *Army in Anguish*. New York, NY: Pocket Books; 1972.

65. Gabriel RA, Savage PL. *Crisis in Command: Mismanagement in the Army*. New York, NY: Hill and Wang; 1978.

66. Cincinnatus. *Self-Destruction: The Disintegration and Decay of the United States Army During the Vietnam Era*. New York, NY: Norton; 1981.

67. Gallup GH. *The Gallup Poll: Public Opinion 1935–1971*. New York, NY: Random House; 1972.

68. Baskir LM, Strauss WA. *Chance and Circumstance: The Draft, the War, and the Vietnam Generation*. New York, NY: Alfred A. Knopf; 1978.

69. Seligman D. A special kind of rebellion. *Fortune*. January 1969: 66–69, 172–175.

70. Binkin M, Eitelberg MJ. From Bunker Hill to Vietnam. In: Binkin M, Eitelberg MJ. *Blacks in the Military*. Washington, DC: Brookings Institution; 1982: 11–38.

71. Mullen RW. *Blacks and Vietnam*. Washington, DC: University Press of America; 1981.

72. Terry W. *Bloods: An Oral History of the Vietnam War by Black Veterans*. New York, NY: Random House; 1984.

73. Terry W. The angry blacks in the army. In: Horowitz D and the editors of Ramparts. *Two, Three . . . Many Vietnams: A Radical Reader on the Wars in Southeast Asia and the Conflicts at Home*. San Francisco, Calif: Canfield Press; 1971: 222–231.

74. Johnston J, Bachman JG. *Young Men Look at Military Service*. Ann Arbor, Mich: University of Michigan, Institute for Social Research; 1971.

75. Bell DB. *Characteristics of Army Deserters in the DoD Special Discharges Review Program*. Arlington, Va: US Army Research Institute; 1979. Report No. 1229.

76. Hayes JH. The dialectics of resistance: an analysis of the GI movement. *J Soc Issues*. 1975;31(4):125–139.

77. O'Donnell JA, Voss HL, Clayton RR, Slatin GT, Room RGW. *Young Men and Drugs: A Nationwide Survey*. Rockville, Md: National Institute on Drug Abuse; 1976. Research monograph No. 5.

78. Greden JF, Morgan DW, Frenkel SI. The changing drug scene: 1970–1972. *Am J Psychiatry*. 1974;131:77–81.

79. Black S, Owens KL, Wolff RP. Patterns of drug use: a study of 5,482 subjects. *Am J Psychiatry*. 1970;127:420–423.

80. Callan JP, Patterson CD. Patterns of drug abuse among military inductees. *Am J Psychiatry*. 1973;130:260–264.

81. Sapol E, Roffman RA. Marijuana in Vietnam. *J Am Pharm Assn*. 1969;9:615–619.

82. Stanton MD. Drugs, Vietnam, and the Vietnam veteran: an overview. *Am J Drug Alcohol Abuse*. 1976;3:557–570. [Reprinted as: Stanton MD. The hooked serviceman: drug use in and after Vietnam. In: Figley CR, Leventman S, eds. *Strangers at Home: Vietnam Veterans Since the War*. New York, NY: Praeger; 1980: 279–292.]

83. Frenkel SI, Morgan DW, Greden JF. Heroin use among soldiers in the United States and Vietnam: a comparison in retrospect. *Int J Addict*. 1977;12:1143–1154.

84. Frank IM, Hoedemaker FS. The civilian psychiatrist and the draft. *Am J Psychiatry*. 1970;127:497–502.

85. Liberman RP, Sonnenberg SM, Stern MS. Psychiatric evaluations for young men facing the draft: a report of 147 cases. *Am J Psychiatry*. 1971;128:147–152.

86. Roemer PA. The psychiatrist and the draft evader [letter]. *Am J Psychiatry*. 1971;127:1236–1237.

87. Ollendorff RH, Adams PL. Psychiatry and the draft. *Am J Orthopsychiatry*. 1971;41:85–90.

88. Moskowitz JA. On drafting the psychiatric "draft" letter. *Am J Psychiatry*. 1971;128:69–72.

89. Lifton RJ. Advocacy and corruption in the healing professions. *Conn Med*. 1975;39:803–813.

90. Spragg GS. Psychiatry in the Australian military forces. *Med J Aust*. 1972;1:745–751.

91. Brass A. Medicine over there. *JAMA*. 1970;213:1473–1475.

92. Maier T. The Army psychiatrist: an adjunct to the system of social control [letter]. *Am J Psychiatry*. 1970;126:1035–1040.

93. Barr NI, Zunin LM. Clarification of the psychiatrist's dilemma while in military service. *Am J Orthopsychiatry*. 1971;41:672–674.

94. APA members hit meeting disruptions in opinion poll results. *Psychiatric News*. March 3, 1971: 6.

95. Psychologists, MH groups attack Vietnam war. *Psychiatric News*. July 5, 1972: 7.

96. Bloch HS. Dr. Bloch replies [letter]. *Am J Psychiatry*. 1970;126:1039–1040.

97. Parrish MD. A veteran of three wars looks at psychiatry in the military. *Psychiatr Opinion*. 1972;2:6–11.

98. Gibbs JJ. Military psychiatry: reflections and projections. *Psychiatr Opinion*. 1973;10:20–23.

99. Bey DR, Chapman RE. Psychiatry—the right way, the wrong way, and the military way. *Bull Menninger Clin*. 1974;38:343–354.

100. Linden E. The demoralization of an army: fragging and other withdrawal symptoms. *Saturday Review*. January 8, 1972:12–17, 55.

101. Gillooly DH, Bond TC. Assaults with explosive devices on superiors: a synopsis of reports from confined offenders at the US Disciplinary Barracks. *Mil Med*. 1973;138:700–702.

102. Cosmas GA, Murray TP. *US Marines in Vietnam: Vietnamization and Redeployment, 1970–1971*. Washington, DC: History and Museums Division, US Marine Corps; 1986: 343–369.

103. Corson WR. The military establishment. In: *Consequences of Failure*. New York, NY: Norton; 1974: 74–105.

104. Jones FD. Disorders of frustration and loneliness. In: Jones FD, Sparacino LR, Wilcox VL, Rothberg JM, Stokes JW, eds. *Military Psychiatry: War Psychiatry*. In: *Textbooks of Military Medicine*. Washington, DC: Office of The Surgeon General, US Department of the Army and Borden Institute; 1995: 63–83.

105. Jones FD. Psychiatric lessons of war. In: Jones FD, Sparacino LR, Wilcox VL, Rothberg JM, Stokes JW, eds. *War Psychiatry*. In: *Textbooks of Military Medicine*. Washington, DC: Office of The Surgeon General, US Department of the Army and Borden Institute; 1995: 3–33.

106. Prugh GS. *Law at War: Vietnam 1964–1973*. Washington, DC: Government Printing Office; 1975.

107. US Army Adjutant General, Casualty Services Division (DAAG-PEC). Active duty Army personnel battle casualties and nonbattle deaths Vietnam, 1961–1979, Office of The Adjutant General counts. February 3, 1981.

108. Bond TC. The why of fragging. *Am J Psychiatry*. 1976;133:1328–1331.

109. Gabriel RA, Savage PL. Cohesion and disintegration in the American Army: an alternative perspective. *Armed Forces Soc*. 1976;2:340–376.

110. Robins LN. A follow-up study of Vietnam veterans' drug use: the transition to civilian life. *J Drug Issues*. 1974;4:61–63.

111. Department of Defense Information Guidance Series. *Drug Abuse in the Military—A Status Report.* Part II. Office of Information for the Armed Forces; August 1972:1–3. No. 5A-18.

112. Ingraham LH. 'The Nam' and 'The World': heroin use by US Army enlisted men serving in Vietnam. *Psychiatry*. 1974;37:114–128.

113. Headquarters, US Army Republic of Vietnam. Drug Rehabilitation/Amnesty Program. [Published as an urgent theater adaptation of Army regulation AR 600-32 (*Drug Rehabilitation/Amnesty Program*) sent to all commands in Vietnam "pending publication of USARV Suppl 1 to AR 600-32." The letter "establishes policies, responsibilities, and procedures for implementation of a Drug Rehabilitation/Amnesty Program in USARV." December 29, 1970 [letter].

114. Lloyd SJ, Frates RC, Domer DC. A clinical evaluation of 81 heroin addicts in Vietnam. *Mil Med*. 1973;138:298–300.

115. Joseph BS. Lessons on heroin abuse from treating users in Vietnam. *Hosp Community Psychiatry*. 1974;25:742–744.

116. Holloway HC, Angel CR, Bardill DR, and the members of work unit 032. Drug abuse in military personnel. In: *Annual Progress Report*. Washington, DC: Walter Reed Army Institute of Research; 1972: 1185–1201.

117. Robins LN, Davis DH, Goodwin DW. Drug use by US enlisted men in Vietnam: a follow-up on their return home. *Am J Epidemiology*. 1974;99:235–249.

118. Ratner RA. Drugs and despair in Vietnam. *U Chicago Magazine*. 1972;64:15–23.

119. Fisher HW. Vietnam psychiatry: portrait of anarchy. *Minn Med*. 1972;55:1165–1167.

120. Stretch RH. Posttraumatic stress disorder among US Army Reserve Vietnam and Vietnam-era veterans. *J Consul Clin Psychol*. 1985;53:935–936.

121. Centers for Disease Control Vietnam Experience Study. Health status of Vietnam veterans. I. Psychosocial characteristics. *JAMA*. 1988;259:2701–2707.

122. Gabriel RA. *No More Heroes: Madness & Psychiatry in War*. New York, NY: Hill and Wang; 1987.

123. Marlowe DH. *Psychological and Psychosocial Consequences of Combat and Deployment, With Special Emphasis on the Gulf War*. Santa Monica, Calif: National Defense Research Institute/Rand; 2001.

124. Dean ET. *Shook Over Hell*. Cambridge, Mass: Harvard University Press; 1997.

125. Veterans Administration. *Myths and Realities: A Study of Attitudes Toward Vietnam Era Veterans*. Washington, DC: Government Printing Office; 1980.

126. Centers for Disease Control and Prevention. *International Classification of Disease, 9th Ed, Clinical Modification*. Available at: http://www.cdc.gov/nchs/icd/icd9.htm. Accessed November 23, 2009.

127. American Psychiatric Association. *Diagnostic and Statistical Manual of Mental Disorders*. 3rd ed (DSM-III). Washington, DC: APA; 1980.

128. Shephard B. *A War of Nerves*. Cambridge, Mass: Harvard University Press; 2000.

129. Kulka RA, Schlenger WE, Fairbank JA, et al. *Trauma and the Vietnam War Generation: Report of Findings From the National Vietnam Veterans Readjustment Study*. New York, NY: Brunner/Mazel; 1990.

130. Holloway HC, Ursano RJ. Viet Nam veterans on active duty: adjustment in a supportive atmosphere. In: Sonnenberg SM, Blank AS Jr, Talbott JA, eds. *The Trauma of War: Stress and Recovery in Viet Nam Veterans*. Washington, DC: American Psychiatric Press; 1980: 321–338.

131. Fleming RH. Post Vietnam syndrome: neurosis or sociosis? *Psychiatry*. 1985;48:122–139.

132. Frueh BC, Grubaugh AL, Elhai JD, Buckley TC. US Department of Veterans Affairs disability policies for posttraumatic stress disorder: administrative trends and implications for treatment, rehabilitation, and research. *Am J Public Health*. 2007;97:2143–2145.

133. Blank AS Jr. Personal communication to author. May 4, 2008.

134. Abse DW. Brief historical overview of the concept of war neurosis and of associated treatment methods. In: Schwartz HJ, ed. *Psychotherapy of the Combat Veteran*. New York, NY: Spectrum Publications; 1984: 1–22.

135. Perlman MS. Basic problems of military psychiatry: delayed reaction in Vietnam veterans. *Int J Offender Ther Comp Criminol*. 1975;19:129–138.

136. Scurfield RM. Posttraumatic stress disorder in Vietnam veterans. In: Wilson JP, Raphael B, eds. *International Handbook of Traumatic Stress Syndromes*. New York, NY: Plenum Publishing; 1993: 285–296.

137. Blank AS Jr. The longitudinal course of posttraumatic stress disorder. In: Davidson JRT, Foa EB, eds. *Posttraumatic Stress Disorder: DSM–IV and Beyond*. Washington, DC: American Psychiatric Press; 1992.

138. Jones FD. Chronic post-traumatic stress disorders. In: Jones FD, Sparacino LR, Wilcox VL, Rothberg JM, Stokes JW, eds. *War Psychiatry*. In: *Textbooks of Military Medicine*. Washington, DC: Office of The Surgeon General, US Department of the Army and Borden Institute; 1995: 409–430.

139. Farrell MJ, Berlien IC. Professional personnel. In: *Zone of the Interior*. Vol 1. In: Glass AJ, Bernucci RJ, eds. *Neuropsychiatry in World War II*. Washington, DC: Government Printing Office; 1966: 41–51.

140. Hauser W. *America's Army in Crisis: A Study in Civil-Military Relations*. Baltimore, Md: Johns Hopkins University Press; 1973.

141. Tureen LL, Stein M. The base section psychiatric hospital. In: Hanson FR, ed. *Combat Psychiatry*. Washington, DC: Government Printing Office; 1949: 105–134. [Also published as a supplement to *Bull US Army Med Depart*. 1949: 9.]

142. Harris FG. Some comments on the differential diagnosis and treatment of psychiatric breakdowns in Korea. In: *Proceedings of Course on Recent Advances in Medicine and Surgery, Army Medical Service Graduate School*. Washington, DC: Walter Reed Army Medical Center; April 30, 1954: 390–402.

143. Lee RA. The Army "mutiny" of 1946. *J Am History*. 1966;53:555–571.

144. Froede RC, Stahl CJ. Fatal narcotism in military personnel. *J Forensic Sci*. 1971;16:199–218.

145. Rose E. The anatomy of a mutiny. *Armed Forces Soc*. 1982;8:561–574.

146. Goffman E. Characteristics of total institutions. In: *Symposium on Preventive and Social Psychiatry, Walter Reed Army Institute of Research*, Washington, DC; April 15–17, 1957: 43–84. Expanded as: Goffman E. *Asylums: Essays on the Social Situation of Mental Patients and Other Inmates*. New York, NY: Doubleday; 1990.

147. Parsons T. *The Social System*. New York, NY: Free Press; 1951.

148. Menninger WC. *Psychiatry in a Troubled World*. New York, NY: Macmillan; 1948.

Chapter 3

PREPARATION FOR DEPLOYMENT: IMPROVING RESILIENCE

PATRICIA WATSON, PhD*; BRETT LITZ, PhD†; STEVEN SOUTHWICK, MD‡; and ELSPETH CAMERON RITCHIE, MD, MPH§

*Assistant Professor, Dartmouth Medical School, 1 Rope Ferry Road, Hanover, New Hampshire 03755-1404; Senior Educational Specialist, Executive Division, Department of Veterans Affairs National Center for Posttraumatic Stress Disorder, White River Junction, Vermont

†Professor, Department of Psychiatry, Boston University School of Medicine, 77 East Concord Street, Boston, Massachusetts 02118; Associate Director, Behavioral Sciences Division, Department of Veterans Affairs National Center for Posttraumatic Stress Disorder, White River Junction, Vermont

‡Professor, Department of Psychiatry, Yale University School of Medicine and Yale Child Study Center, 333 Cedar Street, New Haven, Connecticut 06510; Adjunct Professor, Department of Psychiatry, Mount Sinai School of Medicine, One Gustave L. Levy Place, New York, New York 10029; Deputy Director, Clinical Neurosciences Division, Department of Veterans Affairs National Center for Posttraumatic Stress Disorder, White River Junction, Vermont

§Colonel, US Army (Retired); formerly, Psychiatry Consultant to The Surgeon General, US Army, and Director, Behavioral Health Proponency, Office of The Surgeon General, Falls Church, Virginia; currently, Chief Clinical Officer, District of Columbia Department of Mental Health, 64 New York Avenue NE, 4th Floor, Washington, DC 20002

INTRODUCTION

With ongoing military operations in Afghanistan and Iraq involving multiple deployments for military personnel, there is growing interest in preparatory training activities that can increase service members' resilience to the stress of deployment. Service members are trained in numerous ways that promote adaptation to the stress, strain, and sacrifices of deployments. For example, physical fitness training, mission preparation, specialty role training, experiences that promote confidence in leaders and trust in peers, and messages that emphasize the purpose and function of mission goals are necessary ingredients to successful navigation of various deployment demands. It is not known whether these standard training activities enhance coping capabilities in the face of severe mission demands and traumas. Nor is it known whether existing training regimens effect risk for stress injuries and mental health difficulties linked to deployment stress. Finally, no systematic research has been conducted to date on preparedness interventions specifically designed to build psychological resilience and prevent the development of posttraumatic stress disorder (PTSD) in military personnel.

The lack of empirical literature to support unit preparedness interventions is compounded by the lack of an accepted or unified conceptual framework that defines the necessary and sufficient ingredients for resilience in the face of trauma. In addition, because most research on combat stress has been cross-sectional, little is known about risk, protective, and vulnerability factors, and the mechanisms, processes, and pathways of influence through which they exert their influence on trajectories of adaptation to deployment stress.[1] Unfortunately, the constructs used to define resilience are often extrapolated loosely or interchangeably. Furthermore, research in resilience, hardiness, coping self-efficacy, and biological components of resilience has been conducted within the areas of developmental pathology, trauma, and positive psychology, with little cross-referencing among these disciplines.[2]

Because of the high probability of exposure to severe stress and the extensive motivation to retain a ready and fit fighting force, the military is a natural laboratory to study the effectiveness of resilience-building strategies. What few findings do exist from the adult literature on resilience often come from studies of men in combat. These studies suggest that resilience is related to an ability to bond with a group with a common mission, a high value placed on altruism, the capacity to tolerate high levels of fear and still perform effectively, and psychobiological factors related to a low tendency to dissociate.[3] This chapter will extrapolate from theoretical models about resilience as well as related fields investigating stress, traumatic stress, and recovery from trauma. The goal is to generate an agenda for resilience training that can be examined in future research.

THEORETICAL MODELS OF STRESS, TRAUMA, AND RESILIENCE

It is necessary to first define theoretical models and core constructs related to stress, trauma, and resilience, as well as the implication of these models for preparation and early intervention.

Stress

Research on posttrauma mental health belongs to the broader field of stress research. Stress theory generally assumes that external *demands* (the traumatic event as primary stressor) evoke *responses* that draw on internal and external *resources*. Loss of resources, either concrete (social, financial) or symbolic (beliefs, expectations) may, as secondary stressors, significantly impact the recovery trajectory.[4] Survivors' own responses (anxiety, insomnia, depression) may additionally tax overall resources, becoming tertiary stressors.[5] With sufficient infusion of resources and the passage of time, recovery is the expected outcome of time-limited exposure to a stressor (with great variation depending on the intensity and duration of the stressor[6]). Stress management typically involves identifying and ameliorating those factors that interfere with recovery (lack of supportive others, ongoing stressors, maladaptive beliefs), and providing the resources that help support, organize, and make a plan for survivors.[7]

Trauma

There is no single cause of maladaptive responses to trauma. Traumatic stress theories often draw on psychological and biological research that has identified and mapped processes distinctly reactive to traumatic stress.[8,9] These findings support the proposition that when traumatic responses are overwhelming, uncontrollable, and involve extreme physiological arousal, they may consolidate the link between fear and traumatic recall, leading to avoidance, repeated recall, and ultimately to PTSD. Additional adversity, such as that often seen in the aftermath of extended deployments, can create a chain of mutually reinforcing reactions that may be present forever in a person's memory.

Ehlers and Clark's[10] cognitive model of trauma suggests that preventive interventions focus on reframing negative appraisals of posttraumatic reactions, help individuals to distinguish between past and present threat, and help them process intrusive recollections. Specifically,

- Individuals are at higher risk for persistent PTSD when they make excessively negative appraisals of the trauma and exhibit disturbed memory processes such as poor elaboration and contextualization, strong associative memory, and strong perceptual priming. If individuals appraise their reactions to trauma negatively, they are at risk for enduring PTSD.[11] Therefore, helping individuals to reframe their reactions in a more neutral or positive light should reduce the likelihood of long-term PTSD.
- Because a central process in PTSD is an inability to distinguish past trauma associations of threat with current conditions, Ehlers and Clark advocate interventions that assist with contextual discrimination of past and present circumstances via cognitive therapy.

Intrusive recollections are natural responses to severe and salient life events. Processing (sharing, articulating in a therapeutic manner) incongruous, intrusive, distressful, and unremitting recollections, as well as examining and correcting the cognitive and behavioral responses to them, are the unique factors that should be addressed by trauma interventions above and beyond stress and negative affect management.[12]

Recovery following traumatic stress is promoted by individually chosen disclosure and social support; the perception that the social milieu accepts one's reactions and welcomes disclosure; seeing oneself as a hero or survivor rather than victim; a sense of relationship with "God," a higher power, or some philosophical sense of meaning; and trauma-focused treatment that helps reframe negative reactions, process intrusive recollections, and assist in distinguishing past from present threat.[13] Posttrauma social support and relatively fewer posttrauma negative events may serve as protective factors mediating posttrauma recovery.[14,15]

Resilience

The American Psychological Association Task Force on Promoting Resilience in Response to Terrorism defines resilience as "the process of adapting well in the face of adversity, trauma, tragedy, threats, or even significant sources of stress."[16] It cites many studies showing that the primary factors in resilience are (*a*) caring relationships within and outside the family that create love and trust, provide role models, and encourage and reassure; (*b*) the capacity to make realistic plans and implement them; (*c*) self-confidence; (*d*) communication and problem-solving skills; and (*e*) the capacity to manage emotions. It is generally accepted that resilience is common and derives from the basic human ability to adapt to new situations.[17]

Most research on resilience comes from developmental psychopathology, where initially researchers tried to identify general characteristics associated with resilient recovery from stressors.[18] These general characteristics included hardiness, efficacy (both self and collective), and neurobiological components of resilience.

Hardiness

Research with hardy individuals suggests that they have various personal attributes that may foster resilience. They report seeking help and building large support networks, reframe their experiences more positively (difficulties as leading to benefits); believe they can change a stressor or recover from its detrimental effects; endorse focusing selectively on the positive effects of severe life challenges; view themselves as controlling their fate; are committed to meaningful goals; view stress as a surmountable challenge; are less likely to endorse behavioral disengagement, denial, mental disengagement, and use of alcohol to confront stress; and are more likely to describe themselves as problem solvers.[19–21]

Maddi and Kobasa[22] studied healthy executives to discern the methods they used to increase "mental toughness." They found hardy people were committed to their work (they have a mission they believe in), have a sense of control over what happens in their life, and zestfully seek and take on challenges, feeling they will learn from the experiences. They seldom get sick.

Coping Self-Efficacy

A sense of being able to be effective in the world is the foundation of human agency (the power to originate actions for a given purpose).[23] Unless people believe they can produce desired results and forestall detrimental ones by their actions, they have little incentive to act or to persevere in the face of difficulties. It is partly on the basis of efficacy beliefs that people choose what challenges to undertake, how much effort to expend in the endeavor, how long to persevere in the face of obstacles and failures, and whether failures are motivating or demoralizing. Benight and Bandura[24] recommended that individuals be taught to set achievable goals, which will enable them to have repeated success experiences as well as to establish a sense of environmental control, thus increasing their resilience. Moreover, teaching new problem-solving skills can increase an individual's sense of coping efficacy. A strong sense of coping efficacy, in turn, reduces vulnerability to stress and depression in taxing situations and strengthens resiliency to adversity.

Collective Efficacy

Social cognitive theory extends the conception of individual efficacy to "collective agency,"[25] which is particularly relevant to the military. People's shared belief in their collective power to produce desired results is a key ingredient of collective agency. The findings taken as a whole demonstrate that the stronger the perceived collective efficacy, the higher the group's members aspirations and motivational investment in their undertakings, the stronger their staying power in the face of impediments and setbacks, the higher their morale and resilience to stressors, and the greater their performance accomplishments. Both at the societal and individual level of analysis, a strong perceived efficacy fosters high group effort and performance attainments. Military leaders' efforts to shape collective efficacy require merging diverse self-interests in support of common core values and goals.

Military communities play a proactive role in the resilience-building process by planning and constructing environmental conditions to promote preparedness, leadership, and support.[23,25] Social resources, such as social support, socioeconomic status, and access to services, have shown strong effects on mental health and played a variety of roles in the stress process.[26] Mediational analyses show that social support provides its benefits to the extent that it raises perceived self-efficacy to manage environmental demands.[27]

However, beyond receiving positive social support, a number of research studies indicate that it is not positive social support, but negative social support, that affects recovery. Dunmore, Clark, and Ehlers[28] reported that perception of negative social interactions, rather than perceived positive support, predicts chronic PTSD. It would appear that the military would benefit from programs that build and maintain buddy support (including conflict resolution), model and reinforce social support, and teach strategies for providing support and understanding to those service members, for whatever reason, who express dissatisfaction or show signs of disengagement and withdrawal.

Neurobiological Factors

Neurobiological factors play a central role in the capacity to tolerate stress and trauma. Twin studies have found that overall heritability of PTSD ranges from 28% to 33%.[29] DNA (deoxyribonucleic acid) studies have found that a variety of gene polymorphisms contribute to stress reactivity and possibly the development of trauma-associated psychopathology. Examples include differences in sympathetic nervous system activity (polymorphism of the α-2C-adrenergic receptor gene),[30] cortisol release in response to psychosocial stress (glucocorticoid receptor gene variant),[31] and serotonin metabolism (polymorphism of the serotonin transporter gene).[32]

The role of serotonin metabolism in stress reactivity was studied by Caspi,[32] who found that a functional polymorphism in the promoter region of the serotonin transporter gene moderated the influence of stressful life events on the likelihood of developing depression. Among individuals who had experienced childhood maltreatment, those with two long alleles were significantly less likely to develop depression than those with two short alleles. Thus two long alleles appear to protect against trauma-related psychopathology while two short alleles are associated with vulnerability to trauma. Of note, it appears that environmental factors can serve a protective role even among those with a genetic vulnerability. Kauffman[33] recently found that strong social support protected against the development of depression in traumatized foster children, even among those with genetic vulnerability (ie, two short alleles of the serotonin transporter gene).

A wide variety of hormones, neurotransmitters, and neuropeptides that are known to be activated by stress and trauma are also thought to be associated with resilience. In a comprehensive literature review, Charney[3] highlighted eleven neurochemicals that appear to have particular relevance to the neurobiology of resilience. The evidence posits that resilient individuals will score in the highest range for measures of dehydroepiandrosterone (DHEA), neuropeptide Y (NPY), galanin, testosterone, serotonin (5-HT1a), and benzodiazepine receptor function. These same resilient individuals will score in the lowest range for hypothalamic-pituitary-adrenocortical (HPA) axis, corticotropin-releasing hormone, and locus-caeruleus-norepinephrine activity. The findings are opposite for those individuals vulnerable to stress. For example, NPY is an amino acid that helps to maintain sympathetic nervous system reactivity within an optimal range. Under conditions of danger, the sympathetic nervous system (SNS) releases epinephrine and norepinephrine (NE) as part of the fight–flight response. During these high-stress situations, NPY is also released and helps to inhibit continued release of NE so that the SNS does not overshoot and possibly contribute to anxiety, hypervigilance, and fear. High levels of NPY during extreme training stress have been associated with adaptive performance in Special Forces soldiers. It is likely that robust increases in NE are held in check by similarly robust increases in NPY among these highly resilient soldiers.[3,34,35]

Galanin and DHEA are two other neurochemicals that may enhance resilience by containing or modulating the stress response.[3] For example, cortisol is released during stressful situations and helps to mobilize energy stores and increase arousal, selective attention, vigilance, and consolidation of emotional memory, all of which tend to be adaptive. However, when cortisol remains chronically high and unchecked, it can have toxic effects on the body and brain.[36,37] DHEA, which is released with cortisol, helps to lower levels of cortisol, and thus has protective effects.[35] Like NPY, high DHEA-to-cortisol ratio has been associated with better performance in Special Forces soldiers during high-stress training exercises and may play a role in modulating psychological, physiological, and behavioral responses to stress.

It is likely that individual neurobiological factors by themselves have relatively limited impact on stress resilience. However, in accordance with a model of allostasis,[38] the additive effects of multiple neurobiological factors may have a substantial effect on resilience. Thus, Charney[3] hypothesized that resilient individuals might be those with relatively high stress-induced NPY, galanin, DHEA, and testosterone, and relatively low stress-induced SNS and HPA-axis activation.

Numerous brain regions and neural pathways involved in the processing and regulation of fear, learning, memory, reward, emotion, motivation, and social behavior are also undoubtedly involved in resilience to stress. For example, resilience may be associated with optimal stimulation or inhibition of prefrontal cortical-amygdala circuitry, which would facilitate appropriate and adaptive responses to stressors. Similarly, the capacity for mutual cooperation, social bonding, positive emotions, and hope in the face of adversity, all of which have been associated with resilience, may be dependent on well-functioning reward circuitry involving the nucleus accumbens dopamine system.[3,34]

It is likely that relevant neurotransmitter and hormone systems, as well as neural pathways, can be modified by experience. Developmental studies have shown that early experiences with stress can have long-term effects on behavioral and neurobiological responses to future fear and stress.[38] Thus, uncontrollable or overwhelming stress during infancy can cause exaggerated emotional, SNS, and HPA-axis responsiveness to future stressors even into adulthood. Mild-to-moderate stressors that are controllable can have a "steeling" or stress inoculating effect, where the organism becomes less reactive to future stressors.[39] Although attention and arousal are necessary for survival, going outside an optimal range has detrimental biological effects. During stress, multiple cortical and subcortical brain regions (including sensory, motor, prefrontal and cingulate cortex, hippocampus, amygdala, thalamus, striatum, midbrain, and brain stem monoaminergic nuclei and hypothalamus) become activated. Communication between these regions facilitates evaluation of, psychomotor response to, and memory for stress-related events. Although arousal may be life saving, it has been hypothesized that excessive and sustained arousal following trauma may increase the likelihood of developing PTSD.[5,40,41] Numerous animal studies have shown that extended and excessive states of alarm and arousal may contribute to stress sensitization and long-term potentiation,[42] both of which likely contribute to trauma-related psychopathology.

Understanding and working with biological components of resilience is an area with great potential for intervention. Based on the neurobiological findings on use-dependent neuroplasticity, it is likely that certain preparation and training regimes will alter relevant neural and neurotransmitter systems that are involved in resilience to stress. These include training to regulate emotions, face fear, dispute and reappraise negative cognitions, find positive meaning in adversity, help others in need, and attract social support.

Defining Resilience

Resilience is generally considered to be "multidimensional,"[18] with different characteristics expressed variably across many areas of the individual's life (eg, occupation and social). These "resilient trajectories" may be uneven.[18,43] For example, an individual may function adequately in work settings following a trauma but suffer from interpersonal numbing or withdrawal. Furthermore, the expression of resilience is influenced by context: the quality of the stressor, the individual's traits, and the surrounding culture.[43] Many researchers in this area conclude that resilience is not a fixed attribute but a type of "functional trajectory" dependent on circumstances and individual variations (eg, vulnerability and protective mechanisms) in response to risk. If circumstances change, resilience trajectories can change.[18,44]

Multidimensional analysis indicates that resilient behavior in one domain may extract a price in another; for example, competence in work domains may involve emotional detachment from family problems,[45,46] and at-risk individuals with exemplary behavior may experience internal distress.[47,48] Finally, there has been some acknowledgment that the factors that bolster resilience may not be adaptive in all domains (ie, sociopathy and narcissism[13]).

Experts in the field of resilience hold that all plans for research and intervention should clearly define resilience as a state, not a trait.[18] Therefore, they recommend avoiding the term "resiliency," with its connotation of a trait. Rather, it is recommended to use the phrase "resilient trajectory or adaptation," explaining that these trajectories vary across situations and within individuals at different times.[18]

Indeed, resilience is both a process and an outcome. There are resilient outcomes (eg, in the face of enormous combat traumas, a service member does not develop any mental health problem or significant problems functioning) and there are resilient processes (mechanisms that create resilient outcomes), which change over the life-course, as demands, circumstances, and service members change. The goal of resilience training is to promote or augment existing personal and social resources and create new resources that contribute to adaptation.

EVALUATING RESILIENCE OUTCOMES

Three things are necessary to evaluate resilience as an outcome: (1) the nature of the exposure to trauma; (2) the prevalence of symptoms and problems, with an emphasis on the degree of subjective distress and suffering; and (3) functional capacities in diverse areas (eg, work, leisure, self-care, relationships). However resilience is operationalized, successful adaptation or recovery from deployment trauma within and across service members is dependent on the nature of the trauma and the extent of exposure to war-zone events. It is inappropriate to compare resilience across individuals without accounting for variability in exposure to trauma. In the case of severe and extensive war-zone trauma, resilience should not be narrowly defined as the absence of posttraumatic mental health disorders, such as PTSD. Service members will report a variety of symptoms reflecting the enduring psychological impact of their deployment experiences. What should define resilience is not the mere absence of symptoms, but the degree of subjective distress caused by these problems and, more importantly, the extent to which their functioning is compromised.[49]

In terms of studying resilience as a process, measures need to be developed to evaluate individual differences in protective factors and processes, so that studies can test potential mechanisms mediating exposure to trauma and outcome. Other goals would be to describe the prevalence of various resilience indicators in a given trauma context across time and to evaluate the efficacy of interventions designed to promote resilience. What mechanisms or processes facilitate resilience at a given posttraumatic interval? One way to look at resilience is that resources and strengths in the individual and in the group's culture (eg, a cohesive and supportive squad in the military) outweigh the influence of liabilities and weaknesses. In this context, individual and social resources are used to: (*a*) manage posttraumatic demands; (*b*) find meaning, purpose, and hope; (*c*) reduce or eliminate current adversities and stressors; and (*d*) derive positive feelings from various repertoires of activities (eg, work, leisure). In research on resilience, it is particularly important to recognize that the process of resilience lies in both the individual and in the environment (and the transaction of the two). A thorough evaluation of resilience resources should take into account social-demographic factors, current adversities, social networks, and intimate relationships.

MEASUREMENT OF RESILIENCE FACTORS IN THE MILITARY

The *Deployment Risk and Resilience Inventory* (DRRI)[50,51] treats resilience as an unfolding process and multidimensional construct, with the individual, exposure characteristics, and the social milieu (within the military and in the home) seen as equally important. It was developed based on literature review, survey and focus group input, and confirmatory factor analysis, to assess risk and resilience variables that are related to health and well-being following military deployments. The DRRI assesses risk and resilience in 14 domains, divided into prewar factors, war-zone factors, and postwar factors.

Prewar Factors:

1. Childhood family environment (cohesion, closeness of family)
2. Prior stressors (exposure to highly stressful

or traumatic events)

War-Zone Factors:

3. Preparedness (perceived preparedness, including belief in quality and quantity of equipment, supplies, and training)
4. Combat (exposure to objective warfare experiences)
5. Aftermath of battle (observing or handling remains, dealing with prisoners of war, exposure to devastated communities and refugees)
6. Perceived threat (subjective fear for one's safety and well-being in war zone)
7. Difficult living and working environment (day-to-day pressures, discomfort, deprivation)
8. Concerns about life and family disruptions (career-related concerns, family concerns)
9. Sexual harassment (exposure to unwanted sexual touching or verbal conduct)
10. General harassment (harassment on basis of biological sex or minority status)
11. War-zone social support (assistance and encouragement from leaders, other unit members)
12. Nuclear, biological, and chemical exposures

Postwar Factors:

13. Postwar social support (emotional sustenance and instrumental assistance from family, friends, coworkers and employers, community)
14. Postwar stressors (general stressful events such as accidents, illness; reintegration issues such as job interruption, difficulties reestablishing roles)

Because the DRRI is specifically geared to evaluate adaptation to deployment stress and trauma, and is psychometrically sound, its broad use is recommended. However, the DRRI does not measure individual differences in psychological resilience, which is also an important personal resource. Prior to enlistment, all service members possess varying degrees of an innate and acquired capacity to manage serious life challenges and threats effectively (resilience). Unfortunately, there is no "gold standard" method of evaluating resilience as a individual characteristic, which should not be surprising because there is no unified conceptual or definitional framework. One measure that has been found to have adequate content coverage is the Connor-Davidson Resilience Scale,[52] which is a 25-item questionnaire tapping attitudes about coping with adversity (eg, "having to cope with stress makes me stronger"). Items require respondents to indicate their degree of endorsement on a five-point scale ranging from not true at all to true nearly all the time. Connor and Davidson reported a Cronbach's alpha of .89 in a validation sample of general population subjects, which shows that this instrument is highly likely to elicit consistent and reliable response even if questions were replaced with other similar questions.

The National Center for PTSD is developing a measure called the Response to Stressful Experiences Scale, which seeks to measure resilience. The scale has been structured to cover the following putative mechanisms of resilience:

- **Behavioral**. The actions (active or passive) an individual exhibits in response to an intense life stressor that facilitate a return to psychological baseline functioning or to psychological growth, including actions aimed at marshalling social support.
- **Emotional**. The degree of effectiveness regarding how to use one's emotions to achieve one's goals. This is accomplished by managing emotional reactions in a flexible, situation-appropriate manner.
- **Cognitive**. Conscious thoughts, perceptions, and expectations aimed at adapting to, or overcoming, stressful situations by orienting one's beliefs when useful, to include a realistic and accepting stance about personal vulnerability, the likelihood of future risks, and the ability to achieve personal growth.

It is hoped that by measuring multiple domains, a more useful and accurate level of resilience can be obtained.

INTERVENTIONS FOR BUILDING RESILIENCE AND PREPAREDNESS

It could be argued that the military continuously fosters resilience in service members from recruitment and basic training to retirement. It is beyond the scope of this chapter to catalog and operationally define all the resilience-building efforts in the lifespan of a service member. Instead, this discussion will focus on efforts that occur or should be considered to lessen the mental health impact of various deployment hardships, adversities, and serious traumas (primary prevention).

It is unclear at present whether preparation is likely to inoculate individuals fully against severe trauma. A number of strategies extrapolated from different fields are described as possible components of preparation and prevention. One factor that needs consideration is that preparation requires motivation, foresight, and time and energy, which may not be realistic and cost effective under all circumstances. If preparedness is not feasible, research suggests that preventing resource loss is more efficient in promoting recovery than attempting to introduce additional resources following a traumatic event.[6] Other programs designed to prepare individuals are discussed next.

Toughening Responses to Stress

Can individuals become better prepared for deployment and combat? The literature on "toughness" suggests that under certain conditions, repeated episodes of challenge or threat followed by recovery periods (eg, aerobic exercise and working in cold environments) can "toughen" the neuroendocrine system's response to stress. People who undertook programs of aerobic training, for instance, were subsequently more energetic and more emotionally stable than they were before such an experience.[53] Better performance and learning in even complex tasks was associated with greater adrenergic responsiveness in humans.

Toughness is less relevant, however, to situations experienced as harm or loss, where negative outcomes already have occurred, or where instrumental coping is considered useless (eg, one can overwhelm organisms with excessively intense, extended, or unexpected training; even a single episode of a traumatic stressor can overwhelm). Combining unpredictability with great severity may overwhelm the organism's capacity to recover, leading to weakness rather than toughness.[54]

Building Strengths Through Training Programs

A recent expert panel reached consensus that any intervention program designed for situations of ongoing threat should incorporate elements designed to foster hope, safety, efficacy, calming, and connectedness.[55] Learned optimism and positive psychology models[56,57] incorporate many of these components to build strengths in people at risk. The components they apply to strength building and prevention include: instilling hope; building buffering strengths (ie, interpersonal skill, optimism, perseverance, capacity for pleasure, and purpose); narration, or the telling of stories about one's life to another; and disputing (the skill of recognizing one's own catastrophic and exaggerated thinking and effectively disputing it).

Seligman has found that such training is self-reinforcing and prevents depression and anxiety in children and adults. This training is unique in that it focuses on building strength rather than repairing damage. Seligman's intervention programs are called "training programs" rather than therapy, and yet they have similar beneficial effects as psychotherapy.[57–59]

Building Resilience Through Self-Help Programs

The American Psychological Association has recently placed an online module on building resilience on its self-help Web site.[16] Leading researchers in the field of resilience and posttraumatic growth formed the committee that created the module. The Web site explicates basic self-help steps for improving resilience, based on empirical and consensus information: increasing social support, optimism, realistic appraisal and goal setting, emotional and social balance, and a mix of both problem-focused and emotion-focused coping. Because literature on adult learning suggests that self-paced instruction is important to successful mastery of material, this dissemination strategy may be highly effective in assisting soldiers with their own recovery course, particularly those who are worried about stigma involved with seeking assistance, and whose schedules are busy.

Teaching Skills Commonly Utilized During Survival Situations

Another approach to training resilience is to interview those who have survived highly stressful circumstances to gain an understanding of common factors that are helpful in survival. For instance, a recent case study[60] illustrates that the use of problem-solving techniques in trauma survivors enabled them to retain a sense of efficacy and control during life-threatening situations. Examples of strategies employed by survivors include the following:

- recalling and practicing skills from previous education about the situation they were in (ie, safety and breathing);
- having confidence in friends to help;
- analyzing everything closely, and demanding results;
- dismissing thoughts of death as unconstructive;
- concentrating on how to pacify the person making the threat;
- feeling a sense of control;
- remaining calm;

- thinking of loved ones;
- prayer;
- concentrating on positive coping actions; and
- not letting sounds or sights distract them.

Basic survival skills have been delineated by Gonzales,[61] who conducted case studies and interviews with hundreds of people who had survived life-threatening situations. The following list includes the six factors that are commonly observed across those who survived dangerous situations.

1. Knowing as much as you can about the situation ahead of time, keeping in mind that the forces may be so large (or fast) that they are difficult to imagine.
2. Being adaptive and flexible, based on a true reading of the environment, and changing behavior accordingly.
3. Quickly organizing, setting up routines, and instituting discipline; breaking down very large jobs into small, manageable tasks; setting attainable goals and developing short-term plans to achieve them; and dealing with what is within your power from moment to moment and leaving the rest behind.
4. Knowing your abilities and not over- or underestimating them.
5. Being able to assess and stop if it is clear that the environment does not support going forward, no matter how much you have planned; being realistic about goals and timeframe, then being content with just being in the process.
6. Cultivating a positive mental attitude by:
   - Realizing that life is not always fair.
   - Having fortitude, patience, courtesy, modesty, decorum, and the will (in the worst of situations) to do your best.
   - Celebrating successes, and taking joy in completing tasks, even small ones.
   - Creating an ongoing feeling of motivation, preventing hopelessness, and giving yourself small breaks from the stress of the situation.
   - Being determined to be careful and do your best, and becoming convinced that you will succeed.
   - Not becoming discouraged by setbacks; accepting that the environment is constantly changing; picking yourself up and starting the entire process over again, if necessary, in manageable steps; and embracing the world in which you find yourself and seeing opportunity in adversity.

Military personnel may be better prepared for deployment stresses if they have specific information to help them master life-threatening situations and are instructed in how to use this as part of their problem-solving strategy. In addition to teaching skills for specific situations, it may be important to prepare individuals to cope with unexpected situations where they may feel confused, bewildered, or helpless. Bell's[62] resilience program seeks to address these issues through the use of esoteric training principles, including meditation exercises that develop steadiness, clarity, pliancy, mindfulness, and emotional endurance. These principles, however, have not been tested in situations of traumatic stress.

Reinforcing Skills Through Military Training

Military training focuses on preparation of personnel for battle or other chaotic and disastrous situations. The US military strives to prepare its soldiers for potential exposure to combat, operations other than war, and the stresses of deployment in many ways. In combat units, there are many hours devoted to field training exercises (some quite long), to include exposure to live fire, with reduced sleep, at a high pace of operations. Those trained at the Suvival, Evasion, Resistance, and Escape (SERE) schools undergo extremely stressful mock captures and interrogations at a simulated prisoner-of-war camp. Training in nuclear, biological, and chemical warfare is also standard, including maintenance of the gas mask and donning the mask within 9 seconds. Especially overseas, there are exercises in wearing the chemical protective suit for long periods of time while performing one's job. The constant repetition and standardized measures of mastery are intended to foster a sense of control for the service member, at the same time sending the message that "we are prepared for anything that may come our way down range."

Unit cohesiveness is another critical protective factor in war. Spiegel[63] speculated that it was regard for comrades, respect for leaders, concern for the reputation of the group, and an urge to ensure the success of the unit that kept soldiers fighting in World War II.[64] Furthermore, he identified that when individual's decompensated it was often after a change in the soldier's relation to the group.[63] During the Vietnam War, it was observed that ultimately this unit cohesiveness does not represent an altruism born of interpersonal attraction but rather the realization that a soldier's survival depended upon his ability to make others willing to help him in his own time of need.[65] This cohesiveness can extend throughout an entire organization, with the unit serving as an extension of individual pride. The soldier's self-esteem becomes linked to the reputation of the unit, providing additional motivation. In other words, an individual's identity is not just about self but also incorporates a collective identity that, when well developed, is a protective factor.

Physical fitness is also an essential component of military training. Throughout their career, service members must take a physical fitness test twice a year. This ensures that service members maintain at least a reasonable degree of physical fitness, despite having many other taskings. In the elite units, physical training is a high priority. In addition to preparing soldiers for the physical exertion necessary in battle, physical fitness has also been strongly linked to reductions in stress, anxiety, and depression.[66]

Drills and exercises are another component of preparedness and building resilience. In the Navy, for example, the drills may be centered on reacting to fires, the ship sinking, "man overboard," and other mishaps. These exercises utilize the constructs of stress inoculation, which in the civilian world takes the form of cognitive-behavioral methods to anticipate and diminish responses to anxiety-provoking events, with the aim of reducing the response to a perceived threat.[67] Beyond enhancing cognitive knowledge, exercises in the military encourage bonding and a sense of mastery about disaster. Some of the military survivors of the September 11, 2001, attack on the Pentagon believed that previous drills prepared them for the chaos of the exit, while civilian employees complained that they were underprepared.[68]

Despite the potential benefit of stress inoculation and drills, recent experience has shown that many military members are not prepared for the sights and smells of civilian casualties, nor the experience of handling the bodies of their friends or the enemy. For example, after the USS *Iowa* explosion, when shipmates handled the bodies of their friends, several developed PTSD symptoms.[69] The US Army has developed a pamphlet, *Just the Facts . . . Dealing With the Stress of Recovering Human Dead Bodies*, to provide guidance on how troops should handle remains in order to reduce stress levels.[70] What is not currently known, however, is the best assortment and intensity of stimuli to prepare people, rather than oversensitize them.

In the military, leadership is always emphasized. Military leaders are taught to foster hardiness, unit cohesion, and morale by "leading by example"; facilitating open communication regarding how missions are planned; stating how mistakes or failures are corrected and learned from; seeking out (and creating if necessary) meaningful and challenging group tasks; remaining aware of the basic needs of the team (to include the need for rest); and providing opportunities for all individuals to make use of their unique coping skills (to include prayer or writing letters home). A study conducted with a group of Norwegian navy officer cadets demonstrated that units that increased significantly in cohesion after a stressful exercise also rated their leaders as better skilled and more caring and concerned compared to units that did not increase in cohesion. Individuals who see their leaders as more effective and concerned, even when these leaders are under extreme stress, are in turn more likely to interpret the experience positively. For group tasks, this positive interpretation is reflected in increased group cohesion.

Another component to which the US military pays particular attention in preparation for deployment is the "state of affairs at home," because emotional support has been shown to affect the impact of deployment.[71] Data from the Israeli Defence Forces, for example, show that 30% of their casualties in the Lebanon War were caused by combat stress reactions. The Israeli Defence Forces found that soldiers who had experienced certain marital discord or stress in personal relationships were at high risk of suffering combat stress reactions.[72] Recently, the US Army has developed a vigorous deployment cycle support plan called Battlemind[73] to help reintegrate returning soldiers into their families and society, especially those who have been wounded. The Navy and Marine Corps have developed a multifaceted program centered around acknowledgement that stress reactions, injuries, and illness fall on a dimensional combat and operational stress continnum, with efforts to intervene with both service members and their families early in the continuum to reduce long-term problems.[74–76]

Finally, the military has been increasingly sensitive to properly recognizing the deceased. Following the attack of the USS *Cole* the leadership made a concerted effort to ensure that the deceased were given a proper military burial and that the survivors were allowed to pay their respects. By putting the crew to work to ensure a proper burial, the leader was giving the crew back a sense of control, sending the message to the survivors that each life is valuable and will be treated with due dignity, especially in death, and beginning the mourning process for those more closely linked to those lost.[77]

SUGGESTIONS FOR FUTURE RESEARCH ON RESILIENCE

Primary prevention and training prior to stressful military situations often involves interventions such as teaching problem-solving skills or toughening exercises like those in military training. This form of stress inoculation is designed to foster "resistance." However, by its nature traumatic stress is unpredictable and uncontrollable. Therefore, although stress resistance is related to specific or probable stressors, traumatic stress preparation should be geared more toward preparing individuals for the unexpected, when they may not yet understand what is going on, when conditions are new, and when they may feel confused, bewildered, or helpless.

Another strategy seeks to enhance resilience by teaching certain factors that have worked for others following traumatic or stressful situations, such as social support and self-efficacy or positively changing beliefs or actions. This approach may involve building restorative, replenishing activities into the posttrauma schedule, having individuals try to find what might restore their inherent capacity to thrive, and raising awareness about the cost and benefit of denial at different phases postincident. Programs need to prepare for active outreach and assistance for weeks and months following deployment.

It is important to keep in mind that what works for individuals in one context may not work for the same or other groups in others. A sensible research strategy for maximizing resilient trajectories before, during, and after deployment would be multidisciplinary, multifaceted, and sensitive to the context of the event, as well as to differential exposure and response. There is also a strong need to partner clinicians and researchers in designing and evaluating programs.

It is also important to remain cautious in any statement regarding what interventions can accomplish toward prevention of long-term functional and symptomatic impact. For example, it is unknown whether interventions are associated with significant improvements in functioning. Additionally, care should be taken to include the preferences of soldiers when an intervention is planned. Research on service utilization indicates that the majority of individuals exposed to a traumatic event will not choose to seek mental health services, and therefore a careful study of what interventions are acceptable and supportive of natural recovery trajectories may be called for prior to strong recommendations for any mental health intervention. A more acceptable intervention than individual crisis response might be to provide a "resilience training model" that is implemented as part of basic training for all military personnel, as well as providing family and friends with the tools necessary for helping loved ones more effectively process traumatic or enduring stress.

SUMMARY

This chapter has extrapolated from theoretical models about resilience, as well as related fields investigating stress, traumatic stress, and recovery from trauma, to generate an agenda for resilience training that can be examined in future research. The construct of resilience represents a dynamic process involving protective and vulnerability factors in different risk contexts and developmental stages, and thus is an area of considerable interest and importance to the military. However, the lack of empirical literature to support unit preparedness interventions is compounded by the lack of an accepted or unified conceptual framework that defines the necessary and sufficient ingredients for resilience in the face of trauma or resilience-building interventions to prepare soldiers for deployment.

REFERENCES

1. Layne CM, Warren JS, Watson PJ, Shalev A. Risk vulnerability, resistance, and resilience: toward an integrative conceptualization of posttraumatic adaptation. In: Friedman MJ, Keane TM, Resick PA, eds. *Handbook of PTSD: Science and Practice.* New York, NY: Guilford Press; 2007: 497–520.

2. Luthar SS, Zelazo LB. Resilience and vulnerability: an integrative review. In Luthar SS, ed. *Resilience and Vulnerability: Adaptation in the Context of Childhood Adversities.* New York, NY: Cambridge University Press; 1987: 510–549.

3. Charney DS. Psychobiological mechanisms of resilience and vulnerability: implications for successful adaptation to extreme stress. *Am J Psychiatry.* 2004;161:195–216.

4. Raphael B, Wilson JP, eds. *Psychological Debriefing: Theory, Practice, and Evidence.* Cambridge, UK: Cambridge University Press; 2000.

5. Bryant RA, Harvey AG, Dang ST, Sackville T, Basten C. Treatment of acute stress disorder: a comparison of cognitive-behavioral therapy and supportive counseling. *J Consult Clin Psychol.* 1998;66:862–866.

6. Hobfoll SE. Conservation of resources: a new attempt at conceptualizing stress. *Am Psychol.* 1989;44:513–524.

7. Norris FH, Friedman MJ, Watson PJ, Byrne CM, Diaz E, Kaniasty K. 60,000 disaster victims speak: part I. An empirical review of the empirical literature, 1981–2001. *Psychiatry.* 2002;65:207–239.

8. Pearlin LI, Schooler C. The structure of coping. *J Health Soc Behav.* 1978;19:2–21.

9. Greene GJ, Lee MY, Trask R, Rheinscheld J. How to work with clients' strengths in crisis intervention: a solution focused approach. In: Roberts AR. *Crisis Intervention Handbook: Assessment, Treatment, and Research.* 2nd ed. Oxford, UK: Oxford University Press; 2000.

10. Ehlers A, Clark DM. A cognitive model of posttraumatic stress disorder. *Behav Res Ther.* 2000;38:319–345.

11. Halligan SL, Michael T, Clark DM, Ehlers A. Posttraumatic stress disorder following assault: the role of cognitive processing, trauma memory, and appraisals. *J Consult Clin Psychol.* 2003;71:419–431.

12. Watson, PJ, Shalev A. Assessment and treatment of acute traumatic stress following mass traumatic events. *CNS Spectr.* 2005;10:123–131.

13. Bonanno GA. Loss, trauma, and human resilience: have we underestimated the human capacity to thrive after extremely aversive events? *Am Psychol.* 2004;59:20–28.

14. Brewin C, Andrews B, Valentine J. Meta-analysis of risk factors for posttraumatic stress disorder in trauma exposed adults. *J Consult Clin Psychol.* 2000;68:748–766.

15. King LA, King DW, Fairbank JA, Keane TM, Adams GA. Resilience-recovery factors in posttraumatic stress disorder among female and male Vietnam veterans: hardiness, postwar social support, and additional stressful life events. *J Pers Soc Psychol.* 1998;74:420–434.

16. APA road to resilience Web site. Available at: http://www.apahelpcenter.org/featuredtopics/feature.php?id=6. Accessed July 21, 2009.

17. Masten AS. Ordinary magic. Resilience processes in development. *Am Psychol.* 2001;56:227–238.

18. Luthar SS, Cicchetti D. The construct of resilience: implications for interventions and social policies. *Dev Psychopathol.* 2000;12:857–885.

19. Kobasa SC, Maddi SR, Kahn S. Hardiness and health: a prospective study. *J Pers Soc Psychol.* 1982;42:168–177.

20. Maddi SR, Hightower M. Hardiness and optimism as expressed in coping patterns. *Consult Psychol J.* 1999;51:95–105.

21. Waysman M, Schwarzwald J, Solomon Z. Hardiness: an examination of its relationship with positive and negative long term changes following trauma. *J Trauma Stress.* 2001;14:531–548.

22. Maddi SR, Khoshaba DM. Hardiness and mental health. *J Pers Assess.* 1994;63:265–274.

23. Bandura A. Social cognitive theory: an agentic perspective. *Annu Rev Psychol.* 2001;52:1–26.

24. Benight CC, Bandura A. Social cognitive theory of posttraumatic recovery: the role of perceived self-efficacy. *Behav Res Ther.* 2004;42:1129–1148.

25. Bandura A. *Self-Efficacy: The Exercise of Control.* New York, NY: WH Freeman; 1997.

26. Norris FH, Murrell SA. Protective function of resources related to life events, global stress, and depression in older adults. *J Health Soc Behav.* 1984;25:424–437.

27. Benight CC, Ironson G, Durham RL. Psychometric properties of a hurricane coping self-efficacy measure. *J Trauma Stress.* 1999;12:379–386.

28. Dunmore E, Clark DM, Ehlers A. A prospective investigation of the role of cognitive factors in persistent posttraumatic stress disorder (PTSD) after physical or sexual assault. *Behav Res Ther*. 2001;39:1063–1084.

29. True WJ, Rice J, Eisen SA, et al. A twin study of genetic and environmental contributions to liability for posttraumatic stress symptoms. *Arch Gen Psychiatry.* 1993;50:257–264.

30. Finley PR. Depression and medical comorbidity—treatment considerations. *Rx Consult.* 2004;12:1–8.

31. Wüst S, Federenko IS, van Rossum EF, et al. A psychobiological perspective on genetic determinants of hypothalamus-pituitary-adrenal axis activity. *Ann N Y Acad Sci.* 2003;1032:52–62.

32. Caspi A, Sugden K, Moffitt TE, et al. Influence of life stress on depression: moderation by a polymorphism in the 5-HTT gene. *Science*. 2003;301:386–389.

33. Kaufman J. Stress and its consequences: an evolving story. *Biol Psychiatry.* 2006;60:669–670.

34. Southwick SM, Vythilingam M, Charney DS. The psychobiology of depression and resilience to stress: implications for prevention and treatment. *Ann Rev Clin Psychol.* 2005;27:255–291.

35. Morgan CA 3rd, Wang S, Mason JW, et al. Hormone profiles in humans experiencing military survival training. *Biol Psychiatry.* 2000;47:891–901.

36. Bremner JD, Narayan M, Staib LH, et al. Neural correlates of memories of childhood sexual abuse in women with and without posttraumatic stress disorder. *Am J Psychiatry.* 1999;156:1787–1795.

37. McEwen BS. Allostasis and allostatic load: implications for neuropsychopharmacology. *Neuropsychopharmacol.* 2000;22:108–124.

38. McEwen BS, Stellar E. Stress and the individual. Mechanisms leading to disease. *Arch Intern Med.* 1993;153:2093–2101.

39. Kaufman J, Plotsky PM, Nemeroff CB, Charney DS. Effects of early adverse experiences on brain structure and function: clinical implications. *Biol Psychiatry.* 2000;48:778–790.

40. Brewin CR, Andrews B, Valentine JD. Meta-analysis of risk factors for posttraumatic stress disorder in trauma-exposed adults. *J Consult Clin Psychol*. 2000;68:748–766.

41. Bryant RA, Harvey AG, Guthrie RM, Moulds ML. A prospective study of psychophysiological arousal, acute stress disorder, and posttraumatic stress disorder. *J Abnorm Psychol.* 2000;109:341–344.

42. Blank T, Nijholt I, Eckart K, Spiess J. Priming of long-term potentiation in mouse hippocampus by corticotropin-releasing factor and acute stress: implications for hippocampus-dependent learning. *J Neurosci.* 2002;22:3788–3794.

43. Tusaie K, Dyer J. Resilience: a historical review of the construct. *Holis Nurse Pract.* 2004;18:3–8.

44. Rutter M. Resilience: some conceptual considerations. *J Adolesc Health.* 1993;14:626–631.

45. Anthony EJ, Cohler BJ, eds. *The Invulnerable Child.* New York, NY: Guilford Press; 1987.

46. Werner EE, Smith RS. *Overcoming the Odds: High Risk Children From Birth to Adulthood*. Ithaca, NY: Cornell University Press; 1992.

47. Cohler BJ, Stott FM, Musick JS. Adversity, vulnerability, and resilience. Cultural and developmental perspectives. In: Cicchetti D, Cohen DJ, eds. *Developmental Psychopathology.* Vol 12. *Risk, Disorder, and Adaptation*. New York, NY: Wiley; 1995: 753–800.

48. Luthar SS. Vulnerability and resilience: a study of high-risk adolescents. *Child Dev.* 1991;62:600–616.

49. Litz BT. Has resilience to severe trauma been underestimated? *Am Psychol.* 2005;60:262.

50. King LA, Orcutt HK, King DW, Kimerling R, Ouimette PC, Wolfe J. Gender differences in stress, trauma, and PTSD research: application of two quantitative methods. In: *Gender and PTSD.* New York, NY: Guilford Press, 2002: 403–433.

51. Vogt DS, Pless AP, King LA, King DW. Deployment stressors, gender, and mental health outcomes among Gulf War I veterans. *J Trauma Stress.* 2005;18:272–284.

52. Vaishnavi S, Connor K, Davidson JR. An abbreviated version of the Connor-Davidson Resilience Scale (CD-RISC), the CD-RISC2: psychometric properties and applications in psychopharmacological trials. *Psychiatry Res.* 2007;152:293–297.

53. Dienstbier RA. The effect of exercise on personality. In: Sachs ML, Buffone GD, eds. *Running as Therapy: An Integrated Approach.* Lincoln, Neb: University of Nebraska Press; 1984: 128–135.

54. Dienstbier RA. Arousal and physiological toughness: implications for mental and physical health. *Psychol Rev.* 1989;96:84–100.

55. Hobfoll SE, Watson P, Bell CC, et al. Five essential elements of immediate and mid-term mass trauma intervention: empirical evidence. *Psychiatry.* 2007;70:283–315.

56. Seligman MEP. *What You Can Change and What You Can't.* New York, NY: Knopf; 1994.

57. Seligman MEP, Peterson C. Positive clinical psychology. In: Aspinwall LG, Staudinger UM, eds. *A Psychology of Human Strengths: Fundamental Questions and Future Directions for a Positive Psychology.* Washington, DC: American Psychological Association; 2003: 195–305.

58. Peterson GD. Political ecology and ecological resilience: an integration of human and ecological dynamics. *Ecological Econ.* 2000;35:323–336.

59. Seligman MEP, Schulman P, DeRubeis RJ, Hollon SD. The prevention of depression and anxiety. *Prevention Treatment.* 1999;2(1). Available at: journals.apa.org/prevention/volume2/pre0020008a.html. Accessed December 10, 2004.

60. Ness GJ, Macaskill N. Preventing PTSD: the value of inner resourcefulness and a sense of personal control of a situation. Is it a matter of problem-solving or anxiety management? *Behav Cogn Psychother.* 2003;31:463–486.

61. Gonzales L. *Deep Survival: Who Lives, Who Dies, and Why.* New York, NY: WW Norton; 2003.

62. Bell CC. Cultivating resiliency in youth. *J Adolesc Health.* 2001;29(5):375–381.

63. Spiegel HX. Psychiatry with an infantry battalion in North Africa. In: Mullens WS, ed. *Neuropsychiatry in World War II.* Vol 2. *Overseas Theaters.* Washington, DC: Government Printing Office; 1973: 111–126. GPO Stock No. 0832-00047.

64. Glass AJ. Lessons learned. In: Mullens WS, ed. *Neuropsychiatry in World War II.* Vol 2. *Overseas Theaters.* Washington, DC: Government Printing Office; 1973: 989–1027. GPO Stock No. 0832-00047.

65. Kviz FJ. Survival in combat as a collective exchange process. *J Polit Mil Sociol.* 1978;6:219–232.

66. Salmon P. Effects of physical exercise on anxiety, depression, and sensitivity to stress: a unifying theory. *Clin Psychol Rev.* 2001;21:33–61.

67. Meichenbaum D. *Cognitive-Behavior Modification: An Integrative Approach.* New York, NY: Plenum Press; 1977.

68. Thomas MO. New priorities in evacuation training based on the Pentagon experience. *Mil Med.* 2002;167(9 Suppl):22–23.

69. McCarroll JE, Ursano RJ, Fullerton CS, Liu X, Lundy A. Somatic symptoms in Gulf War mortuary workers. *Psychosom Med.* 2002;64:29–33.

70. Directorate of Health Promotion and Wellness, US Army Center for Health Promotion and Preventive Medicine. *Just the Facts . . . Dealing With the Stress of Recovering Human Dead Bodies.* Available at: http://chppm-www.apgea.army.mil/documents/FACT/36-004-0202.pdf. Accessed November 17, 2008.

71. Bolton E, Litz BT, Glenn DM, Orsillo S, Roemer L. The impact of homecoming reception on the adaptation of peacekeepers following deployment. *Mil Psychol.* 2002;14:241–251.

72. Neumann M, Levy A. A specific military installation for treatment of combat reactions during the war in Lebanon. *Mil Med.* 1984;149:196–199.

73. US Army Medical Department. Battlemind Training. Available at: https://www.battlemind.army.mil. Accessed November 17, 2008.

74. Nash WP, Krantz L, Westphal RJ, Litz B. The evolving challenges of mental health prevention in the military, and two approaches to meet them: Army Battlemind and the Navy–Marine Corps stress continuum. In: Ruzek J, Vasterling, J, Schnurr P, Friedman M, eds. *Posttraumatic Stress Reactions: Caring for the Veterans of the Global War on Terror.* New York, NY: Guilford Press; in press.

75. Ginzburg K, Ein-Dor T, Solomon Z. Comorbidity of posttraumatic stress disorder, anxiety and depression: a 20-year longitudinal study of war veterans. *J Affective Disorders* [Published online]. 2009. Available at: http://www.linkinghub.elsevier.com/retrieve/pii/S0165032709003723. Accessed October 16, 2009.

76. Arik Y. Shalev, MD. Professor and Chairman, Department of Psychiatry, Hadassah University School of Medicine, Jerusalem, Israel. Personal communication, April 18, 2004.

77. Luthar SS, Cicchetti D, Becker B. The construct of resilience: a critical evaluation and guidelines for future work. *Child Dev.* 2000;71:543–562.

Chapter 4

COMBAT AND OPERATIONAL STRESS CONTROL

EDWARD A. BRUSHER, LCSW, BCD*

Lieutenant Colonel, Medical Service Corps, US Army; Deputy Director, Behavioral Health Proponency, Office of The Surgeon General, 5109 Leesburg Pike, Skyline 6, Suite 693, Falls Church, Virginia 22041-3258; formerly, Combat Operational Stress Control Program Manager, US Army Medical Command, Fort Sam Houston, Texas

INTRODUCTION

Combat and operational stress includes all the physiological and emotional stresses encountered as a direct result of the dangers and mission demands of combat and other military operations. Combat and operational stress control (COSC) in the US Army may be defined as programs developed and actions taken by military leadership to prevent, identify, and manage adverse combat and operational stress behavior (COSB) in units. These programs optimize mission performance; conserve fighting strength; and prevent or minimize adverse effects of combat and operational stress reaction (COSR) on soldiers and their physical, psychological, intellectual, and social health. COSC's goal is to return soldiers to duty expeditiously. COSC activities include routine screening of individuals when recruited; continued surveillance throughout military service, especially before, during, and after deployment; and continual assessment and consultation with medical and other personnel from garrison to the battlefield.

Within US military operations historically, COSRs (negative reactions in the spectrum of COSB), have accounted for up to half of all battlefield casualties, depending upon the difficulty of the conditions. Although rates of COSR casualties have remained high in 21st century wars, losses due to COSR have significantly decreased as a result of institutionalizing COSC into military operational functioning. In today's combat environment, military leaders can expect to retain and return to duty (RTD) over 95% of service members who experience COSR. COSC is a tactical consideration that must not be overlooked or minimized. COSC is one of ten identified medical battlefield operating systems (the other nine being command, control, and communication; hospitalization and surgery; preventive medicine; veterinary services; laboratory, blood, and dental services; health service logistics; combat stress control; patient evacuation and regulation; and area medical support).

Service members—especially military leaders—must learn to recognize COSR's symptoms and prevent or reduce its disruptive effects. This chapter provides an overview of the US Army Combat and Operational Stress Control Program as outlined by Field Manual 4-02.51, *Combat and Operational Stress Control* (July 2006)[1] and Field Manual 6-22.5, *Combat and Operational Stress Control Manual for Leaders and Soldiers* (March 2009).[2]

COMBAT AND OPERATIONAL STRESS THREAT

In today's battlefield, everyone is a soldier. Whether serving in the infantry, providing healthcare, or providing logistical support, all military personnel face the threat of attack from a dedicated enemy force. Routine existence in a combat zone places all service members at risk for exposure to a range of significant stressors. In peacetime as well as war, the effects of combat and operational stress are experienced by all soldiers in every type of military operation, including combat-like conditions present throughout the entire spectrum of military operations. These operations range from training, all phases of deployment, peacekeeping, humanitarian missions, stability and reconstruction, and government support missions, to missions that may include weapons of mass destruction or chemical, biological, radiological, nuclear, and explosive weapons.

It is important to understand that combat and operational experiences affect all soldiers and reflect all activities soldiers are exposed to throughout the length of their military service, whether a complete career or single enlistment. Service members continually face the potential for deployment and combat, long and arduous training missions, and separations from families. These stressors are greatest during actual combat, but often begin with notification of a deployment. Combat and operational stress often continues after the fighting is over as the participants deal with the aftermath of deployment, whether they served in support or combat units, were prisoners of war, or experienced severe injuries.

Rigorous research conducted explicitly on the mental health and well-being of service members and families during periods of major military operations is scarce,[3] and most studies on the mental health effects of combat were conducted among veterans years after their military service ended.[4] However, deployment-related stressors have been linked to increased rates of subsequent health problems. Studies have found exposure to severe combat stressors relates to the subsequent development of a range of physiological diseases.[5] Other studies have documented the association between exposure to deployment-related stressors and the development of psychiatric disorders.[4,6–8] Deployment is also associated with increased symptoms of posttraumatic stress disorder,[4] depression,[4,6] and anger problems.[9,10] Furthermore, although symptom reports may be low during the immediate postdeployment period, studies with soldiers have found that these symptoms increase 3 to 6 months later.[11,12] In all, an estimated 20% to 30% of US military personnel returning from current combat operations report significant psychological symptoms.[12]

EXHIBIT 4-1

COMBAT AND OPERATIONAL STRESSORS

Combat Stressors

- Personal injury
- Killing of combatants
- Witnessing the death of an individual
- Death of another unit member
- Injury resulting in the loss of a limb

Operational Stressors

- Prolonged exposure to extreme geographical environments such as desert heat or arctic cold
- Reduced quality of life and communication resources over extended period of time
- Prolonged separation from significant support systems such as family
- Exposure to significant injuries over multiple missions such as witnessing the death of several unit members over the course of many combat missions

Sources of Stress

Combat stressors come from a range of possible sources, including singular incidents with potential to significantly affect the unit or soldiers experiencing them, multiple combat incidents, or prolonged exposures due to continued operations in hostile environments. The effects of these stressors are experienced prior to, during, and after military operations and missions. Sometimes stressors are related to a significant or multiple potentially traumatic events (PTEs). A PTE is an event that causes an individual or group to experience intense feelings of terror, horror, helplessness, or hopelessness, and is perceived and experienced as a threat to one's safety or to the stability of one's world. Guilt, anger, sadness, and dislocation of world view or faith are potential emotional and cognitive responses to PTEs. The combined effect of combat and operational stressors results in COSB (see Exhibit 4-1 for examples of both combat stressors and operational stressors).

Although many stressors in combat situations result from deliberate enemy actions aimed at killing, wounding, or demoralizing US soldiers and US allies, other stressors are due to the natural environment, such as intense heat or cold, humidity, or poor air quality. Still others result from leaders' own calculated or miscalculated choices (for example, decisions about unit strength, maneuvers, the time of an attack, and plans for medical and logistical support). Sound leadership works to keep operational stressors within tolerable limits and prepares troops mentally and physically to endure them. In some cases, however, excessive stress can affect the decision making and judgment of both leader and soldiers, resulting in missed opportunities, or worse, in high casualties or failure to complete the mission.

Finally, some of the most potent stressors are interpersonal in nature and can be due to conflict in the unit or on the home front. Extreme reactions to such stressors may involve harm to self (as in the case of a soldier who becomes suicidal on discovering his wife wants a divorce) or to others (as in the case of a soldier who impulsively fires a weapon at the unit noncommissioned officer out of rage over perceived unfairness). These stressors must be identified and when possible, corrected or controlled.

Mental and Physical Stressors

A mental stressor is one in which the brain receives information about a given threat or demand, but this information results only in indirect physical impact on the body. Instead, its primary effect is to place demands on and evoke reactions from the perceptual, cognitive, or emotional systems of the brain (eg, information overload, perceived lack of control, or grief-producing losses). A physical stressor has a direct, potentially harmful effect on the body. These stressors may be external environmental conditions (such as temperature) or the internal physiologic demands required by or placed upon the human body (such as the need for hydration or an immune response to a viral infection).

Exhibit 4-2 provides examples of the two types of physical stressors (environmental and physiologic) and the two types of mental stressors (cognitive and emotional). Also, physical stressors cause mental stressors when they result in discomfort, distraction, and threat of harm, as well as when they directly impair brain functions. Mental stressors can lead to adaptive or maladaptive stress behaviors that decrease or increase the exposure to physical stressors.

COMBAT AND OPERATIONAL STRESS BEHAVIOR

Stress has both physical and behavioral effects. Stress may increase disease rates by disrupting hygiene and protective measures, as well as impairing the body's immune defenses. Stress may progress to behavioral health disorders, including suicidal or homicidal behaviors. Some stressors contribute to

EXHIBIT 4-2

EXAMPLES OF COMBAT AND OPERATIONAL STRESSORS

Physical Stressors

- Environmental
  - Heat, cold, wetness, dust
  - Vibration, noise, blast
  - Noxious odors (fumes, poisons, chemicals)
  - Directed-energy weapons/devices
  - Ionizing radiation
  - Infectious agents
  - Physical work
  - Poor visibility (bright lights, darkness, haze)
  - Difficult or arduous terrain
  - High altitude
- Physiologic
  - Sleep deprivation
  - Dehydration
  - Malnutrition
  - Poor hygiene
  - Muscular and aerobic fatigue
  - Overuse or underuse of muscles
  - Impaired immune system
  - Illness or injury
  - Sexual frustration
  - Substance use (smoking, caffeine, alcohol)
  - Obesity
  - Poor physical condition

Mental Stressors

- Cognitive
  - Information (too much or too little)
  - Sensory overload or deprivation
  - Ambiguity, uncertainty, unpredictability
  - Time pressure or waiting
  - Difficult decision (rules of engagement)
  - Organizational dynamics and changes
  - Hard choices vs no choice
  - Recognition of impaired functioning
  - Working beyond skill level
  - Previous failures
- Emotional
  - Being new in unit, isolated, lonely
  - Fear and anxiety-producing threats (of death, injury, failure, or loss)
  - Grief-producing losses (bereavement)
  - Resentment, anger, and rage-producing frustration and guilt
  - Inactivity, producing boredom
  - Conflicting/divided motives and loyalties
  - Spiritual confrontation or temptation causing loss of faith
  - Interpersonal conflict (unity, buddy)
  - Home-front worries, homesickness
  - Loss of privacy
  - Victimization/harassment
  - Exposure to combat/dead bodies
  - Having to kill

misconduct that requires disciplinary action and may take a soldier from duty for legal action and incarceration. Stress can also result in battle and nonbattle injuries through inattention, clumsiness, and reckless behavior, including equipment loss and friendly fire incidents. Excessive stress in combat contributes to lapses in operational and tactical judgment and to missed opportunities that could increase the numbers of soldiers injured over time.

"COSB" is the term used to describe the range of reactions, from adaptive to maladaptive, to the full spectrum of combat and operational stress soldiers are exposed to throughout their military experience.[1–14] Figure 4-1 shows how combat and operational stress and PTEs can lead to both adaptive reactions and COSR, as well as postcombat and operational stress (PCOS), which may include either posttraumatic growth (PTG) or posttraumatic stress disorder (PTSD).

Combat and operational experiences impact every soldier in some way, although not everyone handles the stress in the same way. Soldiers surveyed in Iraq indicate that those who experienced the most combat were the most likely to screen positive for a behavioral health (BH) problem, including PTSD. Nearly one third of soldiers operating "outside the wire" (ie, outside the secure area of the base camps) may be experiencing severe negative symptoms related to combat and operational stress exposure, which can potentially affect the unit's mission capability.[14]

In fact, current research shows that soldiers continue to struggle with PCOS symptoms long after deployment. Soldiers *do not* reset quickly after coming home, and up to 17% of returned veterans may continue to struggle with negative PCOS effects even 12 months after coming home.[14] Leaders and soldiers must recognize the continued effects of combat and operational exposure. Understanding these effects will help sol-

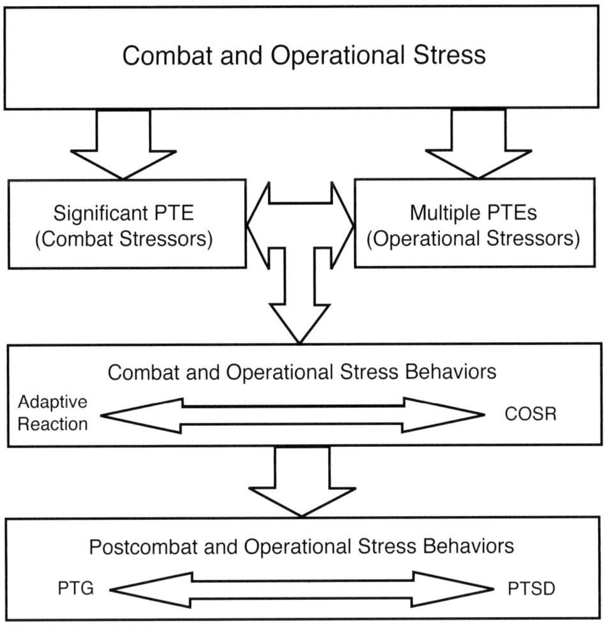

Figure 4-1. Model of stress and its potential soldier and family outcomes.
COSR: combat and operational stress reaction
PTE: potentially traumatic event
PTG: posttraumatic growth
PTSD: posttraumatic stress disorder

diers plan accordingly to support each other and those entrusted to them. This is especially important while sustaining prolonged or multiple deployment rotations as well as combat operations.

Adaptive Stress Reactions

With effective leadership and strong peer relationships, stressors can lead to adaptive stress reactions that enhance individual and unit performance. Examples of adaptive stress reactions include

- horizontal bonding—the strong personal trust, loyalty, and cohesiveness that develop among peers in a small military unit;
- vertical bonding—personal trust, loyalty, and cohesiveness that develop between leaders and their subordinates;
- esprit de corps—a feeling of identification and membership in the larger, enduring organization with understanding of its history and intent (organizations may include the unit [battalion, brigade combat team, regiment, or division], the branch [infantry, artillery, or military police], and the Army); and
- unit cohesion—the binding force that keeps soldiers together and performing the mission in spite of danger and adversity.

Cohesion is a result of soldiers knowing and trusting their peers and leaders and understanding their dependency on one another. It is achieved through personal bonding and a strong sense of responsibility toward the unit and its members. The ultimate adaptive stress reactions are acts of extreme courage and almost unbelievable strength. They may even involve deliberate heroism resulting in the ultimate self-sacrifice.

Combat and Operational Stress Reaction

Focused stress is vital to survival and mission accomplishment. However, stress that is prolonged or too intense results in COSR, which impairs the ability to function effectively. The Army uses the term "COSR" (approved by the Department of Defense) in official medical reports in reference to negative adaptation to high-stress events and PTE exposures. When coded (ie, diagnosed), COSR represents individuals in need of formal or informal COSC support and interventions to identify, treat or normalize, and transition the negative effects of combat and operational stress. Although many reactions look like symptoms of mental illness (such as panic, extreme anxiety, depression, hallucinations), they are actually transient reactions to the traumatic stress of combat and the cumulative stresses of military operations.

Military leaders, soldiers, and medical providers must understand the difference between COSR and PTSD. COSR is *not* the same as PTSD. COSR, representing negative adaptation to high-stress and potentially traumatic events, is considered a subclinical diagnosis with a high recovery rate if appropriate attention and time is provided. PTSD, on the other hand, is an anxiety disorder associated with serious traumatic events and characterized by such symptoms as survivor guilt, reliving the trauma in dreams, numbness and lack of involvement with reality, or recurrent thoughts and images. PTSD is a clinical diagnosis as defined by the *Diagnostic and Statistical Manual of Mental Disorders* and the *International Statistical Classification of Diseases and Related Health Problems*. PTSD is one of many possible long-term outcomes resulting from combat and operational stress exposure (collectively classified as PCOS).

COSR and PTSD may share some common symptoms in presentation; however, COSR is recognizable immediately or shortly after exposure to traumatic events and captures any recognizable reaction resulting from this exposure. PTSD has specific chronological requirements and symptom markers that must be satisfied to diagnose the disorder. PTSD is diagnosable only by a trained and credentialed healthcare provider.

Military personnel and providers must focus their efforts on the management of COSR in an effort to shape the long-term reactions of individual soldiers and their units. Individuals with behavioral disorders that existed prior to deployment or first appeared during deployment may need BH support beyond the interventions for COSR.

Misconduct Stress Behaviors

Misconduct stress behaviors range from minor breaches of unit orders or regulations to serious violations of the Uniform Code of Military Justice and the law of land warfare.[1] Misconduct stress behaviors are most likely to occur in poorly trained, undisciplined soldiers under extreme combat stress. Misconduct stress behaviors may also become a major problem for highly cohesive units with strong esprit de corps. Such units may come to consider themselves entitled to special privileges and, as a result, some members may relieve tension unlawfully when they stand down from military operations. They may resort to illegal revenge when a unit member is lost in combat. Stress-control measures and sound leadership can prevent such misconduct stress behaviors, but once serious misconduct has occurred, soldiers must be punished to prevent further erosion of discipline. Combat stress, even with heroic combat performance, cannot justify criminal misconduct.

Postcombat and Operational Stress

PCOS describes a range of possible outcomes along the continuum of stress reactions that may be experienced weeks or even years after combat and operational stress exposure. PCOS may include PTG (the adaptive resolution), mild COSR, or the more severe symptoms often associated with PTSD. It is imperative to understand this continuum and know the difference between adaptation, COSR, and PTSD.

Posttraumatic Growth

PTG refers to a phenomenon in which positive outcomes occur among survivors of traumatic experiences such as car accidents, fires, sexual abuse or assault, military combat, and being a refugee.[15] PTG among trauma survivors has included improved relationships, renewed hope for life, an improved appreciation of life, an enhanced sense of personal strength, and spiritual development.[16]

Continuum of Combat and Operational Stress Behaviors

The distinctions among adaptive stress reactions, misconduct stress behaviors, COSB, COSR, PTG, and PTSD are not always clear. Indeed, the categories of combat and operational stress behaviors may overlap. Soldiers with adaptive stress reactions may also suffer from COSR. Soldiers in combat experience a range of emotions, usually outside of their daily experience, and their behavior influences the immediate safety of the unit and mission success. Combat and combat-related military missions can also impose combinations of heavy physical work; sleep loss; dehydration; poor nutrition; severe noise, vibration, and blast; exposure to heat, cold, or wetness; poor hygiene facilities; and perhaps exposure to infectious diseases, toxic fumes, or harmful substances. These ranges of emotions and mission-related conditions in combination with other influences, such as concerns about problems back home, affect the ability to manage perceived or real danger, and diminish the skills needed to accomplish the mission. Some reactions sharpen abilities to survive and win; other reactions may produce disruptive behaviors and threaten individual and unit safety. Outstanding combat soldiers who have exhibited bravery and heroism may also commit misconduct stress behaviors.

PCOS may develop after someone has experienced or witnessed an actual or threatened traumatic event. It is common for stress reactions to persist or arise long after exposure to distressing events. If PCOS interferes with the ability to do jobs and enjoy life, and it seems to continually get worse, it could lead to PTSD. Most soldiers do well, but for some, persistent symptoms of postcombat stress may require support or medical care. When there is impairment in social or occupational functioning, a clinical assessment is warranted. COSC is important to sustaining Army strength over the long term and reducing the costs to society, the Department of Defense, soldiers, and families.

COMBAT AND OPERATIONAL STRESS CONTROL

COSC is a full-spectrum behavioral health support program that spans all military operations and deployment cycles, not just in the theater environment. The goal of COSC is to enhance unit cohesion and combat capability in the face of high-stress operational environments and to maximize PTG. COSC is effective when it incorporates not only soldiers but also their extended support system, including significant relationships, families, and external resources. COSC is a comprehensive process that identifies soldiers, Army civilians, and their families who may need assistance with the challenges of deployment, and ensures that they are better prepared and sustained throughout the deployment cycle.[17] Figure 4-2 illustrates the seven stages of deployment cycle support.

The purpose of COSC is to promote soldier and unit readiness by:

- enhancing adaptive stress reactions,
- preventing maladaptive stress reactions,
- assisting soldiers with controlling COSR, and
- assisting soldiers with behavioral disorders.

Battlemind

The term "Battlemind" represents the US Army psychological resiliency building program (see also the attachment to this chapter). The term describes a soldier's resiliency skills or inner strength to face fear and adversity during combat with courage. Battlemind training enhances the psychological readiness of every soldier for a stronger and more resilient force. It targets successful individual and organizational recognition of traumatic brain injury, PTSD, suicide risk, and other predictable stressors from military operations to mitigate the effect on mission and readiness. There are four main objectives of Battlemind training for soldiers and their families: (1) mental preparation for the rigors of combat and military deployments, (2) successful transition back home, (3) effective assistance for "Battlemind buddies" during the transition home, and (4) preparation for the likelihood of deploying again. Battlemind meets these objectives by applying a three-pillar systematic approach: (1) life cycle, (2) deployment cycle, and (3) soldier support.[8]

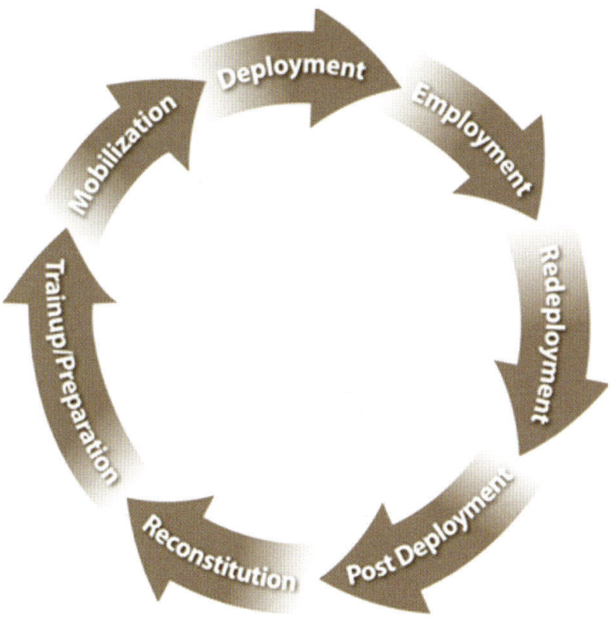

Figure 4-2. Deployment cycle support phases.

Life-cycle training is the long-term institutional initiative to help soldiers and leaders reduce existing behavioral health barriers. It facilitates organizational growth by targeting stigma and institutional barriers through cohesion and progressive leader development training during critical points in a soldier's military career. Deployment-cycle training targets each phase of deployment and builds upon techniques learned during life-cycle training. Combat skills and the battle mindset are what the soldier utilizes to sustain and survive in high-stress operational environments. Battlemind skills help soldiers survive; however, those same skills must be adapted as soldiers transition from a combat or operational mission back to garrison and home environments. Although each soldier makes individual adjustments, the key to a successful transition home is to adapt combat skills so they are just as effective at home as they were in combat. Soldier support training is tailored to special populations, including family systems and military communities. Present day COSC builds on Battlemind skills as proven strengths in the transition to postcombat or operational functioning.

Cohesion and Morale

Cohesion, or the bonds among soldiers, has traditionally been posited as the primary motivation for soldiers in combat.[18] High cohesion and morale enhance adaptive stress reactions in soldiers and organizations and are the best predictors of resiliency within a unit or organization. Units with high cohesion tend to experience a lower rate of COSR than those with low cohesion and morale. Esprit de corps can transcend the problems of race and prejudice. The upkeep of morale and cohesion in combat is recognized as a vital element in the production of combat power in tactical units.[13] Supportive leadership, regardless of whether a soldier has been to combat or not, is related to how well soldiers fare, both at a personal level (personal morale) and at a unit level (unit morale, cohesion, and combat readiness). This is good news for the military, because leaders can be trained to be more supportive and increase the chances of soldiers having higher personal morale, higher unit morale, better unit cohesion, and higher perceptions of combat readiness.[19] In fact, if unit leaders do nothing more under COSC programs integrated in their organization than focus on unit cohesion and morale, they will have met what is known in the US Army as the "80% solution."[18]

Combat and Operational Stress Control as a Function of Leadership

COSC is a command-driven program at all levels. Commanders are assisted by their staff, unit leaders, unit chaplains, and organic medical personnel (ie, those behavioral health and medical personnel assigned directly to the unit). The commander may also receive assistance from organic COSC personnel at brigade level and above, and from corps-level and above medical company or detachment BH personnel. The key concern to combat commanders is to maximize the RTD rate of soldiers who are temporarily impaired or incapacitated with stress-related conditions or diagnosed behavioral disorders.

Combat and Operational Stress Control Professional Disciplines

Five BH professional disciplines and two enlisted specialties support the COSC mission. The professional disciplines include social work, clinical psychology, psychiatry, occupational therapy, and psychiatric or BH nursing; the enlisted specialties are BH and occupational therapy. Although much of the COSC knowledge base and most of the skills are shared by all BH personnel, each discipline brings a unique perspective from its professional training, skills that can only partially be taught to others, and in some cases unique credentials to conduct specific assessments and treatments.

Religious Support for Combat and Operational Stress Control

The US Army Chaplain Corps is an invaluable asset in ongoing COSC support operations. Soldiers often approach chaplains first to obtain resources to address identified COSRs. Soldiers' inner resources are generally rooted in religious and spiritual values. In combat, soldiers often show increased interest in religious beliefs. When religious and spiritual values are challenged by the chaos of combat, soldiers may lose connection with the inner resources that previously sustained them. The unit ministry team is the primary resource available to soldiers experiencing such dilemmas, providing assistance as they seek to refocus their spiritual values. The ministry team provides preventive, immediate, and restorative spiritual and emotional support to soldiers experiencing COSR.

COMBAT AND OPERATIONAL STRESS CONTROL INTERVENTIONS

COSC is performed during all phases of combat operations, stability and reconstruction operations, and support operations. COSC assessments, performed at both the unit and individual level, consider a range of variables according to a model (Figure 4-3) that recognizes the interrelationship of biological, psychological, and social factors. This figure is a conceptual model of stress, its mitigating and aggravating factors, and potential outcomes for soldiers and families. Reviewing these interactions systematically, the COSC assessment identifies which variables can be modified to improve coping or outcome. Based on these assessments, COSC personnel recommend courses of action to the commander to improve unit effectiveness and soldier efficiency and well-being. The stress model can be helpful for designing COSC interventions to improve short-term and long-term outcomes.

Soldier and unit readiness is best achieved through an active, prevention-focused approach. COSC interventions are tailored to the needs of the population, and their application may differ based on a particular level of care and other factors pertaining to the mission, enemy, terrain and weather, troops and support available, time available, and civil considerations (METT-TC). However, all preventive interventions seek to reduce the occurrence or severity of COSR and behavioral disorders, thereby sustaining soldier and unit readiness. COSC interventions can be divided into four categories:

1. **universal** interventions are targeted to the general population or an assigned AO (area of operations);
2. **selective** interventions are targeted to a unit or soldier whose risk is higher than average;
3. **indicated** interventions are targeted to soldiers with COSR or indications of a potential behavioral disorder, and to units showing signs that mission effectiveness is being affected by combat and operational stressors; and
4. **treatment** interventions are targeted to treat and follow up with soldiers with behavioral disorders to prevent their loss from duty.

COSC personnel must identify life- or function-threatening medical, surgical, or psychiatric conditions as soon as possible and provide emergency treatment for those patients.

Combat and Operational Stress Control Management Principles

COSC utilizes the management principles of brev-

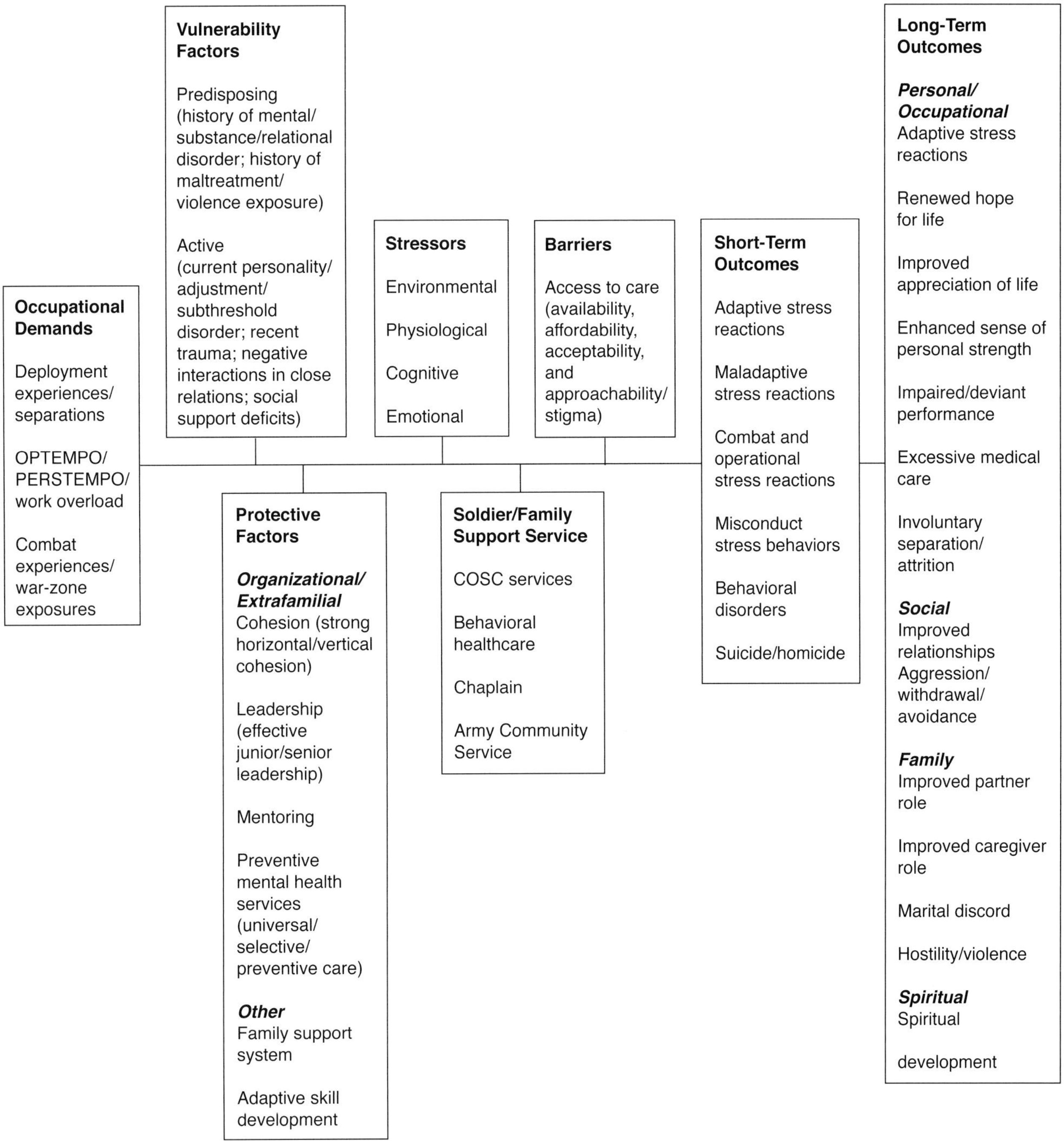

Figure 4-3. Combat and operational stress intervention model.
OPSTEMPO: operations tempo; PERSTEMPO: personnel tempo; COSC: combat and operational stress control

ity, immediacy, contact, expectancy, proximity, and simplicity (BICEPS). Using BICEPS is extremely important in the management of soldiers with COSR or behavioral disorders. COSC personnel in all BH / COSC elements apply these principles to all COSC interventions or activities in theater, although they may be applied differently based on a particular level of care and other METT-TC factors, as described below.

Brevity

Initial rest and replenishment at COSC facilities located close to the soldier's unit should last no more than 1 to 3 days. Those requiring further treatment are moved to the next level of care. Because many soldiers require no further treatment, military commanders expect their soldiers to RTD rapidly.

Immediacy

It is essential that COSC measures be initiated as soon as possible (as soon as symptoms appear) when operations permit.

Contact

Soldiers must be encouraged to continue to think of themselves as warfighters, rather than as patients or sick persons. The chain of command remains directly involved in soldiers' recovery and RTD. The COSC team coordinates with the unit's leaders to learn whether individuals in treatment were good performers prior to the COSR. Whenever possible, representatives or messages from the unit tell these soldiers that they are needed and wanted back. The COSC team coordinates with the unit leaders, through unit medical personnel or chaplains, any special advice on how to assure quick reintegration when the soldier returns to the unit.

Expectancy

Individual soldiers are explicitly told that they are reacting normally to extreme stress and are expected to recover and return to full duty in a few hours or days. A military leader is extremely effective in this role. Of all the things said to a soldier suffering from COSR, the words of the small-unit leader have the greatest effect because of the positive bonding process that occurs. Small-unit leaders should tell soldiers that their comrades need and expect them to return. When they do return, the unit treats them the same as every other soldier and expects them to perform well.

Proximity

Soldiers requiring observation or care beyond the unit level are evacuated to facilities in close proximity to, but separate from, the medical or surgical patients at the battalion aid station or medical company nearest the soldiers' unit. COSRs are often more effectively managed in areas close to the soldier's parent unit. On the noncontiguous battlefield characterized by rapid, frequent maneuvers and continuous operations, COSC personnel must be innovative and flexible in designing interventions that maximize and maintain the soldier's connection to the parent unit. It is best to send soldiers who cannot continue their mission and require more extensive intervention to a facility other than a hospital, unless no other alternative is available.

Simplicity

Brief, straightforward methods should be used to restore physical well-being and self-confidence.

Combat and Operational Stress Control Functional Areas

Combat and operational stress control interventions and activities are organized into nine functional areas. These areas cover the full spectrum of BH care from preventive measures through clinical intervention.

Unit Needs Assessment

Unit needs assessment is the systematic and frequent assessment of supported units to determine the priority and types of BH interventions required.

Consultation and Education

Consultation involves liaison with and preventive advice to commanders, staff of supported units, and soldiers. Education involves training in concepts and skills for increasing soldier resilience to stress.

Traumatic Events Management

Traumatic events management (TEM) blends other COSC functional areas to create a flexible set of interventions specifically focused on stress management for units and soldiers following PTEs. Like other functional areas, COSC providers must tailor TEM to the needs of the unit and the soldier. For military units, TEM is active in all phases of the deployment cycle and across the continuum of military operations, both in garrison and in deployed environments. TEM is a structured unit process designed to mitigate the impact of PTEs and to accelerate normal recovery of personnel involved. The goal of TEM is to enhance PTG and reestablish unit cohesion and structure. Examples of PTEs that might result in a TEM assessment and intervention include

- heavy or continuous combat operations,
- death of unit members,
- accidents,
- serious injury,
- suicide/homicide,
- environmental devastation or human suffering,
- significant home-front issues, and
- operations resulting in the death of civilians or combatants.

If a unit experiences a PTE, unit leadership may request a TEM assessment to determine potential impact. It is recommended that leadership request TEM assessments as close to the specific PTE as practically possible, but there are no time limitations to conducting assessments and implementing TEM interventions in response to PTEs that have had a significant impact on the performance, morale, and cohesion of the effected unit or organization. When requested, the identified TEM team will coordinate an assessment resulting in specific recommendations to address the identified PTE as effectively and efficiently as required. TEM is normally conducted by a team composed of medical officers, chaplains, behavioral health professionals, and other trained unit members.

TEM's main value is to quickly restore unit cohesion and readiness to return to action, through clarifying what actually happened and clearing up harmful misperceptions and misunderstandings. It may also reduce the possibility of long-term distress through sharing and acceptance of thoughts, feelings, and reactions related to the PTE. The TEM process incorporates multiple interventions and clinical strategies to aid the military leader in managing and mitigating the impact of PTEs. TEM responses include

- a needs assessment of the impact of the identified PTE;
- command consultation and education;
- unit and individual education;
- individual supportive intervention and counseling;
- psychological debriefings; and
- leader-led after-action debriefings.

Reconstitution Support

Reconstitution is extraordinary action that commanders plan and implement to restore units to a desired level of combat effectiveness commensurate with mission requirements and available resources. Reconstitution transcends normal daily force sustainment actions, but it uses existing systems and units to do so; no resources exist solely for this function. In reconstitution support, COSC personnel are responsible for providing restoration for soldiers and conducting COSC functions. This support is provided to units following traumatic events and during reconstitution, redeployment, and transition among levels of operational tempo.

Combat and Operational Stress Control Triage

Combat and operational stress control triage is the process of sorting soldiers with COSR or BH disorders based upon where they can best be managed.

Combat and Operational Stress Control Stabilization

Stabilization is the initial management of soldiers with severe COSR or behavioral disorders. Their safety is ensured and they are evaluated for RTD potential or prepared for further treatment or evacuation.

Soldier Restoration

Soldier restoration involves the 1- to 3-day management of soldiers with COSR or behavioral disorders, normally near a medical treatment facility in close proximity to the unit. This approach uses the "5 Rs":

- **R**eassure of normality.
- **R**est (respite from combat or break from the work).
- **R**eplenish bodily needs (such as thermal comfort, water, food, hygiene, and sleep).
- **R**estore confidence with purposeful activities and contact with the soldier's unit.
- **R**eturn to duty and reunite the soldier with the unit.

Behavioral Health Treatment

Patients with identified behavioral disorders receive ongoing evaluation, treatment, and follow-up. This functional area implies a therapist–patient relationship, clinical documentation, and adherence to clinical standards of care.

Soldier Reconditioning

Reconditioning is an intensive program of work therapy, military activities, physical training, and psychotherapy. Reconditioning programs are conducted up to 7 days (or more) in the corps area. Additional reconditioning may be provided in theater outside the combat zone.

SUMMARY

COSC is a joint-service program that affects all service members and their extended support systems in the US military. COSC remains an effective combat multiplier, as it has been in past conflicts. Present-day COSC continues to evolve, incorporating both the lessons of past history and the experiences of current combat. It is strength based, utilizing objective and empirically validated current best practices to enhance and adapt the "battlemind" of the human weapons system. Battlemind is essential to successful military operations, as well as individual adaptive stress reactions and posttraumatic growth. Modern COSC requires close collaboration between military leaders, doctrinal COSC disciplines, chaplains, and the extended medical community. True COSC is only obtained by leadership integration of COSC concepts with the supporting efforts of medical providers and religious support assets.

REFERENCES

1. US Department of the Army. *Combat and Operational Stress Control*. Washington, DC: DA; 2006. Field Manual 4-02.51.

2. US Department of the Army. *Combat and Operational Stress Control Manual for Leaders and Soldiers*. Washington, DC: DA; 2009. Field Manual 6-22.5.

3. Johnson SJ, Sherman MD, Hoffman JS, et al. American Psychological Association Presidential Task Force on Military Deployment Services for Youth, Families and Service Members. *The Psychological Needs of US Military Service Members and Their Families: A Preliminary Report*. Washington, DC: APA; 2007: 5. Available at: http://www.apa.org/releases/MilitaryDeploymentTaskForceReport.pdf. Accessed September 8, 2008.

4. Hoge CW, Castro CA, Messer SC, McGurk D, Cotting DI, Koffman RL. Combat duty in Iraq and Afghanistan, mental health problems, and barriers to care. *N Engl J Med*. 2004;351(1):13–22.

5. Boscarino JA. Diseases among men 20 years after exposure to severe stress: implications for clinical research and medical care. *Psychosom Med*. 1997;59(6):605–614.

6. Jordan BK, Schlenger WE, Hough R, et al. Lifetime and current prevalence of specific psychiatric disorders among Vietnam veterans and controls. *Arch Gen Psychiatry*. 1991;48:207–215.

7. King DW, King LA, Foy DW, Keane TM, Fairbank JA. Posttraumatic stress disorder in a national sample of female and male Vietnam veterans: risk factors, war-zone stressors, and resilience-recovery variables. *J Abnorm Psychol*. 1999;108:164–170.

8. Walter Reed Army Institute of Research—Psychiatry and Neuroscience. *Battlemind Training*. Available at: www.battlemind.army.mil. Accessed July 27, 2009.

9. Adler AB, Dolan CA, Castro CA. US soldier peacekeeping experiences and well-being after returning from deployment to Kosovo. *Proceedings of the 36th International Applied Military Psychology Symposium*. Split, Croatia: Ministry of Defense of the Republic of Croatia. September, 2000; 30–34.

10. McCarroll JE, Ursano RJ, Liu X, et al. Deployment and the probability of spousal aggression by US Army soldiers. *Mil Med*. 2000;165:41–44.

11. Bliese PD, Wright KM, Adler AB, Thomas JL. Psychological screening validation with soldiers returning from combat. In: Roy M, ed. *Novel Approaches to the Diagnosis and Treatment of Posttraumatic Stress Disorder*. Washington, DC: North Atlantic Treaty Organization/IOS Press; 2006: 78–86.

12. Hoge CW, Auchterlonie JL, Milliken CS. Mental health problems, use of mental health services, and attrition from military service after returning from deployment to Iraq or Afghanistan. *JAMA*. 2006;295(9):1023–1032.

13. Cox AA. *Unit Cohesion and Morale in Combat: Survival in a Culturally and Racially Heterogeneous Environment*. Fort Leavenworth, Kan: School of Advanced Military Studies; 1995: 1.

14. Mental Health Advisory Team (MHAT) IV. *Operation Iraqi Freedom 05-07*. Office of the Surgeon, Multinational Force-Iraq, and Office of The Surgeon General, United States Army Medical Command. November 17, 2006. Available at: www.armymedicine.army.mil/reports/mhat.html. Accessed September 4, 2008.

15. Tedeschi RG, Calhoun L. Posttraumatic growth: a new perspective on psychotraumatology. *Psychiatr Times*. 2004;21:4. Available at: http://www.psychiatrictimes.com/p040458.html. Accessed September 8, 2008.

16. Calhoun LG, Tedeschi RG. Posttraumatic growth: future directions. In: Tedeschi RG, Park CL, Calhoun LG, eds. *Posttraumatic Growth: Positive Changes in the Aftermath of Crisis*. Mahwah, NJ: Erlbaum Publishers; 1998: 215–238.

17. Deputy Chief of Staff, US Army G1. *Deployment Cycle Support Process*. Available at: http://www.armyg1.army.mil/dcs/default.asp. Accessed September 8, 2008.

18. Wong L, Kolditz TA, Millen RA, Potter TM. *Why They Fight: Combat Motivation in the Iraq War*. Carlisle Barracks, Penn: Strategic Studies Institute of the US Army War College; 2003: iii.

19. McGurk D, Castro CA, Thomas JL, Messer SC, Sinclair RR. *Leader Behaviors for Combat Veterans and Noncombat Soldiers*. Silver Spring, Md: Walter Reed Army Institute of Research; 2005: 3–4.

BATTLEMIND TRAINING: THE DEVELOPMENT OF THE US ARMY'S INTEGRATED SYSTEM OF MENTAL HEALTH TRAINING

Background

Battlemind training is the US Army's integrated mental health training program. The Battlemind training system encompasses training targeted to all phases of the deployment cycle, as well as to the soldier lifecycle and medical education system. Training is designed for soldiers, leaders, and military spouses. Battlemind training uses a strength-based approach, incorporating "buddy aid" and focusing on the leader's role in maintaining the mental health of all soldiers.

The word "Battlemind" was coined by General Crosby Saint, Commander-in-Chief, US Army, Europe, in a 1992 message titled "Battlemind Guidelines for Battalion Commanders." General Saint's message described Battlemind as "a warrior's fortitude in the face of danger." Thus, Battlemind was originally a concept created by the warfighter for the warfighter. In 1998, then-Major Carl Castro, as commander of the US Army Medical Research Unit–Europe, an overseas laboratory of the Walter Reed Army Institute of Research (WRAIR), read about Battlemind and recognized its relevancy for the Army at large.

Command-Requested Mental Health Training

In 2005 the brigade commander of the 3rd Infantry Division asked Castro (at that time Chief, Department of Military Psychiatry, WRAIR) to present a talk on preparing leaders for combat. Castro's presentation, "10 Tough Facts About Combat and What Leaders Can Do to Mitigate the Risk," incorporated the concept of Battlemind in what later emerged as a module of Battlemind training. This speech was so well received that the brigade developed a brochure summarizing the main points for all its leaders.

Soon after, recognizing the need for training designed for soldiers as well as those in leadership positions, Castro and Colonel Charles Hoge (Director, Division of Psychiatry and Neurosciences, WRAIR) began planning mental health training for soldiers returning from Iraq and Afghanistan. In fact, Castro and Hoge first conceptualized this training, the impetus for what is now Battlemind, while on a plane ride back to Washington, DC, following a briefing to senior Army leaders. Postdeployment Battlemind training, including the creation of the Battlemind acronym, topic areas, and actions, was then developed by Castro, Hoge, Dr Amy Adler (US Army Medical Research Unit–Europe), and Dr Steven Messer (Department of Military Psychiatry, WRAIR).

Postdeployment Battlemind Training Initiated

The first two Battlemind training modules were validated under a WRAIR scientific protocol with soldiers returning from a combat deployment in Iraq. Battlemind training for reintegration (the original Battlemind training) and the postdeployment Battlemind psychological debriefing were both validated in a group randomized trial conducted with a brigade combat team in 2005.[1] Soldiers with high levels of combat experience who received Battlemind training reported better mental health adjustment 4 months after returning from deployment compared to those receiving standard postdeployment stress education. Soldiers in the Battlemind sessions frequently requested that their spouse receive the same training. This led to the development by Castro and Lieutenant Colonel Anthony Cox (Department of Military Psychiatry, WRAIR) of the spouse Battlemind training program (predeployment and postdeployment training designed for individuals or couples).

The original Battlemind training efficacy study was replicated in 2006 with another brigade combat team.[2] Results confirmed that Battlemind training reduced adjustment problems 4 months postdeployment. In addition, while conducting the initial postdeployment Battlemind training, Castro and Adler recognized the need for follow-up training 3 to 6 months later. This recognition was fueled by the intensity with which soldiers described the transition process as well as WRAIR data demonstrating that symptoms increase between return from deployment and 3 to 6 months postdeployment.[3] Battlemind training for the 3- to 6-month postdeployment period was assessed in a group randomized trial in 2005 and 2006.[4] Again, results demonstrated the efficacy of Battlemind training in reducing mental health symptoms. Thus, Battlemind quickly evolved from a one-time intervention to a full program with multiple training modules designed for different points in the deployment and career life cycle.

In addition to PowerPoint presentations, Castro and Colonel Charles S Milliken (Division of Psychiatry and Neurosciences, WRAIR) and Walter Reed Army Medical Center Television created a training video with four scenarios supporting Battlemind training designed for 3 to 6 months postdeployment. Furthermore, Battlemind psychological debriefing techniques were adapted for implementation in-theater and provided to the Army Medical Department Center and School (AMEDD C&S) in February 2007.[5] A Battlemind psychological debriefing training video was then developed by Castro and Major Dennis McGurk (then at the Department of Military Psychiatry, WRAIR), demonstrating the techniques. Battlemind psychological debriefing was integrated into the AMEDD C&S's combat operational stress course by Major Todd Yosick in February 2007. This course is designed for all behavioral health providers and chaplains deploying to Iraq or Afghanistan.

Broadening Battlemind Training

At the same time that postdeployment Battlemind training modules were being studied, predeployment modules were also being developed. Based on perceived need and the findings of the WRAIR Land Combat Study[6] (which evaluated prevalence of posttraumatic stress disorder [PTSD], alcohol abuse, and relationship problems; the impact of operational tempo / combat on these problems; what factors decreased the risk; and the proportion of soldiers and families who are not receiving services for these problems), predeployment training was fielded and assessed for user satisfaction in 2007. Results from the Mental Health Advisory Team (MHAT) V report assessing soldier well-being in Iraq found that those who reported receiving predeployment Battlemind training also reported better mental health adjustment in theater.[7]

As deployment cycle and deployment support cycle programs were being phased into soldier training, other Battlemind modules were also being developed. Specifically, in 2007, Milliken initiated the development of Battlemind First Aid, a training program to provide medics with fundamental skills for identifying mental health and referral needs. This program became the blueprint for what is now Battlemind Warrior Resiliency Training, which targets all Army medical personnel as of 2007.

Each of the new Battlemind modules followed the same fundamental principles. Each module is research-based and rejects a medical or deficit model, focusing instead on soldier strengths. Using examples soldiers can relate to, modules are designed to address misunderstood or conflicted reactions. Each module also identifies specific actions that soldiers can take to maintain their "Battlemind," and emphasizes looking out for oneself, buddies, and subordinates. All training modules were finalized by a team of researchers from both the Department of Military Psychiatry and the US Army Medical Research Unit–Europe.

Battlemind Training and the Army Medical Department

In October and November 2006, a WRAIR team led by Castro and McGurk conducted an MHAT IV assessment of the mental health and well-being of troops deployed to Iraq. A key recommendation of the MHAT IV report was to mandate predeployment and postdeployment Battlemind training. This recommendation was accepted by the US Army surgeon general, the chief of staff of the Army, and the secretary of the Army.

Battlemind training proponency was handed to AMEDD C&S in an operations order (Army Directive 2007-02) signed by the surgeon general on March 26, 2007.[8] Under the provision, the AMEDD C&S officially developed the Battlemind Training System Office to train and maintain the Battlemind mission for the US Army during deployment, the lifecycle, and the soldier support cycle. The office was launched by Major Yosick, Colonel Brian Scott, Colonel Joseph Pecko, and Major Edward Brusher. The operations order also called for the creation of a transition office to serve as an ongoing partner in the continued research and development of Battlemind content; this role was maintained by WRAIR under Lieutenant Colonel Sharon McBride. WRAIR researchers continue to lead the development and validation of Battlemind training.

Current Status

Since the two Battlemind offices were established, other initiatives have been launched, including (*a*) Basic Battlemind, designed for basic training; (*b*) the US Army Training and Doctrine Command's development of "Steel Your Battlemind," a training video for advanced individual training; and (*c*) Battlemind for Leaders, which provides junior leaders with key leadership skills and behaviors and is taught at the Basic Officer Leadership Course and the Warrior Leader Course. As of 2008, other modules under development include (*a*) Battlemind training for senior leaders, (*b*) Battlemind training for Warrior Transition Unit cadres, and (*c*) community Battlemind. Other nations have adapted Battlemind training as well, including Canada (which integrated the training into its Third Location Decompression program) in 2006, and the Netherlands in 2007.

The fact that Battlemind has been readily accepted within the US Army and by other nations reflects the degree to which the training fills an essential need. To remain relevant, the Battlemind system continues to be a dynamic program, creating new modules using the same fundamental principles. Moreover, Battlemind research initiatives at WRAIR are focused on ways to increase the efficacy of the training and ensure its adaptation to operational realities such as multiple deployments. Researchers at WRAIR, WRAIR's transition office, and the AMEDD C&S's Battlemind Office work as a team to ensure the development and implementation of an integrated mental health training program ("armor for the mind") designed to help service members throughout their military career. The evolution of Battlemind concepts continues to influence new initiatives such as the Army Comprehensive Soldier Fitness Office, established in November 2008 under the leadership of Brigadier General Rhonda Cornum, to research resiliency training throughout the Army.

REFERENCES

1. Adler AB, Castro CA, McGurk D, Bliese PD, Wright KM, Hoge CW. Post-deployment interventions to reduce the mental health impact of combat deployment to Iraq: public health policies, psychological debriefing and Battlemind training. Paper presented at: 22nd Annual Meeting of the International Society for Traumatic Stress Studies; November 2006; Hollywood, Calif.

2. Thomas JL, Castro CA, Adler AB, et al. The efficacy of Battlemind at immediate postdeployment reintegration. Paper presented at: 115th Annual Meeting of the American Psychological Association; August 2007; San Francisco, Calif.

3. Bliese PD, Wright KM, Adler AB, Thomas JL, Hoge CW. Timing of post-combat mental health assessments. *Psychol Serv.* 2007;4:141–148.

4. Adler AB, Castro CA, Bliese PD, McGurk D, Milliken C. The efficacy of Battlemind training at 3–6 months postdeployment. Paper presented at: 115th Annual Meeting of the American Psychological Association; August 2007; San Francisco, Calif.

5. Adler AB, Castro CA, McGurk D. *Battlemind Psychological Debriefings*. Heidelberg, Germany: US Army Medical Research Unit–Europe; 2007. USAMRU-E Research Report 2007-001.

6. Walter Reed Army Institute of Research, Department of Military Psychiatry. *Land Combat Study*. Silver Spring, Md: WRAIR. Available at: http://wrair-www.army.mil/Psychiatry-and-Neuroscience/wrair--doms-wwd.htm. Accessed July 24, 2009.

7. Mental Health Advisory Team (MHAT) V Report. *Operation Iraqi Freedom 06-08*. Office of the Surgeon, Multinational Force–Iraq, and Office of The Surgeon General, United States Army Medical Command. February 14, 2008. Available at: http://www.armymedicine.army.mil/reports/mhat/mhat_v/mhat-v.cfm. Accessed June 4, 2009.

8. Geren P, Acting Secretary of the Army. *Deployment Cycle Support (DSC) Directive*. Washington, DC: DA. Memorandum, 26 March 2007. Available at: http://www.apd.army.mil/pdffiles/ad2007_02.pdf. Accessed June 5, 2009.

Chapter 5

WALTER REED ARMY INSTITUTE OF RESEARCH CONTRIBUTIONS DURING OPERATIONS IRAQI FREEDOM AND ENDURING FREEDOM: FROM RESEARCH TO PUBLIC HEALTH POLICY

CHARLES W. HOGE, MD*; AMY B. ADLER, PhD†; KATHLEEN M. WRIGHT, PhD‡; PAUL D. BLIESE, PhD§; ANTHONY COX, MSW¥; DENNIS McGURK, PhD¶; CHARLES MILLIKEN, MD**; AND CARL A. CASTRO, PhD††

*Colonel, US Army (Retired); formerly, Director, Division of Psychiatry and Neuroscience, Walter Reed Army Institute of Research, 503 Robert Grant Avenue, Silver Spring, Maryland 20910

†Research Psychologist, US Army Research Unit—Europe, Walter Reed Army Institute of Research, CMR 442, APO AE 09042-1030

‡Research Psychologist, US Army Medical Research-Europe, Walter Reed Army Institute of Research, CMR 442, Box 94, APO AE 09042; formerly, Deputy Chief, Department of Military Psychiatry, Walter Reed Army Institute of Research, Silver Spring, Maryland

§Colonel, Medical Service Corps, US Army; Director, Division of Psychiatry and Neuroscience, Walter Reed Army Institute of Research, 503 Grant Avenue, Silver Spring, Maryland 20910

¥Lieutenant Colonel, Medical Service Corps, US Army; Social Work Consultant, Great Plains Regional Medical Command; Chief, Social Work, Brooke Army Medical Center, 3851 Roger Brooke Drive, Fort Sam Houston, Texas 78234

¶Major, Medical Service Corps, US Army; Commander, US Army Medical Research Unit—Europe, Walter Reed Army Institute of Research, CMR 442, APO AE 09042-1030

**Colonel, Medical Corps, US Army; Program Director, National Capital Consortium Psychosomatic Medicine/Geriatric Psychiatry Fellowship, Walter Reed Army Medical Center, 6900 Georgia Avenue, NW, Washington, DC 20307; formerly, Principal Investigator, Division of Psychiatry and Neuroscience, Walter Reed Army Institute of Research, 503 Grant Avenue, Silver Spring, Maryland

††Colonel, Medical Service Corps, US Army; Director, Military Operational Medicine Research Program, US Army Medical Research and Material Command, 504 Scott Street, Fort Detrick, Maryland 21702-5012; formerly, Chief, Department of Military Psychiatry and Chief, Soldier and Family Readiness, Walter Reed Army Institute of Research, Silver Spring, Maryland

INTRODUCTION

Research examining the mental health impact of war has typically been conducted years (and often decades) after combat.[1–3] Before Operation Enduring Freedom (OEF) and Operation Iraqi Freedom (OIF), researchers at Walter Reed Army Institute of Research (WRAIR) established an international reputation in deployment psychology. This experience put WRAIR researchers in a position to become leaders in new initiatives to understand the psychological impact of OIF and OEF. During the 1991 Persian Gulf War (Operations Desert Shield and Desert Storm), WRAIR research teams surveyed and interviewed US Army units in theater and postdeployment to assess the psychological impact of deployment to combat.[4–12] WRAIR teams also conducted in-theater research with units deployed to Operation Just Cause in Panama in 1989,[13] Operation Restore Hope in Somalia in 1993,[14] Operation Uphold Democracy in Haiti in 1994,[15] and throughout the Balkans in the mid-1990s in support of Operation Provide Promise in Croatia,[16] Operation Joint Endeavor in Bosnia,[17] and Operation Joint Guardian in Kosovo.[18] When troop mobilizations began for both OEF and OIF in 2002 and 2003, researchers at WRAIR developed and executed a comprehensive research plan to examine the psychological health of soldiers during combat. This program provided real-time data as the war was occurring that led to multiple health policy changes to improve the mental health and well-being of service members and their families. This chapter outlines some of the key mental health research initiatives by WRAIR scientists with a focus on efforts that directly influenced mental health policies, programs, and training for service members serving in war.

WALTER REED ARMY INSTITUTE OF RESEARCH

WRAIR is a premier Department of Defense (DoD) biomedical research center that integrates basic research and advanced technology to protect and sustain military service members. The WRAIR mental health research program is located at two sites: (1) the Department of Military Psychiatry, Division of Psychiatry and Neuroscience, at the main institute in Silver Spring, Maryland, and (2) the US Army Research Unit—Europe in Heidelberg, Germany. Approximately 35 employees work at the two sites. The program is multidisciplinary, including research and clinical psychologists, psychiatrists, social workers, and sociologists, as well as expertise in clinical evaluation and management, organizational psychology, individual and unit performance, leadership, psychiatric epidemiology, and healthcare services research. In addition to military psychology and psychiatry research, the division includes two other world-class research programs, one focused on sustaining performance during sleep deprivation and the other on reducing the impact of battlefield head injuries.

FROM RESEARCH TO PUBLIC HEALTH POLICY

After the events of September 11, 2001, and the onset of the war in Afghanistan, WRAIR researchers embarked on a comprehensive research program to measure the mental health impact of OEF and OIF on military service members. The program, called "Interventions to Enhance Warfighter Psychological Resilience," was predicated on the recognition that few studies examined combat-related mental health problems, posttraumatic stress disorder (PTSD), or healthcare utilization proximal to the time of war. Such population-based health service utilization research had generally been impossible in previous wars, in part because of the lack of integrated electronic databases, which became available only after the Persian Gulf War.

The research program also recognized the need for data to guide public health policies to address war-related mental health problems. The research agenda established by WRAIR focused on three types of products: (1) information products identifying factors that predict high rates of mental disorders, gaps in service delivery, stigma and barriers to care, and the association of mental health with functional impairment and readiness; (2) assessment tools that provide effective methods of conducting psychological health screening in deployed troops; and (3) prevention and early interventions to support psychological adjustment to the demands of combat, prevent stress-related performance degradation, and improve resiliency and health. These tools are the cornerstones of prevention and early intervention efforts. The remainder of this chapter lists WRAIR's significant efforts and accomplishments from this research program.

INITIAL RESEARCH ON THE IMPACT OF MENTAL DISORDERS BEFORE SEPTEMBER 11, 2001

Using population-based healthcare data systems, researchers at WRAIR established baseline prevalence rates of healthcare service use for mental health problems before September 11, 2001.[19–22] These studies, comparing major *International Classification of Disease*, 9th revision, illness categories, established that mental disorders were the most important source of occupational and medical morbidity as measured by use of medical services and attrition from service. The studies demonstrated that 12% of service members utilized mental health services each year, that mental disorders was the leading category of inpatient hospital bed days, and that mental disorders was the disease category most strongly correlated with attrition from military service and attrition from initial entry training. Such results provided a benchmark for understanding the importance of supporting the mental health of service members during the ensuing wars in Iraq and Afghanistan.

MENTAL HEALTH IMPACT OF THE PENTAGON ATTACK

Immediately after the September 11th attack on the Pentagon, the Army Surgeon General's Office established a comprehensive outreach program for Pentagon employees named "Operation Solace" and tasked the US Army Center for Health Promotion and Preventive Medicine to conduct a survey assessing the mental health effects on the employees. WRAIR, together with colleagues at the Center, Uniformed Services University of the Health Sciences, and the Office of The Army Surgeon General, rapidly developed and validated a brief survey instrument and provided descriptive data on the outreach program.[23–25] This survey instrument, along with prototype instruments fielded during deployments in Bosnia and Kosovo, influenced the development of the Post-Deployment Health Assessment (PDHA) implemented by the DoD in 2003 to assess the population-level impact of deployment to a combat zone.

RESEARCH RELATED TO OPERATIONS ENDURING FREEDOM AND IRAQI FREEDOM

In October 2001, the United States and coalition partners initiated OEF combat operations in Afghanistan, followed by OIF, the largest sustained ground operation since the Vietnam War, in Iraq in March 2003. The wars in Afghanistan and Iraq offered a unique opportunity to examine the mental health impact of combat deployment and, in turn, inform military health policy as the wars progressed.

Epidemiological Consultations of Suicide and Homicide Clusters

Just before OIF and OEF, WRAIR investigators established procedures to conduct epidemiological investigations of clusters of serious behavioral health problems, such as suicides or homicides, applying methodology developed for infectious disease outbreaks. Although infectious disease epidemiological consultations (EPICONs) were common in the military and in civilian public health departments, investigations of behavioral health clusters lacked well-established methodology.

The first military behavioral health EPICON to establish the methodology was conducted in 2000. Its objective was to identify correlates of an outbreak of suicidal behaviors and completed suicides among soldiers in basic training at Fort Leonard Wood, Missouri.[26] Since then, WRAIR investigators have been involved as part of Army Medical Department multidisciplinary teams in conducting EPICONS to address clusters of suicides and homicides at other posts. These clusters have been linked primarily to the high operational tempo of combat operations in Afghanistan and Iraq, as well as marital and family stressors.[27–29]

An EPICON that received national media attention pertained to a cluster of suicides and homicides at Fort Bragg, North Carolina, among soldiers involved in operations in Afghanistan.[27] This investigation resulted in recommendations that led to the 2003 establishment of the Army Deployment Cycle Support Program,[30] a comprehensive program designed to support soldiers and family members throughout the deployment cycle and assure that soldiers who return home from the combat environment because of serious family stressors are evaluated upon return to duty.

Land Combat Study

One of the most well known epidemiological surveillance studies pertaining to OIF and OEF is the large-scale, 5-year Land Combat Study. Initiated in 2003, the study involves anonymous cross-sectional and longitudinal surveys that assess the mental health and well-being of service members in combat infantry brigades serving in Iraq and Afghanistan. The surveys use validated measures to assess the mental health and well-being of service members at different points during their deployment cycle (before, during, and after deployment). Surveys have been collected from over 50,000 service members, mostly from Army brigade combat teams but also from Marine Expeditionary Forces and Navy engineers working in ground operational units. Data have also been collected from military spouses.

Data from some of the first units to return from OIF and OEF deployments were rapidly analyzed and published in the *New England Journal of Medicine* in July 2004.[31] This publication provided the first systematic look at the mental health of soldiers and Marines involved in combat operations in Iraq and Afghanistan. The study indicated that 12% to 13% of soldiers and marines from combat units surveyed 3 to 4 months after returning from deployment to Iraq met the screening definition of PTSD, compared with 5% at predeployment. In addition, 15% to 17% of those surveyed at postdeployment met the screening definition of PTSD, major depression, or generalized anxiety disorder, compared with 9% at predeployment.

To maximize specificity for population-level prevalence estimates, investigators used stringent cut-off criteria to determine mental disorders in this study. Using more sensitive criteria widely validated in clinical care settings, the study indicated that 18% to 20% of soldiers returning from combat in Iraq had significant symptoms of PTSD, and 28% to 29% had significant symptoms of PTSD, depression, or anxiety. The study also found deployment to be associated with alcohol misuse: 24% to 35% of subjects reported using more alcohol than intended, and 20% to 29% reported wanting or needing to drink less.

Besides establishing the prevalence of mental health symptoms among military personnel returning from combat, another critical finding identified by this study was the problem with stigma and barriers to care. The study showed that the majority of service members who had significant mental health problems did not receive care, and concerns about stigma and other barriers to care were pervasive. The study led to widespread DoD, public, media, and congressional interest, as well as multiple new clinical, research, and public health efforts throughout DoD and the Veterans Administration to mitigate stigma, remove barriers to care, and improve the screening and treatment of PTSD after deployment.

A subsequent publication from the Land Combat Study assessed the prevalence of mental health problems 12 months postdeployment. In this sample, 17% of service members met the criteria for PTSD, major depression, and/or generalized anxiety using the stringent cut-off criteria.[32] This finding confirmed that no decrease in symptoms occurred during the first year postdeployment. This 1-year period was the same amount of time many units had before rotating back to Iraq or Afghanistan for a subsequent deployment, suggesting that the soldiers had not recovered from the first deployment when they left for their second deployment.

The study also demonstrated that soldiers with PTSD symptoms were much more likely than soldiers from the same deployments who did not have PTSD symptoms to experience lower ratings of general health, more missed work days, higher use of medical services, and higher somatic symptom levels. These findings were independent of being wounded or injured. The study highlighted the comorbidity of PTSD with physical health problems and the need to evaluate veterans who present with somatic concerns for PTSD. This study was one of several that provided data supporting the implementation of new DoD programs to enhance mental health screening and management in primary care settings.[33]

Mental Health Advisory Teams

Another important OIF initiative is the epidemiological assessment of the mental health and well-being of troops during deployment. Each year, the Army surgeon general deploys a team of mental health experts together with researchers from WRAIR to conduct anonymous assessments of the mental health of troops in Iraq. These teams use similar surveys to those administered as part of the WRAIR Land Combat Study research protocol, and also assess the adequacy and distribution of behavioral health resources in theater.[34–37]

Key findings from the mental health advisory team missions included:

- Fifteen to twenty percent of combat troops deployed to Iraq experience significant symptoms of acute stress, PTSD, or depression, and twenty percent of married service members experience marital concerns.
- Longer deployments, multiple deployments, greater time away from the basecamp, and combat frequency and intensity all contribute to higher rates of PTSD, depression, and marital problems.
- Combat frequency and mental health problems are associated with ethical mistreatment

of noncombatants.
- Good unit leadership is key to sustaining mental health and well-being among combat troops.[34–37]

As a result of these findings, the Army revised the combat and operational stress control doctrine and training,[38] mandated stress control training for all deployment mental health professionals, and ensured that sufficient mental health personnel (credentialed providers and mental health technicians) are available in theater. The mental health advisory teams identified an optimal ratio of at least one mental health professional for every 1,000 troops, supporting the Army's effort to ensure optimal distribution and access to services throughout theater. The findings also led to the inclusion of new training initiatives for soldiers and leaders developed by WRAIR researchers.[39]

Research on Deployment Mental Health Screening

Another important WRAIR research initiative has focused on psychological screening. DoD-wide psychological screening began in 1996 with the deployment of US forces to Bosnia and continued as a commander's program with the subsequent deployment to Kosovo.[40] Psychological screening was designed to identify individuals in need of follow-up mental health services and provide a proactive way to link individuals with mental health professionals.

The current DoD screening program was launched in April 2003, a month after the ground war began in Iraq. At that time, the DoD mandated that all service members complete a PDHA immediately upon return from any deployment using a brief screening instrument combined with a clinical interview.[41] Initiated to meet an immediate need, the program generated controversy for being started before any evidence was available to support the effectiveness of such a program.[42,43]

The goal of WRAIR's screening research program has been to validate and improve the screening for mental health problems associated with deployment. In keeping with these goals, WRAIR conducted a series of studies to identify the appropriate content for predeployment and postdeployment screening,[44] the best approach to screening,[45] the psychometrics of the screening instruments,[46] and effective implementation strategies.[47] The results of this research and subsequent program evaluation[48] have influenced the development of the DoD psychological screening program for military personnel returning from Iraq. Three WRAIR studies were particularly notable in guiding the DoD-wide postdeployment screening program.

The first study looked at the timing of the screening process. Shortly after the PDHA was initiated, researchers at the WRAIR unit in Europe determined that soldiers were two to five times more likely to report mental health concerns 4 months after returning from deployment than they were immediately upon return from deployment.[47] The data were communicated to DoD Health Affairs in early 2004 and led to an immediate triservice mandate to expand the PDHA program to include a second screen, the Post-Deployment Health Reassessment (PDHRA), 3 to 6 months after return from deployment.[49]

A second study included a series of analyses that validated the mental health questions used on the PDHA and PDHRA against a "gold-standard" structured diagnostic interview.[46] This study demonstrated that the PDHA questions had acceptable sensitivity and specificity in identifying individuals who needed further evaluation or treatment and contributed to a better understanding of how to score the PDHA and PDHRA questionnaires.

The third study, conducted in collaboration with the Army Medical Surveillance Activity, evaluated the lessons learned from the PDHA program on a population-wide level. The study showed that combat duty in Iraq was correlated with high utilization of mental health services and attrition from military service postdeployment.[48] One third of soldiers returning from OIF utilized mental health services in medical treatment facilities in the year after returning home (including screening, prevention, and treatment services). However, the PDHA was found to have limited utility in predicting the level of mental health services that were needed postdeployment. These data highlight the challenges in ensuring that adequate resources are available to meet the mental health needs of returning veterans. The data also supported the DoD Health Affairs' decision to expand the PDHA program to include the PDHRA 3 to 6 months postdeployment.

Wartime Studies of Leadership and Unit Factors in Operational Units

A unique feature of WRAIR research has been studies of the relationship between mental health and unit factors such as leadership. Studies have collected data from large intact units (eg, brigade combat teams), thereby including responses from members of the same subordinate units (eg, companies and platoons). This sampling strategy provides an opportunity to examine shared collective perceptions of unit members about cohesion and leadership and understand how these perceptions relate to mental health.[50,51] The research has shown that variables of this nature have both main-effect and moderating influences.[52] In terms of main effects, perceptions of leadership, cohesion, and other aspects of the social environment have been shown to be directly related to mental health outcomes. That is, units with positive perceptions of leadership and cohesion also tend to report low levels of psychological problems, and this shared unit effect is often stronger than the effect analyzed as an individual-level relationship.[51,53] Leadership and other unit factors have also been shown to interact with various stressors such that the negative effects of stressors are weakened when unit factors are positive. This finding suggests that leadership, cohesion, and other forms of social climate may serve to protect soldiers from combat stressors. In one example, shared perceptions of leadership provided a protective influence for soldiers deployed to Haiti.[54] As noted, a key finding from the fourth mental health advisory team assessment in Iraq (2006) was that good unit leadership was associated with fewer mental health problems.[37] As a result of these research findings, WRAIR developed training materials to improve leader behaviors and enhance the mental health of units.

Battlemind Training

At the time that the DoD's Deployment Cycle Support Program was initiated, no standardized combat and deployment stress training packages existed to prepare soldiers for the stressors of war, or to facilitate their transition home, and no integrated mental health training occurred across the deployment cycle. Thus, it was up to behavioral health professionals at each military post to come up with their own training material to meet the requirements of the program.

To address this need, WRAIR researchers created a validated standardized mental health risk communication training program called "Battlemind." Battlemind educates soldiers and leaders about

- what to expect at each phase of the deployment cycle,
- how to look out for their own mental health,
- how to help their fellow unit members, and
- resources available for them to get help if they need it during and after deployment.

The content of Battlemind training, based on results and lessons learned from studies of OIF and OEF combat soldiers, focuses on the strengths and skills that help soldiers survive in combat.

Following the piloting of the first Battlemind products in 2005 and 2006, several new products have been developed and disseminated in collaboration with the Army Medical Department (AMEDD) Center and School. Several prototype Battlemind training modules have been developed and piloted for each phase of the deployment cycle. Predeployment training includes a module for soldiers and leaders that builds resilience by anticipating combat stressors and typical reactions while identifying actions that can be taken to meet these challenges. Predeployment modules have also been developed for behavioral health professionals and military spouses.

During deployments in Iraq, mental health professionals are using two types of Battlemind psychological debriefing techniques developed by WRAIR.[55] Event-driven Battlemind psychological debriefing is designed for use after a critical event, and time-driven Battlemind psychological debriefing is designed for use periodically over the course of a 12- or 15-month deployment. Both of these techniques actively integrate Battlemind concepts, using structured group discussion to review key issues, reinforce positive mental health strategies, encourage unit members to look out for one another, and keep individuals focused on professional and ethical conduct.

The practice of psychological debriefing is controversial, and controlled research examining the efficacy of debriefing with at-risk cohesive occupational groups is lacking.[56,57] WRAIR demonstrated the efficacy of postdeployment Battlemind psychological debriefing in a group randomized-control trial in which platoons were assigned to different types of postdeployment transition training.[58] The debriefing techniques used in this study were the basis for in-theater debriefing models and a postdeployment Battlemind psychological debriefing model now integrated into the Combat Operational Stress course taught at the AMEDD Center and School.

In the same study, Battlemind training conducted at reintegration and at 3 to 6 months postdeployment was also found to effectively reduce mental health symptoms over time.[59] These two postdeployment training modules highlight combat skills that can be adapted to facilitate the transition home. A postdeployment Battlemind training module has also been developed for spouses. Additional Battlemind training products under development include a first aid module for medics, basic Battlemind during initial military training, and leadership development courses. Several training DVDs have also been developed to supplement the Battlemind system.

Battlemind training is currently integrated into the Deployment Cycle Support Program directive and is part of the standard training that soldiers receive before and after combat deployment.[30,39] Battlemind training offered for spouses is specifically designed to strengthen their resilience during times of separation due to war. As each Battlemind product is fielded, it has been made available on its Web site, www.battlemind.org. Other nations including Canada, the United Kingdom, and Australia are also adopting Battlemind training.

Army Medical Department General Officers Behavioral Health Summit

In June 2006, WRAIR hosted a general officers summit for the Army surgeon general and the commander of the US Army Medical Research and Materiel Command. The 2-day conference, attended by 20 AMEDD general officers, was conducted with three primary goals: (1) to arrive at a common understanding (or "lexicon") of available data on the mental health impact of combat, (2) to evaluate best practices and lessons learned so that consistent approaches can be established across components and installations, and (3) to establish the AMEDD behavioral health strategy. The conference achieved its goals and led to the publication of a comprehensive report on Army behavioral healthcare strategy.[60]

OTHER WRAIR MENTAL HEALTH RESEARCH INITIATIVES

WRAIR researchers have been involved in a variety of related efforts, including assessing how adverse early childhood experiences affect psychological adjustment following combat,[61] assessing the appropriateness of PTSD diagnostic criteria applied to combat veterans,[62] and developing a conceptual model for understanding the stigma of mental health problems.[63]

The research program has also led to innovations in the development of tools to help unit leaders assess the behavioral health status of their units. WRAIR researchers have used their knowledge of health measures, military norms from the Land Combat Study, and feedback from unit commanders to develop a unit needs assessment program, designed for behavioral health professionals to provide consultation to military units. The program includes tools, scoring guidelines, implementation recommendations, and a briefing template to facilitate the behavioral health assessment of units.

Given the complexities associated with analyzing large data sets collected from soldiers hierarchically nested within military units (squads, platoons, companies, etc), the WRAIR research program has also contributed to innovations in statistical software and statistical techniques. Many of these innovations have been implemented in the open-source statistical language R.[64] For instance, the "lme4" package in R is designed to analyze hierarchical mixed-effects models containing dichotomous outcomes (eg, meeting or not meeting PTSD thresholds). The algorithms used in the lme4 package were developed by the University of Wisconsin and the Toyon Research Corporation (Goleta, Calif) in a Small Business Technology Transfer Program grant managed by WRAIR scientists.

In another example, WRAIR researchers developed and maintain the multilevel package for R, providing a number of routines for determining whether group members significantly agree about shared concepts such as unit leadership or cohesion. Finally, the package "ltm" is designed to perform item response theory analyses on specific survey items to aid in creating scales with good psychometric properties. WRAIR scientists provided funding to expand the ltm package to handle multiresponse items (eg, strongly disagree, disagree, neither, agree, strongly agree). Each of these developments has contributed to the analyses of complex multilevel data sets involving health outcomes.

WRAIR researchers are active in publishing their work in peer-reviewed journals and other outlets. In 2006 the work of several WRAIR researchers was showcased in a four-volume book series, *Military Life: The Psychology of Serving in Peace and Combat*.[65–68] WRAIR research figures prominently throughout this comprehensive examination of the psychological issues facing military personnel and their families. The series also provides an agenda for military psychology research in the coming years.

Finally, WRAIR research has been widely cited by medical policy makers and lawmakers, and has contributed to significant increases in funding for PTSD treatment and research within the DoD and Veterans Administration. The fiscal year 2007 Congressional appropriation, for example, included a total of $450 million for research and treatment initiatives in the area of PTSD, and another $450 million for traumatic brain injury.

SUMMARY

In keeping with its tradition of working directly with military units in times of conflict, WRAIR has been at the forefront of mental health research since the events of September 11, 2001. Researchers have conducted comprehensive analyses of the mental health impact of OIF/OEF, improved deployment-related screening initiatives, and developed interventions to improve the psychological health of US troops. The program has been focused on directly supporting operational units, deploying research teams into Iraq and Afghanistan, generating timely products relevant to current operations, and informing healthcare policies on an Army- and DoD-wide level. Future directions include the development of advanced training modalities to improve resiliency and mitigate the mental health effects of combat, randomized controlled trials to assess early interventions, and studies of the relationship between PTSD and combat injuries, including traumatic brain injuries. Through balancing scientific rigor with the behavioral health needs of military personnel, WRAIR researchers will remain focused on delivering quality information and training products in support of service members and their families.

REFERENCES

1. Prigerson HG, Maciejewski PK, Rosenheck RA. Population attributable fractions of psychiatric disorders and behavioral outcomes associated with combat exposures among US men. *Am J Public Health.* 2002;92:59–63.

2. Kang HK, Natelson BH, Mahan CM, Lee KY, Murphy FM. Post-traumatic stress disorder and chronic fatigue syndrome-like illness among Gulf War veterans: a population-based survey of 30,000 veterans. *Am J Epidemiol.* 2003;157:141–148.

3. Jordan BK, Schlenger WE, Hough R, et al. Lifetime and current prevalence of specific psychiatric disorders among Vietnam veterans and controls. *Arch Gen Psychiatry.* 1991;48:207–215.

4. Martin JA, Vaitkus MA, Marlowe DH, Bartone PT, Gifford RK, Wright KM. Psychological well-being among US soldiers deployed from Germany to the Gulf War. *Army Med Department J.* 1992;Sept/Oct:29–34.

5. Gifford RK, Marlowe DH, Wright KM, Bartone PT, Martin JA. Unit cohesion in Operations Desert Shield/Storm. *Army Med Department J.* 1992;Dec:11–13.

6. Stretch RH, Bliese PD, Marlowe DH, Wright KM, Knudson KH, Hoover CH. Physical health symptomatology of Gulf War-era service personnel from the states of Pennsylvania and Hawaii. *Mil Med.* 1995;160:131–136.

7. Stretch RH, Bliese PD, Marlowe DH, Wright KM, Knudson KH, Hoover CH. Psychological health of Gulf War-era military personnel. *Mil Med.* 1996;161:257–261.

8. Stretch RH, Marlowe DH, Wright KM, Bliese PD, Knudson KH, Hoover CH. Post-traumatic stress disorder symptoms among Gulf War veterans. *Mil Med.* 1996;161:407–410.

9. Rosen LN, Wright K, Marlowe D, Bartone P, Gifford RK. Gender differences in subjective distress attributable to anticipation of combat among US Army soldiers deployed to the Persian Gulf during Operation Desert Storm. *Mil Med.* 1999;164:753–757.

10. Wright KM, Marlowe DH, Gifford RK. Deployment stress and Operation Desert Shield: preparation for the war. In: Ursano RJ, Norwood AE, eds. *Emotional Aftermath of the Persian Gulf War: Veterans, Families, Communities, and Nations.* Washington, DC: American Psychiatric Press; 1996: 283–314.

11. Brandt G, Norwood A, Ursano R, et al. Psychiatric morbidity in medical and surgical patients evacuated from the Persian Gulf War. *Psychiatr Serv.* 1997;48:102–104.

12. Marlowe DH. *Psychological and Psychosocial Consequences of Combat and Deployment.* Santa Monica, Calif: National Defense Research Institute, RAND; 2001.

13. Kirkland FR, Ender MG, Gifford RK, Wright KM, Marlowe DH. Human dimensions in force projection: discipline under fire. *Mil Rev.* 1996;76:57–64.

14. Gifford RK, Jackson JN, DeShazo KB. *Report of the Human Dimensions Research Team: Operation Restore Hope.* Washington, DC: Walter Reed Army Institute of Research; 1993. ADA274340. Available at: http://stinet.dtic.mil/cgi-bin/GetTRDoc?AD=ADA274340&Location=U2&doc=GetTRDoc.pdf. Accessed January 2, 2008.

15. Halverson RR, Bliese PD. Determinants of soldier support for Operation Uphold Democracy. *Armed Forces Soc.* 1996;23:81–96.

16. Bartone PT, Adler AB, Vaitkus MA. Dimensions of psychological stress in peacekeeping operations. *Mil Med.* 1998;163:587–593.

17. Bartone PT. American IFOR experience: stressors in the early deployment period. In: Soeters JL, Rovers JH, eds. *NL Arms: The Bosnian Experience*. Breda, The Netherlands: Royal Netherlands Military Academy; 1997: 133–139.

18. Castro CA, Bienvenu R, Huffman AH, Adler AB. Soldier dimensions and operational readiness in US Army forces deployed to Kosovo. *Int Rev Armed Forces Med Serv.* 2000;73:191–199.

19. Hoge CW, Lesikar SE, Guevara R, et al. Mental disorders among US military personnel in the 1990s: association with high levels of healthcare utilization and early military attrition. *Am J Psychiatry.* 2002;159:1576–1583.

20. Messer SC, Liu X, Hoge CW, Cowan DN, Engel CC. Projecting mental disorder prevalence from national surveys to populations of interest: an illustration using the ECA and US Army. *Soc Psychiatry Psychiatr Epidemiol.* 2004;39:419–426.

21. Pavlin JA, Murdock P, Elbert E, et al. Conducting population behavioral health surveillance by using automated diagnostic and pharmacy data systems. *MMWR Morb Mortal Wkly Rep.* 2004;53(Suppl):166–172.

22. Hoge CW, Toboni HE, Messer SC, Bell N, Amoroso P, Orman D. The occupational burden of mental disorders in the US military: psychiatric hospitalizations, involuntary separations, and disability. *Am J Psychiatry.* 2005;162:585–591.

23. Hoge CW, Engel CC, Orman DT, et al. Development of a brief questionnaire to measure mental health outcomes among Pentagon employees following the September 11, 2001 attack. *Mil Med.* 2002;167(Suppl 9):60–63.

24. Hoge CW, Orman DT, Robichaux RJ, et al. Operation Solace: mental health intervention following the September 11, 2001 Pentagon attack. *Mil Med.* 2002;167(Suppl 9):44–47.

25. Jordan NN, Hoge CW, Tobler SK, Wells J, Dydek G, Egerton WE. Mental health impact of 9/11 Pentagon attack: validation of a rapid assessment tool. *Am J Prev Med.* 2004;26:284–293.

26. Hoge CW, Russell RK, Orman DT, Milliken C, Bliese P. *Final Report of Epidemiologic Investigation of Outbreak of Suicidal Behaviors Among Initial Entry Army Trainees at Fort Leonard Wood, July–October 2000.* Washington, DC: Walter Reed Army Institute of Research, 2001. WRAIR Tech Report.

27. *Fort Bragg Epidemiological Consultation Report*. Washington, DC: Office of the Surgeon General, Department of the Army; 2002.

28. *Epidemiological Consultation Report: Suicides at Fort Hood, Texas*. Washington, DC: Office of the Surgeon General, Department of the Army; 2006.

29. *Epidemiological Consultation Report: Suicides at Fort Riley, Kansas.* Fort Sam Houston, Tex: Great Plains Regional Medical Command, US Army Medical Command; 2005.

30. Army G1 Deputy Chief of Staff for Personnel. Deployment cycle support program. US Army Web site. Available at: http://www.armyg1.army.mil/dcs/default.asp. Accessed January 2, 2008.

31. Hoge CW, Castro CA, Messer SC, McGurk D, Cotting DI, Koffman RL. Combat duty in Iraq and Afghanistan, mental health problems, and barriers to care. *N Engl J Med.* 2004;351:13–22.

32. Hoge CW, Terhakopian A, Castro CA, Messer SC, Engel CC. Association of posttraumatic stress disorder with somatic symptoms, healthcare visits, and absenteeism among Iraq War veterans. *Am J Psychiatry.* 2007;164:150–153.

33. Engel CC. RESPECT-MIL: Bringing best practices and research together in primary care to improve Soldier-centered care. Paper presented at: 2007 Annual Force Health Protection Conference; August 6, 2007; Louisville, Kentucky.

34. *Operation Iraqi Freedom Mental Health Advisory Team (MHAT) Report.* Washington, DC: Department of the Army, Office of the Surgeon General; 2003.

35. *Operation Iraqi Freedom (OIF-II) Mental Health Advisory Team (MHAT-II) Report.* Washington, DC: Department of the Army, Office of the Surgeon General; 2005.

36. Office of the Surgeon, Multinational Forces Iraq, and Office of the Surgeon General, US Army Medical Command. *Mental Health Advisory Team (MHAT-III): Operation Iraqi Freedom 04-06.* Washington, DC: Department of the Army, Office of the Surgeon General; 2006.

37. Office of the Surgeon, Multinational Forces Iraq, and Office of The Surgeon General, US Army Medical Command. *Mental Health Advisory Team (MHAT-IV): Operation Iraqi Freedom 05-07.* Washington, DC: Department of the Army, Office of the Surgeon General; 2007.

38. Headquarters, Department of the Army. *Combat and Operational Stress Control.* Washington, DC: DA; 2006. Field Manual 4-02.51.

39. US Army Medical Research and Materiel Command, Military Operation Research Program. Battlemind. Available at: www.battlemind.org. Accessed July 12, 2007.

40. Wright KM, Huffman AH, Adler AB, Castro CA. Psychological screening program overview. *Mil Med.* 2002;167:853–861.

41. US Department of Defense. *Deployment Health.* Washington, DC: DoD; 2006. DoD Instruction 6490.03. Available at: http://www.dtic.mil/whs/directives/corres/pdf/649003p.pdf. Accessed July 12, 2007.

42. Rona RJ, Hyams KC, Wessely S. Screening for psychological illness in military personnel. *JAMA.* 2005;293:1257–1260.

43. Wright KM, Bliese PD, Adler AB, Hoge CW, Castro CA, Thomas JL. Screening for psychological illness in the military [letter to the editor]. *JAMA.* 2005;294:42–43.

44. Wright KM, Thomas JL, Adler AB, Ness JW, Hoge CW, Castro CA. Psychological screening procedures for deploying US forces. *Mil Med.* 2005;170:555–562.

45. Wright KM, Bliese PD, Thomas JL, Adler AB, Eckford RD, Hoge CW. Contrasting approaches to psychological screening with US combat soldiers. *J Trauma Stress.* 2007;20:965–975.

46. Bliese P, Wright K, Adler A, Hoge C, Prayner R. *Post-Deployment Psychological Screening: Interpreting and Scoring DD Form 2900.* Heidelberg, Germany: US Army Medical Research–Europe, Walter Reed Army Institute of Research; 2005. Research Report 2005-003. Available at: http://www.usamru-e.hqusareur.army.mil/PDHRAResearchReport2005-003.pdf. Accessed July 26, 2007.

47. Bliese PD, Wright KM, Adler AB, Thomas JL, Hoge CW. Timing of post-combat mental health assessments. *Psychol Services.* 2007;4:141–148.

48. Hoge CW, Auchterlonie JL, Milliken CS. Mental health problems, use of mental health services, and attrition from military service after returning from deployment to Iraq or Afghanistan. *JAMA.* 2006;295:1023–1032.

49. Winkenwerder W Jr, Assistant Secretary for Defense (Health Affairs). *Post-Deployment Health Reassessment.* Washington, DC: Department of Defense. Memorandum for Assistant Secretary of the Army, Assistant Secretary of the Navy, Assistant Secretary of the Air Force, March 10, 2005. Available at: http://www.ha.osd.mil/policies/2005/05-011.pdf. Accessed January 3, 2008.

50. Bliese PD, Jex SM. Incorporating a multilevel perspective into occupational stress research: theoretical, methodological, and practical implications. *J Occup Health Psychol.* 2002;7:265–276.

51. Bliese PD. Social climates: drivers of soldier well-being and resilience. In: Britt TW, Castro CA, Adler AB, eds. *Operational Stress*. Vol 2. In: *Military Life: The Psychology of Serving in Peace and Combat*. Westport, Conn: Praeger Security International; 2006: 213–234.

52. Bliese PD, Castro CA. The soldier adaptation model (SAM): applications to behavioral science peacekeeping research. In: Britt T, Adler A, eds. *The Psychology of the Peacekeeper: Lessons From the Field*. Westport, Conn: Praeger Security International; 2003: 185–203.

53. Bliese PD, Halverson RR. Individual and nomothetic models of job stress: an examination of work hours, cohesion, and well-being. *J Appl Soc Psychol*. 1996;26:1171–1189.

54. Bliese PD, Halverson RR. Using random group resampling in multilevel research. *Leadership Q*. 2002;13:53–68.

55. Adler AB, Castro CA, McGurk D. *Battlemind Psychological Debriefings*. Heidelberg, Germany: US Army Medical Research Unit–Europe; 2007. Research Report 2007-001. Available at: http://www.usamru-e.hqusareur.army.mil/Battlemind-PsychDebriefingProcedures2APR07.pdf. Accessed July 16, 2007.

56. Castro CA, Engel CC, Adler AB. The challenge of providing mental health prevention and early intervention in the US military. In: Litz BT, ed. *Early Intervention for Trauma and Traumatic Loss*. New York, NY: Guilford Press; 2004: 301–318.

57. Litz BT, Gray M, Bryant RA, Adler AB. Early intervention for trauma: current status and future directions. *Clin Psychol: Sci Pract*. 2002;9:112–134.

58. Adler AB, Castro CA, McGurk D, Bliese PD, Wright KM, Hoge CW. Post-deployment interventions to reduce the mental health impact of combat deployment to Iraq: public health policies, psychological debriefing and Battlemind training. Paper presented at: International Society for Traumatic Stress Studies; November 2006; Hollywood, Calif.

59. Adler AB, Castro CA, Bliese PD, McGurk D, Milliken C. The efficacy of Battlemind training at 3–6 months postdeployment. Paper presented at: Annual Meeting of the American Psychological Association; August 2007; San Francisco, Calif.

60. *Behavioral Health Strategy for the Way Ahead: Report of Army Medical Department General Officer Behavioral Health Summit, June 20–21, 2006*. Washington, DC: Department of the Army, Office of the Surgeon General; 2006.

61. Cabrera OA, Hoge CW, Bliese PD, Castro CA, Messer SC. Childhood adversity and combat as predictors of depression and post-traumatic stress in deployed troops. *Am J Prev Med*. 2007;33:77–82.

62. Adler AB, Wright KM, Bliese PD, Prayner R, Salvi A, Evans S. Immediate responses to combat-related events: beyond fear, helplessness, and horror. Paper presented at: 114th Meeting of the American Psychological Association; August 2006; New Orleans, La.

63. Greene-Shortridge TM, Britt TW, Castro CA. The stigma of mental health problems in the military. *Mil Med*. 2007;172:157–161.

64. The R Foundation for Statistical Computing. The R project for statistical computing. Available at: http://www.R-project.org. Accessed June 18, 2007.

65. Britt TW, Castro CA, Adler AB, eds. *Military Performance*. Vol 1. In: *Military Life: The Psychology of Serving in Peace and Combat*. Westport, Conn: Praeger Security International; 2006.

66. Britt TW, Castro CA, Adler AB, eds. *Operational Stress*. Vol 2. In: *Military Life: The Psychology of Serving in Peace and Combat*. Westport, Conn: Praeger Security International; 2006.

67. Britt TW, Castro CA, Adler AB, eds. *Military Family*. Vol 3. In: *Military Life: The Psychology of Serving in Peace and Combat*. Westport, Conn: Praeger Security International; 2006.

68. Britt TW, Castro CA, Adler AB, eds. *Military Culture*. Vol 4. In: *Military Life: The Psychology of Serving in Peace and Combat*. Westport, Conn: Praeger Security International; 2006.

COMBAT AND OPERATIONAL BEHAVIORAL HEALTH

Section II: In Theater

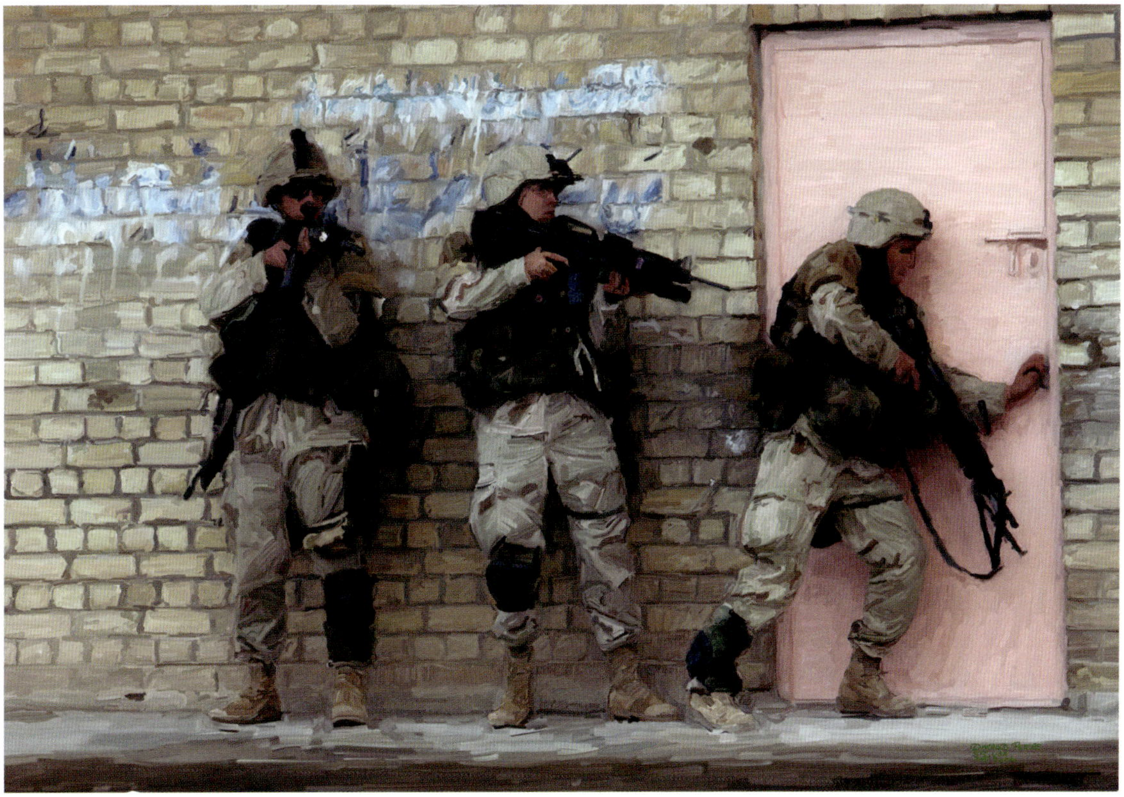

What is Behind the Pink Door, by Darrold Peters, Digital Oils / Corel Painter IX.5, 2006.

Art: Courtesy of the US Army Center of Military History.

Chapter 6

THE DIVISION PSYCHIATRIST AND BRIGADE BEHAVIORAL HEALTH OFFICERS

CHRISTOPHER H. WARNER, MD*; GEORGE N. APPENZELLER, MD†; TODD YOSICK, LISW‡; MATTHEW J. BARRY, DO§; ANTHONY J. MORTON, MD¥; JILL E. BREITBACH, PsyD¶; GABRIELLE BRYEN, MSW, LCSW**; ANGELA MOBBS, PsyD††; AMANDA ROBBINS, PsyD‡‡; JESSICA PARKER, PsyD§§; AND THOMAS GRIEGER, MD¥¥

*Major, Medical Corps, US Army; Chief, Department of Behavioral Medicine, Winn Army Community Hospital, Building 9242, Room 20, 1083 Worcester Drive, Fort Stewart, Georgia 31324; formerly, Division Psychiatrist, 3rd Infantry Division, Fort Stewart, Georgia

†Colonel, Medical Corps, US Army; Commander, US Army Medical Activity, Alaska, 1060 Gaffney Road #7400, Fort Wainwright, Alaska 99703-7400; formerly, Deputy Commander for Clinical Services, Command Group, Winn Army Community Hospital, Fort Stewart, Georgia 31314

‡Major, Medical Service Corps, US Army; Deputy Director, Resilience and Prevention Directorate, Office of the Assistant Secretary of Defense for Health Affairs, Defense Centers of Excellence for Psychological Health and Traumatic Brain Injury, 1335 East-West Highway, Silver Spring, Maryland 20910; formerly, Chief, Battlemind Training Office/Chief, Combat and Operational Stress Control, AMEDD Center and School, Fort Sam Houston, Texas

§Major, Medical Corps, US Army Reserve; Staff Psychiatrist, Rochester Veterans Affairs Outpatient Clinic, 465 Westfall Road, Rochester, New York 14620; formerly, Major, Medical Corps, US Army; Chief of Psychiatric Service USA MEDDAC and 10th Mountain Division Psychiatrist, Fort Drum, New York

¥Major, Medical Corps, US Army; Medical Director, Department of Behavioral Health, Moncrief Army Community Hospital, 4500 Stuart Street, Fort Jackson, South Carolina 29207-5720; formerly, Division Psychiatrist, 1st Armored Division, Wiesbaden, Germany

¶Major, Medical Service Corps, US Army; Neuropsychologist, Department of Psychology, Evans Army Community Hospital, USAMEDDAC, Fort Carson, Colorado; formerly, Group Psychologist, 1st Special Warfare Training Group, Fort Bragg, North Carolina

**Major, Medical Service Corps, US Army; Deputy Chief, Department of Social Work, Womack Army Medical Center, Stop A, Fort Bragg, North Carolina 28310; formerly, Brigade Behavioral Health Officer, 3rd Brigade Combat Team, 4th Infantry Division, Fort Carson, Colorado 80913

††Special Forces Assignment and Selection Psychologist, Special Warfare Center and School, Rowe Training Facility, Building T-5167, 1500 Camp Mackall Place, Marston, North Carolina 28363; formerly, Brigade Psychologist, 3rd Brigade Combat Team, 3rd Infantry Division, Fort Benning, Georgia

‡‡Captain, Medical Service Corps, US Army; Brigade Combat Team Behavioral Health Officer, 4th Brigade Combat Team, 10th Mountain Division, Fort Polk, Louisiana 71459

§§Captain, Medical Service Corps, US Army; Chief, Warrior Restoration Center, Department of Behavioral Medicine, Winn Army Community Hospital, 541 East 9th Street, Building 359, Fort Stewart, Georgia 31314-5674; formerly, Psychology Resident, Traumatic Brain Injury, Brooke Army Medical Center, San Antonio, Texas

¥¥Captain (Retired), US Navy; Associate Professor, Department of Psychiatry, Uniformed Services University of the Health Sciences, 4301 Jones Bridge Road, Bethesda, Maryland 20814

A portion of this chapter has been published as: Warner CH, Breitbach JE, Appenzeller GN, Barry MJ, Morton A, Grieger T. The evolving role of the division psychiatrist. *Mil Med*. 2007;172:918–924.

INTRODUCTION

The psychological effects of warfare have been well documented throughout history, with names such as nostalgia, soldier's heart, shell shock, battle fatigue, and most recently, combat operational stress. In the late 19th and early 20th centuries, military leaders began to recognize the impact of treating and addressing these reactions. This led to an increased presence of mental health providers on the battlefield. Since World War I, the United States Army has been deploying mental health assets to the front line for treatment of combat operational stress and to advise unit commanders on mental health issues and the effect of war on soldiers.[1–3]

The first battlefield psychiatrist for the US Army was Dr Thomas Salmon. During World War I, he noted the value of maintaining a psychiatrist on the division staff who works directly with the surgeon to provide consultation, as well as the importance of the role as a staff officer for the command.[2] Salmon created a successful battlefield management system incorporating treatment, prevention, and consultation. Unfortunately, many of those lessons learned were lost or were deemed unnecessary after the end of the war. It was not until World War II that General Omar Bradley again realized the value of organic mental health assets during the North African campaign of 1943 and reestablished the division psychiatrist position.[3] Since the Korean War, the division psychiatrist has led the division mental health activity (DMHA), both in garrison and during deployment.[1,3] The roles and responsibilities for a division psychiatrist and the DMHA were first outlined in Army Regulation 40-216, *Neuropsychiatry and Mental Health,* in 1957.[4]

The division psychiatrist serves as the leader of the division mental health team whose mission is to assist command in controlling combat operational stress through training, consultation, and restoration.[5] Until recently, the DMHA consisted of three providers (a psychiatrist, a psychologist, and a social worker), complimented by six mental health technicians (Figure 6-1). However, in the midst of the global war on terror, the Army began its largest restructuring since World War II, changing the emphasis from the division to the brigade combat team (BCT).[6] This restructuring effort was designed to make the Army a more modular force, increase efficiency and combat power, and increase the number of BCTs within the force.[6]

In conjunction with the restructuring, there has been a reorganization and an increase in the behavioral health assets assigned to each division. The new force structure eliminated a formal centralized mental health section and created a modular DMHA. The new modular DMHA structure, outlined in Figure 6-2, includes a division psychiatrist and senior noncommissioned officer located with the division surgeon at the division headquarters unit, and a brigade behavioral health officer (BCT BHO; psychologist or social worker) and an enlisted mental health specialist assigned to each BCT. Multiple BCTs are under the control of the division, such that five to six mental health providers (psychiatrists, psychologists, and social workers) can be assigned to a DMHA. This new, modular design yields more providers and allows for projection of resources to commanders at lower levels (ie, battalion and company). With this rapid expansion and evolution of the DMHA, the role of the military mental health provider

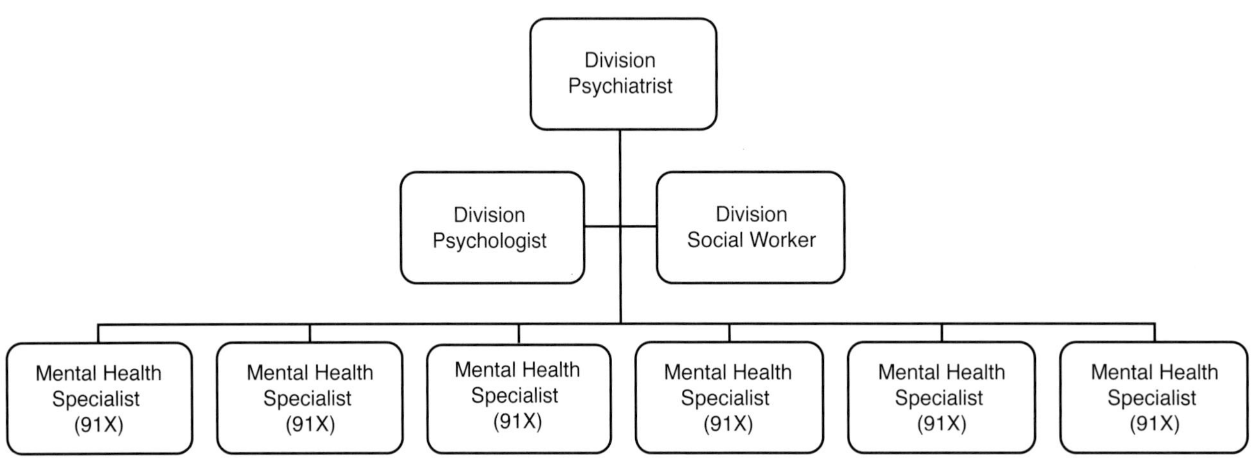

Figure 6-1. Prior structure of division mental health activity.

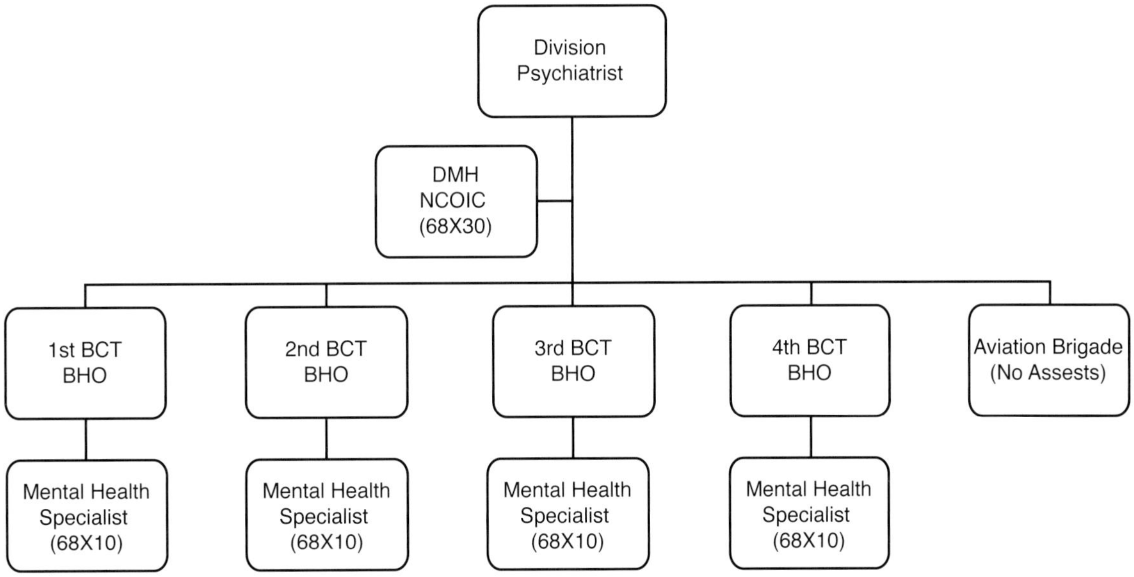

Figure 6-2. Current structure of division mental health activity in the modular Army.
BCT: brigade combat team
BHO: behavioral health officer (psychologist or social worker)
DMH: division mental health
NCOIC: noncommissioned officer in charge

has become more diverse and multifaceted.

The complex effects of combat on soldiers in modern warfare demonstrate the importance of combat and operational stress control during deployment and the need to monitor mental health issues following deployment.[7–11] This has led to recent updates in US Army doctrine, though, unfortunately, little guidance on the specific roles of division mental health has been provided.[12] The purpose of this chapter is to outline the role and utilization of the division psychiatrist and the BCT BHO in both the division and in the DMHA as defined by current military doctrine and based on the more than 10 combined years of deployment experience of the authors.

DOCTRINE

Although much has been published on the psychological consequences of combat and deployment, little has been published on the specific roles of the division psychiatrists, DMHA, or BCT BHOs in garrison or during deployment.[13–20] Army Regulation 40-216, *Neuropsychiatry and Mental Health*, the primary regulation associated with mental healthcare, has not been updated since 1984 and cites only that the division psychiatrist will lead the DMHA, serve as a consultant on neuropsychiatric issues, and in conjunction with the DMHA, provide care to soldiers with neuropsychiatric conditions.[4] Field Manual 8-51, *Combat Stress Control in a Theater of Operations: Tactics, Techniques, and Procedures,* was released in 1994 and updated in 1998.[5] It provided an outline of the overall mission and role of the DMHA and gave some additional insight into the roles and responsibilities of the division psychiatrist as a supervisor. This guidance was recently updated to outline combat and operational stress control (COSC) in Field Manual 4-02.51, *Combat and Operational Stress Control,* but provides little guidance on the operation of a DMHA or on the roles and responsibilities of a division psychiatrist and the BCT BHO.[12]

Lieutenant Colonel Albert Glass defined in his chapter "Lessons Learned" from *Neuropsychiatry in World War II* the need to maintain a strong regiment of active duty psychiatrists, both in war and in peacetime, to manage the operational needs of the armed services. He argued that civilian psychiatric agencies were unable to meet the ongoing demands and maintain the operational preparedness that military psychiatry requires. He also reviewed the complexity of psychiatric diagnosis and screening/selection in wartime, as it effects conservation of the fighting force.[1] In *Combat Psychiatry*, Lieutenant Colonel Glass specifically discussed the role of "Psychiatry at the Division Level." This in-depth review outlined the specific principles for the evaluation, treatment, and disposition of soldiers in a combat environment. Additionally this chapter provided historical data analysis from World War II.[21]

Rock and colleagues discussed the historical development of US Army mental health resources in *War Psychiatry*, in a chapter titled "US Army Combat Psychiatry." This chapter provides insight into changes that were made in doctrine and in the development of division mental health units from World War I through Vietnam. However, as Army mental healthcare evolved into the 1980s, it moved away from the roles of the divisional units and focused on the development of nonembedded combat stress control units.[3] Although both chapters are an excellent source of information on the historical development of military mental health systems and the treatment role of division-level behavioral health officers, they provide little guidance on other duties and responsibilities of these positions.

In 1993, two relevant articles were published in *Military Medicine*. In the first of these, Engel and Campbell addressed the challenges facing a division mental health unit. They discussed the minimal attention focused on their role while not deployed and noted the importance of ongoing preventive missions based on their lessons learned from deployment to Operation Desert Storm.[14] In the second of these, Ritchie and White outlined the guidelines for becoming a successful division psychiatrist, providing practical guidance for preparing psychiatrists who were relatively new to the military on effective means of interacting and engaging with infantry commanders. Additionally, the latter article outlined the various duties and responsibilities of the position including (in their listed order of importance): behavioral health provider, supervisor of other behavioral health providers, educator of division medical providers, administrative psychiatry, consultation to command, planning and oversight of the division mental health section, and serving as an officer in the division.[15] This guidance was recently revised by Hill, Lange, and Bacon. Their focus was on what psychiatry residents should do to prepare for assuming the role.[16] Although these two articles did not deal with the role of the division psychologist or the division social worker, they did outline some of the duties and responsibilities expected of a unit behavioral health leader.

During Operation Iraqi Freedom, Warner, Appenzeller, and colleagues published a group of articles in *Military Medicine* on the roles and responsibilities of division mental health units in the new brigade combat team structure. These articles provided a roadmap of prevention, early identification, and intervention methods for other DMHAs. Additionally, the authors cited several advantages to the new structure, including the increased ability to provide mental health services closer to the front line and the ability to interact and regularly serve as consultants to lower levels of command. Additionally, they noted several limitations of the new structure, including dispersed command and control, increased independence of each provider with decreased supervision, and an increased risk for provider burnout due to the smaller teams. Although there was some discussion about garrison actions required prior to the deployment and the role of the division psychiatrist while in garrison, these articles were predominantly focused on the deployed role.[20,22,23]

Expanding beyond the role of the division psychiatrist to include other mental health providers, *Military Psychiatry: Preparing for Peace in War* addresses the evolving interface between the behavioral health leader and command. Chapter 9 highlights the heightened value by command of services mental health officers offer via command consultation, including cross service consultation needs.[24] Also discussed, in Chapter 10, is the need for mental health providers in recognizing the stressors of those in leadership positions and offering support to build resilience of those in command.[25] Chapters 11 and 12 approach the training needs of mental health workers, emphasizing the value of field training exercises,[26] and proposes a two-part training model to assist medical personnel and command in recognizing combat stress concerns and how to effectively triage combat stress casualties.[27]

PERSPECTIVES ON THE POSITION

According to one division commander, the division psychiatrist and the DMHA are responsible for "maintaining a 'finger on the pulse' of the unit."[28] This guidance provides a global commander's intent to the DMHA, but interpretation and execution of that intent is subject to individual variability.

There are multiple perspectives to consider, as illustrated in Figure 6-3. Division psychiatrists rely on their own perspectives, but must be cognizant of the requirements and expectations of the division surgeon and division commander. Similarly, the BCT BHO must consider the expectations of the division psychiatrist, brigade surgeon, and brigade commander. Additionally, behavioral health providers' different training backgrounds may influence which areas they are both competent and confident to address. For instance, a BCT BHO who is a psychologist has different skill capabilities than a social worker. Despite these training differences, all providers bring their own experiences to the position, which also influences their scope and

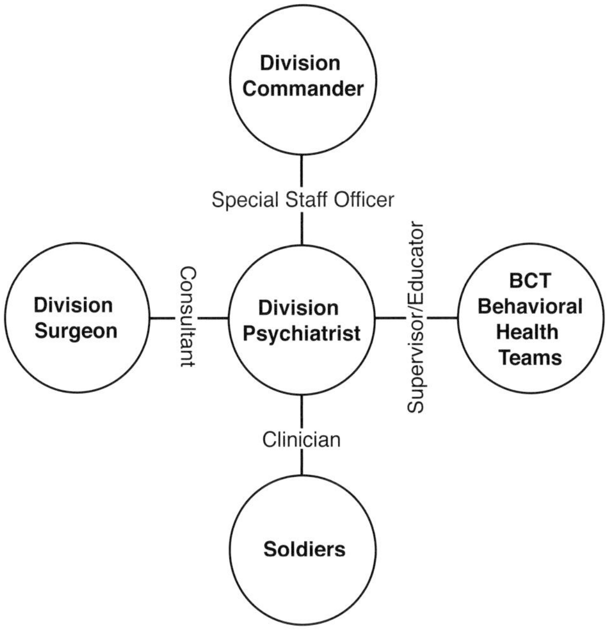

Figure 6-3. Perspectives on the position of the division psychiatrist.
BCT: brigade combat team

breadth of practice.

The division psychiatrist position tends to be assigned to junior officers following completion of their psychiatric residency or fellowship. Many enter the position as a company-grade officer (captain) and are promoted to field grade (major) while in the position. For many incoming division psychiatrists, this is their first opportunity to practice independently. Furthermore, few of the incoming division psychiatrists are familiar with the operation and function of a division staff and most have not attended their branch-specific career course.

Like the psychiatrist, the BCT BHO position tends to be assigned to a junior to mid-level officer. Many enter the position as a company-grade officer and some will be promoted to field grade while in the position. In the past, the psychologists would likely have just completed their internship training and have not done any other operational tour. However, that has changed recently with requirements for licensure for deployability. Currently, most psychologists have completed a 1- or 2-year postinternship tour prior to arriving to the BCT. For social workers, most have completed one tour, generally at a medical center working with a senior social work officer, and then are assigned to an operational billet. For many incoming BCT BHOs, this is their first opportunity to practice without a senior supervisor in their discipline. Like psychiatrists, few of the incoming BCT BHOs are familiar with the operation and function of a brigade staff, and most have not attended their branch-specific career course.

In keeping with their recent training program experience, both incoming division psychiatrists and BCT BHOs tend to focus on their roles as clinicians, and quite possibly, as educators for their enlisted mental health technicians and BCT primary care physicians. They may not rapidly embrace their roles as staff officers, advisors, and consultants to the division or brigade leadership or comprehend how these roles affect care for soldiers. In some instances, division psychiatrists have relinquished their leadership and administrative responsibilities to a brigade BHO to increase time available for their own clinical work. Similarly, for many BHOs, this is their first experience integrating with a line combat unit. The BHO must quickly adjust to training and operation tempo requirements that are expected in these units.

In contrast, division and brigade surgeons expect BHOs to act as advisors and consultants. They envision the psychiatrist or BCT BHO providing assistance in planning for the behavioral health aspects of the entire spectrum of operations and coordinating behavioral health support resources for garrison and deployed activities. They expect their behavioral health consultant to be able to identify the behavioral health threats to the units and make recommendations on preventive mechanisms for the division or brigade. They further expect the BHO to be familiar with the Army Medical Department (AMEDD) principles of treatment, evacuation, and restoration in theater. This includes arranging transportation, coordinating care for evacuated soldiers, and patient tracking.

Additionally, the division psychiatrist expects the BCT BHO to serve as both an advisor and a clinician. In many cases, BCTs are not collocated with their divisions, and division psychiatrists rely on the BCT BHOs to advise them on behavioral health issues that occur within the brigade. Furthermore, they expect the BCT BHO to be the primary provider of behavioral healthcare within the units and to be responsible for evaluating soldiers' behavioral health fitness for duty. Further requirements include training and developing the enlisted mental health technicians and consulting with BCT medical and command personnel.

Both division and brigade commanders expect their staff officers to be able to provide expert advice and alternative courses of action to enable them to make educated decisions in the best interest of the unit. Many commanders see BHOs as an important part of the division or BCT medical team and expect them to be experienced in analyzing behavioral health trends and their potential impacts on unit readiness.

In general, commanders have become very attuned to the behavioral health effects of combat and deployment on their soldiers and look to the unit BHO to provide expert consultation on what they, as commanders, can do to mitigate the inherent stress of deployment, ensure proper surveillance of mental health issues upon redeployment, reduce the stigma of seeking care, and help their soldiers.

Case Study 6-1: During one recent deployment, a division commander told his division psychiatrist that he was "concerned about the mental health of my unit and I want my commanders to know that we as a unit have the resources, ability, and concern to do something to help them." He frequently had the division psychiatrist travel with him throughout the theater of operations to ensure that the behavioral health team was aware of the various conditions soldiers were encountering but also for the subordinate commanders to see the importance that he placed on soldier behavioral health. The division psychiatrist was able to get a "finger on the pulse" of the units that they were visiting, identify the potential risks for combat and operational stress within the unit, and provide the commanders with recommendations on how to mitigate those risks.

These various duties, responsibilities, expectations, and external pressures on unit behavioral health officers pose a formidable challenge for relatively junior officers to properly prioritize their duties. In this setting, optimal performance will be achieved through proper professional development and updated doctrine.

DUTIES AND RESPONSIBILITIES

There are several areas of responsibility of particular importance to these junior officers. These will be discussed in this chapter; a comprehensive listing of the multiple duties and responsibilities of the unit BHO can be found in Exhibit 6-1.

Planning and Oversight for Behavioral Healthcare

The division psychiatrist or BCT BHO is the unit's subject matter expert on the behavioral health effects of combat and other deployments. Therefore, it is imperative that the division psychiatrist or BCT BHO serve as a staff officer within the division or brigade leadership to provide recommendations on the positioning and utilization of behavioral health resources, both in garrison and during deployment.

Prior to deployment the division psychiatrist is responsible for developing and implementing training programs for primary care providers, nonmedical officers, and noncommissioned officers. Training should focus on prevention and management of operational stress and other mental health problems that may be encountered during deployment.

During deployment, it is the responsibility of the division psychiatrist and the BCT BHO to assess the behavioral health threat of the environment and work closely with the command surgeon to review how behavioral health assets are being deployed and utilized within the operational environment. Sources of information include historical data from prior conflicts both in the unit and for that area, rates of combat stress in other units deployed to the conflict, rates of behavioral health issues in the unit in garrison, and effects of psychological profiles related to combat on the fighting strength. The division psychiatrists or BCT BHOs can make recommendations to their respective commands on where to position and how to implement the behavioral resources within the unit. Furthermore, the division psychiatrist should develop standard operating procedures for division mental healthcare, create traumatic event management plans, and provide guidance on the utilization of the Unit Behavioral Health Needs Assessment or other unit evaluation tools. Additionally, it is imperative to coordinate with external assets such as combat stress control units when they are positioned within the area of operations.

Key concepts to be considered when planning the distribution of resources are safety, security, and a close proximity to the units at greatest risk for combat operational stress reactions. This not only involves the division psychiatrist, but also the BCT BHO who must develop plans for allowing outreach from a primary clinic location to extend throughout the unit area of operations that requires logistical support.

Also of significance is the monitoring of, and guidance on, the use of psychotropic medications within the division and brigade, an area that has come under recent public scrutiny. The division psychiatrist needs to work with the medical logistic assets to determine which medications should be used in the area of operations and should help set guidelines for indications, use, and monitoring of psychotropics within the division. In general, use of antidepressants and mild sleep aids is common practice. Use of other psychotropics such as benzodiazepines, stimulants, and antipsychotics should be considered on a case-by-case basis and warrant increased vigilance. This topic is covered in great depth in Chapter 10, Psychiatric Medications in Military Operations, in this volume.

Although BCT BHOs are not credentialed to prescribe medication, they need to be aware of the utilization of psychotropics and their effects on the soldiers within the unit. The BCT BHO needs to work closely

EXHIBIT 6-1

DUTIES AND RESPONSIBILITIES OF THE UNIT BEHAVIORAL HEALTH OFFICER

Planning/Oversight for Division Mental Healthcare

- Plans and coordinates pre- and postdeployment mental health screening
- Provides recommendations on positioning of division mental health assets in garrison and deployment
- Develops division traumatic event management plan
- Consults with combat stress detachment (CSC) commander on placement of resources within division area during deployment
- Monitors and provides guidance on use of psychotropic medications
  - Determines which medications medical logistical personnel need to have on hand during deployments
  - Knows that use of antidepressants and mild sleep aids is common practice; use of other psychotropic medications such as benzodiazepines, stimulants, and antipsychotics should be considered on a case-by-case basis and based on current guidance from higher levels
- Liaisons with other support resources in garrison and during deployment
  - Consults with garrison medical treatment facility, Army Substance Abuse Program, chaplains, Army Community Services, Military OneSource, and local civilian mental health providers and hospitals
  - Works with deployment chaplains, combat stress detachments, and medical providers

Consultant to Commanders and Division Surgeon on Behavioral Health Trends/Issues

- Coordinates behavioral health prevention efforts
  - Provides routine consultative updates on behavioral health threats through monitoring of utilization rates of the division mental health clinic, behavioral health hospitalization rates, child/spouse abuse cases, DUI reports, positive drug test results, and pre- and postdeployment health assessment results
  - Oversees standardized Army Battlemind training for development of mental resiliency of soldiers, spouses, and their families
- Prepares for potentially traumatic events
  - Works with commanders, chaplains, and other medical personnel to develop a unit traumatic event management plan for addressing potentially traumatic events
- Monitors issues of public attention
  - Educates the commander about current ongoing issues of mental health significance and advises commander about potential mental health impacts of varying policy/strategic changes
  - Provides commander with information updates and potential questions/answers for media encounters about mental health prevention and ongoing issues within the unit

Supervisor of BCT Behavioral Health Officers and Enlisted Mental Health Specialists

- Serves as the officer in charge of division mental health
- Establishes the standard of care for practice within the division mental health activity (should be published in some format and reviewed on a regular basis)
- Supervises all BCT behavioral health officers
  - Conducts frequent supervision and chart reviews
  - Ensures that BCT behavioral health officers are adequately supervising their enlisted mental health technicians
- Manages continuing education
  - Develops a continuing education plan for each provider including local training (morning reports, routine training) and other opportunities (combat operational stress course, behavioral health short course)
  - Ensures that all providers are obtaining necessary continuing education requirements and completing necessary tasks for licensure, etc
- Officer and noncommissioned officer development
  - Ensures that all personnel are working towards advancement and achieving necessary requirement to include schooling (captain's career course, NCO Academy) and civilian schooling
  - Serves as a rater for all of the behavioral health officers

Educator of Division Medical Providers

- Ensures that all medical providers are educated about most recent practices in recognition and management of:
  - Posttraumatic stress disorder

(**Exhibit 6-1** *continues*)

Exhibit 6-1 *continued*

- Sleep disorders
- Depression and anxiety
- Psychiatric emergencies
- Traumatic event management
- Use of psychotropic medications during deployment

Clinician

- Serves as a direct provider both in garrison and during deployment
- Understands that care is generally limited to medication management because of limited resources

Administrative Psychiatry

- Performs command-directed evaluations
  - Knows that guidance is provided in Department of Defense Directive 6490.1 and Department of Defense Instruction 6490.4; (can be ordered by the commander or required by Army regulation)
- Performs security clearance evaluations
- Performs forensic exams (sanity boards)
- Writes medical evaluation boards (MEBs)
- Writes Army suicide evaluation reports (ASERs)

Officer and Leader in the Division

- Maintains personal readiness
- Serves as a leader and example for junior officers and enlisted soldiers

ASER: Army suicide evaluation report
BCT: brigade combat team
DUI: driving under the influence
MEB: medical evaluation board
NCO: noncommissioned officer

with the division psychiatrist, BCT providers, and the medical logistic assets as they determine which medications should be used in the area of operations, and know the guidelines for indications, use, and monitoring of psychotropics within the division.

Additionally, the unit behavioral health officer must consider other potential operational activities that might require behavioral health participation, such as detainee operations and preventive training, as well as the soldier resiliency programs. A comprehensive, division level, planning and oversight program, spanning the entire deployment lifecycle, will identify unforeseen obstacles while ensuring that access to care is not impeded by faulty screening programs, unprepared clinical services, or inadequate personnel staffing. At the brigade level it is imperative that a comprehensive planning and oversight program, including brigade behavioral health standard operating procedures (SOPs), be developed within the guidelines of the divisional mental health SOPs.

Attention has been focused on pre- and postdeployment screening by the media and Government Accountability Office for several reasons. These include reports of soldiers being identified during screening but not receiving their consultations or treatment, as well as multiple studies of returning soldiers indicating that rates of reported deployment-related symptoms can increase with time after returning from deployment.[7,9,10,29,30] The responsibility for overseeing an effective screening program (that commanders fully endorse) falls to the division psychiatrist and the DMHA. These plans must focus on education, early identification, and prompt treatment. Additionally, education and coordination must be made with commanders to ameliorate the stigma associated with behavioral healthcare.

Lastly, both during deployment and in garrison, the division psychiatrist must coordinate between, and communicate with, ancillary resources available both within the unit, such as the chaplains and medical providers, and external to the unit. These latter resources include the department of behavioral medicine at the local medical treatment facility and representatives from Military OneSource, Army Community Service, the Army Substance Abuse Program, social work services, garrison chaplain services, and civilian community agencies. Coordination and discussion with these assets arms the psychiatrist with an array of resources available for individual soldiers, families, units, and commanders. In general, for BCTs that are collocated with their division headquarters, the responsibility of coordinating with external resources should fall on the division psychiatrist. However, for BCTs that are in isolated locations, it is the responsibility of the BCT BHO to perform this coordination.

Provide Consultation to Commanders and Command Surgeons on Behavioral Health Trends and Issues

One of the vital roles of unit behavioral health officers is the consultation that they provide to commanders and medical staff. There are many areas on which the psychiatrist or BCT BHO can provide expert advice. Three major areas of concern are prevention, responding to critical events, and dealing with current public affairs issues.

Preventive advice involves prioritizing the threats that have been identified and making recommendations to the medical staff and command on measures to be taken and areas requiring command emphasis. This includes monitoring ongoing trends such as utilization rates of the DMHA, behavioral health hospitalization rates, child and spouse abuse cases, driving under the influence reports, positive drug test results, Army Substance Abuse Program utilization, and pre- and postdeployment health assessment results. Additionally, longitudinal analysis should be made over a significant time frame to visualize current trends and examine behavioral health indicators from current and previous deployments. The outcome of crucial, predictive information could help direct placement and utilization of the limited resources available. Monitoring of these trends should be a regular action and the command should be updated on a monthly basis, in consultation with the command surgeon.

Additionally, a mental health service utilization tracking system that includes the unit, diagnosis, and primary stressor to identify smaller organizational trends, such as at the battalion level, can provide commanders at all levels with valuable information and facilitate targeted interventions.

Case Study 6-2: During a recent deployment, one DMHA was monitoring unit behavioral health trends and noted a significant spike in combat operational stress in a particular battalion. This trend was reported to both the battalion and brigade commander shortly after it developed. The commander then was able to relate that information with safety officer reports of a recent increase in accidents, coupled with a noted decrease in combat effectiveness. This led to the commander switching areas of operation to "give the unit a break" and resulted in both a rapid improvement in combat effectiveness for both units and maintenance of the ongoing combat mission.

In addition to prevention, unit behavioral health officers can have a significant effect in response to potential traumatic events. Working with the unit chaplains, medical resources, and commanders, the division psychiatrist can advise and determine how to respond to deaths, nonbattle injuries, casualties, and other significant events within units. The unit behavioral health officer should develop a traumatic event management plan for advising commanders and responding to soldiers' needs after these occurrences. Being successful in this realm involves good communication, a knowledge and understanding of current medical literature, and good relationships with unit commanders and support resources.

Case Study 6-3: During a recent deployment, one DMHA established a formalized traumatic event management policy. This policy provided clear guidance to the unit commanders and support personnel on how to respond after a potential traumatic event, including contacting the unit mental health and ministry teams to conduct a unit assessment and perform a debriefing if necessary. Additionally, if required, the debriefing would be a joint venture by the behavioral health providers and the chaplains. Whereas during a prior deployment, many of the commanders or chaplains often wanted to conduct sessions immediately upon the return of the unit or conduct full critical incident stress debriefings (which may be harmful), this plan provided clear guidance on how to respond to potentially traumatic events and helped to reduce confusion within the unit.[31] In this case, it was imperative for the BHO to educate command on the importance of the timing and the type of debriefings to reduce potential negative outcomes for the soldiers.

Educating and advising commanders on current ongoing issues of public attention is of critical importance. For example, recent media reports have been critical of the military on such topics as the ability to identify and treat posttraumatic stress disorder and the use of psychotropic medications in combat settings.[30–33] Both the division psychiatrist and BCT BHOs must be aware of these ongoing issues through their own reading and attention. They should be able to advise the commander of any potential questions from media encounters. Identification of these potential topics is accomplished through various sources of information including the unit public affairs officer and review of critical incident reports and serious incident reports. Information can also be gathered from local and national newspaper reports about behavioral health issues in the military and via ongoing communication with the various behavioral health consultants, fellow division psychiatrists, and BCT BHOs about such requests. Responses to media queries should always be coordinated through the unit public affairs officer.

Education of command and support staff can be conducted through various methods: e-mail updates, power-point educational briefings, or prepared commander talking points. The method is at the discretion of the commander and is dependent upon how he or she best processes information. A recommended method is to prepare written talking points in a question-and-answer type format with bulleted responses. It will provide commanders with the information in a succinct format while also preparing them for potential questions from the media.

Supervise the Brigade Combat Team Behavioral Health Officers and Enlisted Mental Health Technicians

The division psychiatrist establishes the standards of care and practices for all the behavioral health providers in the division. The BCT BHO further refines and applies those procedures to the brigade. This task requires the setting of the standards and monitoring practices through ongoing supervision and routine feedback for all BCT BHOs. This is generally done first through a written SOP. Certain taskings or reporting requirements might require a fragmentary order. Areas that require SOPs include operation of the division mental health clinic, record keeping procedures, and management of high-risk personnel. Additionally, the division psychiatrist should establish a supervision policy for chart review and routine feedback, generally conducted on a monthly basis, to all brigade behavioral health officers. For BCTs that are not collocated with the DMHA, it is important for the BCT BHO to obtain the division SOPs and augment them to fit the working environment of the BCT.

Enlisted mental health technicians require ongoing supervision by a licensed provider. Mental health technicians must be supervised at the time of every new soldier encounter and as needed during follow-up evaluations. The supervising provider should use the context of the soldier encounter to teach the enlisted mental health technician about such topics as interviewing techniques, the epidemiology of behavioral disorders, and common adverse medication effects.

Providing this supervision can be challenging with some divisions because not all of the personnel are located at the same installation. Additionally, it is imperative that this feedback and supervision continue throughout deployments, keeping in mind that with the new BCT structure it is likely that BCTs and behavioral health staff from outside the division will be joining the unit during deployment.

An additional responsibility for division psychiatrists is the provision of accruing continuing education for themselves, the BCT BHOs, and the mental health technicians. The BCT BHOs share this responsibility and should be closely involved in the training and education of their assigned technicians. This includes ensuring that there are ongoing training opportunities for educational advancement and access to teaching on the latest information and practices in combat operational stress management. How that is implemented is the responsibility of each division psychiatrist, but consideration can be given to morning reports, monthly training sessions, use of "sergeant's time" training, utilization of local medical treatment facility training, or sending personnel to training conferences or schools.

All behavioral health officers should be encouraged to attend the annual Army Behavioral Health Short Course. This opportunity ensures that behavioral health officers earn sufficient continuing education credits to maintain licensure and promotes professional development, while providing an opportunity for collegiality among officers who are dispersed around the globe. Additionally, all soldiers in the DMHA should attend the combat operational stress course prior to deployment because it provides the most current training on theater policies, lessons learned, and ongoing practices. It also provides an opportunity for teambuilding, predeployment planning, and SOP guidance for those deploying units that are not collocated in garrison.

Lastly, there is the responsibility, as a supervisor, to provide opportunities and advice for career development for BHOs and mental health technicians. This includes counseling soldiers on their duty performance and affording them opportunities to participate in required training, such as the AMEDD career course. Additionally, both the division psychiatrist and the BCT BHOs need to ensure that they develop the writing skills necessary for contributing to, or initiating, developmental counseling forms, officer evaluation reports, noncommissioned officer evaluation reports, and awards.

Educate Division Medical Providers

Because there is only one psychiatrist for a unit of approximately 20,000 soldiers who are, at times, spread over several locations, teaching the unit's primary care providers about key behavioral health issues is imperative, as well as a force multiplier. This can be done through a variety of teaching modalities; creativity is encouraged. Key topics to cover include postdeployment stress, psychiatric emergencies, sleep management, posttraumatic stress disorder, traumatic event management, and depression. This education should include information on recognition, diagnostic evaluation, and pharmacologic management. Pharmacologically, providers should understand the indications for use, common side effects, drug interactions, monitoring requirements, and deployment considerations of each somatic intervention.

The BCT BHO should take responsibility for developing and incorporating this curriculum with the BCT surgeon for providers within the unit. This becomes most important in the deployed environment where the division psychiatrist may not be located close to the brigade. It is incumbent on both the division psychiatrist and the BCT BHO to plan for the continuing curriculum during all portions of the deployment cycle.

Provide Direct Care of Patients

As previously mentioned, the division psychiatrist functions as the senior behavioral health provider for the entire division. Due to other demands, direct clinical opportunities for the division psychiatrist will be limited, and will most often involve brief interventions and medication management. However, to retain skills and credibility, it is important that the psychiatrist continue to maintain practice both during deployment and in garrison.

In garrison the division psychiatrist will be a provider at the consolidated division mental health clinic. Where the division psychiatrist should be located during deployment has been an area of ongoing debate since World War I.[3] With enhanced battlefield communication capabilities offering accessibility to other widely dispersed mental health providers, placing division psychiatrists within the division surgeon section allows them to perform as staff officers and consultants to the command while also providing consultative advice on care, medication management, and other guidance throughout the division via telephonic, e-mail, and, when required, face-to-face evaluations. However, the division psychiatrist should frequently travel to remote sites to provide on-site care, supervision, consultation, guidance, and teaching. This practice not only ensures that the division psychiatrist has a clear understanding of conditions and potential problems throughout the division, but it also enhances visibility from all elements of the forward line units.

The BCT BHO functions as the primary behavioral health provider for the entire BCT. In garrison, BHOs should work in a combined DMHA clinic when possible to help share the workload. When not possible, they are encouraged to collocate with their BCT troop medical clinic because it allows them to maintain close contact with the commanders, medical providers, and soldiers in their units. During deployment, BCT BHOs will routinely locate with their brigade troop medical clinic, but are encouraged to develop close relationships with the combat stress control units supporting their units, which may include collocating clinics.

In both settings, BCT BHOs will be challenged to adapt their schedules and modalities of care, based on the demands of the unit. In general, opportunities for long-term therapy will be very rare. Most interventions will utilize psychoeducation and brief supportive, cognitive, or group therapy modalities.

Fulfill Administrative Psychiatry Requirements

Both the division psychiatrist and the BCT BHO have a large number of administrative responsibilities. Command-directed mental health evaluations are defined in Department of Defense Instructions 6490.4[34] and Directive 6490.1,[35] which outline rules for both command-directed discretionary and nondiscretionary referrals. Nondiscretionary evaluations are those required by regulation, including drill sergeant, recruiter, and sniper evaluations. Additionally, all soldiers undergoing certain administrative ("chapter") separations require mental status evaluations. However, when commanders request evaluations for soldiers who do not require assessment by regulation, they use their discretionary authority to request assessment and feedback. In turn, the qualified unit behavioral health officer provides commanders with feedback and recommendations about their soldiers.

When performing a command-directed evaluation, the evaluator should provide the commander with a formal report of mental status (Department of the Army Form 3822-R, Medical Command Form 699-R) outlining feedback and recommendations. At a minimum, the report should address whether or not a diagnosis exists, a prognosis for the soldier's condition, any duty limitations, review of soldier safety and any safety interventions required, and the soldier's fitness for duty. Regulations require that the commander receive that report no later than 24 hours after completion of the evaluation.

Additionally, BCT BHOs must be familiar with the restrictions that their level of professional degree places on their ability to perform and sign command-directed evaluations. In general, non-PhD social workers are able to perform and sign nondiscretionary evaluations. Discretionary evaluations and those recommending a Chapter 5-13 (personality disorder) or a Chapter 5-17 (failure to adapt) discharge require a PhD-level social worker, or a psychologist, or a psychiatrist. Psychologists who are BCT BHOs are able to perform and sign all forms required for command-directed evaluations.

BCT BHOs who are non-PhD–level social workers should develop contingency plans with their colleagues for performing discretionary command-directed evaluations either in garrison or during deployment. During deployment, this may require coordination with combat stress detachment assets in the area of operations. Additionally, if no psychologists or psychiatrists are available, then a physician (preferably the brigade surgeon) may serve as the signing authority.

At times, military mental health providers may perceive pressure to recommend use of these chapter separations as opposed to a fitness for duty and disability evaluation. This pressure often comes from the patient, the unit, or both who are primarily trying to expedite a rapid exit from the military for varying reasons. These chapter separations are often more expedient, requiring less paperwork and fewer levels of review. However, soldiers who are chapter separated are not afforded medical disability benefits and may reenter military service as early as 6 months after discharge. It is imperative that the military mental health provider conduct a thorough evaluation and ensure appropriate disposition as defined by the current military regulations. It is also important for the service member to understand the meaning and consequences of the evaluation and rationale for separation. This will ensure the best care for the patient, the military, and the society that the soldier may be returning to upon discharge from the military.

In addition, there are a number of other administrative requirements. These include security evaluations for unit soldiers applying for clearance, sanity boards and other forensic psychiatry evaluations when ordered by the courts, and medical evaluation boards when indicated for disposition through medical channels. These assessments all require that the evaluator be either a psychiatrist or psychologist. Lastly, unit behavioral health officers may be asked to perform line-of-duty investigations for those involved in events with unfortunate outcomes, and the Department of Defense suicide event reports when soldiers either make a suicidal gesture or attempt, or complete a suicide. These evaluations can be time consuming, but must be performed expeditiously because they provide commanders and the Army with important information.

Be an Officer and Leader in the Division

Lastly, all BHOs must remember that they are officers in the unit. The Army combat uniform does not display branch insignia; hence, it is imperative that as officers, the division psychiatrists or the BCT BHOs set the standard. They must ensure that they maintain personal readiness and weapons qualification, actively participate in physical training, and attend all functions. It can also be expected that they assume additional taskings; it is their responsibility to perform those duties to the utmost of their ability.

CHALLENGES OF THE POSITION

Balancing the duties and responsibilities of being a division psychiatrist or BCT BHO can be very challenging. There are several other factors that confront those in this position. First, division psychiatrists tend to be junior in rank to other division staff officers. With the recent Modified Table of Organization and Equipment (MTOE) adjustments, the division psychiatrist serves on the staff of the division surgeon (a lieutenant colonel) and works directly with several of the division surgeon's deputies (majors). Additionally, the majority of the officers who directly advise the commanding general are at field-grade level, while the division psychiatrist position has traditionally been filled by individuals shortly after residency who are still at the company-grade (captain) level. This makes it difficult for the individual to gain the trust of the key leaders and advisors. Furthermore, recent changes in assignments have introduced BHOs working for the BCTs who are senior in rank to the division psychiatrist, thus potentially placing psychiatrists in the position of supervising those who are senior to themselves.

The BCT BHO, in turn, serves as a direct advisor to the BCT commander and the BCT surgeon, but is not located within the same unit allocation as those individuals. With the recent MTOE adjustments, the BCT BHO is assigned to the medical company in the brigade support battalion, while the BCT surgeon is assigned to the BCT headquarters unit. This can be very difficult because company and battalion commanders may feel that the BCT BHO "works for them." They may attempt to restrict BHO and enlisted mental health technicians' access to the DMHA and the BCT commander without clearing information through them first. It is the responsibility of the BCT BHOs to work out agreements with their company and battalion commanders about places of duty, interaction with command staff, and required unit activities. BCT

BHOs are reminded to maintain appropriate bearing throughout these interactions and seek the assistance of their division psychiatrists and their BCT surgeons if they are having difficulty.

Access to the enlisted mental health technicians, both in a deployed and garrison environment, can be problematic. This may need to be addressed by the brigade surgeon, the support planning officer, or the division psychiatrist if the BCT BHO is having trouble gaining full use of the mental health technician.

Another challenge is that the BCT BHO works with the BCT surgeon to directly advise the BCT commander about behavioral health issues, but tends to be more junior than other BCT staff officers. In general, both the BCT surgeon and the BCT BHO are junior to mid-level captains or junior majors, while most of the BCT commander's deputies are mid-level to senior majors or other field-grade officers. Being more junior in experience, especially in the operational arena, makes it difficult for the individual to gain the trust of the key leaders and advisors. This requires the BCT BHOs to demonstrate respect, learn about the mission, and develop an understanding of unit capabilities. They must also rapidly adapt to the needs and demands of the BCT commander's staff for updates and information dispersal.

Additionally, both the division psychiatrist and the BCT BHO have to coordinate with other behavioral health resources within the area. While in garrison, the division psychiatrist needs to coordinate resources and the flow of information with the Medical Department activity, medical center, or the local civilian hospitals. This can be difficult at times because many in the hospital positions will not understand the full scope of the division-level BHO's duties and responsibilities. It is possible that they might request that a division psychiatrist, BCT BHO, or enlisted mental health technician work at the local facility and share duty responsibilities. There are no guidelines or specifics on this. Therefore, all such requests should be coordinated locally with the supervising command surgeon.

During deployment, similar coordination will be required. There is potential that a BCT can be spread over a large area through many small forward operating bases, making it difficult for the BCTs limited assets to respond to all of the behavioral health needs. It may be difficult to coordinate with corps-level behavioral health assets for coverage, which will depend on their commanders' opinions on the optimal emplacement of behavioral health resources. In these situations it is vital to have a theater behavioral health consultant who can address these issues.

Another consideration is that, currently, several of the divisions are spread over multiple sites while in garrison. In such situations, it is difficult to both gauge the climate and establish a channel of communication between the BCT BHO and the division psychiatrist. This can create a gap in information flow within the DMHA and can leave a BCT BHO feeling unsupported by the rest of the DMHA. Such a deficiency can persist, and even flourish, during deployment because communications can be unreliable in theater and BCTs may deploy under a different division command than they are assigned to in garrison. It is vital for both the division psychiatrist and the BCT BHO to maintain open communication lines for continued visibility and comprehension of the trends and activities in the units. This provides for continuity of ongoing unit initiatives.

In the theater of operations, assuming unanticipated roles, such as mental health consultant for detainee operations, may present another challenge. In most cases, detainee operations have designated mental health attachments; however, should this service require support of the division psychiatrist, review of local policy, current Army regulations, and Department of Defense guidelines is critical. Comprehensive reference documents would include Army Regulation 190-8, *Enemy Prisoners of War, Retained Personnel, Civilian Internees, and Other Detainees,* and Annex F of the *Mental Health Advisory Team (MHAT) II Report*.[36,37] These, along with current guidance from the US Army surgeon general, can assist the division psychiatrist in ensuring ethical mental healthcare of detainees.

Other stressors in the garrison environment are finances and personnel. The DMHA clinic may be "owned" by the division, where there is little emphasis on workload capture or compensation. Or, as is the case at Fort Drum, New York, DMHA may fold into a larger behavioral health department. Regardless of the specific arrangement, clear boundaries and working agreements must be established between the various organizations to address budgetary, logistical, maintenance, operational, and personnel issues.

There are several possible personnel issues that should be considered. First, in garrison the division resources are limited, as only the maneuver brigades are equipped with BHOs. Units such as the sustainment brigade and combat aviation brigade require support from both division and nondivision resources. Furthermore, it has not been uncommon for BCTs to be missing their full complement of personnel in garrison. This may result in BCT BHOs providing care coverage for soldiers from other brigades at the DMHA clinic or a BCT BHO arriving to the unit shortly before a deployment. During deployment, the division is likely to add BCTs, bringing additional providers who have been working under a different DMHA. It falls upon the division psychiatrist to ensure that all behavioral health providers within the division are properly supervised and educated, and function under the same policies and standards of care.

Lastly, all BCT BHOs should expect to receive supervision, feedback, and information from their division psychiatrist, including those who are not collocated with their divisions. However, under certain circumstances, the BCT BHOs might need to seek supervision from their local Medical Department activity, such as when the division headquarters is deployed while the brigade remains in garrison.

FUTURE DIRECTIONS

With increased public awareness of the behavioral health effects of deployment and the shifting of the Army to a more modular force, the DMHA has many challenging roles. These roles involve a variety of duties and responsibilities that demand a clinically competent provider fluent in the art of multitasking and executive decision making. With the recent Army changes and the increase in size of the division mental health activity, it is imperative that capable, well-prepared psychiatrists, psychologists, and social workers are placed in these positions. With that in mind, several areas of discussion are provided for future consideration.

In the last two decades the US Army has shifted focus away from assets internal to the combat units toward placing emphasis on area support resources (combat support hospitals and combat operational stress control units), which provide coverage based on region rather than units.[3] Furthermore, the combat operational stress control units have larger, more diverse teams normally containing several psychiatrists, psychologists, social workers, and mental health specialists as well as occupational therapists and psychiatric nurses.[11] These units are then spread over a large area providing both preventive and restorative care, often with a centralized restoration center that can provide up to 2 weeks of care.[11]

Many of these units are called to active duty from the Army Reserve or from other branches of service. Few, if any, of these units have had any contact with the units in garrison and thus have not established consultative relationships with the commanders prior to the deployment. Therefore, they do not have the preestablished credibility necessary to provide effective education and consultation to commanders. The essence of this credibility is established in prior demonstration, to command, of the consultant's availability, utility of clinical skills and services, and perception that the consultant is not "investigating or blaming the unit for its problems."[34]

In addition, Department of Defense Directive 6490.5 states that each unit should have training, curricula, and guidance on combat operational stress control with a focus on primary, secondary, and tertiary prevention in garrison.[38] Combat operational stress control units are generally not available in garrison for teaching. Likewise, many medical treatment facilities are not currently capable of providing the primary and secondary prevention and training because of ongoing demands for treatment of soldiers and their family members. This role is, therefore, ideal for the division mental health team and allows for development of strong bonds with units and a sense of ownership among the behavioral teams in their units.

SUMMARY

Now, more than ever, the DMHA is critical. The new modular BCT structure projects mental health resources to lower levels and further toward the front lines. It also allows for development of long-term consultative and treatment relationships at the battalion and company level. This structure can also help to strengthen and emphasize pre- and postdeployment mental resiliency and medical provider training. Maintaining both division and combat stress control mental health resources in a collaborative working environment—where patient-specific issues and policy decisions are jointly determined—allows for continuity of training, education, consultation, and treatment during nondeployed times, with additional mental health resources available during a deployment. Similar lessons are being seen within the US Marine Corps and have led to the development of their Operational Stress Control and Readiness (OSCAR) program. Their program, like that of the US Army, increases the behavioral health resources within the units. That system is placing two psychiatrists within divisions, with one focusing toward the consultative and administrative aspects while the other is leading a multidisciplinary treatment team.

The position of division psychiatrist and BCT BHO presents many challenges, especially in the aspect of balancing responsibilities. The US Marine Corps is the only other US military service that embeds mental health assets with their soldiers and has recognized these same challenges. Because of the complexities of staff, consultant, leadership, teaching, and clinical roles, future assignments to these positions should be based on knowledge, skills, and experience. Preferably, such individuals should be field-grade officers who have served at least one utilization tour after residency to gain experience as a practicing psychiatrist, and are graduates of the AMEDD career course. Additionally, as noted in the 5th iteration of the Mental Health Assessment Team's report, consideration should be given to expanding mental health resources within the divisions, including the addition of an enlisted mental health technician in each battalion and an aeromedically trained psychologist in each combat aviation brigade.

REFERENCES

1. Glass AJ. Lessons learned. In: Anderson RS, Glass AJ, Bernucci RJ, eds. *Neuropsychiatry in World War II. Vol I. Zone of the Interior.* Washington, DC: Government Printing Office; 1966: 735–759.

2. Bailey P, Williams FE, Komora PA, Salmon TW, Fenton N. *Neuropsychiatry.* In: *The Medical Department of the United States Army in the World War.* Washington, DC: Department of the Army, Office of The Surgeon General; 1929: 303–310.

3. Rock NL, Stokes JW, Koshes RJ, Fagan J, Cline WR, Jones FD. US Army combat psychiatry. In: Jones FD, Sparacino LR, Wilcox VL, Rothberg JM, Stokes JW, eds. *War Psychiatry.* In: Zajtchuk R, Bellamy RF, eds. *Textbooks of Military Medicine.* Washington, DC: Department of the Army, Office of The Surgeon General, Borden Institute; 1995: 149–175.

4. US Department of the Army. *Neuropsychiatry and Mental Health.* Washington, DC: DA; June 18, 1959. Army Regulation 40-216.

5. US Department of the Army. *Combat Stress Control in a Theater of Operations: Tactics, Techniques, and Procedures.* Washington, DC: HQDA; 1998. Field Manual 8-51, Change 1.

6. US Department of the Army. *2004 Army Transformation Roadmap*. Washington, DC: DA; July 2004.

7. Hoge CW, Castro CA, Messer SC, McGurk D, Cotting DI, Koffman RL. Combat duty in Iraq and Afghanistan, mental health problems, and barriers to care. *N Eng J Med.* 2004;351:13–22.

8. Hoge CW, Auchterlonie JL, Milliken CS. Mental health problems, use of mental health services, and attrition from military service after returning from deployment to Iraq or Afghanistan. *JAMA.* 2006;295:1023–1032.

9. Southwick SM, Morgan CA 3rd, Darnell A, et al. Trauma-related symptoms in veterans of Operation Desert Storm: a 2-year follow-up. *Am J Psychiatry.* 1995;152:1150–1155.

10. Grieger TA, Cozza SJ, Ursano RJ, et al. Posttraumatic stress disorder and depression in battle-injured soldiers. *Am J Psychiatry.* 2006;163:1777–1783.

11. Appenzeller, GN, Warner CH, Grieger T. Postdeployment health reassessment: a sustainable method for brigade combat teams. *Mil Med*. 2007;172:1017–1023.

12. Department of the Army. *Combat and Operational Stress Control.* Washington, DC: DA; 2006. Field Manual 4-02.51.

13. Jones E, Palmer IP. Army psychiatry in the Korean War: the experience of 1 Commonwealth Division. *Mil Med.* 2000;165:256–260.

14. Engel CC, Campbell SJ. Revitalizing division mental health in garrison: a post-Desert Storm perspective. *Mil Med.* 1993;158:533–537.

15. Ritchie C, White R. Becoming a successful division psychiatrist: guidelines for preparation and duties of the assignment. *Mil Med.* 1993;158:644–648.

16. Hill JV, Lange C, Bacon B. Becoming a successful division psychiatrist: the sequel. *Mil Med.* 2007;172:364–369.

17. Leamon MH, Sutton LK, Lee RE. Graduate medical educators and infantry commanders: working together to train Army psychiatry residents. *Mil Med.* 1990;155:430–432.

18. Deeken MG, Newhouse PA, Belenky GL, Eshelman SD, Parker MT, Jones FD. Division psychiatrists in peacetime. *Mil Med.* 1985;150:455–457.

19. Noy S. Division-based psychiatry in intensive war situations: suggestions for improvement. *J R Army Med Corps.* 1982;128:105–116.

20. Warner CH, Appenzeller GN, Barry MJ, Morton A, Grieger T. The evolving role of the division psychiatrist. *Mil Med.* 2007;172:918–924.

21. Glass AJ. Psychiatry at the division level. In: Anderson RS, ed. *Combat Psychiatry: Experiences in the North African and Mediterranean Theaters of Operation, American Ground Forces, World War II.* Washington, DC: Government Printing Office; 1949: 45–73.

22. Warner CH, Breitbach JB, Appenzeller GN, Yates V, Grieger T, Webster WG. Division mental health in the new brigade combat team structure. Part I. Predeployment and deployment. *Mil Med.* 2007;172:907–911.

23. Warner CH, Breitbach JB, Appenzeller GN, Yates V, Grieger T, Webster WG. Division mental health in the new brigade combat team structure. Part II. Redeployment and postdeployment. *Mil Med.* 2007;172:912–917.

24. McCarroll JE, Jaccard JJ, Radke AQ. Psychiatric consultation to command. In: Jones FD, Sparacino LR, Wilcox VL, Rothberg JM, eds. *Military Psychiatry: Preparing for Peace for War.* In: Zajtchuk R, Bellamy RF, eds. *Textbook of Military Medicine.* Washington, DC: Department of the Army, Office of The Surgeon General, Borden Institute; 1994: 151–170.

25. Kirkland FR, Jackson MA. Psychiatric support for commanders. In: Jones FD, Sparacino LR, Wilcox VL, Rothberg JM, eds. *Military Psychiatry: Preparing for Peace for War.* In: Zajtchuk R, Bellamy RF, eds. *Textbook of Military Medicine.* Washington, DC: Department of the Army, Office of The Surgeon General, Borden Institute; 1994: 171–192.

26. Koshes RJ, Plewes JM, McCaughey BG, Stokes J. Educating mental health workers. In: Jones FD, Sparacino LR, Wilcox VL, Rothberg JM, eds. *Military Psychiatry: Preparing for Peace for War.* In: Zajtchuk R, Bellamy RF, eds. *Textbook of Military Medicine.* Washington, DC: Department of the Army, Office of The Surgeon General, Borden Institute; 1994: 193–213.

27. Lande RG. A model combat psychiatry training program for division personnel. In: Jones FD, Sparacino LR, Wilcox VL, Rothberg JM, eds. *Military Psychiatry: Preparing for Peace for War.* In: Zajtchuk R, Bellamy RF, eds. *Textbook of Military Medicine.* Washington, DC: Department of the Army, Office of The Surgeon General, Borden Institute; 1994: 215–226.

28. Major General WG Webster. Commander, Task Force Baghdad. Personal communication, September 17, 2005.

29. Government Accountability Office. *Post Traumatic Stress Disorder: DoD Needs to Identify the Factors Its Providers Use to Make Mental Health Evaluation Referrals for Servicemembers.* Washington, DC: GAO; May 2006: 1–34. Report No. GAO-06-397.

30. Milliken CS, Auchterlonie JL, Hoge CW. Longitudinal assessment of mental health problems among active and reserve component soldiers returning from the Iraq War. *JAMA.* 2007;298:2141–2148.

31. Jacobs J, Horne-Moyer HL, Jones R. The effectiveness of critical incident stress debriefing with primary and secondary trauma victims. *Int J Emerg Ment Health.* 2004;6:5–14.

32. Chedekel L, Kauffman M. Mentally Unfit, Forced to Fight. *Hartford Courant.* 2006, May 14, 2006. Available at: www.courant.com/news/nationworld/hc-unfit0515.artmay14,0,7374793.story. Accessed April 24, 2009.

33. Thompson M. America's medicated army. *Time.* June 5, 2008. Available at: www.time.com/time/nation/article/0,8599,1811858,00.html. Accessed April 24, 2009.

34. Department of Defense. *Requirements for Mental Health Evaluations of Members of the Armed Forces.* Washington, DC: DoD; August 28, 1998. DoD Instruction 6490.4.

35. Department of Defense. *Mental Health Evaluations of Members of the Armed Forces.* Washington, DC: DoD; October 1, 1997. DoD Directive 6490.1.

36. US Department of the Army. *Enemy Prisoners of War, Retained Personnel, Civilian Internees, and Other Detainees.* Washington, DC: DA; October 1, 1997. Army Regulation 190-8.

37. Mental Health Advisory Team (MHAT-II). *Operation Iraqi Freedom (OIF-II). Annex F: Internment Detainee Facility Assessment of Mental Health Advisory Team (MHAT) II. Report.* The US Army Surgeon General. January 30, 2005. Available at: www.armymedicine.army.mil/reports/mhat.html. Accessed September 4, 2008.

38. Department of Defense. *Combat Stress Control (CSC) Programs.* Washington, DC: Department of Defense; February 23,1999. DoD Directive 6490.5.

Chapter 7

US MARINE CORPS AND NAVY COMBAT AND OPERATIONAL STRESS CONTINUUM MODEL: A TOOL FOR LEADERS

WILLIAM P. NASH, MD*

*Captain, US Navy (Retired); Assistant Clinical Professor, Department of Psychiatry, University of California at San Diego; formerly, Senior Consultant, Defense Centers of Excellence for Psychological Health and Traumatic Brain Injury, Rosslyn, Virginia

INTRODUCTION

In the US military, the overall responsibility for preserving the health of operationally deployed service members is assigned to commanders of combatant commands.[1] Only operational commanders are in a position to balance the evolving tactical requirements that inevitably place service members in harm's way against the enduring strategic imperative to preserve the health of the force. Only line commanders can lead the full spectrum of force health protection activities necessary to "promote, protect, improve, conserve, and restore the mental and physical well being of Service members across the range of military activities and operations."[1(p10)] And only trusted leaders and mentors can reduce the stigma associated with acknowledging mental health problems, and make it acceptable for service members to receive help for them. Even in garrison, line commanders cannot delegate their force health protection responsibilities to medical or religious ministry support personnel, although such support is crucial to accomplishing the health protection mission. The dual goals of force health protection are force conservation and long-term physical and psychological health and well-being for service members and their families.

Military commanders and their health and religious ministry advisors have historically approached psychological health (PH) protection, including combat and operational stress control (COSC), somewhat differently from physical health protection because of the "demedicalized" model of combat stress reactions that has persisted since World War I.[2–4] In this model, combat and operational stress reactions have been viewed not as injuries or illnesses but as temporary and reversible responses to stress over which the individual is believed to retain a significant degree of control. Principles of forward management of stress reactions based on this model, summarized in the acronyms PIES (proximity, immediacy, expectancy, simplicity) and BICEPS (which adds brevity and contact or centrality), recommend that service members suffering from combat and operational stress reactions not be permitted to perceive themselves as sick, ill, or injured (see also Chapter 4, Combat and Operational Stress Control).[5] Early screening and treatment for significant symptoms of mental illness is eschewed in favor of "normalizing" stress reactions and using the power of suggestion ("expectancy") to encourage return to previous occupational functioning. The approach to be taken to service members suffering from combat stress in a war zone, according to this demedicalized model, is summarized in the words of Colonel (Retired) Franklin D Jones, former psychiatry and neurology consultant to the US Army surgeon general, writing in *War Psychiatry* in 1995: "You are neither sick nor a coward. You are just tired and will recover when rested."[5(p9)]

However, evolving scientific thought provides a strong argument, in this author's opinion, for developing a model that bases PH protection and COSC on the same preventive medicine principles that underlie physical health protection. Posttraumatic stress disorder (PTSD), for example, is now known to be a relatively common, potentially disabling, and possibly preventable illness with significant biological, psychological, and social-spiritual components.[6] The risk for PTSD rises in direct proportion to the level of exposure to combat,[7] and the symptoms of PTSD and other stress-related mental disorders are clearly present in personnel in deployed operational settings.[8] Also, the overlap between PTSD and mild traumatic brain injury, both in symptoms and underlying brain pathology, argues for adopting similar approaches to recognizing and managing these two separate but related health problems.[9] Furthermore, PH protection efforts based on previous, demedicalized models have failed to prevent significant postdeployment PTSD in veterans of the wars in Vietnam[10–14] and Iraq.[7,15,16]

In recent years, operational commanders in the US Marine Corps and Navy have collaborated with mental health and religious ministry professionals to develop new PH protection tools for the operating forces. Based on the science of preventive medicine and the art of leadership, these tools have been crafted to fit the needs of commanders and subordinate leaders at all levels. The most basic of these tools is the combat and operational stress continuum doctrinal model (also known as the stress injury continuum model, as described in Chapter 8, Expeditionary Operational Stress Control in the US Navy).

COMBAT AND OPERATIONAL STRESS CONTINUUM

Background and Development

The February 1996 Department of Defense (DoD) inspector general report on combat stress control in the military defined comprehensive COSC as consisting of three key activities—(1) prevention, (2) identification, and (3) treatment—to be applied before, during, and after deployment.[17] Three years later, DoD directed all services to implement COSC programs that included these key activities.[18] However, the imperative to implement PH prevention, identification, and treatment based on the normalizing, demedicalized model has posed two challenges:

1. If all reactions to stress in operational environments are truly "normal," then what is there to prevent and treat? After all, normality is neither prevented nor treated.
2. If all reactions to stress are normal, whereas PTSD and other stress-induced mental disorders are clearly not normal, where is the line to be drawn between them? Where does normality end and pathology begin?

To meet these challenges, the bridging concept of "stress injuries" was developed in the Marine Corps in 2004.[19] Independently, and for similar reasons, the term "operational stress injury" had been established in the Canadian Forces by Lieutenant Colonel Stephane Grenier, a veteran of the 1994 United Nations mission to Rwanda.[20] The validity of the idea that overwhelming or persistent stress can inflict literal injuries to the brain, mind, and spirit is supported by two lines of reasoning. First is the argument that the only alternative to acknowledging that humans can be literally injured by stress is to posit that human brains, minds, and spirits are invincible and unbreakable regardless of the forces acting on them, which cannot be true because the mind and brain are material living systems that are susceptible to damage, senescence, and death. The second argument is based on the assertion that some (though not all) stress responses or outcomes in operational environments fully meet the definitions of the terms "injury" or "wound" as commonly used in medical and nonmedical discourse.[21] In common usage, an injury can be defined as something that

- happens to a person rather than being chosen,
- involves a loss of normal integrity,
- causes at least a temporary loss of function,
- provokes predictable self-protective and healing responses, and
- cannot be undone, although it usually heals over time.

The element of volition in this definition, when applied to stress outcomes, is hard to prove; there is a long tradition of viewing all stress "responses" as chosen by the individual on at least an unconscious level. However, the universal experience of individuals who experience traumatic stress involving terror, horror, or helplessness is one of being acted upon rather than acting. In fact, it may be that the loss of volition during a traumatic event partly defines it as traumatic. Furthermore, the most disabling symptoms of unhealed traumatic stress, such as panic attacks, flashbacks, and rage outbursts, are disabling to the extent they cannot be predicted or prevented by conscious choice.

The second element in the list, loss of integrity, is certainly not externally evident in the same way that loss of the integrity of skin or bone is obvious in the case of physical injury. However, the preponderance of evidence from preclinical studies suggests that acute or chronic stress can cause a loss of the normal integrity of the neurobiological systems necessary for effectively coping with stress, particularly those responsible for regulating arousal and emotional intensity.[6] And the integrity of necessary and deeply held beliefs and attachments are clearly compromised by trauma or loss.[6]

The loss of function caused by a stress injury, the third listed item, is likely the most evident and observable feature, although sometimes only to stress-injured individuals themselves, or those closest to them. Little is known about normal self-protective and healing responses to stress injuries (the fourth item listed), but included in the *Diagnostic and Statistical Manual of Mental Disorders*, 4th edition, diagnostic criteria for PTSD and acute stress disorder are the characteristic avoidance of reminders of traumas and efforts to reduce excessive arousal through isolation.[22]

Finally, the assertion that stress injuries cannot be undone, although also not yet convincingly shown empirically, is strongly supported by the characteristic and lasting vulnerabilities (or increased growth, in many cases) demonstrated by individuals following acute traumatic stress or stress-induced depressive or anxiety disorders.[19] Certainly, traumatic memories and losses of close comrades cannot be undone.

The concept of stress injuries, as a bridging construct between reversible stress reactions at one end of the stress response spectrum and stress illnesses at the other, has gained partial acceptance in the US sea services. Analogous to physical injuries, stress injuries may be seen as less the fault of the individual than how they are considered in the demedicalized model, which implied that disabling and persistent stress reactions were due to preexisting weakness.[3] However, in 2007, the commanding generals of the three Marine Expeditionary Forces expressed concern that a doctrine based on the stress injury conception could be problematic if it did not give sufficient attention to promoting and restoring resiliency before stress reactions progressed to become injuries, or injuries became illnesses. Therefore, in September 2007, the three forces convened a working group including line commanders, senior enlisted leaders, chaplains, medical and mental health professionals, and Marine Corps Headquarters policy makers. The resulting discussion yielded the combat operational stress continuum model, Figure 7-1, which has since become the foundation for all PH and COSC doctrine, training, and early interventions in both the Marine Corps and Navy.[23]

The continuum model is a paradigm that recognizes the entire spectrum of stress responses and outcomes, from adaptive coping and full readiness (color-coded green as the "ready" zone), to mild and reversible distress or loss of function (the yellow "reacting" zone), to more severe and persistent distress or loss of function (the orange "injured" zone), to clinical mental disorders arising from stress and unhealed stress injuries (the red "ill" zone).

Ready: The Green Zone

The green "ready" zone can be defined as encompassing adaptive coping, effective functioning in all spheres, and personal well-being. The green zone is not conceived to represent the absence of stress, but rather its effective mastery without significant distress or impairment. One important goal of all selection, training, and leadership in the military is to promote green zone readiness, or to restore individuals and units to the green zone once they have experienced distress or loss of function because of stress. The ability to remain in the green zone under stress, and to return quickly to it once impaired or injured by stress, are two crucial aspects of resiliency. Both individual service or family members and entire military or family units can be said to operate in the green zone.

The following are some of the attributes and behaviors characteristic of the green "ready" zone:

- remaining calm and steady;
- being confident in self and others;
- getting the job done;
- remaining in control physically, mentally, and emotionally;
- behaving ethically and morally;
- retaining a sense of humor;
- sleeping enough;
- eating the right amount;
- working out and staying fit;
- playing well and often; and
- remaining active socially and spiritually.

Reacting: The Yellow Zone

The yellow "reacting" zone can be defined as encompassing mild and temporary distress or loss of function due to stress. By definition, yellow zone reacting is always temporary and reversible, although while stress reactions are occurring it is hard to know whether they will be temporary and leave no lasting scars. Yellow zone reactions can be inferred by their time course, relative mildness, and commonness. Although no research has yet been done on the prevalence of subclinical distress or loss of function in operational settings, it is likely that such yellow zone stress reactions may be extremely common, if not

READY	REACTING	INJURED	ILL
DEFINITION • Adaptive coping • Effective functioning • Well-being FEATURES • In control • Calm and steady • Getting the job done • Playing • Sense of humor • Sleeping enough • Ethical and moral behavior	DEFINITION • Mild and transient distress or loss of function FEATURES • Anxious • Irritable, angry • Worrying • Cutting corners • Poor sleep • Poor mental focus • Social isolation • Too loud and hyperactive	DEFINITION • More severe and persistent distress or loss of function TYPES • Trauma • Fatigue • Grief • Moral injury FEATURES • Loss of control • Can't sleep • Panic or rage • Apathy • Shame or guilt	DEFINITION • Clinical mental disorders • Unhealed stress injuries TYPES • PTSD • Depression • Anxiety • Substance abuse FEATURES • Symptoms persist > 60 days after return from deployment

Figure 7-1. The combat and operational stress continuum model with its four color-coded stress zones.
PTSD: posttraumatic stress disorder

universal. Figure 7-2 depicts the time course of green zone adaptation and yellow zone reactions in the face of a new challenge such as an operational deployment or combat mission.[19] As depicted in this diagram, the times of greatest risk for yellow zone stress reactions are just before or at the onset of a new challenge, and at the very end or immediately following that challenge.

The following experiences, behaviors, and symptoms may be characteristic of the yellow "reacting" zone:

- feeling anxious,
- worrying,
- cutting corners on the job,
- being short-tempered or mean,
- being irritable or grouchy,
- having trouble falling asleep,
- eating too much or too little,
- feeling apathetic or losing energy or enthusiasm,
- not enjoying usual activities,
- keeping to oneself,
- being overly loud or hyperactive,
- being negative or pessimistic, and
- having diminished capacity for mental focus.

Injured: The Orange Zone

The orange "injured" zone can be defined as encompassing more severe and persistent forms of distress or loss of function that may not completely reverse over time. Whereas yellow zone reactions, by definition, are like a tree branch bending with the wind—always capable of springing back into place once the wind calms—orange zone injuries, by definition, are like a branch breaking, to some extent, because it was bent beyond its limits. Although stress injuries cannot be undone, like physical injuries, their usual course is to heal over time. But as with physical injuries, healed stress injuries may leave behind a "scar"—a mental or physical remnant, vulnerability, or weakness that will likely fade but may never disappear. As with yellow zone stress reactions, the more lasting nature of stress injuries in the orange zone cannot be easily discerned in their early stages. However, stress injuries may be identified in their early stages both by the severity and persistence of the symptoms they provoke and the intensity of the stressors that cause them. Because stress injuries are not clinical mental disorders, they do not require clinical mental health expertise to recognize them, although operational commanders and small unit leaders rely heavily on their chaplains and organic medical personnel to identify and help take care of orange zone stress injuries.

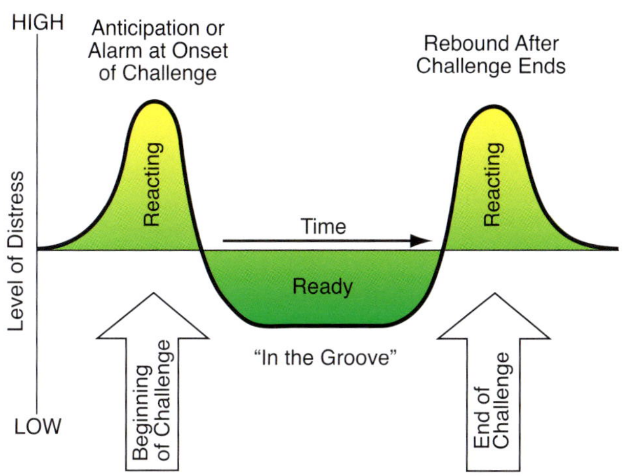

Figure 7-2. Time course of coping and adaptation to a new challenge.

Combat and operational stress injuries have four different possible mechanisms or causes[19]:

1. **Life threat**: exposure to life-threatening situations provoking terror, horror, or helplessness.
2. **Wear and tear**: the accumulation of stress from all causes, including from nonoperational sources, without sufficient sleep, rest, and restoration.
3. **Loss:** separation from cherished people, objects, or portions of oneself.
4. **Inner conflict:** carrying out or bearing witness to acts of omission or commission that violate or disrupt deeply held moral values and beliefs.

Although stress injuries may be caused by one or more of these four different mechanisms, the experiences, behaviors, and symptoms that characterize them are similar regardless of mechanism. They include

- losing control of one's body, emotions, or thinking;
- being frequently unable to fall or stay asleep;
- waking up from recurrent, vivid nightmares;
- feeling persistent, intense guilt or shame;
- feeling unusually remorseless;
- experiencing attacks of panic or blind rage;
- losing memory or the ability to think rationally;

- being unable to enjoy usually pleasurable activities;
- losing grounding in previously held moral values;
- displaying a significant and persistent change in behavior or appearance; and
- harboring serious suicidal or homicidal thoughts.

Ill: The Red Zone

The red "ill" zone can be defined as including all mental disorders arising in individuals exposed to combat or other operational stressors. Because red zone illnesses are clinical mental disorders, they can only be diagnosed by health professionals. However, commanders, other leaders, peers, and family members can and should be aware of the characteristic symptoms of stress illnesses. The most widely recognized stress illness is PTSD. However, stress illnesses may take many different forms, often co-occurring in the same individual at the same time or at different times. Common red zone illnesses include

- PTSD;
- depressive disorders, especially major depression;
- anxiety disorders, including generalized anxiety and panic disorder; and
- substance abuse or dependence.

Although the relationship between orange zone stress injuries and red zone stress illness has not yet been well studied, the presence of a stress illness should be strongly suspected whenever symptoms of a stress injury either do not improve or worsen even after removal of the sources of stress. Specific indicators for possible stress illnesses—and the need for mental health evaluation—include

- stress injury symptoms or behaviors that do not significantly improve within 60 days of returning from operational deployment;
- stress injury symptoms that worsen over time rather than improving;
- stress injury symptoms that return after improving or resolving; and
- significant and persistent distress or loss of function that arises after removal from the sources of stress.

The 60-day duration threshold suggested above for diagnosing stress illnesses is somewhat arbitrary. However, it is believed to represent the best compromise between the competing priorities of quickly identifying problems that may not get better without clinical help, and hesitating to clinically label stress problems that may yet resolve on their own. Again, military leaders need not be concerned about whether particular service members do or do not suffer from diagnosable mental disorders, as much as whether the individuals warrant immediate referral to a mental health professional for evaluation of fitness for duty or treatment requirements.

FIVE CORE LEADER FUNCTIONS FOR PSYCHOLOGICAL HEALTH

The combat and operational stress continuum model is broad in its scope, encompassing all conceivable responses and outcomes to stress, both for service members and their families. Clearly, no one group of individuals can manage the entire stress continuum as defined. At the far left of the continuum—the green and yellow zones—the activities of line leadership predominate to promote resiliency. Here, prevention is paramount. At the far right of the continuum—the orange and red zones—medical and mental health professionals are most critical to providing necessary treatment. Chaplains act in operational units both to promote green zone resiliency and to recognize and respond to yellow, orange, and red zone reactions, injuries, and illnesses, including making appropriate referral decisions, although they usually cannot provide definitive treatment for stress injuries or illnesses. Individual service members and family members bear responsibility for maintaining their own psychological health across the stress continuum, including building their own resiliency, managing their own stress reactions, and recognizing and getting help for stress injuries and illnesses when needed. Even though managing the stress continuum requires the involvement and expertise of several groups of stakeholders, the overall PH promotion effort remains the primary responsibility of operational commanders, as previously stated. Line commanders and their subordinate small unit leaders are responsible for coordinating PH and COSC efforts across the stress continuum to preserve both fighting strength and the long-term health and well-being of service members and families.

The Marine Corps and Navy have identified five core leader functions for the promotion of PH across the stress continuum: (1) strengthen, (2) mitigate, (3) identify, (4) treat, and (5) reintegrate. These five core leader functions are defined below as the context within which the stress continuum model is utilized.

Strengthen Service Members

Building resiliency in individuals, units, and families is the first core PH function of military leaders. Individuals enter military service with a set of preexisting strengths and vulnerabilities based on genetic makeup, prior life experiences, personality style, family supports, and a host of other factors that may be largely immutable. However, centuries of experience in military organizations, as well as a number of research studies, have demonstrated that commanders of military units can do much to enhance the resilience of unit members and their families. Activities available to commanders to strengthen their troops fall into three main categories: (1) training, (2) unit cohesion, and (3) leadership.

Training

Tough, realistic training develops physical and mental strength and endurance, enhances service members' confidence in their ability as individuals and as members of units to cope with the challenges they will face, and inoculates them to future stressors. Exactly how preexposure to stress enhances hardiness is not well understood, but emerging evidence suggests that resilience secondary to stress inoculation has both psychological and biological components. Hardy service members have lower heart rates and higher levels of peptides in the brain that are essential for staying calm in the face of severe stress.[24] They also face familiar challenges with greater confidence and less anxiety-induced loss of mental focus or dissociation.[25] One particular challenge for unit leaders is to deliver training that is tough and realistic enough to build resilience, without making it so tough that it inflicts orange zone injuries on the training field.

Unit Cohesion

Unit cohesion, defined broadly as mutual trust and support in a social group, is developed through sharing adversity over time in a group with a stable membership. Two-way communication, both horizontally among peers and vertically between leaders and subordinates, is essential to unit cohesion. Seamless teamwork is a well-known outcome of unit cohesion. Less well known is how membership in a cohesive unit strengthens unit members against the damaging effects of stress, but it is likely that unit cohesion has both biological and psychological impacts. As psychiatrist and author Jonathan Shay has repeatedly pointed out, "the human brain codes social recognition, support, and attachment as physical safety."[26(p210)] Most leaders know how to build cohesive units given enough time and unit stability, but an all too common challenge is to maintain unit cohesion in the face of rotations into and out of the unit, including casualties and combat replacements. Certainly, the unit rotation policies currently practiced in the US military are more conducive to unit cohesion than the individual rotations common during the Vietnam era, but individual augmentees and members of reserve or National Guard units may still be disadvantaged in this important component of resilience. Another challenge for unit leaders is how to forge mutual trust and peer support among families left behind; they are no less part of the unit than the active duty service members who deploy in cohesive units, but they often have much less opportunity to develop social cohesion with other families.

Leadership

Although complex and multifaceted, leadership is an essential factor for the strengthening of unit members and families. Unit members are strengthened by leaders who teach and inspire them, keep them focused on mission essentials, instill confidence, and provide a model of ethical and moral behavior.[27] Another crucial way in which leaders enhance the resilience of their unit members is by providing a resource of courage and fortitude on which unit members can draw during times of challenge.[28,29] The influence leaders have over their subordinates is a sword that can cut both ways—leaders who are in the yellow, orange, or red zones themselves may become detriments to their units unless their own stress is effectively managed.

Mitigate Stressors

Because no service member, however strong and well prepared, is immune to stress, the prevention of stress injuries and illnesses requires continuous mitigation of the stressors to which individuals and units are exposed. Optimal mitigation of stress requires balancing competing priorities. On one side is the intentional subjection of service members to stress in order to train and toughen them, and to accomplish assigned missions while deployed. On the other side are the imperatives to reduce or eliminate stressors that are not essential to training or mission accomplishment, and to restore the biological, psychological, social, and spiritual resources for resilience that are depleted under stress. As depicted in Figure 7-3, each individual's stores of resources for resilience can be likened to a leaky bucket constantly being drained

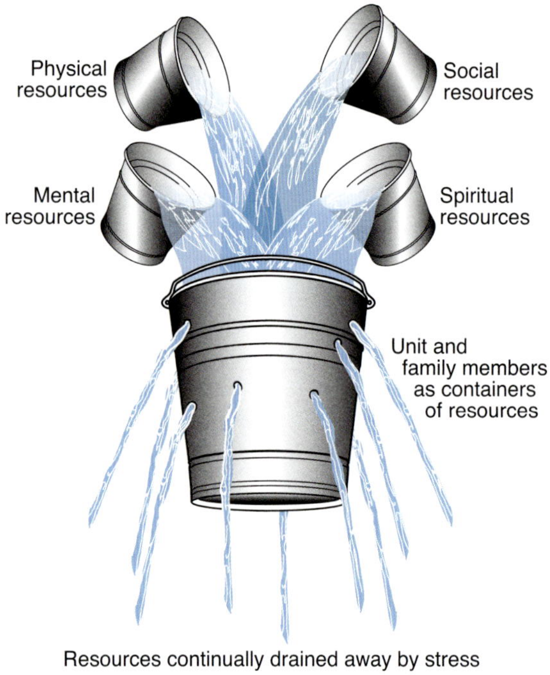

Figure 7-3. "Leaky bucket" metaphor for stress. Each individual's stores of resources for resilience are continually depleted by stress, as if contained in a leaky bucket.

by stress. To keep it from running dry, it must be constantly refilled through sleep, rest, and other forms of replenishment.

Mitigation is a prevention activity, aimed at keeping unit members in the green "ready" zone in the face of operational challenges, and to return them to the green zone after yellow zone reactions. A few of the tactics that can be used by unit leaders to mitigate stress are the following:

- ensure and enforce adequate sleep—7 hours per day for most people;
- ensure physical fitness and recreation;
- encourage spiritual fitness and religious participation;
- enforce ethical standards and the "rules of war";
- rotate units to the rear periodically for rest and replenishment, if possible;
- rotate individual assignments to reduce boredom and complacency;
- protect unit members from scenes of gore whenever possible;
- anticipate and discourage excessive self-blame (guilt or shame); and
- use after-action reviews to give meaning to sacrifices and losses.

Identify Stress Reactions, Injuries, and Illnesses

Even the best PH prevention efforts cannot eliminate all stress problems that might have an effect on occupational functioning or health. Therefore, effective PH protection requires continuous monitoring of stressors and stress outcomes. Operational leaders must know the individuals in their units, including their specific strengths and weaknesses, and the nature of the challenges they face both in the unit and in their home lives. Leaders must recognize when individuals' confidence in themselves, their peers, or their leaders is shaken, or when units have lost cohesion because of casualties, changes in leadership, or challenges to the unit. Most importantly, every unit leader must know which stress zone each unit member is in at every moment, every day. Service members cannot be depended upon to recognize their own stress reactions, injuries, and illnesses, particularly while deployed to operational settings. The external focus of attention and denial of discomfort necessary to thrive in an arduous environment also make it harder to recognize a stress problem in oneself. And stigma can be an insurmountable barrier to admitting stress problems to someone else. Therefore, the best and most reliable method of ensuring that everyone who needs help gets it is for small unit leaders to continually watch out for their subordinates, and for peers to watch out for each other.

To help with this crucial stress zone assessment function, the Marine Corps and Navy have developed the combat and operational stress decision flowchart, Figure 7-4. The flowchart is made up of just four questions. The first is whether there are signs of distress or loss of function, both of which are briefly defined with examples. In the continuum model and decision flowchart, the threshold for recognizing yellow zone reactions is set intentionally low. In other words, to qualify as "distress" or "loss of function," subjective feelings of uneasiness or observable behaviors that interfere with optimal function need not be profound, but merely noticeable. The point is to recognize yellow zone stress reactions early and consistently so they can be monitored and mitigated by leaders, chaplains, and medical support personnel before they progress to orange zone injuries. This is not to say that service members in the yellow zone cannot be pushed harder—just that they may require reassessment and at least stress mitigation as soon as operational requirements permit.

If neither distress nor loss of function is present, then the individual is judged to be in the green zone, and no further action is required other than continuing to monitor for stress. If either distress or loss of

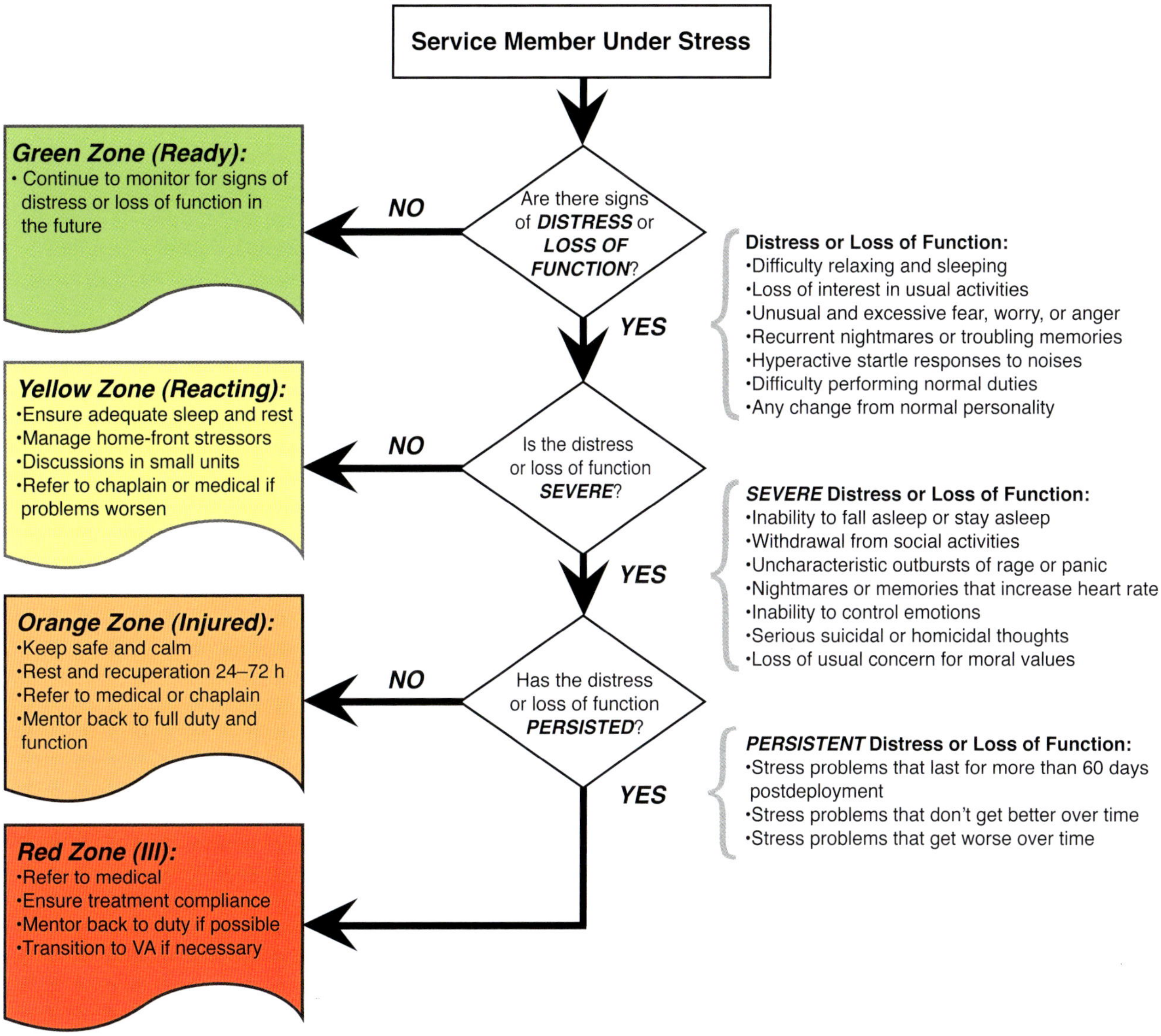

Figure 7-4. The combat and operational stress decision matrix flowchart.
VA: Department of Veterans Affairs

function *is* present, the individual is at least in the yellow "reacting" zone, and the next question to be answered is whether distress or loss of function is *severe*. The decision about whether distress or loss of function is severe is admittedly one of the most challenging judgments to be made in the decision matrix, but it is also one of the most important. By definition, stress responses that involve severe distress or loss of function are at least in the orange zone—at least stress injuries, if not diagnosable stress illnesses. These are stress outcomes that may significantly interfere with effective occupational functioning, may persist or leave a mental or emotional "scar," and may confer increased risk for long-term mental health problems. Because of these risks associated with orange and red zone stress, it is imperative that unit leaders quickly and consistently identify service members with severe distress or loss of function that places them in these two zones. Orange and red zone stress injuries and illnesses all potentially benefit from care and treatment, and all deserve to be closely monitored to ensure recovery.

If severe distress or loss of function is present, the next question—whether these severe stress symptoms have persisted long enough to meet criteria for diagnosis of a clinical mental disorder—is not as crucial for operational commanders to answer. Clinical medical and mental health professionals are normally consulted to help form that judgment. However, the importance to commanders of having a service member in the red zone is significant because a number of important leader decisions follow, including whether the red zone service member is fit to deploy or remain deployed, and whether and how soon the individual can be mentored back to full duty after receiving treatment.

Treat Stress Injuries and Illnesses

As in the case of physical injuries and illnesses, available tools for the treatment of stress injuries and illnesses exist along a broad spectrum, including: (*a*) self- or buddy-applied aid; (*b*) supportive care and advanced aid from a buddy, leader, chaplain, or family member; and (*c*) definitive psychological or medical treatment. Although some of these forms of treatment can clearly be delivered only by a trained medical or mental health provider, others require little special training and can be provided by a small unit leader, peer, or spouse. However, as with the rest of the core functions required to manage the combat and operational stress continuum, the primary responsibility for ensuring that every service member receives the appropriate level of care for orange zone injuries or red zone illnesses rests with operational commanders.

Combat and Operational Stress First Aid

The core principles for immediate, preclinical care of stress injuries, like those for first aid of physical injuries, are built on a simple hierarchy of three priorities: (1) sustain life, (2) minimize further damage, and (3) decide whether further care is needed. For physical first aid, life is sustained through the "ABCs" of basic life support or cardiopulmonary resuscitation—airway, breathing, and circulation—and further damage is minimized through the cleaning and covering of wounds, rest, immobilization, and other basic protective actions. To provide military personnel and their families a set of procedures for the care of stress wounds analogous to those of physical first aid, the Navy, Marine Corps, Defense Centers of Excellence for Psychological Health and Traumatic Brain Injury, and the Veterans Affairs (VA) National Center for PTSD collaborated to develop combat and operational stress first aid (COSFA),[30] based on the evidence-based principles and procedures of psychological first aid previously created by the National Child Traumatic Stress Network and the National Center for PTSD.[31] The seven core components (the "seven Cs") of COSFA are as follows:

1. **Check**: assess continuously for distress or changes in functioning suggestive of a possible stress injury and need for further intervention; reassess after every intervention; continue to assess for delayed or persistent problems.
2. **Coordinate**: continuously inform those who need to know, such as leaders or family members, about identified stress problems; enlist further help from others, as indicated; and ensure that help is obtained.
3. **Cover**: ensure the safety (get to cover) of those experiencing acute distress or alterations in functioning, and ensure the safety of others until normal functioning returns.
4. **Calm**: reduce the intensity of physiological arousal (heart rate and blood pressure) and potentially destructive emotions such as fear or anger; practice deep, diaphragmatic breathing, mental grounding, and other relaxation techniques.
5. **Connect**: ensure peer support in the aftermath of a stress reaction, injury, or illness; restore normal unit or family cohesion as a protective and healing factor; listen empathically and reassure.
6. **Competence**: restore capabilities and effectiveness in all areas of function, including occupational, family, and other social function; mentor back to full duty, if possible.
7. **Confidence**: restore self-esteem and the trust of others in the unit and family in the aftermath of a stress reaction, injury, or illness; restore hope.

Definitive Psychological or Medical Treatment

Definitive clinical care can be delivered in forward operational settings by mental health professionals, such as those attached to Marine Corps Operational Stress Control and Readiness (OSCAR) teams,[32] or it can be delivered in higher echelon treatment facilities in theater or in garrison. The principles of evidence-based care for traumatic stress injuries and illnesses, including PTSD, are contained in the current VA/DoD clinical practice guideline for the treatment of posttraumatic stress.[33] Some of these treatment principles can be applied only by a mental health specialist, but others can be delivered by primary care providers organic to, or in support of, operational units. Regardless of who delivers definitive clinical care, the crucial role of operational commanders and their subordinate small unit leaders in this segment of the treatment continuum is to ensure that treatment is afforded to all service members who need it, and that barriers to care such as stigma and ongoing training or operational time commitments do not preclude care. The earlier stress-injured or ill service members receive definitive clinical care, the more likely they are to recover quickly and fully. Operational commanders bear great responsibility for reducing the stigma associated with receiving mental healthcare because of their influence on the attitudes and behaviors that underlie stigma.

Reintegrate Stress Casualties

As stated above, the normal course for a stress injury, as for a physical injury, is to heal over time. The vast majority of these injuries do heal, with or without treatment. Similarly, the normal course for a stress illness, especially if properly treated, is to improve significantly over time, perhaps even to remit. For example, of all active duty marines diagnosed and treated for PTSD between the start of the war in southwest Asia in 2003 and the end of 2006, fewer than 10% received a medical disability discharge for PTSD.[34] Therefore, operational commanders face one final challenge in their management of service members treated for stress injuries or illnesses—that of continually monitoring their fitness for duty, including worldwide deployment, and mentoring them back to full duty as they recover. This is the challenge of reintegration. For stress casualties to be effectively reintegrated in their units, stigma must be continually addressed. Confidence in stress casualties, both in themselves and their peers and small unit leaders, must be restored. This process may take months to bring to successful conclusion, for recovery from a stress injury or illness can take several months. In cases in which substantial recovery and return to full duty is not anticipated, the challenge for operational commanders is to assist service members as they transition to civilian life and VA care.

SUMMARY

The US Marine Corps and the US Navy, in collaboration with the Defense Centers of Excellence for Psychological Health and Traumatic Brain Injury, have developed and adopted a new model for the promotion of psychological health in service members and operational units based on the health sciences and leadership arts. The core of this new paradigm—the combat and operational stress continuum—recognizes that stress responses and outcomes occur across a broad spectrum, whose zones can be color coded green (for "ready," adaptive coping); yellow (for "reacting," mild and reversible distress or loss of function); orange (for "injured," more severe and persistent distress or loss of function); and red (for "ill," a diagnosable mental disorder). Although chaplains and medical and mental health professionals are important for the management of yellow, orange, and red zone stress, operational commanders and small unit leaders bear primary responsibility for the effective management of the entire stress spectrum. The five core psychological health leader functions developed by the Marine Corps and Navy are: (1) strengthen, (2) mitigate, (3) identify, (4) treat, and (5) reintegrate.

The new PH and COSC model described in this chapter has gained traction in the Marine Corps and Navy partly because it reduces stigma and demystifies aspects of PH promotion. It has also gained acceptance because it forms an effective bridge between the worlds of the troops, the chaplain, the family member, and the medical or mental health professional. Only through a shared language and set of tools can all these stakeholders combine forces to address the challenges posed by warfare to the psychological health of service members and their families.

The stress continuum model and associated core leader functions described in this chapter have not yet been empirically tested, although they are solidly informed by scientific evidence. It is anticipated that empirical evaluation will validate some aspects of the model while suggesting improvements to other aspects. Regardless of these outcomes, the approach to combat and operational stress described here lends itself more fully to empirical assessment than previous models based on a less medical view of adverse stress outcomes.

Acknowledgment

The author wishes to thank Brett Litz, Patricia Watson, Mark Smith, Jeffrey Rhodes, and Eduardo Leardo for helpful comments on the manuscript.

REFERENCES

1. US Department of Defense. *Force Health Protection (FHP).* Washington, DC: DoD; 2004. DoD Directive 6200.04.

2. Shephard B. *A War of Nerves: Soldiers and Psychiatrists in the Twentieth Century.* Cambridge, Mass: Harvard University Press; 2001.

3. Lerner P. *Hysterical Men: War, Psychiatry, and the Politics of Trauma in Germany, 1890–1930.* Ithaca, NY: Cornell University Press; 2003.

4. Wessely S. Risk, psychiatry, and the military. *Brit J Psychiatry.* 2005;186:459–466.

5. Jones FD. Psychiatric lessons of war. In: Jones FD, Sparacino LR, Wilcox VL, Rothberg JM, Stokes JW, eds. *War Psychiatry.* In: Zajtchuk R, Bellamy RF, eds. *Textbook of Military Medicine.* Washington, DC: Department of the Army, Office of The Surgeon General, Borden Institute; 1995: Chap 1.

6. Nash WP, Baker DG. Competing and complementary models of combat stress injury. In: Figley CR, Nash WP, eds. *Combat Stress Injury: Theory, Research, and Management.* New York, NY: Routledge; 2007.

7. Hoge CW, Castro CA, Messer SC, McGurk D, Cotting DI, Koffman RL. Combat duty in Iraq and Afghanistan, mental health problems, and barriers to care. *N Engl J Med.* 2004;351:13–22.

8. US Army Office of the Surgeon General. *Operation Iraqi Freedom Mental Health Advisory Team Report, 16 December 2003.* Washington, DC: OTSG; 2003.

9. Kennedy JE, Jaffee MS, Leskin GA, Stokes JW, Leal FO, Fitzpatrick PJ. Posttraumatic stress disorder and posttraumatic stress disorder-like symptoms and mild traumatic brain injury. *J Rehabil Res Dev.* 2007;44(7):895–920.

10. Kulka RA, Schlenger WE, Fairbank JA. *Trauma and the Vietnam War Generation: Report of Findings From the National Vietnam Veterans Readjustment Study.* New York, NY: Brunner/Mazel; 1990.

11. Dohrenwend BP, Turner JB, Turse NA, Adams BG, Koenen KC, Marshall R. The psychological risks of Vietnam for U.S. veterans: a revisit with new data and methods. *Science.* 2006;313:979–982.

12. Schlenger WE, Kulka RA, Fairbank JA, et al. The psychological risks of Vietnam: the NVVRS perspective. *J Trauma Stress.* 2007;20(4):467–479.

13. McNally RJ. Revisiting Dohrenwend et al's revisit of the National Vietnam Veterans Readjustment Study. *J Trauma Stress.* 2007;20(4):481–486.

14. Kilpatrick DG. Confounding the critics: the Dohrenwend and colleagues reexamination of the National Vietnam Veterans Readjustment Study. *J Trauma Stress.* 2007;20(4):487–493.

15. Hoge CW, Auchterlonie JL, Milliken CS. Mental health problems, use of mental health services, and attrition from military service after returning from deployment to Iraq or Afghanistan. *JAMA.* 2006;295:1023–1032.

16. Smith TC, Ryan MA, Wingard DL, Slymen DJ, Sallis JF, Kritz-Silverstein D. New onset and persistent symptoms of post-traumatic stress disorder self-reported after deployment and combat exposures: prospective population based US military cohort study. *BMJ.* 2008; 336:366–371.

17. US Department of Defense Inspector General. *Evaluation Report on the Management of Combat Stress Control in the Department of Defense.* Arlington, Va: DoD IG; 1996. Report No. 96-079.

18. US Department of Defense. *Combat Stress Control (CSC) Programs.* Washington, DC: DoD; 1999. DoD Directive 6490.5.

19. Nash WP. Combat/operational stress adaptations and injuries. In: Figley CR, Nash WP, eds. *Combat Stress Injury: Theory, Research, and Management.* New York, NY: Routledge; 2007.

20. Grenier S, Darte K, Heber A, Richardson D. The operational stress injury social support program: a peer support program in collaboration between Canadian Forces and Veterans Affairs Canada. In: Figley CR, Nash WP, eds. *Combat Stress Injury: Theory, Research, and Management.* New York, NY: Routledge; 2007.

21. Nash WP. Combat/operational stress injuries (COSIs): fact or fiction? Paper presented at: Marine Corps Combat and Operational Stress Control Conference; June 18, 2007; Arlington, Va.

22. American Psychiatric Association. *Diagnostic and Statistical Manual of Mental Disorders.* 4th ed. Washington, DC: APA; 1994.

23. US Marine Corps. *Tri-MEF Combat Operational Stress Conference.* Camp Pendleton, Calif: I, II, and III Marine Expeditionary Forces. Letter to the Commandant, 12 September 2007. Available at: http://www.mca-marines.org/Gazette/PDF/USMCLetterPP.pdf. Accessed March 30, 2009.

24. Morgan CA 3rd, Wang S, Mason J, et al. Hormone profiles in humans experiencing military survival training. *Biol Psychiatry.* 2000;47:891–901.

25. Morgan CA 3rd, Hazlett G, Wang S, Richardson EG, Schnurr P, Southwick SM. Symptoms of dissociation in humans experiencing acute, uncontrollable stress: a prospective investigation. *Am J Psychiatry.* 2001;158:1239–1247.

26. Shay J. *Odysseus in America: Combat Trauma and the Trials of Homecoming.* New York, NY: Scribner; 2003.

27. US Marine Corps. *Leading Marines.* Washington, DC: Headquarters USMC; 2002. MCWP 6-11.

28. Moran CMW. *The Anatomy of Courage.* Boston, Mass: Houghton Mifflin; 1967.

29. Grossman D. *On Killing: The Psychological Cost of Learning to Kill in War and Society.* Boston, Mass: Little, Brown; 1995.

30. Nash WP, Westphal R, Watson P, Litz B. Combat and operational stress first aid (COSFA): A toolset for military leaders. Presented at: Defence Centers of Excellence Warrior Resilience Conference, November 18, 2008; Vienna, Virginia. Available at: http://www.dcoe.health.mil/event_docs/WRC/COSFA Nash DCoE Conf Nov 08 %5bCompatibility Mode%5d.pdf. Accessed April 29, 2009.

31. Brymer M, Jacobs A, Layne C, et al; National Child Traumatic Stress Network and National Center for PTSD. *Psychological First Aid: Field Operations Guide.* 2nd ed. July 2006. Available at: http://www.ncptsd.va.gov/ncmain/ncdocs/manuals/PFA_2ndEditionwithappendices.pdf. Accessed April 29, 2009.

32. Nash WP. *Operational Stress Control and Readiness (OSCAR): The United States Marine Corps (USMC) Initiative to Deliver Mental Health Services to Operational Units.* Quantico, Va: Headquarters USMC; 2006. NATO RTO-MP-HFM-134-25.

33. Department of Veterans Affairs, Department of Defense. DoD/VA clinical practice guideline for the treatment of posttraumatic stress. 2004. Available at: http://www.oqp.med.va.gov/cpg/PTSD/PTSD_Base.htm. Accessed March 12, 2008.

34. Gaskin TA. US Marine Corps combat/operational stress control program update. Paper presented at: Marine Corps Combat and Operational Stress Control Conference; June 18, 2007; Arlington, Va.

Chapter 8

EXPEDITIONARY OPERATIONAL STRESS CONTROL IN THE US NAVY

ROBERT L. KOFFMAN, MD, MPH*; RICHARD D. BERGTHOLD, PsyD†; JUSTIN S. CAMPBELL, PhD‡; RICHARD J. WESTPHAL, PhD, RN§; PAUL HAMMER, MD¥; THOMAS A. GASKIN, PhD¶; JOHN RALPH, PhD**; EDWARD SIMMER, MD, MPH††; and WILLIAM P. NASH, MD‡‡

*Captain, Medical Corps, US Navy; Director of Deployment Health, Department of the Navy, Bureau of Medicine and Surgery, Deployment Health, 2300 E Street NW, Washington, DC 20372

†Commander, Medical Service Corps, US Navy; Chief of Staff, Wounded, Ill and Injured, Bureau of Medicine and Surgery, 2300 E Street NW, Washington, DC 20372

‡Lieutenant, Medical Service Corps, US Navy; Deployment Health Senior Analyst, Department of the Navy, Bureau of Medicine and Surgery, Deployment Health (M3C3), 2300 E Street NW, Washington, DC 20372

§Captain, Nurse Corps, US Navy; Psychological Health Promotion Programs, Department of the Navy, Bureau of Medicine and Surgery, Deployment Health, 2300 E Street NW, Washington, DC 20372

¥Captain, Medical Corps, US Navy; Director, Naval Center for Combat and Operational Stress Control, 34960 Bob Wilson Drive, Suite 400, San Diego, California 92134-6400

¶Director of Combat Operational Stress Control, US Marine Corps, Manpower and Reserve Affairs, Personal and Family Readiness Division, 3280 Russell Road, Quantico, Virginia 22134

**Commander, Medical Service Corps, US Navy; Director for Mental Health, National Naval Medical Center Bethesda, 8901 Wisconsin Avenue, Bethesda, Maryland 20889; formerly, Officer-in-Command, Presidential Support Program, Marine Barracks, Washington, DC

††Captain, Medical Corps, US Navy; Executive Officer, Naval Hospital, 1 Pinckney, Beaufort, South Carolina 29902; formerly, Senior Executive Director for Psychological Health, Defense Centers of Excellence for Psychological Health and Traumatic Brain Injury, Silver Spring, Maryland

‡‡Captain, US Navy (Retired); Assistant Clinical Professor, Department of Psychiatry, University of California at San Diego; formerly, Senior Consultant, Defense Centers of Excellence for Psychological Health and Traumatic Brain Injury, Rosslyn, Virginia 22209

INTRODUCTION

The diversity of US Naval operations, which span air, land, and sea / subsea dimensions, places extraordinary demands on sailors and their families. Although the US Navy has traditionally been a deployed force, the global war on terror (GWOT) has added to the Navy's list of deployment-related stressors. Stress, as it is referred to in this chapter, is considered as a transactional model[1,2] described as a general strain imposed by the operational milieu that disrupts the physical and psychological equilibrium of sailors, the outcome of which is mediated by a complex interplay between variables specific to the individual, the situation, and the dynamic interaction between the two.

The impact of operational stress upon sailors is manifested in the prevalence of mental health problems among sailors who routinely deploy upon operational platforms. For instance, a study of 782 active duty sailors and marines found the 1-year prevalence of any psychiatric illness to be 21% and the lifetime prevalence to be 40%, based on structured computerized telephone interviews designed to make DSM-III-R (*Diagnostic and Statistical Manual of Mental Disorders*, 3rd edition, revised) psychiatric diagnoses.[3] For those deploying to Operation Enduring Freedom and Operation Iraqi Freedom (OEF/OIF), the risk for having symptoms of either of two illnesses, posttraumatic stress disorder (PTSD) or major depressive disorder, is nearly the same: 20% of these service members reported symptoms of at least one of the two disorders, according to a report from the RAND Corporation's Center for Military Health Policy Research.[4] The dual imperatives of mission effectiveness and moral responsibility for sailor health provide the impetus for the Navy Medicine Support Command to develop and implement programs based on a comprehensive operational stress control doctrine.[5] Discussion of these efforts is the focus of this chapter.

STRESS INJURY CONTINUUM MODEL

Because stress injuries occur across a continuum of severity and settings, Navy stress control doctrine must encompass all sailors regardless of their duty, platform, or assignment (afloat and ashore), not just sailors in specific combat environs. Consequently, Navy leadership (in collaboration with the US Marine Corps) has developed an overarching operational stress control program applicable to the full panoply of Navy missions (see also Chapter 7, US Marine Corps and Navy Combat and Operational Stress Continuum Model: a Tool for Leaders). However, much of the seminal theory and applications for stress control in the military are, as one would expect, derived from stress control practices in the combat environment. In that vein, the doctrine being developed to forge broader Navy stress control initiatives into a more theoretically consistent and unified whole is adapted from the combat stress injury model explicated by Figley and Nash.[1] The starting point for this new paradigm in Navy stress control is the stress injury continuum (SIC) model (see Chapter 7, Figure 7-1 for a description of the model). This chapter will apply the SIC model as the rubric for interpreting extant and future Navy stress control programs.

Adopted because of its ability to educate, acculturate, and engage all sailors in stress control, the SIC paradigm highlights how the onus for stress control is shared among line-duty leadership (eg, squadron commanders, division officers, department heads), the individual sailor, and caregivers (eg, Navy Medicine personnel, the Chaplain Corps). The SIC model charges unit leadership with ensuring that sailors are ready for deployment by fostering an atmosphere within commands that promotes mental health and resilience through realistic training, unit cohesion, and mission focus. Sailors who deploy should be competent, socially supported, and mentally prepared to encounter and adaptively cope with operational stressors.[6] The SIC model contains five functions for leaders that encourage them to (1) strengthen the mental resiliency of sailors through realistic and purposeful training; (2) mitigate physiological stressors by maximizing sailors' access to proper sleep, exercise, and nutrition; (3) develop processes for the early identification of stress reactions and injuries; (4) encourage sailors to care for one another (eg, with "battle buddies"); and (5) remove barriers to care by supporting the transition of stress-injured sailors to higher levels of care and fostering stigma-free reintegration of stress-wounded sailors.

At the first stage of the SIC, sailors are prepared to confront stress. At the second stage, sailors are reacting to the unique operational stressors that challenge their physical and psychological equilibrium. The outcome of this reaction becomes a function of person, situation, and person–situation interactions that influence whether the reaction is mild, transient distress or impairment with associated anxiety, irritability, and unwanted behavioral change. However, each operational milieu has some degree of stress reaction that is normative, which makes distinguishing between normative and abnormal stress reactions a critical consideration for leadership, caregivers, and individual sailors alike. Yet, at the reacting point in the continuum, individual sailors must assume primary responsibility for identifying whether they and their fellow shipmates are effectively coping with the strain of their deployment. Although stress reactions are considered normal reactions to high-stress environments, the severity, persistence, and impairment experienced by some sailors may transcend the reactions experienced by the majority of sailors when perceived through the eyes of leaders, shipmates, caregivers, or reacting sailors themselves.

Rather than establishing clear dividing points, the conceptualization of stress injury as a continuum acknowledges the complex interplay between sailors and situations that must be considered when attempting to ascertain whether an individual's stress reaction has surpassed the normative response and moved from stress reaction to the third stage in the SIC—stress injury. Use of the term "injury" here is important because it conveys to leaders the presence of a more serious threat to both the sailors' individual well-being and operational effectiveness. Sources of stress injury can include trauma from experiencing horror, terror, and helplessness during deployment; fatigue derived from accumulated deployment stressors; grief associated with the loss of a valued person or thing; and moral conflict in belief and value systems.[1]

Although stress-injured sailors are still expected to identify these injuries in themselves and others, Navy Medicine and caregivers begin to play a more prominent role in the stress injury phase of the continuum. At this phase, sailors are not expected to cope with their injury alone, but are empowered to seek help from caregivers, who are the primary support for prevention of permanent, debilitating stress injuries. Once a stress illness (behaviors that fall primarily within diagnostic categories such as PTSD, depression, anxiety, and addiction) is identified in a sailor, treatment becomes the primary responsibility of Navy Medicine. Implementation of the SIC model includes the expectation that all leaders, sailors, and caregivers will be able recognize and respond appropriately to sailors in distress.

The stress injury decision matrix (see Chapter 10, Figure 10-3) is an example of an SIC-based tool designed to help leaders, sailors, and caregivers determine if a sailor is ready, reacting, injured, or ill because of an operational or life stressor. The nascent state of SIC makes it difficult to ascertain the outcomes of the model as a doctrine for combat stress control. However, the model's multidisciplinary and theoretical nature, as well as the incorporation of multiple stakeholders, is a promising feature for establishing doctrine. The multifaceted nature of the SIC model also makes it an ideal context for integrating the various operational stress control programs currently in place.

EXPEDITIONARY MEDICAL PLATFORMS

As alluded to in the SIC model, the Navy as an organization assumes two primary roles in combating stress: (1) preventive consultation and (2) care provision. To keep sailors ready, preventive consultation with line leadership supports development of command policies and procedures that both prepare sailors to face the mental rigors of deployment, and identify, help, and reintegrate sailors who have experienced stress injuries and illness. The more traditional role involves direct healthcare service provision to those with stress injuries and the treatment of those diagnosed with stress illness. Because of the quantity of medical personnel, expeditionary medical platforms offer perhaps the widest range of Navy preventive and direct care services in deployed environments. Expeditionary platforms in the Navy consist of fleet hospital ships and expeditionary medical facilities (EMFs). These platforms are a mixture of specific capabilities that ensure mission flexibility within the logistical constraints of the deployed environment. Expeditionary combat and operational stress control platforms must be capable of performing missions that range from combat service support in GWOT to humanitarian assistance and disaster response. Serving as major instruments of diplomacy, these expeditionary platforms have taken Navy Medicine into Afghanistan, Iraq, and Kuwait while simultaneously providing preventive medicine, combat medical support, health maintenance, medical intelligence, operational planning, and mental health services to military personnel.

Hospital Ships

The fleet of hospital ships consists of the USNS *Mercy* and USNS *Comfort*, which are home ported on the west and east coast of the United States, respectively. The hospital ships have inpatient capabilities comparable to major medical facilities ashore. They each have 12 fully equipped operating rooms, a 1,000-bed hospital facility, radiological services, a medical laboratory, a pharmacy, an optometry laboratory, a computed tomography scanner, and two oxygen-producing plants. Both have a flight deck capable of landing large military helicopters, as well as side ports to take on patients at sea.

Expeditionary Medical Facilities

EMF facilities are designed to approximate the same capabilities as fleet hospital ships, yet maintain a smaller logistic footprint with high mobility. EMFs are fully modular, task-organized structures that can be set up in as little as 48 hours. As EMFs continue to evolve, they will provide more robust medical care for major conflicts, low-intensity combat, operations other than war, and disaster/humanitarian relief operations. As modular expeditionary units, EMFs may be employed independently or in combination with the theater's joint health system for evacuation, medical logistics, medical reporting, and other functions.

Taken together, hospital ships and EMFs are unique among forward-deployed operational stress control platforms with respect to the medical nature of their mission. Perhaps the greatest strength of these platforms is that they include high concentrations of caregivers, providing a versatile mixture of expertise and resources that can anchor both ends of the SIC model.

COMBAT AND OPERATIONAL STRESS CONTROL ELEMENTS

The three combat and operational stress control elements discussed in this section—(1) the Special Psychiatric Rapid Intervention Teams (SPRINT), (2) the carrier psychology program, and (3) the Operational Stress Control and Readiness (OSCAR) program—have arisen within the last 30 years as outgrowths of a larger trend within the US armed services to institutionalize the integration of medical health expertise within operational units. In relation to the SIC model, all three programs are oriented to intervene between the stress injury and illness phases of the continuum. However, the carrier psychology program, and the OSCAR program in particular, also play roles at the readiness end of the stress reaction continuum, through the use of operationally embedded caregivers to provide training and preventive consultation to leaders in supporting individual sailor readiness.

Special Psychiatric Rapid Intervention Teams

History

In 1975 a collision occurred between the USS *Belknap* and the USS *John F Kennedy*, resulting in a significant loss of life and extensive damage to both ships. Subsequently, in 1977, a Navy liberty launch collided with another ship in the Barcelona harbor. In both incidents, the vessels involved were home ported on the east coast, and the psychiatry department at Portsmouth Naval Hospital (now Naval Medical Center, Portsmouth) in Virginia received a significant number of patients presenting with stress symptoms related to the incidents. It became apparent to Navy Medicine that a plan for early intervention to avoid stress illness was needed. The same concepts developed to treat stress in combat were modified for use in early intervention with disasters at sea; the result was the birth of the Special Psychiatric Rapid Intervention Teams—"SPRINT."

Composition and Mission

In 1983 SPRINT teams were formally chartered as one of the Navy's Mobile Medical Augmentation Readiness teams. Navy SPRINT teams are formally organized at Bethesda, Maryland; Portsmouth, Virginia; and San Diego, California. Some informal teams are located at various overseas locations. Since their inception, SPRINT teams have not only provided intervention in maritime mishaps, but also supported military operations other than war, military contingency operations, terrorist attacks, and natural disasters. Each team consist of two psychiatrists, two clinical psychologists, one or two chaplains, two or more psychiatric nurses, one or two clinical social workers, and four or more hospital corpsmen psychiatric technicians. An officer is designated as the team leader, and a senior psychiatric technician serves as the leading petty officer. The SPRINT team's mission is to be trained and immediately available in the event of a contingency to (*a*) assess the psychological effects of traumatic stress, (*b*) offer direct support to individuals and units affected by the event, (*c*) identify and refer those needing psychiatric treatment, and (*d*) consult with commanders and leaders to mitigate the negative impact of the event. From the SIC perspective, SPRINT teams become involved at the reacting stage, the goal being to prevent sailors from moving further along toward the injured and ill end of the spectrum. Teams also provide support to families of active duty members.

Unit leaders are responsible for bringing SPRINT teams into the picture. The teams have limited equipment consistent with their goal of being a rapid-reaction force. Rapid fielding requires that the requesting command or agency provide logistical support (berthing, messing, communications, transportation, etc) to the team. Thus, SPRINT teams are deployable worldwide within 24 hours' notice. Examples of prior SPRINT deployments include Hurricanes Andrew, Ivan, and Katrina; the terrorist attack on the USS *Cole*;

the TWA [formerly Trans World Airlines] Flight 800 disaster; a civilian airline crash in Guam; and severe flooding and landslides in Central America. SPRINT teams also supported the guard force in the early days of the detainee mission at Guantanamo Bay, Cuba. In addition to high-profile events, SPRINT teams also regularly respond to smaller-scale events such as work-related accidents that result in the death of a crewmember, suicides, and aircraft mishaps.

Intervention Strategies

SPRINT does not adhere to any specific professional doctrine on intervention methodology. However, team members are expected to be competent in their respective disciplines and well versed on the latest information in crisis intervention techniques and treatment strategies for acute stress and PTSD. This allows the teams the flexibility to adapt their responses to the demands of a particular situation while ensuring that their methodology is based on best practices and, when possible, evidence-based science. During the 1980s and 1990s, the critical incident stress management (CISM) technique was developed to help emergency service workers, such as firefighters, paramedics, and police officers, address particularly stressful events. Attempts were made to adopt CISM for use in military interventions, but its use has since been officially discouraged because it has not been proven effective in controlled trials, and some evidence shows that it could potentially be harmful.[7–9]

Instead, the current focus is on providing command consultation, psychoeducational intervention, and psychological first aid. The team assists the command in developing a strategy to mitigate the impact of the event on the entire organization; provides timely, targeted, and useful information for command members; briefly contacts as many potentially affected individuals as possible; and supports individuals in acute distress. Every attempt is made to avoid early labeling or diagnoses, even for individuals demonstrating significant stress reactions. Rather, affected individuals are encouraged to mobilize their own and community resources to enhance recovery and restore functioning. SPRINT teams generally provide support rather than treatment. A benefit to adopting the support role is that the teams generally do not contribute documentation to medical records, thereby offering a higher level of confidentiality. It is thought that such confidentiality can reduce the potential stigma associated with seeking mental healthcare.

In addition to maintaining expertise in intervention theory and techniques, SPRINT team members must be proficient serving in diverse operational settings, including surface ships, submarines, and aviation platforms; ground-centric Seabee and marine operating areas; and joint service operations. Team members must also be knowledgeable and comfortable in dealing with various Navy systems, organizations, and structural issues that affect how well a command withstands the impact of a stressful event. Most SPRINT responses are short-term (often only 1 day), but have lasted up to 6 months. In virtually all cases, SPRINT teams work closely with local resources, and turn over functions to the local resources as the situation permits.

Training for SPRINT teams involves a variety of approaches. New members always participate in SPRINT missions under instruction before leading missions. Psychiatric residents and psychology interns are encouraged to participate, under supervision of experienced team members. Psychiatric technician students also receive training in disaster and trauma response. Teams conduct regular refresher training in combat and operational stress first aid (COSFA),[10] and many team members also receive familiarity training in CISM (although CISM's use is discouraged, commanders and others often ask about it, and knowledge of the technique can help to educate them). SPRINT teams remain active during wartime, because natural disasters, maritime accidents, and other noncombat stressful events continue during war, although staffing can be a challenge. The concepts, skills, and techniques developed through the Navy SPRINT teams' experiences in peacetime are invaluable for informing and educating the wider Navy mental health community as a whole and contributing to the overall improvement of stress intervention and treatment of the operating forces.

Carrier Psychology Program

History

Since the mid-1990s, psychologists and psychiatric technicians have served as permanent members of ship's company on all US Navy aircraft carriers. Before the initiation of the carrier psychology program, 25 to 30 sailors were medically evacuated (medevaced) from a carrier for mental health reasons during a 6-month deployment.[11] Since the inception of the program, the number of medevacs has averaged fewer than five per deployment. In 2001 the average fuel/transportation cost of a medevac from a deployed carrier was estimated to be $4,400, suggesting that a typical deployed psychologist saves the Navy at least $110,000 per deployment in prevented medevacs alone.[11] "Prevented medevacs" are defined as situations in which sailors are retained onboard, but due to serious psychological difficulties, would likely not have been retained in the absence of a psychologist. Moreover, this figure ignores the immeasurable costs of losing personnel with valuable experience, and the lowered morale among remaining crew members who are forced to perform extra work to make up for unexpected personnel shortages. Nor does the figure include the cost of providing escorts for medevaced personnel. Additionally, nondeployed carriers report an average of 2.8 prevented medical evacuations per month, thus this cost savings extends throughout the carrier training cycle.

There are numerous examples of this cost savings. Aboard the USS *John F Kennedy* in 1999, 28 sailors were medevaced for psychological problems during a 6-month Mediterranean deployment. In 2001, on the ship's first deployment with a psychologist, there were no psychological medevacs.[12] Similar results were seen aboard the USS *Carl Vinson* in 1999[11] and the USS *Enterprise* in 2001.[13] More recent data continue to support this trend. Through 2006 and 2007, the estimated number of prevented medevacs from deployed carriers averaged slightly more than four per month. (All statistics are derived from monthly reports made by each carrier psychologist; the data are maintained by the Navy clinical psychology community.)

Prevention of Chronic Psychological Problems

Embedded mental health providers are in the unique position of being able to identify problems at early stages in the SIC. By staying abreast of morale and remaining vigilant about the level of stress among unit personnel, carrier psychologists can intervene before problems become severe, either by reaching out to individuals or groups at particularly high risk for mental health problems, or by advising the command on policies to enhance a unit's overall psychological readiness. For many psychological disorders, most notably PTSD, early identification and treatment is essential to avoiding long-term difficulties.

One of the best ways to prevent pathology before it occurs is through education. In this role, carrier psychologists also buttress the work of unit leaders, who ultimately bear the responsibility of readiness within the SIC model. Carrier psychologists and shipboard psychiatric technicians conduct an average of 4.5 prevention-oriented classes per month. Such classes are designed to help service members identify growing psychological problems at an early stage (yellow and orange zone) before they become debilitating. Embedded psychologists can also prevent serious problems from developing through frequent interaction with unit leadership. Carrier psychologists conduct over 40 consultations per month with representatives of their patients' chains of command. These consultations are intended to educate the command, but also to discuss strategies for preventing a worsening of symptoms.

Sailors who are reacting, injured, or ill constitute a considerable responsibility for carrier psychologists and their staff. Carrier psychologists report an average of 105 patient contacts per month, so they are well utilized in the caregiving role. No doubt contributing to the high utilization of carrier psychologist is the fact that they live and work among their patients, frequently encountering them throughout the workday, observing them performing their jobs and interacting with peers. As shipmates, they are able to obtain an in-depth understanding of their patients' daily lives. Given this regular presence, unit members are more likely to utilize mental health services than they would if obtaining such care required a trip to a mental health clinic at a medical facility.

Stigma Reduction

Of all factors obstructing the provision of effective mental healthcare to military personnel, the most powerful may be the lingering perception within many military units that seeking psychological treatment is a sign of personal weakness, or that such care will harm one's military career. One of the major findings of the 2007 Department of Defense (DoD) task force on mental health[14] was that significant stigma remains associated with seeking mental healthcare in the military. A key recommendation, deemed "crucial to the psychological health of service members," was that "the military services should embed mental health professionals as organic assets in line units."[15(p4)]

Three obvious benefits of the SIC model in the carrier psychology program are apparent. First, the familiarity between sailors and the ship's psychologist reduces the stigma associated with seeking help, making it more likely for a sailor to ask for help before a stress injury becomes a stress illness. Second, the proximity of mental health services reduces the temporal distance between recognition of stress injury symptoms and access to care, lessening the need for medical evacuations of sailors who have developed debilitating stress illnesses. Third, psychologists detailed to a carrier are able to support the line leadership in developing a mentally ready force.

Operational Stress Control and Readiness (OSCAR)

History

OSCAR teams and carrier psychologists share many of the same preventive medicine and direct caregiving roles in addressing mental health issues across the spectrum of the SIC. The OSCAR concept was begun in 1999 and piloted as the 2nd Marine Division's operational stress control and restoration program in 2000. Early OSCAR teams included mental health professionals, corpsmen, chaplains, and Marine Corps staff noncommissioned officers in a fully integrated multidisciplinary team. In 2004 the Marine Corps collaborated with the Navy Bureau of Medicine to authorize a 2-year pilot of OSCAR across all three active Marine divisions. Staffing of the OSCAR teams was tenuous due to competing wartime demands for scarce mental health resources, but the pilot team performed well, proving to be a valuable asset to Marine Corps leadership. In 2006 the Center for Naval Analyses[16] evaluated the efficacy of the OSCAR pilot and summarized the model as follows:

> Applying a *community mental health* model to the expeditionary and forward placed nature of Marine life, and taking account of Marine culture, OSCAR is an *organic* program embedded in the units it serves, *expeditionary* (accompanying the unit throughout the deployment cycle), *multidisciplinary* (incorporating a team approach), *preventative* (stressing the full range of primary, secondary, and tertiary prevention measures), and *therapeutic* (providing appropriate mental health services).[16(p1)]

The center deemed the OSCAR pilot and model successful in reaching target audiences and capable of producing expected outputs. OSCAR was recommended for continuation and expansion beyond the active Marine divisions to the air wings, logistics groups, and possibly the drilling reserves.

In 2006 and 2007, the Marine Corps sponsored several working groups to further develop OSCAR capabilities and requirements, with representation from stakeholders including Marine Corps health services, religious programs, training and education, and the operating forces. Optimal OSCAR capabilities were developed. In acknowledgment of the core Marine Corps concept that combat and operational stress control is primarily a leadership responsibility, and should be focused on force preservation and readiness through prevention and early identification more than treatment, the OSCAR program was moved from health services to the Combat Operational Stress Control Program under the deputy commandant for manpower and reserve affairs.

Despite the 2007 DoD report[15] recommending that operational psychological health professionals be embedded in line units, staffing of OSCAR teams by the Navy remained on an ad-hoc basis because of other pressing needs for mental health resources across the system. Sustaining OSCAR became increasingly difficult without a formal requirement from the Marine Corps. In response, the commanding generals of the three Marine expeditionary forces (MEFs) wrote to the commandant of the Marine Corps, stating, "We need . . . OSCAR teams across the three MEFs. We must fully staff, fund, and equip the OSCAR program as soon as possible to support current combat operations."[17] A formal request for OSCAR staffing was sent by the Marine Corps to the Navy in early 2008. Within a few months, the Navy approved funding to permanently staff OSCAR in the Marine divisions and regiments, both active and reserve, starting in 2010.

Capabilities

OSCAR teams provide the following capabilities for operational commanders:

- psychological health surveillance of unit members and units as a whole;
- preventive psychological health training and education when and where needed;
- early interventions to promote recovery in individuals and units from traumatic stressors or losses;
- clinical mental healthcare services in forward operational environments where such services would otherwise be unavailable;
- professional coordination of comprehensive mental healthcare services in garrison before and after deployments to ensure readiness;
- support of spiritual fitness of operational forces throughout the deployment cycle through partnerships between religious ministry and mental health personnel; and
- psychological health support for unit medical and religious ministry personnel who are at high risk for stress-related problems.

OSCAR capabilities are critically dependent on teams being organic, that is, embedded within operational units, much like the traditional model of Navy hospital corpsmen. By placing OSCAR teams within units, team members can fully learn and appreciate the specific missions and cultures of the units they support throughout the deployment cycle: before, during, and after deployment.

The ultimate objectives of OSCAR capabilities in operational units are (*a*) enhanced readiness, (*b*) reduced stress-related decrements to mission effectiveness, and (*c*) enhanced long-term health and well-being of marines, sailors, and their families. OSCAR teams provide psychological health training to marines and Marine leaders, and reduce the stigma associated with receiving mental healthcare. They can assist leaders and marines with informal "hallway consultations" on symptoms and complaints to encourage early mitigation of stress and to promote the earliest interventions when necessary. Team members also serve unit leaders as advisors on how to prevent stress, monitor the psychological health of their units, and take necessary actions to promote healing. Compared to mental health services provided at medical treatment facilities, OSCAR is much more focused on prevention and population-based mental health than on individual clinical care, relying on familiarity between marines and mental health professionals established prior to deployment and maintained through and after deployment. The goal is to increase psychological health awareness and break down barriers to seeking mental healthcare.

Team Design

Marine Corps OSCAR teams provide two licensed mental health professionals and two psychiatric technicians per regiment, or approximately one licensed professional and one psychiatric technician per 2,500 marines. According to the 2007 DoD task force on mental health report to Congress:

> Determining the proper ratio of embedded providers to service members would require additional research; however, evidence from site visits suggested that the Army's ratio of one psychologist or social worker and one psychiatric technician per 5,000 service members is probably not sufficient.[14(p17)]

A team is also attached to each division to provide services to independent battalions and oversight to the regimental OSCAR teams. OSCAR teams are part of each commander's special staff, reporting to the command surgeon. Several different clinical specialties are utilized on OSCAR teams, with a typical team configuration as follows:

- one prescribing, licensed, independent mental health practitioner (psychiatrist, prescribing psychologist, or psychiatric nurse practitioner);
- one nonprescribing, licensed, independent mental health practitioner (psychologist or licensed clinical social worker); and
- two psychiatric corpsmen.

Although still not an ideal ratio of providers to marines to meet the intent of close proximity, familiarity, and trust, this configuration affords OSCAR team members a much larger presence than previously possible. The use of other unit medical professionals, such as physicians and more numerically abundant corpsmen, as OSCAR extenders through training and consultation with team members may be another avenue to improve OSCAR efficacy. The goal is to eventually place teams in all operating units, not only infantry regiments but also air wings and logistics groups.

Although OSCAR may be the newest combat and operational stress control program, it has clearly established itself as an integral component in the Navy's mental health support to the Marine Corps. The SIC model itself is an outgrowth of experiences derived from OSCAR operations. The conceptual link between OSCAR and the SIC model is clear: a shared responsibility between unit leadership and medical/chaplain's corps. This interaction fosters hardiness and resilience within the individual marine, who ultimately must bear the burden of combat and operational stress exposure. Consistent with the core values of the Marine Corps, personal responsibility is a critical component for maintaining mental health readiness, whereas leadership assumes responsibility for cultivating mental health resilience, and medical personnel and chaplains help restore mental health if stress injury or illness overcomes the individual.

EMERGING CHALLENGES FOR OPERATIONAL NAVY MEDICINE

The US military forces have been strained by the GWOT.[4] Despite being a service dedicated to control of the seas, the Navy has stepped forward to share the burden of this prolonged conflict and continues to play a substantial role in ground operations for OIF and OEF. However, the allocation of Navy personnel to ground combat operations remains a nontraditional deployment, resulting in special challenges to combat and operational stress control programs based on the SIC model. Two of the more vexing challenges are detailed below. The first challenge is to provide care for Navy personnel individually assigned to augment positions within combat-deployed Army units, a duty referred to as "individual augmentation" (IA). The second deals with the development of a program to care for a force of medical professionals who, as the OSCAR section explicates, are in high demand, and as a result have sustained a high operational tempo and been exposed to elevated levels of combat.

Individual Augmentation

Although the percentage of sailors assigned to IA duty constitutes approximately 3% of active and reserve duty assignments in the US Navy, the cumulative effect of these deployments has created over 46,000 combat veteran sailors through 2006, with over 7,000 sailors being added to this total annually.[18] The relative obscurity of this duty warrants a description of the IA deployment cycle and the Navy combat and operational stress control programs currently in place to address the unique and diverse mental health needs of "sandbox sailors."

Training and Deployment Cycle

As implied by their name, IA sailors prepare, deploy, and redeploy alone, and for the most part, outside Navy chains of command. Thus, standard Navy medical programs designed to monitor and treat mental health problems are not routinely accessible to IAs during many of the most critical points in their deployments. Before IAs deploy, Navy Medicine personnel conduct a mandatory predeployment health assessment (PDHA). The form used to conduct the PDHA is DD2795. The mental health aspect of the screening consists of the question, "During the past year, have you sought counseling or care for your mental health?" If this question is answered in the affirmative, the physician or healthcare specialist conducting the PDHA may refer the sailor to a mental health provider. Depending on the outcome of the mental health referral, the individual conducting the PDHA can classify the member as either deployable or nondeployable. Once deemed deployable, the IA detaches (either in a temporary duty status or as a permanent change of station, depending on the specific assignment) from the parent command and travels alone to a Navy mobilization processing site for final health, administrative, and legal processing. After spending a week at the processing site, sailors essentially leave Navy culture as they travel to their next destination, which for most is Navy IA combat skills training.

There, a cadre of Army drill instructors teach IAs elementary combat skills such as basic marksmanship, field medical procedures, rules of engagement, convoy operations, and codes of conduct to prepare the IA for integration into an Army-centric combat environment. In addition, most combat gear is provided at this training. Most Navy IAs receive the same training regardless of the duties they will perform when attached to their respective Army unit in theater. Although this broad-based training is beneficial because of the possibility of being remissioned (sometimes more than once) during an IA assignment, some of the missions now taken on by the Navy require competencies that can only be achieved by years of experience.

One such example is detainee operations; although sailors with specific master-of-arms (equivalent to the Army's military police) training are prepared for this duty, the majority of sailors conducting these missions are trained for unrelated positions, such as culinary specialists, machine mates, or yeomen. Within the typical 60-day IA training period, instruction relevant to guard force operations takes 17 days (with a capability for 4 additional days). A lack of confidence in performing a job can increase overall anxiety, and experience and training improve the ability to modulate combat stress (hence the dictum, "fight like you train, train like you fight"). An Army study[19] found that at the start of OIF, 70% of soldiers deploying to Iraq were not psychologically prepared to experience combat trauma.

To address this shortcoming, Navy Medicine has introduced a combat stress component to IA training, the goal of which is to cultivate cognitive coping strategies consistent with Kobasa's stress hardiness cognitive style,[20] characterized by (*a*) recasting challenges as opportunities for growth, (*b*) a commitment to self-improvement, and (*c*) the development of internal locus of control (ie, the ability to control events that affect one's life). Evaluating the influence of this component is essential to refining and maintaining IA combat stress coping training, especially because the empirical data evaluating the efficacy of predeployment stress control programs are inconclusive.[21]

The IA deployment phase starts with transportation to the theater of operations for additional field-based combat skills training for 3 to 4 days. Then the IA platoon is disbanded and individuals are transferred to their ultimate combat duty stations, where, except for rest and recreational leave (up to 14 days), the IAs remain for the duration of their 6-, 9-, or 12-month obligation. At their combat duty station, IAs are under the authority of the requesting service (primarily the Army, although the Marine Corps also utilizes IAs). If necessary, the IA seeks healthcare services, including mental health, from the parent command. However, Navy combat and operational stress control programs reenter the picture as soon as the IA returns to the continental United States. As the IAs transit from their OEF/OIF deployment, they pass through the Navy's Warrior Transition Program (WTP).

The WTP addresses the "four Rs" of operational stress control: (1) *reassurance* that the IAs' response to their deployment is nonpathological; (2) *rest* to compensate for the high operational tempo associated with 14-hour (or more) days, 6 to 7 days a week; (3) *replenishment* in terms of time to leisurely eat and shower; and (4) *restoration* of confidence.[6] Relieving the sailors of their bulky combat gear and completing customs inspections in advance also contribute to rest and replenishment, while reassurance and restoration are initiated with combat stress briefs delivered by mental health and faith-based caregivers. More than a prudent use of logistics, the act of gear turn-in (off-loading of "battle rattle") and the surrendering of issued weapons (after one last ritualistic cleaning) are as symbolic as they are practical. The sudden absence of weapons may produce anxiety, which can be addressed by caregivers as part of the preparatory framework for returning home.

The impetus for this program can be found in the postdeployment experiences of combat veterans like those described in Jonathan Shay's seminal volume, *Achilles in Vietnam*.[22] In his book, Shay explored the need for leadership to provide a sanctioned time for "mutual support and communal reworking of combat trauma,"[22(p61)] which was part of "the long trip home" in World War II but tragically absent in Vietnam. Rather than screen for, or immediately address, combat stress reactions (eg, PTSD), a goal of WTP is to give IA sailors "permission" to grieve and acknowledge the toll of their deployment, while also celebrating successes and gains made during the deployment. These efforts are to help IAs begin integrating potentially fragmented and disassociated deployment experiences into a more coherent and integrated self-script or schema. By institutionalizing time for the IA to acknowledge the psychological effect (positive and negative) of deployment, it is hoped that WTP will reduce the perception of organizational stigma that service members consistently cite as a barrier to accessing mental healthcare.[23] Mental health services are readily accessible during the WTP process.

Analogous to the "third location decompression" process practiced by North Atlantic Treaty Organization countries, WTP takes place at temporal and geographical distance from the deployment site (the potential source of trauma), making it much different from critical incident stress debriefing approaches, which have been found to be ineffective or even detrimental to mental health.[7–9] WTP is more consistent with end-of-tour unit debriefings shown to improve perceptions of organizational support.[24] Nevertheless, because IAs do not participate in WTP with their combat comrades-in-arms, but with other IAs from different deployment locations and experiences, it remains to be seen whether group debriefing works for the IA population. Following WTP, which lasts 3 days, IAs are flown directly home. Upon arrival at their destination airport, parent commands of some IAs may provide formal homecoming ceremonies that help foster reintegration. However, for many IAs, their mission often ends how it started—in isolation.

Isolation Issues

In Vietnam, soldiers trained with one group of people, deployed alone to serve a 1-year combat tour in units of ever-changing composition, and returned home alone to either finish their service commitment or integrate into a new unit.[22] By the 1980s a renewed appreciation for the protective nature of unit cohesion had arisen:

> One of the most significant contributions of World War II and modern warfare was the recognition of the sustaining influence of the small combat unit on the individual member. . . . Interpersonal relationships develop among soldiers and between them and their leaders. . . . It is these relationships which, during times of stress, provide a spirit or force which sustains the members as individuals and the individuals as a working, effective unit.[19(pI-1)]

Recent data indicate that unit cohesion can help reduce factors that place service members at risk for combat-stress–induced mental disorders such as PTSD. Brailey et al[25] evaluated the contribution of unit cohesion to the prediction of PTSD symptoms in a sample of 1,579 nondeployed US Army soldiers. Next to predeployment life trauma, the degree of unit cohesion was the best predictor of predeployment PTSD symptoms.[25] A diagnosis of PTSD or other psychological illness prior to deployment has been shown to put service members at increased risk for future development of PTSD.[26] In another study,[27] a comprehensive metaanalysis of 39 military samples prior to OEF/OIF indicated that unit cohesion was a significant predictor of well-being among a host of other outcomes such as individual performance, job/military satisfaction, retention, and readiness.

Despite the general consensus that mental health in combat-deployed units is bolstered by the social support structures that emerge within cohesive units that train, deploy, and return together, the IA deployment has exposed a new generation of service members to the isolation of Vietnam-style individual deployments. Adding to this problem is the IA's loss of service and professional identity. Data clearly support a link between job satisfaction and work-related stress.[28] A common frustration voiced by IAs is dissatisfaction with the substance of their mission—work that may not utilize their hard-earned Navy designation or operational specialty. Also sometimes lost when sailors go on IA duty is respect for their rank. Each service emphasizes ranks differently. For instance, once enlisted sailors pin on the coveted anchors of a chief petty officer at E7, they become "khaki" (the same uniform officers wear) and are afforded great respect and autonomy within the Navy. However, many IAs indicate that the social status given to E7s in the Navy is equivalent only to that given to an E9 sergeant major in the Army. Data indicate that loss of social rank status is detrimental to mental health and a source of both psychological and physiological stress.[29]

Unfortunately, due to the nascent nature of IA deployment, little or no data are publicly available to evaluate the relative contributions of absent unit cohesion, low job satisfaction, and loss of social rank status in the prediction of combat-related stress reactions. One of the few studies to compare the mental health status of Navy IAs to nondeploying sailors[18] found that in both the enlisted and officer ranks, sailors deployed to an IA billet exhibited significantly more mental health problems, but only if that deployment was to a hostile combat zone. This finding suggests that deployments to the Army have the greatest impact within the combat zone, highlighting the interaction between combat exposure and type of deployment.

Administrative issues can also cause stress for Navy IAs. The handoff from Army to Navy at the end of a deployment is not always well coordinated, and because many Army units are unfamiliar with writing evaluations, fitness reports, or awards for Navy personnel, recognition for IA duty can be lacking (if evaluations and fitness reports are not in a Navy format, they are not accepted by the Navy Bureau of Personnel for inclusion in the service record). The Navy also reviews awards given by the Army, and has occasionally refused to accept or downgraded these awards, with a significant impact on the IA's morale.

An additional issue is family support. Although deployed Army units have robust family support programs, these programs are generally not designed to cross service lines and include the families of assigned Navy personnel. For IAs who are transient between permanent commands, the family may be left with little support. Thus, an area for further attention is ensuring that the families of deployed IAs receive appropriate support and information from the Army unit's family support system.

Adding to problems caused by the unique risks of combat and operational stressors for IA soldiers is the logistical distance between these sailors and the traditional Navy medical infrastructure. Navy Medicine personnel have limited opportunities to share the SIC model with the IA's Army leadership, and thus the model's emphasis on the interaction between unit leadership and caregivers to develop mental health resiliency is difficult to carry out. New initiatives based on IA duty continue to emerge, such as GWOT Support Assignment orders, wherein GWOT requirements are folded into normal permanent change-of-station orders. In response, Navy Medicine has initiated the development of combat and operational stress control programs tailored to meet the evolving needs of the IA mission, with programs at both the predeployment and postdeployment phases that introduce sailors to resilience-inducing cognitive coping skills and provide institutionally sanctioned time to grieve and begin the healing process. However, access to IAs in the combat zone remains a challenge to Navy Medicine and its health surveillance programs.

Care for the Caregiver

Mission and Personnel

Navy caregivers include a broad range of professional and paraprofessional personnel charged with providing care and support to wounded, ill, and injured sailors and marines. Navy caregivers assume a number of roles, both traditional and nontraditional, including corpsmen, chaplains, substance abuse counselors, recovery coordinators, case managers, nurses, clinical support staff, and physicians. Some are civilians and some are contractors.

Operational and occupational stress faced by caregivers is cumulative and extends across the deployment cycle. The acute injuries and chronic illnesses of war are treated across a continuum of care, from the front to hospitals and outpatient centers in the United States. For instance, a corpsman who tended to wounds in Iraq in July may be dressing wounds in San Diego, California in January. Dwell time (ie, the amount of time between deployments) does not necessarily include a respite from exposure to the wounds of war for caregivers. As a result, caregivers have an especially abbreviated opportunity for rest, replenishment, and restoration. The consequences of untreated cumulative stress can result in medical errors; somatic complaints such as changes in eating habits, gastrointestinal distress, headache, fatigue, and sleep disorders; change in work habits such as tardiness and absenteeism; mental and emotional difficulties such as memory disturbances, anger, self-doubt, isolation, and impaired judgment; and accidents.[30–32]

Navy Medicine caregivers are usually deployed as IAs to the combat zone, the exceptions being caregivers who are assigned to embedded duty within operational units (eg, hospital ships, EMFs, SPRINT teams, OSCAR teams). Uniformed caregivers selected for IA duty typically possess specific skill sets that are synergized to form an operational field medical asset. Personnel with combat-essential skills (Fleet Marine Force corpsmen, surgery, anesthesia, critical care, mental health) are particularly likely to deploy, often making multiple deployments within a given tour of duty. IA medical personnel are selected from hospitals and clinics around the world, given "just in time" training, and then configured with other caregivers to form a functional unit. At the end of their deployment, caregivers return as individuals to their hospitals and clinics. The protective connectedness of unit cohesion is lost when they leave their parent command and again when they leave their operational unit. Even more stress may be encountered by those who joined preexisting deployed units, a situation that makes "fitting in" even more difficult.

Trauma Exposure and Intervention Strategies

Providing care in a combat zone increases the likelihood of experiencing direct and secondary exposure to traumatic injuries. Direct exposure constitutes the threat to physical safety from direct and indirect fire, as well as the plethora of fatigue-inducing operational stressors. Secondary trauma can be encountered by working in close contact for extended periods of time with wounded, ill, and injured sailors, the result to caregivers being a phenomenon known as occupational or compassion fatigue. In relation to the SIC model, direct and secondary trauma can, individually or in tandem, contribute to full-blown stress illnesses for Navy caregivers. Stress injury and illnesses can affect mission effectiveness in the form of medical errors, job dissatisfaction, and poor retention.[33]

Part of the responsibility for enhancing the resilience of Navy caregivers rests with the leadership of Navy Medicine itself. Actions are underway within Navy Medicine to implement training based on the SIC model to run through all phases of training for Navy medical personnel. The core leader functions have been applied to day-to-day clinical leadership activities as well as facilitating the transition of Navy Medicine personnel in and out of different operational settings. One key point the SIC model should impart to the leaders of caregivers is that their roles and work environments are inherently stressful, and that stress reactions are common. Many leaders recognize that initial stress reactions increase caregivers' energy and focus their attention on critical changes in a patient's condition, while sustained stress causes a degradation of performance. Leaders should be aware that in caregivers' work environments, occupational stress is endemic and may go unrecognized because such reactions become normalized. A difficult challenge to the leaders of caregivers is reintegrating individually deployed staff into a cohesive unit that did not deploy; the IA caregiver faces the dual task of reintegration while simultaneously letting go of relationships formed during deployment.

The traditional work-stress–response paradigm in both civilian and Navy literature has several common elements: know the sources of job stress, know the signs and symptoms of stress, take care of oneself, and seek help when there is the beginning of impairment in daily life.[5] There are several significant barriers to self-help for caregivers. First, endemic job stress produces some level of stress symptoms in all workers, so that moderate and high stress appear normal. Second, early stress symptoms such as fatigue, impaired sleep, and confusion decrease the self-awareness necessary to initiate self-care. Third, caregivers are "other focused" and may consider self-care unnecessary or antithetical to their goals.

When intervention is necessary, the "five Cs" of COSFA[1]—cover, calming, connectedness, capacity, and confidence—can prove especially helpful. Using the COSFA model, caregivers are encouraged to focus on other caregivers and their shipmates: facilitating connectedness and accessing the healing capability of unit cohesion requires breaking the "code of silence" by asking coworkers questions about their stress coping. Most caregivers do not feel comfortable approaching their peers with questions and concerns about the peer's behaviors. The typical, "How are you doing?" is usually met with a response of, "Fine."

A strategy for facilitating connectedness is based on role expectations of shipmates and uses an "OSCAR" acronym (Exhibit 8-1). The OSCAR communication strategy encourages shipmates to address coworker behavior in five steps. First, observe the behavior, particularly signs of possible impairment, such as poor concentration, looking tired, falling asleep during change of shift, or irritability. Second, state the observation. The observation must be overtly stated because decreased self-awareness is one of the early casualties of a stress reaction. Third, clarify one's role. The roles of shipmate, subordinate, supervisor, friend, and spouse help show why the behavior is being addressed, and help determine which options should

EXHIBIT 8-1

OPERATIONAL STRESS CONTROL ASSESSMENT AND RESPONSE COMMUNICATION

Observation: actively observe behaviors; look for patterns.

State observations: focus all attention on the behaviors; just the facts without interpretations or judgments.

Clarify role: state why you are concerned about the behavior, which validates why you are addressing the issue.

Ask why: seek clarification; try to understand the other person's perception of the behaviors.

Respond: clarify concern if indicated; discuss desired behaviors; state options in behavioral terms.

be used for the shipmate. Fourth, ask the shipmate for personal perception of what the behaviors are. Often, the act of talking about the behavior will allow the individual to clarify how a problem is affecting work behavior. Fifth, respond with guided options that are intended to facilitate change or offer to help the shipmate connect with other resources, such as a leader, chaplain, financial counselor, the Navy-Marine Corps Relief Society, or mental healthcare.

Despite the increased risks of sustaining stress injuries when deployed or in the course of day-to-day work, Navy caregiver duty can be extremely rewarding and satisfying. The Navy "care for the caregiver" concept, based on the SIC model, encourages caregivers to use the same skills they developed to help their patients for helping each other.

SUMMARY

The SIC model represents an ambitious attempt to assimilate the disparate conceptual frameworks of various stress control programs within the Navy, each of which has its own unique history, into a single yet comprehensive operational stress control paradigm. Within this model, three major stakeholders are responsible for supporting sailors and marines faced with the inevitable challenge of sustained operations: (1) leadership, (2) the service member, and (3) the caregiver. Leadership establishes the foundation for effective combat stress control by cultivating a command climate that recognizes the importance of mental health, institutionalizes stress resilience training, and removes barriers to care for those who experience stress reactions and develop illness or injury. Individual service members trained in stress resilience should be capable of developing their own individual stress coping strategies, identifying when their stress reactions are beyond their coping capacity, and knowledgeable and comfortable enough with the care options available to easily seek help when needed. Caregivers must actively pursue a consultative role, working to support the leadership in stress control efforts, yet remaining vigilant to identify sailors who react adversely to stress, and providing quality care to those whose stress reactions lead to illness and injury.

Expeditionary medical platforms, such as hospital ships and EMFs, provide a large, forward-deployed medical capacity for applying the SIC model. However, combat stress control program elements such as SPRINT, carrier psychologists, and OSCAR teams are the best embodiment of the SIC model. In fact, the SIC model itself is an outgrowth of OSCAR philosophy. Unfortunately, both the forward-deployed medical platforms and combat stress control elements are straining to adapt to the burgeoning demands of GWOT that have focused pressure on caregivers themselves, and taken sailors outside of the Navy sphere of influence during the course of IA duty assignments. Building upon the successes of the combat stress control program elements described in this chapter, which arose to meet specific operational demands, Navy medicine can again rise to meet the challenge of caring for combat deployed sailors.

A consistent theme in this chapter has been the utility of mobile and expeditionary Navy Medicine assets. Despite the necessity and quality of the centralized Navy medical capacity, it has been recognized that delivering care within deployed units has reduced the stigma associated with seeking help for stress-related illness. Moreover, the benefit is reciprocal: proponents seem to agree that caregivers themselves benefit from the social cohesion of serving within a unit, a situation that appears to improve caregivers' credibility as well as their overall ability to intervene and treat stress-related injuries.

Each section of this chapter represents cumulative knowledge gleaned from professional training, reviews of the literature, and most importantly, first-hand experiences with Navy combat and operational stress control programs. This chapter should also alert readers to areas where data are needed to evaluate whether the programs discussed are effective in managing combat and operational stress. Despite the myriad models and approaches described, Navy combat and operational stress control programs in their present state are a mission-centered collection of efforts that reflect the multifaceted and dynamic issues associated with stress control in combat and operational environments. The SIC model is a bold, yet necessary, attempt to weave these programs' elements into an overarching Navy combat stress control philosophy.

REFERENCES

1. Figley CR, Nash WP, eds. *Combat Stress Injury: Theory, Research, and Management.* New York, NY: Routledge; 2007.

2. Stokes AF, Kite K. On grasping a nettle and becoming emotional. In: Hancock PA, Desmond PA, eds. *Stress, Workload, and Fatigue.* Mahwah, NJ: Lawrence Erlbaum Publishers; 2001: 107–132.

3. Gunderson E, Hourani LL. The epidemiology of mental disorders in the US Navy: the neuroses. *Mil Med*. 2001; 166:612–620.

4. Tanielian T, Jaycox L. *Invisible Wounds of War: Psychological and Cognitive Injuries, Their Consequences, and Services to Assist Recovery*. Santa Monica, Calif: RAND Corporation; 2008.

5. Cooper CL, Cartwright S. A strategic approach to organizational stress management. In: Hancock PA, Desmond PA, eds. *Stress, Workload, and Fatigue*. Mahwah, NJ: Lawrence Erlbaum Publishers; 2001: 235–248.

6. Lewis SJ. Combat stress control: putting principle into practice. In: Britt TW, Castro CA, Adler AB, eds. *Military Life: The Psychology of Serving in Peace and Combat.* Westport, Conn: Praeger Security International; 2006: 121–140.

7. McNally RJ. Psychological debriefing does not prevent posttraumatic stress disorder. *Psychiatric Times*. 2004;21(4).

8. McNally RJ, Bryant RA, Ehlers A. Does early psychological intervention promote recovery from posttraumatic stress? *Psychol Sci Pub Int*. 2003:42:45–79.

9. Rose S, Bisson J, Churchill R, Wessely S. Psychological debriefing for preventing post traumatic stress disorder (PTSD). *Cochrane Database of Systematic Review*. 2001;4. Art No. CD000560.

10. Nash B, Watson P, Litz B. USN-USMC combat and operational stress first aid (COSFA). Paper presented at: US Marine Corps Combat Operational Stress Control Conference; August 12–14, 2008; San Diego, Calif.

11. Wood DP, Koffman RL, Arita AA. Psychiatric medevacs during a 6-month aircraft carrier battle group deployment to the Persian Gulf: a Navy Force Health Protection preliminary report. *Mil Med*. 2003;168:43–47.

12. Smith D. Taking it to the fleet. *Monitor Psychol*. 2002;33:52–53.

13. Jones DE, Lee JJ. Take the tough cases to sea. *Proceedings*. 2002;128:61–64.

14. US Department of Defense. *An Achievable Vision: Report of the Department of Defense Task Force on Mental Health.* Falls Church, Va: Defense Health Board; 2007.

15. US Department of Defense. *Plan to Achieve the Vision of the DoD Task Force on Mental Health: Report to Congress September 2007*. Washington, DC: DoD; 2007.

16. Harris DM, Edwards JD. *A Preliminary Evaluation of the OSCAR Pilot Program*. Alexandria, Va: Center for Naval Analyses; 2006. Report CRM D0013962.A2/Final.

17. US Marine Corps. *Tri-MEF Combat Operational Stress Conference.* Camp Pendleton, Calif: I, II, and III Marine Expeditionary Forces. Letter to the Commandant, 12 September 2007. Available at: http://www.mca-marines.org/Gazette/PDF/USMCLetterPP.pdf. Accessed March 30, 2009.

18. Andres JM. *Effects of Navy Individual Augmentee Deployments on Mental Health Outcomes* [master's thesis]. Monterey, Calif: Naval Postgraduate School; 2008.

19. US Army Office of the Surgeon General. *Operation Iraqi Freedom Mental Health Advisory Team Report, 16 December 2003*. Washington, DC: OTSG; 2003.

20. Kobasa SC. Stressful life events, personality, and health: an inquiry into hardiness. *J Pers Soc Psychol*. 1979;37:1–11.

21. Sharpley JG, Fear NT, Greenberg N, Jones M, Wessely S. Pre-deployment stress briefing: does it have an effect? *Occup Med (Lond)*. 2008;58:30–34.

22. Shay J. *Achilles in Vietnam: Combat Trauma and the Undoing of Character*. New York, NY: Atheneum; 1994.

23. Hoge CW, Castro CA, Messer SC, McGurk D, Cotting DI, Koffman RL. Combat duty in Iraq and Afghanistan, mental health problems, and barriers to care. *N Engl J Med*. 2004;351:13–22.

24. Adler A, Suvak M, Litz B, et al. A controlled trial of group debriefing in the military: preliminary findings. Poster session presented at: 38th Annual Meeting of the Association for Advancement of Behavior Therapy; August 2004; New Orleans, La.

25. Brailey K, Vasterling JJ, Proctor SP, Constans JI, Friedman MJ. PTSD symptoms, life events and unit cohesion in US soldiers: baseline findings from the neurocognition deployment health study. *J Trauma Stress.* 2007;20:495–503.

26. Ozer EJ, Best SR, Lipsey TL, Weiss DS. Predictors of posttraumatic stress disorder and symptoms in adults: a meta-analysis. *Psychol Bull.* 2003;129:52–73.

27. Oliver L, Harman J, Hoover E, Hayes S, Pandhi N. A quantitative integration of the military cohesion literature. *Mil Psychol.* 1999;11:57–83.

28. Ostroff C. The relationship between satisfaction, attitudes, and performance: an organizational level analysis. *J Appl Psychol.* 1992;77:963–974.

29. DeVries AC, Glasper ER, Detillion CE. Social modulation of stress responses. *Physiol Behav.* 2003;79:399–407.

30. Jacobson BH, Aldana SG, Goetzel RZ, Vardell KD, Adams TB, Pietras RJ. The relationship between perceived stress and self-reported illness-related absenteeism. *Am J Health Promot.* 1996;11:54–61.

31. Barger L, Cade BE, Ayas NT, et al. Extended work shifts and the risk of motor vehicle crashes among interns. *N Engl J Med.* 2005;352:125–134.

32. Gaba DM, Howard SK. Patient safety: fatigue among clinicians and the safety of patients. *N Engl J Med.* 2002;347:1249–1255.

33. Waterman AD, Garbutt J, Hazel E, et al. The emotional impact of medical errors on practicing physicians in the United States and Canada. *Jt Comm J Qual Patient Saf*. 2007;33(8):467–476.

Chapter 9

PROVISION OF MENTAL HEALTH SERVICES IN OPERATION IRAQI FREEDOM 05-07

MARC A. COOPER, MD*; SHARON M. NEWTON, MHS†; AND JEFFREY S. YARVIS, MSW, PHD‡

*Chief, Community Mental Health Service, Moncrief Army Community Hospital, 4500 Stuart Street, Fort Jackson, South Carolina 29207; formerly, Major, Medical Corps, US Army; OIF 05-07 Theater Mental Health Consultant, Task Force 30th Medical Brigade, Baghdad, Iraq

†Lieutenant Colonel, Medical Specialist Corps , US Army; Command Inspector General, 30th Medical Command, CMR 442, APO AE 09042; formerly, Theater Consultant for Combat and Operational Stress Control, Iraq

‡Lieutenant Colonel, Medical Service Corps, US Army; Chief, Behavioral Health, Department of Psychiatry, Borden Pavilion, Walter Reed Army Medical Center, 6900 Georgia Avenue NW, Washington DC 20307; formerly, Director of Social Work, Uniformed Services University of the Health Sciences, Bethesda, Maryland

INTRODUCTION

During Operation Iraqi Freedom (OIF) 05-07, the third anniversary of combat operations in Iraq was observed. The battlefield had changed dramatically since US forces first invaded Iraq in March 2003. Open fighting along the routes into major cities had been replaced with door-to-door city fighting. The enemy had changed from a visible fighting force into a largely unseen guerilla force. As the battlefield transformed, so did the provision of mental health services. Mental health providers still supported soldiers, but this task evolved, resulting in the improvement of earlier operations, the incorporation of new missions, and an increased emphasis on data collection. Being in country for 3 years and utilizing the widespread availability of computerized technology, military mental health provision developed to a level of sophistication never before seen in a theater of operations.

This chapter will explore how duration of the conflict affected the provision of mental health services during OIF 05-07. It will look at factors that influenced the entire military that had consequences for mental health providers, such as facing a more sophisticated enemy, living on more developed bases, and implementing new Department of Defense policies. It will also look at ways in which mental health services expanded based on lessons learned from OIF-I and OIF-II. Finally, the length of the conflict and the increasing number of casualties amplified media interest in the conflict and in mental health services available to soldiers in combat. This chapter will discuss the influence of the media on the provision of mental health services during OIF 05-07.

CHANGING DYNAMICS OF THE CONFLICT

A More Sophisticated Enemy

In March 2003, the enemy was clear—the Iraqi Army commanded by Saddam Hussein. After Hussein's troops surrendered in April 2003, defining the "enemy" became more complicated. Pockets of insurgent groups coupled with sectarian violence began producing coalition casualties through various guerilla warfare tactics. During the ensuing years, these tactics became more sophisticated, using the skills of sharpshooters and explosives experts. These deadly encounters with insurgents resulted in the decision by the US military that there had to be increased preparedness for all deployed soldiers. Consequently, one of the improvements made during OIF 05-07 was that all soldiers already deployed, as well as those soon to deploy, were given protective equipment that was normally provided only to combat units. In addition to the Army combat uniform and improved Kevlar helmets, all soldiers were also issued "hemcon" (hemorrhage control) bandages, which were a vast improvement over the previous field bandage. Soldiers received deltoid and axillary protector plates, and enhanced small arms protective insert plates, aimed at providing better protection. However, these protective measures also significantly increased the weight each soldier had to carry. This extra weight, especially in the hot summer months, was an added stressor for all soldiers, including the combat operational stress control providers during travel outside the forward operating base (FOB).

Travel between FOBs was improved during OIF 05-07. During the first half of OIF-I, travel was in soft-sided vehicles for the simple reason that there were no up-armored vehicles. The dangers of ground travel (ie, improvised explosive devices, rocket-propelled grenades, suicide bombers) became more common and deadlier, necessitating the requirement that all vehicles traveling outside the FOB be up-armored. In general, although more travel now occurs via aircraft than during OIF-I (where nearly all travel was by ground convoy), most combat stress control teams continue to travel by convoy.

Another area in which there was improvement as the conflict continued was the standardization of convoy procedures. During OIF-I, depending on the location of the team and its higher headquarters, there was a wide variation in procedures. Some teams traveled by nontactical vehicle, while other teams were required to be in a convoy of at least three vehicles, with a specified number of crew-served weapons. Although the standardization of convoy procedures was developed to enhance safety, this more-involved process has created frustrations for the combat stress control teams who regularly need to leave a FOB to provide services to a supported unit.

More Developed Forward Operating Bases, More Developed Mental Health Services

The living and working conditions improved considerably by OIF 05-07. During OIF-I, soldiers (including mental health personnel) lived and worked out of tents for the most part, using burnout latrines, field-expedient showers, and meals, ready-to-eat. Conditions began to improve even before the end of the OIF-I rotation, and the improvements continued through each rotation. During OIF 05-07, the majority of personnel lived and worked in trailers or buildings that were climate controlled and had electricity, including hygiene facilities with running water. Even the presence of beds instead of an Army cot contributed to the overall improvement in the standard of living. Obviously, these improvements affected the level of stress perceived by the supported soldiers as well as the mental health personnel providing the support.

One observation of the 30th Medical Brigade (TF30 Med) mental health personnel is that subordinate units seemed to be reporting more psychiatric patients than expected by combat operational stress control (COSC) doctrine. A rough comparison was made of the average monthly number of new psychiatric contacts to the average monthly number of new combat stress contacts from the Combat Operational Stress Control Workload Activity Reporting System (COSC-WARS) reports from OIF-I, OIF-II, OIF 04-06, and OIF 05-07. The average number of new psychiatric contacts rose disproportionately higher than the average number of new combat stress contacts from OIF-I to OIF 05-07. (Only a rough estimate is possible as data collection during the early part of the conflict was obviously not the priority.) The reasons for the increase are not clear. Among possible explanations are improved workload reporting procedures, an increase in the population at risk or the number of soldiers deploying with psychotropic medications, or providers more willing to use medication to treat combat stress and thus convert what would have traditionally been a new combat stress contact into a psychiatric contact. Providers were likely more comfortable prescribing medication because the living environment was more stable and better follow up was available; thus soldiers would not need to be sent out of the theater for treatment.

There was a very clinical feel to many of the services provided during OIF 05-07. (One benefit that comes from a longer conflict is that better working conditions develop.) During OIF-I, tents were the norm. By OIF 05-07 the tents had been replaced by buildings—working in buildings instead of working outside the same tent where one lives lends itself to a more clinical feel. Additionally, more combat stress control (CSC) units had teams collocated with a combat support hospital (CSH) compared to OIF-I.[1] These teams would frequently provide primarily mental health services. Often times, this was out of necessity, as they were the only mental health providers on the FOB, or the CSH did not have the personnel due to split-base operations. Sometimes this was the choice of the provider, the combat stress control commander, or the CSH commander.

This is not to say that COSC personnel were not providing preventive outreach services. As alluded to earlier, many of the division mental health personnel had a preventive focus, as did the mental health personnel from echelons above division beyond those in the CSC units. All teams from the CSC units did some form of outreach through classes, consultation, and education, as well as regular outreach by walking around and talking to the supported units.

By OIF 05-07, theater mental health assets had learned the basics of their jobs in a combat environment and began to expand their roles into more forensic and administrative psychiatry services, which would not normally be associated with combat psychiatry. Sanity boards and mental status evaluations are not even mentioned in the COSC field manual[2] or the two psychiatry volumes in the *Textbooks of Military Medicine* series.[3,4] It is unclear if the requests for these specialty services had any relationship to the fact that mental health services were being offered in more clinical environments, and thus providers were more able or prepared to fulfill these requests.

The fact that commanders and soldiers were requesting these services while deployed to a combat zone merits discussion. The Mental Health Advisory Team (MHAT) IV found that soldiers who had deployed to Iraq more than once were more likely to screen positive for depression, acute stress, anxiety, or other mental health problems. It also reported that soldiers who screened positive for a mental health problem were twice as likely to engage in unethical behavior as those who did not screen positive.[5] The number of moral waivers for felonies given to recruits increased from 459 in 2003 to 1,002 in fiscal year 2006.[6] Thus, whether due to a mental health problem or a history of illegal behavior, it appears that the longer this conflict continues, the greater the chances are that soldiers will be acting out while deployed, and there will be an ever-increasing need for sanity boards or command-directed mental health evaluations performed in theater.

Established mental health clinics during OIF 05-07 also managed to work out logistical problems that plagued clinics at the start of the conflict. One of the biggest improvements was the formulary, which now contains a broader spectrum of antidepressant medication and stimulants, two concerns brought up by providers during OIF-I.[7] The formulary was frequently reevaluated, as the Multi-National Force–Iraq (MNF–I) pharmacists held quarterly meetings that allowed providers to make suggestions for additions or substitutions.

Despite great interest in knowing how many psychotropic prescriptions were written in theater, several mechanisms make this data difficult to accurately report. First, most established psychiatric patients deploy with a 90-day supply of medication from their home duty station or soldier readiness processing site. The TRICARE mail-order pharmacy was also frequently used for established psychiatric patients and those stabilized on medication in theater. Theater pharmacies ordered their own stocks of medications and kept their own records of prescriptions written for each psychotropic. Thus, centralized order tracking would only reflect shipments to theater pharmacies, not how much of those shipments were actually being prescribed.

Another advance that occurred in theater was the increased availability and usage of Composite Health Care System-Interactive Training Tool (CHCS-ITT), the deployment electronic medical record. Because CHCS-ITT is linked with the computerized medical record system utilized in garrison, provider notes written in the combat zone can be accessed at any military treatment facility in the world. This system greatly improved continuity of care between the Iraq Theater of operations and the medical facilities where soldiers were being treated and reduced the biggest risk of paper documentation—misplacement. Unfortunately, the only facilities that had reliable electricity, computer access, and CHCS-ITT trainers were the Level III CSHs and Level II battalion aid stations. Unless they were collocated in one of these facilities, the CSC teams did not have access to the CHCS-ITT system.

The debate that had occurred in garrison mental health clinics was subsequently heard in theater. This debate centered on the inclusion of mental health notes in the general medical record and the lack of privacy of the computerized mental health record. The CHCS-ITT "sensitivity feature" was nonfunctional in theater. This sensitivity feature, also known as the "break the glass" feature, keeps record of all users accessing any clinical notes labeled as "sensitive." Prior to accessing a sensitive note, medical providers are warned with a pop-up message that they are about to read sensitive data and they will be audited. For CHCS-ITT, in-theater providers could designate a note as sensitive, but there was no record created of who accessed a sensitive note and there was no warning pop-up message. To use the system while protecting patient privacy, some providers opted to keep all their records electronically unsigned, which kept the encounter in an "open" status and prevented other providers from being able to read the notes, but still allowed treating providers to write up a summary of their encounter with the patient and print it out. The disadvantage of this was that future mental health providers could not access these notes because they were never closed, and open encounters significantly downgraded the entire system so that all notes in all clinics on that particular network took longer to write.

With more established FOBs offering more services, KBR (formerly Kellogg Brown & Root, the largest civilian contractor in Iraq at the time), and the Army and Air Force Exchange Service required more civilian employees during OIF 05-07 than in OIF-I. Problems arose when these employees, who were supposed to be psychiatrically cleared prior to their deployment, showed up at military mental health clinics in need of treatment. This put military providers in an uncomfortable position for several reasons: *(a)* military malpractice did not cover the care of contractors, *(b)* contractors were not eligible for care and so prescriptions would be difficult to fill, and *(c)* if the contract agency found out that an employee was receiving mental healthcare, the employee would be sent home, so when contractors presented to mental health clinics, they asked the providers not to report them. KBR brought its own employee assistance program counselors to Iraq, which was helpful when KBR employees were involved in a casualty-producing incident, because their own counselors could offer debriefings or counseling. However, KBR had no physicians or psychiatrists on staff. Because only physicians can initiate air evacuation requests, military psychiatrists were tasked with authorizing all KBR psychiatric emergencies requiring evacuation from theater.

Developed FOBs brought with them communication systems that were vastly improved from OIF-I. This had several implications for the mental health community. First, most FOBs now had widespread Internet access and phone centers, which enabled soldiers to call home more regularly. Mental health providers in theater considered this a mixed blessing—soldiers could receive additional support or they could receive devastating news, yet they were still expected to perform the mission.

Another consequence of improved communication, especially the ability to send US mail across FOBs fairly reliably, was that the design for MHAT IV could be simplified. Rather than having a team of researchers come into theater and travel across FOBs administering the surveys, the surveys were sent by express mail to the theater. They were then mailed to the mental health assets organic to the FOBs where the participating units were stationed. The surveys were administered by each unit's mental health asset and then mailed back to the MNF–I surgeon's office, where MHAT IV was housed. This new process allowed for a reduction in the number of researchers needed to deploy to theater. The mission now focused more on data analysis rather than survey administration. Although this expanded the mission of the theater mental health provider, it gave units an opportunity to interact with their own mental health assets, rather than with a group of outsiders. It also decreased the need for travel across FOBs by MHAT personnel, a process with its own inherent risks. Ultimately, there were delays in the mail system, so MHAT personnel did more travel than was originally planned, but this was still far less than previous MHAT teams.

Increased Multiple Deployers

Clearly, with each additional year of the conflict, the chances increase that the population of deployed soldiers will contain greater numbers of multiple deployers. The increased number of multiple deployers during OIF 05-07 was not unique to soldier patients seeking mental healthcare. Many healthcare providers were also affected. It is not unusual to have COSC providers return from a deployment only to discover the need to prepare for the next deployment. They may not have had sufficient time to recover from the first deployment. The very nature of providing COSC services in a combat theater means repeated exposure to stress and hearing the tragedies of those being supported. Twenty-one percent of OIF 05-07 behavioral health providers reported high or very high levels of burnout.[5] It is unclear how many of these providers had had multiple deployments. An area of further research might be to look at the long-term effect of multiple deployments on behavioral health providers, especially with little time between each one.

Ongoing provision of mental health service would have resulted in rotation through Army providers more quickly had it not been for the US Air Force and Navy contributing greater mental health assets than in previous OIF years. The Air Force deployed its mental health providers for 4 months at a time. They were placed in CSC teams or in the Air Force hospital in central Iraq. The Navy deployed its mental health providers in support of Marine line units, but also filled some of the rotating reservist slots of the CSC units.

New Department of Defense Policies

As after-action reports and other reported difficulties from OIF-I and OIF-II made their way through the top levels of the military, new policies made their way down in an attempt to make needed improvements. One such policy concerned treating victims of sexual assault. This policy originated as a result of an inquiry made by the Secretary of Defense (then Donald Rumsfeld) in February 2004 over concerns of sexual assault allegations made by soldiers deployed to Iraq and Kuwait.[8] A task force that was formed to investigate these allegations found inconsistency in sexual assault prevention programs across the services. The task force reported that barriers to reporting sexual assault were significant in the military environment and that without an advocate looking out for the victim, it was easy to overlook a victim's rights and needs. Among the task force's recommendations was the establishment of a Department of Defense policy addressing sexual assault prevention and response, and the creation of a task force that would oversee this policy. After receiving congressional approval, Department of Defense Directive 6495.01, the Sexual Assault Prevention and Response Program, was published in October 2005. It outlined the treatment and care for victims of sexual assault and required that provisions be made for theater operations. The Army published its policy in Army Command Policy, Army Regulation 600-20, which was first published February 1, 2006, and revised June 7, 2006.

The Sexual Assault Prevention and Response Program affected theater mental health providers because it potentially added further missions. First, behavioral health personnel were often tasked with acting as the unit's victim advocates due to their demonstrated ability to empathize. Even if they were not victim advocates, however, mental health personnel had the potential for greater contact with sexual assault victims, because the new policy required immediate availability of mental health services for all victims presenting to a medical treatment facility. Alternatively, a mental health visit could be the first contact a sexual assault victim had with the medical community. Thus providers had to know about the new reporting options, which were restricted reporting and unrestricted reporting. In restricted reporting, only the treatment community is authorized to know the victim's identity (the victim's chain of command is never told about the assault). In unrestricted reporting, the victim's chain of command is informed and an official Criminal Investigation Division inquiry is opened. Finally, sexual assault review boards were now meeting in theater and behavioral health chiefs were a required component of these boards.

The other policy that had a significant effect on the mental health mission during OIF 05-07 took effect June 1, 2006, when the Army revised its deployment drug testing procedures. The main changes involved giving more responsibilities to deployed units.[9] This included medical personnel because medical review officer (MRO) services now had to be available in the deployed environment. An MRO is a physician appointed to determine if a urinalysis positive for opiates, barbiturates, steroids, or stimulants is the result of a legitimate prescription or illegitimate use.[10] In garrison, MROs are trained through a medical command course and are certified after passing an examination.

An informal survey of division surgeons and the CSHs indicated that there were not enough certified MROs in theater to handle this new tasking. Ultimately, the decision was made to have two MROs appointed at each Level III CSH, two at the multifunctional medical battalion, and additional MROs as needed in the divisions. The Army Forensic Drug Testing Program then distributed training CDs to theater. Commanders appointed MROs, the CDs were reviewed, and MROs took the certifying exam via e-mail. The majority of newly appointed MROs were psychiatrists, although some of the CSHs appointed family practice physicians.

In addition to the MRO mission, the new drug testing policy also affected the mental health community by identifying more substance abusers in theater. Unfortunately, the Army Substance Abuse Program did not formally exist in theater, thus treatment and rehabilitation options for those identified were extremely limited. Some of the larger FOBs had Alcoholics Anonymous meetings, but for the most part, any drug and alcohol counseling was left to chaplains and the mental health community.[11]

Improvements in Command and Control of Echelon-Above-Division Stress Control Personnel

As the theater matured, so did the ability to command and control COSC personnel in the echelon-above-division units. At the start of combat operations, there were many changes in command structure, supporting units, who would support whom, and so forth.[1] During OIF 05-07, not only was there only one medical headquarters in theater, but it was stationary. There was no longer a need to move north as the conflict progressed.

Each rotation made improvements, and by OIF 05-07 the medical headquarters had a firm foundation on which to build. The introduction of a mental health consultant at the Multi-National Corps–Iraq (MNC–I) level continued during OIF 05-07 as a dual role position with the TF30 Med mental health consultant. This permitted a single medical headquarters to coordinate plans with the divisions and other separate brigades, as well as ensure the MNC–I and MNF–I commanders and command surgeons were kept informed. The result was an enhanced ability for greater situational awareness and coordination of COSC/mental health needs and services.

This enhanced situational awareness also assisted in planning for coverage. Because of improved communication systems, a stationary headquarters, and solid foundation from previous rotations, planning was able to be more deliberate and organized, obtaining input from multiple sources. As the theater changed, so did the method of estimating COSC coverage. In OIF-I, one CSC unit provided coverage to a specific division; there was one preventive team per brigade. By OIF 05-07, area support was the norm. COSC coverage was divided more by geographic location than strictly by division.

Situational Awareness

Managing and directing the COSC medical functional area in a theater of operations requires accurate and up-to-date situational awareness. This required verification of the location of COSC personnel in theater, by clinical specialty. Fortunately, a listing that included MH personnel from the divisions, KBR, the Air Force, the Navy, and the Marine Corps Operational Stress Control and Readiness (OSCAR) teams already existed. A database was developed, adding clinical specialties at each location, and updated regularly. This listing proved to be extremely helpful and provided the situational awareness required for optimal management of COSC resources. Not only did it help to identify the proper unit to task when specific missions were requested, but it also assisted in the planning process by ensuring minimal duplication of services among the various mental health resources on an FOB.

Planning Process

Even though the theater had evolved considerably since the start of the conflict, having the right number of people in the right place was always a challenge. Because planning did not have to occur as troops were on the move, as at the beginning, it was possible to use a very thorough planning process. TF30 Med developed a process that utilized a historical review of workload and operational tempo, COSC doctrine, and a staffing model. (The staffing model that was used was based very closely on one proposed by the second MHAT.[12] It considered three primary categories of services: (1) clinical, (2) unit outreach, and (3) the restoration center. The clinical usage was calculated based on the average of the percentages that want help, need help, and use help. Some of the assumptions were corrected to reflect current processes, and items were modified to be applicable in the deployed environment.)

This was the "science" of operational planning. The "art" of operational planning was then employed by comparing the requirements from the different methods, considering input from the CSC unit commanders, and applying the technical knowledge and expertise of the staff officer. The result was a proposed realignment plan. Mental health personnel in TF30 Med were always cognizant of their role as consultants, and not the final decision makers. Therefore, this recommended plan was presented throughout the chain of command and others involved in providing COSC/mental health services. Because this process may be different from what is experienced by most mental health providers, it bears explanation. The plan was initially reviewed and approved within TF30 Med—

from clinical operations, through G3 (operations), to the commander/theater surgeon. It was then staffed through TF30 Med's direct reporting units—the commanders, the operations officers (S3s), and of course the CSC unit leadership. The units being supported were part of the divisions, so the plan was briefed to the division surgeons and medical planners as well. Additionally, the equivalent personnel from the US Navy were included in the discussion. Changes were made at each step, based on input and needs identified. The final product was published in a fragmentary order. Even then, it specified only the minimal number of personnel at each FOB—by unit—and the location of the restoration centers. The CSC unit commanders were still responsible for determining the correct specialty and personnel to place at each location.

Coordination and planning was continuous. Distribution of COSC personnel changed and adapted as situations changed or divisions made requests. This involved TF30 Med working in partnership with MNC–I mental health consultant, and coordinating closely with the senior mental health personnel of both divisions and Marine Expeditionary Forces on the placement of CSC units—fostering cooperation and minimizing duplication of services.

As previously alluded to, provision of services involved planning and anticipating needs for the future as well. During OIF 05-07, this included coordinating with the US Air Force, which was compiling a CSC for a follow-on rotation. TF30 Med invited an Air Force representative to attend the COSC conference held in theater and meet other CSC commanders, discuss the mission, and get questions answered. The commander of the CSC unit that the Air Force team would be replacing also provided vital input to smooth the transition. After the visit, the utilization of the Air Force liaison officer in country proved invaluable in fine-tuning the coordination, planning, and preparation for the incoming team.

Another manner in which command and control was improved was in the redistribution of the CSC units. After extensive mission analysis and communication with all involved, including the incoming medical headquarters, the CSC units were placed under the command and control of the newly formed provisional multifunctional medical battalion. One of the benefits to having all the CSC units under the same battalion was the enhancement of the ability to coordinate among all of these units. It was now easier to maintain situational awareness across the theater, task the most appropriate unit for any missions that arose, and simplify communication. An illustration of this was when the members of a specific brigade combat team (BCT) were told that they were going to be extended. The extension meant the BCT would need to relocate, and would involve a change in COSC team as well. Due to the ease in communication under one battalion, the efforts of each of the CSC units was well-coordinated and they were able to ensure a minimal disruption of services and affect on the soldiers in the BCT. This also included TF30 Med coordination with the BCT's organic mental health personnel.

Challenges

As with previous rotations, the OIF 05-07 rotation faced several challenges. One of these was the rotation of the divisions midway through the tour of the combat stress control unit supporting them. When the new division arrived, it would sometimes want to change the number or specialty of the mental health personnel on different FOBs. Different mental health personnel may vary on how to implement COSC/mental health services. The challenge presented itself in that the CSC team had already established trust and rapport with the supported units. Changing COSC personnel would affect continuity of care. This was not a problem for the division soldiers as they were leaving, but the supported population included soldiers from the echelon-above-division units as well. It was easier to address this challenge because of the open lines of communication between the CSC units, their battalion headquarters, and the TF30 Med.

Another challenge was in the coordination of who would provide services on a particular FOB. Because the method of team placement emphasized minimizing duplication of services, the only mental health support might be through the division team. This would often require the division mental health personnel to perform COSC and mental health activities to both echelon-above-division and division soldiers. Naturally, the reverse occurred when a CSC unit team was the only mental health asset at a location.

Standardization of Practices

The better-established theater provided the opportunity for the standardization of policies and procedures, and quality control. There are certain issues that seemed to be prevalent in providing COSC services, spanning the OIF rotations. Topics such as how to document contacts, how to measure workload, what is required to evacuate a soldier, and even interpretation of COSC doctrine were addressed. Standardization was difficult when personnel brought with them different levels of training in COSC and differing individual comfort levels with the prevention and outreach focus of COSC. COSC doctrine addressed these topics, but finding the answer was cumbersome at best. To alleviate this, TF30 Med simplified the search by addressing these topics in the COSC annex to the operation orders for both TF30 and MNC–I. This annex established consistent policies and practices theater-wide.

Documentation

One of the main principles behind COSC is to maintain a nonclinical approach when managing soldiers with combat and operational stress reaction (COSR).[2] However, COSC personnel perform interventions and activities not only for soldiers with COSR, but also those with diagnosable psychiatric conditions. What, constitutes appropriate documentation for a soldier with COSR? Does the documentation differ from that for mental health treatment of a psychiatric disorder? Where is this documentation kept, and for how long? Based on COSC doctrine found in Field Manual 4-02.51, a policy was established based on whether or not a soldier would be placed in a COSR restoration program.

Care for a soldier participating in a restoration program for COSR was tracked from the initial contact until the soldier was released from the program. It included the COSC interventions and activities provided, soldier response, and a summary of COSC services provided. This record, or file, was kept separate from the soldier's outpatient treatment record or deployment health record, and safeguarded on premises. As outlined by the Patient Administration Systems and Biostatistics Activity, this file was kept by the CSC unit for 5 years, and destroyed in December of the fifth year.[13] Only a notation of the dates and the CSC unit providing the services was entered into the soldier's official record.

Care for soldiers with COSR, but not participating in a restoration program, was documented according to the level of intervention and severity of COSR. One level was a soldier who was experiencing normal stress reactions, and received only brief supportive "therapy," skill acquisition, or "psychoeducation" to normalize the response. These contacts did not require documentation. However, the soldier who was experiencing a more severe, yet normal, stress reaction would require a notation in the outpatient treatment record. These reactions are described in Field Manual 4-02.51 as "maladaptive stress behaviors."[2] Documentation was also required if the COSR was interfering with the soldier's ability to function. The notation included the CSC unit, a statement that there were no safety issues, and no medication was needed. At the soldier's request, the provider would document any of the above situations. Care for soldiers with psychiatric disorders was documented the same as if the care was provided in garrison. The standards outlined in Army Regulation 40-66 apply on deployment, too.[14]

Reporting Workload

Keeping accurate records is important in identifying any potential trends in healthcare use, incidence of disease, and injury rates. Current methods in force health protection and healthcare include reporting disease nonbattle injuries, surgery hours, and hospital inpatient occupancy. The types of interventions and activities performed in COSC do not fit well into these types of reporting methods. As a result, the COSC-WARS was developed. Because the OIF units were the only ones using the COSC-WARS, permission was received to revise the form. During OIF 05-07, the COSC-WARS summary report was modified twice in an effort to ensure the data collected were sufficient to answer requests from a variety of sources. The final version contained data that allowed accurate responses to requests from the Government Accountability Office, Office of The Surgeon General consultants, and the command surgeons at all levels—MNF–I, MNC–I, and TF30. This form also provided data that proved to be invaluable in the planning process. It is important to note that this process also utilized input from the users of the form—the COSC personnel. The latest version of the COSC-WARS summary report was on a Microsoft Excel worksheet that was easier for the units to complete, and with nearly zero errors. The report was also easier for TF30 staff to collect and enter error free into the summary worksheet. Automatic totals made responding to inquiries and analyzing data almost effortless. Due to the elimination of specific identifying information, units could submit the report over nonsecured means.

Completing the COSC-WARS summary report often seemed a daunting task because of the length. However, COSC personnel were provided with various methods of explanation that included a decision diagram and line-by-line explanations. The more problematic terms such as "walk-about" and "COSR contact" were also explained.

Keeping Statistics

Psychiatric casualty statistics were frequently requested from all levels of leadership, from TF30 Med through MNF–I. Prior to OIF 05-07, most casualty statistics that were reported were based on the daily figures from the Level III hospitals, which included inpatient hospitalizations and inpatient and outpatient evacuations. This resulted in underreporting the number of evacuations, as outpatient evacuations also occurred from the divisions and Level II clinics. This realization led to the creation of a new database, the Mental Health Casualty Tracker for OIF (MHCTO) during OIF 05-07. The MHCTO utilized six sources of information: (1) the daily inpatient census report for theater, (2) the daily inpatient census report for garrison, (3) the US Transportation Command Regulating and Command and Control Evacuation System, (4) the Joint Patient Tracking Application, (5) the Command Critical Intelligence Requirements, and (6) the MNC–I casualty report. Combining these separate data sources into one database allowed for the tracking of all inpatient mental health admissions in theater, all inpatient and outpatient air evacuations, and all suicide completions and suicide attempts that resulted in hospitalization or air evacuation. Because all the notes were electronic and had to be read to fill in the data fields, this also served as a quality assurance measure for all air evacuations.

Suicide statistics were also frequently requested. In addition to tracking the raw numbers, it became apparent that there was a lot of useful information available in the Army Suicide Event Reports (ASER) that had already been completed for suicide events occurring in Iraq. The TF30 Med mental health consultant was able to analyze the raw data on all ASERs submitted for the Iraq theater of operations. As a result of this analysis, it was clear that providers had different interpretations of certain questions, which resulted in lower quality data. The TF30 Med mental health consultant made the ASER a higher priority and took a more proactive stance toward completed ASER submissions for all suicide attempts. With the help of the MHCTO, suicide attempts were now easier to track, so corresponding mental health providers were now contacted and informed of the expectation that the ASER would be submitted. Certain providers even sent ASER drafts to the mental health consultant to ensure accuracy. With more providers submitting more accurate ASERs, the accuracy of the suicide statistics for OIF 05-07 was greatly improved over previous years. Additionally, in the clinical background information gathered from the MHCTO and the ASER it was possible to read about actual incidents in which buddy aid—the basis for Army suicide prevention programs—was successfully administered and resulted in a saved life. Every month, a new vignette was chosen and disseminated at the TF30 Med Battle Update Brief.

Quality Assurance

Having standardized practices and theater-wide policies in place was the first step toward assuring that quality care was consistently being provided across theater. The next logical step was to devise a way to ensure these policies were available and understood by those to whom they applied. By OIF 05-07 the electronic communication systems had been greatly improved and allowed wide dissemination of information. It was now possible to send the policies, through command channels, all the way down to the individual provider. Additionally, the TF30 Med chief of professional services held a regular teleconference in which the deputy chiefs of clinical services from all the CSHs and the multifunctional medical brigade, in addition to the division surgeons, were invited. The mental health consultant regularly disseminated new theater-wide mental health policies through this manner, which allowed for a dynamic discussion to take place prior to the implementation of new policies.

One such policy that was initiated during OIF 05-07 was the guidelines for psychotropic prescribing in theater. The purpose of the guidelines was threefold. First, they set a standard with which most psychiatrists should already be familiar, but primary care providers may not. Secondly, they clearly stated that psychiatrists and certain psychiatric advanced nurse practitioners were the only mental health providers credentialed to prescribe psychotropic medication. (Anecdotally, medical providers had asked social workers and psychologists to write prescriptions, unaware that this was not within their scope of practice.) Finally, the guidelines offered an information paper for commanders, who frequently asked providers which of their soldiers were taking psychotropic medications. There seemed to be a misperception that starting someone on an antidepressant would lead the soldier to be nonmission capable. (Also anecdotally, many soldiers reported feeling more mission capable once their depressive or anxiety symptoms were under better control from medication.)

Another method used to support subordinate units in ensuring quality of care was the staff assistance visit (SAV). TF30 Med conducted SAVs to gain a first-hand awareness of "best practices," make recommendations where indicated, and answer questions. It provided the valuable opportunity to get to know the combat stress control teams and COSC/mental health personnel, their locations, and so forth. A checklist was developed to standardize the questions asked during the visit and to help clarify TF30 Med's priorities. The visit was not meant to be punitive, but rather to offer assistance in meeting expectations outlined in TF30 Med policies and procedures. The SAV was coordinated with the direct reporting unit commanders or deputy chiefs of clinical services, allowing a visit to each CSC unit headquarters and restoration center, mental health personnel at the CSHs, and some area support medical company mental health personnel. It also allowed the headquarters to obtain input from subordinates. In conjunction with these visits, TF30 Med personnel acted as an advocate for COSC/mental health at higher levels. A good example of this occurred after an SAV to one of the CSHs. Based on input from the mental health personnel, the TF30 Med mental health officer could ensure that the need of CSH mental health personnel for appropriate space was heard at brigade headquarters. This included current and future facility needs.

Toward the end of its rotation, TF30 Med decided to institute more regular, formalized, quality control through the establishment of monthly mental health chart reviews. Up until this point, peer reviews were inconsistently being done and most were informally conducted, usually consisting of case discussions. The first question to be addressed was which encounters were to be reviewed: COSR, psychiatric mental disorder (PMD), or both. Because providers were presumably more familiar with the behavioral health standards of the Joint Commission, and because there was more ambiguity in the COSR charting requirements, it seemed reasonable to start with chart reviews on the PMD charts rather than the COSR charts. The next issue was determining a standard for mental health charting in theater. The MNC–I surgeon/TF30 Med commander's directive was that the standards in theater be the same as those for garrison. Even though the Joint Commission would never visit the combat zone, its standards were based on patient safety issues, which still applied in theater. A garrison mental health chart review was then e-mailed to all the CSHs and CSC commanders for feedback on which standards did not apply to the theater. After a consensus was reached, the next step was to determine how isolated clinics could perform the review. It was decided that if there was only one provider at a certain location, that provider was expected to have another medical provider conduct the chart review. This only happened on rare occasions because of the frequency of CSC commander SAVs. The results of the reviews were then e-mailed to the mental health consultant, who could verify to the TF30 Med commander that they were being done.

As a result of the mental health peer review, there was now one standard for mental health charting in the combat zone. This brought up some issues that were previously not being addressed. First, it became apparent that most reserve providers were unaware of the requirement for cosigning the notes of their mental health technicians. Not having a civilian equivalent of an outpatient mental health technician, this was understandable. Additionally, more questions were being asked about what was in a specific provider's scope of practice, such as whether or not a psychiatric nurse practitioner was able to prescribe medications. Finally, as mentioned previously, with more forensic psychiatry requests, there was an increased likelihood that psychiatric charts could be subpoenaed. Chart reviews indicated that this, along with limits of confidentiality, was not always discussed with patients.

Another quality assurance initiative developed by TF30 Med involved a review of the scope of practice of unlicensed providers, such as medics and other health technicians. Upon learning that there were unlicensed psychologists in theater who required regular supervision, the TF30 Med commander began discussions with the Office of The Surgeon General and Medical Command about this practice. Ultimately, the decision was made that no further unlicensed psychologists would deploy to the Iraq theater of operations. The mental health community was not prepared for this policy change. In the immediate aftermath of this, major changes had to be made in assignments. The result was an acute shortage of psychologists, which led to psychiatrists or psychiatric nurse practitioners being used to fill vacant deployment psychologist slots. According to the director, Behavioral Health Proponency, Office of The Surgeon General,[15] training for psychologists in the last year has been extended to 2 years to prevent unlicensed psychologists from being assigned to deployable positions.

ROLE OF THE MEDIA

The quality of information provided to the media is important and can have widespread effect on the mission. To this end, the TF30 Med COSC and mental health consultants worked closely with the task force in developing a Public Affairs Office policy as it related to COSC operations in theater. This ensured the protection of the service members being supported, and provided guidelines for the providers on releasing information. This policy also covered any articles or research requests from providers in theater. Headquarters has a broader awareness of events across the theater, is in a better position to ensure the information is consistent with the overall mission objectives of OIF, and that release of this information is compliant with operational security requirements. By having TF30 Med answer incoming questions, it allowed providers in the field to focus on their mission of providing COSC/mental health services to the force.

Although it is impossible to determine exactly how much the media influenced the daily operations of mental health providers during OIF 05-07, there were headlines that commanded the attention of soldiers and military leadership alike. These media reports ultimately translated into combat mental health practices being more carefully scrutinized and greater accountability of mental healthcare providers, neither of which is necessarily a negative result. In this section a closer look will be taken at some of the more significant headlines during OIF 05-07 and how they potentially impacted the mental health community.

Reporting Increase in Suicide Rates

In April 2006, the 2005 Army suicide rate was released and became widely quoted in the press, the media, and on the Internet. The Associated Press reported that 83 soldiers killed themselves in 2005, the greatest number of Army suicides since 1993.[16] The following month, *The Hartford Courant* ran a series entitled "Mentally Unfit, Forced to Fight." In an article in the series, titled "Potent Mixture: Zoloft and a Rifle," the authors discuss case reports of soldiers prescribed medication in a combat zone who later committed suicide. The article suggested that psychotropic medications were being prescribed too freely in theater and were related to suicides.[17]

The release of the 2005 suicide rate generated considerable interest in the topic of suicide and, specifically, how it applied to the conflict. In "Zoloft and a Rifle," the authors used the increased suicide rate to criticize the combat effort and point out flaws with military mental health. The article sent a mixed message to soldiers in theater—the authors cared about soldiers and wanted to honor those who committed suicide, yet if they were having problems, health providers in theater would only make them worse. Little attention was paid to the theater suicide prevention programs already in existence, or the power of buddy aid.

As the reporting of the increase in the suicide rate spread throughout the media, TF30 Med and MNC–I received additional inquiries related to suicide statistics. By April, the MHCTO was fully operational, which enabled the TF30 Med to support the requests for information. As mentioned previously, studying the ASERs also provided valuable information about theater suicides that was frequently requested by mental health providers and was presented at theater mental health conferences.

Although dramatic, "Zoloft and a Rifle" did bring up a valuable point regarding how nonpsychiatrists were treating mental illness. An informal survey of physician assistants in theater demonstrated that comfort levels with the use of psychotropics varied greatly. This prompted the MNC–I surgeon to commission the psychotropic prescribing guidelines, which came out as a MNC–I fragmentary order during the summer of 2006. The guidelines were meant to assist providers in better understanding psychotropic prescribing in the combat zone and included information about monitoring laboratory reports, side effects, drug interactions, standard of care for treating psychiatric disorders, and what to tell commanders requesting information about their soldiers.

Airing the *Baghdad ER* Special

Baghdad ER is a Home Box Office special that aired May 21, 2006. It is a graphic and emotional account of the realities of combat through the experiences of a CSH. Yet graphic documentaries also have other implications. They can serve as powerful reminders or "triggers" for soldiers who have been exposed to trauma. *Baghad ER* is indeed a harsh reminder of the brutal realities of combat.

Lieutenant General Kevin Kiley, then the Army Surgeon General, directed Army mental health experts to prepare for the impact of *Baghdad ER*. Said Kiley, "This film will have a strong impact on viewers and may cause anxiety for some soldiers and family members."[18] He suggested that mental health facilities should extend their treatment hours and reach out to the troops proactively. The Army recognized that it had to address the near-term implication of the program and also recognized that the families and soldiers who might be traumatized by this media event might also have on-going psychological issues.

The theater mental health consultant wrote the following talking points,which were disseminated in theater prior to the airing of the program.

1. Most soldiers returning from deployment seek to avoid images and media coverage related to the global war on terrorism. Soldiers in theater will have limited access to the HBO special. The greatest impact will likely be on soldiers' families, brought about by fears raised from direct viewing or the publicity afterwards.
2. Technology has significantly altered communications with the home front, with increased accessibility and frequency. Mental health providers have noticed spouses who are coping poorly can significantly affect the morale of their deployed soldier.
3. In the days and weeks following the program airing, commanders should:
   - Check in with their soldiers to see how their spouses are coping.
   - Consider limiting contact immediately before a mission or have mental health assets or chaplains available during popular calling periods.
   - Be aware of common warning signs of

increased stress, such as soldiers becoming isolated, becoming easily angered, or seeming distracted, and a change in work performance.
- Encourage soldiers to talk with their peers, chaplains, or mental health providers if they start to feel more stressed after talking with family members.

4. There are assets available in stay-behind elements to assist family members coping with a soldier's deployment, such as TRICARE and Military OneSource. Additionally, commanders should encourage active participation in family readiness groups, as this provides a unique opportunity for families with a common interest to support each other.[19]

Based on conversations with CSC providers, the aftereffects from *Baghdad ER* were not as intense in theater as was expected. Nevertheless, the event was a clear example of how the media influenced mental health providers in theater during OIF 05-07.

Media Coverage of Civilian Deaths in Haditha

In November 2005, Marines killed 24 Iraqi civilians in the town of Haditha, Iraq. Specifics of the story were not immediately available, but eventually it was reported that the killings were in retribution for a roadside bomb in which a Marine had been killed. *The Washington Post* wrote that "[t]wo US military boards are investigating the incident as potentially the gravest violation of the law of war by US forces in the 3-year-old conflict in Iraq."[20]

Haditha was a complex media event because it lasted for months, as each new revelation had its turn in the media frenzy that followed. Mental health experts were often interviewed to try to make sense of the killings. The psychiatrist Robert Jay Lifton explains that "atrocity is a group activity." Therefore, he writes at *Editor & Publisher* "[t]o attribute the likely massacre at Haditha to 'a few bad apples' or to 'individual failures' is poor psychology and self-serving moralism."[21] Lifton says that the Haditha incident can be understood as what he calls "an atrocity-producing situation," which he defines as "one so structured, psychologically and militarily, that ordinary people, men or women no better or worse than you or I, can commit atrocities."

Interest in combat ethics grew substantially during OIF 05-07 as a result of the killings in Haditha. All subsequent war misbehavior was often presented in comparison to that event. MHAT-IV was commissioned by the MNF–I commander with the request to investigate combat ethics. The MHAT-IV accomplished this through survey questions and focus group discussions. The final report includes information about behaviors during deployment and discusses ideas for teaching ethics. Recommendations include incorporating battlefield ethics in all behavioral health counseling and anger management classes, especially when conducted in a combat zone.[5] These recommendations could substantially increase the scope of duties of deployed mental health providers.

SUMMARY

This chapter has explored how the provision of mental health services advanced during OIF 05-07 as a result of a more mature battlefield. Without having to worry about basic necessities or establishing new clinics, mental health providers were able to take on additional missions, such as serving as MROs or on sexual assault review boards, responding to the media, and meeting standards of care that were the same as garrison mental health clinics. The provision of mental health consultation to TF30 Med, MNC–I, and MNF–I leadership was also able to advance because providers had become adept at mastering the basics. Although not mentioned specifically in this chapter, brevity, immediacy, contact, expectancy, proximity, and simplicity (BICEPS) remained as the cornerstone of mental health services in the combat zone during OIF 05-07. The fact that they did not require alterations speaks to their universality. As future battlefields will likely look as different from OIF as OIF does from World War II, it is reassuring to know that there will be at least one constant in the provision of mental health services. That constant is the BICEPS approach to combat and operational stress reactions.

REFERENCES

1. Caravalho J. *30th Medical Brigade After-Action Review for OIF-I.* October 16, 2004. 30th Medical Brigade Lessons Learned Database. Accessed December 11, 2006.

2. US Department of the Army. *Combat Stress Control.* Washington, DC: DA; June 6, 2006. Field Manual 4-02.51.

3. Jones F, Sparacino L, Wilcox V, Rothberg J, Stokes J, eds. *War Psychiatry*. In: Zajtchuk R, Bellamy RF, eds. *Textbooks of Military Medicine.* Washington, DC: Department of the Army, Office of The Surgeon General, Borden Institute; 1995.

4. Jones F, Sparacino L, Wilcox V, Rothberg J, eds. *Military Psychiatry: Preparing in Peace for War*. In: Zajtchuk R, Bellamy RF, eds. *Textbooks of Military Medicine.* Washington, DC: Department of the Army, Office of The Surgeon General, Borden Institute; 1994.

5. Mental Health Advisory Team (MHAT) IV. *Operation Iraqi Freedom 05-07.* Office of the Surgeon, Multi-National Force-Iraq, and Office of The Surgeon General, United States Army Medical Command. November 17, 2006. Available at: www.armymedicine.army.mil/reports/mhat.html. Accessed September 4, 2008.

6. Tan M. Gangs in uniform. *Army Times*. September 3, 2007:14.

7. Mental Health Advisory Team (MHAT). *Operation Iraqi Freedom (OIF). Report.* The US Army Surgeon General and HQDA G-1. December 16, 2003. Available at: www.armymedicine.army.mil/reports/mhat.html. Accessed September 4, 2008.

8. United States Department of Defense Sexual Assault Prevention and Response Web site. Available at: http://www.sapr.mil. Accessed September 9, 2008.

9. All Army Activity (ALARACT) Message No. 087/2006. *Drug Testing During Deployments*. April 26, 2006.

10. US Army Medcial Command Military MRO Information Pamphlet, May 30, 2006.

11. Chagalis GP. *Army Substance Abuse Program Guidance for Deployed Commanders*. Information Paper, April 6, 2004. Available at: www.sbasap.com/files/deployed_cdrs.pdf. Accessed September 9, 2008.

12. Mental Health Advisory Team (MHAT-II). *Operation Iraqi Freedom (OIF-II). Report.* The US Army Surgeon General. January 30, 2005. Available at: www.armymedicine.army.mil/reports/mhat.html. Accessed September 4, 2008.

13. Patient Administration Systems and Biostatistics Activity Memorandum. *Consolidation of Deployment Medical Documentation*. October 21, 2005.

14. US Department of the Army. *Medical Record Administration and Health Care Documentation*. Washington, DC: DA; June 17, 2008. Army Regulation 40-66.

15. Ritchie EC. Colonel, Medical Corps, US Army. Personal communication, February 2009.

16. Army suicides hit highest level since 1993. *Associated Press*. April 21, 2006. Available at: http://www.msnbc.msn.com/id/12428185. Accessed September 9, 2008.

17. Chedekel L, Kauffman M. Potent mixture: Zoloft & a rifle. *Hartford Courant.* May 16, 2006:A1.

18. Starr B. Army: HBO documentary could trigger stress disorder [transcript]. *Entertainment.* CNN television. May 15, 2006.

19. Cooper MA. Major, Medical Corps, US Army. Personal communication, November 2008.

20. Knickmeyer E. In Haditha, memories of a massacre: Iraqi townspeople describe slaying of 24 civilians by Marines in Nov. 19 incident. *Washington Post.* May 27, 2006:A01. Available at: http://www.washingtonpost.com/wp-dyn/content/article/2006/05/26/AR2006052602069.html. Accessed September 9, 2008.

21. Lifton RJ. The psychology of atrocity. *Editor and Publisher.* June 4, 2006.

Chapter 10

PSYCHIATRIC MEDICATIONS IN MILITARY OPERATIONS

BRETT J. SCHNEIDER, MD*; JOHN C. BRADLEY, MD†; CHRISTOPHER H. WARNER, MD‡; AND DAVID M. BENEDEK, MD§

*Lieutenant Colonel, Medical Corps, US Army; Deputy Chief, Department of Psychiatry, Building 61, Child and Adolescent Psychiatry Clinic, Walter Reed Army Medical Center, 6900 Georgia Avenue NW, Washington, DC 20307

†Colonel, Medical Corps, US Army; Chair, Department of Psychiatry, Borden Pavilion, Room 2022, Walter Reed Army Medical Center, 6900 Georgia Avenue NW, Washington, DC 20307; Psychiatry Consultant, North Atlantic Regional Medical Command and Vice Chair, Department of Psychiatry, Uniformed Services University of the Health Sciences, Bethesda, Maryland

‡Major, Medical Corps, US Army; Chief, Department of Behavioral Medicine, Winn Army Community Hospital, Building 9242, Room 20, 1083 Worcester Drive, Fort Stewart, Georgia 31324; formerly, Division Psychiatrist, 3rd Infantry Division, Fort Stewart, Georgia

§Colonel, Medical Corps, US Army; Professor and Deputy Chair, Department of Psychiatry, Uniformed Services University of the Health Sciences, 4301 Jones Bridge Road, Bethesda, Maryland 20814

A portion of this chapter has been published as: Benedek DM, Schneider BJ, Bradley JC. Psychiatric medications for deployment: an update. *Mil Med*. 2007;172:681–685.

INTRODUCTION

Until the mid-1990s, psychotropic medication use for the treatment of ongoing mental disorders during combat operations was uncommon. Stimulants and other psychotropic medications were used, at times, to enhance the vigilance and performance of fatigued service members. However, in the mid-1990s the introduction of medications with more favorable side-effect profiles—particularly the selective serotonin reuptake inhibitors (SSRIs)—revolutionized the role of medications in the practice of military operational psychiatry. The widespread incorporation of these medications into civilian and military garrison psychiatric practice has resulted in an evolution in operational practice such that medication use in combat operations now focuses on the capacity for soldiers with symptoms of psychiatric illness to return to their premorbid level of functioning, rather than on efforts to "enhance" baseline performance.

Before the current conflicts in Iraq and Afghanistan, recent experiences either predated the current usage patterns of medications in psychiatric care, or were limited in duration (the Persian Gulf War) or scope (Bosnia, Kosovo, Somalia), so that few service members were affected. As a result, comprehensive experience and doctrine for the use of psychotropic medications consistent with current practice patterns in psychiatry were not feasible. This chapter will focus on the use of psychotropic medications during deployment. An overview of the history of the usage of medications will highlight the doctrinal evolution. Current practice guidance will be outlined and as yet unresolved questions addressed.

HISTORY OF PSYCHOTROPIC MEDICATION USE IN DEPLOYMENT

The ancient Assyrians, Egyptians, and Greeks reportedly used opiates before and during battles to sustain or enhance bravery and courage.[1] Other drugs studied or used to enhance combat performance include ergot alkaloids, cannabis, amphetamines, and other stimulants; Dramamine (McNeil-PPC Inc, Morris Plains, NJ) and other antihistamines; benzodiazepines; and L-tryptophan.[1] The most extensive modern use of performance-enhancing drugs occurred during World War II by German, Japanese, and English soldiers.[2] Amphetamines were noted to be useful not only to stave off fatigue and drowsiness but also to improve memory, concentration, physical strength, and endurance.[3–5]

During the Vietnam conflict, methylphenidate (Ritalin [Novartis AG, Basel, Switzerland]) and sometimes dextroamphetamine (Dexedrine [GlaxoSmithKline, Philadelphia, Pa]) were standard-issue drugs carried by long-range reconnaissance patrol soldiers, who reported the drugs' usefulness when they developed fatigue at the end of missions and had to return rapidly to base camp. Mild rebound depression and fatigue after discontinuation were the only reported adverse effects.[1] Sedatives were also explored as a method to improve performance in anxiety-producing situations, such as paratroopers making low-altitude jumps, or to reduce the emotional tension of young soldiers when guns were fired.[6]

Although the concept of using medications for performance enhancement remains an area of ongoing research, the documented usage of psychotropic medications to treat symptoms associated with current psychiatric diagnoses in soldiers actively involved in combat is limited. In earlier conflicts, limited experience using psychotropic medications to treat anxiety symptoms has been reported. These conditions have been treated with sedatives ranging from chloral hydrate and bromides in World War I to barbiturates in World War II and self-prescribed alcohol, cannabis, and heroin in Vietnam.[1] However, discussions of usage commented mostly on the medications' unwanted side effects, such as sedation, and the concern that their usage would lead to the fixation of a sickness role suggested by taking medication.

In 1978 Datel and Johnson[7] reviewed the usage of psychotropic medications by physicians deployed to Vietnam in 1967. They surveyed a group of mostly primary care physicians about how they prescribed 28 different psychotropic medications, including "major tranquilizers," "minor tranquilizers," antidepressants, stimulants, and sedatives for a 30-day period during the summer of that year. The most commonly utilized "psychotropic medication" was Compazine (GlaxoSmithKline) for gastroenteritis, and anxiety and insomnia were the most frequent mental health reasons for prescribing medications. Minor tranquilizers such as Equanil (Wyeth, Madison, NJ); Librium (Hoffman-LaRoche Inc, Nutley, NJ); Valium (Hoffman-LaRoche Inc); and Vistaril (Pfizer Inc, New York, NY) were most frequently prescribed for symptoms of anxiety, with Librium accounting for the majority of prescriptions (65%) and Thorazine (GlaxoSmithKline) accounting for most of the major tranquilizer prescriptions (86%). The authors noted that a "surprisingly low frequency" of depression was an indication for the usage of psychotropic medications. In general, the drugs that were utilized were perceived by the prescribing physicians as being quite efficacious.[7] Six medications (Prolixin [Bristol-Myers Squibb, Princeton, NJ];

Vesprin [Bristol-Myers Squibb]; Nardil [Pfizer]; Parnate [GlaxoSmithKline], Taractan [Hoffman-LaRoche Inc]; and desipramine) were not prescribed by any of the reporting physicians.

The first Israeli reports of operational use of tricyclic antidepressants in combat soldiers occurred during the 1982 war with Lebanon. Belenky noted that in 1973 the Israelis created a policy prohibiting forward use of medications and even hypnosis, expressing concern about the potential effect of this policy on battle fatigue return-to-duty rates.[8,9] Belenky advocated for longer-term military treatment facilities in theater, but cautioned against placing soldiers on psychotropic medications in forward deployed areas because of the possibility of side effects that might interfere with psychomotor performance or impair judgment in dangerous situations. He also noted potential medical risks from side effects in the field environment and problems with resupply.[8]

No reports have been published on the utilization rates or rationale for usage of psychotropic medications during the Persian Gulf War (1991), possibly because of the lack of prolonged combat exposure, or possibly because the military stress control doctrine at the time emphasized triage and normalization, discussing the use of psychotropic medications only in emergency situations. Staudenmeier and Bacon[10] reviewed the history and role of combat stress units during deployments and noted that one unit, the 528th, conducted 514 psychiatric evaluations during the Persian Gulf War. Of those evaluated, 24% were held for treatment and 3.5% were evacuated. Although this information demonstrated that combat stress units were being utilized, no data were given on the usage of medications among service members identified for treatment or evacuation.[10]

Ritchie[11] described a decision-making process for choosing which psychotropic medications to bring and use in Somalia during Operation Restore Hope (1993). Ritchie recommended considering two broad categories: emergency and maintenance medications. The former group included benzodiazepines (diazepam and lorazepam) and neuroleptics (haloperidol). The latter included antidepressants ("one tricyclic antidepressant and one SSRI"); anxiolytics (buspirone, benzodiazepines, or antidepressants); and sedatives (temazepam, triazolam, and trazodone). The rationale for bringing just one tricyclic antidepressant and one SSRI mirrored clinical practice at the time, which suggested that patients being treated by one antidepressant could be switched to another with little problem. Subsequently, practitioners have recognized that frequently patients only respond to a particular antidepressant or have side effects with one SSRI but not another. Ritchie recommended that medications such as lithium, carbamazepine, valproic acid, and all monoamine oxidase inhibitors be avoided during deployment because of problems with safety and monitoring.[11]

Pincus and Benedek[12] summarized the integrated use of combat stress detachments and division mental health (DMH) assets during Operation Joint Endeavor in Bosnia during 1995. The article does not specifically discuss medication usage in detail, but it considered the mission, a year-long peacekeeping operation, as more similar to the practice of garrison mental health than to other deployment environments.[12] Garrison mental health in 1995 typically consisted of a DMH team providing routine outpatient mental healthcare, including using psychotropic medications as indicated for the treatment of disorders seen in routine outpatient clinics. This practice suggests that mental health assets deployed during Operation Joint Endeavor utilized psychotropic medications routinely during the more than 3,000 outpatient contacts made over the year-long deployment. The authors acknowledged use consistent with garrison psychiatric practice in subsequent descriptions of their deployments.[12]

Warner et al[13] reviewed the utilization of one DMH activity during deployment to Operation Iraqi Freedom (OIF) in 2005. The authors noted 5,542 clinical contacts, of which 29.8% were for psychiatric mental disorders and the other 70.2% were for combat operational stress reactions. The top two psychiatric mental disorders in theater were generalized anxiety disorder (42.4%) and major depressive disorder (33.4%). The authors defined a "mature theater" as permitting the ongoing management of psychiatric disorders with psychotropic medications, although personnel were generally restricted to the use of SSRIs and mild hypnotics in theater. The article did not report rates of how many soldiers were prescribed or took the medications in theater; however, the account demonstrated the incorporation of practice patterns established in more recent peacekeeping operations (Bosnia) into psychiatric practice in the combat environment, with service members receiving treatment for ongoing mental health issues beyond the scope of combat operational stress.[13]

In July 2007, Schneider, Bradley, and Benedek[14] revisited the question of a rationale for choosing a psychotropic formulary for military operations. Recommendations were based on a combined 18 months of experience by the authors as psychiatrists deployed with combat stress control detachments during the first and third rotations to Iraq. The authors discussed the evolution of treatment of combat operational stress casualties from triage and nonpharmacologic, treatment-forward psychiatry principles to a role more consistent with contemporary outpatient psychiatric practices, noting some caveats related to environmental and operational concerns. From their perspective, the nature of combat had changed. The idea that soldiers could be removed from the front lines and treated in the rear echelons no longer worked, because no true rear echelons exist in Iraq. It was now important to treat some mood and anxiety disorders as far forward as possible.[14]

Schneider and colleagues also noted that the increased dependence on National Guard and Reserve soldiers meant that the Army was receiving personnel who were treated according to civilian community standards rather than military readiness standards concerning prescriptions for SSRIs, atypical antidepressants, and antianxiety medications. This resulted in an increased requirement for available medications in theater. They suggested that most routine outpatient psychiatric conditions might be managed with medications and therapy in the combat zone, with the caveat of factoring in the "limitations inherent in the operational environment,"[14(p685)] such as military occupation, travel limitations for follow-up, and the restricted ability to educate the soldier and command about the medications' potential risks, benefits, side effects, and possible effect on mission requirements. They proposed a psychotropic formulary of at least 24 medications under the categories of antidepressants/antianxiety medications, benzodiazepines, antipsychotics/antimanics, sleep medications, adrenergic agents, and attention deficit hyperactivity disorder medications (Table 10-1).[14]

The level of comfort with the use of psychotropic medications in combat has mirrored trends in the larger US society. The change in psychotropic medication use from the last major extended US conflict (Vietnam) to current operations in Afghanistan and Iraq is well illustrated by a comparison between Datel and Johnson's questionnaire and the recent recommended psychotropic formulary for OIF by Schneider, Bradley, and Benedek. The only medications common to both documents are Ritalin and Dexedrine.[7,14]

DOCTRINE AND POLICY

US Army doctrine on the use of psychotropic medication has evolved significantly in the last 20 years. The initial Army field manual (FM) on combat stress control, *Combat Stress Control in a Theater of Operations* (FM 8-51),[15] published in 1994 and updated in 1998, focused on triage and nonpharmacologic interventions aimed at normalizing and minimizing combat stress. Little guidance was provided on the role and usage of psychotropic medications. The word "medication" occurs 25 times in this document, which contains 9 chapters. Most of these references discuss the use of medications in emergency situations when medication might be needed to calm an agitated service member. Chapter 3, section 8, states that "medication is prescribed sparingly and only when needed to temporarily support sleep or manage disruptive symptoms."[15(p3-8)] Chapter 6, section 3, discusses how to manage a service member who deploys after having been "diagnosed with psychiatric disorders by a civilian physician," advising the clinician as follows:

> These soldiers may hide the fact that they are taking psychotherapeutic medication to keep the diagnosis off their military record. Once in the theater they may experience a relapse or self-refer themselves to an MTF [medical treatment facility] when their medication supply is exhausted. The evaluating psychiatrist must determine if the soldier can function without the medication. If the soldier requires medication, can he be re-stabilized on a drug which can be provided in the theater? Can the drug be given without risk of harmful side effects? If the alternatives are not feasible, the soldier must be evacuated out of the theater.[15(p6-13)]

During the spring and summer of 2004, the Army mental health community recognized, based on experience in the first year of OIF, that the FM required some revisions based on the changes in overall Army doctrine and lessons learned from the first long-term sustained conflict in more than 30 years. In the new manual, *Combat and Operational Stress Control* (FM 4-02.51),[16] published in 2006, the word "medication" occurs 30 times in an 11-chapter manual. Although the overall number of times medication usage is discussed barely eclipses the number of times it was mentioned in the previous manual, a change in the accepted role of medications can be seen. Three sections in the new manual highlight the gradual move towards acceptance of psychotropic medication usage in a combat zone. Section 8-21 discusses how a service member may have both a combat stress reaction and a mental disorder, and directs clinicians to use clinical judgment and consultation to help "distinguish among these sometimes overlapping conditions."[16(p8-6)] When a service member presents with reemerging symptoms of a previously diagnosed mental disorder or for refill of previously prescribed psychotropic medication, "deferral of diagnosis is preferred, but diagnosis can be considered."[16(p8-6)] Sections 9-8 and 11-1 outline doctrinal changes in the role of medication in treating service members diagnosed with mental disorders while deployed. Section 9-8 states:

> Ongoing treatment and/or therapeutic modalities are essential to improving a Soldier's chances to RTD [return to duty] whether in theater or af-

TABLE 10-1

EXAMPLE PSYCHIATRIC FORMULARY FOR DEPLOYMENT

Medication	Amount
Antidepressants/Antianxiety Medications	
Citalopram 20 mg	15 bottles
Sertraline 100 mg	30 bottles
Prozac* 10 mg	5 bottles
Paroxetine 20 mg	5 bottles
Venlafaxine XR 37.5 mg	10 bottles (good for initiating treatment)
Venlafaxine XR 150 mg	10 bottles
Bupropion XL 150 mg	10 bottles (more if planning to do smoking cessation)
Bupropion XL 75 mg	10 bottles (good for initiating treatment)
Mirtazapine 20 mg	10 bottles
Benzodiazepines	
Lorazepam 1 mg tablets	30 bottles
Clonazepam 1 mg tablets	30 bottles
Lorazepam 2 mg injectable	30 dosages (must be refrigerated)
Antipsychotics/Antimanics	
Risperidone 1 mg tablets	10 bottles
Quetiapine 100 mg tablets	30 bottles (can be used off-label for PTSD, insomnia)
Olanzapine 5 mg tablets	10 bottles
Haloperidol injectable	30 dosages
Sleep Medications	
Trazodone 100 mg tablets	30 bottles
Zolpidem 10 mg tablets	30 bottles
Adrenergic Agents	
Clonidine 0.1 mg tablets	10 bottles (may be better for startle, flashbacks in PTSD)
Prazosin 1 mg tablets	10 bottles (may be better for nightmares in PTSD)
Propranolol 20 mg tablets	10 bottles
ADHD Medications	
Atomoxetine 20 mg tablets	10 bottles
Methylphenidate or Dexedrine†	10 bottles (may want to have combination of long-/short-acting forms)

*Eli Lilly and Company, Indianapolis, Ind
†GlaxoSmithKline, Philadelphia, Pa
ADHD: attention deficit hyperactivity disorder
PTSD: posttraumatic stress disorder
Reproduced from: Schneider BJ, Bradley JC, Benedek DM. Psychiatric medications for deployment: an update. *Mil Med*. 2007;172:683.

ter evacuation. Therapeutic modalities are similar to those used on inpatient units, but must remain consistent with COSC [combat operational stress control] principles. These modalities include medication, individual psychotherapy, group psychotherapy, and appropriate therapeutic occupations.[16(p9)]

Section 11-1 states:

> Behavioral health treatment is provided for Soldiers with behavioral disorders to sustain them on duty or to stabilize them for referral/transfer. This is usually brief, time-limited treat-

ment as dictated by the operational situation. Behavioral health treatment includes counseling, psychotherapy, behavior therapy, occupational therapy, and medication therapy.[16(p11)]

Despite this subtle but real evolution of the role of psychotropic medications, in the fall of 2006—only 4 months after the FM was released—the Department of Defense developed criteria for psychiatric medications use in deployment. The policy was initially released in November 2006 in a memorandum titled *Policy Guidance for Deployment-Limiting Psychiatric Conditions and Medications*,[17] in response to a congressional directive[18] after several media reports of deployed mentally ill soldiers who were unstable or taking medications without follow-on care. The memorandum outlined the restrictions and minimum mental health deployment criteria for all soldiers. Exhibit 10-1 lists key factors related to medications in the policy. Although the policy does not address how long a soldier on a medication for anxiety, depression, or insomnia should be monitored, at least 1 month prior to deployment is a good time frame for consideration.

Current military operations in war zones such as Iraq or Afghanistan no longer have true "rear" areas to which soldiers can be evacuated and treated away from the threat of attack. The ability to provide more definitive treatment to soldiers with certain mood or anxiety disorders as far forward as possible is increasingly important in these operations. For most soldiers, this means that a battalion aid station, DMH element, or a combat stress team is the most easily accessible location for treatment that could allow the soldier to remain mission capable.

EXHIBIT 10-1

KEY POINTS IN THE NOVEMBER 2006 POLICY GUIDANCE FOR DEPLOYMENT-LIMITING PSYCHIATRIC CONDITIONS AND MEDICATIONS

- Soldiers currently being treated for psychosis or bipolar disorder are not deployable.
- Soldiers who are taking medications that require laboratory monitoring, such as lithium or valproic acid, are not deployable.
- Soldiers who are taking antipsychotic medications to control psychotic, bipolar, or chronic insomnia conditions are not deployable.
- The continued use of psychotropic medications that are clinically and operationally problematic during deployments, including short half-life benzodiazepines and stimulants, should be balanced between the necessity for successful functioning in the theater of operations and the ability to obtain the medication, the potential for withdrawal, and the potential for abuse.
- If a soldier is placed on a psychotropic medication within 3 months of deployment, then he/she must be improving, stable, and tolerating the medication without significant side effect to deploy.

Data source: Assistant Secretary of Defense. *Policy Guidance for Deployment-Limiting Psychiatric Conditions and Medications*. Washington, DC: Department of the Army; 2006.

PREDEPLOYMENT ACTIONS

It is imperative that all military primary care and mental health providers know where a soldier under treatment is in the deployment cycle. The stage of the deployment cycle can play a major role in the selection of particular medication choices. Communication among the soldier, medical and mental health providers, and the brigade surgeon and brigade behavioral health officer is essential to ensure that treatment plans are developed without creating additional unnecessary limitations for the soldier. Two key actions required before deployment are (1) determining if soldiers currently taking psychotropic medications meet the minimum mental health fitness standards for deployment, and (2) choosing the medications to make available during deployment.

Psychiatric Medication Clearance for Deployment

To determine if soldiers meet the minimum mental health standards for deployment outlined in Exhibit 10-1, units have added mental health medication screening to the predeployment medical screening process. In one recently deploying brigade combat team, screening questions were added to the face-to-face interview by a primary care provider; all soldiers taking psychotropic medications were required to meet with a behavioral health provider to ensure they met deployment requirements.

Case Study 10-1: A deploying brigade combat team of 3,312 soldiers implemented the process described above. The brigade identified 143 soldiers (4.3%) who were or had recently been under the care of a mental health provider, and 86 (2.6%) who were currently taking a psychotropic medication. Of those taking psychotropic medications, 53 (1.6%) used antidepressant medications; 11 (0.3%) used medications other than antipsychotics for chronic insomnia or sleep disturbances; 11 (0.3%) used stimulants for attention deficit problems; 8 (0.2%) used antipsychotic medications for chronic insomnia; 2 (0.06%) used benzodiazepines for chronic anxiety symptoms; and 1 (0.03%) used Depakote (Abbott Laboratories, Abbott Park, Ill) for bipolar disorder. Of the group on medication, 68 (2.1%) required mental health clearance for deployment; of the 68, 4 (0.1%) were delayed 1 to 2 months before deploying for medication stabilization, and 3 (0.09%) were not cleared for deployment because of their medications (a tricyclic antidepressant, an antipsychotic, and a mood stabilizer). An additional 19 soldiers (0.6%) were deemed unqualified for deployment because of their current medication even though they were stable and performing required duties without impairment.[19]

For soldiers who are stable but on medications that disqualify them from deployment, such as a stimulant for attention deficit hyperactivity disorder or a low-dose antipsychotic for chronic insomnia, a waiver may be requested. The process is instituted through unit medical channels and is requested through the combatant command surgeon—the senior ranking command surgeon in theater. In most cases, if a unit provides a justification, plan for continuation of treatment, and safety assessment, the waiver is likely to be granted. Medications generally eligible for a waiver are benzodiazepines used for anxiety, stimulants for treatment of attention deficit disorder, nonlaboratory monitoring mood stabilizing agents for impulse control and nonbipolar mood management, and low-dose antipsychotics for sleep and anxiety symptoms. In deciding whether to request a waiver, a unit should consider the duties and responsibilities the soldiers will hold and ensure that they will have ongoing access to mental healthcare throughout deployment. The final decision on the waiver is at the discretion of the combatant command surgeon.

Case Study 10-2: The 19 soldiers deemed unqualified from the brigade combat team in Case Study 10-1 were eligible for waivers. Many were taking stimulants for attention deficit problems or low doses of atypical antipsychotics for chronic insomnia. The unit leadership deemed that most of the soldiers were critical to the mission, and waivers were requested for all of them. The waiver requests outlined length of time on the medication and how the soldier would be followed by mental health services during deployment. All soldiers received waivers and deployed. The DMH team and the brigade surgeon ensured that each of the soldiers was seen on a regular basis (monthly), and after 6 months of deployment, all remained in theater, stable, and functioning well in their duties.[19]

Psychopharmacologic Planning for Deployment

A psychiatrist assigned to a DMH or combat stress control (CSC) unit must determine what type of psychotropic medications, and how much of each, to obtain for use in a deployment. For most brigade combat teams, the individual who makes these decisions is the brigade surgeon; the surgeon often acts on the advice of the brigade behavioral health officer or the division psychiatrist. Factors to be considered are the current medications used by soldiers within the unit, the availability of medications in theater, and the maturity of the theater. Medications are class VIII in the military supply classification system, and most medical/mental health units deploy with an initial supply stock.

The brigade surgeon can determine which medications soldiers are currently taking by asking them during the predeployment screening program or consulting the local medical treatment facility pharmacist. Medication availability is determined by the local theater. The brigade medical supply officer can provide a standard formulary for the region in which the unit is deploying. For example, in the current conflicts in Iraq and Afghanistan, the medications available for resupply are determined by the central command pharmacy review committee. In preparation for deployments, brigade surgeons should ensure that local home station providers have the theater formulary, and that they utilize the listed medications as the first choice.

The maturity of theater plays a key role in the amount of medications a unit needs to take with it. An important finding of the original mental health assessment team (MHAT) in the first year of OIF was that psychotropic medications were not adequately available in theater and resupply was not effective.[20] However, the theaters in Iraq and Afghanistan have now become more mature, and resupply channels are clearly established and effective. The formulary provided by Schneider et al[14] (see Table 10-1) delineates initial planning guidance, but it should be modified based on the factors outlined above.

DISPENSING PSYCHIATRIC MEDICATION IN THEATER

Multiple factors affect the dispensing of medications in the deployed environment. Providers must be able to support follow up for individuals who are started on medications and ensure that resupply is available. A number of options for resupply of medications are available in theater. DMH units are generally located with Level-II aid stations, and CSC units may have relationships with local unit medical clinics. CSC units can also establish medication resupply channels with medical logistics units. Psychiatrists must maintain ongoing communication with their resupply sources to ensure availability as well as to report utilization trends, which allows medical supply officers to effectively maintain supplies.

Once medications have been obtained, their storage and security are the next consideration. Although most medications are stable compounds, checking package inserts or asking the pharmacist or pharmaceutical company about any problems with keeping the specific compounds in the deployment environment is advisable. Deploying behavioral health units that intend to maintain their own medication supply should consider obtaining a small refrigerator for storage, taking into account the availability and source of power in theater. Medications such as benzodiazepines and stimulants are controlled substances with the potential for abuse. These medications must be securely maintained under clear standard operating procedures that fall within military regulations for maintenance of controlled substances.

Methods for dispensing psychotropic medications in theater will be determined by several factors, including the soldier's access to mental health services, the soldier's reliability, and the proximity of other pharmacy services. In current operations in Iraq, multiple methods have been utilized, including providing soldiers with a supply of medication, providing a starting dose and a prescription to take to the local aid station or pharmacy, or providing only a prescription for the patient to have filled locally. In general, soldiers should be provided no more than a 1-month supply of medication. Additionally, in 2006 the Army opened the TRICARE mail order pharmacy program, which allows soldiers to have refills shipped directly to them.

PHARMACOLOGIC TREATMENT OF MENTAL HEALTH CONDITIONS DURING DEPLOYMENT

Clinicians must make decisions regarding the extent of services they can safely and effectively provide within their units. Potential pharmacological interventions, such as medication for posttraumatic stress disorder (PTSD), attention deficit hyperactivity disorder, or smoking cessation fall into a "gray area" of in-theater treatment considerations. The decision to continue treatment or evacuate patients with these conditions depends on which medications are available, how significant the symptoms are, how the soldier initially responds to treatment, and how significantly the symptoms interfere with the soldier's assigned duties.

Mood Disorders

Bipolar Disorder

Bipolar disorder requires evacuation from the combat zone, especially if the soldier presents in the midst of a manic or hypomanic episode. Because the number of manic or hypomanic patients likely to present during military operations is minimal, psychiatrists should select medications useful for multiple situations. Because only acute and emergent management are conducted in theater, the most practical course of action is to stock at least two atypical antipsychotic agents, such as olanzapine, quetiapine, risperidone, aripiprazole, and ziprasidone. All of these medications are effective in treating acute mania and have multiple additional indications (mood instability, anxiety, agitation, psychosis, and augmentation strategies for depression).

Major Depressive Disorder and Dysthymic Disorder

In planning for the treatment of new-onset depressive disorders, clinicians should request a considerable quantity of the SSRI they are most comfortable prescribing. They should request the largest amount of an SSRI that is also indicated for new-onset anxiety disorders. Zoloft (sertraline [Pfizer-Roerig, New York, NY]) and Celexa (citalopram [Forest Pharmaceuticals, Saint Louis, Mo]) are reasonable first choices because neither interacts significantly with other medications through the cytochrome P450 enzyme system, and both are usually well tolerated by both depressed and anxious patients.[21,22] The long half-life of fluoxetine offers an advantage; however, its tendency to be more activating than other medications makes its use for both anxiety and depressive disorders less favorable.[23] Paroxetine's potential for a discontinuation syndrome if doses are missed could prove problematic in a combat zone.[24] Additionally, paroxetine's anticholinergic properties may prove problematic in Iraq, where temperatures often reach 140°F. Nonetheless, a small supply of all of the SSRIs mentioned above should be secured, because these medications are so commonly prescribed that clinicians will surely encounter patients who either are currently receiving them or have responded favorably to them in the past.

Clinicians should also consider keeping at least two non-SSRI antidepressants in the formulary (see Table 10-1). Some deployed psychiatrists have selected bupropion and venlafaxine because they have different mechanisms of action than the SSRIs and both can be used for more than treatment of depression (bupropion for attention deficit hyperactivity disorder and smoking cessation, and venlafaxine for generalized anxiety disorder), allowing for maximal flexibility and economy.[25,26] Other potential choices include Cymbalta (duloxetine [Eli Lilly and Company, Indianapolis, Ind]) and Remeron (mirtazepine [Organon USA, West Orange, NJ]). The recently released Cymbalta has a mechanism of action similar to that of venlafaxine with less reported risk of causing hypertension, and Remeron treats insomnia, which is nearly ubiquitous during deployments.[27,28] Not recommended are tricyclic antidepressants, which have anticholinergic properties, and nefazadone, because of the potential need for laboratory monitoring with liver function tests.

Anxiety Disorders

SSRIs are the mainstay of treatment for various anxiety disorders because they have demonstrated efficacy in panic disorder, PTSD, obsessive-compulsive disorder, and generalized anxiety disorder.[29–31] Clinicians should consider having one SSRI in large quantities to be used for both depressive and anxiety disorders. Benzodiazepines may be helpful for panic disorder and acute stress disorder because they improve sleep and decrease general anxiety symptoms, although they may increase the severity of PTSD, especially if used for long periods.[29] Venlafaxine may be useful in treating generalized anxiety disorder. A useful adjunct in the treatment of acute stress disorder and PTSD is an α-adrenergic or β-adrenergic receptor antagonist to target the autonomic symptoms and nightmares that may be associated with these disorders. Prazosin is a medication in this group with preliminary data supporting its usefulness in treating trauma-related nightmares.[32]

Psychotic Disorders and Acute Agitation

Injectable haloperidol and lorazepam remain excellent choices for management of acutely agitated, violent, or psychotic patients.[33] Although injectable forms of both Geodon (ziprasidone [Pfizer-Roerig]) and Zyprexa (olanzapine [Eli Lilly and Company]) are now available that may have better side-effect profiles, including decreased risk of extrapyramidal symptoms, both require preparation (being mixed with sterile water for 1–5 minutes) before use.[34,35] Additionally, DMH sections and CSC units have a limited number of psychiatrists and psychiatric clinical nurse specialists. Physician's assistants, general medical officers, flight surgeons, and others who transport soldiers between echelons of care often have limited experience with these medications and may be more comfortable with Haldol (haloperidol [Ortho-McNeil Inc, Titusville, NJ]) as the antipsychotic agent for treating acute mania, agitation, or psychosis in a combat zone.[33]

The authors recommend that deploying psychiatrists' formulary include two orally administered atypical neuroleptic agents, one injectable typical neuroleptic agent (most likely haloperidol), one injectable benzodiazepine (most likely lorazepam), and injectable Benadryl (diphenhydramine [Pfizer]). The latter is useful to treat agitation and some acute side effects (such as dystonic reactions) of neuroleptic agents.

Insomnia

Insomnia was the most common symptom reported by soldiers presenting for care at the 528th CSC during the first year of OIF.[14] Clinicians treating soldiers with insomnia must initially decide whether the problem is part of a major psychiatric disorder, a symptom of operational stress, or an adjustment disorder. In the absence of other symptoms, behavioral interventions such as education on sleep hygiene may be the preferred initial intervention because of the possibility that prescribed medications will cause drowsiness during missions or difficulty awakening during times of peril. The decision to use medications should include consideration of the soldier's military occupational specialty, current duties, comorbid symptoms, substance use history, and estimated ability to adhere to instructions and the recommended dosing schedule. Potential deployment formulary medications for the treatment of insomnia include trazodone, zolpidem, lorazepam, clonazepam, prazosin, and quetiapine.[14]

Trazodone is particularly useful for patients with difficulty staying asleep throughout the night.[36] To maximize its successful use, clinicians must spend extra time educating patients about how to take this medication in a field environment. One disadvantage of trazodone is its tendency to cause morning sedation or sluggishness, particularly if the dose is too high. Frequently, the standard dosage (50 or 100 mg with subsequent 50- to 100-mg increments) leaves a patient either undermedicated or overmedicated. Because the 528th CSC prescribed this medication only for sleep, patients there were given a range of pill strengths (usually between 25 and 200 mg) and flexible dosing instructions. They were encouraged to take the initial moderate dose to assess their individual response and then titrate the dosage up or down within the predetermined dosage range until they could (*a*) fall asleep within 1 hour of taking the medication, (*b*) sleep all night, and (*c*) wake up without feeling groggy.

Lorazepam and clonazepam proved most useful in treating patients at the 528th CSC with prominent anxiety symptoms in addition to insomnia. These medications were practical for patients who presented with panic attacks and insomnia because they could be taken in divided doses to treat both problems, sparing the soldier a more complicated treatment regimen. However, clinicians must carefully evaluate a patient's need to take these medications for extended periods to prevent physiological dependence, which could lead to withdrawal if refills are unavailable. Patients who have a history of substance abuse or are thought to be at risk for abuse should generally not be prescribed benzodiazepines in theater. Clinicians must use care to ensure that patients taking benzodiazepines are closely monitored. It is prudent to inform someone in the soldier's chain of command (with the soldier's consent) when sleep medications are prescribed because they may affect the soldier's ability to perform duties during the first few days while the dosage is being adjusted.

Ambien (zolpidem [Sanofi-Aventis, Bridgewater, NJ]) is particularly useful for treating patients with initial insomnia as an isolated symptom or in the context of a mood disorder.[37] Prazosin, although not yet extensively studied, has received increasing attention for helping to alleviate nightmares brought on by traumatic experiences.[32] Seroquel (quetiapine; AstraZeneca US, Wilmington, Del) may also be useful in this population, as well as for patients with bipolar II disorder, both as a treatment for insomnia and as a mood stabilizer.

ETHICAL ISSUES

The conflicts in Iraq and Afghanistan present for the first time since the advent of "biological psychiatry" a situation in which a large part of the military is forward deployed for extended periods. In addition, many service members are returning to combat zones for second or third tours of duty. The risks of keeping service members diagnosed with psychological problems in theater, or redeploying these patients a second or third time, presents a worrisome ethical question. Medication use may inform this discussion.

The most prevalent disorders in theater are anxiety and depressive disorders. Most of the disorders in these two categories respond to treatment with psychotropic medications. If a soldier has a mood or anxiety disorder and a desire or duty to deploy to a combat zone, and a provider believes medication will help resolve the symptoms and contribute to successful performance, then perhaps the ethical decision is to provide the treatment. Historically, large numbers of service members who required evacuation for psychiatric symptoms never returned to their units and, unfortunately, developed chronic dysfunction and guilt.[38] Although mere presence in a combat zone is a risk factor for psychological sequelae, experience has shown that failing to successfully negotiate, process, and come to proper closure with an experience as emotional as a deployment may also present long-term challenges.[6] Modern psychotropic medications can clearly reduce psychiatric symptoms of many disorders in the combat theater. The extent to which medication and treatment may facilitate successful negotiation and processing of combat experience and thus reduce long-term morbidity, however, remains an open question.

SUMMARY

The use of psychotropic medications in combat has evolved significantly, mirroring changes in psychiatric practice and use of these medications in the military garrison environment and the civilian sector. Many disorders are now being successfully treated with medications in theater. Psychiatrists must prepare a deployment formulary before departure, and consider the individual circumstances as well as guidelines for pharmaceutical usage in theater. Factors such as the nature of the conflict, duration of deployment, size of deploying force, and guidance of military doctrine and policy will continue to inform and shape the use of psychotropic medications in combat zones.

REFERENCES

1. Jones FD. Sanctioned use of drugs in combat. In: Pichot P, Berner P, Wolf R, Thau K, eds. *Psychiatry: The State of the Art.* New York, NY: Plenum; 1985: 489–494.

2. Cornum R, Caldwell J, Cornum K. Stimulant use in extended flight operations. *Airpower.* 1997;1153–1158.

3. Weiss B, Laties VG. Enhancement of human performance by caffeine and the amphetamines. *Pharm Rev.* 1962;14:1–36.

4. Hauty GT, Payne RB. Mitigation of work decrement. *J Exp Psych.* 1955;49:60–67.

5. Seashore RH, Ivey AC. Effects of analeptic drugs in relieving fatigue. *Psychol Monogr.* 1953;67:1–16.

6. Jones FD. Psychiatric principles of future warfare. In: Jones FD, Sparacino LR, Wilcox VL, Rothberg JM, Stokes JW, eds. *War Psychiatry*. In: Zajtchuk R, Bellamy RF, eds. *Textbooks of Military Medicine*. Washington, DC: Department of the Army, Office of The Surgeon General, Borden Institute; 1995: 113–132.

7. Datel WE, Johnson AW Jr. *Psychotropic Prescription Medication in Vietnam*. Washington, DC: Walter Reed Army Institute of Research; 1978.

8. Belenky GL. Military psychiatry in the Israeli Defence Force. In: Gabriel RA, ed. *Military Psychiatry: A Comparative Perspective*. Westport, Conn: Greenwood Press; 1986: 147–179.

9. Howe EG, Jones FD. Ethical issues in combat psychiatry. In: Jones FD, Sparacino LR, Wilcox VL, Rothberg JM, eds. *Military Psychiatry: Preparing in Peace for War*. In: Zajtchuk R, Bellamy RF, eds. *Textbooks of Military Medicine*. Washington, DC: Department of the Army, Office of The Surgeon General, Borden Institute; 1994: 115–131.

10. Bacon BL, Staudenmeier JJ. A historical overview of combat stress control units of the US Army. *Mil Med*. 2003;168;689–693.

11. Ritchie EC. Psychiatric medications for deployment. *Mil Med*. 1994;159:647–649.

12. Pincus SH, Benedek DM. Operational stress control in the former Yugoslavia: a joint endeavor. *Mil Med*. 1998;163:358–362.

13. Warner CH, Breitbach JE, Appenzeller GN, Yates V, Webster WG. Division mental health in the new brigade combat team structure: part I. Predeployment and deployment. *Mil Med*. 2007;172:907–911.

14. Schneider BJ, Bradley JC, Benedek DM. Psychiatric medications for deployment: an update. *Mil Med*. 2007;172:681–685.

15. US Department of the Army. *Combat Stress Control in a Theater of Operations*. Washington, DC: DA; 1994 [updated 1998]. Field Manual 8-51.

16. US Department of the Army. *Combat and Operational Stress Control*. Washington, DC: DA; 2006. Field Manual 4-02.51.

17. Assistant Secretary of Defense. *Policy Guidance for Deployment Limiting Psychiatric Conditions and Medications*. Washington, DC: Department of the Army; 2006.

18. The National Defense Authorization Act for Fiscal Year 2007. Pub L 109-364.

19. Warner CH. Division mental health throughout the deployment cycle. In: *Proceedings of the Multi-National Corps Surgeon Conference, 12–13 November 2007, Camp Victory, Iraq*. Baghdad, Iraq: Multi-National Corps–Iraq Surgeon's Office; November 2007.

20. *Operation Iraqi Freedom Mental Health Advisory Team (MHAT) Report*. Washington, DC: Office of The Surgeon General, Department of the Army; 2003.

21. Zoloft (sertraline HCl) [product information]. New York, NY: Pfizer-Roerig; 2005. Available at: http://www.zoloft.com/pdf/ZoloftUSPI.pdf. Accessed February 14, 2008.

22. Celexa (citalopram) [product information]. Saint Louis, Mo: Forest Pharmaceuticals; 2005. Available at: http://www.celexa.com/pdf/celexa_pi.pdf. Accessed February 14, 2008.

23. Prozac (fluoxetine) [product information]. Indianapolis, Ind: Eli Lilly and Company; 2005. Available at: http://pi.lilly.com/us/prozac.pdf. Accessed February 14, 2008.

24. Paxil (paroxetine) [product information]. Research Triangle Park, NC: GlaxoSmithKline; 2005. Available at: http://us.gsk.com/products/assets/us_paxil.pdf. Accessed February 14, 2008.

25. Wellbutrin XL (bupropion) [product information]. Research Triangle Park, NC: GlaxoSmithKline; 2005. Available at: http://us.gsk.com/products/assets/us_wellbutrinXL.pdf. Accessed August 25, 2009.

26. Effexor XR (venlafaxine) [product information]. Philadelphia, Pa: Wyeth Pharmaceuticals; 2005. Available at: http://www.wyeth.com/content/ShowLabeling.asp?id=100. Accessed February 14, 2008.

27. Cymbalta (duloxetine HCl) [product information]. Indianapolis, Ind: Eli Lilly and Company; 2005. Available at: http//pi.lilly.com/us/cymbalta-pi.pdf. Accessed February 14, 2008.

28. Remeron (mirtazapine) [product information]. West Orange, NJ: Organon USA Inc; 2005. Available at: http://www.remeronsoltab.com/Authfiles/Images/292_73428.pdf. Accessed February 14, 2008.

29. American Psychiatric Association. Practice guidelines Web site. Practice guideline for the treatment of patients with acute stress disorder and posttraumatic stress disorder. Available at: http://www.psychiatryonline.com/content.aspx?aid=52257. Accessed February 14, 2008.

30. Stahl SM. *Essential Psychopharmacology*. 2nd ed. Cambridge, United Kingdom: Cambridge University Press; 2000: 237.

31. Ball SG, Kuhn A, Wall D, Shekhar A, Goddard AW. Selective serotonin reuptake inhibitor treatment for generalized anxiety disorder: a double-blind, prospective comparison between paroxetine and sertraline. *J Clin Psychiatry*. 2005;66(1):94–99.

32. Raskind MA, Peskind ER, Kanter ED, et al. Reduction of nightmares and other PTSD symptoms in combat veterans by prazosin: a placebo-controlled study. *Am J Psychiatry*. 2003;160(2):371–373.

33. Haldol (haloperidol) [product information]. Raritan, NJ: Ortho-McNeil Pharmaceuticals; 2001. Available at: http://www.ortho-mcneil.com/products/pi/pdfs/haldol.pdf. Accessed January 19, 2007.

34. Olanzapine (zyprexa) [product information]. Indianapolis, Ind: Eli Lilly and Company; 2007. Available at: http://pi.lilly.com/us/zyprexa-pi.pdf. Accessed February 14, 2008.

35. Geodon (ziprasidone) [product information]. New York, NY: Pfizer-Roerig; 2005. Available at: http://www.pfizer.com/brands/geodon.jsp. Accessed November 18, 2008.

36. Schwartz T, Nihalani N, Virk S, et al. A comparison of the effectiveness of two hypnotic agents for the treatment of insomnia. *Int J Psychiatr Nurs Res*. 2004;10(1):1146–1150.

37. Ambien (zolpidem) [product information]. Bridgewater, NJ: Sanofi-Aventis; 2008. Available at: http://products.sanofi-aventis.us/ambien_cr/ambiencr.html. Accessed February 14, 2008.

38. Jones FD. Lessons of war for psychiatry. In: Pichot P, Berner P, Wolf R, Thau K, eds. *Psychiatry: The State of the Art*. Vol 6. New York, NY: Plenum; 1985: 515–519.

Chapter 11

THE ROLE OF CHAPLAINS IN THE OPERATIONAL ARMY

PETER FREDERICH, MDIV*; THOMAS C. WAYNICK, MDIV†; JASON E. DUCKWORTH, DMIN, MDIV‡; AND JEFF VOYLES, MDIV§

*Lieutenant Colonel, Chaplain Corps, US Army; Family Ministries Officer, Directorate of Ministry Initiatives, US Army Chief of Chaplains Office, 1421 Jefferson Davis Highway, Suite 10600, Arlington, Virginia 22202; formerly, Director, US Army Family Life Chaplain Training Center, Fort Benning, Georgia

†Lieutenant Colonel, Chaplain Corps, US Army; Command Chaplain, Family, Morale, Welfare, and Recreation Command, 4700 King Street, Alexandria, Virginia 22301; formerly, Director and Clinical Supervisor, US Army Family Life Chaplains' Training Program, Fort Benning, Georgia 31905

‡Lieutenant Colonel, Chaplain Corps, US Army; Garrison Chaplain, Religious Support Office, US Army Garrison, Heidelberg, Germany, CMR 419 Box 1876, APO AE 09102; formerly, Training Developer, Chaplain Basic Officer Leader Course, US Army Chaplain Center and School, Fort Jackson, South Carolina 29207

§Lieutenant Colonel, Chaplain Corps, US Army; Director and Clinical Supervisor, Chaplain Family Life Training Program, Building 2606 Collins Loop, Fort Benning, Georgia 31905

INTRODUCTION

In the US Army's current care structure, chaplains are frequently first responders to the personal and psychological problems of soldiers. This is a long tradition. Long before mental health providers existed in the ranks, chaplains were available to soldiers as pastors, lending a listening ear and wise counsel. Today, maintenance of the soul of the soldier is the primary mission of the military chaplaincy. Wherever faith and life intersect, the chaplain is present. Chaplains, like their civilian counterparts, play a defined role in rites and rituals celebrating the meaningful passages of life from birth to the grave. Their calling is to the development and growth of the soul, both temporally and eternally. These activities inherently support the mental health of soldiers and their family members, and make the chaplain a natural partner to military psychiatric caregivers.

THE CHAPLAIN AS PASTORAL COUNSELOR

Vignette 11-1: Private Sam Jones doesn't really know what to do or think. Four months into his first Iraq deployment, he's afraid his marriage is falling apart—he feels helpless and desperate. Married just over a year to Sarah, his high-school girlfriend, he thought they were the picture of a great young Army couple. Sarah had written him faithfully while he was in basic and advanced individual training, and when he proposed during the Christmas break she'd said yes. They had a wonderful holiday, showing family and friends her engagement ring and making plans for the future. There wasn't a lot of time or money, no big wedding or a honeymoon, but by summer they had moved into a small apartment outside Fort Bragg, North Carolina. Sarah started taking classes at the local community college, got pregnant, and made some friends.

And then came Iraq. They both put on a brave face, but both were scared. The baby would be born while he was in Iraq. She had friends, but not necessarily the kind to help when a baby comes, so they decided she would move back home until he returned. And so, a month before his departure, Sam took a week's leave, loaded up a rented trailer, and drove Sarah home. As he watched her waving goodbye, he knew this was going to be a long haul. But he was confident they'd get through this, raise kids, and grow old together. They were so in love.

But things didn't go as planned. With perverse precision, Sarah miscarried the baby on the last day of the first trimester while Sam was actually in the air, flying to the Middle East. It was 4 days before he got the news, and even though his commander found him a phone and a quiet place to call right away, it was days late for Sarah. The call didn't go well. To Sam, it seemed like Sarah blamed him for the miscarriage, and couldn't understand why Sam's unit didn't send him home. What was supposed to be a loving call of support turned into a frustrating exchange that was mercifully cut off by a break in the lines.

Somehow the phone just didn't work for them. Calls were characterized more by silences and anger than by love and affection. E-mail, while better, couldn't patch it up. Then, it seemed like he could never find her at home. He'd wait in line an hour for a phone, only to leave a message on an answering machine. Worse, e-mails stopped being regularly answered. Before long, weeks passed with no contact between them.

Now Sam is sitting staring at his computer screen in despair. A well-intentioned friend just sent an e-mail telling Sam he'd seen Sarah at a movie with her old boyfriend, a week after he saw the pair sitting in a car outside the Denny's she and Sam used to frequent as a couple. He's telling Sam this because he "doesn't want to see you get hurt."

Suddenly it all makes sense to Sam and it seems hopeless and more than he can bear. In his mind he sees some really ugly pictures of Sarah with her new friend. And it seems like there's nothing he can do—how can he win her back when she doesn't even answer his calls? Sam doesn't know what to think, but he knows this: he doesn't want to live if he can't be with Sarah. Looking over his shoulder, Sam sees his M4 rifle: clean, loaded, and ready for action. Just three steps, pick it up, pull the charging handle, rotate, and fire. All this pain would be over, and Sarah would be so sorry . . .

In the future Sam would always look back to that moment and wonder if it was just coincidence, or the hand of God. But as the thoughts of suicide came through his mind, so did the sound of a knock at the door of the squad "hooch" where Sam was sitting. A moment later Chaplain Watson walked through the door. Strange thing. The chaplain didn't come every day, but more than once a week he'd come through, handing out candy, care packages, or something else. Sometimes he seemed out of his element in the rough atmosphere of the forward operating base, but he came by anyway. And whether it was his jump shot (he'd played NCAA Division-III basketball in college and was a solid addition to any platoon's pick-up team) or his insistence on regularly, voluntarily joining squads on patrols, he was a respected member of the battalion, even among soldiers who couldn't find the chapel.

It didn't take the chaplain long to pick up the cues from Sam's feeble answers to his standard "How's it going?" questions. He sat down on the bed next to the computer desk, and asked for more information. Before he knew it, Sam was roughing out the details of his situation and finding someone who'd heard it before, cared, had hope, and had a plan. "Let's go find out what's happening and figure out what to do." The chaplain invited Sam back to the chapel, where there was a class-A line (a line that connects to phones outside the military installation) and plenty of privacy to start the process of pulling things back together.

With only simple changes to the details, Sam's story could be retold tens of thousands of times every decade. In the Western world soldiers for centuries have looked to clergy to help them sort through problems and answer the deeper existential questions of the soul. The US Army's Chaplain Corps was established at the Army's inception by General George Washington.

Pastoral Care and Counseling in the Chaplain Corps

Chaplains draw from a centuries-old tradition of pastoral care. Historically, and throughout the first centuries of American colonial and national history, pastors of various denominations lived or sometimes "circuit rode" between tiny, agrarian communities, leading worship, caring for the sick, and often burying the dead. With college and frequently seminary degrees, these clergymen were often the most highly educated and widely experienced in their communities, and were called on to perform many helping tasks, sometimes even including medical care, for their isolated charges. "Pastoral care" developed a very wide range of activities during this period.[1]

Following this historic pattern, today's clergy often see the role of pastoral counseling as part of their scriptural injunction to take oversight of the flock by caring for one another's burdens.[2] Chaplains do their trade well when they follow recognized principles of spiritual leadership regarding the care of another's soul—personal concern, faith in the value and meaning of life, and hope.[3] These values are typically shared by most counseling modalities—pastoral or not.

Although chaplains collectively represent many faiths, each individually comes from one particular faith group.[4] Each chaplain is endorsed by a specific denomination, but the task is to minister to every soldier in the command. Consequently, chaplains have diverse responsibilities. Besides conducting the rituals, rites, and sacraments (referred to above) and public worship services (their most common responsibility), chaplains also provide pastoral care and counseling. It is in the pastoral relationship that the work of chaplains overlaps most closely with military psychiatry. As a result, military mental health workers commonly find that they are partnered with chaplains in areas such as resiliency in preparation for combat, stress control in combat, suicide prevention, wounded soldier recovery, soldier reintegration, trauma recovery, family issues, and care for the caregiver.

All chaplains have rudimentary training in care and counseling. However, skill and education levels cover a broad range. Actual training in counseling may vary from a couple of seminary courses to a doctorate in clinical psychology. Recognizing this range, and attempting to ensure that every chaplain has a basic workable skill set, the Chaplain Corps has been proactive in raising the standard of care in pastoral counseling. The heart of this effort is focused on the family life chaplain and hospital chaplain programs.

For over 30 years, the Chief of Chaplains has sponsored an advanced civilian schooling program for midcareer chaplains. Chaplains selected for this program attend a 15-month masters degree course in pastoral counseling and, upon graduation, are assigned to Family Life Centers spread throughout the Army in garrisons and divisions. Many graduates from this program become licensed as marriage and family therapists or professional counselors.

The chaplaincy has also continued to raise the level of pastoral care through its clinical pastoral education programs. Located in major medical centers, these programs train chaplains to do ministry in the hospital environment where the basic skills of listening and self-awareness are tantamount to quality care. Once in positions in Family Life Centers or military hospitals, these chaplains provide care as well as training in pastoral counseling for unit chaplains. Under a new initiative, both family life and hospital chaplains will be used to mentor young chaplains in "battlefield pastoral education"—a program designed to raise the quality of care and counseling across the Chaplain Corps.

The ministry of care and counseling to the greater community begins with the chaplain and chaplain assistant. They make up the unit ministry team (UMT) in the Army and the religious support team in joint environments. UMTs are assigned down to battalion level, so there is typically one UMT for every 600 soldiers. Because the UMTs are assigned to the unit, there is generally a very close relationship between the team and the unit. That close relationship makes chaplains and their assistants ideal "first responders." Because soldiers trust the UMT, they are likely to respond positively when its members advise them to talk to someone else in the helping professions, such as mental health providers. Additionally, because chaplains and assistants live and work closely with soldiers, they make ideal follow-on caregivers for soldiers and family members who are in parallel treatment with military medical providers. A time-honored best practice is for UMTs and military mental health practitioners to build and maintain robust relationships in order to facilitate early recognition and integrated treatment for military constituents.

Chaplains and Confidentiality

One unique aspect of the chaplain–penitent relationship is the nature and extent of confidentiality. In order to best partner with chaplains, mental health providers must become comfortable with this unique aspect of the chaplain–soldier–family-member relationship. Society has long recognized the need for certain relationships, such as marriage, to be protected by confidential communication. The main reason for protecting communication within a marriage is to promote absolute trust in the marital bond. Society has decided that a husband and wife should be able to communicate freely about even the most sensitive issues without the threat of that communication being used against them in a legal setting.

Similarly, the communication between an attorney and a client has also traditionally been protected by confidential communication so that the client can receive accurate legal advice. The conversations between patients and their healthcare providers have also been protected, most recently in the 1996 Health Insurance Portability and Accountability Act. Patients need to know their conversations with healthcare providers are protected so they can make a full disclosure of their history and symptoms without fearing that others will have access to this information.

As for these other relationships, long tradition has held that conversations between a member of the clergy and a parishioner or penitent have also been protected so that the matters of soul and conscience can be fully and freely discussed without fear of these conversations becoming public. The concept of the privilege of confidential communication between a member of the clergy and a penitent has been around for almost two centuries. It was first introduced in the United States in New York in the early 19th century. Every state and the District of Columbia have enacted laws that protect this relationship.[5] On the federal level, in *Trammel v US* (1980),[6] the US Supreme Court recognized "the human need to disclose to a spiritual counsel, *in total and absolute confidence*, what are believed to be flawed acts or thoughts and to receive priestly consolation and guidance in return." In a case 5 years later, the court stated that

> [t]he privilege regarding communications with a clergyman reflects an *accommodation* between the *public's right to evidence* and the *individual's need* to be able to speak with a spiritual counselor, in absolute confidence, and disclose the wrongs done or evils thought and receive spiritual absolution, consolation, or guidance in return.[7]

The US military also has regulations that govern confidential communications. Military rule of evidence (MRE) 503 covers confidential communications to members of the clergy.[8] The general rule of privilege in MRE 503 states:

> A person has a privilege to refuse to disclose and to prevent another from disclosing a confidential communication by the person to a clergyman or a clergyman's assistant, if such communication is made either as a formal act of religion or as a matter of conscience.[8(pIII-23)]

It is significant that the privilege belongs to the declarant. The chaplain is bound by this privilege, and is not free to waive it. It also states that a chaplain assistant is bound by the privilege. Thus, if an individual is speaking to a chaplain or chaplain assistant, and believes the conversation is in confidence, it is a protected communication. As used in this rule, a "clergyman" is a minister, priest, rabbi, chaplain, or other similar functionary of a religious organization, or an individual reasonably believed to be so by the person consulting the clergyman. MRE 503 also states that a communication is "confidential" if made to a clergyman in the clergyman's capacity as a spiritual advisor or to a clergyman's assistant in the assistant's official capacity. MRE 503 makes all communications to a chaplain in this role privileged. As such, they are not admissible in court. Further policies interpret this privilege broadly, making chaplain–parishioner privilege "nearly absolute." As a result, the chaplain is often viewed as a safe place to go by both soldiers and the command. Soldiers can go to the chaplain to have their problems addressed without the matter being made known to their units.

This relationship has been repeatedly tested in court, and as recently as 2007 was clarified by the chief of chaplains. The term that has typically been connected to this relationship is "absolute confidentiality." The bottom line guidance given to chaplains and their assistants is this: the privilege that soldiers and family members own as a result of the relationship is absolute. It cannot be waived for any reason (to include threat of harm) unless the soldier or family member waives it.

Although this absolute privilege has been viewed with angst by many professionals, in practice the safety that soldiers thereby attach to the relationship is virtually always positive. The hypothetical situations of danger (eg, a chaplain remaining quiet in the case of child abuse or some other heinous situation) are grist for interesting legal discussions, but virtually never come to reality. In fact, a multiyear search done by the chiefs of chaplains across the Department of Defense did not find a single instance where harm ensued as a result of a chaplain or assistant holding confidence. However, the search uncovered many instances where the perceived safety of the relationship enabled chaplains and assistants to gain early access to dangerous situations and prevent harm. The bottom line for mental health professionals is this: the privilege attached to the soldier–chaplain relationship makes the chaplains and chaplain assistants in the military extremely valuable partners in the care of soldiers and their family members.

The Chaplain as Facilitator of Religious Strength

The free exercise of religion has been the source of the chaplain's ability to be a facilitator of religious strength. This has

> corresponded well with the intent of the Founding Fathers and the Constitution of the United States. . . . Long before the Constitution was framed, a distinct tradition of free exercise of religion developed within the army by necessity. The pattern for chaplain ministry to soldiers of different religious backgrounds was set in the seventeeth century, from the time of the first militia units drilled at Jamestown, Plymouth, Boston, and New York.[9]

Today's Army maintains a Chaplain Corps for the primary reason of ensuring a soldier's free exercise of religion. However, the motivation at the operational level may be different. In the Army, everything must support the soldier on the front line. Logisticians ensure that the infantry on the front have beans and bullets. The Signal Corps supports the fight by providing clear means of communication. The Medical Command attends to the health of the soldier. The chaplain is seen as a force health contributor by supporting the spirit of the individual soldier, enabling the soldier to be resilient in the fight.

But how does religion support the soldier? The answer to that question is threefold. It has to do with the nature of belief systems, which bring meaning to life. First, belief systems support soldiers throughout combat. Before the battle, belief systems aid the process of convictions in just and right causes. In the midst of the chaos and horror of combat a belief system can sustain an individual. After the battle the application of meaning to the traumatic event can help restore not only a sense of order and meaning, but also a renewed calling to life. Secondly, belief systems offer rites, rituals, and sacraments that provide healing, cleansing, and restoration that can be very important to the wounded soul of the warrior. Thirdly, chaplains perform a symbolic role, referred to by the Chaplain Corps as the "ministry of presence." The chaplain is perceived by some as the embodiment of God's presence in the midst of soldiers.

Some commanders feel that a chaplain accompanying troops during the mission is more important than the current doctrine of locating chaplains at the aid station. These commanders believe that a chaplain's presence, a symbol of God's closeness with the troops, is an encouragement to soldiers in the field. These officers are not alone in their convictions that belief in God sustains a person in combat. In an address at Trinity College in Hartford, Connecticut, in 1941, General George C Marshall said these words:

> The soldier's heart, the soldier's spirit, the soldier's soul, are everything. Unless the soldier's soul sustains him he cannot be relied on and will fail himself and his commander and his country in the end. . . . It is morale that wins the victory. . . . The French never found an adequate "dictionary" definition for the word. . . . It is more than a word—more than any one word, or several words, can measure. Morale is a state of mind. It is steadfastness and courage and hope. It is confidence and zeal and loyalty. . . . It is élan, esprit de corps and determination. It is staying power, the spirit which endures to the end—the will to win. With it all things are possible, without it everything else, planning, preparation, production, count for naught. I have just said it is the spirit which endures to the end. And so it is.[10]

Dynamics of Faith in Soldier Resilience and Recovery

The chaplain may or may not be a symbol of God's presence to the individual soldier. The greater question is how does individual belief, religion, or faith promoted and supported by the chaplain enable soldiers first to stay in the fight and then return to the fight after being wounded in body or spirit? Anecdotal accounts and folk wisdom have supported the belief that religious faith adds a profound dimension to the emotional resilience and recovery capabilities of people under stress. One example comes from World War II in this report of the country's response to the invasion of Normandy:

> The whole country knew on June 6 that something dire, something that might fail, was taking place . . . in a Brooklyn shipyard, welders knelt on the decks of their Liberty ships and recited the Lord 's Prayer. At the opening, the New York Stock Exchange observed two minutes of silent prayer. All over America church bells tolled, and the Liberty Bell was rung in Philadelphia. In Columbus, Ohio, at 7:30 in the evening, all traffic stopped for five minutes while people prayed in the streets.[11(p37)]

Another example is the nation's spiritual reaction to the attacks of September 11, 2001. In the days after the fall of the World Trade Center, church prayer services were well attended, crosses and other religious symbols were erected, and memorial events such as Oprah Winfrey's grand prayer service at Yankee Stadium to commemorate the victims were celebrated. Even years later it is not uncommon for a soldier to tell a chaplain that God called him or her into the military in response to September 11.

A growing amount of empirical research supports the concept that for many individuals faith is a resource for resiliency and recovery. Pargament's seminal work, *The Psychology of Religion and Coping*, encapsulates much of the research on religion and resiliency of the previous decade. He writes:

> A number of studies have compared the frequencies of religious and nonreligious forms of coping and found that religion looms large. For example, McCrae (1984) studied the coping mechanisms reportedly used by a community sample of men and women faced with events categorized as losses, threats, or challenges. Of the 28 coping mechanisms, "faith" was the second most frequently used for dealing with threats (72%), and the third most frequently used for dealing with losses (75%). Faith was less frequently used in coping with challenges (43%). Conway (1885–1986) interviewed black and white urban elderly women who had experienced stressful medical problems in the past year. Asked how they coped with their medical problems, prayer was selected by 91% of the sample; it was the most frequently reported of all coping mechanisms including seeking information, resting, treatment, prescription drugs, and going to a doctor.[12(pp137–138)]

In a more recent work, *Learning from Resilient People: Lessons We Can Apply to Counseling and Psychotherapy*, Glicken refers to the following studies:

> Gartner, Larson, and Allen reviewed over 200 psychiatric and psychological studies and concluded that religious involvement has a positive impact on both health and mental health, while Ellison and colleagues indicate that "there is at least some evidence of mental health benefits of religion among men and women, persons of different ages and racial and ethnic groups, and individuals from various socioeconomic classes and geographical locations. Further, these salutary effects often persist even with an array of social, demographic, and health-related statistical controls."[13(p23)]

If there is, as the research and recent history indicate, a connection between faith resources and a soldier's ability to be resilient and recover from the traumas of military life, then the role of the chaplain as pastoral counselor is an important resource to be accessed by those involved with operational psychology. (For further discussion, see Waynick and colleagues, "Human Spirituality, Resilience, and the Role of Military Chaplains."[14])

CHAPLAINS AS PARTNERS IN OPERATIONAL PSYCHOLOGY

Chaplains are partners with other military helping personnel in the overall psychological well-being of soldiers. Because they are typically assigned at battalion level, chaplains often handle the day-to-day bulk of basic issues faced by soldiers. This often consists of straightforward "problem solving" related to professional issues, relationships, life choices, and spirituality. Chaplains provide proximity, immediacy, and expectancy in their basic counseling services—they have the ability to work with soldiers within the unit and meet their needs quickly. This is an important operational concept because when soldiers are sent away for help, there is a reduced expectancy of their return.

Because chaplains are an integral part of their units, they are often familiar with the home situations of the soldiers. Chaplains can provide a "reach-back" capability to soldiers, contacting other chaplains who are collocated with family members. Thus the deployed chaplain often bridges the gap on issues caused by family separations. Rear detachment chaplains often find themselves tasked by command to react to family crises and provide crisis intervention counseling.

It is important to reiterate that chaplains are not mental health professionals (the exception being licensed family life chaplains); their primary role is that of pastor. As such they do pastoral counseling, which includes serving as first responders to crisis events as well as making good and timely referrals to mental health and other agencies for the well-being of the soldier. After some initial counseling a chaplain may decide that the combat stress control team (CSCT) or other professionals may be better suited to help a particular individual. At this point the chaplain will often refer the person to the CSCT. Depending on the nature of the issue, the chaplain may personally escort the person, have a noncommissioned officer escort the person, or suggest the person seek additional help from the CSCT unaccompanied. It is important for the mental health team to know that chaplains do not perceive this as a "hand off." Chaplains are typically eager to continue the pastoral relationship and play an adjunct role in the healing of the soldier. Some past tension between mental health professionals and the chaplaincy resulted from a perceived message that once the soldier is in the medical chain there is no need for the pastoral role, as if mental health somehow trumped all other care giving. Chaplains as a whole come from theological communities that believe human beings function best when they have multiple supportive resources.

A prime example of chaplains partnering with mental health personnel is occurring during critical incidents in both Iraq and Afghanistan. Unlike chaplains, the CSCT is usually assigned at brigade level, although sometimes at forward operating bases controlled by a single battalion. Typically both the CSCT and the chaplain respond to the same client during the same events, such as a significant amount of combat loss, but each in their own role. Chaplains often respond immediately to a critical incident with a pastoral presence on the scene. The CSCT often follows up by triaging those involved and treating the emotional aftermath of the traumatic experience. Chaplains trained in crisis processing often perform critical incident stress ministry shortly after the event. Mental health professionals respond in similar fashion. Chaplains then continue follow-up care by checking in with the soldiers while living and working with them on a daily basis. Chaplain assistants can also participate in the contacting, assessing, and referral process. Unit leaders recognizing the teamwork of UMTs and CSCTs often advise or direct soldiers to talk with personnel in one or the other group.

Another area where mental health practitioners and chaplains work hand in hand is in suicide prevention. The Army suicide prevention program has four elements: (1) primary prevention through life and relationship skills training, (2) awareness training, (3) intervention training, and (4) treatment for suicidal soldiers.[15] Whereas mental health providers have the task of diagnosis and treatment, chaplains are the primary vehicle for prevention and awareness education. UMTs are often the first to identify a soldier in need of psychological evaluation for suicidal or homicidal ideations. This is particularly important downrange, where perceptive chaplains can expedite, on the basis of their position, a soldier being taken to receive mental healthcare.

In March 2007, the US Army Center for Health Promotion and Preventative Medicine released a new suicide awareness program for soldiers and Army leaders. Urging soldiers to "get help" if needed and "protect your buddy," this training emphasizes practical protective steps. This program is now the Army standard for suicide awareness training.[16] UMTs train their units in suicide awareness under the Deployment Cycle Support program, as well as providing periodic retraining of soldiers and leaders.

A less talked about role chaplains play in operational psychology is serving as a personal resource for mental health providers. Being connected, but not in the same professional community, many mental health providers find chaplains to be safe friends and confidants to process their own experiences. Mental health providers also play this role for chaplains. Both professions speak a similar language and have similar goals in ensuring the well-being of soldiers. Mental health providers enjoy the same "absolute privilege" as chaplains, which can be very advantageous in the close quarters of deployments.

Chaplains and CSCTs should work together and be aware of the workloads each is carrying. Equitable distribution of work is part of taking care of the caregiver. Chaplains have been, and will continue to be, available as a resource to all those who work in operational psychology. Chaplains also must take care of themselves and each other if they are going to take care of the soldier. Consequently, for many chaplains and CSCTs, it has become a best practice to maintain mutually supportive relationships in which each tracks the physical and emotional fitness and workload of the other, and which provide informal support and care. The nuanced nature of both spiritual and psychiatric care requires providers to remain emotionally sound. For many deployed chaplains and mental health professionals, the personal relationships they share and the supportive interactions they sustain in the midst of the struggle have become a keystone of their ability to stay healthy and effective through the trials of long deployments.

SUMMARY

Today's military Chaplain Corps is an expression of millenia-long traditions of pastoral practice that include the practice of worship and sacramental rites as well as a tradition of personal soul care. Responding to this tradition, US military chaplains are ubiquitous among soldiers and their family members, leading worship and prayer, and listening, comforting, and providing guidance. In support of this tradition, military chaplains receive extensive training in supportive counseling, personal resilience, and family health promotion. Consequently, chaplains support the mission of military healthcare providers and are natural partners in pursuit of soldier and family mental health. Additionally, as a caring professional functioning outside normal medical channels, the chaplain is a "safe resource" for mental health providers and a good fit for providers seeking a means to support their own personal emotional health. As a result of this alignment and shared mission, many mental health providers find it a best practice to build and maintain rich, supportive relationships with chaplains in their area of action. This partnership has for many been a source of increased effectiveness, durability, and, ultimately, better health for the soldiers and family members whose welfare they support.

REFERENCES

1. Schuetze AW, Habeck IJ. *The Shepherd Under Christ–A Textbook for Pastoral Theology.* Milwaukee, Wisc: Northwestern Publishing House; 1974.

2. Galatians 6:2. Available at: http://scriptures.lds.org/gal/6. Accessed April 20, 2009.

3. Nouwen HJM. *The Wounded Healer.* Garden City, NY: Image Books; 1979: 70–76.

4. US Department of the Army. *Chaplain Activities in the United States Army.* Washington, DC: DA; 2004. Army Regulation 165-1.

5. Broyde M, Reiss Y, Diament N. Confidentiality and rabbinic counseling: an overview of Halakhic and legal issues. *Jewish Law Articles*. Available at: http://www.jlaw.com/Articles/RabbinicCounseling1.html. Accessed December 16, 2009.

6. *Trammel v US*, 445 US 40 (1980).

7. *US v Moreno*, 20 MJ 623, 626 (ACMR 1985).

8. US Department of Defense. Military rules of evidence, section 503, communications with clergy. *Manual for Courts-Martial, United States.* Washington, DC: DoD; 2000: III-23.

9. Brinsfield JW. Our roots for ministry: the Continental Army, George Washington, and the free exercise of religion. *Mil Chaplain's Review.* 1987;Fall:25.

10. The Marshall Papers. Speech at Trinity College, June 15, 1941. The George C Marshall Foundation. Available at: http://www.marshallfoundation.org/Database.htm [Note: search for "zeal"; select #2-484]. Accessed September 15, 2009.

11. Fussell P. How the leaders led. *Newsweek.* May 23, 1994:36–38.

12. Pargament KI. *The Psychology of Religion and Coping.* New York, NY: Guildford Press; 1997.

13. Glicken D. *Learning From Resilient People: Lessons We Can Apply to Counseling and Psychotherapy.* Thousand Oaks, Calif: Sage Publications; 2006.

14. Waynick T, Frederich P, Scheider D, Thomas R, Bloomstrom G. Human spirituality, resilience, and the role of the military chaplain. In: Adler A, Castro C, Britt T, eds. *Operational Stress.* Vol 2. In: *Military Life—The Psychology of Serving in Peace and Combat.* Westport, Conn: Praeger Security International; 2006: 173–199.

15. US Department of the Army. *Army Health Promotion.* Washington, DC: DA; 2004. Army Regulation 600-63, Chapter 5.

16. US Department of the Army, Chief of Chaplains. *The New Army Standard Suicide Awareness Program*. Information paper to all Army Chaplains, April 27, 2007.

Chapter 12

PSYCHIATRIC CONSULTATION TO COMMAND

CHRISTOPHER H. WARNER, MD[*]; GEORGE N. APPENZELLER, MD[†]; JILL E. BREITBACH, PsyD[‡]; JENNIFER T. LANGE, MD[§]; ANGELA MOBBS, PsyD[¥]; AND ELSPETH CAMERON RITCHIE, MD, MPH[¶]

INTRODUCTION

ORIGIN AND HISTORY OF PSYCHIATRIC COMMAND CONSULTATION

FACTORS ASSOCIATED WITH COMMAND CONSULTATION

PERFORMING THE CONSULTATION

DETERMINING FITNESS FOR DUTY AND DEPLYOMENT CLEARANCE

COMMAND-DIRECTED EVALUATIONS

RISKS TO THE CONSULTANT AND ETHICAL ISSUES IN CONSULTATION

NOTABLE CONSULTATIVE POSITIONS IN THE ARMY

SUMMARY

Major, Medical Corps, US Army; Chief, Department of Behavioral Medicine, Winn Army Community Hospital, Building 9242, Room 20, 1083 Worcester Drive, Fort Stewart, Georgia 31324; formerly, Division Psychiatrist, 3rd Infantry Division, Fort Stewart, Georgia

†Lieutenant Colonel, Medical Corps, US Army; Commander, US Army Medical Activity, Alaska, 1060 Gaffney Road #7400, Fort Wainwright, Alaska 99703-7400; formerly, Deputy Commander for Clinical Services, Command Group, Winn Army Community Hospital, Fort Stewart, Georgia 31314

‡Major, Medical Service Corps, US Army; Neuropsychologist, Department of Psychology, Evans Army Community Hospital, USAMEDDAC, 1650 Cochrane Circle, Fort Carson, Colorado 80913; formerly, Group Psychologist, 1st Special Warfare Training Group, Fort Bragg, North Carolina

§Lieutenant Colonel, Medical Corps, US Army; Medical Director, Behavioral Health Clinic, Department of Psychiatry, Walter Reed Army Medical Center, 6900 Georgia Avenue NW, Washington, DC 20307-5001

¥Captain, Medical Service Corps, US Army; Special Forces Assignment and Selection Psychologist, Special Warfare Center and School, Rowe Training Facility, Building T-5167, 1500 Camp Mackall Place, Marston, North Carolina 28363; formerly, Brigade Psychologist, 3rd Brigade Combat Team, 3rd Infantry Division, Fort Benning, Georgia

¶Colonel, US Army (Retired); formerly, Psychiatry Consultant to the Army Surgeon General, and Director, Behavioral Health Proponency, Office of The Surgeon General, Falls Church, Virginia; currently, Chief Clinical Officer, District of Columbia Department of Mental Health, 64 New York Avenue, NE, 4th Floor, Washington, DC 20002

INTRODUCTION

The psychological effects of warfare have been well documented throughout history. Since World War I, the US Army has been deploying behavioral health assets to the front line for treatment of combat operational stress and to advise unit commanders about combat stress and its effects on soldiers. Currently, commanders of combat units are being encouraged to attend to the overall health of their soldiers, including consulting with behavioral health professionals about the psychiatric well-being of their soldiers. One of the many challenges that behavioral health professionals are confronted with is the need to educate commanders about the role of psychiatric command consultation. This chapter outlines the many responsibilities of this role.

ORIGIN AND HISTORY OF PSYCHIATRIC COMMAND CONSULTATION

Whereas mental health evaluations are typically thought of in terms of an encounter between a provider and a patient, a psychiatric command consultation occurs when a military commander desires to know mental health information or factors about an individual, unit, or command, and how to improve overall behavioral health. Historically, psychiatric command consultation has occurred in two different capacities: (1) attempts to screen for vulnerability and determine fitness for duty, and (2) preventive psychiatry. Previous overviews have described the history related to these components in depth. It is important to know how these roles have developed when outlining the future of psychiatric command consultation.[1] Additionally, although "psychiatric consultation" will often be performed by psychiatrists, other behavioral health professionals will also perform these consultations, thus, the term "behavioral health professionals" is used in discussion of consultations. For guidance regarding the specific roles of psychiatrists, psychologists, social workers, and technicians, the reader is encouraged to explore their individual discipline regulations.

Screening for Vulnerability and Determining Fitness for Duty

For individuals desiring to enter the military, their first encounter with medical personnel will generally be at the Military Entrance Processing Station. Here new recruits complete a thorough medical evaluation that includes answering questions regarding mental health. Certain individuals may be barred from entry to service or require further evaluation prior to entering the military. This process, a reflection of the recognized need to screen military personnel for psychiatric vulnerabilities, dates back to the mid-18th century.

"Nostalgia," which was the recognized ailment defined by Aurenbrugger in 1761, was the term used to describe the "disease" where soldiers lost hope, became sad, isolative, inattentive, and apathetic—what today is commonly termed "combat stress."[2] French physicians of the Napoleonic era recognized factors associated with producing and preventing nostalgia, and began screening soldiers accordingly.[2]

The US military began psychological screening in the early 20th century. During World War I, the famous Army Alpha and Beta testing and psychiatric interviews were applied to screen the massive influx of military recruits needed to fight the war.[3] At that time, the personality and estimated intellectual functioning of each individual was assessed, and recommendations regarding suitability for military service and service specialties were made. The decisions made concerning suitability largely reflected the belief that psychiatric symptoms and illnesses reflected a "weak personality"; individuals with psychoneurotic illness were not normal, and thus not capable of marshalling defenses needed to serve during war.[3] This method of screening military soldiers for service is largely viewed by historians as a failure.[4] However, as a consequence of the efforts, the perception of psychology as a valuable science capable of producing results of immediate and practical significance to command was substantially bolstered.[5]

In 1941, Harry Stack Sullivan was appointed as a psychiatric consultant to the Selective Service Program and helped develop a more comprehensive system that incorporated screening interviews.[6] However, over the course of World War II, attitudes changed about the effectiveness of these screening methods and many began to view them as excessive, ineffective in accurately predicting the resilience of individuals to withstand the risks of war, and resulting in a substantial and excessive loss of potential soldiers.[6–8] After World War II, psychiatric screening methods were modified to focus on identifying and disqualifying only gross psychiatric disorders. This process has remained in place since then, with varying modifications over time.

Although the screening purpose has remained relatively unchanged, the debate continues over the role that preexisting medical and psychiatric conditions have in making individuals more vulnerable to negative outcomes in times of stress. Conflicting data continue to exist as to whether preexisting psychological conditions are a contributing factor to psychiatric attrition in a combat zone.[9–18] This debate is especially salient given the estimated rates of depression, anxiety, and posttraumatic stress disorder in returning Operation Iraqi Freedom and Operation Enduring Freedom veterans.[19]

What remains unclear is what number of service personnel experiencing psychiatric problems upon return from combat had preexisting mental health conditions before deployment and, more specifically, what number had conditions that existed prior to entry into the service. The psychiatric conditions that should perhaps preclude service because of vulnerability under stress, which may only have minimal effects on the well-being of soldiers in combat, are not yet understood.

Since the establishment of the Office of Strategic Services in World War II, screening processes have also been conducted in soldiers seeking special duties. Through the years, the role of behavioral health professionals has evolved with expansion of special operations and special missions. Not only do psychologists screen applicants for suitability for special operations, they also monitor progress throughout special operations training.[20] After training has been completed, psychologists screen soldiers for special missions, which requires these behavioral health professionals to carefully assess the "biopsychosocial fit" of individuals to their specified mission tasks. Mental health providers must become familiar with the demands that will be placed on the soldier (ie, isolation from others, exposure to extreme conditions), and work intimately with command regarding the establishment of desired competency for the mission. This aspect of command consultation is unique in that the commander of the mission will often dictate aspects of required competencies. It is the job of the mental health professional to apply these principles in a psychiatric framework for screening. Assessments are presently performed for a variety of special missions (special operations service members) or specialty job requirements (security clearance evaluations, intelligence positions, nuclear weapons specialists).

Preventive Psychiatry

Military psychiatrists were the first to focus on the total social environment of the individual in establishing programs not only for the treatment, but also the prevention, of mental illness.[11] This shift in focus came in 1944, when the Army began using psychiatrists in a preventive fashion, morphing the role of psychiatry from overseeing straight disposition of personnel into recommending how to use marginal personnel and implementing mental hygiene training programs.[21] Furthermore, the Vietnam War provided a unique opportunity to understand combat, from which significant understanding of the individual's response to extreme conditions was gained.[11] Thus, the role of psychiatry in providing primary, secondary, and tertiary prevention training based on understanding the biopsychosocial influences on behavior was established. The effectiveness of preventive psychiatry was later shown by the Group for the Advancement of Psychiatry when it reported that preventive psychiatry could reduce combat ineffectiveness through early recognition and prompt outpatient treatment of emotional difficulties during combat and noncombat situations.[22]

Much of what is understood about prevention of psychiatric casualties comes from the work of William C Menninger, who identified the failure to meet basic needs (such as food, water, sleep, social interaction, and recreation) as a significant contributor to the incidence of psychiatric casualties in combat.[7] Likewise, unit cohesion and morale have repeatedly been found important in supporting individual coping behavior and unit performance, both in wartime and in peacetime.[23,24] Although morale remains difficult to operationally define, it may be considered to represent the general sense of unit cohesion, confidence in ability, and overall well-being of a unit. Failure to experience positive morale in a group (because of a lack of order and security, a lack of fusion with the group, having insufficient leadership, or lack of absorption into the unit's work) has been associated with increased psychiatric referral, at least upon initial deployment.[23] Morale and unit cohesion are often synonymous; one of the greatest defenses against breakdown in combat is the development and reinforcement of group cohesiveness.[25]

Additionally, it has been well documented throughout history that the time spent exposed to combat correlates with the number of psychiatric casualties.[21–26] This was perhaps most salient in the Vietnam War, where soldiers knew that if they could survive for 12 months, their removal from combat was assured. The rest-and-recreation policy, which sought to reduce continued exposure, was also widely implemented. The effect of time on psychiatric visits has also been seen in recent conflicts, where multiple studies have noted an increase in combat operational stress reactions after 6 months of deployment.[26,27] Understanding these factors, as well as their historical context, provides a framework for application of current principles and avoidance of prior pitfalls.

FACTORS ASSOCIATED WITH COMMAND CONSULTATION

As the consultant prepares to perform an evaluation, there are several factors that must be considered. These include the environment, the nature of the request, and the proximity of the consultant to the unit or individual being evaluated.

Deployed Versus Garrison

Consultations can vary significantly depending on the environment. In a garrison environment, commanders are generally looking for risk reduction methods and to determine if a soldier is fit for duty or deployment. During deployment, commanders are more focused on interventions for maintaining their combat power and assessing the levels of unit cohesion and soldier quality of life to maintain soldier readiness.

Level of Preventive Consultation

Preventive consultative advising involves using the threats identified during the planning and oversight phases of operations and making recommendations to the medical staff and command on measures to be taken and areas requiring command emphasis. Three categories of prevention can generally occur both in the garrison and deployed environment: (1) primary prevention, (2) secondary prevention, and (3) tertiary prevention. These prevention activities are especially critical in the deployed environment given that resources may be limited.

Primary Prevention

Primary prevention generally comes in the form of education. Most units regularly employ periodic training on topics such as prevention of sexual assault, suicide, and substance abuse. These training sessions allow behavioral health professionals an opportunity to gain visibility with command and soldiers alike. Furthermore, behavioral health professionals can play key advisory roles in preparation for deployment, as well as during deployment, in such areas as training (including training schedules), personnel issues, discipline, crosscultural issues, and, most importantly, the morale of the unit. All preventive services provided in garrison and during deployment establish credibility with the command.

Recently, in response to evolving technology and the recognition that soldiers and commanders are presented with differing stressors throughout the deployment cycle, the Army Medical Department designed an educational series called "Battlemind" training.[28] These modules were designed for specific portions of the deployment cycle, to build upon a soldier's strength, help soldiers develop resiliency in stressful situations, and to teach soldiers how to utilize their strengths during times of transition. Modules for both soldiers and their families were designed for predeployment, reintegration (immediate return from a deployment), and reconstitution (90–180 days after return from deployment).[28] Initial research on the effectiveness of "Battlemind" training appears promising; this effectiveness will continue to be explored.[26,29]

Secondary Prevention

Secondary prevention involves identifying as early as possible those soldiers who are at risk to develop mental health problems and intervening to prevent the development or worsening of symptoms after exposure. These types of procedures are accomplished both through individual and unit-level screening and also through traumatic event management.

Postdeployment psychological screening has been growing in importance since Operation Desert Storm in 1991 and became mandatory in 1997.[30,31] Shortly thereafter, the Department of Defense introduced the Post-Deployment Health Assessment, which screened soldiers for physical and mental health problems upon return from deployment. It was a method for early identification of problems and for decreasing the stigma associated with behavioral healthcare. However, few studies have looked at validating the postdeployment screening instrument against other measures or functional outcomes.[32,33] Furthermore, experiences from other samples of returning soldiers indicate that rates of reported deployment-related symptoms increased with time after returning from deployment.[19,34,35] This led to an extension of the Post-Deployment Health Assessment program to include a reevaluation (the Post-Deployment Health Reassessment) at 3 to 6 months after return from a combat zone.[36] These programs allow for early identification; however, there has been notable criticism that effective follow-up of the concerns identified has not occurred.[37] It is important that consultants be engaged throughout these screening processes and that commanders be very involved. Both occurrences will increase soldier participation and help decrease the potential for soldiers to "fall through the cracks."[38]

Other assessment methods allow for broad unit-wide assessments rather than individual screenings. An example of this type of method is the Unit Behavioral Health Needs Assessment. This tool allows the consultant to take a sampling of a unit, employing a standardized survey that assesses areas such as morale, cohesion, ongoing stressors, and soldier concerns, as well as current levels of need and barriers to care. This allows the consultant to provide the commander with clear objective findings and provide customized recommendations specific to the unit. Additionally, the Unit Behavioral Health Needs Assessment has comparison data that have been collected from multiple units at varying stages throughout Operation Iraqi Freedom to serve as a gauge.[39]

Another area of secondary preventive psychiatric consultation is that of traumatic event management (TEM). TEM involves intervening after a potentially traumatic event has occurred, with the purpose of seeking to decrease the effect of the event and prevent long-term negative consequences. Considerable debate continues between both military and civilian behavioral health providers about the utility and efficacy of debriefings (which are traditionally part of an overall TEM strategy) as preventative interventions. Traditionally, the TEM process is conducted at the request of a unit supervisor to begin the process of integrating a traumatic experience into the individual and group experience. Debriefings involve a structured meeting of all parties directly involved with a traumatic event. Members of the group tell their individual stories about what happened in the presence of trained behavioral health providers or chaplains, followed by processing of the cognitive and emotional components of the event.

Currently there are many different models for debriefings. Most evolved out of Marshall's work in World War II when he attempted to record accounts of unit operations for historical purposes.[40] Interestingly, these initial sessions were not for the expressed purpose of psychological benefits to the involved parties. Marshall noted, however, that during the process of debriefing many misperceptions were corrected by other individuals involved in the traumatic event, and the debriefing appeared to render social support and decrease the development of combat stress reactions.[40]

Although debriefings have been used throughout military conflicts, their effectiveness has not been well documented in research studies and they have not been proven to prevent posttraumatic stress disorder.[41–44] Part of the problem in examining the utility of debriefings is the evolution of what TEM actually entails. In fact, "debriefings" are now thought to take many forms commonly used by all military personnel, to include after-action reviews, which are now a standard operating procedure for all US Army teams and small units following any training exercise.[40] Other forms of debriefings include defusing, critical event debriefing, critical incident stress debriefing, psychiatric debriefing, historical debriefing, and intelligence debriefing. Thus, one of the inherent problems in determining the effectiveness of TEM is the lack of consistent standardized protocols across providers and across organizations. Furthermore, what constitutes a debriefing, or what form of a debriefing to use for a particular circumstance, often varies.

Despite all of the inherent problems in TEM definition, standardization, and demonstrable utility, TEM nonetheless remains a common consultation task that is expected of behavioral health providers, and thus it is imperative that behavioral health providers be proficient in TEM. US Army Field Manual 4-02.51, *Combat and Operational Stress Control*,[45] provides a standardized outline and structure for current TEM operations. The Army has recently introduced Battlemind psychological debriefings.[46] These debriefings take into account military rank and structure and incorporate resiliency based educational principles that help to build upon the soldier's strengths during the process. As with other debriefing methods, the effectiveness of this process is not known at this time.

Tertiary Prevention

Disease nonbattle injuries—specifically combat operational stress and psychiatric casualties—have long accounted for vast numbers of non–mission-capable soldiers. Indeed, one of the defining principles of history's victorious commanders has been to "break the enemy's will to fight," and thus produce combat stress and psychiatric casualties in the opposing force. History has revealed consistent themes in soldiers who persevere in combat compared with those who break down in combat, with the difference in outcome often being reduced to adaptability and cohesion.[23,24] Tertiary prevention involves the treatment of those who have ongoing issues, with the goal to return soldiers to duty and to advise commanders on who should be removed from the combat operations.

Internal (Division Mental Health) Versus External (Combat Stress Detachment) Resources

The primary resources responsible for preventive psychiatry missions and the control of combat operational stress during both garrison and deployment are the combat stress control (CSC) and division mental health (DMH) units. These units establish a diplomatic relationship with command to earn credibility in the consultative role. Preventive missions of both of these units are defined by US Army doctrine as the following: consultation-liaison services; reorganization and reconstitution support; proximate neuropsychiatry triage; and stabilization, restoration, and reconditioning and retraining.[23]

Although the mission is the same, the two units have notable differences that present varying challenges. DMH units are organic to the organization and have been deploying in that structure since World War II.[47,48] Recently, the transformation of the US Army from a division-centric focus to one in which the brigade combat team is the primary unit of action has resulted in the expansion of the DMH organization and mission. (In this volume, Chapter 6, The Division Psychiatrist and Brigade Behavioral Health Officers, discusses DMH and the positions within it at much greater length.) DMH units are with the larger organization both in garrison and during deployment and thus have the ability to establish long-term relationships with commanders and implement long-term prevention plans. These units, however, tend to be smaller and more limited in capability than CSC units.

Like DMH units, CSC detachments have been evolving for quite some time in the US Army. They first appeared during the Korean War when Colonel Albert Glass established these teams to augment existing DMH assets.[47] Glass, drawing on his own experiences from World War II, organized what were called "KO" teams (the "KO" designation refers to one in a series of hospital augmentation detachments). They provided mobile consultation throughout the corps and US Army areas.[47] The first KO teams were deployed to Korea; CSCs have augmented organic mental health assets in every major conflict since that time. They officially became known as CSCs in the mid-1980s. Presently, the CSC model remains largely unchanged from that originally established by Colonel Glass; however, the mission has expanded to include additional preventive psychiatric care and restoration capabilities. Today, CSC detachments and companies traditionally provide US Army Echelon II or III care during deployed operations and are external to the brigade, division, or other unit.[45]

Local Versus Remote Behavioral Health Resource

The type of consultation may dictate the use of a local versus a remote behavioral health resource. For issues that will require ongoing follow-up and will require a relationship with a commander, it is best to use local resources. These individuals are more apt to have some familiarity with the systems, personnel, and processes involved and can develop ongoing relationships with the commanders and provide follow-up.

An excellent example of this process is the use by a brigade behavioral health officer of a unit behavioral health needs assessment within a battalion. The officer may have only a limited relationship with that commander but has some familiarity with the brigade. The officer performs the assessment and informs the command of the key findings and recommendations. As a local resource, the brigade behavioral health officer is then able to follow up with the unit and continue to both monitor and reassess the situation to provide continued feedback to the leadership. These processes allow for identification of such items as barriers to care, stigma about using mental healthcare, and leadership issues.

In contrast, remote consultations will generally require mobilization of a team to conduct an evaluation, make recommendations, and then return to its home station, likely not to follow up again or with limited follow-up. These types of consultations tend to occur in units that have minimal mental health contacts or desire an independent assessment from someone who has minimal to no knowledge of the unit or its experiences.

Examples of these types of consultation can be seen in the site assistance visit or with the epidemiologic consultation team evaluations of suicide behaviors that have occurred at several sites throughout the Army in the past several years. In these cases, the team arrives, does a thorough analysis of potential factors, interviews individuals from the unit, and then provides a report of its findings and recommendations. It is left to the unit and local personnel to enact and follow up those recommendations.

PERFORMING THE CONSULTATION

Forming a Consultative Team

A consultation can be completed by either an individual clinician or by a team. If forming a team, the lead consultant should seek individuals who either have areas of expertise that will be needed to answer the consultation question, or with similarities in experience or background to the group requesting the consult. When assembling a team, it is also important to ensure it can work cohesively. The lead consultant must make clear the roles and duties of each team member. This can be especially difficult if the members have not worked together before and are coming together solely for the purpose of a consultation. It is often immediately evident if a team is or is not working together. Team cohesion will often determine success of the consultation process and whether the consultation is performed adequately, effectively, and efficiently.

Formulating the Consultation Question

Prior to performing the consultation, the clinician should ensure that the question being asked has been clarified. For instance, the consultative question can concern clinical care requirements or the deployability of a particular soldier, or it may include a broader question of unit policy, behaviors, or actions. The consultative team needs to ensure that it focuses its efforts to meet the needs of the requesting commander. The team should only give additional information about individuals on a need-to-know basis. Once the nature of the request is determined, specific goals of the consultation must be established. Often command and other military personnel are unclear of their desired "goals," and are best able to describe a "desired end state." Setting specific goals at the onset of the consultation will ensure that expectations are met. It will also help prevent any misperceptions of what the consultative team is doing or its capabilities. In addition to setting goals, it is also important to explain the limitations of the consultative team. One specific difficulty can arise if the requesting commander believes that a consultation also provides treatment. An illustration of this misperception is discussed below.

Case Study 12-1: A company commander came to the brigade behavioral health office during a deployment in Iraq. He stated that one of his route clearance platoons was recently having behavioral problems. It was also failing to find as many improvised explosive devices as it had on previous missions. After the brigade behavioral health officer went on a route clearance mission with the platoon members, it became evident they were fatigued—arguing with each other instead of focusing on the mission—and frustrated about not having had a day off in weeks. When this information was shared with the company commander, the command expressed confusion with regards to the outcome of the consultation. Specifically, the command in this instance had expected the brigade behavioral health officer would "fix" the soldiers by just spending time with them. Instead, the behavioral health officer had taken the consultative question and developed recommended changes in the soldiers' schedules. This example highlights the need for the consulting provider to clarify the request, set clear goals, and explain the limitations of the consultation services. Attention to these processes can ensure both parties are clear about the goals of the consultation and satisfied with its outcome.

Gaining Entry to the Unit

A consultation generally occurs at the request of the unit's commander. First and foremost, an appropriate member of the chain of command must request the consultation. During deployments, this can be difficult, because many individuals, especially those in combat stress detachments, want to assist the unit. However, if their participation is not invited, the "consultation" may develop into a confrontational relationship with the commander.

Additionally, the consultation team must establish rapport with the soldiers being evaluated. It should be clear that the team is there to help the unit, not to blame or hold certain members responsible for any problems that the unit may have. Demonstrating that the team cares and wants to make improvements will increase the willingness of the unit to disclose factual as well as emotional material, thus providing information that may assist in answering the consultation question.

It is important that the unit views the consultant as someone who is genuine; available not only in the moment, but for future involvement; supportive of their needs; and perceived as someone recognized in the field in which the consultant is asked to evaluate. Additionally, being someone who has provided assistance previously or spent time with members of the unit helps to establish an early rapport. By ensuring the behavioral health consultant possesses these qualities, there is an increased likelihood of being asked into the unit, as well as ensuring the consultant will be used again in the future.

In Case Study 12-1, concerning the evaluation of the route clearance platoon, the consultant had previously gone on a few route clearance missions with the soldiers for no other reason than to understand what their mission was and experience what it was like. Not only did this permit the consultant to earn the respect of the soldiers, it also solidified the consultant's credibility with command and led to numerous consultations in which the consultant was able to assist the unit.

Explaining the Purpose of the Consultation

Before gathering information from soldiers, it is necessary to explain the purpose of the consultation, including who requested it, what information is being gathered, and what will be done with that information. It is imperative for all parties in the evaluation to be clear about all the issues involved, including legal and ethical ones, and potential consequences. Knowing the basic legal rights of the individuals undergoing the process, as well as to whom to refer service members if issues arise, is also important. Furthermore, walking the involved parties through a step-by-step overview of the process and then performing a "back brief" will also ensure that command understands the consultation process. Finally, clarifying the scope of the consultation process as it is occurring is essential.

Cross-Service Consultations

In some cases, individuals may be required to perform consultations for another US military service. The consultative team should review the doctrine, regulations, and mission-specific goals for sister services and their units because there may be significant differences in how information is gathered, what documents are used, and how information is shared. Additionally, consultants should take time to learn about the differences in a particular service's systems, as well as the differences in unit functions. Consultants can demonstrate interest by explaining what information they have already learned, then asking questions that may assist in better understanding the sister branch. This process will likely guide the consultation while building rapport.

Uniform

One of the greatest challenges for a consultative team is to establish trust and mutual respect with the leadership requesting the consultation. To further this end, team members should determine the current uniform status of the unit to which they are consulting and dress accordingly. For example, if the consultative team was meeting with a number of line commanders in a field environment, the Army Class B uniform would not be appropriate.

Additionally, members of the consultative team need to ensure that they display the proper wear, fit, and appearance of the uniform. Commanders may see it as a sign of disrespect and lack of concern about their military mission if consultative team members do not pay attention to what is the proper uniform; this can have a negative effect on the relationship developed between the team and the command. In a deployment setting, knowing what the proper uniform is and wearing it appropriately may also be a safety concern because some locations are at high-risk for attacks, therefore requiring more extensive gear and protective wear. Moreover, it can provide yet another segue in building rapport with the unit by showing interest in how it operates, while decreasing the psychological distance between the consultant and unit members.

Language

The consultative team members should identify the common terminology, slang, and descriptive terms that are frequently used by the organization requesting the consult and adapt their own language to those with whom they are speaking. Not only does this require adapting to the language of the command, but also to that of the members of the unit. Speaking in simple language, minimizing medical jargon, and not using "psychobabble" are recommended. However, when trying to adapt one's own communication style to that of the group, do not use obscene or coarse language that may jeopardize professional credibility.

Understanding Unit Structures and Functions

Prior to providing a unit with recommendations for intervention and ideally prior to beginning the consultation, consulting clinicians should educate themselves about the unit or organization requesting the consultation. Understanding the unit and its mission will guide how the consultant engages with the participating soldiers and the interventions that might be recommended. It is helpful to know the formal and informal structure of the unit and how it directly and indirectly affects the unit. Relying solely on an organizational chart of the unit would be remiss. Many subgroups and personalities frequently play a significant role in how the unit runs and operates. Gaining knowledge on how communication is relayed and who has the power in the unit is also of utmost significance. Making assumptions due to rank (enlisted or officer) and branch could lead to false or inappropriate conclusions. Additionally, the consultant must be cognizant of the limitations that these functions place on their recommendations; otherwise, it may set the unit up for failure or not have the intended result.

Case Study 12-2: A company commander at a patrol base in Iraq stated that morale was down and he wasn't exactly sure why. He asked the brigade behavioral health officer if she could assess the situation and give him some feedback and recommendations. After surveying the unit and talking to the soldiers at length, the consultant determined that the soldiers were frustrated with their leadership because they felt they were not receiving information on missions and they were doing missions that were not necessary, thus putting them in harm's way. This information was back briefed to the commander. When the situation was reassessed a week later, nothing had changed; the soldiers continued to be frustrated and unmotivated. During the reassessment, the behavioral health officer determined that the first sergeant was failing to provide information to the soldiers, leading to a breakdown in information flow within the unit. Until the first sergeant was briefed directly, none of the feedback from the consultation had been discussed or implemented at his level. Once he fully understood the recommendations, he began making changes on the patrol base and morale began improving.

Engaging With Soldiers

Consultants need to be cautious about how they begin a visit. Many times the participating soldiers will decide within the first 5 minutes whether they feel the effort of talking with a consultant is relevant to them and if they will participate. It is the job of the consultant to get service members to "buy in" to the consultation process. Many times it is effective to begin by opening with a question and seeking the participants' responses and input rather than talking to them at length. Zeroing in on key leaders and getting them engaged in the process will lower the barriers and intimidation of other soldiers who may be reluctant to get involved. Consultants should inform the unit of how they want to help the unit and the soldiers, while telling the soldiers that they are the true experts and allowing them to inform the consultant. Taking the time to sit back and listen to them in their element (ie, motor pool, guard towers, etc) will assist in making soldiers feel comfortable and further reinforce how the consultant values their opinions and knowledge. Soldiers are trained and conditioned to listen and take orders, so when somebody sits back and genuinely listens, a lot of valuable information and insight can quickly and easily be gathered.

Interventions

The consultant must consider realistic interventions that are not only applicable to the current conditions, mission, operational tempo, and resources available, but also with realistic implementation strategies. As one division commander in combat expressed to a visiting consultation team, "Don't tell me it's hard here or that conditions suck, we all know that. Don't give me platitudes, give me clear and specific guidance that my commanders can actually use to help my soldiers."

To meet these goals, the consultant must consider realistic interventions that will address function as opposed to pathology. These include educating the unit as well as the command on how the intention of the intervention is to keep soldiers ready to fight and make them more productive for the mission; briefing the commander with simple, objective, and clear-cut ways that the situation can be improved using clearly defined recommendations that can be easily implemented; and reinforcing in a step-by-step method how the recommendations will be executed and how they will ultimately improve the unit's ability to accomplish its mission. Once the interventions have been made, it is imperative that the consultant remains available to clarify any ambiguities or address any questions that arise during the implementation process.

Terminating the Consultation

The type of consultation determines the number of sessions required. Some consultations will be over after one visit, others might last several months. As part of terminating the consultation, a final report should be provided to the requestor, the participants should be thanked, and those who may have developed relationships during the consultation experience should have an opportunity to say goodbye. Consultants must ensure all of their questions have been addressed, and make certain they have provided information for future contacts while imparting other resources that may be of assistance. It is preferable that the consultants talk to all parties involved in the consultation process to close all the loops of communication. Consultants use valuable unit resources such as time, energy, and information. Therefore, it is important to include the contributing parties in the termination process.

A good consultation can be ruined by a poor termination. If consultants leave the group feeling "used" or "no longer important" then they will lose credibility. It is probable that the long-term benefit of their interventions will fail because they are likely to lack unit acceptance. Additionally, it can make it more difficult to gain access to future groups for establishing consultative relationships.

Reporting the Consultation

As part of the termination process, a report should be given to the requestor. This may not initially be in written form, but should at least be via a back brief and then followed at a later date by a written brief with recommendations. A formal out brief should always be offered to the commander who has allowed access into the unit. This not only shows respect and understanding of the command relationship, it also provides access to the person who can implement the recommendations and programs suggested. Furthermore, it is an opportunity to gain insight into areas that may have been missed or may require further study. This should be followed by sending a written brief subsequent to the back brief, which guarantees that consultants have had time to reflect and consider all aspects of the group; think things through more carefully; and consult with a trusted colleague if any reservations have arisen.[49] It will also provide the consultant with an opportunity to ensure that the consultation question has been answered clearly and concisely while ensuring the commander's objectives were met.

Additionally, if the consultant intends to use the information from this report for any other endeavor, such as publication or report to any outside agencies, then permission should be gained from the unit.

DETERMINING FITNESS FOR DUTY AND DEPLOYMENT CLEARANCE

At times, consultants are requested by commanders to determine if a soldier is fit for continued military service or deployment. There are several aspects associated with determining fitness for duty and deployment clearance.

Disqualifying Conditions

The first step is to have a thorough and detailed understanding of Army Regulation 40-501, *Standards of Medical Fitness,* particularly Chapters 3 and 7.[50] Chapter 3 outlines the standards for medical fitness and separation. Chapter 7 provides guidance on profiling.[50] Current Army regulations require soldiers with disorders with psychotic features not caused by organic pathology or toxic substances to undergo a medical board to determine fitness for continued service in the military. This includes bipolar disorder and schizophrenia or any other mental disorder that causes gross impairment in reality testing. There is further guidance regarding other diagnoses and the criteria for referral to a medical board. In general, mood, anxiety, somatoform, and dissociative disorders are disqualifying if they necessitate recurrent hospitalization, persistently limit duty, or interfere with effective military performance.[50]

Personality, substance-related, and adjustment disorders are generally not disqualifying through the physical disability system, but may be cause for administrative separation. Before recommending administrative separation for these conditions, a detailed exploration for potential posttraumatic stress should be performed, particularly in previously deployed soldiers with changes in behavior patterns, because the outcome of the evaluation may significantly affect postseparation benefits and access to ongoing medical care.

Medical Profiling

Army Regulation 40-501, Chapter 7, details physical profiling and is an area of ongoing confusion and contention among soldiers, providers, and commanders.[50] A thorough knowledge of the regulations will enable providers to clearly articulate both the limitations of the profile and the regulatory responsibilities of command, and ensure expectation management on the part of the profiled soldier.

The profile serial system (P-U-L-H-E-S, which stands for **P**hysical capacity or stamina; **U**pper extremities; **L**ower extremities; **H**earing and ears; **E**yes; and p**S**ychiatric) is used to define the effects of a soldier's medical condition in relation to the performance of duties. Psychiatric disorders are denoted in the "S" section and rated from 1 to 4. This rating is to provide an assessment of overall functioning and is not based on the diagnosis itself. When determining the rating, the provider must consider the type, severity, and duration of symptoms, amount of external stressors, predisposition, intelligence, prior psychiatric history, and current duty performance. Additionally, the regulation provides some specific guidance for conditions that require a particular rating to be given, including when (*a*) no psychiatric pathology is evident; (*b*) there is a history of recovery of an acute psychotic reaction from external but non–substance-abuse-related cause; (*c*) there has been remission of a mental health disorder that is not otherwise disqualifying, but requires either limitations of assignments or duties; and (*d*) a rating of "3" cannot be met.[50] Assignment of a permanent S3 or S4 rating requires a medical board to be performed.

The specific limitations recommended on the profile are as important as the profile designator. According to Army Regulation 40-501, the condition itself should not be the sole consideration when recommending limitations. The profiling officer must also consider the prognosis, the possibility of aggravation, and the effects the profile will have on the soldier's ability to perform required duties.[50] The regulation states specifically that profiles "must be realistic."[50(p73)] Profiles are required to be specific and written in lay terms.[50]

It should be clearly articulated to a soldier being profiled that determination of duties, assignments, and deployment are command matters. Given this, profiles such as no deployment, no field duty, or no overseas duty are "not proper medical recommendations"[50(p73)] to be written on a profile. It is incumbent upon the profiling officer to provide adequate and clear recommendations so the commander can make an informed decision based on medical limitations and capacities, duty requirements, assignment limitations, mission requirements, and duties of the soldier among other command and mission-related issues.

If the commander does not feel the soldier can perform within the profile, reconsideration can be requested. If requested, reconsideration must be accomplished and will either amend the profile or revalidate it. This can be requested for both temporary and permanent profiles.

Deployment Clearance

In the fall of 2006, the Assistant Secretary of Defense for Health Affairs and The Surgeon General, US Army, provided guidance on the minimum mental health standards for deployment.[51] This policy was outlined in a memorandum, "Policy Guidance for Deployment Limiting Psychiatric Conditions and Medications." This guidance came in response to a congressional directive[52] after several media reports stated that mentally ill soldiers were being deployed who were unstable or taking medications without follow-on care. Additionally, some media reports cited soldiers being started on medications shortly before deployment and receiving a year supply of medication without monitoring.

Key factors in the policy related to mental health conditions and medications included: (*a*) soldiers currently being treated for psychosis or bipolar disorder were not deployable; (*b*) soldiers who were taking medications that require laboratory monitoring, such as lithium or valproic acid, were not deployable; (*c*) soldiers who are taking antipsychotic medications to control psychotic, bipolar, or chronic insomnia conditions were not deployable; (*d*) the continued use of psychotropic medications that are clinically and operationally problematic during deployments, including short half-life benzodiazepines and stimulants, should be balanced between the necessity for successful functioning in the theater of operations and the ability to obtain the medication, the potential for withdrawal, and the potential for abuse; (*e*) soldiers with significant mental health conditions require 3 months of stability prior to deployment; and (*f*) if a soldier is placed on a psychotropic medication within 3 months of deployment, then that soldier must be improving, stable, and tolerating the medication without significant side effects to deploy.[51] Although not articulated in the policy, consideration should be given to monitoring, for at least 1 month prior to deployment, any soldier on medication for anxiety, depression, or insomnia.

Screening for conditions that preclude deployment as part of the predeployment health process enables identification of soldiers not meeting minimum criteria for deployment. The screening process in one deploying unit prior to Operation Iraqi Freedom in 2007 consisted of an initial survey that was filled out concurrently with the predeployment health assessment. This process identified any soldier who was currently on any psychiatric medication, under psychiatric care, or experiencing significant stressors. Soldiers who screened positive were referred to mental health services for an evaluation for deployability based on the outlined minimum standards for deployment. Those who met standards were cleared. Those who did not were either referred to a medical board or the provider met with command to discuss limitations. Soldiers were then either left on rear detachment (delayed in deployment until stable on medications [typically 1–2 months]) or a waiver was granted through the combatant command surgeon. In general, the number of soldiers requiring clearance was minimal (less than 20 / 3,500 soldiers) because the majority who were unable to deploy were identified prior to beginning the predeployment screening process. However, this is an important safety mechanism that is recommended to all deploying units, and it is likely that a standardized procedure and survey will be implemented in the near future.[53]

Separation From the Military

At times soldiers may have mental health conditions that make them unfit for duty, although they do not require a medical board per se. These conditions are defined in Army Regulation 635-200, *Enlisted Separations*.[54] Although these separations are primarily a command function, an evaluation and diagnosis by an appropriately credentialed provider is required. Functional knowledge of these chapters and the separation process will enable consultants to counsel commanders—who may be junior or facing other more pressing issues—regarding the appropriate and judicious use of these actions, thus avoiding unnecessary delays, misdiagnoses, inappropriate separations, and potential procedural errors.

Mental health providers will predominantly be involved with Chapter 5-13 (personality disorders) and Chapter 5-17 (other mental or physical disorders).[54] Both of these chapters require that the soldier not have a condition that amounts to disability, and both require that the soldier be formally counseled and afforded "ample opportunity to overcome those deficiencies."[54(p56)] These mechanisms should not be used in lieu of judicial actions or other administrative separations.

Chapter 5-13 states that a soldier can be separated for personality disorder if the condition severely impairs the soldier's ability to function in the military environment. It further states it must be a long-standing and deeply ingrained condition.[54] This is particularly important when dealing with the postdeployment soldier who may have confounding posttraumatic stress issues, mild traumatic brain injury, or acute situational issues.

Chapter 5-17 deals with physical or mental issues that "potentially interfere with assignment to or performance of duty"[54(p57)] and are not covered under other areas of the separation regulations. This includes conditions such as claustrophobia; disturbances of perception, emotional control, or behavior; dyslexia; sleepwalking; or other disorders that may significantly impair the performance of military duties.

COMMAND-DIRECTED EVALUATIONS

Command-directed mental health evaluations are defined in DoD Instruction 6490.4,[55] DoD Directive 6490.1,[56] and US Army Medical Command Regulation 40-38,[57] which outline rules for both discretionary and nondiscretionary command-directed referrals. Nondiscretionary evaluations are those required by regulation to include the positions of drill sergeant, recruiter, and sniper. Additionally, all soldiers undergoing certain chapter separations require mental status evaluations. However, when commanders request evaluations for soldiers who do not require assessment by regulation, they use their discretionary authority to request evaluation and feedback.

When performing a command-directed evaluation, commanders should be provided a formal "Report of Mental Status" outlining feedback and recommendations. At a minimum, the report should address if a diagnosis exists, a prognosis for the soldier's condition, any limitations, a review of soldier safety and any safety interventions required, and the soldier's fitness for duty. Regulations require that the commander receive that report no later than 24 hours after completion of the evaluation.

Additionally, evaluating providers must be familiar with the restrictions that their level of professional degree places on their ability to perform and sign command-directed evaluations. In general, non–doctoral-level social workers are able to perform and sign nondiscretionary evaluations. Discretionary evaluations and those recommending a Chapter 5-13 (personality disorder) or Chapter 5-17 (failure to adapt) discharges require a doctoral-level social worker, a psychologist, or a psychiatrist. If there is a condition in which the only available mental health provider does not have signing authority, such as during a deployment or in a remote location, then a physician may serve as the signing authority.

RISKS TO THE CONSULTANT AND ETHICAL ISSUES IN CONSULTATION

As previously mentioned, serving in the role of a command consultant is very different from a typical doctor–patient encounter. The role of the consultant can at times present ethical challenges and difficult situations.

Double Agency

In command consultation, the military mental health provider is frequently called upon to simultaneously address the needs of both the unit and the soldier-patient. This dual responsibility is termed "double agency." Sometimes in command consultation, the only "patient" is the unit, and there is not an identified soldier of concern. In other cases, a soldier is identified as the patient, and the provider has a responsibility to provide treatment and, at the same time, to advise the commander regarding the military's most favorable course of action. The two are synchronous a majority of the time: that is, what is good for the soldier is also good for the military. For example, a soldier with permanent cognitive impairment from a brain injury should not remain in the military, because it would not be safe for that soldier to function in combat. Thus, the soldier is recommended for a medical evaluation board to determine the level of disability and ensure that this individual receives the appropriate long-term medical and financial benefits. Additionally, the unit's needs are met because having an impaired soldier in combat poses greater risk for fellow soldiers, and by medically boarding such a soldier, the unit is able to receive a healthy replacement.

However, a mutually beneficial course of action does not always exist. Such is the case when a dysfunctional soldier will suffer financial hardship, or the family will lose needed medical benefits due to separation from the military. When making recommendations concerning treatment, limitations, or separation/evacuation, the behavioral health officer must keep in mind the soldier's ability to perform assigned tasks in a combat environment. This becomes more difficult in the case of soldiers who are struggling with the psychological effects of combat. The provider may find it very difficult to determine when is the proper time to remove a soldier from continued combat exposure while also keeping in mind the unit's mission and current needs.

These situations must be carefully examined and, as with many ethical issues, there is no single correct answer. Discussion with colleagues or senior behavioral health providers, including the theater mental health consultant, can be helpful in processing these issues and is recommended.

Confidentiality

The commander has a right to know a soldier's diagnosis, prognosis, treatment plan, and duty limitations. Beyond these concise details, the behavioral health providers must be very careful concerning what information is provided to the commander. However, the commander is under no such restriction and can provide a great deal of information to the behavioral health provider, including reports about the soldier's ability to function at work, relationships with peers and supervisors, past occupational counseling, and the "other side" of the story. If viewed as partners on a team, rather than as adversaries, the consulting relationship between behavioral health providers and commanders can be mutually beneficial to each party, as well as to soldiers. Frequently, both the commander and the behavioral health provider can work together to help a soldier function better.

Thus, even though a commander has a right to know a soldier's diagnosis, prognosis, treatment plan, and duty limitations, behavioral health providers certainly do not contact every patient's commander with that information. If soldiers have mild symptoms that neither impair their functioning at work nor require duty limitations, there is no need to contact the commander. However, if there is risk to the unit, mission, or soldier, it is incumbent upon the provider to be certain that command is aware to ensure the ongoing safety and treatment of the patient, as well as that of the unit.

Objectivity Versus Intimacy

When the mental health provider is closely integrated into the unit, ongoing relationships are established with commanders that significantly improve the effectiveness of the consultative process. However, because of this intimacy, some objectivity may be lost. The behavioral health provider needs to continually ask the question, "What is my role in this situation?" to ensure that appropriate impartiality is being maintained. As a result of the intimacy, the provider is also vulnerable to the same stressors and tragedies as the unit. Closely aligned behavioral health providers can still be able to help the unit during times of crisis, but also need to be aware of their own stressors and limitations. In some circumstances, behavioral health providers may need their own treatment or intervention as a part of the unit.

Short Versus Long Consultations and the Development of Relationships

Some consultation relationships exist over an extended period of time, such as that of DMH officers with the commanders in their division. Others by nature are of a limited or one-time duration, such as a soldier who is seen for a command-directed mental health evaluation. Although a behavioral health provider may only plan to see a particular soldier for a single evaluation, frequently the provider ultimately has further contact with the command regarding other soldiers. This fosters the long-term consultative relationship.

Every interaction with a commander has the potential to help a particular soldier, but also to "take the pulse" of the unit's climate, to cultivate future cooperative relations, and to educate commanders about leader actions for decreasing combat operational stress within their units. The behavioral health provider's conscious grooming of this relationship allows commanders to begin to feel more comfortable accepting behavioral health interventions for their soldiers, as well as for themselves.

Investigation Verus Consultation

It can be easy for commanders to feel that they or their practices are being investigated during the information-gathering portion of a consult. This can feel intrusive and cause anxiety. For example, a commander in Iraq referred a soldier who had allegedly assaulted the unit's first sergeant. The soldier reported having assaulted the first sergeant only after the first sergeant had pushed him against the wall in a chokehold. This situation required a careful consultative approach to balance advocating for the soldier, defusing tension at the unit, and promoting future consultation. Generally, approaching the situation from a shared problem-solving stance, rather than seeking to find blame, is more productive.

Impact of HIPAA on Command Consultation

Aspects of the Health Insurance Portability and Accountability Act (HIPAA) address safeguarding the security and privacy of protected health information, including names, Social Security numbers, dates of birth, and other patient identifying data. Soldiers are commonly designated on military records by this information. Military hospitals and clinics are required to comply with HIPAA, and generally have the required safeguards in place. Providers need to ensure that any protected health information sent electronically to commanders is either sent over a closed network, or that some form of encryption is used. Routine measures for HIPAA compliance ensuring patient privacy include placing computer workstations out of the public view and locking them when not in use, securing charts behind locked doors, and protecting identifying information on charts from being seen by others during an office visit.

NOTABLE CONSULTATIVE POSITIONS IN THE ARMY

Most military behavioral health providers will be placed in a command consultative role at some time in their careers, whether it is simply to evaluate one soldier or to provide an overview of a large unit. Three particular consultative roles merit further discussion: (1) Consultant to The Surgeon General of the Army; (2) member of a Mental Health Advisory Team (MHAT); and (3) division psychiatrist/brigade behavioral health officer.

Consultant to The Surgeon General, US Army

This assignment is generally a 4-year tasking, which the consultant undertakes in addition to usual assigned duties. In behavioral health, these consultant positions include research and clinical psychology, social work, psychiatric nursing, and occupational therapy. There are four consultant positions in psychiatry: general, child, forensics, and addiction. There is also a consultant for the Exceptional Family Member Program, which usually is either a pediatrician or a psychiatrist. Functionally, the consultant positions in general and child psychiatry, research and clinical psychology, social work, and psychiatric nursing contribute to assignment determinations for personnel in these specialties.

For the last 20 years, these behavioral health consultants have been located throughout the United States, although principally at the US Army Medical Command Headquarters in San Antonio, Texas. After the attacks on September 11, 2001, the respective behavioral health consultants spent numerous weeks and months at the Office of The Surgeon General in Washington, DC. In 2007, a new Proponency for Behavioral Health was established, solidifying a requirement for a behavioral health consultant at the Office of The Surgeon General.

Key functions of the behavioral health Consultants to The Surgeon General of the Army include assignments, taskings for deployment, review of records, and strategic communications.

Assignments

The most important function of a Consultant to The Surgeon General is the task of assignments. The consultant recommends assignments to the specialty branch manager who makes the assignment decision. In general, the recommendations of the consultant are followed. The assignment process, however, involves several matrices. The current psychiatry consultant, for instance, asks graduating residents and staff who are eligible to move for a list of ten desired assignments as well as any family considerations. The consultant then generates a list of potential assignments. Additional related issues, such as whether candidates are medically deployable, are also considered. (It is essential to put deployable psychiatrists and other behavioral health assets in divisions and CSC units.) Following the Graduate Medical Education Selection Board and the Officer Distribution Plan conference (where Board decisions are made and announced), the draft assignments can be distributed. Request for orders and the actual orders subsequently follow. These orders may be modified in the event of unanticipated personnel changes or in the event of new, emergent missions.

The priorities for assignment are: first the needs of the Army and second the needs of the soldier. Army needs include the two graduate medical education programs (National Capital Area and Tripler Army Medical Center) and power projection platforms, such as Fort Hood, Texas; Fort Benning, Georgia; Fort Riley, Kansas; Fort Stewart, Georgia; and Fort Bragg, North Carolina.

Many assignment choices are dominated by family needs. Those couples with small children usually want to live as close as possible to their extended families. Spouses who are employed usually want to be able to find good career-related jobs. Some have aged parents or ill siblings to tend for. The consultant works to take all these needs into account, but the needs of the Army are still paramount.

Tasking for Deployment

For "Tier I specialties," including psychiatry, psychology, and social work, the consultant is now intimately involved in deciding who will be tasked to deploy. The "cardinal rule" for the Medical Command is that no one should go twice until all have gone once. The deployment decisions are now made at the Professional Officer Filler Information System support conference, with the input of the regional medical consultants. However, it is not infrequent that last-minute taskings will arise due to unforeseen illness, injury, or other factors that make a projected officer unable to deploy, requiring the consultant to review the entire provider inventory and adjust priorities of need.

Review of Records

Another function of the psychiatry consultant is to review mental health records. These are received for a multitude of purposes, including: (*a*) waivers for accessions to both the officer and enlisted ranks; (*b*) determinations on line-of-duty investigations, especially following suicides; (*c*) review of completed investigations; and (*d*) review of cases where there is a question as to whether someone should have received a medical board or chapter.

Strategic Communications

The consultant functions in numerous roles to include reviewing scientific papers, answering media inquiries, advising on the suitability of others to participate in media interviews, and advising the public affairs officer. The position presents numerous challenges. A major one is that of recruiting and retaining medical personnel with the Army's current operation tempo.

Mental Health Advisory Team Member

Since 2003, the Army Surgeon General has annually deployed an MHAT at the request of the US Central Command commanding general to evaluate the behavioral health needs of soldiers during deployment. The initial team performed their evaluation during Operation Iraqi Freedom 1 after there were reports of elevated suicide rates in theater. More recently, MHAT teams have focused on the quality of care provided and the behavioral healthcare system of delivery within the theater of operations.

The MHATs have varied in their composition, at times consisting of large multidisciplinary mental health teams while more recent MHATs have only had a few research psychologists. The MHAT teams utilize methods of paper surveys and focus groups, and each year issue a report of findings with recommendations. Key recommendations have included the establishment of a theater suicide prevention program, implementation of "Battlemind" training, institution of unit behavioral health needs assessments, and battlefield ethics training. The MHAT teams and their recommendations are discussed in greater detail in Chapter 5, Walter Reed Army Institute of Research Contributions During Operations Iraqi Freedom and Enduring Freedom: From Research to Public Health Policy, in this volume.

Division Psychiatrist/Brigade Behavioral Health Officer

Chapter 6, The Division Psychiatrist and Brigade Behavioral Health Officers, in this volume details the role of these mental health specialists. However, this unique position places a behavioral health officer within a combat unit working directly as an ongoing consultant to a combat commander rather than working for the medical command. This position entails continuing responsibilities to the command as a consultant on issues such as how and where to deploy behavioral health resources, methods and techniques for controlling combat operational stress, and determining plans for prevention of behavioral casualties.

SUMMARY

Military mental health professionals provide critical consultation to command when psychiatric casualties are seen in garrison or during deployment. The challenge to the mental health consultant is to balance the need of the unit with what is in the best interest of the soldier's short-term and long-term mental health. Commanders have the utmost concern for their soldiers; it is therefore imperative that they trust the judgment of their consulting behavioral health officer in the decisions that they are making on the treatment of their soldiers. In addition, these same challenges exist in garrison because the consultant has to determine if a soldier is no longer fit to continue in service and requires a medical evaluation board or if this soldier might have a more favorable prognosis for recovery and continued military service.

REFERENCES

1. McCarroll JE, Jaccard JJ, Radke AQ. Psychiatric consultation to command. In: Jones FD, Sparacino LR, Wilcox VL, Rothberg JM, Stokes JW, eds. *War Psychiatry*. In: Zajtchuk R, Bellamy RF, eds. *Textbooks of Military Medicine*. Washington, DC: Department of the Army, Office of The Surgeon General, Borden Institute; 1995: 151–170.

2. Rosen G. Nostalgia: a "forgotten" psychological disorder. *Psychol Med*. 1975;5:340–354.

3. McGuire F. Army Alpha and Beta tests of intelligence. In: Sternberg RJ, ed. *Encyclopedia of Intelligence.* Vol 1. New York, NY: Macmillan; 1994: 125–129.

4. Spring JH. Psychologists and the war: the meaning of intelligence in the Alpha and Beta tests. *Hist Educ Q.* 1972;12:3–15.

5. Page GD. Clinical psychology in the military: developments and issues. *Clin Psychol Rev.* 1996;16:383–396.

6. Berlien IC, Waggoner RW. Selection and induction. In: Glass AJ, Bernucci RJ, Anderson RS, eds. *Neuropsychiatry in World War II.* Vol 1. *Zone of the Interior.* Washington, DC: Office of The Surgeon General; 1966: 153–191.

7. Menninger WC. *Psychiatry in a Troubled World.* New York, NY: MacMillan; 1948: 289.

8. US Department of the Army. *Induction Station Neuropsychiatric Examination.* Washington, DC: DA; April 1944. Technical Bulletin (TB MED).

9. Brill NQ, Beebe BW. *Veterans Administration Medical Monograph: A Follow-Up Study of War Neuroses.* Washington, DC: US Government Printing Office; 1955.

10. Plag JA, Arthur RJ. Psychiatric re-examination of unsuitable Naval recruits: a two-year follow-up study. *Am J Psychiatry.* 1965;122:534–541.

11. Bourne PG. Military psychiatry and the Vietnam experience. *Am J Psychiatry.* 1970;127:481–488.

12. Lachar D, Sparks JC, Larsen RM, Bisbee CT. Psychometric prediction of behavioral criteria of adaptation for USAF basic trainees. *J Community Psychol.* 1974;2:268–277.

13. McCraw RK, Bearden DL. Personality factors in failure to adapt to the military. *Mil Med.* 1990;155:127–130.

14. United States General Accounting Office. *Military Attrition: DoD Needs to Better Understand Reasons for Separation and Improve Recruiting Systems.* Testimony before the Subcommittee on Personnel, Committee on Armed Services, US Senate, March 4, 1998. Available at: http://www.gao.gov/archive/1998/ns98109t.pdf. Accessed February 4, 2010.

15. Williams RA, Hagerty BM, Yousha SM, Hoyle KS, Oe H. Factors associated with depression in Navy recruits. *J Clin Psychol.* 2002;58:323–337.

16. Martin PD, Williamson DA, Alfonso AJ, Ryan DH. Psychological adjustment during Army basic training. *Mil Med.* 2006;171:157–159.

17. Warner C, Warner C, Matuszak T, Rachal J, Flynn J, Grieger T. Disordered eating in entry-level military personnel. *Mil Med.* 2007;172(2):147–151.

18. Warner CM, Warner CH, Breitbach JE, Rachal J, Matuszak T, Greiger TA. Depression in entry-level military personnel. *Mil Med.* 2007;172(8):795–799.

19. Hoge CW, Castro CA, Messer SC, McGurk D, Cotting DI, Koffman RL. Combat duty in Iraq and Afghanistan, mental health problems, and barriers to care. *N Engl J Med.* 2004;351:13–22.

20. Stokes JW, Jones FD. Combat stress control in joint operations. In: Jones FD, Sparacino LR, Wilcox VL, Rothberg JM, Stokes JW, eds. *War Psychiatry.* In: Zajtchuk R, Bellamy RF, eds. *Textbooks of Military Medicine.* Washington, DC: Department of the Army, Office of The Surgeon General, Borden Institute; 1995: 243–270.

21. Appel JW. Preventive psychiatry. In: Glass AJ, Bernucci RJ, Anderson RS, eds. *Neuropsychiatry in World War II.* Vol 1. *Zone of the Interior.* Washington, DC: Office of The Surgeon General; 1966: 373–416.

22. Group for the Advancement of Psychiatry. *Preventive Psychiatry in the Armed Forces: With Some Implications for Civilian Use.* New York, NY: Group for the Advancement of Psychiatry; 1960. Report 47.

23. Tischler GL. Patterns of psychiatric attrition and of behavior in a combat zone. In: Bourne PG, ed. *Psychology and Physiology of Stress*. New York, NY: Academic Press; 1969: 19–44.

24. Gal R, Jones FD. A psychological model of combat stress. In: Jones FD, Sparacino LR, Wilcox VL, Rothberg JM, Stokes JW, eds. *War Psychiatry*. In: Zajtchuk R, Bellamy RF, eds. *Textbooks of Military Medicine*. Washington, DC: Department of the Army, Office of The Surgeon General, Borden Institute; 1995: 133–148.

25. Glass AJ. Lessons learned. In: Glass AJ, Mullins WS, eds. *Neuropsychiatry in World War II*. Vol 2. *Overseas Theaters*. Washington, DC: Office of The Surgeon General; 1973: 989–1027.

26. Mental Health Advisory Team IV. *MHAT IV Operation Iraqi Freedom 05-07 Final Report*. Washington, DC: US Army Surgeon General; November 17, 2006.

27. Warner CH, Breitbach JE, Appenzeller GN, Yates V, Grieger T, Webster WG. Division mental health in the new brigade combat team structure. Part 1: Predeployment and deployment. *Mil Med*. 2007;172:907–911.

28. Walter Reed Army Institute of Research. Psychiatry and Neuroscience. Battlemind training. Available at: http://www.battlemind.org. Accessed February 4, 2010.

29. Warner CH, Appenzeller GN, Mullen K, Warner CM, Greiger T. Soldier attitudes toward mental health screening and seeking care upon return from combat. *Mil Med*. 2008;173(6):563–569.

30. Hyams KC, Riddle J, Trump DH, Wallace MR. Protecting the health of United States military forces in Afghanistan: applying lessons learned since the Gulf War. *Clin Infect Dis*. 2002;15:S208–S214.

31. US Department of Defense. *Implementation and Application of Joint Medical Surveillance for Deployments*. Washington DC: Department of Defense; August 7, 1997. Instruction 6490.3.

32. Bliese PD, Wright KM, Adler AB, Hoge C, Prayner R. *Post-Deployment Psychological Screening: Interpreting and Scoring DD Form 2900*. Walter Reed Army Institute of Research-Europe: Heidelberg; Research Report #2005-003. Available at: https://www.battlemind.army.mil/assets/files/PDHRAResearchReportwithAppendices.pdf. Accessed February 4, 2009.

33. Hoge CW, Auchterlonie JL, Milliken CS. Mental health problems, use of mental health services, and attrition from military service after returning from deployment to Iraq or Afghanistan. *JAMA*. 2006;295:1023–1032.

34. Southwick SM, Morgan CA 3rd, Darnell A, et al. Trauma-related symptoms in veterans of Operation Desert Storm: a 2-year follow-up. *Am J Psychiatry*. 1995;152(8):1150–1155.

35. Grieger TA, Cozza SJ, Ursano RJ, et al. Posttraumatic stress disorder and depression in battle-injured soldiers. *Am J Psychiatry*. 2006;163:1777–1783.

36. Secretary of the Army. *Post Deployment Health Re-Assessment*. Washington, DC: Department of the Army; January 23, 2006.

37. US Government Accountability Office. *Post Traumatic Stress Disorder: DoD Needs to Identify the Factors Its Providers Use to Make Mental Health Evaluation Referrals for Servicemembers*. Washington, DC: GAO, Report to Congressional Committees; 2006: 1–34. GAO-06-397.

38. Appenzeller GN, Warner CH, Grieger T. Post deployment health reassessment: a sustainable method for brigade combat teams. *Mil Med*. 2007;172:1017–1023.

39. Mental Health Advisory Team III. *MHAT III Operation Iraqi Freedom 04-06 Final Report*. Washington, DC: US Army Surgeon General; May 29, 2006.

40. Koshes RJ, Young SA, Stokes JW. Debriefing following combat. In: Jones FD, Sparacino LR, Wilcox VL, Rothberg JM, Stokes JW, eds. *War Psychiatry*. In: Zajtchuk R, Bellamy RF, eds. *Textbooks of Military Medicine*. Washington, DC: Department of the Army, Office of The Surgeon General, Borden Institute; 1995: 271–290.

41. Rose S, Bisson J, Churchill R, Wessely S. Psychological debriefing for preventing post traumatic stress disorder (PTSD). *Cochrane Database Syst Rev.* 2002;2:CD000560.

42. MacDonald CM. Evaluation of stress debriefing interventions with military populations. *Mil Med.* 2003;168:961–968.

43. Jacobs J, Horne-Moyer HL, Jones R. The effectiveness of critical incident stress debriefing with primary and secondary trauma victims. *Int J Emerg Ment Health.* 2004;6:5–14.

44. Mitchell SG, Mitchell JT. Caplan, community, and critical incident stress management. *Int J Emerg Ment Health.* 2005;8:5–14.

45. US Department of the Army. *Combat and Operational Stress Control.* Washington, DC: Headquarters, DA; 2006. Field Manual 4-02.51.

46. Alder AB, Castro CA, McGurk D. *Battlemind Psychological Debriefings.* Heidelberg, Germany: Walter Reed Army Institute of Research-Europe; 2007. Research Report 2007-001.

47. Rock NL, Stokes JW, Koshes RJ, Fagan J, Cline WR, Jones FD. US Army combat psychiatry. In: Jones FD, Sparacino LR, Wilcox VL, Rothberg JM, Stokes JW, eds. *War Psychiatry.* In: Zajtchuk R, Bellamy RF, eds. *Textbooks of Military Medicine.* Washington, DC: Department of the Army, Office of The Surgeon General, Borden Institute; 1995: 149–175.

48. Jones E, Wessely E. "Forward psychiatry" in the military: its origin and effectiveness. *J Trauma Stress.* 2003;16:411–419.

49. McCarroll JE, Ursano RJ. Consultation to groups, organizations, and communities. In: Ritchie EC, Watson PJ, Friedman MJ, eds. *Interventions Following Mass Violence and Disasters: Strategies for Mental Health Practice.* New York, NY: Guilford Press; 2006: 193–205.

50. US Department of the Army. *Standards of Medical Fitness.* Washington, DC: Headquarters, DA; 2007. Army Regulation 40-501.

51. Assistant Secretary of Defense, US Department of Defense. *Policy Guidance for Deployment-Limiting Psychiatric Conditions and Medications.* Washington, DC: Department of the Army; November 7, 2006. Memorandum. Available at: http://www.ha.osd.mil/policies/2006/061107_deployment-limiting_psych_conditions_meds.pdf. Accessed February 4, 2010.

52. National Defense Authorization Act for Fiscal Year 2007. Pub L No. 109-364, Section 738.

53. Warner CH, Appenzeller GN, Mobbs A, Grieger T. Division mental health through the deployment cycle. Paper presented at: Force Health Protection Conference; August 13, 2008; Albuquerque, NM.

54. US Department of the Army. *Active Duty Enlisted Administrative Separations.* Washington, DC: Headquarters, DA; 2005. Army Regulation 635-200.

55. US Department of Defense. *Mental Health Evaluations of Members of the Armed Forces.* Washington, DC: Department of Defense; October 1, 1997. Directive 6490.1.

56. US Department of Defense. *Requirements for Mental Health Evaluations of Members of the Armed Forces.* Washington, DC: Department of Defense; August 28, 1998. Instruction 6490.4.

57. US Army Medical Command. *Command Directed Mental Health Evaluations.* Fort Sam Houston, Tex: Headquarters, MEDCOM; 1999. US Army Medical Command Regulation 40-38.

COMBAT AND OPERATIONAL BEHAVIORAL HEALTH

Section III: The Road Home

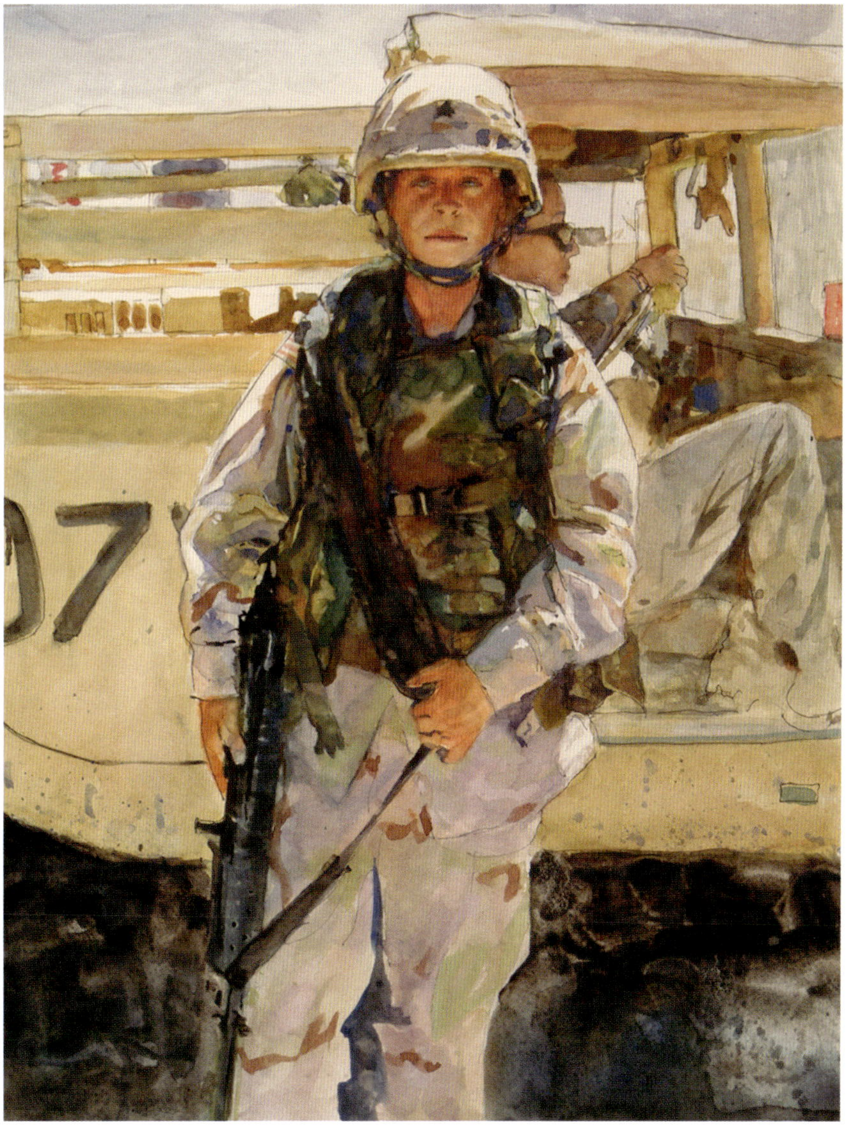

SGT Vickie Hodge, 3d ID, Baghdad Airport, by Elzie Golden, watercolor/ink on paper, 2005.

Art: Courtesy of the Army Art Collection, US Army Center of Military History.

Chapter 13

THE AEROMEDICAL EVACUATION

ALAN L. PETERSON, PhD, ABPP*; KELLY R. MCCARTHY, MA†; DANIEL J. BUSHEME, MA, LCDC‡; RICK L. CAMPISE, PhD, ABPP§; AND MONTY T. BAKER, PhD¥

*Professor, Department of Psychiatry, Mail Code 7792, University of Texas Health Science Center at San Antonio, 7703 Floyd Curl Drive, San Antonio, Texas 78229; formerly, Chair, Department of Psychology, Wilford Hall Medical Center, San Antonio, Texas
†Captain, Nurse Corps, US Air Force; Historian, Peterson Air Force Base, 150 Vandenberg, Suite 110S, Peterson Air Force Base, Colorado 80914; formerly, Chief, Behavioral Health Nursing Management, Life Skills Center, United States Air Force Academy, Colorado Springs, Colorado
‡Lieutenant Colonel, Nurse Corps, US Air Force; Chief, Mental Health Nursing, US Air Force Medical Operations Agency, 485 Quentin Roosevelt Road, Suite 400, San Antonio, Texas 78226-2017; formerly, Deputy Squadron Commander and Inpatient Mental Health Flight Commander, Travis Air Force Base, California
§Colonel, Biomedical Sciences Corps, US Air Force; Commander, 559th Medical Group, 1920 Biggs Avenue, Lackland Air Force Base, Texas 78236; formerly, Commander, 1st Medical Operations Squadron, Langley Air Force Base, Virginia
¥Major, Biomedical Sciences Corps, US Air Force; Director of Clinical Research, Warrior Resiliency Program, San Antonio Military Medical Center, 2200 Bergquist Drive, Suite 1, Lackland Air Force Base, Texas 78236; formerly, Element Leader, Mental Health Clinic, 59th Military Health System, Lackland Air Force Base, Texas

INTRODUCTION

Aeromedical evacuation is the movement of patients under medical supervision to and between medical treatment facilities by air transportation.[1] The global war on terror has been the largest sustained combat operation by the US military since the Vietnam War. Almost 2 million US military personnel have deployed to support Operation Iraqi Freedom (OIF) and Operation Enduring Freedom (OEF). The current aeromedical evacuation system used in support of OIF/OEF is one of the factors that is credited for the greatly improved survival rate for combat-wounded personnel in Iraq.[2] The current survival rate is approximately 90%, and it is the highest in recorded history; it is a significant increase from the 74% to 75% survival rate of wounded personnel in the wars in Korea, Vietnam, and the Persian Gulf.[2]

This chapter will review the aeromedical evacuation of patients from military battlefield locations and other operational locations, to include the types of aircraft used, the functioning of contingency aeromedical staging facilities (CASFs), guidelines and principles for evacuation of medical and psychiatric patients, and the pertinent military regulations and instructions that guide the evacuation process. A particular emphasis of the chapter is on aeromedical evacuation in support of OIF and OEF.

EVOLUTION OF MILITARY MEDICAL EVACUATION

A Brief History of Military Medical Evacuation

Throughout history many different approaches have been used to evacuate combat casualties from the battlefield to receive medical care. In the United States, the earliest recorded reports of the need for a military medical evacuation system occurred during the American Revolutionary War.[3] In April of 1777, the US Congress passed a bill recommending that "[a] suitable number of covered and other wagons, litters, and other necessaries for removing the sick and wounded, shall be supplied by the Quartermaster or Deputy Quartermaster General; and in case of their deficiency, by the Director or Deputy Director General."[3(p36)] However, there are no records that indicate that any such vehicles were actually built or supplied at that time.

The first reports of the actual use of a medical evacuation system occurred during the American Civil War,[4] which resulted in many battle-injured patients who challenged the military medical community.[5] As a result, significant changes were made in how soldiers were evacuated. During this time, at least 10 different designs were proposed for ambulance wagons that were to transport sick and wounded military personnel. Dr Jonathan Letterman was the first to create an organized system of medical evacuation during the Civil War. His pioneering work formed the basis for the present military medical evacuation system. President Lincoln commissioned railroads and riverboats during the Civil War for the medical transport of patients.[6]

The invention of automobiles was followed shortly thereafter by the invention of motorized ambulances to transport emergency medical patients.[7,8] More than 2 years prior to the United States' formal entry into World War I, teams of US military surgeons and their support personnel had already been deployed to France.[9] The collaboration of military and civilian surgeons at the Ambulance Americaine in Paris led to the use of ambulances to evacuate injured military personnel throughout Europe during World War I.

The invention of aircraft led to evolutionary changes in the medical evacuation of military patients throughout the 20th century.[10] The potential use of aircraft for the medical evacuation of injured military personnel was conceptualized in the early 1900s.[11,12] Marie Marvingt, a French nurse, was one of the most influential and effective proponents for the use of aircraft to evacuate the wounded in combat settings.[13] In 1913, Colonel Samuel F Cody demonstrated the potential use of a biplane as an air ambulance at Farnborough, England.[14] The initial conversion of military aircraft into air ambulances by the US Army occurred during the period from 1918 to 1924.[15] However, the concept of aeromedical evacuation of military medical patients did not gain widespread acceptance until World War II.[16] At that time, naval vessels were the most common form of transport for movement of military personnel to and from the war zone. Ships were also the most common means of transporting casualties to the United States for more definitive medical care. However, transport by ship could take weeks; there was a need to provide faster medical evacuation for more seriously injured military personnel. Subsequently, extensive use of military aircraft for patient evacuation began during 1945 when approximately 625,000 casualties (25% of all patients) were aeromedically evacuated to the United States.[16]

The first widespread use of helicopters for aeromedical evacuation occurred during the Korean War.[17] Use of helicopters was instituted because of the necessity to move patients rapidly from the battle area over rugged and inhospitable terrain. Helicopter evacuation

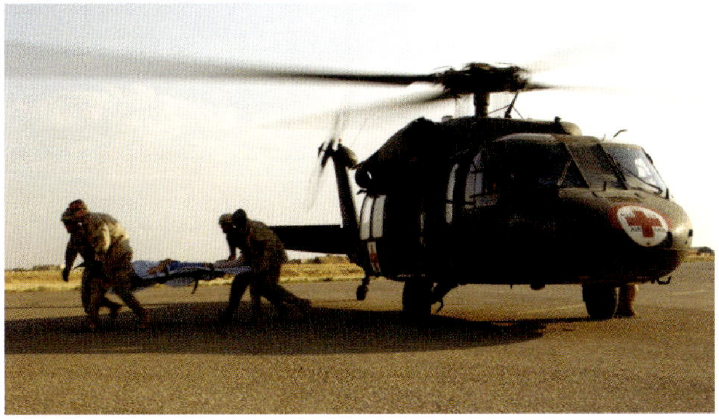

Figure 13-1. The UH-60 Black Hawk. The UH-60 Black Hawk can hold up to six litters for patient transport and is the Army's front-line helicopter for aeromedical evacuation in Iraq and Afghanistan.
Reproduced from: US Air Force Link photo library. www.af.mil/shared/media/photodb/photos/030822-F-7709W-005.jpg.

led to the successful transport of nearly 22,000 patients and is attributed to a reduction in the casualty mortality rate.[17] The combat experiences of the United States in Korea, the British in Malaya, and the French in Indochina proved that rotary-wing aircraft were invaluable in reducing battlefield death rates.[18] During the Vietnam conflict helicopters were firmly established as an essential component of aeromedical evacuation on the modern battlefield.[18] Operations Desert Shield and Desert Storm involved the deployment of 1,950 aeromedical evacuation personnel to support medical airlift.[19] Aircrews were deployed to 17 locations in the region and more than 12,500 patients were successfully airlifted using converted cargo aircraft.[19] The majority of these patients were general medical patients and not battle-related injuries.

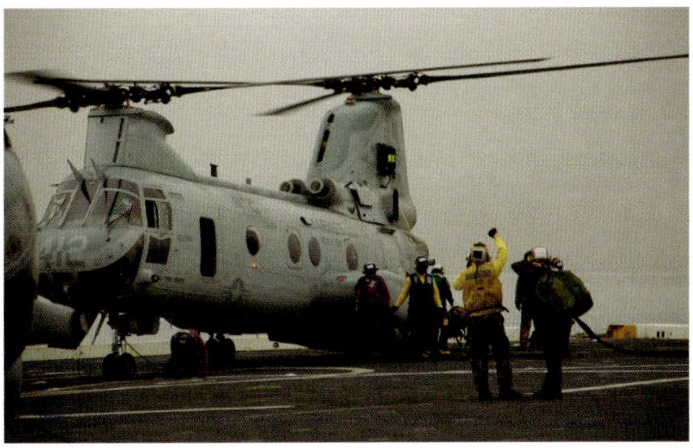

Figure 13-2. The CH-46 Sea Knight. The CH-46 can accommodate up to 15 patients and was used extensively by the Marines during the battle of Fallujah in November 2004. Here, Marine Reserves—the "Moonlighters" from Marine Medium Lift Helicopter Squadron 764, based at Edwards Air Force Base, Calif—pause for refueling and servicing by the US Navy flight deck crew aboard the USS *New Orleans*, participating in a nine-country training excercise called Partnership of the Americas, July 3, 2010. Photographer: MSgt Peter C Walz.
Reproduced from: US Marines Web site. www.marines.mil/unit/marforsouth/PublishingImages/NewsStoryImages/2010/100703-M-3168W-008.jpg.

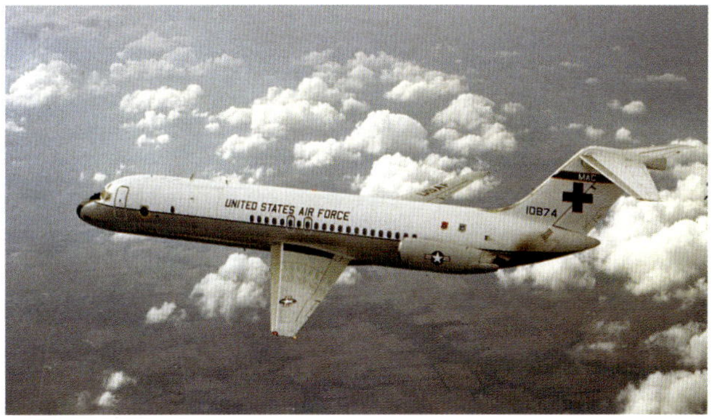

Figure 13-3. The C-9 Nightingale. The C-9 is the only military aircraft that was specifically designed for the aeromedical evacuation. Nicknamed the "Cadillac of Medevac," the C-9 was the workhorse of medical evacuation. It was phased out in 2003.
Reproduced from: US Air Force Link photo library. www.af.mil/shared/media/photodb/photos/021202-O-9999G-007.jpg.

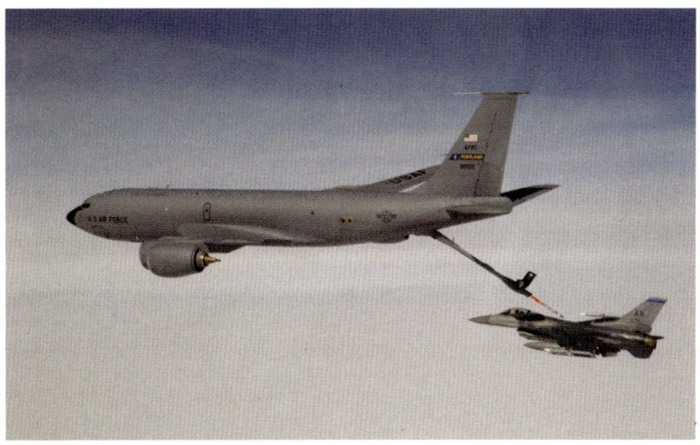

Figure 13-4. The KC-135 Stratotanker. The KC-135 is used primarily for air refueling, but it can be configured with patient-support pallets and used for aeromedical evacuation.
Reproduced from: US Air Force Link photo library. www.af.mil/shared/media/photodb/photos/ 060613-F-4192W-808.jpg.

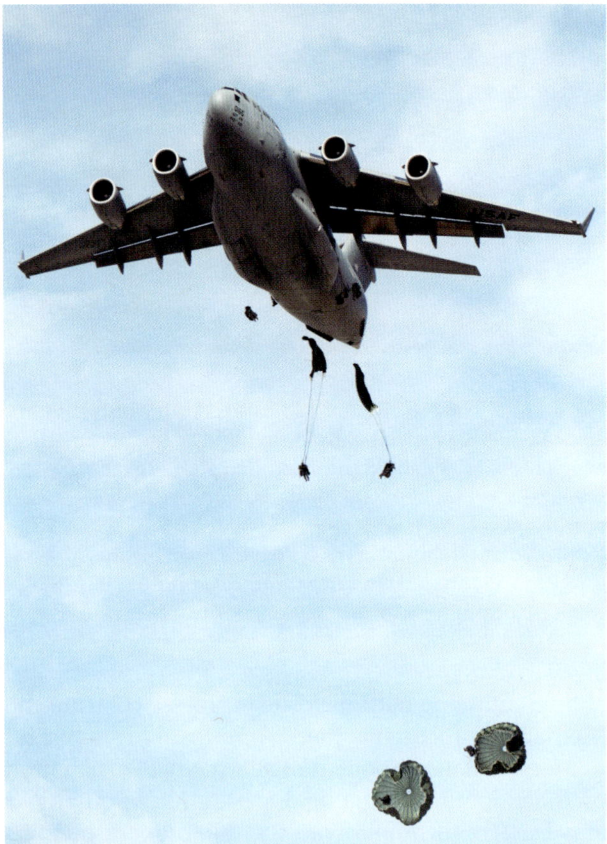

Figure 13-5. The C-17 Globemaster III. The C-17 is the most commonly used fixed-wing aircraft for aeromedical evacuation out of the combat theater to military medical centers.
Reproduced from: US Air Force Link photo library. www.af.mil/shared/media/photodb/photos/091118-F-3431H-513.jpg.

Currently, the military uses a variety of vehicles for transport of patients to include medical ground vehicles, nonmedical ground vehicles, watercraft, rail transport, and sometimes whatever vehicle of convenience is available.[20] However, today virtually 100% of casualties requiring transport away from areas of insurgent activities or out of the war zone are moved by aircraft.

Aircraft Used for Aeromedical Evacuation

Rotary wing aircraft are the primary vehciles used for casualty evacuation from the battlefield. These aircraft, in addition to improved body armor and advancements in casualty care, are thought to contribute to the increased survival rate that has occurred during the military actions in Iraq and Afghanistan.[2]

The Army and Marines operate most of the rotary wing aeromedical evacuation aircraft. The UH-60 Black Hawk (Figure 13-1), the Army's front-line utility helicopter, is used for air assault, air cavalry, and aeromedical evacuation. The UH-60 can hold up to six litters for patient transport. UH-60s can travel at high speeds, land on rough terrain in remote locations, and evacuate most injured patients for emergency department care within one hour—"the golden hour"[21] of critical importance to casualty survival. The CH-46 Sea Knight (Figure 13-2) is a larger twin-engine heavy-lift helicopter similar to the CH-47 Chinook and can accommodate up to 15 litters. CH-46s and CH-47s are vital aircraft dur-

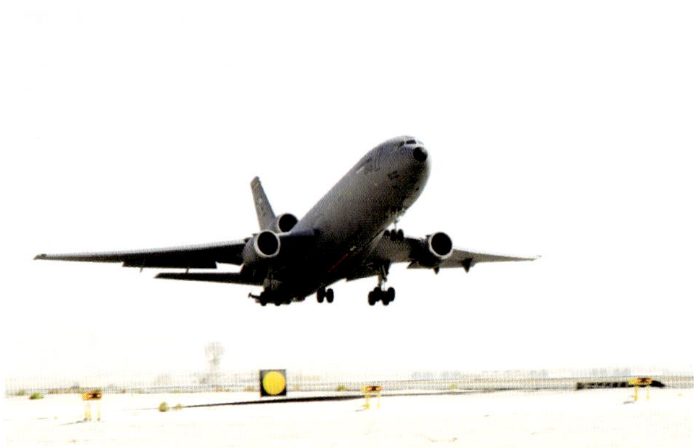

Figure 13-6. KC-10A Extender. The KC-10A is another air refueler that can be configured for aeromedical evacuation when loaded with patient-support pallets.
Reproduced from: US Air Force Link photo library. www.af.mil/shared/media/photodb/photos/091013-F-3140L-112.jpg.

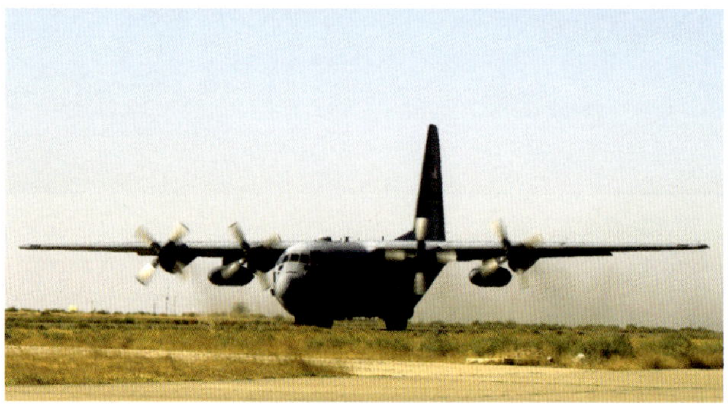

Figure 13-7. The C-130 Hercules. The C-130 is the most versatile fixed-wing aircraft used for aeromedical evacuation. It can carry up to 70 litters and can operate in austere locations.
Reproduced from: US Air Force Link photo library. www.af.mil/shared/media/photodb/photos/031030-F-9629J-005.jpg.

ing intense offensive military assaults when potentially large numbers of casualties need aeromedical transport during a short period of time. The AH-1W Cobra is an attack helicopter that often provides in-flight protection for rotary wing evacuations.

Fixed-wing aircraft are the primary means of aeromedical evacuation out of theater and from outside the continental United States (OCONUS) to the continental United States (CONUS) medical facilities. These are controlled by the Air Force. The C-9 Nightingale was introduced in 1968 and is the only military aircraft that was specifically designed for the aeromedical evacuation (Figure 13-3). However, the C-9 was phased out in 2003 and all medical evacuations now utilize "aircraft of opportunity." The development of patient-support pallets has increased the ability of alternative aircraft to be used for aeromedical evacuation. PSPs are built on a standard cargo pallet that can be loaded onto a variety of mobility aircraft. They provide support for six litters or a combination of three airline seats and three litters. The KC-135 Stratotanker (Figure 13-4) and KC-10A Extender (Figure 13-6) are aircraft used for air refueling that can be configured for aeromedical evacuation when loaded with patient-support pallets.

The C-17 Globemaster III (Figure 13-5) is the newest and most flexible long-range mobility aircraft. It was designed to support aeromedical evacuation as a secondary mission. The operational and tactical capabilities of the C-17 aircraft have led it to become the primary aircraft for airlift out of Iraq and Afghanistan. The design of the C-17 allows it to land on austere airfields. It can take off and land on runways as narrow as 90 feet and as short as 3,000 feet. It can be configured to carry 48 litters and 40 ambulatory patients. The C-17s are used to transport patients from theater to Landstuhl Army Regional Medical Center in Germany to Andrews Air Force Base in Washington, DC.

The C-130 Hercules (Figure 13-7) is a four-turboprop aircraft. First used by the Air Force in the 1950s, it is the oldest aeromedical evacuation aircraft. Its versatility, reliability, and capability of operating from rough, dirt strips make it an invaluable resource in deployed settings. Within theater, the C-130 Hercules can carry 70 all-litter loads, or a combination of 50 litters and 27 ambulatory patients. In Iraq, C-130s are often used for intratheater missions to Qatar and Kuwait.

THE DEPARTMENT OF DEFENSE PATIENT MOVEMENT SYSTEM

The mission of the Department of Defense Patient Movement System is to transport US military casualties and other medical patients from combat zones to field hospitals or other fixed medical treatment facilities located in or out of the combat theater.[22] Medical evacuation of military personnel injured in combat begins on the battlefield. Patients are assessed and treated across echelons of care. After combat life-saving care or forward surgical team intervention is provided at the initial injury site, the next echelon of care is often at an Army combat support hospital or an Air Force theater hospital. Navy medical hospital ships, such as the USNS *Comfort* (T-AH 20) or USNS *Mercy* (T-AH 19), are also sometimes available as a first echelon of care in deployed locations. Patients not expected to be able to return to duty within 7 days (or the established combat theater evacuation policy standard) will normally be evacuated to the next level of care once they are approved for aeromedical evacuation.

If patients require further evacuation, they are transported by fixed wing aircraft, rotary wing aircraft, or ground vehicle to a CASF, where they are prepared for aeromedical evacuation out of theater. Table 13-1 includes a summary of primary aeromedical evacuation instructions, regulations, and reference guidelines.

Patient movement is tracked through a computerized system at entry and during transit, and completed at exit from the aeromedical evacuation system. Patient movement requirements (PMRs; also called "patient movement requests" and "patient movement records") are medical requests to transport a patient to a higher echelon of care. The US Transportation Command is responsible for intertheater patient movement. Patients who require intertheater aeromedical evacuation are entered into the US Transportation Command Regulating and Command and Control Evacuation System (TRAC2ES), which allows their movement to be tracked by various facilities and the Joint Patient Movement Requirement Centers. The Global Patient Movement Requirements Center (GPMRC) is an organizational element of US Transportation Command that manages patient movement. The GPMRC integrates intertheater and CONUS medical regulation services, mission requirements, clinical validation, and related activities that support patient movement requests. Using TRAC2ES, the GPMRC and the Theater Patient Movement Requirements Center receives, consolidates, and processes PMRs to coordinate aeromedical evacuation requirements with available airlift operations, health service support capabilities, and available bed space.

Aeromedical Evacuation Movement Precedence

When a patient requires aeromedical evacuation, the attending physician is responsible for determining the

TABLE 13-1

AEROMEDICAL EVACUATION PUBLICATIONS

Title	Publication Date	Brief Description
Air Force Policy Directive 41-3 *Worldwide Aeromedical Evacuation*	July 29, 1994	Establishes responsibilities and authorities for aeromedical evacuation with the Air Force Surgeon General, Air Mobility Command, Air Combat Command, and the surgeon generals of the US Air Force Reserves and National Guard.
Air Force Instruction 41-301 *The Worldwide Air Medical Evacuation System*	August 1, 1996	Provides an overview of the entire aeromedical evacuation process.
Air Force Instruction 41-303 *Aeromedical Evacuation Dietetic Support*	March 27, 1995	Provides guidance and procedures for dietetics departments in medical treatment facilities that feed patients in the aeromedical evacuation system during peacetime and contingency operations.
Air Force Instruction 41-305 *Administering Aeromedical Staging Facilities*	December 1, 1997	Delineates requirements to set up and operate a contingency aeromedical staging facility including staffing and equipment lists.
Air Force Instruction 41-307, Attachment 6 *Aeromedical Evacuation Patient Considerations and Standards of Care*	August 20, 2003	Provides information on nursing care requirements and general guidelines for aeromedical evacuation of psychiatric patients. Includes descriptions of flight-specific medical issues, such as Boyle's Law. Outlines the special considerations for psychiatric patients.
Air Force Instruction 41-309 *Aeromedical Evacuation Equipment Standards*	November 1, 2001	Provides a listing of approved Air Force Research Laboratory and US Army Aeromedical Research Laboratory medical equipment, which can be used on fixed and rotary wing aircraft.
Air Force Joint Instruction 41-315 *Patient's Regulated to and Within the Continental United States*	March 30, 1990	Prescribes uniform procedures and establishes responsibilities during peacetime and contingencies for regulating the transfer of patients from overseas to the CONUS, the transfer of patients between uniformed services, VA, or civilian medical treatment facilities within the CONUS, and the assignment of beds in VA Medical Centers for members of the uniformed services who will require further hospitalization or nursing home care after separation or retirement from all military services.
DoD Directive 4500.9E *Transportation and Traffic Management*	February 12, 2005	Establishes DoD policy for transportation and traffic management. States that DoD transportation resources should be used for official purposes only. DoD transportation resources may be used to move non-DoD traffic only when the DoD mission will not be impaired and movement of such traffic is of an emergency or life-saving nature, specifically authorized by statute, in direct support of the DoD mission, or requested by the head of an agency of the government.
DoD Directive 6000.12 *Health Services Operations and Readiness*	January 20, 1998	Establishes patient movement policy and assigns the Commander, US TRANSCOM responsibilities as the DoD single manager for patient movement, other than intratheater patient movement. The Commander, US TRANSCOM is responsible for establishing and maintaining a system for medical regulating and movement.
DoD Regulation 4515.13-R *Air Transportation Eligibility*	April 9, 1998	Implements DoD policies governing the use of DoD-owned or DoD-regulated aircraft and establishes criteria for passenger and cargo movement. Chapter 5, "Aeromedical Evacuation" of DoD Regulation 4515.13-R is used to determine eligibility for patient movement.

(**Table 13-1** *continues*)

Table 13-1 *continued*

DoD Instruction 6000.11 *Patient Movement*	September 9, 1998	Establishes procedures for the movement of patients, medical attendants, and related patient movement items on DoD-provided transportation. Addresses the evacuation of patients through the Air Force fixed-wing aeromedical evacuation system and the medical regulating of patients to appropriate locations of care. Establishes aeromedical evacuation patient priorities that are used by competent medical authorities to classify a patient as a candidate for patient movement.
Joint Pub 4-02.2 *Joint Tactics, Techniques and Procedures for Patient Movement in Joint Operations*	December 30, 1996	Delineates requirements and considerations for joint patient movement planning. Includes special aspects of special operations and military operations other than war. Describes doctrine of the exercise of command and control by joint force commanders engaged in all types of operations and exercises.
Army Technical Manual MED 289 *Aeromedical Evacuation: A Guide for Health Providers* (also known as Armed Forces Pamphlet 164-4)	November 1, 1991	Provides guidance to physicians and other healthcare providers who select and prepare patients for transport on all types of aeromedical evacuation aircraft. It applies to all DoD facilities using the aeromedical evacuation system, including Air National Guard and Air Force Reserve units and members.
United States Naval Flight Surgeon Handbook	1998 (2nd ed)	Provides a brief summary of aeromedical evacuation as it applies to Navy medical personnel. It includes details on patient movement, patient classification, movement precedence, and special in-flight considerations regarding physicians and patients.

CONUS: continental United States
DoD: Department of Defense
MED: medical
Pub: publication
TRANSCOM: US Transportation Command
VA: Veterans Affairs

movement precedence, in accordance with the urgency for transport, to the destination medical facility.

Urgent. The urgent precedence applies when immediate aeromedical evacuation is required to save life, limb, or eyesight or prevent complications of serious illness. The attending physician is required to coordinate with an accepting physician at the destination facility for urgent patients.

Priority. A priority precedence is used when there is the need for prompt medical care not available locally. Similar to urgent cases, the attending physician must coordinate directly with the accepting physician for priority patients and the goal is to transport the patient within 24 hours.

Routine. The routine precedence applies to all other patients.

Patient Classification Codes for Aeromedical Evacuation

A patient classification code is used as a management tool to track types of aeromedical evacuation patients. Table 13-2 includes the patient classification codes for aeromedical evacuation. Mental health patients are classified in several different categories based on their diagnosis and risk prior to being manifested on an aeromedical evacuation flight. Attachment 6 of Air Force Instruction 41-307, *Aeromedical Evacuation Patient Considerations and Standards of Care,*[23] outlines the aeromedical evacuation psychiatric categories. The psychiatric patient categories include:

- *Category 1A.* This category is for the severely ill psychiatric patient who requires close supervision during the entire aeromedical evacuation process. Category 1A patients should be transported wearing hospital clothing or physical training gear. They should be chemically sedated and restrained on a dressed litter during the flight. These patients are required to have a medical attendant with a minimum rank of E-5 (sergeant). To help ensure patient safety, medical attendants for category 1A patients must be trained in neurological and circulatory checks and the proper use of restraints.

TABLE 13-2

AEROMEDICAL EVACUATION PATIENT CLASSIFICATION CODES

Code	Classification
1 (Psychiatric)	
1A	Severe psychiatric patient
1B	Intermediate psychiatric patient
1C	Moderate psychiatric patient
2 (Litter)	
2A	Immobile patient
2B	Mobile patient
3 (Ambulatory)	
3A	Nonpsychiatric, non–substance-abuse patient going for treatment
3B	Recovered patient returning home
3C	Drug or substance abuse patient going for treatment
4 (Infant)	
4A	Infant or child under 3 years old in bassinette or car seat
4B	Recovered infant or child requiring seat
4C	Infant in incubator
4D	Child under 3 years old on a litter
4E	Outpatient under 3 years old
5 (Outpatient)	
5A	Ambulatory, nonpsychiatric, or substance abuse outpatient going for treatment
5B	Ambulatory, psychiatric, or substance abuse outpatient going for treatment
5C	Psychiatric outpatient going for treatment and/or evaluation
5D	Outpatient on litter for comfort and/or safety going for treatment
5E	Outpatient returning on litter for comfort and/or safety
5F	All other returning outpatients
6 (Attendant)	
6A	Medical attendant
6B	Nonmedical attendant

- *Category 1B*. Category 1B is for moderately to severely ill psychiatric patients. These patients also should be chemically sedated, wear hospital clothing or physical training gear, and be transported on a litter. However, restraints are not routinely applied for Category 1B patients. A set of restraints must be readily available during the aeromedical evacuation flight and should be secured to the litter or maintained by the patient's attendant.
- *Category 1C*. Cooperative, reliable, and moderately severe psychiatric inpatients traveling in ambulatory status are placed in Category 1C. These patients may wear their military uniforms and may have a medical or nonmedical attendant. They may administer their own medication based on the evaluation by the mental health provider and flight surgeon.
- *Category 3C*. This category is for ambulatory patients who are being evacuated for inpatient treatment for substance use disorders. These patients wear their military uniforms during aeromedical evacuation. A nonmedical attendant usually accompanies them.
- *Category 5B*. Ambulatory patients evacuated for outpatient treatment for substance use disorders are placed in Category 5B. A nonmedical attendant usually accompanies them.
- *Category 5C*. This category is for outpatient mental health patients evacuated for evaluation or treatment of psychiatric disorders. This category is rarely used when transporting a patient from the area of responsibility. It is more common when patients are transferred from Germany (OCONUS) to CONUS locations.

Completion of Patient Movement Records

The *Aeromedical Evacuation Patient Record* (Air Force Form 3899) is used for the initiation of an aeromedical evacuation. In most deployed locations, the PMR is completed in a handwritten format. A sample PMR is included in Exhibit 13-1. The Air Force Form 3899 includes information pertaining to treatment, diagnosis, medication, status as an inpatient or an outpatient, and the attending physician. Although PMRs are required to be signed by an attending physician, in many deployed locations where a psychiatric patient requires aeromedical evacuation, a mental health provider will complete a draft of the PMR and have it cosigned by the attending physician.

An electronic version of the PMR has recently been developed. This form was previously only available on

EXHIBIT 13-1

SAMPLE PATIENT MOVEMENT REQUEST

PATIENT MOVEMENT REQUEST
DATA PROTECTED BY PRIVACY ACT OF 1974

Created on: Lo-Side **Run Date:** 079 2007

PATIENT DEMOGRAPHICS Cite # 0630746017

Patient Name:
Status: A11
ID:
Grade: E02
Age: 22 Year
Nationality: UNITED STATES
Tracking Number: .
Cite Number: 0630746017
Gender: Male
Will Return: U
Precedence: Routine
Classification: 1A
Special: N
CCATT: N

ADMINISTRATIVE DATA Cite # 0630746017

Originating MTF: 28th CSH - BAGHDAD
Destination MTF: LANDSTUHL REGIONAL MED CTR GE
Appt:
Casualty Event: OIraqF-Disease/NonBI
Origination ICAO: ORBD
Destination ICAO: ETAR
Transport Mode: MA
Planned Departure Date:
Ready Date: 307 2006
Reason Regulated: CC
Source System: T-WEB
Planned Arrival Date:

Attending Physician:
Ward Name: .
Last PMR State Changed by:
Accepting Physician: .
Max Stops: .
Max RONs:
DSN Phone: .
DSN Phone: .
DSN Phone: .
DSN Phone: .
Altitude Restriction: .
Com Phone: .
Com Phone: .
Com Phone: .
Com Phone: .
Comm Travel?: .

CLINICAL DATA Cite # 0630746017

Primary Med Spec: Psychiatry (Male General Care)
Secondary Med Spec: Neurosurgery
Other Med Spec: .
Primary Diagnosis: BP I DISORD,1 MNIC EPISD,UNSPC
Secondary Diagnosis: BACKACHE NOS
Other Diagnosis: .

Patient History: Pt is 22yo MWM E-2/PV2 with 1yr TIS, 1yr TIU with 3mo TIC on first deployment as 91W/line medic. For past few weeks he has been experiencing SI and has been put his weapon in his mouth 4-5 times with safety off. Pt stated his plan was to committ suicide by gunshot or pills or with the Morphine he carries as a line-man. He also expresses HI to his peers b/c he stated, "they call me 'fat-boy' , 'Pog' and alot of name calling. Pt states for the past 2 weeks he has only had 2hours sleep each night. He states he has very little interaction with others b/c his only friend was airevaced out b/c he was hit with an IED. Pt denies any feelings of guilt. He admits to being "cynical, reckless, and disrespectful" to his Platoon SGT. He admits to dangerous display of behavior by kicking an IED and laughing. He stated during this event he was praying for death. He admits hedoes not feel safe, has continued SI/HI and is unable to contract for safety. Denies AH/VH. Pt stated he would be cooperative with the airevac process. VS within normal limits. 4 pt litter restriant; q15min restraint checks; q2hr vitals; q1hr offer food/water/hygiene needs; do not remove restraints during transport. The attendant is a psyc tech and can administer meds to patient. *please see remark section for FS update.

MEDICATIONS (5 Rows) Cite # 0630746017 IV's (0 Rows) Cite # 0630746017

Medication Name	Dose	Frequency	IV Location	IV Type	Solution	Rate cc/hr
Valium	5-10 mg	Q 4-6 PRN sedation	.	.	.	.
Motrin	800mg	TID prn pain with food				
haldol	5mg	PRN agitation				
ativan	2mg	PO IM PRN agitation				
benadryl	50mg	PO IM PRN agitation				

Special Diet: .
Amount: .
Allergies:
N-NKDA
Formula: .
Infusion Rate: .

VITAL SIGNS, LABS AND ARTERIAL BLOOD GASES: CITE # 0630746017

Temperature: 97.9 F **Pulse:** 80 **Respiratory:** 16 **BP:** 128 /70 **Wt:** 220.0 lbs **Oxygen Rate:** .
HGB: **HCT:** **WBC:** **Date Taken:** 307 2006 **Oxygen Mode:** .
SPO2 Rate: 99 **FIO2:**

Drainage (0 Rows) Cite # Orthopedic (0 Rows) Cite #

Drainage Location	Type	Suction Type	Suction Amount	Type	Location

PMI DATA CITE # 0630746017

Cardiac Monitor: N **Suction:** N **Pulse Ox:** N **Incubator:** N
Ventilator: N **Pump:** N **Stryker:** N **Traction:** N

TRANSPORTATION INFORMATION: CITE # 0630746017

Orig Transport Name: . **POC:** . **Com Phone:** . **DSN Phone:** .
Dest Transport Name: . **POC:** . **Com Phone:** . **DSN Phone:** .

MOVEMENT INFORMATION: CITE # 0630746017

Transport ID: .
Transport Origin: . **Transport Destination:** .
Movement Remarks:
.

ADMIN REMARKS:

1A: Pt will be in pajamas or PT gear, will be sedated and on a litter with restraints in place. Pt can only carry small amount of money ($25), ID, ring and watch. Attendant is familiar with keys and opening restraints in case of emergency. JD 307, 3 NOV 06, 1830z BALAD FS update: 22y.o medic with increased levels of SI/HI. Unable to contract for safety. No pain currently. No current backpain. Alert, awake, NAD. A/p Depression with active SI, agree with 1A routine status. Stops OK, no alt restrictions. Medicate assist/ egress. Cleared CASF & AE to LRMC. -Dr. . JPMRC UPDATE-AE crew will manage psychiatric patients in accordance with AFI 41-307, atch 6. Pt will be sedated and restrained prior to flight. Cleared for Routine AE/skc.

ATTENDANTS (1 Rows) Cite # 0630746017

Attendant Name	Status	Grade	Age	Gender	Type
	Army Active Duty	Enlisted Grade E5	0 Year	Male	Psychiatric Technician

paper, which sometimes resulted in clerical errors or loss of information. The electronic version of the PMR developed at Landstuhl is automatically populated with data from the European Composite Health Care System on a daily basis. All aeromedical evacuation personnel working at the first geographic CONUS sites encountered in patient transport (eg, Andrews Air Force Base, Landover, Maryland; the National Naval Medical Center [known locally as "Bethesda"], Bethesda, Maryland; and Walter Reed Army Medical Center, Washington, DC) can access a real-time version of the electronic PMR.

AEROMEDICAL STAGING FACILITIES

Aeromedical staging facilities (ASFs) are medical facilities similar to a medical passenger terminal that are used to stage patients prior to aeromedical evacuation. Some ASFs are permanent facilities that operate in peacetime as well as times of military conflict (eg, ASF at Andrews Air Force Base). Contingency aeromedical staging facilities (CASFs) are temporary facilities placed at strategic locations to facilitate the aeromedical evacuation of patients. The mission of a CASF is the safe medical airlift of combat- and noncombat-related casualties from deployed locations to a higher echelon of medical care. CASFs operate around the clock to reassess, stabilize, stage, and transport US military medical patients. Other patients are sometimes transported through CASFs, including coalition military personnel, Department of Defense civilians, and patients engaged in humanitarian missions.

The typical staffing composition of a CASF includes 60 military medical personnel: 45 nurses, 2 flight surgeons, 6 administrative personnel, 3 mental health staff, and 1 individual from each of the logistics, bioenvironmental engineering, pharmacy, and nutritional medicine specialty areas. The CASF mental health team includes one officer and two enlisted mental health technicians. The officer position is usually filled by a psychiatric nurse or advanced practice psychiatric nurse. However, the specific staffing composition and requirements may be modified depending on the location and mission of the CASF.

Aeromedical evacuation personnel provide medical care and treatment to patients during aeromedical evacuation flights according to published guidelines. Prior to cosigning the PMR and writing medication orders, a flight surgeon must ensure the patient is physically stable for flight. The aeromedical evacuation of psychiatric patients includes additional medical and logistical issues that must be considered for the safety of patients and aircrew members.[24] Psychiatric patients should be given special consideration and attention during all phases of the aeromedical evacuation to safeguard their personal dignity and to help ensure respect for cultural, psychological, and spiritual values. The overall goal is to use the safest and least restrictive measures to control behavior of psychiatric patients during aeromedical evacuation. However, some psychiatric patients may place the aircraft, crew, and other patients at risk. The use of in-flight restraints is sometimes necessary for patients who present a clear risk to flight safety.[23] A physician's order is required for restraints and their use should be limited to cases in which there is a clear indication of a flight safety risk. Restraints should not be used merely for the convenience of the aeromedical evacuation crew.

Mental health staff members play an important role in advising the flight surgeon regarding the patient's mental health diagnosis, prognosis, and the need for aeromedical evacuation for psychiatric reasons. When a patient is manifested for aeromedical evacuation, a psychiatric category is determined depending on the severity of the illness, diagnosis, and mental status. It is the responsibility of the CASF mental health team to regularly reassess the patient to ensure that the assigned psychiatric category is appropriate. The CASF staff should alert the flight surgeon if a category requires changing or if other modifications are needed regarding medications, need for restraints, appropriateness for flight, and need for a medical or nonmedical attendant. Almost all mental health patients require either a medical or nonmedical attendant prior to entering the aeromedical evacuation system. Nonmedical attendants are usually a member of the patient's military unit and are required to be the same gender and of higher military rank. Nonmedical attendants are assigned to accompany stable and cooperative mental health patients during the aeromedical evacuation. Medical attendants can include mental health technicians, mental health nurses, or other medical personnel who accompany more severe mental health patients during aeromedical evacuation. CASF mental health personnel ensure the patient's attendant is briefed and educated on the responsibilities prior to the aeromedical evacuation flight. Furthermore, psychiatric patients are often asked to complete a behavioral contract form agreeing to comply with aeromedical evacuation system standards.

Contingency Aeromedical Staging Facilities

To provide medical support for operational missions, CASFs are positioned in key locations to facilitate the aeromedical evacuation of patients. For OIF, a CASF was initially established in Baghdad adjacent to the Baghdad International Airport. The CASF was moved from this location because Baghdad International Airport was converted back to commercial use. The 332nd CASF was established at Joint Base Balad, which became the primary air hub in the region for all US operations. At Balad, about 25% of patients are direct transfers from one of several CSHs located throughout the area of responsibility. The largest proportion of the patients at the Balad CASF is first transferred to the Air Force Theater Hospital at Balad, where the patients are screened and treated prior to transfer to the CASF. A small number of stable patients not requiring medical screening are transferred directly to the CASF. Aeromedical evacuations from Balad depart for Germany several times per week. The frequency of flights depends on the number of medical patients requiring transport; more frequent flights are arranged when necessary. Critical care air transport flights are mobilized for the most seriously injured or ill patients who require urgent aeromedical evacuation after initial patient stabilization. The critical care air transport team consists of a physician, a nurse, and a cardiopulmonary technician, which allows ventilated patients to be evacuated. Burn patients are often evacuated on these critical care transport missions.

The CASF at Kuwait has a significantly smaller mission than the Balad CASF. Patients with less severe injuries or ones who can be adequately treated in Kuwaiti hospitals are evacuated to the Kuwait CASF. Many of these patients are ones who are expected to be able to return to duty in the deployed setting after their medical care.

Currently, there is no CASF to support the transport of medical patients at Bagram Air Base in Afghanistan. Patients requiring aeromedical evacuation from Afghanistan are transferred to Bagram using rotary or fixed-wing aircraft. Patients are then transported to the CASF at Ramstein Air Base, Germany, on C-17 aircraft.

Patients evacuated from the combat zone in Iraq and Afghanistan are received at Landstuhl. Once there, patients are reassessed and may undergo additional surgery or medical treatments prior to aeromedical evacuation to CONUS.

The Ramstein Air Base Contingency Aeromedical Staging Facility

The 435th CASF at Ramstein Air Base, Germany, is staffed by a contingency of 96 medical personnel. This includes two flight surgeons, 18 registered nurses, and 76 medical technicians and administrative support staff. The medical staff is responsible for receiving patients aeromedically evacuated from all OIF and OEF locations. The ambulatory patients are housed in the CASF, which has a 60-bed capacity. Ambulatory patients are transported to CONUS on the next available flight. The more critically injured patients are transferred via ambulance bus from Ramstein Air Base to Landstuhl Army Regional Medical Center. Once patients are treated and stabilized at Landstuhl, a small proportion of them are returned to duty at their deployed location. Most patients, however, are medically evacuated to CONUS after treatment at Landstuhl.

Those patients who require CONUS evacuation are transported to the Ramstein CASF. Patients are then sent to receiving hospitals within CONUS for further treatment and disposition. In most cases, patients from Landstuhl are first transported to the Andrews Air Force Base ASF and then to Walter Reed Army Medical Center. However, patients are also sent to a variety of military hospitals around CONUS, depending on the medical needs of the patient and the availability of medical care resources.

Between March 2003 and March 2007 approximately 62,000 patients were seen at the Ramstein CASF as part of OIF and OEF. About 40,000 of these patients arrived at Landstuhl from OIF/OIF, and about 22,000 of them were transported to CONUS. Differences in the inbound and outbound patient numbers reflect that slightly less than half of the patients who arrived were transported back to theater or to other locations through nonmedical transportation methods. Overall, battle-injured patients have accounted for about 21% of the total number of patients transported.

The Andrews Air Force Base Aeromedical Staging Flight

The ASF at Andrews Air Force Base plays a critical role in the aeromedical evacuation process of patients during both war and peace. Andrews' ASF is the first stop into the United States for all patients from the European theater, OIF, and OEF. The Andrews ASF is operated by 31 permanent party members and 33 augmentees. In addition, the ASF has one marine and three soldiers permanently assigned to the unit to assist with the transition of marines and soldiers. The Air Force Family Liaison Officer program is also used to meet patient needs. To perform their mission, the ASF is equipped with six "ambuses" (medium-size buses equipped to carry litters), three ambulances, one box truck, one step van, and two patient-loading systems. On average, each month the ASF assists about 800 inbound and outbound patients.

In Germany, the Joint Patient Movement Requirement Center coordinates with the GPMRC to establish CONUS destinations for patients who are grouped into mission loads based upon the bed availability at Landstuhl and patient care movement requirements. Aeromedical evacuation missions are launched three times per week from Germany, with other missions added as needed depending upon Landstuhl's capacity or patient acuity.

The mission operations component of the Andrews ASF receives information regarding the mission and its patient load. The PMR information obtained via TRAC2ES' Web-based electronic record describes clinical information, equipment, staffing, and other operational information on every patient. This information is available to Walter Reed, Bethesda, and the Andrews ASF at the same time through TRAC2ES. The TRAC2ES system is also used in the area of responsibility and is the key communication link to the Theater Patient Movement Requirements Center in Qatar.

A typical mission load is 25 to 30 patients with a variety of diagnoses, medical conditions, and levels of acuity. These may include critical care, amputations, head injuries, psychiatric conditions, cardiac complications, diabetes, and eye injuries. An example of a mission package is as follows: "Mission K-6 includes 12 litters, 17 ambulatory, 4 medical/nonmedical personnel arriving at 1600 hours at Andrews AFB [Air Force Base] on Julian date 214." The mission load is further broken down to reveal which patients will be transported to Walter Reed or Bethesda, and which will need to remain overnight at Andrews prior to transport to another medical facility.

During the 24-hour period prior to a plane's arrival at Andrews, much preparatory work is accomplished. Rooms are readied, meals are ordered, clinical information is reviewed, the flight line crews are alerted, and leaders are notified of mission and other pertinent clinical and administrative information.

Three hours before the plane's arrival, the ASF flight line nurse arrives to review the latest information received from Germany on the patients' conditions after the plane departed. A typical report might contain information such as the number of patients added or cancelled and reason for cancellation; number of critical care air transport (CCAT) cases; if blood was transfused en route; the need for an ambulance on arrival; patients with conditions requiring special room accommodations or care; family member traveling with a patient; amputee needs for wound wash or operating room visit for dressing change; and if a psychiatric patient is to be admitted at Walter Reed. In summary, to be properly prepared for the arrival of a mission, all staff members involved in each aspect of Andrews ASF review the latest available information regarding vital clinical and administrative information before the aeromedical evacuation mission arrives.

Prior to the plane's landing, transport vehicles from Walter Reed Army Medical Center and the National Naval Medcial Center (Bethesda, Md) are positioned to move designated patients to their respective facilities based upon TRAC2ES information and any updates and changes from GPMRC. Sometimes patient destinations are changed while the plane is in the air due to changes in patient condition, medical capability changes, and other administrative reasons. All of this is done in the best interest of patient care.

Two hours before the plane's arrival, all flight line personnel report to duty. This usually includes about 10 personnel from the ASF, Walter Reed, and Bethesda; the Army and Marine liaisons; and volunteers. During the first hour, refresher training is conducted on the litter carry, and mission planning is performed to identify vehicles, drivers, spotters, and other necessary personnel. During the second hour, a mission brief is given on the latest clinical picture and an ASF flight surgeon is present to clarify any clinical questions.

At the flight line landing zone, the ground crew coordinator interacts with the medical crew director and loadmasters to arrange the vehicles in the best manner to expedite the offload and transport of patients from the plane to the waiting motor vehicles. Priority is given to the CCAT patients. Usually, the Walter Reed and Bethesda buses are loaded prior to the Andrews bus, because they have a 40- to 50-minute travel time to their respective hospitals. During this transition period, a flight surgeon or other physician completes an assessment of every patient onboard. The flight surgeon can evaluate, stabilize, and arrange transportation for the patient to the emergency room at Andrews if needed.

Once the patients arrive at their designated medical facilities, additional personnel process them based on their ward destinations. After treatment at Walter Reed or Bethesda, many patients are transferred to other hospitals depending on the specific needs of the patient. Patients are often transferred to hospitals or clinics near their home military station or near their hometown once they have become medically stable. The time frame for these transfers varies widely. The aeromedical evacuation process varies somewhat for special patient categories such as burn patients. Brooke Army Medical Center at Fort Sam Houston in San Antonio, Texas, is the Department of Defense Burn Center. Burn patients are transferred to Brooke as soon as they are stable enough for aeromedical evacuation. Some patients are flown directly to the burn unit from the area of responsibility or from Landstuhl.

Patients remaining at Andrews Air Force Base are housed in the ASF, which has 32 beds and an expansion capability to 45. The next morning, missions are launched to transport patients to their various CONUS destinations. Ultimate destinations are determined by clinical needs and facilities' capabilities.

AEROMEDICAL EVACUATION OF PATIENTS IN SUPPORT OF OPERATION ENDURING FREEDOM AND OPERATION IRAQI FREEDOM

As of January 2009, there had been over 65,000 hostile and nonhostile US military casualities in Iraq, including over 4,000 fatalities and almost 30,000 wounded in action.[25] About 70% of the wounded were treated in theater and returned to duty without the need for evacuation for additional medical care. However, about 45,000 US military personnel required aeromedical evacuation out of Iraq, including about 9,000 wounded, 9,000 with nonhostile injuries, and 26,000 with other medical conditions.

Significantly fewer aeromedical evacuations have been required for patients deployed to Afghanistan in support of OEF.[26] As of January 2009, over 9,000 US military personnel were evacuated, including about 1,400 wounded, 2,000 with nonhostile injuries, and 5,500 with other medical conditions requiring care outside the area of responsibility. There were over 600 US fatalities in OEF during this same time period.

Recent publications have underscored the potential mental health impact of the military operations in Iraq and Afghanistan on personnel.[27–29] Since 2003, all personnel returning from deployment complete a Post-Deployment Health Assessment.[30] A review of 303,905 of these health assessments showed that over 19% of soldiers and marines who returned from OIF met risk criteria for a mental health concern. However, only 18.4% of these "at risk" soldiers were referred for mental health treatment. In addition, posttraumatic stress disorder symptoms are associated with lower general health ratings, more primary care visits, and missed workdays among military personnel during the year following deployment.[31]

Several recent journal articles have evaluated the aeromedical evacuation of psychiatric patients from OIF/OEF.[32–35] Turner and colleagues[35] evaluated 116 British military personnel who were evacuated between January 2003 and October 2003 to the United Kingdom for admission at a military inpatient psychiatric facility. The majority of the psychiatric patients (69%) were noncombatants, and 21% were Reserve personnel. A large percentage (37%) had a previous mental health history.

Harman and colleagues[32] completed a descriptive analysis of 11,183 US military patients who were aeromedically evacuated from Iraq between January 2003 and December 2003. Of those patients evacuated, the most common patient categories were orthopaedic surgery (21.5%) and general surgery (13.3%). Psychiatric patients were the third most common patient category, comprising 6.9% of all evacuees.

Two articles reviewed US military patients evacuated from both OIF and OEF. Stetz and associates[34] evaluated 5,671 OEF/OIF patients evacuated from March 2003 to September 2003. Out of all patients aeromedically evacuated, 386 (6.8%) were psychiatric patients. Seventy-three patients (19%) were diagnosed with psychotic disorders, 242 (63%) were nonpsychotic disorders, and 60 (15%) had either DSM-IV (*Diagnostic and Statistical Manual*, 4th revision) V-codes or a deferred diagnosis. About 13% of patients had suicidal ideations or self-injurious behaviors.

Rundell[33] conducted the most comprehensive review of psychiatric patients evacuated from OIF/OEF. He included data from 1,264 US military psychiatric patients who were evacuated to Landstuhl Army Medical Center in Germany between November 4, 2001 and July 30, 2004. The psychiatric patients were about 10% of the total population of 12,480 patients evacuated to Landstuhl. A retrospective review of the psychiatric clinical records was conducted to characterize the demographic composition, clinical diagnoses, and clinical dispositions given to the patients. A psychiatrist or clinical psychologist evaluated all patients according to a single, standardized clinical process.

The results indicated that women were twice as likely to be psychiatric patients compared to the percentage of female medical patients (19% vs 10%). Psychiatric patients were more likely to be younger, enlisted, Reserve or National Guard members, and African-American or Hispanic. The majority of psychiatric patients were Army personnel (86%), which most likely reflects the higher proportion of deployed Army personnel during that time. About half of the psychiatric patients (49%) were evacuated during the first 3 months of their deployment. Another third of the patients (33%) were evacuated during the second 3 months of deployment.

The most frequent psychiatric diagnostic categories were adjustment disorders (34%), mood disorders (22%), personality disorders (16%), and anxiety disorders (15%). Of the patients diagnosed with anxiety disorders, 36% were diagnosed with acute stress disorder and 29% with posttraumatic stress disorder. About 6% were diagnosed with a psychotic disorder, 4% with bipolar disorder, and 5% with a substance abuse disorder.

After psychiatric hospitalization at Landstuhl, most patients (81%) were sent back to their home stations for outpatient mental health treatment, and 14% were transferred to other inpatient psychiatric settings. Only about 5% of these patients were returned to duty in a deployed location after successful treatment at Landstuhl. The long-term disposition of the psychiatric patients evacuated from OEF/OIF is not known. However, previous research has shown that about two thirds of active duty military members who are hospitalized for a mental health condition are discharged from active duty within 2 years of the initial hospitalization.[30,36]

BEHAVIORAL HEALTH CONSULTATION FOR MEDICAL PATIENTS

The primary mission of mental health staff members involved in the aeromedical evacuation process is the screening and preparation for evacuation of psychiatric patients. However, psychiatric patients are usually less than 10% of all patients evacuated, and it is known that a much larger percentage of patients have had some type of combat or other trauma exposure.[34]

Military personnel who sustain combat-related physical injuries are at increased risk for developing combat-related stress disorders. A recent study[37] evaluated the relationship between combat-related physical injuries and posttraumatic stress disorder in 60 combat-injured soldiers. A matched group of 40 soldiers who took part in the same combat situations but were not injured was used as a comparison group. The study found that 16.7% of the combat-injured soldiers met diagnostic criteria for posttraumatic stress disorder as compared to 2.5% in the noninjured comparison group. Another recent study found that a large percentage of combat-injured personnel have a delayed onset of combat stress symptoms.[38] Almost 80% of combat-injured patients who initially screened negative for posttraumatic stress disorder or depression at the 1-month point after the injury were later found to screen positive at the 7-month point. These results suggest that brief contact of combat-injured personnel by mental health staff during the aeromedical evacuation process may be warranted. This may be important even if combat stress symptoms are not present at the time of the aeromedical evacuation.

Many locations across the aeromedical evacuation continuum have implemented programs using a behavioral health consultation model to provide for brief contact and screening of all medical patients by mental health staff members. Various versions of behavioral health consultation programs are currently being used at the Air Force theater hospital and CASF at Balad,[39] at Landstuhl, and at Walter Reed Army Medical Center.[40]

Brief contact with at-risk medical patients has allowed mental health providers to expand their role and be actively involved with all patients being evacuated for medical or nonpsychiatric reasons. This approach has been used successfully in primary care settings where many patients have significant behavioral health risk factors or are at risk for comorbid psychiatric conditions.[41–45] A similar model was used with approximately 700 military personnel who were deployed to work at the Armed Forces Mortuary at Dover Air Force Base, Delaware, to process the human remains from the 189 individuals killed in the terrorist attacks at the Pentagon.[46]

The behavioral health consultation model involves brief individual consultation with all medical patients. The goals are to assess for trauma or combat stress exposure, normalize combat stress symptoms, initiate positive contact with mental health staff, and describe symptoms that might emerge in the future that would indicate that follow-up with a mental health provider might be helpful.[39] It is helpful to provide patients with a description of the normal course of trauma-related symptoms and how some symptoms can have a delayed onset.

SUMMARY

The US military aeromedical evacuation system is one of the primary contributors to the significantly improved survival rate in patients injured in support of OIF/OEF. Its ability to transport a patient from point of injury to specialized hospital trauma care is currently unsurpassed. The professionals who maintain this system continue to make strides to improve safety, comfort, and speed. Military mental health professionals play an important role in the aeromedical evacuation of medical and mental health patients from a war zone. Mental health professionals are actively involved in all aspects of the aeromedical evacuation system, including screening of psychiatric patients, making recommendations of psychiatric patient category, preparing patients and attendants for the aeromedical evacuation flight, and providing organizational consultation to aeromedical evacuation medical staff. Nonpsychiatric medical personnel often have little or no experience in working with severe psychiatric cases. The placement of mental health professionals as part of the aeromedical evacuation system is a significant relief to medical staff.

The Department of Defense patient movement and aeromedical evacuation system involves a complex interaction between patients, healthcare providers, patient movement administrators, aircraft, and computer tracking systems. In this chapter, an overview of the entire aeromedical evacuation process was provided with as much accuracy as possible. However, as with many complex systems, changes in the aeromedical evacuation process occur on a regular basis depending on local conditions, operational requirements, and changing priorities. Therefore, it is likely that some of the specific details contained in this chapter may have changed since the time that the chapter was written. Nevertheless, it is hoped that this chapter will serve as a general guide for the military aeromedical evacuation system and a helpful tool for military personnel involved in the aeromedical evacuation of patients in both deployed and nondeployed locations.

REFERENCES

1. Teichman PG, Donchin Y, Kot RJ. International aeromedical evacuation. *N Engl J Med.* 2007;356:262–270.
2. Gawande A. Casualties of war—military care for the wounded from Iraq and Afghanistan. *N Engl J Med.* 2004;351:2471–2475.
3. Brown HE. *The Medical Department of the United States Army From 1775 to 1873.* Washington, DC: Surgeon General's Office; 1873.
4. Nolan DL, Pattillo DA. The Army Medical Department and the Civil War: historical lessons for current medical support. *Mil Med.* 1989;154:265–271.
5. Blansfield JS. The origins of casualty evacuation and echelons of care: lessons learned from the American Civil War. *Int J Trauma Nurs.* 1999;5:5–9.
6. Bollet AJ. *Civil War Medicine: Challenges and Triumphs.* Tucson, Ariz: Galen Press; 2002.
7. Larcan A. History and tradition of the military service of ambulance transportation. *Bull Acad Natl Med.* 1994;178:1695–1713.
8. McKenny EM. History of the motorized ambulance transport. *Mil Med.* 1967;132:819–822.
9. Rutkow EI, Rutkow IM. George Crile, Harvey Cushing, and the Ambulance Americaine: military medical preparedness in World War I. *Arch Surg.* 2004;139:678–685.
10. Bricknell MC. The evolution of casualty evacuation in the 20th century. 4: an international perspective. *J R Army Med Corps.* 2003;149:166–174.
11. Hall WF. Air evacuation. *JAMA.* 1951;147:1026–1028.
12. Hall WF, Nolan JD. Advantages of air transportation of patients. *U S Armed Forces Med J.* 1950;1:115–118.
13. Lam DM. Marie Marvingt and the development of aeromedical evacuation. *Aviat Space Environ Med.* 2003;74:863–868.
14. Gibson TM. Samuel Franklin Cody: aviation and aeromedical evacuation pioneer. *Aviat Space Environ Med.* 1999;70:612–617.
15. Lam DM. Kelly's hospital ship. *Aviat Space Environ Med.* 1992;63:1115–1117.
16. Mabry EW, Munson RA, Richardson LA. The wartime need for aeromedical evacuation physicians: the US Air Force experience during Operation Desert Storm. *Aviat Space Environ Med.* 1993;64:941–946.

17. Driscoll RS. New York Chapter History of Military Medicine Award. US Army medical helicopters in the Korean War. *Mil Med.* 2001;166:290–296.

18. Meier DR, Samper ER. Evolution of civil aeromedical helicopter aviation. *South Med J.* 1989;82:885–891.

19. Howell FJ, Brannon RH. Aeromedical evacuation: remembering the past, bridging to the future. *Mil Med.* 2000;165:429–433.

20. Mclaren CAB, Guzzi LM, Bellamy RF. Military medical evacuation. In: Zajtchuk R, Grande CM, eds. *Anesthesia and Perioperative Care of the Combat Casualty*. In: Zajtchuk R, Bellamy RF, eds. *The Textbooks of Military Medicine*. Washington, DC: Department of the Army, Office of The Surgeon General, Borden Institute; 1995: 751–785.

21. Lerner EB, Moscati RM. The golden hour: scientific fact or medical "urban legend"? *Acad Emerg Med.* 2001;8:758–760.

22. Department of Defense. *Report on the DoD Patient Movement System*. Washington, DC: Office of the Inspector General; July 2005. Report D-2005-095.

23. US Department of the Air Force. *Aeromedical Evacuation Patient Considerations and Standards of Care.* Washington, DC: USAF; 2003. Air Force Instruction 41-307, Attach 6. Available at: http://www.e-publishing.af.mil/pubfiles/af/41/afi41-307/afi41-307.pdf. Accessed December 26, 2006.

24. Ritchie EC, Morse JH, Brewer PG. Surviving the "air evac": medical and logistical issues of evacuating psychiatric patients by air from Korea to the United States. *Mil Med.* 1996;161:298–302.

25. Defense Manpower Data Center. Data, Analysis and Programs Division. Global War on Terrorism, Operation Iraqi Freedom, by Casualty Category Within Service, March 19, 2003 Through January 3, 2009. Available at: http://siadapp.dmdc.osd.mil/personnel/CASUALTY/OIF-Total.pdf. Accessed January 18, 2009.

26. Defense Manpower Data Center. Data, Analysis and Programs Division. Global War on Terrorism, Operation Enduring Freedom, by Casualty Category Within Service, October 7, 2001 Through January 3, 2009. Available at: http://siadapp.dmdc.osd.mil/personnel/CASUALTY/WOTSUM.pdf. Accessed January 18, 2009.

27. Friedman M. Posttraumatic stress disorder among military returnees from Afghanistan and Iraq. *Am J Psychiatry.* 2006;163:586–593.

28. Jones S. Paying the price: the psychiatric cost of war. *Arch Psychiatr Nurs.* 2004;18:119–120.

29. Lamberg L. Military psychiatrists strive to quell soldiers' nightmares of war. *JAMA.* 2004;292:1539–1540.

30. Hoge CW, Auchterlonie JL, Milliken CS. Mental health problems, use of mental health services, and attrition from military service after returning from deployment to Iraq or Afghanistan. *JAMA.* 2006;295:1023–1032.

31. Hoge CW, Terhakopian A, Castro CA, Messer SC, Engel CC. Association of posttraumatic stress disorder with somatic symptoms, health care visits, and absenteeism among Iraq war veterans. *Am J Psychiatry.* 2007;164:150–153.

32. Harman DR, Hooper TI, Gackstetter GD. Aeromedical evacuations from Operation Iraqi Freedom: a descriptive study. *Mil Med.* 2005;170:521–527.

33. Rundell JR. Demographics of and diagnoses in Operation Enduring Freedom and Operation Iraqi Freedom personnel who were psychiatrically evacuated from the theater of operations. *Gen Hosp Psychiatry.* 2006;28:352–356.

34. Stetz MC, McDonald JJ, Lukey BJ, Gifford RK. Psychiatric diagnoses as a cause of medical evacuation. *Aviat Space Environ Med.* 2005;76(7 suppl):C15–C20.

35. Turner MA, Kiernan MD, McKechanie AG, Finch PJ, McManus FB, Neal LA. Acute military psychiatric casualties from the war in Iraq. *Br J Psychiatry.* 2005;186:476–479.

36. Hoge CW, Lesikar SE, Guevara R, et al. Mental disorders among US military personnel in the 1990s: association with high levels of health care utilization and early military attrition. *Am J Psychiatry.* 2002;159:1576–1583.

37. Koren D, Norman D, Cohen A, Berman J, Klein EM. Increased PTSD risk with combat-related injury: a matched comparison study of injured and uninjured soldiers experiencing the same combat events. *Am J Psychiatry.* 2005;162:276–282.

38. Grieger TA, Cozza SJ, Ursano RJ, et al. Posttraumatic stress disorder and depression in battle-injured soldiers. *Am J Psychiatry.* 2006;163:1777–1783.

39. Peterson AL, Baker MT, McCarthy KR. Combat stress casualties in Iraq. 1: Behavioral health consultation at an expeditionary medical group. *Perspect Psychiatr Care.* 2008;44:146–158.

40. Wain H, Bradley J, Nam T, Waldrep D, Cozza S. Psychiatric interventions with returning soldiers at Walter Reed. *Psychiatr Q.* 2005;76:351–360.

41. Cummings N, Cummings J, Johnson J, eds. *Behavioral Health in Primary Care: A Guide for Clinical Integration.* Madison, Conn: Psychosocial Press; 1997.

42. Hunter CL, Peterson AL. Primary care psychology training at Wilford Hall Medical Center. *Behav Therapist.* 2001;24:220–222.

43. Isler WC, Peterson AL, Isler D. Behavioral treatment of insomnia in primary care settings. In: James LC, Folen RA, eds. *The Primary Care Consultant: The Next Frontier for Psychologists in Hospitals and Clinics.* Washington, DC: American Psychological Association; 2005: 121–151.

44. Strosahl K. Confessions of a behavior therapist in primary care: the odyssey and the ecstasy. *Cogn Behav Pract.* 1996;3:1–28.

45. McDaniel S. Collaboration between psychologists and family PCMs: implementing the biopsychosocial model. *Prof Psychol Res Pr.* 1995;26:117–122.

46. Peterson AL, Nicolas MG, McGraw K, Englert D, Blackman LR. Psychological intervention with mortuary workers after the September 11 attack: the Dover Behavioral Health Consultant model. *Mil Med.* 2002;167:83–86.

Chapter 14

BEHAVIORAL HEALTHCARE AT LANDSTUHL REGIONAL MEDICAL CENTER

JEFFREY V. HILL, MD*; DAVID REYNOLDS, PHD†; AND RONALD CAMPBELL, MD‡

*Lieutenant Colonel, Medical Corps, US Army; Chief, Child and Adolescent Psychiatry, Landstuhl Regional Medical Center, CMR 402 Box 1356, APO AE 09180; formerly, Chief, Outpatient Psychiatry, Landstuhl Regional Medical Center

†Major, Biomedical Sciences Corps, US Air Force; Mental Health Element Leader, Department of Psychology, Malcolm Grow Medical Center, 1050 West Perimeter Road, 779 MDOS/SGOH, Andrews Air Force Base, Maryland 20762; formerly, Chief, Department of Health Psychology, Landstuhl Regional Medical Center, Landstuhl, Germany

‡Chief, Inpatient Psychiatry Service, Department of Behavioral Health, Landstuhl Regional Medical Center, CMR 462, APO AE 09180

INTRODUCTION

The mission of Landstuhl Regional Medical Center (LRMC) is to provide world-class comprehensive and compassionate care to the nation's warriors, their families, retirees, and all other patients as directed, while maintaining unit and personal readiness to meet the demands of the United States. This is accomplished by maintaining a trained and ready healthcare force that seeks, thrives on, and embraces change while accomplishing the healthcare mission, utilizing outcomes to drive medical decisions.

LRMC sits on a hill overlooking the German city of Landstuhl. The garrison belongs to the Kaiserslautern military community, which consists of several military bases scattered in the Kaiserslautern area. Landstuhl is a city of 20,000 located in the Rheinland-Pfalz province of Germany, about 30 miles east of the French border, near the town of Kaiserslautern and Ramstein Air Force Base. US Army outpatient psychiatric care in Germany catchment areas consists of the Wurzburg area in the southeast, the Heidelberg area in the south-central region, and LRMC, covering outpatient psychiatric care in southwest Germany (Figure 14-1).[1]

This US Army facility is the largest American hospital outside the United States and the only American tertiary (specialty) care hospital in Europe, serving 245,000 beneficiaries within the European command, of which 100,000 are primary care beneficiaries. Landstuhl also supports active duty service members, their family members, and other beneficiaries in Africa and Asia. About half of the LRMC permanent staff is civilian, with Army personnel making up the next largest group, and the remainder being US Air Force and small percentages of Navy personnel. Some personnel are borrowed from local units. There are also global war on terror augmentees (including civilians). In total, about 2,800 personnel are assigned to work at LRMC, with about 2,200 permanent party. A typical day at LRMC in Fiscal Year 2008–2009 will see 20 admissions, 14 operating room cases, an intensive care unit (ICU) census of 6.4, 2.5 births, and an average length of stay of 3.2 days.[1]

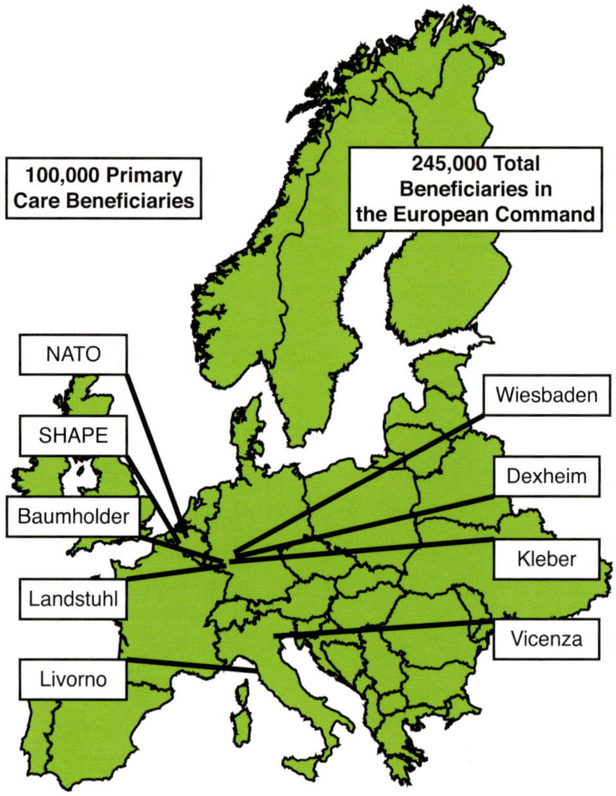

Figure 14-1. Landstuhl Regional Medical Center and outlying clinics as of 2007.
NATO: North Atlantic Treaty Organization
SHAPE: Supreme Headquarters Allied Powers Europe

ROLE OF LANDSTUHL REGIONAL MEDICAL CENTER IN WARTIME

LRMC serves as the primary evacuation center for Central Command, thus the majority of Operation Iraqi Freedom (OIF) and Operation Enduring Freedom (OEF) evacuees pass through LRMC. (Table 14-1 details the impact of OIF/OEF on the patient load at LRMC.[1]) Nearly every day a transport aircraft lands at Ramstein Air Force Base near the city of Frankfurt and unloads medical evacuees who are then transported to LRMC. As they arrive, medics, nurses, physicians, and other clinicians gather in front of the emergency room. The patients are unloaded from the back of the bus, some walking, others on stretchers. As of November 24, 2008, over 51,750 OIF and OEF service members have been treated at LRMC (10,575 battle injuries, 41,178 nonbattle injuries). Of these, 35,939 were outpatients; the remaining 15,814 were inpatients.[1] Over 9,000 were returned to duty in Central Command.[1]

Initial Assessments

Staff members triage the patients, taking the most seriously injured to the ICU or surgery. The less seriously wounded and injured are taken to the medical and surgical wards, where they share rooms with other, similarly injured patients. The psychiatric patients are quickly evaluated and either sent to the

TABLE 14-1

IMPACT OF OPERATIONS IRAQI FREEDOM AND ENDURING FREEDOM ON PATIENT LOAD: A TYPICAL DAY AT LANDSTUHL. COMPARISON BETWEEN 2001 AND 2006

	2001	2006	Change
Admissions	16	23	+ 43%
Operating Room Cases	9	16	+ 73%
Intensive Care Unit			
Census	3	9	+ 300%
Overall Acuity	2.7	5.01	+ 85%
Meals	800	1,178	+ 47%
Births	3	2.3	- 23%
Average Length of Stay (days)	4.6	3.4	- 27%
Pharmacy Products	1,026	1,589	+ 54%

outpatient clinic or seen in the emergency room by the mental health team after hours. All psychiatric evacuations are seen, evaluated, and have their dispositions determined the day of their arrival. Many are on medications; most have been traveling for hours, some for days, and may be tired and hungry.

While psychiatric patients are at LRMC, the Deployed Warrior Medical Management Center (DWMMC) tracks their progress and provides logistical support, including briefings, housing, food, finance, and other needed support. Each soldier is assigned a DWMMC case manager, a liaison from the service member's unit or service, and given access to primary care physicians. DWMMC has other staff members, nurses, and medics or corpsmen, to assist as needed. The case managers and liaisons manage service members with the full spectrum of illness, from the severely injured to stable routine patients.

Until 2007, outpatient evacuees from OIF/OEF usually stayed at another military base within the Kaiserslautern military community. Due to concerns about supervision and access to the hospital, a new facility known as the Medical Transient Detachment was opened in 2007, allowing many outpatients (especially psychiatric) to stay next to the hospital on the Landstuhl base. These patients fall under a military command organization with regular formations and accountability. During their free time they may engage in on- and off-post activities such as visiting the gym and the post exchange, or engaging in activities on the local economy. Patients treated at LRMC are usually discharged or complete their course of treatment within a week, thereafter returning to theater, the United States, or their home station. Many leave within 72 hours of arrival.

Medical and Surgical Evacuees

All patients evacuated to LRMC for medical and surgical reasons are screened for mental health issues by their primary physicians both downrange and upon arrival at LRMC. Most inpatients are briefly screened by members of the outreach team, which is separate from the consultation team and consists of multidisciplinary healthcare professionals, chaplains, and technicians trained to provide proactive mental health outreach to wounded warriors. Chaplains brief all arriving soldiers on combat operational stress awareness. Many primary care providers also include brief education and screening for combat-related emotional problems. Medical staff members are constantly trained to recognize and provide basic levels of care for combat stress and other combat-related symptoms. Few of these patients evacuated for medical or surgical reasons demonstrate significant psychiatric symptoms. Those demonstrating significant psychiatric symptoms are referred to behavioral health providers after ruling out medical etiologies. Inpatients in emotional distress or with symptoms secondary to emotional distress are referred to the behavioral health inpatient consultation team. Outpatients are referred to the outpatient behavioral health team. The inpatient consultation team consists of multidisciplinary behavioral healthcare workers (social workers, psychiatric nurses, psychologists, psychiatrists, counselors, and mental health technicians) who provide consultation and management suggestions to primary medical staff.

Psychiatric Evacuees

Most arriving psychiatric casualties are triaged through either the outpatient behavioral health clinic, consisting of a multidisciplinary team of technicians, psychiatrists, psychologists, and social workers, or the after-hours on-call emergency clinicians. After-hours services are provided through the combined efforts of the LRMC and Ramstein Air Force Base psychiatrists, social workers, psychologists, nurses, and mental health technicians.

Characteristics of Psychiatric Evacuees

Landstuhl supports various coalition countries. Foreign service members are rare in the outpatient

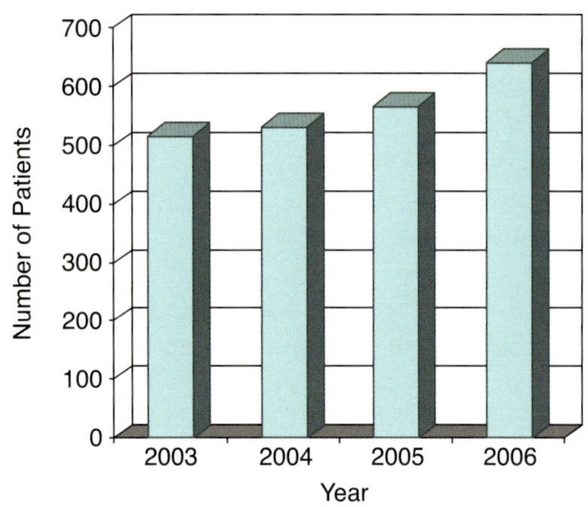

Figure 14-2. Operation Iraqi Freedom / Operation Enduring Freedom evacuations by year. Those seen in the Landstuhl Regional Medical Center outpatient clinics represent the majority, but do not include those admitted to the psychiatric ward in the evening or on the weekend.

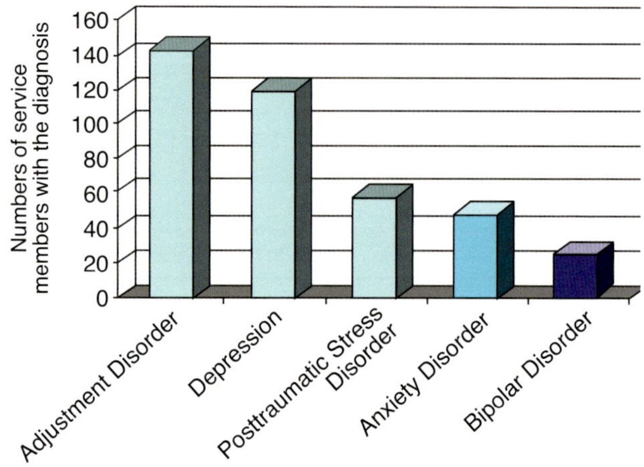

Figure 14-3. Top five Landstuhl Regional Medical Center outpatient psychiatry diagnoses for Operation Iraqi Freedom / Operation Enduring Freedom evacuations during 2005 (563 patients, diagnosis known on 507). Anxiety includes acute stress disorder / acute stress reaction.

mental health setting but are often seen in medical and surgical wards. The number of OIF / OEF patients evacuated to LRMC has steadily increased since the war began (Figure 14-2). This influx of battle-zone patients significantly affects the daily mission at LRMC. Figure 14-3 demonstrates the top five diagnoses given to OIF / OEF evacuees by outpatient psychiatry during a 1-year period: (1) adjustment disorder, (2) depression, (3) posttraumatic stress disorder (PTSD), (4) anxiety disorder, and (5) bipolar disorder.

Dangerous Patients

One notable characteristic of a majority of patients evacuated for psychiatric reasons is concern for dangerousness to self or others. Patient Movement Requests are the documents the evacuating physician completes in the combat theater when evacuating a service member from the combat environment. Each request contains a brief paragraph about the concerns leading to the evacuation. In a 3.5-month review of all available Patient Movement Requests of psychiatric patients evacuated to LRMC, the evacuating physician had concerns about suicidality or homicidality in nearly 60%. By the time of arrival at LRMC, however, active suicidal or homicidal thoughts diminish considerably. Less than 3% of OEF / OIF service members reported active suicidal or homicidal thoughts on presentation at LRMC in the psychiatric intake paperwork. Nevertheless, patient safety cannot be assumed; each evacuee receives a clinical assessment for dangerousness to self or others. When the evaluating provider deems a patient at-risk for harm to self or others, the patient is admitted to the inpatient psychiatry service.

CHALLENGES TO PROVIDING PSYCHIATRIC CARE TO EVACUEES

Patient Actions and Behaviors

Patients who are evacuated for psychiatric reasons often have behavioral components to their illness. As described above, a high proportion are evacuated because of potential for harming themselves or others. They may be in the midst of an emotional crisis when they arrive at LRMC. Sometimes their efforts are manipulative attempts to avoid combat or simply to go home.[2] They often do the unexpected. By policy, if the assessing clinician has doubt about the patient's ability to function in the outpatient setting, the pateint is admitted to LRMC Inpatient Psychiatry.

Minimally Supervised

Until the establishment of the Medical Transient Detachment, evacuees were minimally supervised. Now there is a chain of command that increases supervision substantially. However, determined service members have accessed alcohol and weapons. Case Study 14-1 describes the potential problem of an unsupervised patient stay at LRMC.

Case Study 14-1: Two service members in their early twenties were evacuated from theater with adjustment disorder symptoms and triaged to outpatient evacuation to the United States. The evening after their evacuation they returned to the barracks and immediately booked a hotel in downtown Kaiserslautern, where they spent the next 2 days drinking local beer and missing medical and accountability formations. This resulted in delays in the soldier's treatment. The soldiers' down-range rear detachment commands were notified.

Potential Harm to Self or Others

Frequently by the time service members arrive at LRMC they expect to be sent home to the United States. They no longer consider returning to duty an option. When clinicians attempt to send such service members back to combat duty, it almost always leads to a worsening of symptoms with frequent acting out. Case Study 14-2 describes such a case.

Case Study 14-2: A 25-year-old active-duty male soldier became involved in a love triangle with his girlfriend and her other boyfriend in the deployment environment. An altercation ensued in which the patient was attacked. Shortly afterwards he described symptoms of acute stress disorder relating to the attack. He was evacuated to LRMC after mentioning suicidal thoughts. On arrival at LRMC he related that the treating clinicians in theater had told him he would be going home. By the time he arrived at LRMC he demonstrated no symptoms. When told he would be returning to duty he became extremely anxious and all his symptoms of flashbacks, reported dissociation, dreams, and jumpiness returned. The following morning he presented to the emergency room after superficially cutting both his wrists. The treating clinician continued the air evacuation to the continental United States (CONUS) for treatment and disposition there.

Case Study 14-3 describes the interaction of two soldiers who arrived at LRMC for different reasons requiring psychiatric evaluation and shared quarters while awaiting their evaluations.

Case Study 14-3: Soldier #1 is a 30-year-old seasoned veteran, family man with several young children, on his third deployment. In prior deployments he had been personally involved in some of the most notable battles with intense urban warfare, including hand-to-hand fighting. He witnessed multiple deaths and maimings of both friendly and enemy forces. He presented to Landstuhl cardiology for onset of chest pains. There were no medical findings and he was referred to psychiatry for evaluation.

His roommate, Soldier #2, a 24-year-old junior noncommissioned officer (NCO) on his first combat tour, had flown to the forward operating base on a helicopter, had never been outside the perimeter, never seen any combat action, nor witnessed trauma of any sort. He was anxious and reported vague suicidal ideation contingent on his return to theater.

The two soldiers arrived together at the psychiatry clinic. Soldier #2 was evaluated first. The clinician felt that he presented too much risk for acting out if returned to duty and decided to return him as an outpatient to the United States. On his way out he met Soldier #1, the veteran war fighter, and gloated over the psychiatrist's decision to send him home. He was happy and felt he got what he desired.

After Soldier #1's evaluation the clinician informed him he would be returned to duty. The chest pain was likely related to stress. Though he had some combat-related symptoms, the clinician felt he could be returned to duty with continued mental healthcare in theater. The veteran NCO pleaded with the evaluator not to send him back to combat. He cited past experiences, heroic actions, and circumstances contrasting with those of his "suicidal" roommate. He related how he knew his roommate was just lying to get out of duty. He stated he could never harm himself or lie about suicidality to get out of duty, but cited the unfairness of the situation where someone who had truly sacrificed and experienced much was returned to harm's way, while someone who had never faced any danger would be spared threat. He further stated that after doing more than his share of combat he had been having premonitions that he would be killed in action, leaving his family alone and his wife widowed. The provider empathized with the soldier, but could not justify removing him from combat. In the end, the heroic NCO, Soldier #1, was returned to duty while Soldier #2 (most likely malingering) was taken out of theater.

Similar situations repeat themselves nearly every day at LRMC and most likely throughout the military. Soldiers and other service members who have already sacrificed much are required to give more. Many other soldiers are returned to CONUS for suicidal ideation based solely on anxiety about returning to combat. Often the providers suspect malingering as a cause but are unable to act on mere suspicions and are unwilling to risk repercussions of a bad outcome due to the provider taking a risk returning such a patient to combat.

Because of such incidents and the lack of supervision and control of return-to-duty patients while they await return to their units, most clinicians are not willing to send such patients back to the combat environment. In many cases such service members are using statements of self-harm to manipulate the system or go home early.[3] An unfortunate aspect of their evacuation is that other soldiers, who will not go to the extremes of manipulation and may have some symptoms, will return to duty while those manipulating the system will achieve their exit from the situation. In this embroiled climate, clinicians are likely to continue exercising conservative judgment such that many patients will be sent to CONUS instead of returning to duty in Iraq or Afghanistan. The return-to-duty rate for OIF/OEF mental health evacuees at LRMC varies between 3% and 6%. Even when it is clear that a service member is malingering, the risks of that soldier acting out if forced to return to duty may necessitate continued air evacuation to the home station (Figure 14-4).

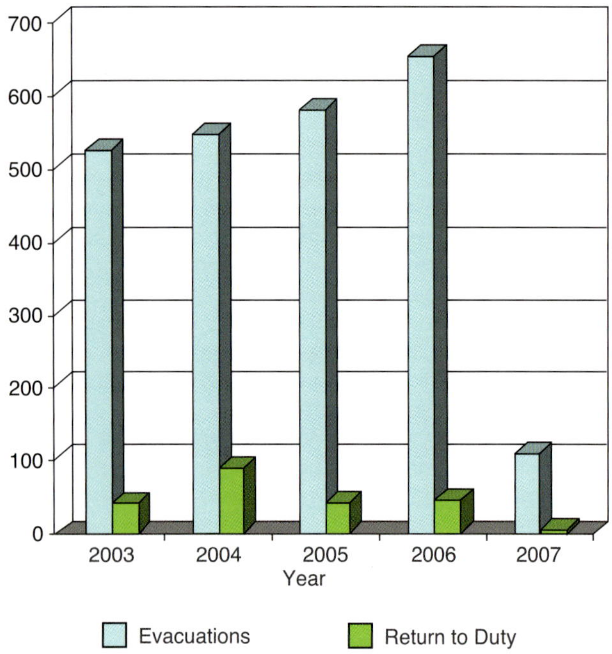

Figure 14-4. Operation Iraqi Freedom/Operation Enduring Freedom total evacuations compared to return to duty by year until February 2007. Those seen in Landstuhl Regional Medical Center outpatient clinic represent the majority, but do not include those admitted to the psychiatric ward in the evening or on weekends.

Circumvention of Evacuation Channels

Many service members are evacuated to LRMC for routine medical evaluation. Often they present to LRMC's behavioral health division as a self- or clinician referral. For the most part they have not yet been treated by behavioral health personnel in theater.[3] Clinicians noted that this population's return-to-duty rates were especially low. Often the mental symptoms increased after arrival at LRMC and even further after presenting to behavioral health. They are especially challenging to treat, given their isolation from sources of support and unit supervision.[4] Some were expecting to be sent to CONUS for treatment of their medical symptoms, but instead were found medically able to return to the combat zone. In essence, they skip in-theater mental health resources and become a rear-echelon psychiatric evacuation upon presentation at LRMC.

Clinicians observe that with this rear-echelon presentation, service members' chances of return to duty are considerably less than if they first presented in theater (95%–99% vs 3%).[5] It seems that with each passing moment at LRMC, it becomes more difficult to return such a soldier to the combat zone. Living in a safe environment, along with a lowered expectancy of returning to combat duty, decreases levels of vigilance and combat mind frame, and alters one's view of oneself. Often such service members develop ever-increasing psychiatric symptoms as their return-to-duty day draws near (see Case Study 14-2 and Case Study 14-3). One potential factor contributing to these mental symptoms is the loss of expectancy that they will return to duty. Such loss of expectancy has been found to be related to worse outcomes.[6]

One controversial approach, based on the assumption that these service members' units and social supports are better in theater, is to return such soldiers to their combat duty stations to receive their care. They are triaged for dangerousness, and evaluation and treatment at LRMC are minimized. They are expected to return to duty and get further care in theater. Appropriate mental health resources are usually available through combat stress control or other behavioral health personnel in theater. This approach not only maintains the fighting force but potentially improves the long-term prognosis for those treated in theater. In a sense, without the presence of fellow soldiers to provide social support and a leadership role in a service member's care, they will actually receive a lower level of care at LRMC than they would in theater with such peer support.[3,4,6–8] It is assumed that many service members with similar emotional symptoms are functioning in the combat zone. Their presentation at Landstuhl behavioral health, rather than at their in-theater mental health service, is determined solely by their need for a medical evaluation, which should not determine the level of mental healthcare required.

This approach, however, is not entirely without risk. Some of the potential hazards are that the service members may act out at LRMC, there may not be adequate care available for them in their combat duty stations, and they may perceive that they are being denied care at LRMC. The alternate approach of thoroughly evaluating and treating each such soldier is risky and may cause unnecessary delays in return to duty and thus lessen overall return-to-duty rates (Figure 14-5).

Staff Characteristics and Actions

Rotating Staff

To meet the additional duty of immediately evaluating all OIF/OEF mental health evacuees, LRMC is augmented with clinicians who have been rotating to LRMC for the majority of the wars. Though the augmentees are vital to performing the LRMC OEF/OIF mission, the rotations are not always predictable.

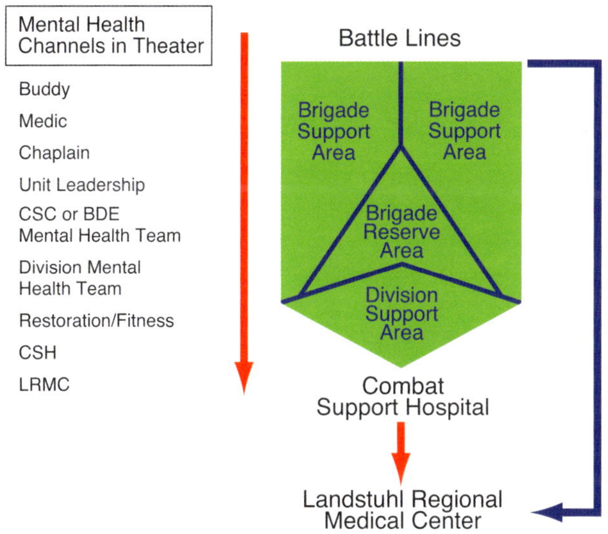

Figure 14-5. Circumventing mental healthcare in theater. Soldiers evacuated for medical reasons who then present at Landstuhl for mental health reasons may have skipped all mental health resources in theater and, in essence, become rear-echelon psychiatric casualties (with rear-echelon return-to-duty rates).
BDE: brigade; CSC: combat stress control; CSH: combat support hospital; LRMC: Landstuhl Regional Medical Center.

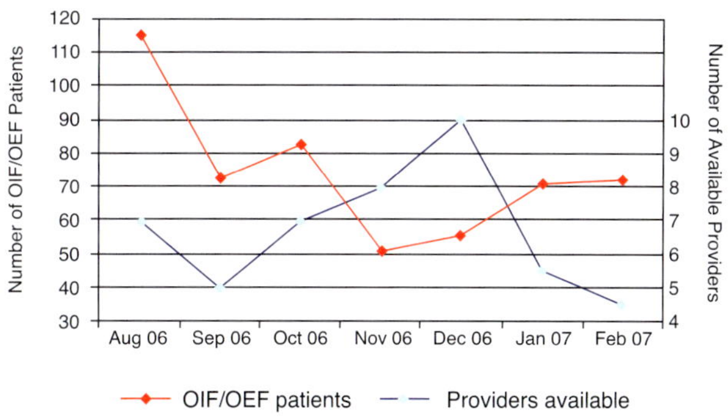

Figure 14-6. Comparison between Operation Iraqi Freedom/Operation Enduring Freedom evacuations and available clinicians at Landstuhl Outpatient Behavioral Health Clinic.

Sometimes the clinicians scheduled to arrive never show up. Usually this is due to an administrative or mobilization problem. Sometimes the rotation schedule is manipulated, bringing a clinician to LRMC either later or earlier than expected, thereby creating overlap or underlap and resulting in too many clinicians at some times and too few at others.

Augmentees are generally Army, Navy, or Air Force reservists. Usually they are clinically adept. They share the latest skills and knowledge from the civilian world, keeping the staff current. Some understand principles of combat operational stress control while others do not. They often need extensive training and supervision as they take on the relatively unique role of OIF/OEF evaluation and disposition. Figure 14-6 demonstrates a 5-month period in which the numbers of OIF/OEF patients are graphed compared with the number of available providers in the clinic. The number of clinicians available does not always correlate with the number of OIF/OEF evacuations. In some instances it is almost an inverse relationship. The unpredictable OIF/OEF load and the unpredictable augmentee support challenge the ability of the clinic to provide cohesive, continuous mental healthcare to those living in the local area.

The primary difficulty lies in maintaining adequate clinician availability to meet the surges of OEF/OIF patients without wasting clinician time or tying them down with excessive case loads. The need to maintain this reserve challenges measures of provider performance and productivity with the ever-looming threat that future personnel allocations will be based on that productivity.

Outreach to Wounded Warriors

As already mentioned, the majority of OIF/OEF evacuees sent to LRMC will stay only a couple of days. Concerned clinicians have consistently pondered the question, "What can we do to help the mental health of these patients?"[9] Concerns expressed by clinicians interacting with the wounded warriors include concern about harming the soldiers' mental recovery (perhaps by making them talk about their experience before they are ready, or by creating or worsening symptoms through conscious or unconscious suggestion during interactions) and concern about loss of follow-up care.

More than one soldier has stated that discussing the problem once was hard enough. There was no desire or intent to discuss it with another professional later. The relationship that is formed when a soldier discusses trauma is often intense and trusting, and may be ill-timed given that the soldier will leave within the next couple of days. Thus the mental health professional may have concerns about consciously or unconsciously pathologizing or labeling the patient's symptoms, or concerns about stigmatizing service members as either "crazy" or weak.[10]

Development of an Emergency Mental Health Model

The majority of clinicians serving in this capacity

at LRMC have supported an emergency mental health model with the following key components:

- **Avoid stigmatizing service members.** Avoid diagnostic labeling,[11] and do not single out any one soldier. For example, clinicians could say: "Hello, I'm a psychiatrist working with your medical team. Every patient gets 'top-to-bottom' care."
- **Look after basic needs.** Many patients are less than 2 days out from a major traumatic event, though many of them have been having traumatic events for months in the deployment setting. Ensure that their physical needs (rest, food, medical care) are being met.
- **Help them learn to ask for help and to communicate their needs.** Let them know that the more comfortable they are, the sooner they will heal. Observe comfort measures—pain control, room temperature, hydration, nutrition, sunlight, and privacy.
- **Ask about their pain and comfort.** Using a 0-to-10 pain scale (with 10 being the most pain possible and 0 being no pain), ask soldiers how they would rate the pain and at what level they would call the nurses. Catching the pain early may reduce the total amount of pain medication required.
- **Help them answer questions about what happened.** The most common questions asked by wounded service members at Landstuhl concern the status of their buddies, what happened, what weapons were involved, and whether they were personally responsible for what happened.
- **Connect them with their unit if indicated.** The unit may provide information to clarify the event and prevent solidification of false impressions or memories.
- **Normalize reactions.** Educate patients on symptoms they may experience.
- **Refrain from making statements indicating that they are ill,** or even that they scored higher than others on various screening tools.
- **Talk about normal things**—sports, football, or their hometown.
- **Assess them for posttraumatic stress symptoms.**
- **Help service members take charge of their medical care.** Ensure that they know what they need to about their condition and options, give them a sense of control, explore their knowledge of their injury, and help them understand the injury.
- **Help them know when they can expect to fly and where they will be transferred.** Many are anxious about the next step in their evacuation.
- **Follow up on their care.** Communicate to receiving physicians about service members demonstrating psychological symptoms.
- **Instill hope by discussing others who have recovered from similar events.**
- **Sincerely express appreciation for what they have gone through.** Add value and meaning to their experience.

Case Study 14-4: A 22-year-old soldier lost his vision in an explosion and was evacuated to LRMC. One of the outreach team members entered his room and noticed that the soldier's lips were parched and dry. The team member asked him if he was thirsty. The soldier replied "Yeah, I guess I could use a drink." There was a glass of ice water sitting a few inches away from where the soldier was resting his hand. The team member gave him the water then took his hand and showed him where the water was placed. During the ensuing conversation the team member mentioned that all the soldier needed to do is ring for a nurse to help him with his needs. The soldier replied, "I know that, but they are busy and there are a lot of us here."

Case Study 14-5: A 23-year-old soldier lost his leg in an explosion in Iraq. When he arrived at LRMC he was agitated and anxious to know if his gunner had survived the explosion. His primary physicians were unsure whether

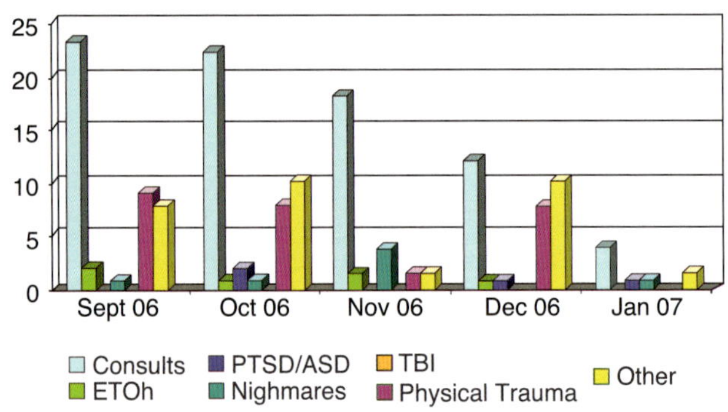

Figure 14-7. Landstuhl Regional Medical Center psychiatric consultation to medical and surgical wards, September 1, 2006, to February 1, 2007. By November 2006, the multidisciplinary Combat and Operational Stress/Staff Resiliency team and patient outreach teams were effectively established throughout the hospital. There was a significant drop in official consultations as informal, nonstigmatizing outreach efforts proceeded. Data are from 236 inpatient consultations. ETOh: ethanol (alcohol abuse); PTSD/ASD: posttraumatic stress disorder/acute stress disorder; TBI: traumatic brain injury.

they should tell him that the gunner, a close friend of his, had died. They contacted the behavioral health consultation team. In discussing his desire to know about his friend with the treating physicians, chaplains, and members of the soldier's unit (by telephone), the team decided on an appropriate time and place to let him know the bad news. The team arranged for the service member to speak to his unit members by telephone during the meeting. The soldier was notably saddened by the news but stated that the additional support of his unit by telephone helped him "drive on."

Case Study 14-6: A 25-year-old squad leader lost several squad members during a firefight and blamed himself for not reacting appropriately during the action. Regardless of what the physician and nursing staff told him, he continued to hold himself responsible for actions over which he had no real control. The outreach team arranged a telephone consultation with the soldier's command and fellow unit members. During the conversation, the events of the firefight were related and the squad leader realized that he did not cause the deaths of his subordinates, but rather that he acted as any other NCO would have done.

Local Area Support

One of the greatest challenges of the LRMC behavioral health division is to maintain consistent, continuous, mental health support to its catchment area despite unpredictable surges in staffing and patient load (Figure 14-7). Eight outlying clinics—(1) North Atlantic Treaty Organization, Holland; (2) Supreme Headquarters Allied Powers Europe, Belgium; (3) Vicenza, Italy; (4) Livorno, Italy; (5) Kleber, Germany; (6) Dexheim, Germany; (7) Wiesbaden, Germany; and (8) Baumholder, Germany—fall under the LRMC support area, which covers approximately 100,000 primary care beneficiaries (see Figure 14-1). In addition to the primary care mission, the tertiary care mission includes approximately 245,000 total beneficiaries in the European command. Many service members in the LRMC support area have served in OIF/OEF and experience ongoing sequelae of their time there,[1,12] resulting in additional combat-related patients for the psychiatry service.

INPATIENT PSYCHIATRY AT LANDSTUHL REGIONAL MEDICAL CENTER, 2003–2007

Increasing Patient Load

The inpatient psychiatry service maintains an 18-bed service for all active duty service members and beneficiaries throughout Europe, Asia, Africa, and the Middle East. Criteria for admission are similar to those in the civilian world. However, given the limited supervision of patients treated and evacuated in the outpatient setting, if an evaluating provider has concerns about safety, including the patient's potential to abuse substances, then the patient is admitted, usually for continued evacuation in the inpatient setting. In 2003 there were 382 OIF/OEF service members admitted; in 2004 there were 269; in 2005 there were 346; in 2006 there were 408; in 2007 there were 563; and as of October 2008 there were 481 OIF/OEF admissions. As for total admission numbers, which include OIF/OEF as well as other patient populations (family members, local military), there were 902 total in 2006, 990 total in 2007, and 822 (as of Oct 2008) in 2008.

The majority of OIF/OEF patients admitted remain in the inpatient setting for evacuation to the United States. Most OIF/OEF admissions continue their evacuation within a couple of days, leading to extremely rapid turnover on the ward. Contacting an accepting physician in the United States can be challenging, especially given the 6- to 9-hour time difference and sheer volume of turnaround. This is partially resolved by the ability to send patients on to Army hospitals with an "open OIF/OEF" status that does not require physician-to-physician discussion to establish an accepting physician. However, such is not the case with accepting hospitals from sister services, which often require physician-to-physician establishment of acceptance.

Prior to 2003, the 18-bed inpatient psychiatry service had averaged about 675 admissions per year. By June 2003, it was admitting 100 patients per month (1,200 annualized rate). As many of the admissions seemed inappropriate, a 100% screening was implemented for patients arriving from OIF. This helped, but in 2005, for example, 902 patients were still admitted (Figure 14-8 and Figure 14-9). The 100% screening, in turn, caused its own problems. It became necessary to change the psychiatry call schedule to accommodate the numbers of OIF patients who were arriving and needed screening. The inpatient psychiatrists were augmented by outpatient psychiatrists and further augmented by the local Air Force providers.

The ward itself was augmented by a succession of reservists. The nursing personnel came for a year at a time. Their "train up" required an intensive schedule of activities before they could begin to "orient." Even after the formal train-up activities, the nursing personnel required considerable time to make them comfortable in handling all the nuances of the inpatient ward.

The psychiatrists who came to augment LRMC were there for only 90 days. They varied greatly in experience levels, ranging from current active duty to reserv-

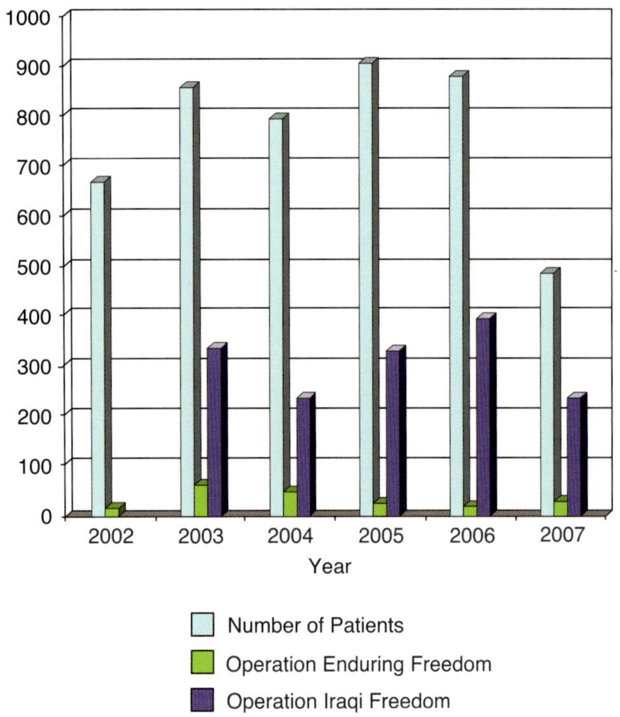

Figure 14-8. Landstuhl Regional Medical Center inpatient admissions, 2002 through July 2007.

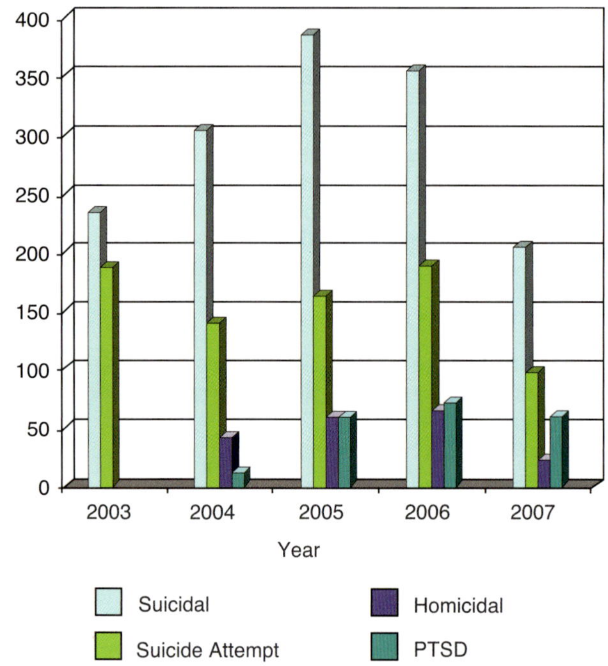

Figure 14-9. Landstuhl Regional Medical Center (LRMC) inpatient admissions, 2003 through July 2007. LRMC began tracking homicidal ideations and posttraumatic stress disorder (PTSD) in 2004.

ists who had never been activated. Some were quickly able to absorb the complexities of the rapid turnover of patients, while others could master only a portion of the tasks at hand. The Composite Health Care System electronic medical record used throughout the military proved to be a record-keeping system that many inexperienced physicians could not master.

The effect of the patient volume can be understood by dividing 902 admissions in 2006 by the number of inpatient beds available: 18. The result, 50.1, is the number of times that a bed was turned over during the year. Dividing that 50 into 365 yields a theoretical length of stay of slightly over 7 days.

Receiving patients, screening them, stabilizing them on the ward, and placing them on an aeromedical evacuation became the routine. With increased OIF/OEF workload, the ward was frequently too full to accept nonactive duty patients. The "available to nonactive duty" measure (over 90% on an annual basis during the pre-OIF period) decreased to approximately 60% once casualties from OIF began arriving (meaning that there were spaces available to nonactive duty personnel only 60% of the time.)

With the slowly increasing census of inpatients since 2003, air evacuation flights from Landstuhl to CONUS became more and more crowded. Beginning in November 2006 and continuing regularly over the next several months, the inpatient team encountered difficulties getting patients out on air evacuation flights fast enough to have beds available for incoming service members. Service members coming from garrisons in Europe were diverted to German hospitals. Such diversions of active-duty soldiers to German hospitals usually lasted only a few hours to a couple of days, but demonstrate that the 18-bed inpatient psychiatry ward is insufficient to handle both local support and air evacuation missions during wartime.

Psychological Stressors and Staff Resilience

The daily psychological stressors for LRMC team members are significant. A recent article in a German newspaper described LRMC's role as being at the outer perimeter of the Iraq battlefield.[13] Indeed, in previous wars many of the casualties arriving at LRMC would not have made it out of theater. Now, however, modern transportation and stabilization capabilities bring the battle to LRMC's front door,[13] exposing many LRMC staff to trauma of combat casualties on a daily basis. In previous wars the patients seen at LRMC would probably have been seen in a hospital much closer to the battlefield. The Combat and Operational Stress Response/Staff Resilience Program at LRMC was developed to address the short- and long-term consequences of this experience with casualties.

Compassion Fatigue

In its present-day connotation, compassion fatigue refers to the deleterious effect on caregivers of repeated exposure to physically or psychologically traumatized patients. Compassion fatigue was initially construed as a secondary trauma experienced by those treating PTSD patients, who have experienced primary trauma.[14] The symptoms are similar. And although it has been called various things (secondary traumatic stress disorder or compassion stress), the main point is that anyone in a care-giving or helping profession—from psychotherapists to nurses to police—can experience acute and chronic stress reactions in the course of their duties. So, too, may they experience symptoms as a result of their own primary trauma or occupational burnout.

Specific to LRMC, compassion fatigue results from caregivers' repeated exposure to soldiers with severe burns, amputated limbs, or traumatic brain injury. With the exception of those staff who have worked in major metropolitan trauma centers, most have not been exposed to this frequency and severity of wounds. Because LRMC is the deployed location for many of its personnel (ie, the Navy and Army reservists who deploy to Landstuhl to help with the wartime mission), many staff who are actually deployed personnel will face deployment-related stressors such as being away from home and loved ones.

Combat and Operational Stress Reaction

Army Field Manual 4-02.51, *Combat and Operational Stress Control,*[15] redefines soldiers' negative reactions to combat and support operations (previously known as "battle fatigue") as combat and operational stress reactions (COSR). This new term considers soldiers who are not directly involved in battle but nonetheless develop stress-related symptoms (loss of appetite, increased irritability, or a desire to smoke), as having a normal reaction to a potentially hostile environment and the related demands that this entails (high operations tempo, living in austere conditions, and extensive separations from family).

Resiliency

Just as two soldiers can be involved in the same firefight and one develop COSR while the other does not, so, too, can two providers treat a similar number and type of patients and one develop compassion fatigue while the other remains intact. The mechanism that allows this has come to be called "resilience." *Combat and Operational Stress Control*[15] mentions resilience as something that is desirable and can be increased, but does not describe how this can be accomplished.

Resilience as a phenomenon has been studied in the civilian population, including in children who suffer physical and emotional abuse or neglect,[16] adult victims of crime,[17] and people exposed to natural disasters.[18] Proposed factors leading to individual resilience are physical (exercise, nutrition), emotional (social support, optimism), psychological (attributional style), and spiritual (a life meaning or purpose). Unit morale and cohesion are additional factors within the military social context that may lead to resiliency among troops.

DEVELOPMENT OF LANDSTUHL'S STAFF RESILIENCY PROGRAM

Precipitating Event and Command Response

Following a series of patient fatalities in LRMC's ICU in July 2005, the hospital commander contacted the on-call chaplain to discuss what could be done to alleviate some of the providers' stress. After that discussion (and the resulting actions taken to help reduce the effect of these ICU deaths on the staff), a team was formed to address this overlooked need among physicians, nurses, and their technical staff.

A consultative team approach was deemed the best way to deal with these operational stressors. Although various agencies (chaplaincy, employee assistance program, behavioral health) already existed to help LRMC staff cope with stress or PTSD symptoms, these services were not accessed by those in need for various reasons (eg, stigma, availability). The plan was to provide outreach by chaplains and behavioral health staff who typically worked in close proximity with LRMC staff to address their concerns and direct them toward the best resources.

Structure and Focus of Program

In November 2006, the compassion fatigue team changed its name to "Combat and Operational Stress/Staff Resiliency" (COSR/SR). This is not merely semantics. Rather, the scope of concern has been widened beyond compassion fatigue (trauma secondary to care giving) to include COSR, acute or chronic reactions to primary trauma (ie, PTSD), burnout, and efforts to restore or improve resiliency. In addition to physicians and nurses in the ICU, COSR/SR consultation now includes all LRMC staff, from those who carry litters and help move patients, to the finance staff who hear soldier's stories as they help with pay and benefits.

Program Director

Prior to August 2006, LRMC's COSR/SR team utilized an informal committee led by a behavioral health provider. Funding was secured to hire a clinical psychologist to fill the position of program director. This individual leads the team and, more importantly, serves as the main point of contact for COSR/SR-related questions. This program director is tasked to conduct a majority of the brief consultations and office visits.

Team Membership

The COSR/SR team is composed of chaplains, nurses, and behavioral health providers in officer ranks or their civilian equivalent. Team members voluntarily take on—as an additional duty—reaching out to LRMC personnel who might not otherwise access services for symptoms that develop as a result of treating severely wounded soldiers and operations in support of this mission. They also make short presentations at various venues—newcomers' orientation, professional and clinic staff meetings, and for new leadership. Additional ways of "getting the word out" about the program include a trifold brochure that outlines the program. A business card listing online and local resources is also used. Finally, e-mail messages distributed to LRMC staff describe sponsored events (sleep hygiene or stress-management classes) and highlight the COSR/SR program.

Confidential Visits

In an attempt to circumvent the often-noted stigma associated with seeking help, LRMC's COSR/SR team allows for two consultation meetings that are highly confidential. If there is no diagnosis, there is no documentation. As always, domestic violence, child abuse, and intent to harm oneself or others must be reported. Although previously one "free" visit had been advertised, the hope was that a second such visit would allow for additional assessment of any advice or suggestions given. If the problems were continuing, this second visit would give the COSR/SR team member a better opportunity (because of increased rapport) to encourage entry into some form of treatment or referral to an appropriate resource.

The goal is for LRMC staff to feel comfortable in reaching out to COSR/SR team members, knowing they can get some advice on psychological or emotional symptoms they may experience as a result of their work at LRMC or from other situations. Some of the symptoms LRMC staff may experience include poor sleep, increased irritability, and hypervigilance. The key is that LRMC staff must have confidence that their personal affairs will remain private and their careers will not be put in jeopardy. In those cases where minor support and guidance is not enough, COSR/SR team members will point the LRMC staff member in the right direction and, perhaps, answer some questions of concern such that, in most cases, their anonymity is protected.

Hallway Consultation Versus Office Visit

In an attempt to track the utility of LRMC's COSR/SR program, short, informal consultations were differentiated from longer, sit-down sessions. This differentiation is useful to characterize support and minimal advice-giving from processing and intervention. For example, during October through December 2006, 65 LRMC staff were provided hallway consultation and four were seen in an office visit. Of these, 20% were later seen in formal treatment. Due to a multitude of changes from one month to the next, these visits fluctuate. In March and April 2007, for example, the COSR/SR team had 38 hallway consultations and 46 office visits. In part due to the increase in office visits, the follow-on to treatment rate dropped to 10%.

In addition to tracking hallway consultation versus office visits, COSR/SR team members collect information on the staff member's ward or clinic. By learning about the events and environment of wards and clinics throughout the hospital, the COSR/SR team is able to understand the experiences and conditions of most of the hospital workers. The COSR/SR team can then reallocate resources to those areas most needing them. When the mental health needs, working environment, or experience of the staff dictates, consultation with the clinic or service chief may prove beneficial.

Debriefs

Critical incident stress management defusings and debriefings appear to have fallen out of favor. However, hospital staff can still benefit from a chance to process their experiences in a safe, nonjudgmental setting. LRMC's COSR/SR team attempts to provide this environment. A prime example of where this appears to be helpful is with the personnel team, which provides litter bearers and evacuation personnel for the incoming and outgoing flights. Many of these team members are exposed to physically traumatized, wounded, maimed, and dying service members. These LRMC staff are at substantial risk for mental and emotional problems. At the end of each team's 1-month rotation, a debrief is held during which a chaplain, supported by another COSR/SR team member (typically a behavioral health staff member), leads the members through mental processing. Most of the manpower team members feel the experience is meaningful and generally positive. Often they develop a greater appreciation for the positive factors in their lives, such as health, well-being, and a supportive family. Occasionally problems with the system are discussed in the debriefings. Problems (with the personnel system or other units debriefed) that can be remedied by command action are anonymously conveyed to command staff who may act to correct the situation.

In the months of March and April 2007, 134 LRMC staff were debriefed in some capacity, either because of a critical event (death of a patient who was on the ward for an unusually long time) or a chronic stressor (higher than average number of amputees). One example of the latter is a young troop member who, while replacing equipment in a wounded soldier's room, was affected by the smell of the patient's burn wound. He said that on and off for several nights afterward he dreamt of the event. By addressing how the human brain processes trauma to self or others, and normalizing his reaction, he was able to quickly return to his previously high-functioning status.

DAILY OPERATIONS

Member Dispersal

Team members are dispersed throughout the hospital to consult on COSR/SR as needed. Additionally, members take part in hospital committees and functions to ensure that system-wide efforts are made to reduce stress or provide input to command staff on actionable items. The main point is that the COSR/SR team attempts to address issues not only on a one-on-one basis, but also at higher levels within the organization, by consulting with supervisors and commanders. In large part this is due to research suggesting that unit morale and cohesion are factors of resiliency, which should be addressed at all levels by everyone involved.

Committee Meetings

The multidisciplinary COSR/SR team convenes weekly to discuss consultation trends and upcoming issues, either in terms of wards or units affected, or the types of stressors reported. The meeting is vital to disperse information and provide emotional and leadership support to team members. Based on the feedback from the team members, an accurate picture can be developed of the emotional status throughout the hospital and resources can then be allocated to those areas needing them. A forum is provided where advice dealing with particular situations can be asked for and shared. Additional planning is also coordinated at these meetings to ensure continued advertising and coverage for clinic debriefs or presentations.

Surveys

In an attempt to keep pace with LRMC as a dynamic organization, the COSR/SR team periodically surveys various wards or sections on stress levels, morale, and general knowledge of the program.

CHALLENGES AND FUTURE DIRECTIONS

Program Director

Presently [in 2007], the COSR/SR program has funds for a 1-year program manager position, someone solely dedicated to advancing the program and working with staff. Although additional funds will be requested, it is difficult to find potential candidates willing to relocate to Germany, knowing their position is time-limited. Other options, such as using interns or community volunteers, are being considered. Additionally, there is some debate whether the ideal candidate for the position of COSR/SR program director should be a psychiatrist, psychologist, or social worker, with or without experience in community or system-wide interventions. Ideally the candidate would be familiar with the military and its deployment process as well as the healthcare system in general and work at a major medical hospital, specifically.

Personnel

The Mental Health Advisory Team II noted that

20% to 30% of behavioral health personnel reported burnout, low motivation, or some form of impairment related to deployment.[19] Thus, it will be important to assess COSR/SR team members and provide respite or resiliency support to avoid their becoming overwhelmed.[19] Consideration is being given to the use of enlisted medical technicians to work with enlisted LRMC staff seeking access to the COSR/SR program. Additionally, peer support personnel may be culled from LRMC's wards and clinics to help augment the COSR/SR team. Within the framework of focusing on building and supporting staff resiliency, clinic chiefs and NCOs may be encouraged to identify those subordinates they see as "resilient" and match them up with those deemed "at risk."

Central Point of Contact

One difficulty noted is that hospital staff may not know who to contact, especially given the need for team members to rotate on-call availability. Asking around to find the appropriate person may feel uncomfortable. It also decreases the anonymity of the person seeking help. Efforts are being made to simplify the process by establishing a designated cell phone number to be carried by the COSR/SR team member on duty. That cell phone number could be published throughout the hospital, thus ensuring that hospital workers know how to access the team.

Stigma

Recent surveys of LRMC staff show continued evidence of a stigma against seeking help from any official program. The COSR/SR team continues to advertise the difference between COSR help and being "crazy" (ie, psychotic), as well as the likelihood of career impact from voluntarily seeking behavioral health counseling versus being command directed to seek such help. These data collection points will be included on future surveys.

Data Collection

The aforementioned surveys used a modified form of the Secondary Trauma Cost-of-Caring scale[20] with unknown validity and reliability. Future efforts will go toward securing or developing a sound psychometric tool with which to assess COSR/SR. Ideally such measures would include objective indicators of the organization's health as a whole. For example, days missed from work or number of letters of counseling or reprimand might be useful signs of organizational distress, which could then be tracked.

Types of Stressors

In an effort to obtain more data to form more precise interventions, LRMC's COSR/SR team has begun to collect information about the types of stressors addressed—operational, organizational, occupational, home front, interpersonal, or other. The pace of one's duty is an example of an operational stressor. An organizational stressor could be the impact of staff turnover during the permanent-change-of-station season. Occupational stressors include burnout and the effect of a specific duty (working with amputees or burn victims). Home front and interpersonal issues are self-explanatory and take the form of relationship problems or parenting issues, and communication or teamwork in the workplace, respectively. Considered in the "other" category are attempts by COSR/SR team members to reassure staff that psychotherapy works, addressing how confidential sessions really are, or defining various diagnostic categories (ie, "Am I dealing with acute stress disorder or PTSD and what does that mean?").

SUMMARY

The COSR/SR team at LRMC has grown from a "psych–spiritual" dyad, consisting of a behavioral health provider and chaplain supporting ICU staff, to a full compliment of providers from several disciplines and branches dispersed throughout the hospital, to include the much-appreciated ancillary and support services such as finance and personnel teams. The scope of concern has been widened from provider secondary trauma (ie, compassion fatigue) to all stress reactions produced by operating in a major medical facility that receives nearly every OEF/OIF casualty. This adaptive contingent of professionals will be bolstered by additional direction and support from higher command levels (in terms of funding and personnel), and will lean towards becoming a proactive (rather than a reactive) force, perhaps through a newcomer's combat and operational stress assessment and resiliency development plan, yet to be created. Work remains to be done, but the underlying concept of the COSR/SR team approach is sound and of value to the LRMC staff and the patients they serve.

Acknowledgment

Thanks to Major Michael McBride, MD, who made many contributions to the outreach team protocols and developed many of the interventions discussed in this chapter.

REFERENCES

1. Lein B. Colonel, Medical Corps, US Army. Command brief, Landstuhl, Germany, November 24, 2008.

2. Ritchie EC, Keppler WC, Rothberg JM. Suicidal admissions in the United States military. *Mil Med*. 2003;168(3):177–181.

3. Forsten R, Schneider B. Treatment of the stress casualty during Operation Iraqi Freedom One. *Psychiatr Q*. 2005;76(4):343–350.

4. Hill JV, Johnson RC, Barton RA. Suicidal and homicidal soldiers in deployment environments. *Mil Med*. 2006;171(3):228–232.

5. Mental Health Advisory Team (MHAT). *Operation Iraqi Freedom (OIF). Report.* The US Army Surgeon General and Department of the Army G-1. December 16, 2003. Available at: www.armymedicine.army.mil/reports/mhat.html. Accessed September 4, 2008.

6. Solomon Z, Benbenishty R. The role of proximity, immediacy, and expectancy in frontline treatment of combat stress reaction among Israelis in the Lebanon War. *Am J Psychiatry*. 1986;143(5):613–617.

7. Hassinger AD. Mentoring and monitoring: the use of unit watch in the 4th Infantry Division. *Mil Med*. 2003;168(3):234–238.

8. Bacon BL, Staudenmeier JJ. A historical overview of combat stress control units of the US Army. *Mil Med*. 2003;168(9):689–693.

9. Ritchie EC, Owens M. Military issues. *Psychiatr Clin North Am*. 2004;27:459–471.

10. Greene-Shortridge TM, Britt TW, Castro CA. The stigma of mental health problems in the military. *Mil Med*. 2007;172(2):157–161.

11. McDuff DR, Johnson JL. Classification and characteristics of Army stress casualties during Operation Desert Storm. *Hosp Community Psychiatry*. 1992;43(8):812–815.

12. Blackwell J. Captain, US Army. Chief, Managed Care Division, Landstuhl Regional Medical Center. Personal communication, May 2007.

13. Fichtner U. The German front in the Iraq war: a visit to the US military hospital at Landstuhl. *Spiegel Online International*. March 14, 2007. Available at: http://www.spiegel.de/international/germany/0,1518,471654,00.html. Accessed September 3, 2008.

14. Figley CR, ed. *Compassion Fatigue: Coping With Secondary Traumatic Stress Disorder in Those Who Treat the Traumatized.* New York, NY: Brunner/Mazel; 1995.

15. US Department of the Army. *Combat and Operational Stress Control.* Washington, DC: DA; July 6, 2006. Army Field Manual 4-02.51.

16. Daigneault I, Hébert M, Tourigny M. Personal and interpersonal characteristics related to resilient developmental pathways of sexually abused adolescents. *Child Adolesc Psychiatr Clin N Am*. 2007;16(2):415–434.

17. Winkel FW, Blaauw E, Sheridan L, Baldry AC. Repeat criminal victimization and vulnerability for coping failure: a prospective examination of a potential risk factor. *Psychol Crime Law.* 2003;9(1):87–95.

18. Tang CS. Trajectory of traumatic stress symptoms in the aftermath of extreme natural disaster: a study of adult Thai survivors of the 2004 Southeast Asian earthquake and tsunami. *J Nerv Ment Dis.* 2007;195:54–59.

19. Mental Health Advisory Team (MHAT-II). *Operation Iraqi Freedom (OIF-II). Report.* The US Army Surgeon General. January 30, 2005. Available at: www.armymedicine.army.mil/reports/mhat.html. Accessed September 4, 2008.

20. Motta RW, Hafeez S, Sciancalepore R, Diaz AB. Discriminant validation of the Modified Secondary Trauma Questionnaire. *J Psychothera Independent Pract*. 2001;2(4):17–24.

Chapter 15

TRAUMATIC BRAIN INJURY IN THE MILITARY POPULATION

LOUIS M. FRENCH, PsyD*; KATHERINE H. TABER, PhD†; KATHY HELMICK, MS, CNRN, CRNP‡; ROBIN A. HURLEY, MD§; and DEBORAH L. WARDEN, MD¥

*Director, Traumatic Brain Injury Service, Defense and Veterans Brain Injury Center and Department of Orthopaedics and Rehabilitation, Walter Reed Army Medical Center, 6900 Georgia Avenue NW, Washington, DC 20307; Department of Neurology, Uniformed Services University of the Health Sciences, Bethesda, Maryland 20814

†Research Health Scientist, Department of Research and Education, WG Hefner Veterans Affairs Medical Center, Mailstation 11M, 1601 Brenner Avenue, Salisbury, North Carolina 28144; formerly, Research Fellow, School of Health Information Sciences, University of Texas at Houston

‡Senior Executive Director, Traumatic Brain Injury, Defense Center of Excellence for Psychological Health and Traumatic Brain Injury, 1335 East-West Highway, 9th Floor, Suite 700, Silver Spring, Maryland 20910; formerly, Deputy Director, Defense and Veterans Brain Injury Center, Walter Reed Army Medical Center, Washington, DC

§Associate Director, Education, WG Hefner Veterans Affairs Medical Center (Mailcode 11F), 1601 Brenner Avenue, Salisbury, North Carolina 28144; formerly, Associate Director, Mental Health, WG Hefner Veterans Affairs Medical Center, Salisbury, North Carolina

¥Formerly, National Director, Defense and Veterans Brain Injury Center Headquarters; Departments of Neurology and Psychiatry, Walter Reed Army Medical Center, 6900 Georgia Avenue NW, Washington, DC 20307; Departments of Neurology and Psychiatry, Walter Reed Army Medical Center, 6900 Georgia Avenue NW, Washington, DC 20307-5001

INTRODUCTION

Traumatic brain injury (TBI) is a very significant public health issue and the leading cause of death and disability in young people. The Centers for Disease Control and Prevention (CDC)[1] estimates that 1.4 million individuals sustain a TBI in the United States annually, with 50,000 deaths. About 80,000 to 90,000 individuals suffer permanent disability. The monetary cost to society is almost $50 billion annually when treatment costs, lost wages, disability, and death are considered.[2,3] Even more significant, at its most severe, TBI robs individuals of important aspects of their relationships, well-being, and happiness.

Service in the military, which includes both rigorous and often dangerous training, and exposure to the combat environment, places individuals at greater risk than the general population. Surprisingly, young adult men (the group with the highest rate of TBI in the civilian population), have about the same rate of TBI as young women in the military, a figure that underscores the inherent risk in service.[4] However, Ivins and colleagues,[5] in a recent paper examining trends in TBI-related hospitalizations in the active duty US Army during the 1990s, reported that the Army's TBI-related hospitalization rates decreased for all severity levels, both sexes, and all age categories during that decade. The paper also indicated that in the first half of the 1990s, many of the Army's adjusted TBI-related hospitalization rates, including the overall rate, were higher than the rates for US civilians 17 to 49 years of age. In the second half of the 1990s, most of the Army's adjusted TBI-related hospitalization rates, including the overall rate, were lower than civilian rates, with a 75% reduction overall. These decreases resulted in a relative improvement in the Army's TBI-related hospitalization rates over civilian rates by the late 1990s. This may be related to successful educational efforts or other factors.

Somewhat more difficult to quantify is the effect of TBI on military readiness. Because some potential consequences of TBI include slowed reaction, reduced speed of cognitive processing, and mood changes, the effects of even transitory symptoms could have implications for the deployability or fighting effectiveness of the service member. Additionally, there is the risk that the TBI, especially at the milder end of the spectrum, will be unrecognized. This chapter will describe (*a*) what TBI is, (*b*) how severity is determined, (*c*) common consequences of the injury, and (*d*) some treatment strategies. Furthermore, the identification and management of TBI in a military operational setting will be discussed. Although the entire spectrum of brain injury severity will be discussed, the focus of the chapter is on those with mild TBI (mTBI), as that is the population that is most likely to come to the attention of the military behavioral health provider. Additionally, the overlap of typical postconcussive symptoms with symptoms of mood, anxiety, or other disorders may make referral to such providers probable when an individual with such symptoms of unclear etiology is recognized.

The current conflicts in Iraq (Operation Iraqi Freedom) and Afghanistan (Operation Enduring Freedom) are different than past wars in terms of the survival rates of those injured. The current wounded-to-killed ratio in Iraq is more than 9:1,[6] compared to less than 3:1 in Vietnam and Korea, and approximately 2:1 in World War II.[7] This increased survival of wounded personnel is related to numerous factors including advanced in-theater medical care and superb protective equipment. With these new survival rates come increased numbers of those who may have experienced a TBI. Because the most common injury mechanism in the current conflict is blast, there are possibilities for TBI either through direct blast effect or secondary or tertiary blast effects. It is essential for the healthcare provider to be aware of the possibility that an injured service member may also have sustained a TBI. In many cases, this identification is early after the injury. There is greater potential, however, for more delayed recognition of such an injury, especially if the TBI is at the milder end of the severity spectrum. These "silent injuries" may have implications for functioning over the short or long term, and may affect recovery and rehabilitation of other more visible injuries.

ETIOLOGY AND DIAGNOSIS OF TRAUMATIC BRAIN INJURY

TBI is described as either penetrating or closed. A penetrating brain injury occurs when a foreign object or bone penetrates the dura surrounding the brain. (In the military setting, the object is most commonly a bullet or fragment.) In a closed TBI, penetration does not occur, but forces acting on the head cause damage to the brain. Although there is some variability in the definition of TBI, especially at the milder end of the spectrum, most accepted definitions (CDC,[8] American Congress of Rehabilitative Medicine [ACRM],[9] American Psychiatric Association [APA],[10] and World Health Organization [WHO][11]) have common elements. The Defense and Veterans Brain Injury Center (DVBIC) defines mTBI in a military operational setting as an injury to the brain caused by an external force, with either an acceleration or deceleration mechanism (or both in some instances), from an event such as a blast, fall, direct impact, or motor vehicle accident. This trauma causes an alteration in mental status, typically resulting in the temporally related onset of symptoms such as headache, nausea, vomiting, dizziness or balance problems, fatigue, insomnia or other sleep disturbances, drowsiness, sensitivity to light or noise, blurred vision, and difficulty remembering or concentrating.

This operational definition of mTBI was established in 2006 by a workgroup of experts in the field of military operational medicine and TBI.[12] They drew from widely accepted definitions, such as those already mentioned (CDC, ACRM, APA, and WHO), as well as the National Athletic Trainers' Association position statement on management of sport-related concussion,[13] and the Prague sports concussion guidelines,[14] incorporating common criteria. These established definitions endorse biomechanical forces as the cause of concussion that results in an alteration of consciousness (AOC), including loss of consciousness (LOC), posttraumatic amnesia (PTA) or retrograde amnesia, or being dazed or confused at the time of the injury. An important aspect of this new operational definition of TBI is that LOC is not a required characteristic of concussion. That is, a service member does not have to have an LOC to have sustained a concussion or mTBI (these terms are used interchangeably). The group acknowledged the continued usefulness of these parameters and adopted them with a few changes. Variations from the established definitions included adding common combat-related mechanisms such as exposure to blast as a possible mechanism of injury, as well as adding a comprehensive list of TBI-related symptoms.

The majority of TBI experts in this workgroup agreed that symptoms are common following mTBI, but the presence of these symptoms is not mandatory to establish the diagnosis of mTBI. That is, although concussion to the brain may have occurred, it does not always result in self-reported symptoms. In some circumstances there may be measurable changes in functioning or performance, such as increased latency of response on measures of reaction time, even in the absence of changes noticeable to the injured individual.[15] It should be noted that wide consensus among the members of the workgroup supported the inclusion of an AOC in the definition of mTBI, including reports of feeling "dazed and confused" after a traumatic event. There are instances, both in the sports literature and military arena, of individuals who were involved in a traumatic event but did not report any AOC, yet these patients subsequently developed symptoms consistent with concussion, with onset temporally related to the event. Given these cases, a conservative approach might be that those individuals involved in events with an associated high risk for TBI, who report subsequent symptoms, be evaluated further. However, without supporting diagnostic evidence, these individuals do not meet the criteria for having sustained an mTBI. More research is needed to better characterize this group.[13]

Closed-TBI severity is characterized by duration of length of LOC and PTA, and initial, postresuscitation Glasgow Coma Scale (GCS) score (Table 15-1). Those individuals who meet these criteria as having sustained an mTBI, but have positive findings on imaging of the brain, are classified as having suffered a TBI of moderate severity, as these individuals are known to have outcomes similar to those who meet criteria for moderate TBI on the basis of length of coma or duration of LOC.[16,17] It is important to note that these designations describe the severity of the brain injury itself, and do not necessarily describe clinical outcomes or functionality in the future. Although there is greater chance for persisting problems as injury severity increases, many patients at the more severe end of the spectrum can have good outcomes, while some patients who were initially diagnosed as having a "mild" TBI go on

TABLE 15-1

TRAUMATIC BRAIN INJURY DESCRIPTION

Severity	GCS*	LOC	PTA
Mild	13–15	< 20 min–1 h	< 24 h
Moderate	9–12	1–24 h	24 h– < 7 days
Severe	3–8	> 24 h	> 7 days

GCS: Glasgow Coma Scale
LOC: loss of consciousness
PTA: posttraumatic amnesia
*The Glasgow Coma Scale (GCS) is the most commonly used scale to determine the severity of a brain injury. It must be noted, however, that a GCS score signifies the patient's "best" response. A patient could have a serious deficit that is not indicated by the GCS. Also, the score does not indicate the amount of stimulation required to get the patient to score at that level. A severe brain-injured patient usually has a GCS score of 3–8 and presents with a significant neurological deficit. The lowest GCS score is 3 (no neurological functioning). A patient with a severe brain injury also will experience loss of consciousness for more than 1 hour. Posttraumatic amnesia (PTA) refers to the loss of memory of events immediately following the injury. A typical question to ask to assess for PTA is, "What is the first thing you remember after your injury?" If the first memory occurred more than 24 hours after the injury, then, by definition, the patient has suffered a moderate-to-severe traumatic brain injury.

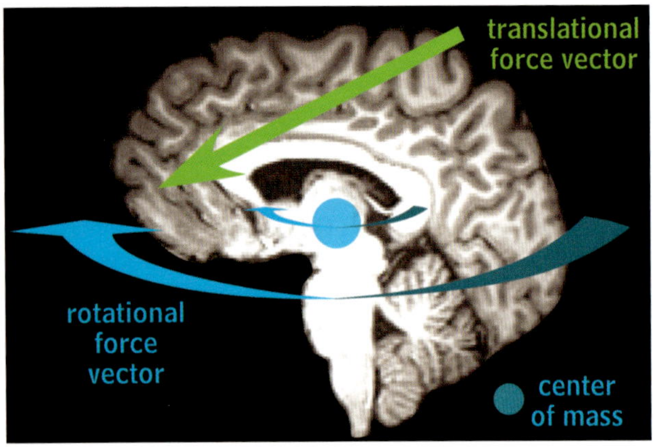

Figure 15-1. The physical forces exerted on the brain during most of the events that can cause traumatic brain injury are reasonably well understood. Both linear (green) and rotational (blue) forces can arise. The brain can be physically displaced within the skull. It can also be rotated or twisted. Rotational forces make the lower-density tissues (eg, cerebral cortex) move more quickly than the higher-density tissues (eg, subcortical white matter), resulting in stretching and shearing forces.

to have seemingly catastrophic changes in personal, social, and occupational functioning. Persistent postconcussional syndromes are discussed more fully later in this chapter.

Forces That Cause Traumatic Brain Injury

Traumatic brain injury may arise from many causes, including accidents, assaults, falls, and exposure to explosions. The physical forces exerted on the brain during most of the events that can cause TBI are reasonably well understood (Figure 15-1). The brain can be physically displaced within the skull by linear forces. It can also be rotated or twisted by angular or rotational forces. These forces make the lower-density tissues, particularly the outer layer of the brain (the cerebral hemispheres), move more quickly than the higher-density tissues that make up the core of the brain. They can also twist the brain around its central axis. Both types of movement result in stretching and shearing forces within the brain. Explosion-related brain injury is a new area of investigation. Although it is not yet proven that the changes in pressure that characterize the blast wave directly injure the brain as they do other parts of the body (eg, air-filled organs such as the lungs, tympanic membrane, and abdominal viscera), preliminary evidence suggests that this can occur.[18] It is clear that both the blast wave and the blast wind propel objects, including people, with sufficient power to cause TBI due to both linear and angular forces.

Vulnerable Areas and Injury Evolution

The most common primary injuries in TBI are traumatic axonal injury (TAI), contusion (bruising), and subdural hemorrhage. Movement of the brain within the skull can tear the surface veins that bridge from the brain to the dural venous sinus, resulting in a traumatic subdural hemorrhage (Figure 15-2).[19] The most common locations are the frontal and parietal convexities on the same side as the injury.[20] Subdural hemorrhage is crescent shaped on neuroimaging and conforms to the cerebral surface.[19,20] Its spread is limited by the dural reflections, and it rarely crosses the midline. When the brain moves within the skull enough to impact bone,

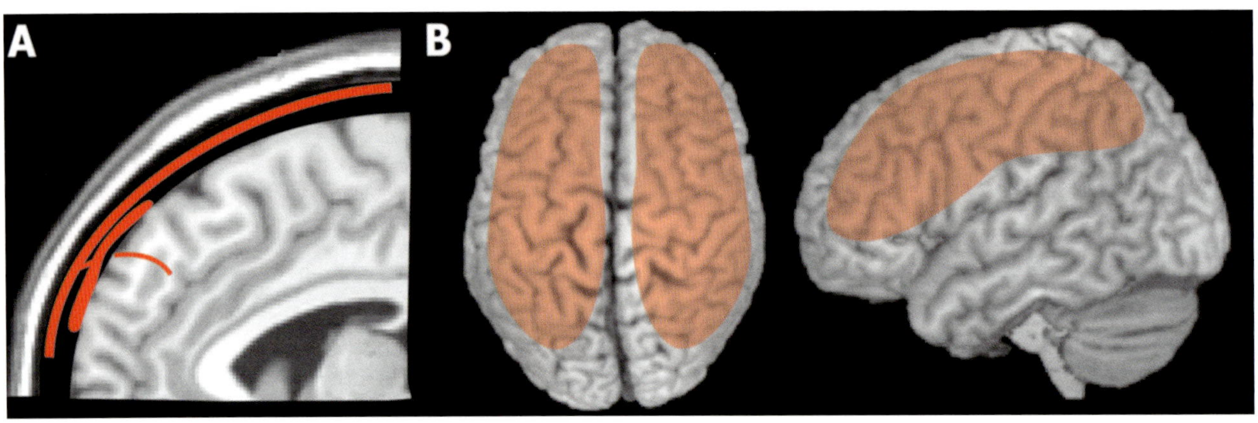

Figure 15-2. Traumatic subdural hemorrhage occurs when the brain moves within the skull enough to tear the vessels that bridge from the brain surface to the dural venous sinus (**a**). The most common locations are the frontal and parietal convexities on the same side as the injury (**b**).

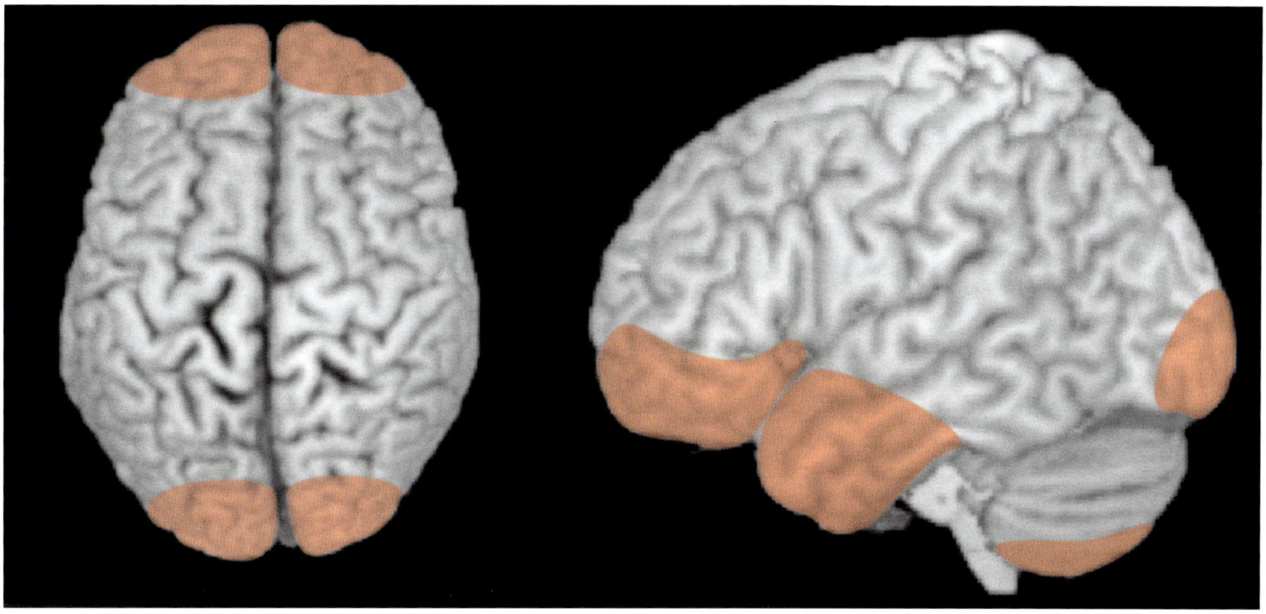

Figure 15-3. Contusions occur when the brain moves within the skull enough to impact bone, causing bruising. The most common locations are the superficial gray matter of the inferior, lateral, and anterior aspects of the frontal and temporal lobes, with the occipital poles or cerebellum less often involved.

it can cause contusion of the brain parenchyma (Figure 15-3). The most common locations are the superficial gray matter of the inferior, lateral, and anterior aspects of the frontal and temporal lobes; the occipital poles or cerebellum are less often involved.[20]

The most likely injury to occur in mTBI is TAI, also called diffuse axonal injury. Certain areas of the brain are particularly vulnerable to TAI (Figure 15-4). One is the corticomedullary (gray matter–white matter) junction, particularly in the frontal and temporal lobes. Areas of very concentrated white matter, such as the corpus callosum and internal capsule, are also quite vulnerable. Finally, the deep gray matter and upper brainstem are also frequent sites of TAI.[20] TAI is the result of shearing, stretching, or angular forces pulling on axons and small vessels.[21]

The old view of TAI was that these forces produced mechanical tearing of axons. Although this can occur, it is now considered to be unusual. The present understanding is that TAI is a progressive injury.[22,23] Stretching of the axon and its enclosing myelin sheath results in increased permeability, allowing an influx of calcium. This, in turn, triggers events that loosen the normally tight myelin sheath in the vicinity of the injury and also cause damage to the axon's cytoskeleton (a complex network of microtubules and neurofilaments that form the internal supporting structure for neurons).

The integrity of the cytoskeleton is essential for many vital functions, including transport of substances from the cell body out to the axon and dendrites

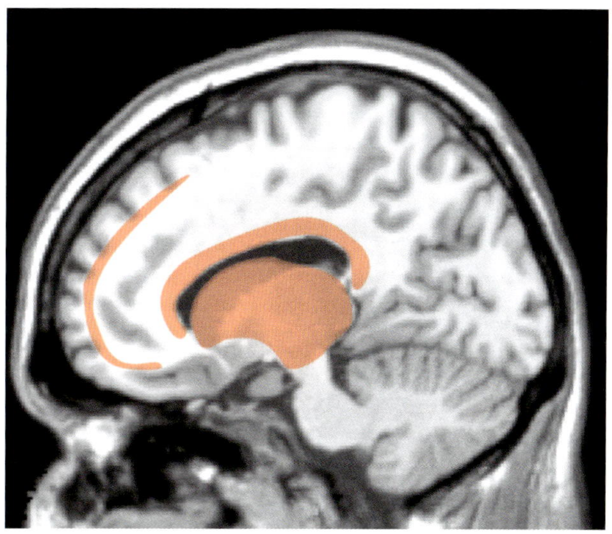

Figure 15-4. Traumatic axonal injury (TAI) results when shearing, stretching, or angular forces pull on axons and small vessels. Impaired axonal transport leads to focal axonal swelling and (after several hours) may result in axonal disconnection. The most common locations are the corticomedullary junctions (particularly frontotemporal), internal capsule, deep gray matter, upper brainstem, and corpus callosum.

(axoplasmic transport). Breakdown of the cytoskeleton disrupts transport of materials within the axon. Material collects proximal to the injury, leading to focal axonal swelling. If the swelling continues to progress, the axon eventually detaches. The proximal end seals and continues to swell, leading to the formation of the classic axonal retraction ball. The distal portion of the axon undergoes Wallerian degeneration, a process that can take several months in humans.[24] (This account is based primarily on the study of heavily myelinated, large-diameter axons, such as those that make up the majority of the corpus callosum and internal capsule.)

Growing evidence suggests that the injury cascade may be quite different in other populations of axons (eg, small-diameter, unmyelinated axons) and vulnerable areas (eg, injuries close to cell bodies, as occurs at the corticomedullary junction and in deep gray matter).[24] This has important implications both for neuropathological identification of TAI and for potential therapeutic targets.[24] Secondary processes can cause further brain injury.[24–27] For example, there may be a widespread release of glutamate (an excitatory neurotransmitter), with the potential for lethal overstimulation of neurons (excitotoxicity). Release of blood into brain tissue has toxic effects, including the possibility of triggering cerebral vasospasm, which increases the risk for ischemia.

DETERMINING SEVERITY OF TRAUMATIC BRAIN INJURY

Structural Neuroimaging

TAI is characterized by multiple small injuries, often widely dispersed in the brain rather than clustered. As a result, its identification on structural neuroimaging can be quite challenging. Although magnetic resonance imaging (MRI) is more sensitive than computed tomography in detecting this type of brain injury, even MRI is often negative.[20,22,28–31] Gradient-echo MRI is especially useful because it can visualize even very small areas of hemorrhage, as often occur in conjunction with axonal injury.[32–36] This type of MRI is sensitive to alterations in magnetic susceptibility. Presence of blood within tissue creates a local magnetic field disturbance, causing a decrease in signal intensity in the area containing blood. Areas of TAI not containing hemorrhage are better seen on T2*-weighted spin-echo MRI, where they will appear bright. Particularly useful is the FLAIR (fluid attenuated inversion recovery) sequence, in which the normally high signal intensity of cerebrospinal fluid is suppressed, making lesions near the ventricles much easier to identify.[37] A newer method of MRI that shows great promise for improved imaging of TAI is diffusion tensor imaging, in which the image is made sensitive to the speed and direction of water diffusion.[38,39] In gray matter and fluid, water diffuses at the same speed in all directions (isotropic diffusion). In white matter, water diffuses much more quickly along the length of axons (fibers, tracts) than across them (anisotropic diffusion). Thus, diffusion tensor imaging provides a way to examine the structural integrity of the white matter.

Combat-Related Traumatic Brain Injury

There is increasing evidence that combat-related TBIs are a frequent occurrence. Approximately one half of combat-related injuries, many a result of explosions, involve the head or neck.[40,41] Several studies from the DVBIC document the presence of TBI in soldiers returned from Afghanistan or Iraq.[42–45] Common postconcussive symptoms included headache (47%), irritability or aggression (45%), difficulty with memory (46%), and difficulty with concentration (41%).[43] Studies of active duty soldiers suggest that the majority of brain injuries would be classified as mild, as indicated by either no or only brief LOC.[44,46] In most cases these less severe injuries would not have required medical evacuation.[45]

It is well known that mTBI in civilians is underrecognized by both medical personnel and patients, resulting in significant underreporting.[47,48] A similar situation exists in the military in that combat-related mTBI may often be unrecognized by both medical personnel and service members.[44,46,49] DVBIC has recently released a new assessment tool—the Military Acute Concussion Evaluation (MACE)—to facilitate identification and evaluation of postconcussive symptoms following combat-related brain injuries. The literature on concussion strongly supports the need to fully evaluate anyone experiencing alteration in mental status (eg, dazed, confused, "saw stars," LOC) as a result of exposure to conditions that can injure the brain.[26] Of particular importance is evaluation of memory, as presence of PTA appears to be associated with higher rates of cognitive difficulties during the first few weeks after injury.[49]

Postconcussive symptoms may include altered consciousness (drowsiness, confusion, lethargy), headache, amnesia, nausea or vomiting, fatigue, irritability, restlessness, auditory or vestibular disturbances (balance problems, ringing in the ears, dizziness, hearing changes, sensitivity to noise), visual disturbances (blurred vision, sensitivity to light, double vision), gait abnormalities, and problems sleeping.[50,51] Although most patients recover well from mTBI, the rate of recovery is highly variable. During this period of healing individuals are likely to perform below their normal level on both physical and cognitive tasks. Evidence also suggests that the brain is more vulnerable to reinjury during this period. Therefore, in the context of active combat, premature return to duty increases risks for both the individual and the team.[26]

Many mild brain injuries will not become evident until after the service member returns home. Although the majority of people recover well following mTBI, a significant minority do not.[25] Common problems in the chronic phase following TBI include headaches, dizziness, fatigue, sleep disturbances, spasticity, vestibular impairments, visual difficulties, personality changes, and cognitive or emotional deficits. Some studies indicate that as many as one third of these patients may have psychiatric symptoms within the first year postinjury.[52–54]

COMMON COGNITIVE SEQUELAE

An examination of cognitive dysfunction following TBI must take into account myriad factors, including severity and nature of the injury (focal vs diffuse), time since injury, motivation of the subject, and other injuries. In the case of mTBI, there is agreement that there are short-term cognitive consequences of the injury, affecting various aspects of attention, speed of processing, and other cognitive domains. Even in the absence of self-reported cognitive dysfunction or other symptoms, decrements in reaction time have been reported.[14] The longer-term cognitive consequences from mTBI are less clear.

Iverson and colleagues[55] report data on a group of young adult patients seen in the trauma service of a Pennsylvania general hospital (1991–1994) with mTBIs (based on postinjury GCS scores) who completed neuropsychological testing within the first week postinjury. Those who met severity inclusion criteria and were under age 40 accounted for 484 of the 1,695 total patients. Most were men, with motor vehicle accidents being the most common cause of injury. Most patients (82%) had GCS scores of 15, with the remaining ones having GCS scores of 14. About 56% had known LOC, with about 18% negative, and the rest unclear or unknown. The prevalence of intracranial abnormalities on day-of-injury computed tomography was 11.8%. The rest of these patients had negative (68.6%) or missing (19.6%) results. The patients were split into two groups on the basis of differences on the Galveston Orientation and Amnesia Test (GOAT). The groups were relatively evenly split by scores above 90 and those below (range 0–100). Scores between 90 and 75 are not low enough to indicate frank PTA, but do suggest some ongoing confusion. All those patients were administered a brief (30–45 minutes) but wide-ranging neuropsychological test battery. Overall, the results suggested that when trauma patients are evaluated shortly after an mTBI, the presence of posttraumatic confusion is related to worse short-term neuropsychological outcome in that subjects with lower GOAT scores had significantly worse scores on measures of simple attention, verbal learning, verbal and visual memory, and some aspects of executive functioning than did subjects in the above-90 range on GOAT. Furthermore, brief traumatic LOC (less than 5 minutes) is not related to short-term neuropsychological outcome (there were no significant differences in scores based solely on whether or not there was brief LOC).

Belanger and colleagues[56] conducted a metaanalysis of the relevant literature based on 39 studies involving 1,463 cases of mTBI and 1,191 control cases to determine the impact of mTBI across nine cognitive domains—(1) global cognitive ability, (2) attention, (3) executive functions, (4) fluency, (5) memory acquisition, (6) delayed memory, (7) language, (8) visuospatial skill, and (9) motor functions. The overall effect of mTBI on neuropsychological functioning was moderate ($d = .54$). However, findings were influenced by cognitive domain, time since injury, patient characteristics, and sampling methods. Acute effects (less than 3 months postinjury) of mTBI were greatest for delayed memory and fluency. In unselected or prospective samples, the overall analysis revealed no residual neuropsychological impairment by 3 months postinjury. In contrast, clinic-based samples and samples including participants in litigation were associated with greater cognitive sequelae of mTBI.

In another metaanalysis focused on the sports concussion literature, the authors reviewed studies from 1970 to 2004 from which 21 studies met inclusion criteria, with 790 cases of mTBI and 2,016 control cases.[57] The overall effect for size of concussion on cognition was 0.49, with delayed memory, memory acquisition, and global cognitive functioning showing the greatest effects acutely. No residual effects were found from the group tested over 1 week postinjury.

Postconcussive Disorder

A WHO analysis of outcome in mTBI concludes that although acute symptoms are common, the vast majority of individuals have good resolution of their mTBI symptoms by 3 months postinjury and many quite sooner.[58] The authors acknowledge (and this is consistent with clinical practice in both military and civilian settings) that there are individuals who show persistent symptoms. The fourth edition of the *Diagnostic and Statistical Manual for Mental Disorders* proposed diagnostic criteria for a postconcussional disorder in its appendix of provisional diagnostic criteria sets.[10] Diagnosis of a postconcussional disorder required a "significant cerebral concussion" with measured cognitive deficit and the presence of at least three of eight symptoms—(1) fatigue, (2) sleep disturbance, (3) headache, (4) dizziness, (5) irritability, (6) anxiety/depression, (7) personality change, and (8) apathy—with onset after injury and persistence past 3 months. (See Exhibit 15-1 for full criteria for postconcussional disorder.) Criteria have also been included in the *International Classification of Diseases, 10th Revision* (ICD-10).[59] These criteria require a history of TBI and the presence of three of eight symptoms—(1) headache, (2) dizziness, (3) fatigue, (4) irritability, (5) insomnia, (6) concentration problems, (7) memory difficulty, and (8) reduced tolerance of stress, emotion, or alcohol.

Boake et al[60] compared these two diagnostic sets and concluded that there was a large difference between the prevalence of postconcussive syndrome using these two criteria sets, with the ICD-10 criteria being more inclusive. The differences suggest that there could be disagreement in diagnosis depending on which criteria set is used. Furthermore, they concluded that both criteria sets had limited specificity to TBI (if the history of TBI itself was removed as a criteria), as the other criteria could be met after general trauma, whether or not the brain was injured. The authors point out that this finding is supportive of previous CDC recommendations—namely that postconcussional symptoms in themselves are not sufficient to make a diagnosis of mTBI. Iverson and colleagues,[61] in a review article on outcome from mTBI, also report that postconcussion symptoms are common in healthy subjects, those without a history of TBI, and in various patient groups.

The existence of a group of patients with persistent symptoms has been controversial. The scope of the problem itself is difficult to determine (clinical lore has set the figure at 10%–20% although it is likely less than 5% of the total number of individuals who suffer mTBI; see Iverson[55] for a complete discussion). There is also disagreement concerning the cause of these persistent symptoms. Various authors have attributed them to different causes, some believing them to reflect the injury itself, and others attributing these symptoms to a multicausal etiology, with premorbid personality characteristics, social-psychological factors, and exaggeration

EXHIBIT 15-1

RESEARCH CRITERIA FOR POST-CONCUSSIONAL DISORDER

A. History of closed head injury:
- Causing cerebral concussion
- Symptoms include:
  - loss of consciousness
  - posttraumatic amnesia
  - posttraumatic onset of seizuers (less common)

B. Difficulty (based on cognitive evaluation) in:
- attention, such as:
  - concentration
  - shifting focus of attention
  - performing simultaneous cognitive tasks

  or
- memory, such as:
  - learning
  - recalling information

C. Three or more of the following occuring post-trauma (and lasting 3 or more months):
- easy fatigue
- disordered sleep
- headache
- vertigo/dizziness
- irritability/aggression on little or no provocation
- anxiety/depression/affective lability
- changes in personality
- apathy/lack of spontaneity

D. "B" and "C" symptoms:
- have onset following head trauma

  or
- represent a substantial worsening of preexisting symptoms

E. Disturbance causes significant impairment/significant worsening in:
- social/occupational functioning (adults)
- school/academic performance (school-age children)

F. Symptoms do not meet criteria for/not better accounted for by:
- dementia due to head trauma
- another mental disorder such as:
  - amnestic disorder due to head trauma
  - personality change due to head trauma

Adapted with permission from American Psychiatric Association. *Diagnostic and Statistical Manual*. 4th ed. Washington, DC: APA; 2000: 761–762.

(either conscious or unconscious) playing a role.

The Relationship Between Posttraumatic Stress Disorder and Traumatic Brain Injury

Posttraumatic stress disorder (PTSD) can result from highly stressful experiences, such as being in combat or being injured in combat. Hoge and colleagues[62] reported that for all groups surveyed after their deployment, there was a strong relationship between intensity of combat experiences (killing the enemy, being shot at) and exposure to traumatic combat-related events (handling dead bodies, knowing someone who was killed), and the prevalence of PTSD. Among service members in OIF, the prevalence of PTSD increased with the number of firefights during deployment (with increases to 19.3% for those involved in more than five firefights). The rates of PTSD were significantly associated with having been wounded or injured (odds ratio for those deployed to Iraq, 3.27; odds ratio for those deployed to Afghanistan, 2.49). This is consistent with the findings of Koren et al[63] in a small but well-designed study looking at rates of PTSD in injured Israeli war veterans. That study clearly indicated that bodily injury is a risk factor for PTSD, with odds of developing PTSD following traumatic injury approximately eight times higher than following injury-free emotional trauma. The authors suggest that even this rather high figure might be an underestimate of the rate because 35% of these injured combat veterans had refused to participate in the study.

Controversy exists, however, regarding the rate and risk factors for PTSD following TBI. Bombardier and colleagues[64] report a cumulative rate of 11.3% in a mixed sample of those with TBI ranging from mild to severe over a 6-month period. Furthermore, their findings were consistent with those of previous studies suggesting that more severe TBI may be protective with regard to the development of PTSD, that is, the AOC or LOC associated with TBI may lessen the individual's ability to reexperience the trauma.[65] Risk factors for developing PTSD following TBI include having less education, feeling terrified or helpless, and having major depression.[64]

In-Theater Management

The in-theater management of TBI depends on its severity. (There are guidelines recently released on the management of more severe combat TBI,[66] but in-depth discussion of these guidelines is beyond the scope of this chapter.) The clinical management of the mTBI patient in a military occupational setting was addressed in the 2006 DVBIC workgroup. A graphical representation of the level-I practice guideline is shown in Figure 15-5. This guideline relies on the use of the MACE (see Exhibit 15-2 for full instrument), a tool developed by the DVBIC. The MACE has both a history and evaluation component. The history component can confirm the diagnosis of mTBI after establishing that a trauma has occurred and during the course of this traumatic event, the service member experienced an AOC. An AOC can be defined on a continuum from "dazed and confused," to not remembering the injury, to an LOC. The evaluation component, designed to be easily used by medics and corpsmen, can be administered within 5 minutes. It utilizes the Standardized Assessment of Concussion[67] to preliminarily document neurocognitive deficits in four cognitive domains: (1) orientation, (2) immediate memory, (3) concentration, and (4) delayed recall.

The Relationship Between Substance Abuse and Traumatic Brain Injury

The relationship between TBI and substance use and abuse is an important one that presents a number of complexities for understanding their interrelatedness. Intoxication is in itself a risk factor for TBI. That is, TBI can result from unintentional alcohol-related causes such as motor vehicle accidents or falls while intoxicated. More intentional alcohol-related TBI can result from other causes such as assault while intoxicated (both on the part of the victim and perpetrator), mate-related abuse, and direct self-harm such as suicide attempts.[1] Savola, Niemelä, and Hillbom[68] investigated the relationship of different patterns of alcohol intake to various types of trauma. They examined the alcohol consumption in a series of 385 consecutive trauma admissions. On admission, 51% of the patients had alcohol in their blood. Binge drinking was the predominant (78%) drinking pattern of alcohol intake, and assaults, falls, and biking accidents were the most frequent causes of trauma. Dependent alcohol drinking and binge drinking were found to be significantly more common among patients with head trauma than in those with other types of trauma. The relative risk for head injury markedly increased with increasing blood alcohol levels.

A TBI can also exacerbate previous substance abuse or lead to behavioral and personality changes that could lead to alcohol or drug misuse. Prior history of a substance abuse disorder is a risk factor for greater morbidity[69] and excessive use following TBI.[70] Substance-use disorders following TBI adversely affect neuropsychological functioning, subjective well-being, employment, and involvement with the criminal justice system.[71–74]

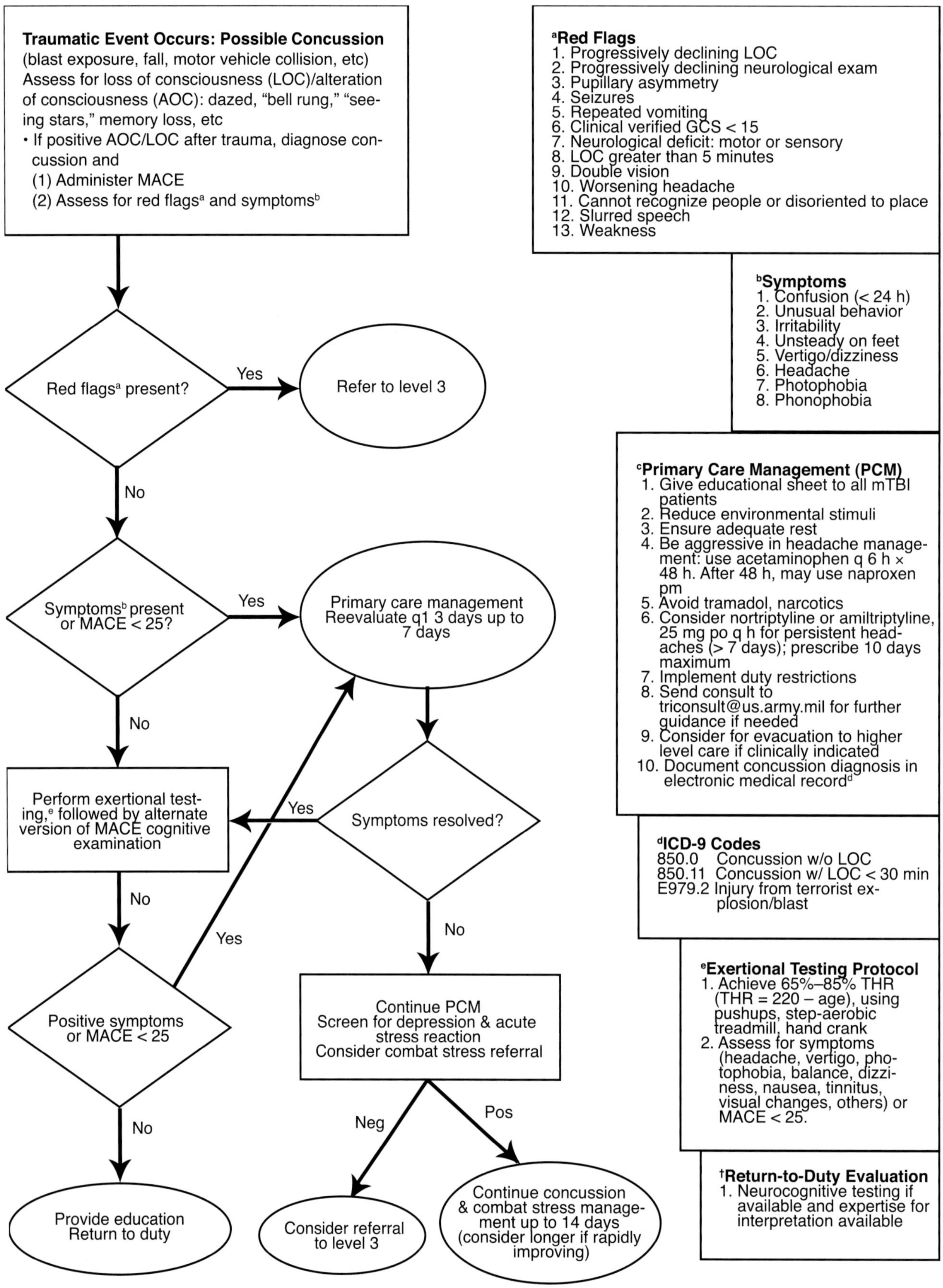
Traumatic Event Occurs: Possible Concussion
(blast exposure, fall, motor vehicle collision, etc)
Assess for loss of consciousness (LOC)/alteration of consciousness (AOC): dazed, "bell rung," "seeing stars," memory loss, etc
• If positive AOC/LOC after trauma, diagnose concussion and
(1) Administer MACE
(2) Assess for red flags[a] and symptoms[b]
Red flags[a] present?
Yes
Refer to level 3
No
Symptoms[b] present or MACE < 25?
Yes
Primary care management Reevaluate q1 3 days up to 7 days
No
Symptoms resolved?
Yes
Perform exertional testing,[e] followed by alternate version of MACE cognitive examination
No
Yes
Positive symptoms or MACE < 25
No
Provide education Return to duty
No
Continue PCM
Screen for depression & acute stress reaction
Consider combat stress referral
Neg
Pos
Consider referral to level 3
Continue concussion & combat stress management up to 14 days (consider longer if rapidly improving)
[a]Red Flags
1. Progressively declining LOC
2. Progressively declining neurological exam
3. Pupillary asymmetry
4. Seizures
5. Repeated vomiting
6. Clinical verified GCS < 15
7. Neurological deficit: motor or sensory
8. LOC greater than 5 minutes
9. Double vision
10. Worsening headache
11. Cannot recognize people or disoriented to place
12. Slurred speech
13. Weakness
[b]Symptoms
1. Confusion (< 24 h)
2. Unusual behavior
3. Irritability
4. Unsteady on feet
5. Vertigo/dizziness
6. Headache
7. Photophobia
8. Phonophobia
[c]Primary Care Management (PCM)
1. Give educational sheet to all mTBI patients
2. Reduce environmental stimuli
3. Ensure adequate rest
4. Be aggressive in headache management: use acetaminophen q 6 h × 48 h. After 48 h, may use naproxen pm
5. Avoid tramadol, narcotics
6. Consider nortriptyline or amiltriptyline, 25 mg po q h for persistent headaches (> 7 days); prescribe 10 days maximum
7. Implement duty restrictions
8. Send consult to triconsult@us.army.mil for further guidance if needed
9. Consider for evacuation to higher level care if clinically indicated
10. Document concussion diagnosis in electronic medical record[d]
[d]ICD-9 Codes
850.0 Concussion w/o LOC
850.11 Concussion w/ LOC < 30 min
E979.2 Injury from terrorist explosion/blast
[e]Exertional Testing Protocol
1. Achieve 65%–85% THR (THR = 220 – age), using pushups, step-aerobic treadmill, hand crank
2. Assess for symptoms (headache, vertigo, photophobia, balance, dizziness, nausea, tinnitus, visual changes, others) or MACE < 25.
[f]Return-to-Duty Evaluation
1. Neurocognitive testing if available and expertise for interpretation available

Figure 15-5 (left page). Initial management of concussion in a deployed seting. Defense and Veterans Brain Injury Center decision algorithm for battlefield mild traumatic brain injury at a Level I setting. Definitive assessment and care is given by providers to include a more detailed assessment, management recommendations, and consideration for evacuation to a higher level of care.

AOC: alteration of consciousness
GCS: Glasgow Coma Scale
HS: at bedtime
ICD-9: International Statistical Classification of Diseases, 9th edition
LOC: loss of consciousness
MACE: Military Acute Concussion Evaluation
mTBI: mild traumatic brain injury
po: by mouth
q: every
THR: target heart rate
w/: with
w/o: without

Reproduced from: US Army Institute of Surgical Research. Joint Theater Trauma System Web site. Available at: http://www.usaisr.amedd.army.mil/cpgs/mTBIDplydSet0811.pdf. Accessed December 15, 2009.

SYMPTOM TREATMENT

Symptom treatment for mTBI can be discussed from four areas: (1) pharmacologic management, (2) educational interventions, (3) rest/return-to-duty decisions, and (4) targeted therapies. An extensive discussion of the pharmacologic interventions in TBI is beyond the scope of this chapter. The reader is referred to reviews of the evidence for various pharmacologic interventions.[45,73–76] In general, however, symptomatic treatment strategies can be the most effective, including regulation of sleep through pharmacologic and nonpharmacologic strategies,[77] headache management,[78] pain management,[79] and treatment of depression.[80] Treatment of all of these has been associated with improved quality of life or outcomes.

Educational Interventions

Educational and psychological therapies have also proven effective in mTBI. Mittenberg et al[81] compared two mTBI groups: a treatment group (n = 29) and a control group (n = 29). The treatment group received a printed manual and met with a therapist prior to hospital discharge to review (*a*) the nature and incidence of expected symptoms, (*b*) the cognitive-behavioral model of symptom maintenance and treatment, (*c*) techniques for reducing symptoms, and (*d*) instructions for gradual resumption of premorbid activities. The control group received routine hospital treatment and discharge instructions. After 6 months, the treated patients reported significantly shorter average symptom duration (33 days vs 51 days) and significantly fewer symptoms at follow-up. The conclusion was that brief, early psychological interventions are effective in reducing the incidence of postconcussive symptoms. Ponsford and colleagues[82] have shown similar results in a group of individuals with mTBI. Those who were seen at 1 week postinjury and given informational material reported fewer symptoms overall and were significantly less stressed at 3 months after the injury than a group that did not receive the same education. A number of educational materials effective for individuals with brain injuries and their families are available at a number of sources including the Defense and Veterans Brain Injury center Web site (www.dvbic.org/cms.php?p=Education).

Rest and Return-to-Duty Issues

Other palliative interventions such as bed rest have been shown to have some efficacy in treating postconcussive symptoms over the short term (eg, decreased dizziness), but have not proven to have long-term outcomes better than individuals who did not get such rest.[83] Return-to-duty issues in the military operational setting are addressed in the algorithm above (see Figure 15-5). Most of the decisions are based on the resolution of self-reported TBI symptoms as well as the integration of clinical data based on testing a service member to see if symptoms may return when physically stressed.

SUMMARY

In modern warfare, TBI is a common occurrence that has significant implications for the health and welfare of the troops, as well as overall fighting effectiveness. Early identification of less obvious (usually milder) TBI is important, as is a basic understanding of when individuals may be treated in situ and ways to maximize recovery. Even in peacetime, there are concerns about TBI because it occurs at high rates in the military. It is essential, therefore, that healthcare providers and the fighting force both have a basic understanding of the need for prevention of these injuries, and early identification when they do occur.

EXHIBIT 15-2

MILITARY ACUTE CONCUSSION EVALUATION FORM

Military Acute Concussion Evaluation (MACE)

Defense and Veterans Brain Injury Center

Patient Name: ______________________

SS#: ______-______-______ **Unit:** __________

Date of Injury: ____/____/____

Time of Injury: __________

Examiner: ______________________

Date of Evaluation: ____/____/____

Time of Evaluation: __________

History: (I – VIII)

I. **Description of Incident**

Ask:

a) What happened?

b) Tell me what you remember.

c) Were you dazed, confused, "saw stars"?

❒ Yes ❒ No

d) Did you hit your head? ❒ Yes ❒ No

II. Cause of Injury (Circle all that apply):

1) Explosion/Blast 4) Fragment

2) Blunt object 5) Fall

3) Motor Vehicle Crash 6) Gunshot wound

7) Other ______________

III. Was a helmet worn? ❒ Yes ❒ No

Type ______________

IV. Amnesia Before: Are there any events just BEFORE the injury that are not remembered? (Assess for continuous memory prior to injury)

❒ Yes ❒ No If yes, how long ________

V. Amnesia After: Are there any events just AFTER the injuries that are not remembered? (Assess time until continuous memory after the injury)

❒ Yes ❒ No If yes, how long ________

VI. Does the individual report loss of consciousness or "blacking out"?

❒ Yes ❒ No If yes, how long ________

VII. Did anyone observe a period of loss of consciousness or unresponsiveness?

❒ Yes ❒ No If yes, how long ________

VIII. Symptoms (circle all that apply)

1) Headache 2) Dizziness

3) Memory Problems 4) Balance problems

5) Nausea/Vomiting 6) Difficulty Concentrating

7) Irritability 8) Visual Disturbances

9) Ringing in the ears 10) Other __________

Examination: (IX – XIII)

Evaluate each domain. Total possible score is 30.

IX. Orientation (1 point each)

Month:	0	1
Date:	0	1
Day of Week:	0	1
Year:	0	1
Time:	0	1

Orientation Total Score ____/5

08/2006 DVBIC.org 800-870-9244

This form may be copied for clinical use.

(Exhibit 15-2 *continues*)

Exhibit 15-2 *continued*

Military Acute Concussion Evaluation (MACE)

Defense and Veterans Brain Injury Center

X. Immediate Memory:

Read all 5 words and ask the patient to recall them in any order. Repeat two more times for a total of three trials.

(1 point for each correct, total over 3 trials)

List	Trial 1		Trial 2		Trial 3	
Elbow	0	1	0	1	0	1
Apple	0	1	0	1	0	1
Carpet	0	1	0	1	0	1
Saddle	0	1	0	1	0	1
Bubble	0	1	0	1	0	1
Trial Score						

Immediate Memory Total Score ______/15

XI. Neurological Screening

As the clinical condition permits, check

Eyes: pupillary response and tracking

Verbal: speech fluency and word finding

Motor: pronator drift, gait/coordination

Record any abnormalities. **No points are given for this.**

XII. Concentration

Reverse Digits: (go to next string length if correct on first trial. Stop if incorrect on both trials.) 1 pt. for each string length.

4-9-3	6-2-9	0	1
3-8-1-4	3-2-7-9	0	1
6-2-9-7-1	1-5-2-8-5	0	1
7-1-8-4-6-2	5-3-9-1-4-8	0	1

Months in reverse order:

(1 pt. for entire sequence correct)

Dec-Nov-Oct-Sep-Aug-Jul

Jun-May-Apr-Mar-Feb-Jan 0 1

Concentration Total Score ____/5

XIII. Delayed Recall (1 pt. each)

Ask the patient to recall the 5 words from the earlier memory test (Do NOT reread the word list.)

Elbow	0	1
Apple	0	1
Carpet	0	1
Saddle	0	1
Bubble	0	1

Delayed Recall Total Score ____/5

TOTAL SCORE ______/30

Notes: ______________________________________

____

____

____

____

____

____

Diagnosis: (circle one or write in diagnoses)

No concussion

850.0 Concussion without

Loss of Consciousness (LOC)

850.1 Concussion with

Loss of Consciousness (LOC)

Other diagnoses ____________________________

____

McCrea, M., Kelly, J. & Randolph, C. (2000). *Standardized Assessment of Concussion (SAC): Manual for Administration, Scoring, and Interpretation.* (2nd ed.) Waukesa,WI: Authors.

Defense & Veterans Brain Injury Center
1-800-870-9244 or DSN: 662-6345

Reproduced from: Defense and Veterans Brain Injury Center, Walter Reed Army Medical Center. Military Acute Concussion Evaluaton (MACE) form.

REFERENCES

1. Langlois JA, Rutland-Brown W, Thomas KE. *Traumatic Brain Injury in the United States: Emergency Department Visits, Hospitalizations, and Deaths.* Atlanta, Ga: Centers for Disease Control and Prevention, National Center for Injury Prevention and Control; 2004.

2. Lewin I. *The Cost of Disorders of the Brain*. Washington, DC: The National Foundation for the Brain; 1992.

3. Centers for Disease Control. *Traumatic Brain Injury in the United States: A Report to Congress*. Atlanta, Ga: Centers for Disease Control; 2001.

4. Ommaya AK, Ommaya AK, Dannenberg AL, Salazar AM. Causation, incidence, and costs of traumatic brain injury in the US military medical system. *J Trauma*. 1996;40(2):211–217.

5. Ivins BJ, Schwab KA, Baker K, Warden DL. Hospital admissions associated with traumatic brain injury in the US Army during peacetime: 1990s trends. *Neuroepidemiol*. 2006;27:154–163.

6. Operation Iraqi Freedom (OIF) US casualty status. Available at http://www.defenselink.mil/news/casualty.pdf. Accessed May 16, 2007.

7. Armonda RA, Bell RS, Vo AH, et al. Wartime traumatic cerebral vasospasm: recent review of combat casualties. *Neurosurg*. 2006;59(6):1215–1225.

8. Langlois JA, Rutland-Brown W, Thomas KE. Traumatic brain injury in the United States: emergency department visits, hospitalizations, and deaths. Atlanta, Ga: US Department of Health and Human Services, Centers for Disease Control and Prevention; 2004.

9. Kay T, Harrington DE, Adams R, et al. Definition of mild traumatic brain injury. *J Head Trauma Rehabil*. 1993;8:86–87.

10. American Psychiatric Association. *Diagnostic and Statistical Manual of Mental Disorders*. 4th ed. Washington, DC: APA; 1994.

11. Borg J, Holm L, Peloso PM, et al. Non-surgical intervention and cost for mild traumatic brain injury: results of the WHO Collaborating Centre Task Force on Mild Traumatic Brain Injury. *J Rehabil Med*. 2004;43(Suppl):76–83.

12. Helmick K, Guskiewicz K, Barth J, et al. Acute management of mild traumatic brain injury in military operational settings. *Clin Pract Guide*. December 2006. Available at: http://www.dvbic.org. Accessed June 1, 2007.

13. Guskiewicz KM, Bruce SL, Cantu RC, et al. National Athletic Trainers' Association position statement: management of sport-related concussion. *J Athl Train*. 2004;39(3):280–297.

14. McCrory P, Johnson K, Meeuwisse W, et al. Summary and agreement statement of the 2nd International Conference of Concussion in Sport, Prague 2004. *Clin J Sport Med*. 2005;15(2):48–55.

15. Warden DL, Bleiberg J, Cameron KL, et al. Persistent prolongation of simple reaction time in sports concussion. *Neurol*. 2001;57:524–526.

16. Williams DH, Levin HS, Eisenberg HM, et al. Mild head injury classification. *Neurosurg*. 1990;27(3):422–428.

17. Hsiang J, Yeung T, Yu AL, Poon WS. High-risk mild head injury. *J Neurosurg*. 1997;87(2):234–238.

18. Taber KH, Warden DL, Hurley RA. Blast-related traumatic brain injury: what is known? *J Neuropsychiatry Clin Neurosci*. 2006;18:141–145.

19. Taber KH, Hayman LA, Diaz-Marchan PJ, Rauch RA. Imaging of intracranial blood. In: Latchaw RE, Kucharczyk J, Moseley ME, eds. *Imaging of the Nervous System: Diagnostic and Therapeutic Applications*. Philadelphia, Penn: Elsevier Mosby Inc; 2005: 555–575.

20. Gutierrez-Cadavid JE. Imaging of head trauma. In: Latchaw RE, Kucharczyk J, Moseley ME, eds. *Imaging of the Nervous System: Diagnostic and Therapeutic Applications*. Philadelphia, Penn: Elsevier Mosby Inc; 2005: 869–904.

21. Mendez CV, Hurley RA, Lassonde M, Zhang L, Taber KH. Mild traumatic brain injury: neuroimaging of sports-related concussion. *J Neuropsychiatry Clin Neurosci.* 2005;17:297–303.

22. Hurley RA, McGowan JC, Arfanakis K, Taber KH. Traumatic axonal injury: novel insights into evolution and identification. *J Neuropsychiatry Clin Neurosci.* 2004;16:1–7.

23. Povlishock JT, Katz DI. Update of neuropathology and neurological recovery after traumatic brain injury. *J Head Trauma Rehabil.* 2005;20:76–94.

24. Büki A, Povlishock JT. All roads lead to disconnection?—traumatic axonal injury revisited. *Acta Neurochir (Wien).* 2006;148:181–193.

25. Bazarian JJ, Blyth B, Cimpello L. Bench to bedside: evidence for brain injury after concussion—looking beyond the computed tomography scan. *Acad Emerg Med.* 2006;13:199–214.

26. Lovell M, Collins M, Pardini JE, Parodi A, Yates A. Management of cerebral concussion in military personnel: lessons learned from sports medicine. *Oper Tech Sports Med.* 2005;13:212–221.

27. Yi JH, Hazell AS. Excitotoxic mechanisms and the role of astrocytic glutamate transporters in traumatic brain injury. *Neurochem Int.* 2006;48:394–403.

28. Le TH, Gean AD. Imaging of head trauma. *Semin Roentgenol.* 2006;41:177–189.

29. Brandstack N, Kurki T, Tenovuo O, Isoniemi H. MR imaging of head trauma: visibility of contusions and other intraparenchymal injuries in early and late stage. *Brain Inj.* 2006;20:409–416.

30. Kurca E, Sivák S, Kucera P. Impaired cognitive functions in mild traumatic brain injury patients with normal and pathologic magnetic resonance imaging. *Neuroradiol.* 2006;48:661–668.

31. Shin YB, Kim SJ, Kim IJ, et al. Voxel-based statistical analysis of cerebral blood flow using Tc-99m ECD brain SPECT in patients with traumatic brain injury: group and individual analyses. *Brain Inj.* 2006;20:661–667.

32. Tong KA, Ashwal S, Holshouser BA, et al. Hemorrhagic shearing lesions in children and adolescents with posttraumatic diffuse axonal injury: improved detection and initial results. *Radiol.* 2003;227:332–339.

33. Kuzma BB, Goodman JM. Improved identification of axonal shear injuries with gradient echo MR technique. *Surg Neurol.* 2000;53:400–402.

34. Huisman TA, Sorensen AG, Hergan K, Gonzalez RG, Schaefer PW. Diffusion-weighted imaging for the evaluation of diffuse axonal injury in closed head injury. *J Comput Assist Tomogr.* 2003;27:5–11.

35. Yanagawa Y, Tsushima Y, Tokumaru A, et al. A quantitative analysis of head injury using T2*-weighted gradient-echo imaging. *J Trauma.* 2000;49:272–277.

36. Scheid R, Preul G, Gruber O, Wiggins C, von Cramon DY. Diffuse axonal injury associated with chronic traumatic brain injury: evidence from T2*-weighted gradient-echo imaging at 3 T. *Am J Neuroradiol.* 2003;24:1049–1056.

37. Paterakis K, Karantanas AH, Komnos A, Volikas Z. Outcome of patients with diffuse axonal injury: the significance and prognostic value of MRI in the acute phase. *J Trauma.* 2000;49:1071–1075.

38. Taber KH, Pierpaoli C, Rose SE, et al. The future for diffusion tensor imaging in neuropsychiatry. *J Neuropsychiatry Clin Neurosci.* 2002;14:1–5.

39. Sundgren PC, Dong Q, Gómez-Hasssan D, Mukherji SK, Maly P, Welsh R. Diffusion tensor imaging of the brain: review of clinical applications. *Neuroradiol.* 2004;46:339–350.

40. Murray CK, Reynolds JC, Schroeder JM, Harrison MB, Evans OM, Hospenthal DR. Spectrum of care provided at an echelon II Medical Unit during Operation Iraqi Freedom. *Mil Med.* 2005;170:516–520.

41. Gondusky JS, Reiter MP. Protecting military convoys in Iraq: an examination of battle injuries sustained by a mechanized battalion during Operation Iraqi Freedom II. *Mil Med.* 2005;170:546–549.

42. Okie S. Traumatic brain injury in the war zone. *N Engl J Med.* 2005;352:2043–2047.

43. Warden DL, Ryan LM, Helmick KM, et al. War neurotrauma: the Defense and Veterans Brain Injury Center (DVBIC) experience at Walter Reed Army Medical Center (WRAMC). *J Neurotrauma* 2005;22:1178.

44. Schwab KA, Baker G, Ivins BJ, Sluss-Tiller M, Lux W, Warden DL. The Brief Traumatic Brain Injury Screen (BTBIS): investigating the validity of a self-report instrument for detecting traumatic brain injury (TBI) in troops returning from deployment in Afghanistan and Iraq. *Neurology.* 2006;66:A235.

45. Warden DL. Military TBI during the Iraq and Afghanistan wars. *J Head Trauma Rehabil.* 2006;21:398–402.

46. Ivins BJ, Schwab KA, Warden D, et al. Traumatic brain injury in US Army paratroopers: prevalence and character. *J Trauma.* 2003;55:617–621.

47. Langlois JA, Rutland-Brown W, Wald MM. The epidemiology and impact of traumatic brain injury: a brief overview. *J Head Trauma Rehabil.* 2006;21:375–378.

48. Setnik L, Bazarian JJ. The characteristics of patients who do not seek medical treatment for traumatic brain injury. *Brain Inj.* 2007;21:1–9.

49. Drake AI, McDonald EC, Magnus NE, Gray N, Gottshall K. Utility of Glasgow Coma Scale-Extended in symptom prediction following mild traumatic brain injury. *Brain Inj.* 2006;20:469–475.

50. Kennedy JE, Lumpkin RJ, Grissom JR. A survey of mild traumatic brain injury treatment in the emergency room and primary care medical clinics. *Mil Med.* 2006;171:516–521.

51. Potter S, Leigh E, Wade D, Fleminger S. The Rivermead Post Concussion Symptoms Questionnaire: a confirmatory factor analysis. *J Neurol.* 2006;253:1603–1614.

52. Fann JR, Burington B, Leonetti A, Jaffe K, Katon WJ, Thompson RS. Psychiatric illness following traumatic brain injury in an adult health maintenance organization population. *Arch Gen Psychiatry.* 2004;61:53–61.

53. Deb S, Lyons I, Koutzoukis C. Neuropsychiatric sequelae one year after a minor head injury. *J Neurol Neurosurg Psychiatry.* 1998;65:899–902.

54. Deb S, Burns J. Neuropsychiatric consequences of traumatic brain injury: a comparison between two age groups. *Brain Inj.* 2007;21(3):301–307.

55. Iverson GL, Lange RT, Gaetz M, Zasler ND. Mild TBI. In: Zasler ND, Katz DI, Zafonte RD, eds. *Brain Injury Medicine: Principles and Practice.* New York, NY: Demos Medical Publishing; 2006: 333–371.

56. Belanger HG, Curtiss G, Demery JA, Lebowitz BK, Vanderploeg RD. Factors moderating neuropsychological outcomes following mild traumatic brain injury: a meta-analysis . *J Int Neuropsychol Soc.* 2005;11(3):215–227.

57. Belanger HG, Vanderploeg RD. The neuropsychological impact of sports-related concussion: a meta-analysis . *J Int Neuropsychol Soc.* 2005;11:345–357.

58. Carroll LJ, Cassidy JD, Peloso PM, et al. Prognosis for mild traumatic brain injury: results of the WHO Collaborating Centre Task Force on Mild Traumatic Brain Injury. *J Rehabil Med.* 2004;36:84–105.

59. World Health Organization. *The ICD-10 Classification of Mental and Behavioural Disorders: Clinical Descriptions and Diagnostic Guidelines*. Geneva, Switzerland: WHO; 1992.

60. Boake C, McCauley SR, Levin HS, et al. Diagnostic criteria for postconcussional syndrome after mild to moderate traumatic brain injury. *J Neuropsychiatry Clin Neurosci*. 2005;17:350–356.

61. Iverson GL, Zasler N, Lange RT. Post-concussive disorder. In: Zasler ND, Katz DI, Zafonte RD, eds. *Brain Injury Medicine: Principles and Practice.* New York, NY: Demos Medical Publishing; 2006: 373–405.

62. Hoge CW, Castro CA, Messer SC, McGurk D, Cotting DI, Koffman RL. Combat duty in Iraq and Afghanistan, mental health problems, and barriers to care. *N Engl J Med.* 2004;351:13–22.

63. Koren D, Norman D, Cohen A, Berman J, Klein EM. Increased PTSD risk with combat-related injury: a matched comparison study of injured and uninjured soldiers experiencing the same combat events. *Am J Psychiatry.* 2005;162:276–282.

64. Bombardier CH, Fann JR, Temkin N, et al. Posttraumatic stress disorder symptoms during the first six months after traumatic brain injury. *J Neuropsychiatry Clin Neurosci.* 2006;18:501–508.

65. Warden DL, Labbate LA, Salazar AM, et al. Posttraumatic stress disorder in patients with traumatic brain injury and amnesia for the event? *J Neuropsychiatry Clin Neurosci.* 1997;9:18–22.

66. Brain Trauma Foundation. *Guidelines for the Field Management of Combat-Related Head Trauma. 2005.* Available at: http://www.braintrauma.org/guidelines/. Accessed August 31, 2009.

67. McCrea M, Kelly J, Randolf C. *Standardized Assessment of Concussion (SAC): Manual for Administration, Scoring, and Interpretation.* 2nd ed. Waukesa, Wisc: Comprehensive Neuropsychological Services; 2000.

68. Savola O, Niemelä O, Hillbom M. Alcohol intake and the pattern of trauma in young adults and working aged people admitted after trauma. *Alcohol Alcohol.* 2005;40(4):269–273.

69. Corrigan JD. Substance abuse as a mediating factor in outcome from traumatic brain injury. *Arch Phys Med Rehabil.* 1995;76(4);302–309.

70. Horner MD, Ferguson PL, Selassie AW, Labbate LA, Kniele K, Corrigan JD. Patterns of alcohol use 1 year after traumatic brain injury: a population-based, epidemiological study. *J Int Neuropsychol Soc.* 2005;11(3):322–330.

71. Sherer M, Bergloff P, High W Jr, Nick TG. Contribution of functional ratings to prediction of long-term employment outcome after traumatic brain injury. *Brain Inj.* 1999;13(12):973–981.

72. Corrigan JD, Smith-Knapp K, Granger CV. Validity of the functional independence measure for persons with traumatic brain injury. *Arch Phys Med Rehabil.* 1997;78(8):828–834.

73. Kreutzer JS, Witol AD, Marwitz JH. Alcohol and drug use among young persons with traumatic brain injury. *J Learn Disabil.* 1996;29(6):643–651.

74. Kreutzer JS, Wehman PH, Harris JA, Burns CT, Young HF. Substance abuse and crime patterns among persons with traumatic brain injury referred for supported employment. *Brain Inj.* 1991;5(2):177–187.

75. Neurobehavioral Guidelines Working Group. Warden DL, Gordon B, McAllister TW, et al. Guidelines for the pharmacologic treatment of neurobehavioral sequelae of traumatic brain injury. *J Neurotrauma*. 2006;23(10):1468–1501.

76. Lee HB, Lyketsos CG, Rao V. Pharmacological management of the psychiatric aspects of traumatic brain injury. *Int Rev Psychiatry.* 2003;15(4):359–370.

77. Thaxton L, Myers MA. Sleep disturbances and their management in patients with brain injury. *J Head Trauma Rehabil.* 2002;17(4):335–348.

78. Walker WC, Seel RT, Curtiss G, Warden DL. Headache after moderate and severe traumatic brain injury: a longitudinal analysis. *Arch Phys Med Rehabil.* 2005;86(9):1793–1800.

79. Young JA. Pain and traumatic brain injury. *Phys Med Rehabil Clin N Am*. 2007;18(1):145–163, vii–viii.

80. Alderfer BS, Arciniegas DB, Silver JM. Treatment of depression following traumatic brain injury. *J Head Trauma Rehabil*. 2005;20(6):544–562.

81. Mittenberg W, Tremont G, Zielinski RE, Fichera S, Rayls KR. Cognitive-behavioral prevention of postconcussion syndrome. *Arch Clin Neuropsychol*. 1996;11(2):139–145.

82. Ponsford J, Willmott C, Rothwell A, et al. Impact of early intervention on outcome following mild head injury in adults. *J Neurol Neurosurg Psychiatry*. 2002;73:330–332.

83. de Kruijk JR, Leffers P, Meerhoff S, Rutten J, Twijnstra A. Effectiveness of bed rest after mild traumatic brain injury: a randomised trial of no versus six days of bed rest. *J Neurol Neurosurg Psychiatry*. 2002;73:167–172.

Chapter 16

PSYCHIATRIC INTERVENTION FOR THE BATTLE-INJURED MEDICAL AND SURGICAL PATIENT FOLLOWING TRAUMATIC INJURIES

HAROLD J. WAIN, PHD*; SCOTT C. MORAN, MD†; MARVIN OLESHANSKY, MD‡; ANDREE BOUTERIE, MD§; AND CHRISTOPHER L. LANGE, MD¥

*Chief, Psychiatry Consultation Liaison Service, Building 2, Room 6238, Walter Reed Army Medical Center, 6900 Georgia Avenue NW, Washington, DC 20307-5100

†Major (P), Medical Corps, US Army; Psychiatry Residency Training Program Director, Psychiatry Consultation Liaison Service, Building 6, Room 2060, Walter Reed Army Medical Center, 6900 Georgia Avenue NW, Washington, DC 20307-5100

‡Colonel, US Army (Retired); Staff Psychiatrist, Psychiatric Outpatient Service, Department of Psychiatry, Tripler Army Medical Center, 1 Jarrett White Road, Honolulu, Hawaii 96822; formerly, Staff Psychiatrist, Psychiatry Consultation Liaison Service, Walter Reed Army Medical Center, Washington, DC 20307-5100

§Staff Psychiatrist, Psychiatry Consultation Liaison Service, Walter Reed Army Medical Center, 6900 Georgia Avenue, NW, Washington, DC 20307-5100

¥Lieutenant Colonel, Medical Corps, US Army; Program Director, National Capital Consortium Forsenic Psychiatry Fellowship Program, Department of Psychiatry, Walter Reed Army Medical Center, 6900 Georgia Avenue NW, Building 6, Room 3038, Washington, DC 20307; formerly, Staff Psychiatrist, Psychiatry Consultation Liaison Service, Walter Reed Army Medical Center, Washington, DC

INTRODUCTION

Trauma, whether resulting from the actions of humans or nature, as a precipitant of medical and surgical injuries can be emotionally overwhelming, not only for the patient dealing with the medical issues, but for the family and caregivers as well. Each will have to cope with the trauma of the event leading to the injury as well as the subsequent psychological sequelae. In the hierarchy of needs regarding patient care, stabilization of the medical physical injury of the patient takes precedence. However, often ignored are the psychiatric after-effects that traumatic injury may elicit.

For years the Psychiatry Consultation Liaison Service (PCLS) at Walter Reed Army Medical Center (WRAMC) has been helping patients deal with the psychiatric and psychological consequences of medical and surgical disease. Since the beginning of the global war on terror in 2001, the goal for the psychiatry consultation liaison service at Walter Reed has been two-fold: (1) decrease the psychiatric manifestations of trauma that may disrupt medical treatment, and (2) decrease the chronic and disabling psychiatric disorders that may occur as a result of trauma. Several chapters and articles describing in detail the PCLS approach to meet these goals have been published, including discussions of Gulf War I,[1] the Pentagon attacks,[2] the bombings of the US embassy in Nairobi,[3] and the current wars in Afghanistan and Iraq.[4] Since 2003, PCLS has seen over 3,000 battle-injured patients using the methods described in these chapters.

One of the main features of effective mental health intervention in polytrauma (or any consultation-liaison psychiatry setting for that matter) is for mental healthcare providers to ally themselves with the patient, the patient's family, and the patient's treatment team. Since the start of the global war on terror, PCLS has been a routine part of trauma care at WRAMC. Immediately following the attack on the Pentagon on 9/11, casualties who required extended inpatient management of their injuries were admitted to civilian hospitals closer to the Pentagon than WRAMC. During that time, PCLS deployed teams to these facilities to assist in their clinical management. The PCLS teams were recognized consultants to the endogenous medical team of the local hospitals.

Trauma patients are routinely seen upon arrival at WRAMC and followed with the trauma team throughout the hospital stay as integral part of the medical care. Mental health interventions are provided to assist these patients in processing their trauma and its aftermath, support the family members who provide critical emotional support to these patients, and facilitate interactions with their treatment team for an optimal clinical outcome. All this happens as the patients undergo medical and surgical care and seek to adapt physically and mentally to the new realities imposed upon them by their traumatic injuries. Thus, a comprehensive program designed to help the medical institution as a whole respond to the psychological demands of a traumatic event must take into account the needs of not only the patients, but also the patients' families and medical staff involved in their care.

This chapter focuses on the psychological and psychiatric issues of medical and surgical patients suffering from traumatic injuries. This approach to care for these patients, their family members, and medical care providers, was developed by the PCLS, and is based on the experience of the authors and their colleagues in the care of these patients, family members, and treatment teams at WRAMC over the past 30 years.

INJURIES AND THE STRESS OF TRAUMA

Soldiers wounded in combat in Operation Enduring Freedom (OEF) and Operation Iraqi Freedom (OIF) receive immediate lifesaving intervention on the battlefield or in the battalion aid station by a combat medic, further treatment at a combat surgical hospital, and then aeromedical evacuation to Landstuhl Regional Medical Center. The military air evacuation system facilitates transfer of the patient to WRAMC following injuries in theater and stabilization at Landstuhl. Because of advances in medical care on the battlefield and through far-forward surgical interventions and advances in critical care transport, casualties survive wounds that in previous wars would have lead to certain death. Casualty rates have dropped from 1 in 2 in the American Civil War to 1 in 16 in OIF. This means many more patients survive to deal with the psychological after-effects of traumatic injury.

The nature and severity of traumatic injuries vary depending on the inciting event. Terrorist attack victims suffer from injuries that include severe and extensive burns, blunt trauma, multiple wounds from fragments or broken glass, and smoke inhalation injuries. Combat trauma includes gunshot wounds, fragment wounds, abdominal wounds, brain and spinal cord injuries, and amputations. Many of the soldiers injured in OIF and OEF have multiple categories of wound and are referred to as polytrauma patients.

The resulting injuries from the traumatic event often

represent the end of life as the patient knew it, and the beginning of a painful and arduous ordeal with an uncertain outcome. The surviving patient is subject to a broad range of psychological stresses throughout the process of recovery. Pain is exacerbated by frequent wash-outs and debridement, dressing changes, skin grafts, plastic surgery, and the need to exercise damaged limbs to avoid contractures. Medical treatments, including the use of narcotics, can often interfere with patients' motivation. The patient may need to be isolated until the danger of infection has passed, and extensive bandaging further reduces environmental contact, especially for facial or ocular wounds. A tracheotomy or traumatic brain injury (TBI) may interfere with communication.

Initial medical and surgical care is essential for the recovery of the trauma victim. The patient and the family report that this clinical care is often experienced as a significant ongoing stressor, and, in severe cases, as an extension of the trauma itself. The mental healthcare provider must take into account not only the effects of the traumatic event, but also the effect of the stressors arising from their medical and surgical management in the wake of trauma, in order to prevent or minimize psychological sequelae and to optimize clinical outcome.

Neurological and physiological disturbances and behavioral changes often follow traumatic injury that has resulted in amputations, brain injury, spinal cord injury, facial disfigurement, burns, blindness, and mutilating and castrating wounds of the external male genitalia.[5] Stressors including pain, complications arising in the course of the patient's treatment and recovery, infection, the need for repeated incision and drainage or revision of surgical wounds, development of decubiti in the bedridden, side effects from medications, hospital-acquired infections, delays in recovery and prolonged hospital stays, and uncertainty in the outcome and time course are just a few of the emotional and psychological effects on the patient.

The Effect of Trauma

Trauma results in the normal adaptive mechanisms being compromised when psychological defenses cannot be employed.[6] Self-integrity, self-confidence, and self-esteem may be undermined as a consequence of trauma. Trust of others is diminished, critical judgment is suspended, feelings of helplessness, dependency, and regression may occur. Feelings of rage, anger, and frustration may also result. Personality structures and defenses are pushed to their limits. Trauma may also recreate previous maladaptive patterns of behavior that had been dormant.

To facilitate patient care it is critical to obtain a good biopsychosocial and developmental history. The patient or the patient's family, or both, may have previous trauma or mental health issues that affect the response to trauma following injury. It is facilitative if the clinicians are aware of the underlying personality structures and defense mechanisms that the patient utilizes to personal advantage to help facilitate mental health interventions. The method of gaining this information needs to be different than traditional approaches with nontraumatized patients. A directive approach may cause a revivification of the trauma and contribute to regressive behavior that may disrupt medical care. A normal supportive conversational tone with humor (if possible, and if the provider is comfortable) is advocated.

Traumatic injuries may result in both short- and long-term emotional trauma, most of which are acute stress reactions and posttraumatic stress disorder (PTSD). Studies conducted at WRAMC have shown that the level of physical severity of injury may be correlated with the development of depression and PTSD following traumatic injury.[7] It has also been well documented that traumatic injury in the civilian healthcare setting often results in stress disorders.[8,9] Rates of PTSD following traumatic injury vary from 12% to 30%, but at WRAMC battle-injured service members had a 4% prevalence at 1 month, and 12% prevalence at 7 months following injury.[7] Trauma victims may also experience a variety of psychological responses that occur independently or simultaneously with the above disorders. Other diagnoses, including affective, anxiety, and somatoform spectrum disorders as well as TBI, may also occur.[10] Some of these responses that have been observed by the authors include separation anxiety, grief, anger, rage, fear, frustration, regret, shame, dissociation, regression, denial, and shattered ego integrity.

Soldiers in combat have a battle mindset while in theater. This mindset includes many psychological symptoms that, although helpful in a war zone, are not helpful when returning home or following evacuation for injury, as many of these symptoms may mimic acute stress disorder. These may include difficulty sleeping, irritability, hypervigilance, exaggerated startle response, and motor restlessness. Other symptoms that may develop (and that can be detrimental) are poor concentration, fear, helplessness, horror, anxiety, detachment, absence of emotions, numbing, and anxiety. Cognitive symptoms may consist of recurrent dreams, thoughts, and flashbacks. Behavioral symptoms can include avoiding people, places, activities, thoughts, emotions, conversations, or television programs reminiscent of the event. Typically these resolve over a period of time, but may persist after the initial trauma is over in a significant percentage of patients, and do not rise to the level of clinical diagnosis of acute stress disorder or PTSD.

PCLS routinely assesses patients for these symptoms and provides psychoeducational interventions, normalization of the responses, and empathic exposure as a means to develop resiliency and return patients to mental health. The clinician's awareness of the effect of these responses to the patient facilitates the development of therapeutic alliances with the patient that improve treatment outcomes and reduce stigma associated with mental health providers.

The severity of the injury and body part affected may also help to determine the patient's response to the traumatic injury. Injury to parts of the body with real or perceived significance may increase the patient's stress.[11] Therefore, PCLS routinely assesses patients for body image and physical integrity issues following trauma. Phantom limb pain is often treated with a combination of medications and hypnotherapy performed at the patient's bedside. Patients are also taught self-hypnosis techniques to manage their pain. Patients with facial disfigurement and spinal cord injuries often have the most severe body image reactions to their injury. PCLS providers attempt to address these issues early in the course of treatment. In addition to the patient's emotional reaction to these types of injuries, medical and surgical providers also have difficulty with these types of injuries.

Trauma patients who experience severe pain are less likely to be amenable to psychotherapeutic interventions. Schreiber and Galai-Gat[12] identify uncontrolled pain as a stressor that, if not treated effectively, may result in the development of PTSD. Uncontrolled pain may also lead to the development of anxiety, depression, loneliness, hostility, and sleep disturbances.[13] Studies at WRAMC have also demonstrated that increased pain may be a predictor for the development of PTSD and depression in battle-injured soldiers.[14] PCLS uses many interventions to reduce or eliminate pain. As mentioned above, hypnotherapy is often practiced at the bedside. Other therapies—such as cognitive reframing, antidepressant medications, and stimulants—are recommended to the treating trauma team as adjuncts to manage pain.

Physical loss of a limb brings with it the added anxiety of potential social and interpersonal difficulty. Trauma patients are described by Blum[15] as experiencing a loss of identity, self-confidence, self-esteem, self-reliance, and ideal self. Horowitz[16] and Landsman and colleagues[17] noted that patient's reactions to traumatic injury can be similar to bereavement. In addition to concern regarding physical appearance, patients sustaining an amputation may be concerned with the reactions from peers, the ability to earn a living,[11] socialization, dating, and sexual behavior.[10] Trauma victims are at risk for developing psychiatric illnesses based on these factors: exposure to trauma, intensity of exposure, psychiatric history, gender, and level of education.[18]

The need for early psychiatric intervention was recognized following the attacks on 9/11.[4,19,20] Hoge and colleagues[21] demonstrated that the greatest deterrent to soldiers exposed to trauma who may need psychiatric intervention is their perception of psychiatry. To destigmatize mental health for the battle-injured soldier, the PCLS service was redesignated as Preventive Medical Psychiatry (PMP) to gain greater acceptance by patient, family, and staff alike. This change addressed the need for the mental health team to be seen as any other medical service,[20] and ensured that every patient from OIF/OEF hospitalized on a medical surgical unit at WRAMC was evaluated and followed. Integrating psychiatry into the trauma team and providing routine preventive psychiatric interventions with trauma patients may prevent psychiatric symptoms from becoming disabling. The benefit of this program is demonstrated by the fact that the rate of PTSD development among medically injured patients treated at WRAMC is lower than noninjured soldiers exposed to trauma.[7,21] Furthermore, early psychiatric intervention may also alleviate the stigma associated with being a psychiatry patient and allow appropriate psychiatric intervention to occur when necessary, often after the patient has left the hospital.

Hospitalization and the Meaning of Injury

In the period immediately following injury, patients often report a sense of shock, denial, and disbelief. The feeling of being dependent on others can become intimidating and overwhelming. Fear over loss of life, limb, or capability, as well as a feeling of loss of control is a common occurrence. Apprehension of being abandoned prior to regaining control or receiving help can be very overpowering. Once help has arrived and the fear of being alone is relieved, a sense of initial comfort develops, along with potential dependency needs. Based on the severity of the injury, patients may not be aware of all that has transpired until they awake in the hospital. Some patients are initially elated at being alive. After a time, however, the elation may fade and anxiety and depressive symptoms may appear. Others who suffer brain injuries or loss of consciousness may never remember the event or the trauma and wait for others to fill in the gap.

In general, a patient who is exposed to trauma can

experience a threat to both physical and emotional integrity. Loss of body parts and threat of death or annihilation are also significant fears for these patients. They become vulnerable and dependent, a state many patients have not experienced in many years. Fear or discomfort with strangers may also become prominent because of the unknown effect of the disfigurement on the new relationship. Fear of not having as many loved ones around and leaving a safe environment are also major concerns for patients being discharged from the hospital. Patients' perceptions can result in childlike patterns of behavior, which lead to conflicts with the nursing and medical staff. Regression and dependency needs are frequently observed in traumatically injured patients, and an overwhelming sense of narcissistic injury is frequently present.

Complicating these factors are the anxieties of the patient's loved ones. The family's needs must be addressed so that their anxieties do not affect the patient and thus exacerbate an already emotionally complicated situation. For example, family members often choose to sleep in the patient's room rather than leaving them alone at night. This, however, can result in the patient later having difficulty sleeping if someone isn't in the room.

An individual's adaptive functioning may be compromised by the traumatic event. Most patients eventually find ways to deal with the emotional effects of traumatic injury, and although personality features that have been effective as coping styles in the past may become overwhelmed initially, patients usually self-correct. Patients with poor or disordered personality structures may have conflicts with staff or families and are at risk for developing maladaptive behaviors or psychiatric illnesses. These patients may respond in a less-than-optimal manner because medical or traumatic injuries can be an overwhelming stressor. These patients and families are vulnerable and need support and guidance from caring individuals. Developing a therapeutic relationship with them is imperative. Utilizing warmth, caring, empathy, and support can go a long way when attempting to form an alliance with the family and the patient, and can facilitate healthy behaviors and responses.

The Role of Psychiatry Following Trauma

Nearly all survivors exposed to traumatic events briefly exhibit one or more stress-related symptoms.[22] In many instances these symptoms dissipate within a reasonable amount of time. However, symptoms persisting for a prolonged period following a traumatic event increase the probability of developing PTSD or other stress-related psychiatric disorders. Koren[8] found that injured soldiers were more than five times as likely to develop psychiatric symptoms than were those only exposed to trauma. Though the initial goal of the mental health team is to facilitate medical treatment, a secondary goal is to prevent or decrease the probability of chronic debilitating psychiatric symptoms. To meet these goals in treating the medical-surgical patient following a traumatic injury, new approaches were adapted at WRAMC.[2,10]

Rather than waiting for consultations to be received before intervention occurs, the PMP at WRAMC developed a therapeutic interaction to overcome the stigma of being seen by psychiatry. Overcoming this obstacle is important because many patients tend to downplay their distress and underreport their symptoms for fear of being labeled a psychiatric patient. (As discussed above, the PMP was developed to decrease the stigma associated with mental health and psychiatry).

Case Study 16-1: A 36-year-old soldier with a soft-tissue injury to the right eye, fractures to the left femur and tibia, and a right-leg below-the-knee amputation (BKA) responded in a sullen manner to his orthopaedic and physical therapy teams. Upon the initial visit by a psychiatrist he denied any problems as a result of the improvised explosive device (IED) blast. He claimed he did not need psychiatric intervention and was upset that the team referred him. When he became aware that the psychiatry approach was routine and preventive in nature, he began describing his concerns about his decision-making process while in theater that may have led to his unit receiving the blast it sustained. He continued to describe his concerns, and the psychiatry team worked to reframe what had happened while maintaining an advocacy role. As he accepted the routine of the psychiatry approach, he began to respond more favorably, assimilated the intervention, and cooperated more fully with his rehabilitation.

THERAPEUTIC INTERVENTION FOR THE PREVENTION OF PSYCHIATRIC STRESS DISORDERS

The PMP service at WRAMC employs the Therapeutic Intervention for the Prevention of Psychiatric Stress (TIPPS) disorders model.[10] The approach draws upon many tools used by the mental health provider in the consult–liaison setting. This intervention was developed to address the psychological needs of trauma victims, provide support to the individuals and their families, assess psychiatric status, provide early intervention when needed without stigmatization of the patient, and support the staff. To help with the clinical process, objective instruments are given to patients while they are in the hospital. The questionnaires are helpful in providing objective data and facilitating follow-up.

The major components of the TIPPS approach are mental health becoming a routine part of trauma care, empathetic exposure therapy, developing a strong therapeutic alliance with the patient and family, normalizing the experience and the psychological response to the trauma, reinforcing resiliency, and promoting positive coping behaviors. TIPPS has been used successfully at WRAMC since the attacks on the Pentagon on September 11, 2001. Studies infer the effectiveness of this approach for reducing the prevalence of mental health disorders in battle-injured soldiers treated at WRAMC.[7] Other significant components of the intervention include recognizing personality styles and psychological defenses, countertransference and transference issues, normalizing events, cognitive reframing, educating patients and families, prescribing appropriate psychopharmacology, and utilizing hypnotic and relaxation techniques. Reinforcing patients' strengths regarding their survival was also a primary theme of this approach. A review of some of the principles of TIPPS follows.

Routine Consultation and Therapeutic Alliance

The patients are initially approached with an informal style and avoidance of traditional psychiatric jargon. A typical introduction may begin by saying, "Hello, I'm Dr ____ from Preventive Medical Psychiatry. Welcome back. We are sorry you had to experience your injury and we all thank you for what you did. You took care of us by being there. It is now our turn to take care of you." Family members are also greeted in a similar manner if they are present. The provider is introduced to the family as staff of the PMP service. The provider also lets the soldier and the soldier's family know that mental health assessment is part of the routine care for returning OIF/OEF patients. This approach frequently sets patients and families at ease. Providers are trained to be cognizant of the variety of reactions to mental healthcare that patients and families may have and adjust their approaches accordingly.

The therapeutic alliance is built with the patient and families over time, as patients are seen briefly several times per week. PMP involves the entire family unit in adjusting to, and recovering from, the traumatic event. The family may be seen separately from the patient as well as together. Understanding their position and problems is necessary. PMP social workers also follow patients and their family members twice a week. The child and adolescent psychiatry service joins the PMP for rounds and sees families with children of injured soldiers to assess the family support structure and to help the family deal with the effect of trauma.

Patients are asked to rate how they are feeling, their pain, and their sleep, and if they are having any nightmares or feelings about the trauma. The development of the therapeutic alliance cannot be underestimated. It facilitates the assessment of psychological symptoms and treatment while in the hospital and allows for easier follow-up treatment if problems arise for patients or their families upon discharge. This helps ensure that patients feel comfortable approaching psychiatry for help, if needed.

Transference and Countertransference in the Therapeutic Relationship

Understanding the interpersonal interaction between clinician and patients facilitates evaluation and treatment.[20] Patients' responses to clinicians will often be expressed in various manifestations of transference. At times the transference can be modified by the actual behavior of the therapist. The need to elicit a therapeutic alliance and a positive transference from the trauma patient is crucial. This will likely occur when the clinician is perceived as both good and helpful in the here-and-now situation. Negative transferences are more likely to recreate spontaneous reenactments due to rapidly shifting mood, affect deregulation, and disconnection within self. The potential for revictimization may be enhanced or diminished by the negative transference experience of the patient. With a negative transference, the trauma patient may come to categorize the clinician as a past perpetrator. This occurrence may likely contribute to a regression or oppositional style to medical treatment. This is detrimental in particular for the wounded soldier because medical stabilization and recovery is of necessity. It is clearly essential for the clinician to recognize the significance of the transference responses and react in an appropriate therapeutic manner. During the early stages of therapy with trauma patients, the immediate goal is to establish the holding milieu for the emergence of positive transference.

Clinicians can also develop countertransference issues that need monitoring. Clinician overindulgence of patients' needs, silence, avoidance, and overidentification with the patient or family members can cause disruption in the recovery of the patient. The concept of neutrality can be lost and patients can feel revictimized. In general, being aware of patients' transference or countertransference issues and the effect on the therapeutic process allows for greater clinical clarity and appropriate interventions. Awareness of countertransference issues also allows the PMP clinician to be a more effective clinician and consultant. Knowledge of these skills can help colleagues in other services in their interactions with their patients.

INDIVIDUAL THERAPEUTIC COMPONENTS

Empathic Exposure

Providers allow the patient to process the trauma through empathic supportive exposure therapy. In other words, in an empathic manner, patients are asked to reflect on their traumatic experiences, suggesting that description at present is helpful in the future. Empathic exposure may help them integrate the past trauma into their present stream of consciousness. Patients are usually seen three times per week for 15 to 20 minutes. The frequency of this empathic exposure appears to allow for the normalization of the event and consolidation of the experience in the patient's memory.

Providers are trained to offer rapid empathic responses to patients' recall of their trauma and injuries. As the patients continue to relate their trauma, empathic reinforcing statements are made about their psychological assets. These statements reinforce their positive behaviors during their descriptions. Nonthreatening techniques are employed and confrontational approaches are avoided. Comments that demonstrate patients' positive assets are quickly reinforced, such as, "How did you know to do that?" or, "Where did you learn that?" Traditional psychotherapeutic interventions aid the provider in supporting the trauma patient. Acceptance, respect, empathy, warmth, advice, praise, affirmation, and a sense of hope are qualities and characteristics the clinician is encouraged to display while working with these patients. Providers need to be viewed as genuine in their concern and support of the patient, while offering empathic validation and encouraging patients to elaborate on reactions relevant to the trauma. These techniques reinforce the therapeutic alliance and treatment. In summary, while the patients are relating their traumas, clinicians find a way of reinforcing their assets. Providers continue this procedure each time they see these patients. Supportive reinforcing statements regarding their assets while they are describing their trauma may help them integrate the conflict in a more productive manner.

Hypnotherapy

Hypnotic techniques are taught while the patients are in their beds. Providers have them practice breathing and then utilize a rapid hypnotic induction that patients can repeat to themselves. This can, at times, allow for management and control over symptoms such as pain, hypervigilance, and anxiety. It may also allow for distancing from the trauma—giving patients some control in finding a safe mental place where they can begin processing thoughts and feelings about the trauma. The clinician can facilitate the patient's going to the imaginary safe place to process and reframe traumatic events. Subsequently these patients can get to their safe place on their own. These techniques can also be an outstanding adjunct to help pateints integrate their conflicts with phantom-limb pain, sleep, and smoking cessation in a facilitative manner. Many of the trauma patients at WRAMC smoke even when they know smoking disrupts wound healing.

Group Therapy

As a supplement to individual therapy, groups can provide beneficial support and help many of the patients begin working through the process. Group therapy was demonstrated as an effective technique for treating Vietnam-era veterans with PTSD.[23] At WRAMC, groups are held twice a week in the hospital ward and led by providers. The groups are open to the medical and surgical injured patients. Topics such as anger, expectations, recognition of limitations, sexual fears, separation anxieties, survivor guilt, losses, family concerns, and public responses are discussed after initiated by a patient.

Pharmacological Interventions

Pharmacological approaches are often used to facilitate mental health recovery from traumatic injury. Physical trauma results in significant somatic pain and, according to Schreiber and Galai-Gat,[12] uncontrolled pain may result in the development of PTSD. Some patients associate pain with the severity of their injury, which may also lead to the development of anxiety, depression, loneliness, hostility, and sleep disturbances.[11,13] Studies at WRAMC have demonstrated that patients with increased levels of physical injury are more likely to develop PTSD and depression following injury.[7] Furthermore, patients experiencing pain are less likely to respond to traditional psychotherapeutic interventions.[13] Thus, prompt pain control is critical in trauma patients and must be addressed early with judicious use of analgesics. PMP often recommends several adjunct treatments to the trauma team to manage pain, including tricyclics and other antidepressants, hypnotherapy, and relaxation therapy. Myriad pharmacological interventions are available to treat patients with psychiatric diagnoses or symptoms such as agitation, anxiety, or perceptual disturbances. Some of the agents utilized are antipsychotics, atypical antipsychotics, selective serotonin reuptake inhibitors (SSRIs), and serotonin-norepinephrine reuptake inhibitors.

Insomnia

Insomnia in the polytrauma patient is a near universal observation. Insomnia can be attributed to delirium, nursing care interventions, lab draws, pain, fever, and doctors' rounds, among other things encountered in the hospital. Benzodiazepines, anticholinergic medications, and antidepressants can interfere with clarity of thought and prevent psychological integration of the traumatic event, as well as foster the development of a delirium. Insomnia in the trauma patient is treated with a variety of interventions. First, orders are reviewed to ensure that nursing care interventions (such as q4 hour vitals) are not still ordered when no longer necessary. Patients are given permission to close their doors and put signs up instructing that they not be disturbed. The nursing staff is encouraged to allow for uninterrupted sleep. Patients are also educated on sleep hygiene, and relaxation techniques are taught to help them rapidly induce sleep.

Often, however, these measures are insufficient. Medications for insomnia can be extremely useful in the hospitalized setting. The choice of medication is often based on the patient's symptoms, medical condition, and preference. For nightmares and sleep maintenance problems, Seroquel (quetiapine; AstraZeneca US, Wilmington, Del) is often used in low doses, 25–100 mg. There has only been one small open-label study published looking at Seroquel and sleep quality, which showed effects on nightmares and sleep maintenance. The experience at WRAMC shows this approach to be effective and well-tolerated by patients. However, there have been a few patients who experienced elevations in their liver-associated enzymes due to Seroquel. There are other drawbacks. Seroquel is expensive and is an atypical antipsychotic; there is debate about its cost effectiveness and the risks of dyslipidemia, blood-sugar abnormalities, and extrapyramidal symptom disruptions. In treating thousands of patients at WRAMC with this medication, there have not been observed instances of these problems. Other antipsychotics have been employed somewhat successfully for the treatment of sleep disturbances with nightmares. Other medications may be indicated in the presence of flashbacks or disorientation and emotional dysregulation from multiple or high-dose pain medications or other medical issues.

Ambien (zolpidem; Sanofi-Aventis, Bridgewater, NJ) has not been found to be as useful as Seroquel in patients at WRAMC. The half-life of Ambien is short and patients quickly develop a tachyphylaxis. Also, Ambien does not seem to work as well for stress-induced insomnia. When insomnia is associated with anxiety or depression, mirtazapine can offer relief. Nightmares, when overwhelming, have been reported to respond well to prazosin, though caution should be exercised due to its hypotensive properties. One small study of 10 patients showed some alleviation from nightmares in patients with PTSD using prazosin. A discussion on the use of pharmacotherapy is provided elsewhere in this volume.

TREATMENT

As described earlier, a variety of psychotherapeutic and psychopharmacologic interventions, techniques, and styles are utilized. In the PMP service, the mechanism of normalization of feelings is a fundamental aspect of treatment. Soldiers in the initial phases of trauma recovery are not generally willing to discuss their feelings with the providers, but with the mandatory screening and monitoring that the service provides, patients become "used to" someone coming in and normalizing some of their "potential" emotional responses. After some time, they may often choose to speak more freely, knowing they are going to be listened to and understood.

The first step is to allow these patients to fully describe their losses. It is only through this step that the necessary information can be gathered to determine if their depression is from grieving, from a sense of helplessness in not knowing how they are going to handle a change of life as a result of their injury, or if there is a truly endogenous depression. In these initial few sessions, mental health professionals can learn a great deal about value systems, usual responses to adverse life events, and expectations and fantasies of what would happen in the next few months of these patients' lives.

These soldiers, regardless of the etiology of their situations, must be given a chance to mourn their losses. An essential aspect of working through this is identifying the loss, the importance of that loss in their lives, and its effect. In each of these "grieving sessions," the psychiatrist needs to focus on the recurrent themes and begin to lay foundations for growth and resiliency *despite* the loss. As these patients discover that life does not halt because of the loss, they realize that the traumatic incident is another chapter in the rest of their lives. They can then begin to recover their sense of purpose and well-being. Some soldiers, despite psychotherapeutic interventions, continue to have depressive or anxiety symptoms, and require pharmacological interventions. Fortunately, soldiers in these situations typically respond well to the usual treatment course of antidepressants.

Depression and Mood Disturbances

Being a patient often precipitates a sense of loss that many cannot verbalize. Because soldiers are taught throughout their military training to "bottle up" their feelings, their sense of loss can manifest itself though behavioral problems. This section addresses the various ways that loss can be experienced by these patients, how the process of normalization of experiences can allow them to work through their sensations, and effective treatment strategies for the more recalcitrant cases.

From the very beginning, battle-injured soldiers will generally indicate that they are simply "happy to be alive." However, this statement is often followed by a second statement: "I guess I was lucky." The progression of this thought is stunning; soldiers will seem genuinely relieved at their fortune, but an overriding sense of guilt actually visibly appears to overtake them, and they must attribute this fortune to luck to again regain their emotional control over survivor guilt. The reality of survivor guilt has been well established in patients who are covictims in traumatic events. In soldiers, this guilt is intensified by the ubiquitous code of teamwork that military service requires of its members. This feeling is often stronger in those patients who have minimal injuries compared to the death or severe maiming of their peers.

Loss of functioning goes well beyond the mere physical loss of limbs. Many of these soldiers tend to be athletic and active in their preinjury lives. They perceive their lives as "forever changed" because of the amputations, and frequently believe they will have no ability to engage in their former activities. Although there is some basis in reality with this thought, unless they move through this phase, they will not be able to see the abilities they still have or may regain.

Case Study 16-2: AB was a 22-year-old Army sergeant. He was the team leader for four other infantry soldiers. The unit had been together in theater for 7 months when they were attacked by an IED on a routine patrol. AB was knocked unconscious by the blast, but awoke with a BKA of his left leg. He learned that two members of his team had perished in the blast, another had an amputation of his right arm and leg, and the fourth one had suffered a TBI and his status was unknown to the patient. AB spent 3 weeks in a facility before being transferred to WRAMC. In that time he had minimal exposure to mental healthcare, primarily because of his statements that he was "doing fine." However, after his air evacuation to the United States, AB stated that he was "surrounded by the reminders of his loss," and became tearful during his history and physical with his primary team. They requested a consultation. AB spoke of his loss of his own limbs, but realized that he was "lucky." However, this conflicted with his sensation that he "should" feel more for his soldiers than for his own self. He stated that this was the reason that he spoke little of his feelings in his previous hospitalization, believing that if he focused on himself, he would be perceived as weak. AB was deeply troubled at his change of lifestyle, but extremely worried that he would need to "forever show his grief" when he was at his unit to pay homage to his team soldiers. Determining that he would "never be happy," he fell into a state where he would not participate in activities, have outside visitors, or speak with his unit liaisons as they visited in the hospital.

Anxiety

During the acute period of hospitalization of battle-injured soldiers, the PMP service observes a range of symptoms in the anxiety spectrum of disorders. Most commonly seen are those symptoms that are consistent with acute stress reactions. In particular, the reexperiencing of traumatic events through nightmares, flashbacks, intrusive thoughts, and recurrent images are common. Equally common are symptoms related to hyperarousal, such as difficulty falling or staying asleep, hypervigilance, increased startle response, irritability, and poor concentration. Obsessive rumination themes in the injured soldiers include worries regarding the threat to physical integrity, the effect on current and future functioning, and the effect on family members and friends. Soldiers removed from theater often worry about unit members left behind and are distressed by their perceived inability to help their friends in the field. Many soldiers hear the sound of the blast or the gunshot that injured them replayed over and over either in their minds or in dreams. Others may ruminate over the death of friends and are overcome by survivor guilt. Very frequently battle scenarios are reviewed over and over and soldiers wonder what they might have done differently to have effected a different outcome. Some of the most distressing memories for patients include seeing fellow soldiers die, seeing dead children, and exposure to body parts. Finally, shame may lead to emotional conflicts that may ultimately feed anxiety.

In the absence of traumatic or anoxic brain injuries, where patients have no recollection of traumatic events secondary to organic causes, few patients seem concerned about overt dissociative symptoms (such as not recalling important aspects of the trauma or a feeling of emotional numbing or detachment) in the acute period. Indeed, it appears that most patients, at least in the initial period of hospitalization, seek to reconnect with family members and loved ones and are particularly comforted by contact with commanders and unit members still in the field. Although some hospitalized soldiers may avoid television or movies that remind them of traumatic events, it is less common for patients to overtly avoid reexperiencing the traumatic events by refusing to discuss the trauma, or feelings and thoughts about the trauma. When this overt avoidance occurs, it should be particularly worrisome to the mental health provider and consideration for further intervention should be given.

In addition to symptoms that are consistent with acute stress disorder, anxiety may manifest in the form of specific fears or phobias, such as a fear of falling asleep (usually reported as fear of dreaming), fear of being alone (separation anxiety), or fear of being in the dark. Overt anxiety and panic attacks are observed infrequently. Often these are aggravated in soldiers with prior personal or family histories of anxiety disorders.

Rapid eye movement sleep behavior disorders are not uncommon where patients report acting out combat-related scenes, presumably during rapid-eye-movement sleep. Hypnogogic and hypnopompic phenomena and other perceptual disturbances may occur and may represent hyperarousal symptoms. The service member has just traveled across multiple time zones and may be undergoing frequent painful surgical procedures and necessary nursing interventions throughout the day and night (which continue to promote disturbance of the sleep–wake cycle). The utility of other treatments, such as image rehearsal therapy (where dream endings are more positively construed), are also being explored to address sleeping concerns and nightmares.

In the acute treatment setting, when these symptoms appear, it may be difficult to make a specific anxiety-disorder diagnosis, given that very frequently the service member does not meet full criteria for any one specific diagnosis. Additionally, there are many confounding factors, such as pain, pain medications (opiates, benzodiazepines, or anesthetics) or other medications or substances, head injuries, and other treatment factors that may account for, exacerbate, or create any of the aforementioned symptoms. Above all else, it is important to determine whether a general medical condition, particularly associated with delirium, is not causing or contributing to the anxiety symptom. For this reason, very frequently a diagnosis of anxiety disorder not otherwise specified may be given if one or more symptoms are particularly apparent and troublesome but the patient does not meet full criteria for a specific diagnosis. Additionally, a diagnosis of adjustment disorder with anxiety may be made, although in some cases it is difficult to deem that one person's response is in excess of what might be expected for such an extreme situation.

Later in the course of medical stabilization, almost all of these symptoms lessen for most patients but may persist for a few. For example, patients may continue to reexperience traumatic events, particularly through nightmares. Likewise, new anxiety symptoms may emerge as patients are exposed to new situations outside of the hospital room. Another common example is when they may realize that they have less ability to emotionally connect with others and may have more social withdrawal, such as difficulty tolerating crowded areas. In a few cases, patients have refused to leave their hospital rooms altogether when medically deemed physically capable. As patients physically heal and develop more cognitive reserve, more standardized treatment strategies may be utilized (such as more formalized cognitive behavioral therapy) for the identified disorder. They may then participate in supportive group therapies or perhaps engage in psychodynamic therapy if more developmental and interpersonal concerns appear to be affecting the current condition. The importance of early and consistent treatment of these disorders is borne out by the fact that between 12.2% and 12.9% of soldiers at WRAMC with serious combat injuries returning from OIF or OEF will go on to manifest full criteria for PTSD, with the injury itself being a major risk factor for ultimate development of the disorder.[7] Without these interventions it is likely that these numbers would be even higher.

The general approach to the acutely battle-injured soldier with anxiety begins, as for all patients, with an empathic stance that focuses on the building of a therapeutic alliance. Building early rapport helps the patient identify mental health specialists as part of the medical team and facilitates patient comfort with providers. Additional social assistance is provided where necessary to mobilize and establish a support network and resources for the patient in the hospital. The medical needs of the patient are reviewed and an understanding of the illness or injuries or both from the patient's perspective is explored to help identify beliefs and concerns (and perhaps any doubts or misgivings) that the patient may have regarding care or prognosis.

Psychoeducation is provided to help build a framework for treatment and to normalize current feelings and emotions. Supportive psychotherapy is offered to identify and engage patient strengths and to bolster ego defenses. Patients are encouraged to discuss the trauma "when they are ready," at which time providers reinforce what the patient did well throughout the traumatic event. Cognitive techniques are employed to help patients reframe thoughts about traumatic experiences so that anxiety is better understood and tolerated. Relaxation techniques may be taught and, in certain instances, hypnosis may be added to help patients achieve a deeper sense of relaxation and mastery of emotions. Particular attention is paid to pain control and sleep, as any inadequacy in these areas may hinder the patient's ability to employ effective coping strategies. For this purpose, recommendations for the adjustment of pain medications or for the addition of new ones may be made to the primary medical team. Prior to making any medication recommendations, it is important to consider the patient's underlying medical condition, current medications, and allergies. Medication interaction checks should always be performed, given that most psychoactive medications have the propensity for interactions with multiple other drugs and antibiotics.

SSRIs remain the drugs of first choice for PTSD, generalized anxiety disorder, panic disorders, and social phobia. They may also be utilized for severe, prolonged acute stress, and for adjustment disorders, although some of the newer non-SSRI antidepressants such as venlafaxine and mirtazapine have also been used successfully. Of the SSRIs, sertraline and citalopram are generally preferred given their tolerability and relatively decreased potential for drug–drug interactions. Benzodiazepines are generally avoided where possible, particularly in PTSD, given the lack of data to support their use and the potential for addiction and worsening of PTSD in the long term. They are, however, occasionally used for the temporary relief of severe anxiety and panic attacks. Frequently, patients will already have benzodiazepines prescribed for other indications such as muscle spasms or phantom limb pain. In this latter case, patients should be educated on the effect of benzodiazepines on anxiety and the effects should be monitored. Treatment for persistent conditions may ultimately extend beyond the period of hospitalization. It is therefore important on a consult-liaison service to work closely with the medical team on aspects of discharge planning so that there is a seamless transition of care between inpatient and outpatient mental health providers.

Cognitive Disorders

Approximately one third of service members injured in OIF and requiring medical evacuation to WRAMC are found to have a TBI. Of these, about half are classified as mild TBIs and the other half are rated as moderate to severe. Many of the TBIs occur in the setting of polytrauma. All service members with an injury history that may be associated with a TBI (such as an IED blast exposure, a moving vehicle accident, or falls) are screened during the initial phase of their hospitalization for a TBI by a specialized team from the Defense Veterans Brain Injury Center. Additionally, as part of the routine screening by PCLS/PMP of all injured service members who are admitted to WRAMC, a further psychiatric assessment of these inpatients is performed. A multidisciplinary team from neurology, physical medicine and rehabilitation, psychiatry, physical therapy, occupational therapy, and speech pathology provide ongoing assessment and treatment of these patients.

The role of the PMP includes clinical assessment of the TBI and treatment of associated behavioral sequelae. This begins in the intensive care unit (ICU) for more severely injured service members who arrive at WRAMC on ventilator support. In addition to the common problems of disorientation and frank delirium seen in patients with polytrauma as they are weaned from sedation, patients with TBIs may take considerably longer to wake up, may be more agitated and disorganized, and are generally less able to participate in their own care. Family members of injured service members with TBI are provided information that the prognosis for moderate-to-severe TBI is hard to predict and may be very frightening and upsetting to loved ones. In addition, therapeutic nihilism in staff members treating severe TBIs is not uncommon and frequently needs to be addressed by the consultation liaison psychiatrist. Recommendations for treatment of delirium and agitation often involve modification of the intravenous pain regimen, minimization of external stimulation, addition of neuroleptic medication, and restraint when other modalities fail. Sleep disruption is common and may be associated with other symptoms of hyperarousal. Preemptive treatment of sleep disruption with low-dose atypical neuroleptics has proven to be especially effective in decreasing hyperarousal.

On the medical and surgical wards, psychiatric evaluation of TBIs focuses on the ongoing assessment of cognitive function and the emotional adjustment of service members to their wartime experiences, their injuries, and their futures. The interplay of cognitive deficits and organic mood and personality changes with acute and posttraumatic stress disorders provides diagnostic and therapeutic challenges. Conversion disorder is not uncommonly seen in the context of mild TBI and takes the form of embellishment and exaggeration of cognitive deficits, sensory and motor abnormalities, gait disturbances, and stuttering.

Case Study 16-3: GQ is a 32-year-old active duty E6 with 13 years in service. He was injured by an IED explosion while on a mission in OIF that resulted in a penetrating head injury. At a combat support hospital in Iraq, he underwent a left frontoparietal craniectomy for removal of an embedded fragment and duraplasty, and placement of an intracranial pressure (ICP) monitor. The patient was then transferred to Landstuhl Regional Medical Center in Germany where his ICP was noted to be increased to 15–22 mm Hg, but interval head computed tomography (CT) was unchanged. Patient was noted to be combative when attempts were made to wean him off sedation. Once his ICP stabilized and the monitor was removed, the patient was transferred to WRAMC, where he arrived intubated and sedated. Following the patient's admission to the WRAMC ICU, his wife was seen daily at his bedside by the PCLS staff. Several days into the hospital stay, his wife became extremely distraught. She reported that she had been told by the ICU house staff that her husband's prognosis was guarded. Additionally, she was shown his head CT scan and interpreted the large area of skull loss from the craniectomy as massive brain loss. She did not know if she could live with her husband "being a vegetable." A meeting with the patient's wife, PCLS, and the ICU team was useful in correcting her misunderstanding of the CT scan and providing her with a better understanding of his prognosis. The patient was subsequently extubated and was initially agitated and moving only his left side. Over the next month he made a gradual recovery, with resolution of posttraumatic amnesia and return of speech and full motor activity. He denied flashbacks, hyperarousal, anxiety, depression, or other symptoms of acute stress disorder, with the exception that he had difficulty sleeping. He was treated with increasing doses of Seroquel up to 75 mg for his sleep difficulty. He actively participated in physical therapy, occupational therapy, and cognitive therapy with speech pathology, and was transferred to a Veterans Administration center for cognitive rehabilitation. He made an excellent recovery, had a cranioplasty for his skull defect, and eventually resumed working in his previous capacity, albeit in a nondeployable status.

Follow-Up Contact

All patients are given a contact number and encouraged to call the PMP office at WRAMC should concerns develop for the patients or their families. They are also called 30, 90, and 180 days following discharge from the hospital. One of the early goals has been to make psychiatry an ally to the patient. When patients have returned to their homes they have found it easier responding and receiving intervention, and when crises occur they appear more willing to accept referral recommendations. In general, patients who need treatment upon leaving WRAMC are referred to resources within the military, veteran's health system, or civilian community.

The Trauma Patient's Family

Family members also experience psychological trauma as a result of the injury of their loved ones.[24–27] Families typically know little about the extent of the injuries or their prognosis, and therefore experience more anxiety and feelings of helplessness.[11] Crisis intervention for the family members of trauma victims may be needed.

It is difficult to predict how family members will react to the trauma and the injuries sustained by the patient. The experience of having a family member injured may exacerbate family malfunctioning.[17] However, the interventions to assist these families in coping with the traumatic event may lessen the family member's chance of developing secondary PTSD.[26] Trauma patients need as much support as possible, and family members are often better at providing emotional support and reassurance to the trauma patients than the staff.[24] Effective therapeutic family interventions may not only help the family members cope with the traumatic events but may help the patient as well. The family's anxieties tend to exacerbate the patient's conflict. Negative family behavior may also have a deleterious effect on the nursing staff. But if the family remains stable and supportive, the patient's anxiety is decreased and outcome is improved. The family's built-in support system may need to be augmented with professional help.[28] The purpose of the family crisis intervention is to build up the family's coping skills and resolve symptoms associated with psychological trauma. Sharing meals with families of other trauma patients, for example, also provides the family with additional support.[26]

Initially it is important that family members of the injured soldier have access to food, clothing, and shelter. A family assistance center is available 24 hours a day at WRAMC. This alleviates any additional stress and allows the family to focus its attention on the patient and deal with the ongoing events.[26] Each institution needs to provide personnel to help with this task. At WRAMC, PMP social workers are advocates for patients and their families.

Brief supportive counseling has also been proven effective at reducing anxiety in family members of trauma victims.[11] PMP staff will often spend time with family members interviewing and supporting them emotionally. Support groups formed specifically to assist these families provide an outlet for them to address their needs and feelings.[28] When developing family groups, Harvey and colleagues[28] found that families were more willing to attend when the group focus was on education and families sharing their stories. Families attending these support groups realized that they were not alone and were able to support each other. Additional benefits the families received from attending these groups included the ability to share feelings, reduce anxiety, instill hope, and gain a better understanding of their family members' injuries, medical treatments, and hospital procedures. PMP social workers also started a group for spouses and other family members of injured soldiers to allow for empathetic sharing and support. Groups are offered twice weekly for spouses and other family members. Topics include fear, frustration, the need to protect the injured patient, depression, anger, education, coping with disabled spouses, and feelings of alienation and disappointment.

Based on experiences at WRAMC, families are also seen by a provider in PMP in the hospital. Family members are assessed to determine how their children are adjusting, and how parents educate their children about the patient's injury. Many of the techniques used with patients are often effective with families. Empathic listening, reassurance, and normalization are usually enough to help family members through their initial emotional response to the trauma. Staff members of the child and adolescent psychiatry service routinely see the families and assess their psychological response to the trauma. Education and support to the children is provided as needed.

***Case Study 16-4*:** BB is a 35-year-old male with BKAs from injuries sustained in OEF. The patient was flown to Germany and then air evacuated to WRAMC. Initially his wife was very supportive and attentive, but as the rehabilitation progressed, greater frustration was observed. Ambivalence about her role and problems with her in-laws became prominent. Therapeutic interventions were undertaken and as a result she began to understand the normalcy of her behavior. This allowed her to understand her conflict and recommit herself to the marriage. The wife was given the PMP phone number for follow-up.

SUPPORTING MEDICAL STAFF WHO CARE FOR THE MEDICALLY INJURED TRAUMA VICTIM

There has been relatively little research conducted regarding the psychological impact that working with trauma victims has on medical staff[29,30] and the resources available to them. Taylor[31] suggests that, on average, there are three major disasters per week worldwide. By responding to the needs of these disaster victims, nurses and clinicians may be placing themselves at risk of experiencing secondary trauma. Dyergrov[32] suggests that among disaster workers, 80% are likely to experience emotional disturbances following the event, although only 3% to 7% are likely to experience significant psychological disruptions.

The myth that those in the helping profession are somehow immune to the stresses experienced by those they help, and therefore are unaffected, was debunked by Bamber.[33] Professionals, however, may be reluctant to seek help.[34] To help destigmatize mental health, PMP has routine visits with the clinical staff. For example, groups have been established in which nurses share their conflicts. Mutual support is also received. Nurses are included as team members in PMP and visit the wards to work with the nursing staff. Education about stress and responses are given when appropriate, and formal lectures are also provided.

Often overlooked is the stress the physicians experience, which may be exhibited during "curb-side" conversations.[35] Colleagues at times are wary about intervening and invading another's privacy. Providers are often concerned that their records or promotions will be affected if they seek help from the PMP. They also worry that others might see them as "weak." For instance, a surgeon walking in the hallway asked, "Can I ask you a question about one of my colleagues? He is not sleeping and has been irritable. What can I give or tell him?" While the psychiatrist should respond as if the advice is for the surgeon's colleague, there should be an awareness that the question may be about the surgeon. After maintaining the relationship, the surgeon could be asked if the conversation was really about a colleague. The psychiatrist could then offer to see the surgeon in the PMP office. In general, offering support and time to talk is necessary.

Physicians are, at times, reluctant to talk about their fears and frustrations. Giving lectures to the medical staff and maintaining a professional, empathetic relationship are essential to medical and surgical providers seeing mental health as a resource for themselves. At times, it has been helpful to hold groups for physicians prior to their morning rounds, where support is offered and difficult cases are discussed. E-mail messages and notes about stress are also distributed via department channels. These approaches have been extremely helpful.

A similar approach has been undertaken with administration and command staff. Maintaining a close working relationship with command is imperative for the needs of the service and for its commander's needs as well. Many forget that the commanders are under stress and may not have any outlet. Keeping them informed, as well as being available for their concerns, will help contribute positively to a successful approach.

Last, but not least, the mental health providers also need support. Reinforcement of their skills and keeping them educated about providing new approaches is helpful. Maintaining a positive esprit de corps and sensitivity to each other's needs also helps. Giving them time off and the use of humor, lunches, and dinners may also help. It is imperative that leaders keep an open door and be sensitive to the frustrations and countertransference issues of the providers. In particular, this is important with younger physicians and other staff that may be deployed. Sensitivity to these concerns is incumbent upon members of the PCLS/PMP staff.

SUMMARY

Physical injury as result of a trauma is an overwhelming experience that results in a life-changing event. Exposure to the trauma of war may result in psychiatric sequelae, but exposure to both physical and emotional conditions can have a geometric effect on psychiatric symptoms. Though most trauma patients adjust well and recognize that symptoms dissipate, others need psychiatric intervention. Based on past experiences, psychiatry staff at WRAMC developed an early intervention treatment plan for responding to injured soldiers. Traditional debriefing (classical incidence stress debriefing) interventions were not effective in this population. A new approach, under the umbrella of therapeutic intervention for prevention of psychiatric stress symptoms, was developed. This program entails intervening early without a formal consultation, destigmatizing mental health, adhering to a biopsychosocial approach, recognizing the importance of the therapeutic alliance using condensed aspects of traditional psychotherapeutic techniques, reinforcing patient assets, using relaxation or hypnotic techniques, prescribing appropriate pharmacology, and using empathic exposure. Though the goal is to avoid inappropriate pathologizing, treating psychiatric symptoms is necessary.

In an attempt to destigmatize mental health, a subsection (PMP) of the psychiatry service was created. Other goals of the intervention are to decrease the effect of disabling psychiatric symptoms, facilitate a speedy recovery, initiate integration of trauma into a normal stream of consciousness, ease symptoms, teach mastery or control techniques, and recognize and treat psychiatric illnesses early. Being able to refer patients for treatment if required after they leave the hospital is also a major component of this intervention. The development of a program for combat casualties necessitates the inclusion of patients' family members, hospital staff, and hospital leadership, as well as the mental health team serving this population. Besides the immediate positive therapeutic outcomes, a therapeutic alliance facilitates the acceptance of referrals by patients and family members upon discharge from the hospital.

Finally, based on the experience at WRAMC, becoming a part of a trauma team and being seen as member of PMP further expedited intervention and allowed psychiatry assistance for the patient without the typical stigmatization. Walking rounds further solidified patients, family members, and staff seeing PMP service staff as members of the trauma team. A similar plan can be developed at any hospital treating large volumes of trauma patients.

REFERENCES

1. Wain HJ, Jacaard JT. Psychiatric intervention with medical and surgical patients of war. In: Ursano RJ, Norwood AR, eds. *Emotional Aftermath of the Persian Gulf War: Veterans, Families, Communities, and Nations.* Washington, DC: American Psychiatric Press; 1996: 415–442.

2. Wain HJ, Grammer GG, Stasinos JJ, Miller CM. Meeting the patients where they are: consultation-liaison response to trauma victims of the Pentagon attack. *Mil Med.* 2002;167(9 suppl):19–21.

3. Wain HJ, Stasinos J. Response to bombing victims. Presentation at the State Department, Washington DC; 1999.

4. Wain HJ, Grammer G, Stasinos J, DeBoer C. Psychiatric intervention for medical surgical patients following traumatic injuries. In: Ritchie EC, Watson PJ, Friedman MJ, eds. *Interventions Following Mass Violence and Disasters: Strategies for Mental Health Practice.* New York, NY: Guilford Press; 2006: 278–298.

5. Weinstein EA. Disabling and disfiguring injuries. In: Jones FD, Sparacino LR, Wilcox VL, Rothberg JM, Stokes JW, eds. *War Psychiatry.* In: Zajtchuk R, Bellamy RF, eds. *Textbook of Military Medicine.* Washington, DC: Department of the Army, Office of The Surgeon General, Borden Institute; 1995: 353–381.

6. Furst SS, ed. *Psychic Trauma.* New York, NY: Basic Books; 1967.

7. Grieger TA, Cozza SJ, Ursano RJ, et al. Posttraumatic stress disorder and depression in battle-injured soldiers. *Am J Psychiatry.* 2006;163:1777–1783.

8. Koren D, Norman D, Cohen A, Berman J, Klein EM. Increased PTSD risk with combat-related injury: a matched comparison study of injured and uninjured soldiers experiencing the same combat events. *Am J Psychiatry*. 2005;162(2):276–282.

9. Ursano RJ, Norwood AR, eds. *Emotional Aftermath of the Persian Gulf War: Veterans, Families, Communities, and Nations*. Washington, DC: American Psychiatric Press; 1996.

10. Wain HJ, Grammer G, Cozza SJ, et al. Treating the traumatized amputee. *Iraq War Clinician Guide.* 2nd ed. Palo Alto, Calif: National Center for Posttraumatic Stress Disorder; 2004: 50–57.

11. Lenehan GP. Emotional impact of trauma. *Nurs Clin N Am*. 1986;21(4):729–740.

12. Schreiber S, Galai-Gat T. Uncontrolled pain following physical injury as the core-trauma in post-traumatic stress disorder. *Pain*. 1993;54:107–110.

13. Mohta M, Sethi AK, Tyagi A, Mohta A. Psychological care in trauma patients. *Injury*. 2003;34:17–25.

14. Grieger TA. Early predictors of later PTSD and depression in battle-injured soldiers. Paper presented at: American Psychiatric Association Meeting; May 24, 2006; Toronto, Canada.

15. Blum HP. Psychic trauma and traumatic object loss. *J Am Psychoanal Assoc*. 2003;51(2):415–432.

16. Horowitz MJ. Psychological processes induced by illness, injury, and loss. In: Milton T, Green C, Meagher R, eds. *Handbook of Clinical Health Psychology*. New York, NY: Plenum; 1982: 53–67.

17. Landsman IS, Baum CG, Arnkoff DB, et al. The psychosocial consequences of traumatic injury. *J Behav Med*. 1990;13(6):561–581.

18. Armfield F. Preventing post-traumatic stress disorder resulting from military operations. *Mil Med*. 1994;159(12):739–746.

19. Wain HJ, Bradley J, Nam T, Waldrep D, Cozza S. Psychiatric interventions with returning soldiers at Walter Reed. *Psychiatr Q*. 2005;76(4):351–360.

20. Wain HJ, Gabriel GM. Psychodynamic concepts inherent in a biopsychosocial model of care of traumatic injuries. *J Am Acad Psychoanal Dyn Psychiatry*. 2007;35(4):555–573.

21. Hoge CW, Castro CA, Messer SC, McGurk D, Cotting DI, Koffman RL. Combat duty in Iraq and Afghanistan, mental health problems, and barriers to care. *N Engl J Med*. 2004;351:13–21.

22. Morgan CA 3rd, Krystal JH, Southwick SM. Toward early pharmacological posttraumatic stress intervention. *Biol Psychiatry*. 2003;53(9):834–843.

23. Brende JO. Combined individual and group therapy for Vietnam veterans. *Int J Group Psychotherapy*. 1981;31(3):367–378.

24. Solursh DS. The family of the trauma victim. *Nurs Clin North Am*. 1990;25:155–162.

25. Brown V. The family as victim in trauma. *Hawaii Medical J*. 1991;50(4):153–154.

26. Flannery RB Jr. Treating family survivors of mass casualties: a CISM family crisis intervention approach. *Int J Emerg Ment Health*. 1999;1:243–250.

27. Alexander DA. The psychiatric consequences of trauma. *Hosp Med*. 2002;63:12–15.

28. Harvey C, Dixon M, Padberg N. Support group for families of trauma patients: a unique approach. *Crit Care Nurse*. 1995;15(4):59–63.

29. Robbins I. The psychological impact of working in emergencies and the role of debriefing. *J Clin Nurs*. 1999;8:263–268.

30. Salston M, Figley C. Secondary traumatic stress effects of working with survivors of criminal victimization. *J Trauma Stress*. 2003;16(2):167–174.

31. Taylor SE. Adjustment to threatening events: a theory of cognitive adaptation. *Am Psychol*. 1983;38:1161–1173.

32. Dyergrov A. Caring for helpers in disaster situations: psychological debriefing. *Disaster Manage*. 1989;2:25–30.

33. Bamber M. Providing support for emergency service staff. *Nurs Times*. 1994;90(22):32–33.

34. Collins S. What about us? The psychological implications of dealing with trauma following the Omagh bombing. *Emerg Nurse*. 2001;8(10):9–13.

35. Wain HJ, Grammer G, Cozza SJ, et al. Caring for clinicians who care for traumatically injured patients. *Iraq War Clinician Guide*. 2nd ed. Palo Alto, Calif: National Center for Posttraumatic Stress Disorder; 2004: 62–65.

Chapter 17

ORAL HEALTH EFFECTS OF COMBAT STRESS

GEORGIA DELA CRUZ, DMD, MPH*; AND PAUL COLTHIRST, DDS, MS†

*Lieutenant Colonel, Dental Corps, US Army; Office of The Surgeon General, US Army, 5109 Leesburg Pike, Suite 682, Falls Church, Virginia 22041

†Major, Dental Corps, US Army; Dental Public Health, Department of Leadership Development, US Army Medical Department Center and School, 2250 Stanley Road, Fort Sam Houston, Texas 78234-6100; formerly, Staff Officer, Dental Command Headquarters, Fort Sam Houston, Texas

The average American, if not prepared, will cope with distress by eating more junk food, drinking more alcohol, smoking more cigarettes, taking more over-the-counter drugs, or under-the-counter drugs. We are a society that copes with distress with some form of oral behavior.

—JO Prochaska, PhD, developer of the Trans-Theoretical Model of Behavior Change
(interview available at: mms://mediastream.buffalo.edu/content/nur/Part1a.wmv, accessed July 13, 2010)

INTRODUCTION

Approximately 5% to 10% of disease and nonbattle injuries among service members result from oral diseases or injuries.[1] The rate of dental emergencies is higher for units whose soldiers deploy with poor oral health. Oral diseases can cause impaired duty performance, work loss, restricted activity, poor diet, difficulty pronouncing words, inability to sleep, and excruciating pain. If they are not prevented or treated early, oral diseases can cause severe, life-threatening illness and may even require medical evacuation from theater. One recent study of US Army soldiers (regular Army, reserve, and National Guard) medically evacuated from the Central Command area of responsibility during 2003 and 2004 found that oral disease accounted for 42% of oral-facial evacuations.[2]

STRESS AND ORAL HABITS

Many Americans have a low level of health literacy and perceive oral health as less important and separate from general health.[3] Advances in dental research since the 1950s have shown that nearly all oral disease is preventable, yet many people continue to have a fatalistic view that "dental problems" are inevitable, of mysterious origin, and can be ignored as long as they are not unaesthetic or painful. Many service members join the military with these erroneous beliefs about oral diseases, viewing oral hygiene as mainly cosmetic and unnecessary during field training or operations.

The primary causes of oral diseases during deployment are bacterial or viral infections that are initiated or exacerbated by the effects of poor oral hygiene, poor diet, or substance use. Self-care and hygiene habits are often the first things to break down when a soldier is deployed to an austere environment or experiences overwhelming stress. Many of these soldiers also turn to harmful oral habits such as using tobacco or eating and drinking nutrient-poor beverages and foods that are high in simple carbohydrates.

According to the 2006 Department of Defense Survey of Health-Related Behaviors in the Reserve Component,[4] nearly 45% of service members admitted to eating as a way to cope with stress. Women were significantly more likely than men to eat as a coping strategy (51.8% vs 42.5%), while more men than women reported using cigars or smokeless tobacco (11.4% vs 3.6%). Reserve-component men and women were similar in their use of cigarettes (19.4%) and alcohol (24.9%) for coping. Results of the 2008 Department of Defense Survey of Health-Related Behaviors Among Active Duty Military Personnel[5] shows that men were significantly more likely to smoke cigarettes (28.6%) or drink alcohol (34.5%) for coping than were women (21.0% and 25.2%, respectively). Comparisons between the services show that more service members in the Marine Corps (39.9%), the Army (35.6%), and the Navy (33.7%) have a drink to cope with stress than do service members in the Air Force (25.0%). The same pattern is seen for smoking, with 33.2% of Marine Corps, 30.8% of Army, 27.9% of Navy, and 18.8% of Air Force service members lighting up a cigarette to cope with stress. Women, on the other hand, are still significantly more likely to use eating as a coping mechanism (56.2%) than are men (45.7%). Service members in the Navy and Army are significantly more likely to use eating as a coping mechanism (49.6% and 48.2%, respectively) than those in the Air Force or Marine Corps (45.1% and 44.5%, respectively). The combination of poor oral hygiene with harmful oral habits such as tobacco use and increased intake of refined carbohydrates causes oral disease (Figure 17-1).

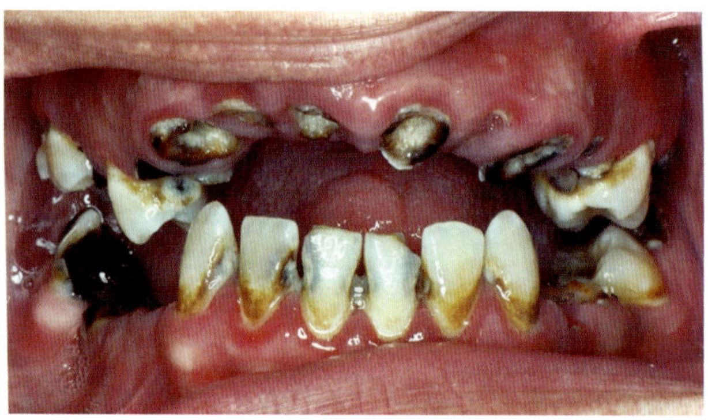

Figure 17-1. Plaque accumulation, tobacco staining, gingival inflammation, and generalized caries resulting from a combination of inadequate oral hygiene, tobacco use, and refined carbohydrate intake.

Changes in diet during deployment or other stressful situations can cause service members to suffer from dehydration and micronutrient deficiencies that can lead to skin conditions, stress fractures, anemia, and other conditions.[6–11] Because the oral epithelium has a high rate of cellular turnover, these same deficiencies can affect oral health by preventing the oral epithelium from renewing or repairing itself. As a result, the first signs of micronutrient deficiency can appear in the mouth, and may present as glossitis, angular cheilitis, stomatitis, and gingivitis. Undernutrition can also exacerbate oral infections and has been associated with increased progression of periodontal disease.[12] Vitamins A, C, D, E, B_2, B_6, B_{12}, niacin, and folic acid, and minerals such as zinc, iron, magnesium, and calcium are essential for repairing oral epithelium, maintaining periodontal attachment, preventing demineralization of bones and teeth, and ensuring an adequate amount of saliva of sufficient quality to protect the oral cavity. In addition to enabling taste, mastication, and digestion, saliva is critical for defense against oral diseases. Compromised saliva composition or flow impairs or eliminates its antifungal, antiviral, and antibacterial activities and prevents it from protecting the teeth from demineralization by acids from oral bacteria or foods and beverages.

STRESS AND DENTAL HARD-TISSUE DISEASES

When eating is used as a coping mechanism for stress, it often involves the frequent consumption of foods containing organic acids and simple carbohydrates such as sugar and starch. Between-meal consumption of these foods or beverages (ie, sports drinks, energy drinks, or soda) promotes dental caries and dental erosion.

Dental Caries

The majority of dental emergencies during deployment have been for conditions resulting from dental caries.[13–18] Exact incidence of new disease is unknown, but a pilot study[19] of soldiers deployed in Operation Iraqi Freedom for 6 months during 2003 found that the number of carious lesions increased by 156%, and the severity of disease, as measured by the number of tooth surfaces involved, increased by 183% over predeployment statistics.

Dental caries is caused when poor oral hygiene allows uncontrolled growth of bacteria in dental plaque on tooth surfaces (Figure 17-2). The bacteria rapidly metabolize the simple carbohydrates (starches or sugars) in the diet into destructive acids (lactic acid). Fermentable carbohydrate metabolism supports the colonization of more bacteria on the tooth surface, further increasing the amount of acid produced. Following exposure to fermentable carbohydrates, plaque pH falls below 5.5, the critical pH for maintaining the structural integrity of the mineralized dental tissue. It can take 30 to 40 minutes for the pH to rise again, depending on the flow rate and buffering capacity of the individual's saliva. As a result, the amount of bacterial acid produced in any 24-hour period mirrors the frequency and duration of exposure to fermentable carbohydrates more closely than the total amount of carbohydrate consumed.

Starches do not directly serve as substrate for oral bacterial fermentation. Starch granules in grains, vegetables, potatoes, and beans are damaged when they are subjected to heat and mechanical forces, producing a gelatinized starch. This starch is further broken down by salivary and bacterial amylases into sucrose, maltose, and maltotriose—substances that are available for bacterial acid production.[20] As a result, untreated whole grains and raw vegetables have lower caries-promoting potential than heat-processed foods like white breads, crackers, chips, snacks, and dry cereal. Foods that contain sugar plus starch destroy dental enamel more rapidly than pure sugar foods because the starch acts like digestible glue, keeping the sugar in close contact with the tooth surface for longer periods of time. Teeth that have low levels of fluoride in the enamel are more vulnerable to these acids, and decay can begin and progress quite rapidly. Without regular exposure to fluoride, sugar consumption is a strong indicator of caries risk.[21]

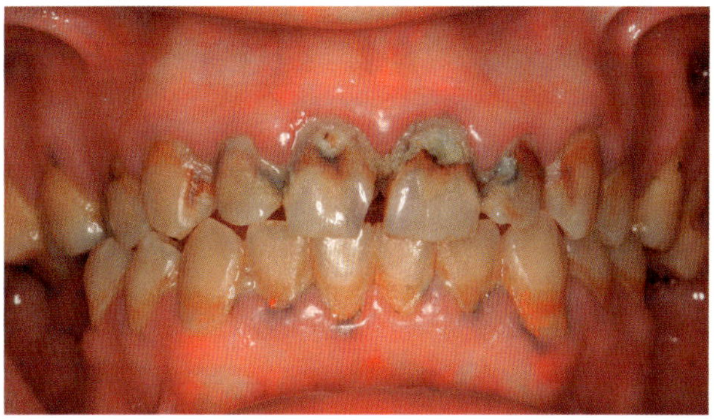

Figure 17-2. Extensive accumulation of bacterial plaque after cessation of oral hygiene. Gingiva is inflamed and several carious lesions are evident.
Photograph: Courtesy of Captain Andrew Marshall, US Army Dental Corps.

Dental Erosion

Dental erosion, or erosive tooth wear, is described as "the loss of dental hard tissue either through chemical etching and dissolution by acids of nonbacterial origin or by chelation."[22(p243)] The prevalence of dental erosion is increasing, particularly in younger populations.[23,24] Nonbacterial acids that cause erosion primarily come from two sources: gastric acids or diet. Caffeinated sodas, sports drinks, and energy drinks are commonly used in theater for hydration, to maintain alertness, or for simple enjoyment. These flavored beverages often contain polybasic organic acids such as citric acid, phosphoric acid, malic acid, and tartaric acid. Popular beverages that fall into this category include soft drinks, sports drinks, energy drinks, and sweetened, bottled tea blends. Other types of acidic drinks include apple or citrus fruit juice. Acidic foods include citrus, pineapple, and sour candies. Any of these acidic foods and beverages can accelerate the progression of dental caries. Organic acids accelerate the progression of decay by chemically eroding the dental enamel[25] (Figure 17-3). Polybasic acids have a unique buffering capacity and can maintain an acidic pH even with marked dilution. This high titratable acid level multiplies the actual number of hydrogen ions available for interaction with the tooth surface, and is thought to be an important reason for their erosive properties. The chemical structure of polybasic organic acids also gives them the ability to chelate calcium at higher pHs, so they can erode dental enamel even in a neutral environment.[26]

Exposure to gastric acids is caused by either gastroesophageal reflux disease (GERD) or eating disorders that involve self-induced vomiting. Exposure to gastric acids is one of the most destructive processes that can affect the teeth. Stomach acids demineralize the outer layers of tooth enamel, leaving behind the protein matrix, which is then easily removed with brushing. GERD is the most common gastrointestinal-related diagnosis given during office visits, and affects somewhere between 10% to 20% of the Western population.[27] The disorder causes erosion of the lingual and occlusal surfaces of the teeth, affecting the posterior teeth most severely. In the early stages, affected teeth exhibit a smooth, glazed appearance. Damage generally progresses to the development of a "dished out" appearance and the exposure of the dentin layer (Figure 17-4). Over time the affected teeth can become weakened and may develop thermal sensitivity.[28] Patients with GERD are usually prescribed proton pump inhibitors and must avoid eating certain foods, as well as sleeping within a few hours of eating, exercising, or bending over. Disruption of dietary or medication routines by high operations tempo or combat situations may cause recurrence of GERD symptoms and repeated exposure of the dentition to gastric acids.

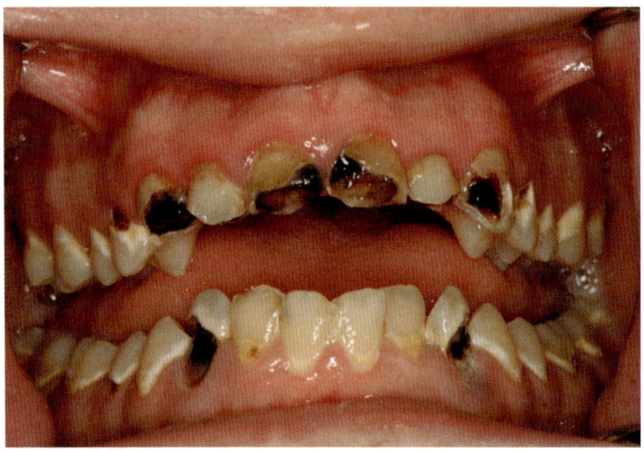

Figure 17-3. Generalized demineralization and loss of enamel on the facial surfaces of teeth just above the gingival margin in the absence of gingival inflammation is often an indication of frequent use of sugared beverages that contain organic acids.
Photograph: Courtesy of Captain Andrew Marshall, US Army Dental Corps.

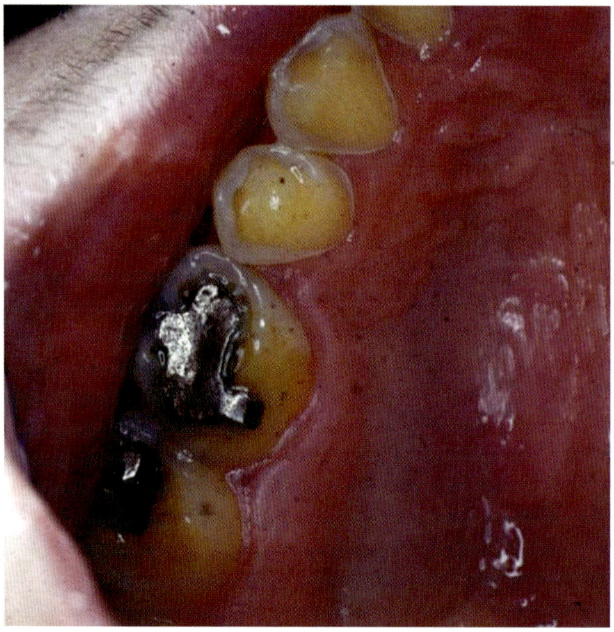

Figure 17-4. Erosion of enamel and exposure of the dentin layer in a patient with gastroesophageal reflux disease.
Photograph: Courtesy of Bennett T Amaechi, Associate Professor and Director of Cariology, University of Texas Health Science Center at San Antonio.

Eating Disorders

In most cases, dental hard-tissue damage is unlikely to signify anorexia or bulimia, except in those with an already established diagnosis who experience a recurrence under stress. Oral manifestations associated with eating disorders may include one or more of the following[29]:

- smooth erosion of the enamel or perimylolysis,
- traumatized oral mucosal membranes and pharynx,
- variations in the periodontium,
- enlargement of the parotid or submandibular salivary glands,
- xerostomia (dry mouth due to reduced salivary flow), and
- dental caries.

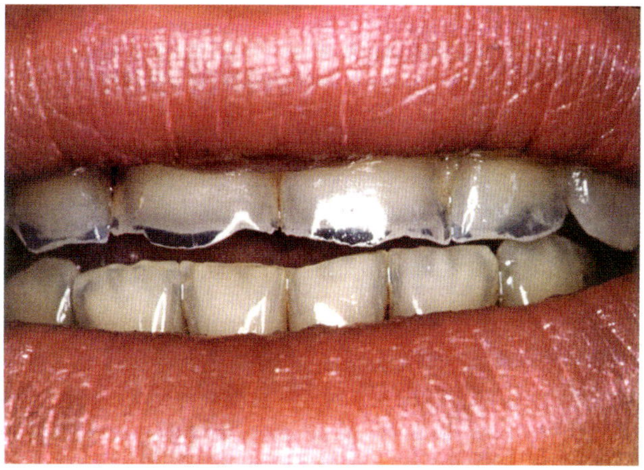

Figure 17-6. Translucency of the maxillary central incisors due to erosion in a patient with bulimia.
Photograph: Courtesy of cosmetic dentist Dr Craig Mabrito, Houston, Texas.

When vomiting occurs repeatedly over time, tooth enamel becomes thin and eroded, resulting in a smooth, glassy appearance. In the case of eating disorders, these changes are most commonly seen on the lingual, occlusal, and incisal surfaces of the maxillary teeth. When confined to these areas, the condition is termed "perimylolysis" (Figures 17-5 and 17-6). These areas of the teeth are more susceptible to erosion due to the combined chemical and mechanical effects of regurgitated gastric acids and their retention on the surface of the tongue. Erosion is usually not clinically detectible until vomiting behavior has occurred for about 2 years. However, the daily frequency of self-induced vomiting is one of the main determinants of the rate of progression and degree of dental erosion. As is the case with GERD, erosion may eventually affect the occlusal and facial surfaces of teeth, resulting in exposure of the underlying dentin and decreased vertical dimension (overclosure; Figure 17-7).

Patients with eating disorders may also develop diet-caused dental erosion in other areas of the teeth. Several studies have reported that people with restrictive anorexia tend to favor highly acidic, low-

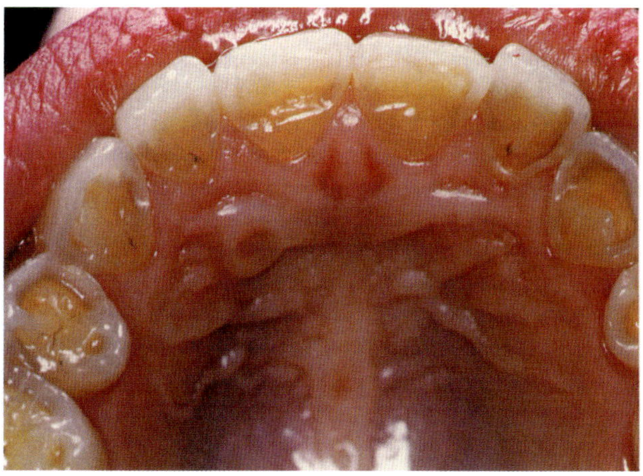

Figure 17-5. Erosion of the lingual, occlusal, and incisal surfaces of the maxillary teeth in a patient with bulimia.
Photograph: Courtesy of cosmetic dentist Dr Craig Mabrito, Houston, Texas.

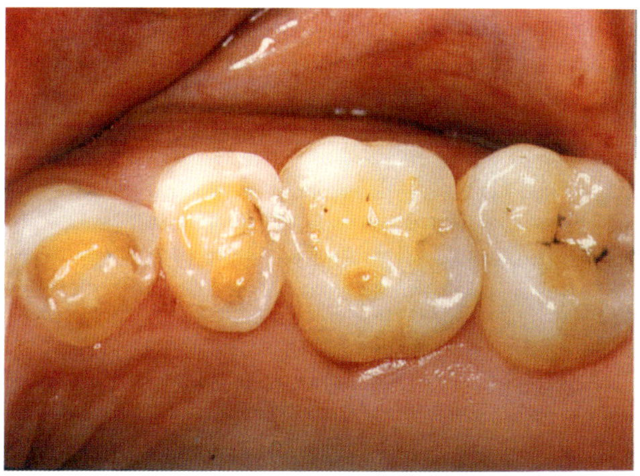

Figure 17-7. Occlusal wear and dentin exposure due to erosion in a patient with bulimia.
Photograph: Courtesy of cosmetic dentist Dr Craig Mabrito, Houston, Texas.

calorie foods, particularly raw citrus.[29–31] If exposure is frequent, these foods tend to cause erosion on the buccal or facial surfaces of the tissue, in contrast to perimylolysis (Figure 17-8).

Stomach acids may irritate the gingival tissue if exposure is frequent, but controlled studies of gingival inflammation in patients with eating disorders have produced conflicting results.[32,33] A more common cause of gingival inflammation in patients with eating disorders appears to be a lack of interest in oral hygiene, which can accompany depression. Also, alveolar bone support of the teeth may be compromised in some patients. Patients with severe disease experience early bone loss or osteoporosis as a result of changes in their estrogen and cortisol levels, and are probably at risk for accelerated alveolar bone loss.

Trauma to the oral mucous membranes or the oropharynx may also occur in patients who engage in binge eating or self-induced vomiting. The rapid ingestion of food associated with binge eating may cause trauma, as may the force of regurgitation. Objects used to induce vomiting may also injure the soft palate.

Salivary gland enlargement is seen in approximately 10% to 50% of patients who binge eat and purge by vomiting. The gland most frequently involved is the parotid gland, and swelling usually occurs 2 to 6 days after bingeing/purging behavior. The enlargement often becomes persistent as the eating disorder progresses. The swelling may give a square, widened appearance to the mandible. However, the involved gland is usually soft and painless upon palpation and has a patent duct, normal salivary flow, and an absence of inflammation, both clinically and histologically. Other histological characteristics include greater acinar size, increased secretory granules, fatty infiltration, and fibrosis. The exact cause of the enlargement is not known, but individuals who purge by methods other than vomiting do not experience salivary gland enlargement. Hypothesized reasons include autonomic stimulation of the glands by activation of the taste buds or cholinergic stimulation of the glands during vomiting.[29]

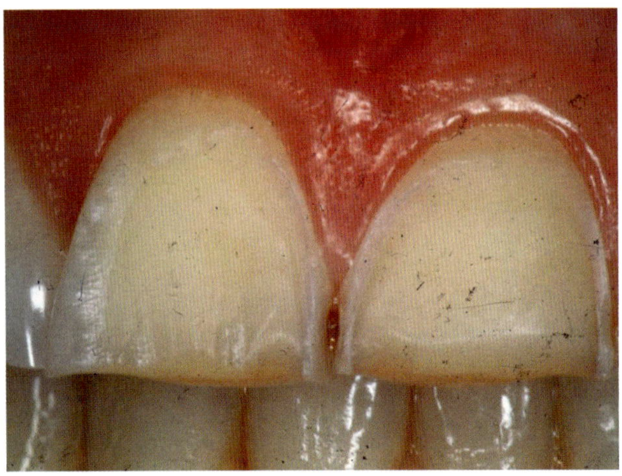

Figure 17-8. Erosion of the facial enamel and exposure of the underlying dentin.
Photograph: Courtesy of Bennett T Amaechi, Associate Professor and Director of Cariology, Department of Community Dentistry, University of Texas Health Science Center at San Antonio.

Antidepressants, which are frequently used to treat anorexia nervosa, usually cause xerostomia, and patients with xerostomia are more susceptible to developing carious lesions. Risk for dental caries may also be increased in patients whose bingeing episodes frequently involve high-calorie, high-carbohydrate foods. As a general rule, however, patients with eating disorders who primarily practice restriction or self-induced vomiting do not experience an increase in caries rates.[29]

Prevention

Nearly all dental caries is preventable with the use of good personal health habits (proper diet and nutrition, oral hygiene, and avoiding substance use). Daily oral hygiene is essential for the removal of harmful microorganisms and maintenance of oral health. Soldiers must be trained in proper field oral hygiene. Brushing after meals with fluoride toothpaste is the most effective caries prevention method. Soldiers who have been diagnosed with GERD should attempt to maintain or reestablish medication and dietary restrictions.

To prevent tooth decay, soldiers must use combat stress control techniques to help cope with the stresses of deployment, rather than relying on harmful dietary habits. Techniques such as talking, exercise, quick relaxation, deep relaxation, and cognitive exercises can all be used to relieve combat stress without harming oral health.[34,35]

Use of gum or mints that contain xylitol as the first ingredient, three to five times a day, between meals or after snacks also prevents dental decay.[36] Xylitol is a naturally occurring sweetener found in fruits, vegetables, and some other plants. It has about half the calories of sugar but is just as sweet. Xylitol prevents harmful bacteria from using starchy or sugary food particles to create acids that cause dental caries. It works synergistically with fluoride to prevent decay and promote remineralization of damaged tooth structure. Xylitol gum is distributed in theater dining facilities in the accessory pack of the MRE (meal, ready-to-eat). Chewing xylitol gum for about 5 minutes regularly after meals and snacks should help prevent decay.

For both oral health and weight management, free sugar intake from foods and beverages should be less than 10% of energy intake (less than 41 g/day).[37] On average, people who consume over 55 grams of sugar a day are at high risk for dental caries. The frequency of free sugar intake should be less than five times a day. Cariogenic foods and beverages can be combined with protective foods (cheese, tea, protein, high-fiber foods, etc) to prevent dental caries.[38] Soldiers should be encouraged to drink fluoridated water for hydration between meals, and limit consumption of foods and drinks that contain harmful polybasic organic acids to mealtimes. Soldiers can also mitigate the effects of foods and beverages that have a high organic-acid or refined-carbohydrate content by rinsing their mouths with water after ingestion.

Patients who experience xerostomia are at increased risk for dental caries, and should be advised to use artificial saliva preparations to lubricate the oral tissues, avoid cariogenic foods or drinks, and use sugarless or xylitol-containing candies or mints. Sucking on these items can stimulate increased salivary flow, which may buffer oral acids. Increased saliva flow also increases the concentration of calcium, phosphate, and hydroxyl ions, which may aid remineralization of early carious lesions. Xylitol may also be beneficial because of its bacteriostatic properties.

Treatment

Patients should be referred to a dentist for treatment of dental caries. Soldiers who experience recurrence of GERD symptoms for any reason should be seen by a dentist as soon as possible. To prevent chemical damage to dental hard tissues by stomach acids, dentists may fabricate a thin plastic stent that covers the dentition. The stent is to be worn at night or at times when reflux symptoms are most likely to occur. Early referral of eating-disorder patients to a psychiatric therapist can reduce the risk of further damage to the teeth and the oral cavity. Patients should be referred to a dentist for an evaluation of dental erosion, salivary flow rate, and oral mucosa condition. Comprehensive dental procedures should not be performed until vomiting behavior is significantly improved or the patient has recovered completely; until then, proper home care is the best treatment.

All patients whose oral cavity is exposed to gastric acid should be counseled on several important principals of home care[29,33]:

- Toothbrushing should never be performed immediately after the mouth is exposed to stomach acid because demineralized enamel has been shown to be vulnerable to removal by abrasive forces.
- Following acid exposure, patients should rinse with a buffering or alkaline solution to neutralize the acid and allow the saliva to remineralize the teeth, thereby reducing damage from demineralization. Options include 0.5% sodium fluoride sodium bicarbonate in water, liquid antacids, slightly alkaline mineral water, or plain water.
- If acid exposure happens repeatedly on a daily basis, a neutral sodium fluoride mouth rinse or prescription fluoride gel may be necessary to prevent dental erosion.
- Acidic foods and drinks should be avoided, including citrus, pineapple, and lemon candies; apple or citrus fruit juice; alcohol (particularly white wine); and drinks that contain polybasic organic acids such as citric, phosphoric, malic, and tartaric.[10,11]
- Patients who experience xerostomia should be advised to use artificial saliva preparations to lubricate the oral tissues, avoid cariogenic foods or drinks, and use sugarless or xylitol-containing candies or mints. Sucking on these items can stimulate increased salivary flow, which may buffer oral acids.

STRESS AND PERIODONTAL DISEASES

Gingivitis

Neglect of oral hygiene is common in stressful operational environments. Failure to properly remove plaque from the teeth and gums for a week or more usually results in the development of gingivitis in response to bacteria (Figure 17-9). The previously mentioned evaluation of soldiers deployed to Iraq showed that these service members experienced a significant worsening of their average periodontal screening and recording scores after 6 months of deployment.[19] If left untreated, gingivitis associated with tenderness and bleeding gums may discourage soldiers from performing normal oral hygiene.

Acute presentations of gingivitis can be managed by improved oral hygiene and the use of an antimicrobial mouth rinse. Soldiers with extreme gingival tenderness may be encouraged to reestablish oral hygiene proce-

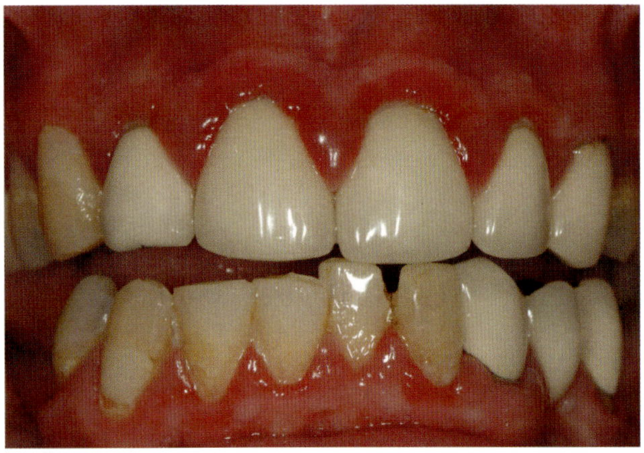

Figure 17-9. A case of gingivitis.
Photograph: Courtesy of Colonel Dave Reeves, US Army Dental Corps, Consultant to The Surgeon General for Periodontology, and Chief, Periodontics, Fort Hood, Texas.

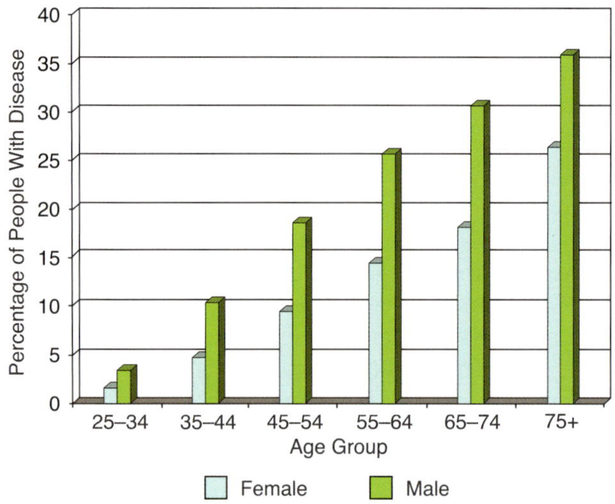

Figure 17-11. Prevalence of periodontal disease. Males are more likely than females to have at least one tooth site with 6 mm or more of periodontal loss of attachment.
Adapted from: US Department of Health and Human Services. *The Surgeon General's Report on Oral Health*. Washington, DC: USDHHS; 2000: 65.

dures using viscous lidocaine on their toothbrushes rather than a dentifrice.

Periodontitis

Untreated gingivitis may progress to periodontal disease (Figure 17-10). The risk of periodontal disease has been studied for both men and women (Figure 17-11), and several risk factors have been identified,[39–42] such as gram-negative anaerobic bacteria, smoking, diabetes mellitus, a genetic tendency to produce increased levels of proinflammatory mediators, and use of hormone-mimicking medications.

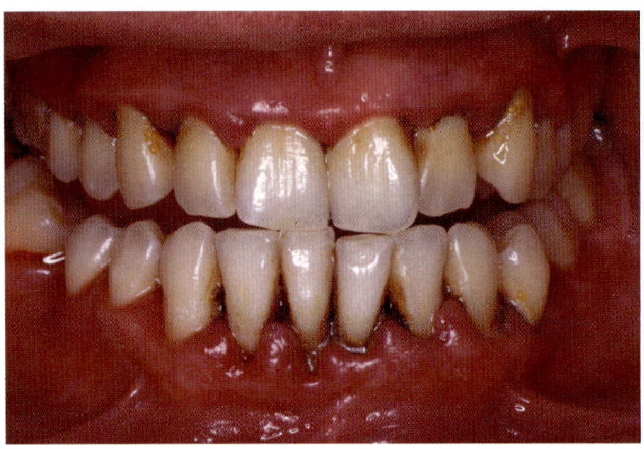

Figure 17-10. Gingival erythema, edema, and recession in conjunction with blunting of the interdental papilla are evident in this patient with periodontal disease.
Photograph: Courtesy of Lieutenant Colonel Georgia dela Cruz, US Army Dental Corps, Falls Church, Va.

Periodontitis has been described as "a complex disease in which disease expression involves intricate interactions of the oral biofilm with the host immunoinflammatory response and subsequent alterations in bone and connective tissue homeostasis."[43(p1560)] Classification of periodontal disease is based on two clinical factors: inflammation and loss of supporting tissue.[44] Inflammation features typically seen are redness, edema, and bleeding on probing. Loss of supporting tissue is usually measured as increased probing depth, decreased attachment level, or alveolar bone loss. Even with the presence of periodontal pathogens, the pathogenesis of periodontitis cannot occur without immune and inflammatory responses, which are in turn shaped by both intrinsic (eg, genetics, age, systemic disease) and extrinsic (eg, toxins, tobacco, plaque) host factors[45] (Figure 17-12). How much bone loss occurs depends largely on the level of inflammatory mediators present in gingival tissue.

Alveolar bone destruction occurs after activation of the pathogenesis pathways and the penetration of inflammatory mediators deep into gingival tissue, near alveolar bone. Several proinflammatory cytokines are responsible for bone resorption, such as interleukin-1, -6, -11, and -17; tumor necrosis factor-α; leukemia inhibitory factor; and oncostatin M.[45] When an inflammatory response occurs, periosteal osteoblasts are stimulated by proinflammatory cytokines and other mediators. Once the osteoblasts are stimulated,

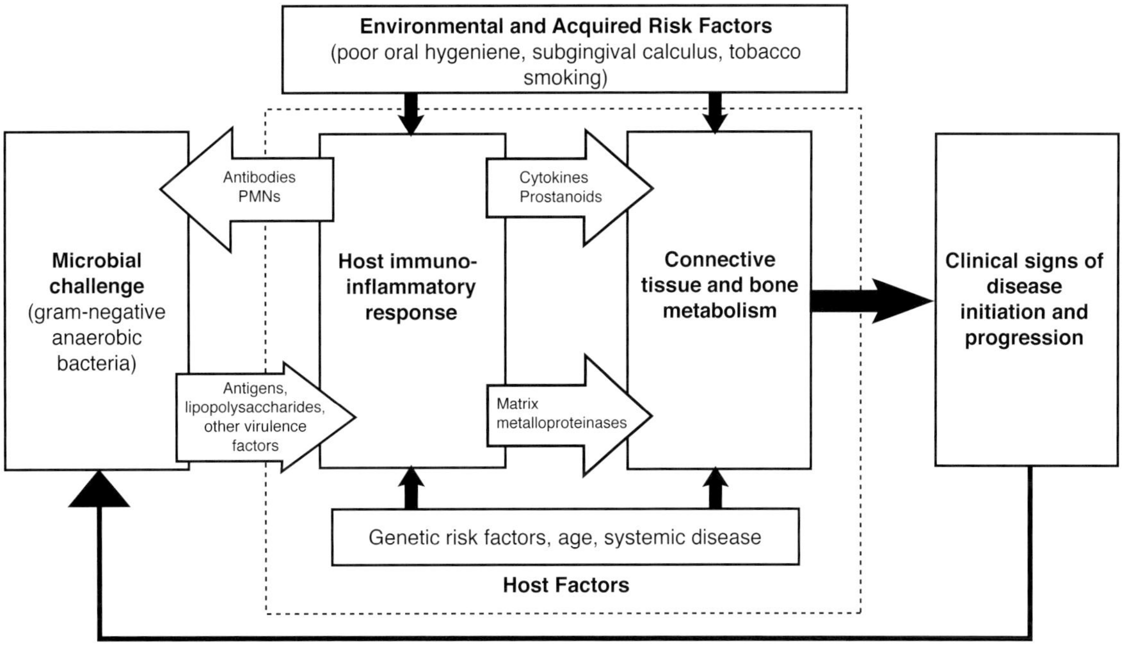

Figure 17-12. Model of periodontitis depicting the multifactorial nature of periodontal disease. A change in any one factor can result in clinical signs of the disease.
PMN: polymorphonuclear leukocytes
Data sources: (1) Page RC, Kornman KS. The pathogenesis of human periodontitis: an introduction. *Periodontology 2000*. 1997;14:9–11. (2) US Department of Health and Human Services. *The Surgeon General's Report on Oral Health*. Washington, DC: DHHS; 2000. (3) Gluck G, Morganstein W. *Jong's Community Dental Health*. 5th ed. St Louis, Mo: Mosby; 2003: 185–187.

changes in the overall cell surface occur that increase the expression of a protein called "receptor activator of nuclear factor-κ B ligand (RANKL)."[45] RANKL can be found on the surface of many other cells, including fibroblasts, T lymphocytes, and B lymphocytes. In the noninflammatory state, there is a balance between osteoclastic and osteoblastic processes determined by the proportion of RANKL. However, during an active inflammatory response, the proinflammatory mediators increase the expression of RANKL while at the same time decreasing other surface protein production in osteoclast precursor cells, triggering the formation of mature osteoclasts. Alveolar bone resorption by these osteoclasts leads to destruction of the supporting structures of the teeth, which, in the absence of intervention, leads to tooth loss.[45]

Women's risk of developing gingival inflammation or periodontal problems may be increased by the higher levels of estrogen and progesterone associated with the menstrual cycle and use of oral contraceptives.[46,47] Gingival tissues may become tender and swollen, and may bleed during brushing. Human gingiva has specific high-affinity estrogen receptors and can function as an estrogen target tissue. The stratified squamous epithelium of the oral mucosa and gingiva responds to ovarian hormone levels, with alterations in maturation and keratinization. Estrogen is involved in the regulation and maintenance of collagen synthesis and has been associated with gingival hyperplasia.

Estrogen and progesterone also promote changes in the microcirculatory system of the gingiva. The endothelial cells and pericytes of the venules swell, granulocytes and platelets adhere to the vessel walls, microthrombi form, and perivascular mast cells are disrupted.[46] The microvasculature proliferates and becomes more permeable, causing gingival edema and increasing the flow of gingival crevicular fluid. The resulting fluid also contains elevated levels of sex hormones, polymorphonuclear leukocytes, and increased levels of prostaglandin E_2. Anaerobic bacteria (eg, *Bacteroides melaninogenicus, Prevotella intermedia,* and *Porphyromonas gingivalis*) may be present and proliferate under these conditions.

The increase in bacteria production is a result of two factors: (1) some bacteria associated with gingival inflammation are able to metabolize steroid hormones and use them for energy production, thereby directly increasing their numbers; and (2) increased estrogen and progesterone levels also depress T-cell responses and decrease neutrophil chemotaxis and phagocytosis. This impaired immune response allows bacteria in the gingival crevice to proliferate without restraint.

Proliferating bacteria can cause increased levels of bacterial endotoxins, which can increase inflammation and trigger bone loss from the periodontium. Oral contraceptives, especially those containing progesterone, have been associated with an increased risk of periodontal bone loss.[47,48] No studies have been done on Depo-Provera (medroxyprogesterone acetate [the Upjohn Company, Kalamazoo, Mich]) and periodontal bone loss.

Necrotizing Ulcerative Gingivitis

When soldiers are placed under severe stress, increased cortisol levels can compromise immune function. Under these conditions, gingivitis can progress to acute necrotizing ulcerative gingivitis, an extremely painful inflammation accompanied by necrosis of the interdental gingiva and a fetid odor (Figure 17-13).

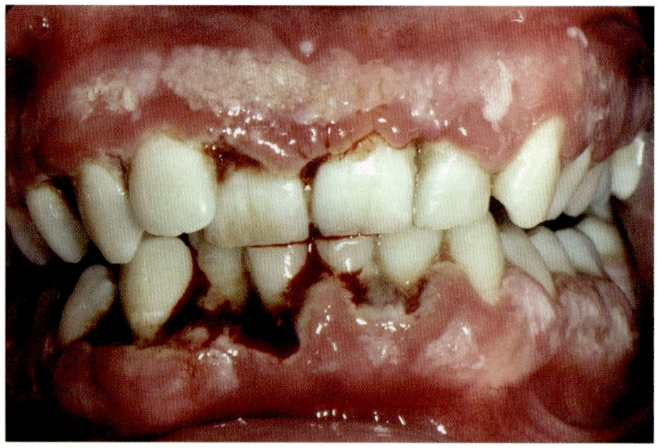

Figure 17-13. Gingival edema, erythema, and cratering of the interdental papilla and purulent exudate are visible in this patient with acute necrotizing ulcerative gingivitis.
Photograph: Courtesy of Dr Carl Allen, Professor and Director, Oral and Maxillofacial Pathology, Ohio State University College of Dentistry.

Prevention

Noncommissioned officers should ensure that the oral hygiene routine of all troops includes the following:

- toothbrushing, once daily at a minimum, preferably twice daily, with fluoride toothpaste to prevent dental caries and gingival problems;
- flossing daily, which is also effective in preventing gingival or periodontal problems; and
- rinsing several times a week with an antimicrobial mouthwash containing thymol or chlorhexidine gluconate (for those with chronic periodontal conditions).

Treatment

Acute presentations of necrotizing periodontitis should be referred to a dental professional. In addition to reestablishing oral hygiene procedures with viscous lidocaine hydrochloride and an antimicrobial mouthwash, acute periodontal disease usually requires the removal of plaque-retentive factors, such as calculus or defective restorations, from the crown and root surfaces of the teeth.

TEMPOROMANDIBULAR DYSFUNCTION

Stress can produce temporomandibular dysfunction (TMD) symptoms when it causes patients to clench or brux their teeth more frequently, either at night or during the day. Masticatory muscle spasms and pain may result. Other known causes of TMD symptoms include injury to the temporomandibular joint from blunt force to the face, arthritis, joint overload, or repetitive loading (usually because of bruxism or grinding of the teeth).

Although the overall incidence of the condition is low, TMD affects both men and women. According to a 1994 triservice recruit comprehensive oral health survey,[49] approximately 3.5% of female recruits were found to have some type of orofacial pain or limited mandibular movement sufficient to require referral or treatment for TMD. The incidence for women was significantly higher than that for men (1.5%). Civilian studies[50,51] have consistently shown an increased incidence of TMD (1.5- to 2-fold higher) in women compared with men, and most patients treated for TMD are women (80%). Age plays a strong role in women. Symptoms begin after puberty and peak during the reproductive years, with prevalence highest among women aged 20 to 40. Gender and age distributions of TMD expression strongly suggest a link to the female hormonal system. Some studies[51–53] have shown that women who use oral contraceptives may be at increased risk compared with women who do not. TMD pain levels increase during menstruation.[54,55] Current studies investigating the relationship of increased risk with the presence of estrogen receptors in the temporomandibular joint structures (particularly the synovial lining cells, the articular disc, and the chondrocytes) have produced contradictory results.[56,57]

Prevention

TMD can be prevented by avoiding opening the mouth too wide during eating or yawning, and avoiding frequent, prolonged masticatory activity associated with pervasive oral habits such as jaw clenching, gum chewing, cheekbiting, or nailbiting.

Treatment

Acute open lock (an internal joint derangement that prevents closing the mouth) can cause extreme pain and should be immediately referred to a dental provider for reduction of the dislocation. If the provider is unable to reduce the dislocation due to severe muscle spasm or extreme pain, then the patient must be referred to an oral and maxillofacial surgeon for sedation prior to reduction of the dislocation. An acute closed lock (where the mouth is prevented from opening) warrants an immediate referral for evaluation by an oral and maxillofacial surgeon or an orofacial pain specialist because early intervention beyond conservative therapy (such as arthrocentesis) may be necessary. For all other cases, conservative therapy for an acute condition should focus on reducing joint loading and inflammation. Attempts should be made to relax the muscles as much as possible. The patient should use ice or cold packs for the first 24 to 48 hours, adhere to a soft diet, and avoid gum chewing. After the first 24 to 48 hours, the patient should apply moist heat several times a day. Gentle stretching exercises of the mastication muscles should be performed after heat application. The patient should continue to avoid gum chewing and adhere to a soft diet for several days to limit masticatory activity.

Pharmacological interventions should begin as soon as possible with analgesics, preferably nonsteroidal antiinflammatory analgesics. Patients with more severe TMD may also require short-term use of skeletal muscle relaxants. Because low-dose tricyclics improve sleep, they may be effective in decreasing pain from nocturnal bruxism. If symptoms recur, the patient should initiate moist heat application, stretching therapy, and use of nonsteroidal antiinflammatory drugs. Normally, this treatment prevents the development of more severe problems.

Ideally, TMD patients should be referred to a dentist for a comprehensive evaluation of contributing factors from diet, occlusion, oral habits, and stress. However, because no national standards exist for TMD curricula at the predoctoral level, finding a knowledgeable practitioner may be difficult.[58] Initial evaluation for acute TMD pain from trauma must rule out fractures, tears, and articular disc displacement. Examination of the occlusion and oral habits may show whether the patient would benefit from wearing an appliance (eg, a bite plate) every night to prevent or minimize the effects of jaw movements during sleep.

If symptoms do not resolve, patients should be referred to an orofacial pain specialist, who can determine if the patient would also benefit from cognitive-behavioral skills training and biofeedback (eg, relaxation techniques) to decrease muscle jaw tension, decrease stress, increase awareness, and prevent diurnal tooth grinding or clenching incidents. Studies have shown that early intervention using a biopsychosocial approach is effective in reducing TMD pain and decreasing the progression of the disorder to chronic stages, as well as decreasing depression, increasing positive coping behaviors, and significantly reducing TMD-related healthcare costs.[59,60]

SUMMARY

The stress of deployment can cause serious oral health problems. Soldiers should be trained in stress-reducing techniques to avoid these problems (as well as the many other negative effects of combat stress). However, once problems occur, they should be treated with self-care techniques; more serious conditions necessitate attention from oral care practitioners.

REFERENCES

1. Darakjy S, Marin RE, Knapik JJ, Jones BH. Injuries and illnesses among armor brigade soldiers during operational training. *Mil Med*. 2006;171(11):1051–1056.

2. Mitchener TA, Hauret KG, Hoedebecke EL, Darakjy S, Jones BH. Air medical evacuations of soldiers due to oral-facial disease and injuries, Operations Enduring Freedom/Iraqi Freedom. *Mil Med*. 2008;173(5):465–473.

3. US Department of Health and Human Services. *National Call to Action to Promote Oral Health*. Rockville, Md: USDHHS, Public Health Service, National Institutes of Health, National Institute of Dental and Craniofacial Research; 2003. NIH Publication 03-5303.

4. Hourani LL, Bray RM, Marsden ME, et al. *2006 Department of Defense Survey of Health Related Behaviors in the Reserve Component*. Research Triangle Park, NC: RTI International; 2007.

5. Bray RM, Hourani LL, Rae-Olmsted KL, et al. *2008 Department of Defense Survey of Health Related Behaviors Among Active Duty Military Personnel*. Research Triangle Park, NC: RTI International; 2009.

6. McClung JP, Marchitelli LJ, Friedl KE, Young AJ. Prevalence of iron deficiency and iron deficiency anemia among three populations of female military personnel in the US Army. *J Am Coll Nutr.* 2006;25(1):64–69.

7. McClung JP, Scrimgeour AG. Zinc: an essential trace element with potential benefits to soldiers. *Mil Med.* 2005;170(12):1048–1052. Review.

8. Halliday AW, Vukelja SJ. Neurologic manifestations of vitamin B-12 deficiency in a military hospital. *Mil Med.* 1991;156(4):201–204.

9. Friedl KE, Evans RK, Moran DS. Stress fracture and military medical readiness: bridging basic and applied research. *Med Sci Sports Exerc.* 2008;40(11 suppl):S609–S622.

10. Lappe J, Cullen D, Haynatzki G, Recker R, Ahlf R, Thompson K. Calcium and vitamin D supplementation decreases incidence of stress fractures in female navy recruits. *J Bone Miner Res.* 2008;23(5):741–749.

11. Scrimgeour AG, Lukaski HC. Zinc and diarrheal disease: current status and future perspectives. *Curr Opin Clin Nutr Metab Care.* 2008;11(6):711–717. Review.

12. Moynihan PJ. The role of diet and nutrition in the etiology and prevention of oral diseases. *Bull World Health Organ.* 2005;83:694–699.

13. Dunn WJ, Langsten RE, Flores S, Fandell JE. Dental emergency rates at two expeditionary medical support facilities supporting Operations Enduring and Iraqi Freedom. *Mil Med.* 2004;169(7):510–514.

14. Simecek JW. Estimation of nonpreventable dental emergencies in US Marine Corps personnel. *Mil Med.* 2008;173(11): 1104–1107.

15. Deutsch WM, Simecek JW. Dental emergencies among Marines ashore in Operations Desert Shield/Storm. *Mil Med.* 1996;161(10):620–623.

16. Moss DL. Dental emergencies during SFOR 8 in Bosnia. *Mil Med.* 2002;167(11):904–906.

17. Mahoney GD, Coombs M. A literature review of dental casualty rates. *Mil Med.* 2000;165(10):751–756.

18. Teweles RB, King JE. Impact of troop dental health on combat readiness. *Mil Med.* 1987;152(5):233–235.

19. dela Cruz G. US Army Center for Health Promotion and Preventive Medicine. Unpublished study on degradation of oral health of soldiers deployed to Iraq, March 2004.

20. Mobley CC. Nutrition and dental caries. *Dent Clin North Am.* 2003;47(2):319–336. Review.

21. Burt BA, Satishchandra P. Sugar consumption and caries risk: a systematic review. *J Dent Educ.* 2001;65(10):1017–1023.

22. Amaechi BT, Higham SM. Dental erosion: possible approaches to prevention and control. *J Dent.* 2005;33(3):243–252.

23. Lussi A, Hellwig E, Zero D, Jaeggi T. Erosive tooth wear: diagnosis, risk factors and prevention. *Am J Dent.* 2006;19(6): 319–325.

24. Young A, Amaechi BT, Dugmore C, et al. Current erosion indices—flawed or valid? Summary. *Clin Oral Invest.* 2008;12 (suppl 1):S59–S63.

25. von Fraunhofer JA, Rogers MM. Effects of sports drinks and other beverages on dental enamel. *Gen Dent.* 2005;53(1):28–31.

26. von Fraunhofer JA, Rogers MM. Dissolution of dental enamel in soft drinks. *Gen Dent.* 2004;52(4):308–312.

27. Sharma P, Wani S, Romero Y, Johnson D, Hamilton F. Racial and geographic issues in gastroesophageal reflux disease. *Am J Gastroenterol*. 2008;103(11):2669–2680.

28. Huber MA. Gastrointestinal illnesses and their effects on the oral cavity. *Oral Maxillofacial Surg Clin N Am.* 2008;20:625–634.

29. Studen-Pavlovich D, Elliott MA. Eating disorders in women's oral health. *Dent Clin North Am*. 2001;45(3):491–511.

30. Hurst PS, Lacey LH, Crisp AH. Teeth, vomiting and diet: a study of the dental characteristics of seventeen anorexia nervosa patients. *Postgrad Med J.* 1977;53(620):298–305.

31. Brown S, Bonifazi DZ. An overview of anorexia and bulimia nervosa, and the impact of eating disorders on the oral cavity. *Compendium*. 1993;14(12):1594, 1596–1602, 1604–1608; quiz 1608. Literature review.

32. Montecchi PP, Custureri V, Polimeni A, et al. Oral manifestations in a group of young patients with anorexia nervosa. *Eat Weight Disord*. 2003;8(2):164–167.

33. Sundaram G, Bartlett D. Preventative measures for bulimic patients with dental erosion. *Eur J Prosthodont Restor Dent*. 2001;9(1):25–29.

34. US Department of the Army. *Combat Stress*. Washington, DC: DA; 2009. Field Manual 6-22.5.

35. US Army Center for Health Promotion and Preventive Medicine. *Guide to Coping With Combat and Deployment Stress*. Aberdeen Proving Ground, Md: USACHPPM; 2008. TG 320.

36. Ly KA, Milgrom P, Rothen M. Xylitol, sweeteners, and dental caries. *Pediatr Dent*. 2006;28(2):154–163.

37. Sheiham A. Dietary effects on dental diseases. *Public Health Nutr*. 2001;4(2B):569–591. Review.

38. Moynihan P. Foods and dietary factors that prevent dental caries. *Quintessence Int*. 2007;38(4):320–324.

39. Page RC, Kornman KS. The pathogenesis of human periodontitis: an introduction. *Periodontol 2000*. 1997;14:9–11.

40. US Department of Health and Human Services. *Oral Health in America: A Report of the Surgeon General*. Washington, DC: USDHHS, National Institute of Dental and Craniofacial Research, National Institutes of Health; 2000: 39–42.

41. US Department of Health and Human Services. *Healthy People 2010: Understanding and Improving Health*. 2nd ed. Washington, DC: US Government Printing Office; November 2000: 41.

42. Gluck GM, Morganstein WM, eds. *Jong's Community Dental Health*. 5th ed. St Louis, Mo: Mosby; 2003: 185–187.

43. Kornman KS. Mapping the pathogenesis of periodontitis: a new look. *J Periodontol*. 2008;79(8):1560–1568.

44. Offenbacher S, Barros SP, Beck JD. Rethinking periodontal inflammation. *J Periodontol*. 2008;79:1577–1584.

45. Cochrane DL. Inflammation and bone loss in periodontal disease. *J Periodontol*. 2008;79:1569–1576.

46. Krejci CB, Bissada NF. Women's health issues and their relationship to periodontitis. *J Am Dent Assoc*. 2002;133:323–329.

47. Knight GM, Wade AB. The effects of hormonal contraceptives on the human periodontium. *J Periodont Res*. 1974;9:18–22.

48. Tilakaratne A, Soory M, Ronasinghe AW, Corea SM, Ekanayake SL, de Silva M. Effects of hormonal contraceptives on the periodontium, in a population of rural Sri-Lankan women. *J Clin Periodontol*. 2000;27:753–757.

49. Tri-Service Comprehensive Oral Health Survey Working Group. *1994 Tri-Service Comprehensive Oral Health Survey—Active-Duty Report*. Washington, DC: Department of Defense, Office of the Assistant Secretary of Defense for Health Affairs; June 1995. Naval Dental Research Institute. PR 9503.

50. Dworkin SF, Huggins KH, LeResche L, et al. Epidemiology of signs and symptoms in temporomandibular disorders: clinical signs in cases and controls. *J Am Dent Assoc*. 1990;120:273–281.

51. Warren MP, Fried JL. Temporomandibular disorders and hormones in women. *Cells Tissues Organs*. 2001;169:187–192.

52. Bragdon EE, Light KC, Costello NL, et al. Group differences in pain modulation: pain-free women compared to pain-free men and women with TMD. *Pain*. 2002;96:227–237.

53. Nekora-Azak A. Temporomandibular disorders in relation to female reproductive hormones: a literature review. *J Prosthet Dent*. 2004;91:491–493.

54. LeResche L, Mancl L, Sherman JJ, Gandara B, Dworkin SF. Changes in temporomandibular pain and other symptoms across the menstrual cycle. *Pain*. 2003;106:253–261.

55. Isslee H, De Laat A, De Mot B, Lysens R. Pressure-pain threshold variation in temporomandibular disorder myalgia over the course of the menstrual cycle. *J Orofac Pain*. 2002;16:105–117.

56. Campbell JH, Courey MS, Bourne P, Odziemiec C. Estrogen receptor analysis of human temporomandibular disc. *J Oral Maxillofac Surg*. 1993;51:1101–1105.

57. Abubaker AO, Raslan WF, Sotereanos GC. Estrogen and progesterone receptors in temporomandibular joint discs of symptomatic and asymptomatic persons: a preliminary study. *J Oral Maxillofac Surg*. 1993;51:1096–1100.

58. Klasser GD, Greene CS. Predoctoral teaching of temporomandibular disorders: a survey of US and Canadian dental schools. *J Am Dent Assoc*. 2007;138:231–237.

59. Gatchel RJ, Stowell AW, Wildenstein L, Riggs R, Ellis E 3rd. Efficacy of an early intervention for patients with acute temporomandibular disorder-related pain: a one-year outcome study. *J Am Dent Assoc*. 2006;137(3):339–347.

60. Stowell AW, Gatchel RJ, Wildenstein L. Cost-effectiveness of treatments for temporomandibular disorders: biopsychosocial intervention versus treatment as usual. *J Am Dent Assoc*. 2007;138:202–208.

COMBAT AND OPERATIONAL BEHAVIORAL HEALTH

Section IV: Reunion and Reintegration

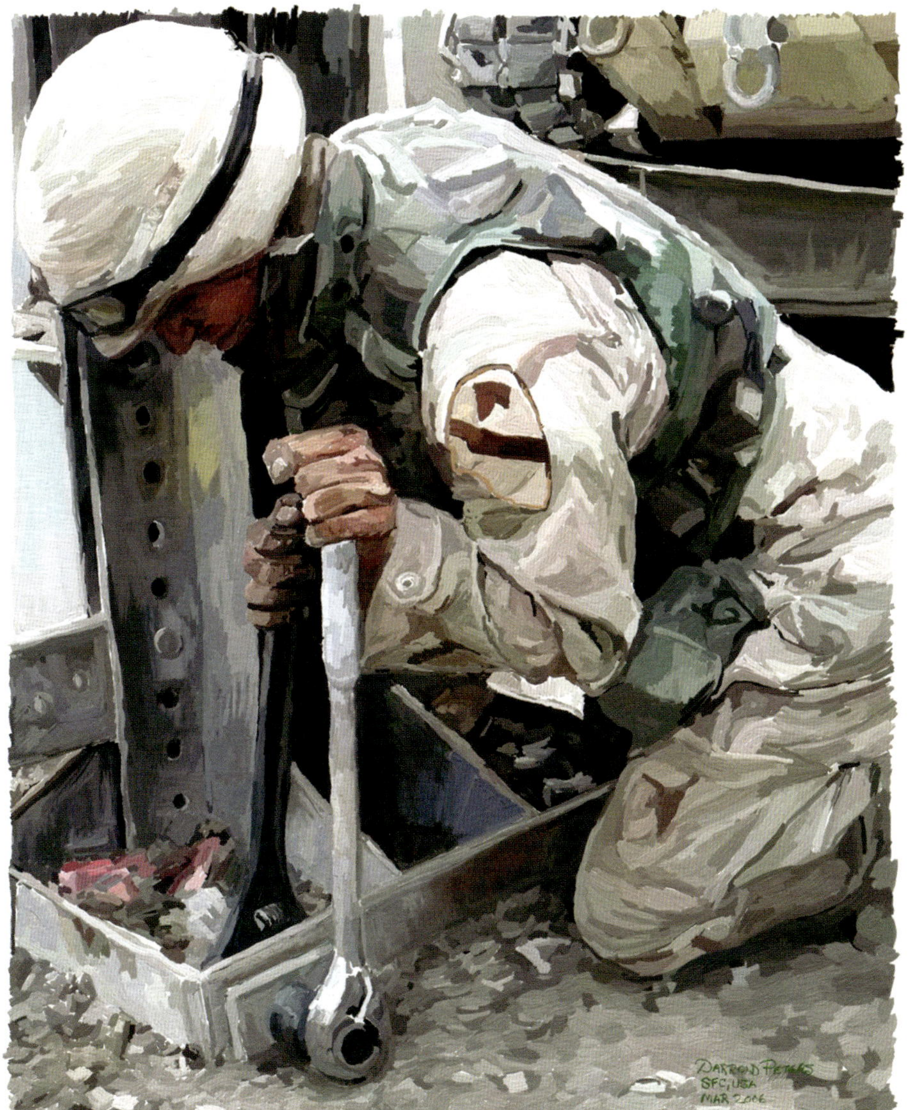

Fix It, Sarge, by Darrold Peters, Digital Oils/ArtRage 2.0, 2006.

Art: Courtesy of the US Army Center of Military History.

Chapter 18

RESETTING THE FORCE: REENTRY AND REDEPLOYMENT

KRIS A. PETERSON, MD*; AND MICHAEL E. DOYLE, MD†

*Colonel, Medical Corps, US Army; Chief, Department of Psychiatry, Madigan Army Medical Center, Tacoma, Washington 98431; formerly, Child and Adolescent Psychiatry Consultant to The Surgeon General, US Army

†Lieutenant Colonel, Medical Corps, US Army; Deputy Commander for Clinical Services, USAMEDDAC West Point, 900 Washington Road, West Point, New York 10996

This chapter was previously published as: Doyle ME, Peterson KA. Re-entry and reintegration: returning home after combat. *Psychiatric Quarterly*. 2005;76:361–370. Adapted with permission of Springer.

The capacity of Soldiers for absorbing punishment and enduring privations is almost inexhaustible so long as they believe they are getting a square deal, that their commanders are looking out for them, and that their own accomplishments are understood and appreciated.

—General Dwight D Eisenhower, 1944

INTRODUCTION

Soldier life in the US Army is structured by the cycles of predeployment, deployment, and postdeployment. Management of behavioral health in each phase is a continuous process, with features unique to each phase. Soldiers redeploying from combat to their home units face a number of stressors that may affect postdeployment adjustment. Among the factors that influence stress levels are the nature of the conflict, level of national support, family support and family stability, and the soldier's component (regular Army, National Guard, or US Army Reserve).

"Resetting the force"—reentry, reintegration, recovery, and reconstitution—has become an essential operation of the postdeployment phase of the cycle. Resetting the force can be thought of as personal or soldier maintenance. Just as equipment needs to be repaired or refurbished after deployment, and maintained throughout its use to prevent breakdown, so, too, do soldiers need "maintenance" in the form of support before, during, and after deployment. This chapter will look at processes developed by the military over the course of the global war on terror (GWOT) to reset the force by assisting soldiers in reentry and reintegration.

Resetting the force includes many concepts; for example, implicit in maintaining a ready deployable force is making soldiers available for contingency operations while simultaneously sustaining garrison operations. Early inclusion of families and communities into the planning for reentry and reintegration, normalization (nonmedicalization of distress), destigmatization of behavioral health problems, and assistance for behavioral health needs, including easy access to a behavioral health professional and education of soldiers and families on resources and benefits, are other essential elements in this process.

The military recognizes resetting the force as a vital part of the return to readiness, as important as preparing soldiers for deployment. This concept acknowledges that recovery after a deployment maintains the soldier and is part of the preparation process for future deployments. Soldiers recover and return to combat readiness as the next round of deployments approaches. The effectiveness of the reintegration process strongly affects the state of individual and unit readiness. Thus, stakeholders include the soldier; the soldier's family, unit, and local community; the Army; and all of US society. These identified stakeholders provide context to resetting the force and shape its outcome.

Recognizing this, Army leadership (under G1), in concert with behavioral health professionals, developed an intensive program to reach all returning soldiers—active duty, reserve, and National Guard—who were mobilized and deployed to combat zones. The Deployment Cycle Support Program (DCSP) directs as much attention to the postdeployment phase as the Army historically has to the actual deployment and run-up to it. The DCSP brings balance to the varying soldier, unit, and family needs within the deployment cycles or continuum.

BACKGROUND

Accounts of wars throughout recorded history frequently include descriptions of the physical and emotional suffering of the combatants. The GWOT, Operation Iraqi Freedom (OIF), and Operation Enduring Freedom (OEF) will likely continue this trend. Scientific study of the emotional and psychiatric impact of combat operations is extensive up to and including the Persian Gulf War. Publications since then include numerous reports on peacekeeping operations[1,2] and a recent article on symptoms of posttraumatic stress disorder in OIF/OEF soldiers and marines.[3]

For OIF/OEF, reentry—or returning home after combat—and reintegration have received attention in the media, but rigorous scientific study has not yet occurred. Moreover, the media attention has been primarily negative: individual incidents of criminal behavior with deployment experience implicated as the cause, an anticipated epidemic of posttraumatic stress disorder as thousands of service members demobilize following the war, and problems with soldiers' follow-up medical care, infrastructure at major medical centers, and the physical disability system.

In the 1995 textbook *War Psychiatry*,[4] Faris Kirkland discusses at length the impact on soldiers primarily, and on society to a lesser extent, of troops returning home after conflict. Kirkland divides US involvement in numerous conflicts and armed interventions into three categories: major wars, limited actions, and rapid-deployment operations. Major wars are those defined by large-scale mobilizations against a defined, "evil" and dehumanized enemy, fought by "champions of the people" for the greater good, in which reentry of the combatant into civilian life is accomplished by demobilization. Demobilization places responsibility for reentry and reintegration squarely on society at large, making it "a societal, not military problem." In major wars the soldier and family impact involves less conflict. The societal embrace of soldiers doing their duty in the face of a dehumanized enemy, fighting for a greater good, validates the soldier's actions and modifies the negative psychological sequelae of combat. Resetting via acknowledgment of meaningful actions and sacrifices "not in vain" is more readily accomplished.[4]

Limited wars are those requiring only a fractional commitment of national resources; they are conducted in a different psychopolitical climate than major wars.[4] National interests frequently serve as the pretext for action, civilian inconvenience and involvement are modest, and ambivalence about the cause pervasive. Numerous factors complicate reentry of service members, significantly, the absence of national consensus, lack of validation of soldiers' efforts, and the return of soldiers individually from theater. "Soldiers were not able to process their experiences with the comrades with whom they had trained and fought."[4(p293)] Reentry management in modern limited wars has been shouldered by society. Following the Korean War, soldiers met indifference; following Vietnam, hostility.[4] Thus far public ambivalence has greeted returning OIF and OEF troops: praise for heroism, countered by belief in the moral injustice of the war, coupled with the portrayal of soldiers as pawns trapped in a commitment to serve.

In limited wars, wherein society does not identify with the soldier and is neutral or even negative toward a soldier's sacrifice, the psychological impacts land more heavily upon both soldier and society. "Psychiatric casualties increase greatly when the soldier feels isolated, and psychological and social isolation from home and society was one of the results of the growing antiwar sentiment in the United States," such as during the Vietnam War.[5] Furthermore, in Vietnam, one consequence of soldiers' alienation was an increase in "Dear John" letters.[5] OIF and OEF reflect similar dynamics; the divorce rate for soldiers, and the officer corps in particular, rose rapidly in the first 3 years of the conflict, leveled off, and then rose again.

Psychiatric casualty rates in Vietnam "were similar to home-front approval ratings for the war, and an argument can be made that psychiatric casualties can be impacted by public disapproval."[5(p278)] In multiple studies two factors show up again and again as critical to the magnitude of the posttraumatic response. First and most obvious is the intensity of the initial trauma. The second, and less obvious but absolutely vital, factor is the nature of the social support structure available to the traumatized individual.[5] Society accepting as necessary soldiers' behavior in combat—killing, managing violence—vitalizes resetting the force and mitigates the psychological impact of combat. In contrast, the decline in public support for the war in Iraq as well as negative media attention may contribute to difficulties in reentry and reintegration for redeploying and demobilizing service members. Leaders and citizens, locally and nationally, who comment that a war is unjust, based on a lie, or in vane, make the soldier's task to refit and reset more difficult. It is consequently important for leaders to speak up about the justness of the fight, identify what the country is fighting for, and outline the strategic successes. Reset must encompass not just an acceptance of but accolades for soldiers' accomplishments.

The third form of combat, the rapid-deployment operation, is enacted for national interest by a professional military cohort that has trained together but must rapidly transition from training to combat mode and back again to prepare for the next deployment scenario.[4] Soldiers involved in these actions seldom have time to consider or internalize virtues of the cause, but instead must rely on horizontal and vertical cohesion

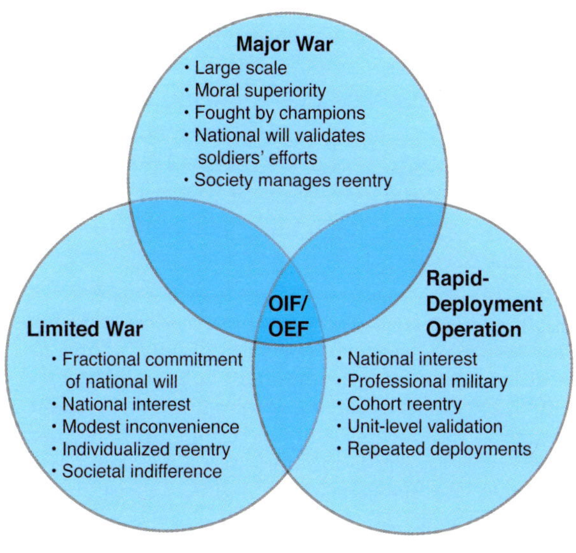

Figure 18-1. The characteristics of major wars, limited wars, and rapid deployment operations overlap in Operation Iraqi Freedom (OIF) and Operation Enduring Freedom (OEF).

within their units for validation.[4] Responsibility for reentry and reintegration rests primarily on the unit and military. The ability of these soldiers to rely on unit cohesiveness and esprit de corps significantly impacts deployment readiness.[4]

Special forces operations employed in GWOT as well as during the Cold War fall under this construct. The resetting of these combat teams is made easier through the unit cohesion and esprit de corps developed during their specialized training. Conversely, frequent deployments, toxic environments, and combat losses take a toll. The stigma of having a behavioral health problem is amplified because these soldiers may feel they cannot rely upon distressed members. Consequently, seeing behavioral health practitioners for assistance in a reset is made even more difficult in this group. Typically, special forces soldiers reach out to chaplains and leaders for these needs. Increasingly, however, regular forces follow the same behavior pattern, and the factors that mitigate distress in the special operations population may not exist as robustly in the regular forces community.

History may determine where GWOT, OIF, and OEF fall among the models discussed. These related conflicts have been framed as a major war against a great evil but executed as a limited war by an increasingly professional and full-time military that must prepare for return-to-combat while planning its return home. OIF and OEF also entail the largest call-up of reserve forces since World War II, with 18-month mobilization orders for the National Guard, and 2- to 3-year mobilizations for reservists. These groups also face the increasing pressures of the deployment cycle. Figure 18-1 depicts this overlap between major, limited, and rapid deployment operations, with elements of each apparent in OIF and OEF.

REENTRY CHALLENGES BY POPULATION

The unusual spectrum of the GWOT, OIF, and OEF conflicts presents multiple challenges to reentry and reintegration for the three separate populations of regular Army soldiers, National Guard and reserve soldiers, and family members.

Regular Army

The DCSP, resulting from the peacekeeping operations of the 1990s and the development of concepts based on expeditionary force practices among Army leadership, reflects recognition that in the post-Cold War era, soldiers are in predeployment, deployed, or postdeployment states at any given time. And so are family members. The DCSP plan, dated May 2, 2004, disseminated and operationalized Army-wide, includes a return-to-readiness—termed "recovery" or "reconstitution"—period (Figure 18-2). The plan is intended to assist soldiers in reentry and reintegration and restore them and their units to combat readiness:

> Reintegration training for both the Soldier and his/her family is an essential task for all units' return to readiness plans. It is as important as any other training or personnel action the Soldier undertakes. Reintegration entails three components; the single Soldier and his/her assimilation back into a garrison environment; the married Soldier and his/her assimilation with his family; and the family of the deployed Soldier.[6]

Reintegration training is not a single session but a continuous and, at times, parallel process:

- Reintegration training occurs in advance of soldiers' return to home station, often in-theater or at the location to which soldiers have been deployed.
- Rear detachment leaders coordinate with the installation to provide reintegration training to families of deployed soldiers as well. Although the training is voluntary for family members, units encourage participation. Units publicize training sessions and conduct them at times that allow maximum family member participation. The training also includes take-home information about what families might expect during the homecoming of their combat veteran.[6]
- The reconstitution phase starts upon a soldier's arrival at home station after deployment. Commanders establish a half-day schedule to "facilitate family reintegration and to commence administrative tasks required upon return."[6] Half-days occur through the first 10 days, and during this time the soldier's duties entail "administrative functions, Soldier and leader professional education, and family reintegration."[6]

Rear detachment commanders and personnel provide support and training resources for reintegration in advance of the unit's return. They ensure that "suitable time is allocated for family reintegration activities both for the married and single Soldier."[6] Leaders will "execute family reintegration counseling for all redeploying Soldiers. To the greatest extent

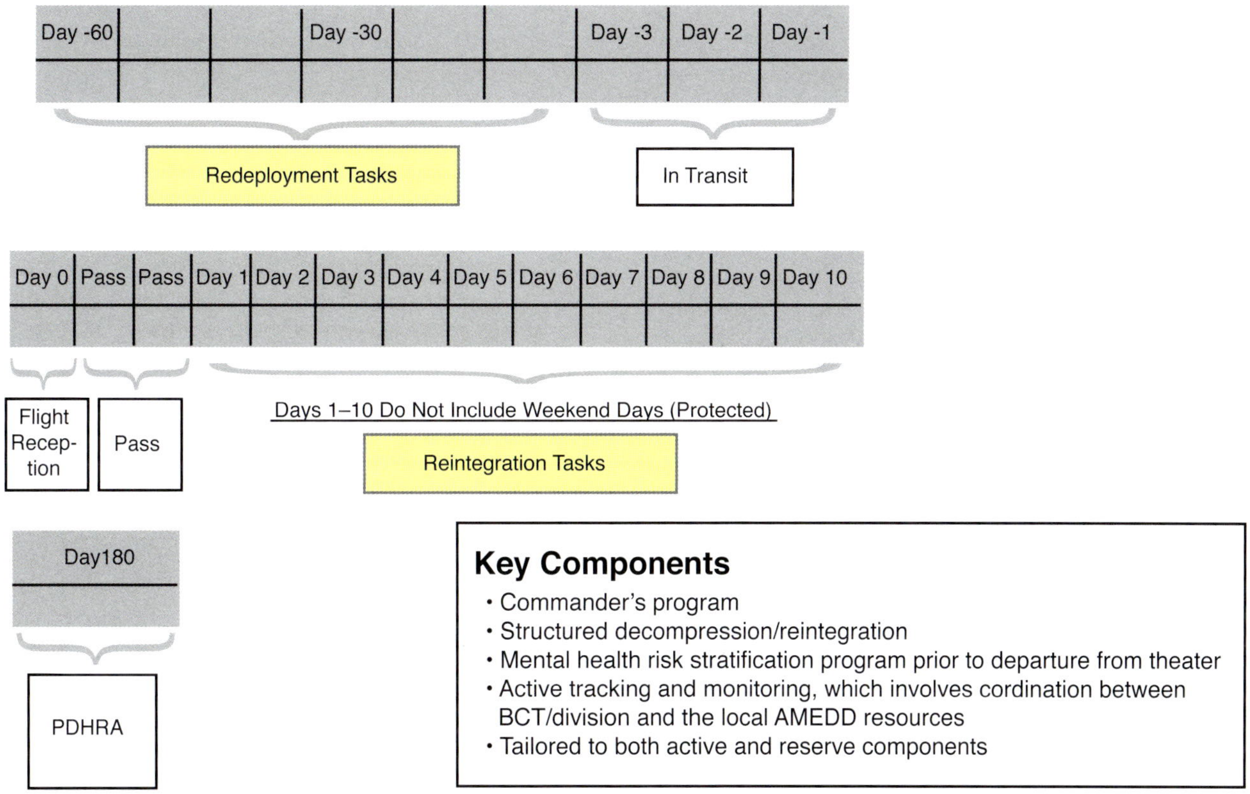

Figure 18-2. Key components in decompression and reintegration.
BCT: brigade combat team
AMEDD: Army Medical Department
PDHRA: Post-Deployment Health Re-Assessment

possible, this counseling will occur in theater, prior to the Soldiers redeploying."[6] Units are expected to sustain needed family reintegration training following soldiers' return, based on unit sensing sessions, command climate surveys, and feedback to the unit leadership from installation support agencies and healthcare providers.

At-risk soldiers are identified by commanders prior to returning home to "ensure that they receive tailored training and/or assistance based on their particular circumstances."[6] The Army identifies soldiers-at-risk by marital difficulties or difficulties with fiancés, financial difficulties, problems with alcohol or substance abuse, medical problems, and problems such as depression or anxiety reported by the soldier during pre- and postdeployment screening. This list is not all-inclusive and other issues might identify a soldier as at risk as well.[6]

Lastly, as directed March 26, 2007,[7] all redeploying soldiers undergo a health reassessment 3 to 6 months after redeployment. This reassessment includes general health questions, seeking to address medical issues not identified at the initial screening, but also presents soldiers with the opportunity to seek treatment for any behavioral health concerns that may have arisen since the initial screening.

National Guard and Army Reserve

As advocated by the "One Army" concept of seamlessness among components, requirements of the DCSP apply equally across active duty, National Guard, and reserve units. Reserve and National Guard soldiers are demobilized, like soldiers from World War II or Korea; their reentry and reintegration is largely shouldered by their communities; and medical care is provided by the Department of Veterans Affairs (VA) hospital nearest their home.

Reentry anxieties abound among these soldiers. Many have lost their jobs or fear the possibility of job loss, despite legislative protections. Sole proprietors and small-business owners are particularly at risk. A frequently noted concern is that soldiers feel different than they did before deployment. Other issues faced by demobilizing reservists and Guard members include a sense of isolation from peers, estrangement from family and friends, and a loss of common purpose. The bonds forged in combat and other operations may remain if the Guard unit has a localized base; however, this is often not the case.

Case Study 18-1: Specialist A presented for care shortly after being notified of his imminent release from active duty. The soldier expressed fears that he would respond negatively or even violently in his work environment when confronted with inevitable conflicts. "I'm not ready to go home. Most of the guys where I work are Middle Eastern; I'm afraid I will go off on them."

Demobilizing reservists and National Guard personnel often return to their home unit stations as soon as 4 days after arriving at the demobilization site. This facilitates a quick reunion for them and their families; however, follow-up care and monitoring may be scarce in the home communities. Thus, these soldiers may find themselves in a difficult situation: either remain on active duty, separated from family and loved ones, to address medical questions, or ignore the medical issues and return home. Washington state sought to redress these issues in November 2004 when it established a memorandum of agreement with multiple federal agencies to

> augment the ongoing, comprehensive effort to ensure military service members and their families are honored for their valuable and honorable service to our country. It is recognized that the Department of Defense and the U.S. Department of Veterans Affairs are providing world-class transition service . . . to deal with the multitude of medical and mental conditions associated with war. This agreement will focus primarily on "after active-duty" and deal with problems and issues military members often face several months or years following military service.[8]

This agreement and its accompanying programs aim to shore up local reintegration and reentry of returning service members. Features include

- ensuring that each returning veteran receives a letter from the governor, the adjutant general, and the director of the Washington State Department of Veterans Affairs thanking them for their service and encouraging them to seek their various veteran benefits and entitlements;
- follow-up letters at 3 and 6 months;
- a family activity day, held within 3 to 6 months following return, conducted by teams consisting of representatives from the VA, Veterans Benefits Administration, Veterans Health Administration, and Washington Employment Security Department; accredited veteran services officers; and mental health professionals for the purpose of providing information to assist veterans and their family members with reintegration; and
- a family support program providing education about VA services and benefits in classes for family members of deployed service members, conducted by accredited veteran services officers at local armories and sponsored by the command.[8]

Like those on active duty, reserve component soldiers receive the health reassessment screening at 3 to 6 months postdeployment. Specific questions on the screening aim to measure the presence and impact of posttraumatic stress disorder. If the reassessment identifies healthcare needs, soldiers are offered care through military medical treatment facilities, VA medical centers or veterans' centers, TRICARE providers, or community-based healthcare organizations established by the Army. Part of this intervention plan are behavioral healthcare providers, who further assess soldiers' needs and ensure that care is offered.

Family Members of Regular Army, Reservists, and National Guard Members

The Deployment Health Clinic at Madigan Army Medical Center, Tacoma, Washington, like similar clinics at other military treatment facilities, recognizes that family preparedness for deployment is essential to ensuring soldier readiness for deployment. With this in mind, the Deployment Health Clinic developed the Army Family Readiness Course, which is an online resource for soldiers and family members. This has evolved over time into additional resources for soldiers and family members now embodied in the efforts of the Technology and Telehealth Initiative from the Department of Defense.

Case Study 18-2: Ms B is a 32-year-old spouse of an infantryman. The couple arrived at Fort Lewis, Washington, 3 months prior to his deployment to Iraq. His previous assignment was in Korea, where his 12-month tour had been extended to 15 months. Ms B presented feeling overwhelmed at being separated from her spouse so soon and for yet another year. The couple had four children, ages 3 to 13. Ms B had significant back pain, anxiety, and a history of depression. Following her spouse's return from Iraq, where he had served as a squad leader for an infantry squad with numerous combat encounters, she reported, "He tells me everything. I thought he'd keep it inside. I thought I'd be better when he came home, but I still can't sleep."

During deployment, family members of regular Army soldiers usually have the benefit of support from the on-post community, support that is often not available for National Guard members or reservists. However, family members of National Guard and reserve soldiers may have greater access to family and long-standing community relationships that regular Army families do not. Regardless of component, home-front stability is key to soldier readiness. Family instability, which generally increases at deployment, distracts the service member, and absence of a family care plan often results in administrative separation of deploying soldiers.

Often, however, the greatest challenge to families is the return of the deployed soldier. When the returning soldier reclaims prior responsibilities, the spouse may be left feeling that his or her efforts during deployment are invalidated. Months of adaptation and coping are upended, giving rise to such questions as:

- Who now pays the bills, takes out the trash, mows the lawn?
- Who disciplines the children? How?
- Who gets the remote?
- Are there problems with intimacy?[9]

REDEPLOYMENT PROGRAMS

Commanders' plans for resetting the force have varied, but they generally intend to provide a broad-based and inclusive assessment of the mental well-being of soldiers deploying to and returning from combat. In the Army's first resetting iteration, the Walter Reed Army Institute of Research developed a postdeployment questionnaire that was filled out by soldiers upon or near redeployment and often in theater. This questionnaire became known as the Health Risk Appraisal questionnaire (HRA I). Subsequently, many local institutions and commands broadened the questionnaire and, through consensus, standardized its contents to create the HRA II. Soldiers completed the HRA II prior to deployment and upon return from a combat theater. Based on these assessments, interventions could be carried out to assist resetting soldiers in need. For example, a soldier who started smoking in the combat theater might express interest in smoking cessation. The request would be identified on the HRA II, and follow-up contact and treatment interventions arranged.

Further evolution of the resetting efforts occurred over time, with different programs being implemented on different military posts. Ultimately, Army leadership adopted a standardized schedule and format for the predeployment and postdeployment assessments and the postdeployment health reassessment (see Attachment). In addition to the health assessments administered upon deployment, redeployment, and 3 to 6 months postdeployment, the DCSP supports behavioral health by surveillance for trends and compliance, treatment referrals when indicated, and, most importantly, making it mandatory that soldiers have the opportunity to complete all assessments (although completion is voluntary).

The Army initially delegated treatment decisions to local medical treatment facilities. Arguably the most comprehensive of these efforts is a program called the Soldier Wellness Assessment Pilot Program (SWAPP), deployed initially at Fort Lewis, Washington (Exhibit 18-1).

In general, military treatment facility reintegration programs operate as follows: Returning soldiers are assigned a care manager (usually a social worker) if medical or behavioral health issues are identified on the postdeployment health screening. The care manager assists the soldier in scheduling needed follow-up and then in keeping those appointments. This often requires coordination with the soldier's command to ensure that the needed time is given. Those who need ongoing care are assigned case managers, who monitor the progress of the soldier's therapy with a goal of full return to duty. Soldiers with identified behavioral health concerns that may limit duty are assisted by case managers in concert with behavioral health professionals.

However, soldiers may also present with behavioral health concerns to the local behavioral health clinic, where those recently deployed are offered a wide variety of therapeutic modalities. These may include one-to-one supportive, insight-oriented, or cognitive/behavioral therapy, as well as group therapies such as postdeployment adjustment groups, interpersonal process groups, depression groups, groups focused on adjustment to military life, or groups focused on life skills or anger management. Marital and family therapies are also offered in a variety of modalities. Medication management is also available when appropriate. Treatment for posttraumatic stress disorder, consistent with treatment guidelines based on the literature, is also offered.[10]

The expectation of wellness and recovery remains an integral part of any treatment program. For many, use of reassurance is efficacious. Practitioners should use language such as: "What you are experiencing now is an expected consequence of your combat tour. It will get better with time. However, the following may be helpful in this process. . . ."

EXHIBIT 18-1

SOLDIER WELLNESS ASSESSMENT PILOT PROGRAM

Interventions to reset the force have been in development since soldiers began redeploying to combat operations in Afghanistan and Iraq. A program that has gained significant acceptance and captured the commander's intent is the Soldier Wellness and Assessment Pilot Program (SWAPP) at Fort Lewis, Washington. SWAPP is a useful model built on the Deployment Cycle Support Program's intents to

- standardize predeployment and postdeployment health risk assessments, with an identical process before and after deployment;
- encompass a broad definition of health and wellness, including physical, emotional, spiritual, financial, and legal needs;
- make data transparent to commanders and medical staff; and
- ensure a face-to-face encounter with a licensed provider for each soldier assessed.

Participation in SWAPP is voluntary. Many commanders and soldiers view the program as an opportunity to establish a broad-based overview of physical, emotional, and spiritual wellness. The assessment is scheduled for completion between 90 and 180 days after return, and 45 to 125 days prior to departure. As seen in Figure 18-3, soldiers check in and begin with a face-to-face encounter that introduces aspects of the program and attempts to destigmatize the resetting process. It is made clear that the process is voluntary.

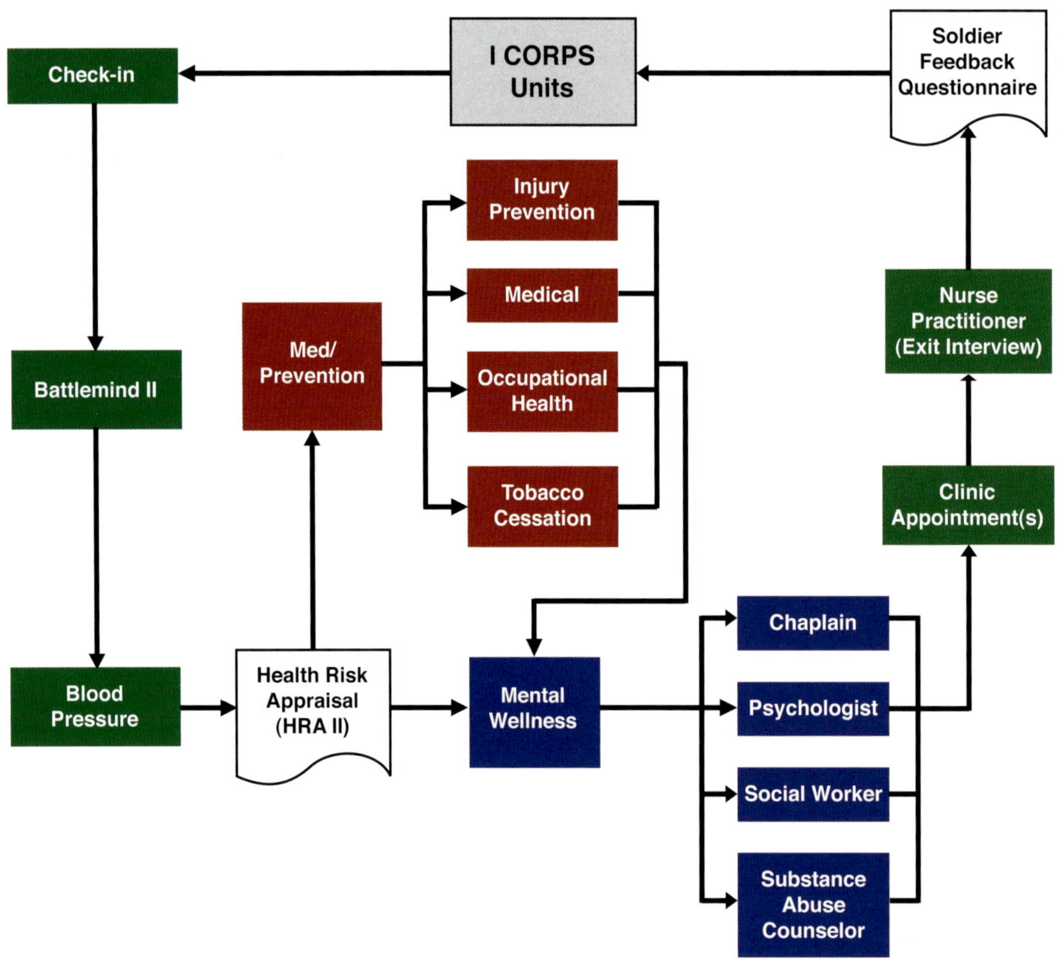

Figure 18-3. Soldier Wellness and Assessment Pilot Program flow chart.

(**Exhibit 18-1** *continues*)

Exhibit 18-1 *continued*

Soldiers complete the health risk appraisal (HRA II) questionnaire in several venues, administered on computer kiosks, and results are forwarded to providers. The questions encompass the postdeployment health reassessment questions in form DD 2900 (see Attachment). HRA II has 76 questions used to identify risk in soldiers, who are categorized as being at high, moderate, and low risk for disease or mental health conditions. If soldiers are high risk, 60 minutes is allotted for a face-to-face meeting with a credentialed provider, and a soldier at moderate risk is allotted 30 minutes. Credentialed providers include psychologists, psychiatrists, social workers, psychiatric nurse practitioners, and chaplains. Licensed practical nurses and occupational and preventive medicine professionals are also on site to assess needs unrelated to mental health, such as tobacco cessation and medical referrals.

As the program matures, its data will be accessible, comparable, and transparent, allowing for longitudinal follow-up. Currently data pertaining to form DD 2900 are sent to the Army Medial Surveillance Activity to be entered into the Defense Medical Surveillance System. Feedback from this system is sent to commanders via a Web-based report that is compliant with the Health Insurance Portability and Accountability Act of 1996. The data provided to commanders include diagnoses by type and prevalence, deployment-related conditions, safety issues, legal and financial problems, and the overall state of morale.

As Figure 18-3 demonstrates, SWAPP is resource intensive. Though it is not used Army-wide, its elements are encompassed in return processing at other duty stations, and it serves as a model for many other programs in the military. Initial feedback and response from commanders and soldiers alike has been positive. Efforts to expand the SWAPP program to other Army posts are underway.

Case Study18-3: Staff Sergeant C had recently been evacuated from Iraq following an improvised explosive device explosion in which he sustained an injury to his leg. His physical recovery was progressing well and he was hopeful for a full recovery. However, he complained of increasing awareness of disrupted sleep due to nightmares. He stated that he'd had them start before being injured and leaving Iraq and thought they'd go away once he was home. But now, some 2 months later, the nightmares persisted. Typically they involved combat operations and often centered on having to make a choice such as kill or be killed, killing, and then discovering the victim was a child.

Other soldiers often complain of hypervigilance while driving—fearing every piece of trash is an improvised explosive device or other drivers are potential suicide bombers. For many, the lack of sleep alone, without nightmares, represents a problem; often soldiers' spouses report these concerns. Recognizing a more pervasive need to normalize experiences and assist redeploying soldiers in adapting what is a normal and acceptable behavior and response in the combat zone to what is normal and acceptable at home, the Army developed and introduced Battlemind training.

The Battlemind program (Exhibit 18-2) is another intervention with a renewed emphasis on normalizing anticipated feelings and reactions during the deployment cycle. "Battlemind" is the soldier's inner strength and ability to face fear and adversity in combat with courage. Components are designed to build self-confidence and mental toughness. However, although Battlemind skills are helpful in combat, they may cause problems on returning home; for example, tactical awareness in a combat zone might become hypervigilance at home. Battlemind training is a method of aiding soldiers in transitioning to home-front living. Battlemind training emphasizes that

EXHIBIT 18-2

BATTLEMIND

Buddies (cohesion)

Accountability

Targeted aggression

Tactical awareness

Lethally armed

Emotional control

Mission operational security

Individual responsibility

Nondefensive (combat) driving

Discipline and ordering

Adapted from: US Army. Battlemind Web site. http://www.Battlemind.army.mil. Accessed March 31, 2010.

- Battlemind "injuries" (ie, a maladaptive response to a formerly dangerous situation) can occur in any soldier when combat skills are not adapted to the home;
- getting help for a Battlemind injury is NOT a sign of weakness; and
- it takes courage to ask for help and it takes leadership to help a fellow soldier get help.

The training, conducted upon redeployment, initially consists of an educational brief that emphasizes Battlemind concepts. Retraining after 3 to 6 months includes scenario-driven vignettes and videos that recreate typical situations experienced by redeployed soldiers and suggested ways of handling these issues.

The programs and procedures outlined above work towards improving communication between soldiers and family members in an effort to resolve crises and mitigate distress. The inclusion of these programs in command-sponsored and command-driven operations plans and memoranda of understanding highlights a number of important considerations:

- Planners must integrate families and communities early into the planning for reentry and reintegration.
- Distress during this time is expected and should not be medicalized.
- Behavioral health professionals should be available to soldiers and families following return from combat.
- Education of families about available resources and benefits is as important as training soldiers.

Services for family members need to be easily accessible, perhaps even more so when the soldiers are deployed. Families with preexisting mental health needs frequently have increased demands, and those who did not demonstrate preexisting problems might also need services. Often sources in the community are not readily available or sufficient, even in more populated areas. With active duty mental health professionals deployed, the increased demand for services from family members at home may tax behavioral health resources beyond capabilities. For example, at the Madigan Army Medical Center outpatient psychiatry clinic, patient contacts for fiscal year 2001 numbered approximately 8,000; the same number was logged during just the first 6 months of 2005.

SUMMARY

In current and projected future operations, the burden of soldier reentry and reintegration will be borne equally by the Army and society, who must collaborate to ensure that maximal benefits to the soldier, family members, and society are realized. Since the beginning of GWOT, OEF, and OIF, the US Army has developed and refined its efforts to reset the force, reaching out to all returning and redeploying service members with a variety of mental and behavioral health initiatives. How well these efforts are working must be tracked and analyzed, so that the programs may continue to evolve to serve the changing needs of soldiers, families, the Army, and US society.

REFERENCES

1. Adler AB, Castro CS. *US Soldiers and Peacekeeping Deployments*. Heidelberg, Germany: US Army Medical Research Unit-Europe; 2001. Research Report.

2. Schumm WR, Bell DB, Knott B. Characteristics of families of soldiers who return prematurely from overseas deployments: an assessment from Operation Restore Hope (Somalia). *Psychol Rep*. 2000;86(3 Pt 2):1267–1272.

3. Hoge CW, Castro CA, Messer SC, et al. Combat duty in Iraq and Afghanistan, mental health problems, and barriers to care. *N Engl J Med*. 2004;351(10):13–22.

4. Kirkland FR. Postcombat reentry. In: Jones FD, Sparacino LR, Wilcox VL, Rothberg JM, Stokes JW, eds. *War Psychiatry*. In: Zajtchuk R, Bellamy RF, eds. *Textbooks of Military Medicine*. Washington, DC: Department of the Army, Office of The Surgeon General, Borden Institute; 1995: 291–317.

5. Grossman D. *On Killing: The Psychological Cost of Learning to Kill in War and Society*. New York, NY: Little Brown and Company; 1995.

6. I (US) Corps OPLAN 04-10 (Return to Readiness). Unclassified. Fort Lewis, Wash. April 2004.

7. Peter Geren, Acting Secretary of the Army. *Deployment Cycle Support (DCS) Directive*. Washington, DC: US Department of the Army. Memorandum, March 26, 2007. Available at: http://www.armyg1.army.mil/dcs/docs/DCS%20Directive.pdf. Accessed September 15, 2009.

8. Memorandum of Understanding Between Washington State Military Department, Washington State Department of Veterans Affairs, Washington State Employment Security Department, US Department of Veterans Affairs, Benefits Administration, US Department of Veterans Affairs, Health Administration, US Department of Labor, Association of Washington Business, Governor's Veterans Affairs Advisory Committee, November 2004.

9. Robertson M, Humphreys L, Ray R. Psychological treatments for posttraumatic stress disorder: recommendations for the clinician based on review of the literature. *J Psychiatr Pract.* 2004;10:106–118.

10. *Getting Back Together (Homecoming/Reunion)* [videotape]. Washington, DC: US Army; 1994. US Army training video TVT20-1048.

ATTACHMENT: HEALTH ASSESSMENT FORMS

33823

PRE-DEPLOYMENT Health Assessment

Authority: 10 U.S.C. 136 Chapter 55. 1074f, 3013, 5013, 8013 and E.O. 9397

Principal Purpose: To assess your state of health before possible deployment outside the United States in support of military operations and to assist military healthcare providers in identifying and providing present and future medical care to you.

Routine Use: To other Federal and State agencies and civilian healthcare providers, as necessary, in order to provide necessary medical care and treatment.

Disclosure: **(Military personel and DoD civilian Employees Only)** Voluntary. If not provided, healthcare WILL BE furnished, but comprehensive care may not be possible.

INSTRUCTIONS: Please read each question completely and carefully before marking your selections. Provide a response for each question. If you do not understand a question, ask the administrator.

Demographics

Last Name

Today's Date (dd/mm/yyyy) __ / __ / ____

First Name **MI**

Social Security Number ___ - __ - ____

Deploying Unit

DOB (dd/mm/yyyy) __ / __ / ____

Gender
- ○ Male
- ○ Female

Service Branch
- ○ Air Force
- ○ Army
- ○ Coast Guard
- ○ Marine Corps
- ○ Navy
- ○ Other

Component
- ○ Active Duty
- ○ National Guard
- ○ Reserves
- ○ Civilian Government Employee

Pay Grade
- ○ E1 ○ E2 ○ E3 ○ E4 ○ E5 ○ E6 ○ E7 ○ E8 ○ E9
- ○ O1 ○ O2 ○ O3 ○ O4 ○ O5 ○ O6 ○ O7 ○ O8 ○ O9 ○ O10
- ○ W1 ○ W2 ○ W3 ○ W4 ○ W5 ○ Other

Location of Operation
- ○ Europe
- ○ SW Asia
- ○ SE Asia
- ○ Asia (Other)
- ○ South America
- ○ Australia
- ○ Africa
- ○ Central America
- ○ Unknown

Deployment Location (IF KNOWN) (CITY, TOWN, or BASE):

List country (IF KNOWN):

Name of Operation:

Administrator Use Only

Indicate the status of each of the following:

Yes	No	N/A	
○	○	○	Medical threat briefing completed
○	○	○	Medical information sheet distributed
○	○	○	Serum for HIV drawn within 12 months
○	○	○	Immunizations current
○	○	○	PPD screening within 24 months

33823

DD FORM 2795, MAY 1999

ASD (HA) APPROVED SEPTEMBER 1998 Ver 1.3

Reset

Adobe Professional 7.0

33823

PLEASE FILL IN SOCIAL SECURITY # ☐☐☐-☐☐-☐☐☐☐

Health Assessment

1. Would you say your health in general is: ○ Excellent ○ Very Good ○ Good ○ Fair ○ Poor
2. Do you have any medical or dental problems? ○ Yes ○ No
3. Are you currently on a profile, or light duty, or are you undergoing a medical board? ○ Yes ○ No
4. Are you pregnant? (FEMALES ONLY) ○ Don't Know ○ Yes ○ No
5. Do you have a 90-day supply of your prescription medication or birth control pills? ○ N/A ○ Yes ○ No
6. Do you have two pairs of prescription glasses (if worn) and any other personal medical equipment? ○ N/A ○ Yes ○ No
7. During the past year, have you sought counseling or care for your mental health? ○ Yes ○ No
8. Do you currently have any questions or concerns about your health? ○ Yes ○ No

   Please list your concerns: ______________________

I certify that responses on this form are true. Service Member Signature

Pre-Deployment Health Provider Review (For Health Provider Use Only)

After interview/exam of patient, the following problems were noted and categorized by Review of Systems. More than one may be noted for patients with multiple problems. Further documentation of problem to be placed in medical records.

REFERRAL INDICATED

○ None
○ Cardiac
○ Combat / Operational Stress Reaction
○ Dental
○ Dermatologic
○ ENT
○ Eye
○ Family Problems
○ Fatigue, Malaise, Multisystem complaint
○ GI
○ GU
○ GYN
○ Mental Health
○ Neurologic
○ Orthopedic
○ Pregnancy
○ Pulmonary
○ Other ______________

FINAL MEDICAL DISPOSITION: ○ **Deployable** ○ **Not Deployable**

Comments: (If not deployable, explain)

____

I certify that this review process has been completed.

Provider's signature and stamp:

Date (dd/mm/yyyy) ☐☐/☐☐/☐☐☐☐

End of Health Review

Reset

33823

DD FORM 2795, MAY 1999 ASD (HA) APPROVED SEPTEMBER 1998 Ver 1.3

33348

POST-DEPLOYMENT Health Assessment

Authority: 10 U.S.C. 136 Chapter 55. 1074f, 3013, 5013, 8013 and E.O. 9397

Principal Purpose: To assess your state of health after deployment outside the United States in support of military operations and to assist military healthcare providers in identifying and providing present and future medical care to you.

Routine Use: To other Federal and State agencies and civilian healthcare providers, as necessary, in order to provide necessary medical care and treatment.

Disclosure: (Military personnal and DoD civilian Employees Only) Voluntary. If not provided, healthcare WILL BE furnished, but comprehensive care may not be possible.

INSTRUCTIONS: Please read each question completely and carefully before marking your selections. Provide a response for each question. If you do not understand a question, ask the administrator.

Demographics

Last Name ______________

Today's Date (dd/mm/yyyy) __ / __ / ____

First Name ______________ **MI** __

Social Security Number ___ — __ — ____

Name of Your Unit or Ship during this Deployment ______________

DOB (dd/mm/yyyy) __ / __ / ____

Date of arrival in theater (dd/mm/yyyy) __ / __ / ____

Date of departure from theater (dd/mm/yyyy) __ / __ / ____

Gender
- ○ Male
- ○ Female

Service Branch
- ○ Air Force
- ○ Army
- ○ Coast Guard
- ○ Marine Corps
- ○ Navy
- ○ Other

Component
- ○ Active Duty
- ○ National Guard
- ○ Reserves
- ○ Civilian Government Employee

Pay Grade

○ E1	○ 001	○ W1
○ E2	○ 002	○ W2
○ E3	○ 003	○ W3
○ E4	○ 004	○ W4
○ E5	○ 005	○ W5
○ E6	○ 006	
○ E7	○ 007	○ Other
○ E8	○ 008	
○ E9	○ 009	
	○ 010	

Location of Operation

○ Europe	○ Australia	○ South America
○ SW Asia	○ Africa	○ North America
○ SE Asia	○ Central America	○ Other ______
○ Asia (Other)	○ Unknown	______

To what areas were you mainly deployed:
(mark all that apply - list where/date arrived)

○ Kuwait ______	○ Iraq ______
○ Qatar ______	○ Turkey ______
○ Afghanistan ______	○ Uzbekistan ______
○ Bosnia ______	○ Kosovo ______
○ On a ship ______	○ CONUS ______
	○ Other ______

Name of Operation: ______________

Occupational specialty during this deployment (MOS, NEC or AFSC) ______

Combat specialty: ______________

Administrator Use Only

Indicate the status of each of the following:

Yes	No	N/A	
○	○	○	Medical threat debriefing completed
○	○	○	Medical information sheet distributed
○	○	○	Post Deployment serum specimen collected

33348

Reset

DD FORM 2796, APR 2003 PREVIOUS EDITION IS OBSOLETE. ASD(HA) APPROVED

Please answer all questions in relation to THIS deployment

1. Did your health change during this deployment?

○ Health stayed about the same or got better
○ Health got worse

2. How many times were you seen in sick call during this deployment? [|] No. of times

3. Did you have to spend one or more nights in a hospital as a patient during this deployment?

○ No
○ Yes, reason/dates: ______________

____

____

4. Did you receive any vaccinations just before or during this deployment?

○ Smallpox (leaves a scar on the arm)
○ Anthrax
○ Botulism
○ Typhoid
○ Meningococcal
○ Other, list: ______________
○ Don't know
○ None

5. Did you take any of the following medications during this deployment?
(mark all that apply)

○ PB (pyridostigmine bromide) nerve agent pill
○ Mark-1 antidote kit
○ Anti-malaria pills
○ Pills to stay awake, such as dexedrine
○ Other, please list ______________
○ Don't know

6. Do you have any of these symptoms now or did you develop them anytime during this deployment?

No	Yes During	Yes Now	
○	○	○	Chronic cough
○	○	○	Runny nose
○	○	○	Fever
○	○	○	Weakness
○	○	○	Headaches
○	○	○	Swollen, stiff or painful joints
○	○	○	Back pain
○	○	○	Muscle aches
○	○	○	Numbness or tingling in hands or feet
○	○	○	Skin diseases or rashes
○	○	○	Redness of eyes with tearing
○	○	○	Dimming of vision, like the lights were going out

No	Yes During	Yes Now	
○	○	○	Chest pain or pressure
○	○	○	Dizziness, fainting, light headedness
○	○	○	Difficulty breathing
○	○	○	Still feeling tired after sleeping
○	○	○	Difficulty remembering
○	○	○	Diarrhea
○	○	○	Frequent indigestion
○	○	○	Vomiting
○	○	○	Ringing of the ears

7. Did you see anyone wounded, killed or dead during this deployment?
(mark all that apply)

○ No ○ Yes - coalition ○ Yes - enemy ○ Yes - civilian

8. Were you engaged in direct combat where you discharged your weapon?

○ No ○ Yes (○ land ○ sea ○ air)

9. During this deployment, did you ever feel that you were in great danger of being killed?

○ No ○ Yes

10. Are you currently interested in receiving help for a stress, emotional, alcohol or family problem?

○ No ○ Yes

11. Over the LAST 2 WEEKS, how often have you been bothered by any of the following problems?

None	Some	A Lot	
○	○	○	Little interest or pleasure in doing things
○	○	○	Feeling down, depressed, or hopeless
○	○	○	Thoughts that you would be better off dead or hurting yourself in some way

33348

Reset

DD FORM 2796, APR 2003

12. Have you ever had any experience that was so frightening, horrible, or upsetting that, IN THE PAST MONTH, you ....

No	Yes	
O	O	Have had any nightmares about it or thought about it when you did not want to?
O	O	Tried hard not to think about it or went out of your way to avoid situations that remind you of it?
O	O	Were constantly on guard, watchful, or easily startled?
O	O	Felt numb or detached from others, activities, or your surroundings?

13. Are you having thoughts or concerns that ...

No	Yes	Unsure	
O	O	O	You may have serious conflicts with your spouse, family members, or close friends?
O	O	O	You might hurt or lose control with someone?

14. While you were deployed, were you exposed to:
(mark all that apply)

No	Sometimes	Often	
O	O	O	DEET insect repellent applied to skin
O	O	O	Pesticide-treated uniforms
O	O	O	Environmental pesticides (like area fogging)
O	O	O	Flea or tick collars
O	O	O	Pesticide strips
O	O	O	Smoke from oil fire
O	O	O	Smoke from burning trash or feces
O	O	O	Vehicle or truck exhaust fumes
O	O	O	Tent heater smoke
O	O	O	JP8 or other fuels
O	O	O	Fog oils (smoke screen)
O	O	O	Solvents
O	O	O	Paints
O	O	O	Ionizing radiation
O	O	O	Radar/microwaves
O	O	O	Lasers
O	O	O	Loud noises
O	O	O	Excessive vibration
O	O	O	Industrial pollution
O	O	O	Sand/dust
O	O	O	Depleted Uranium (If yes, explain) ____________
O	O	O	Other exposures ____________

15. On how many days did you wear your MOPP over garments?

[ ][ ] No. of days

16. How many times did you put on your gas mask because of alerts and NOT because of exercises?

[ ][ ] No. of times

17. Were you in or did you enter or closely inspect any destroyed military vehicles?

O No O Yes

18. Do you think you were exposed to any chemical, biological, or radiological warfare agents during this deployment?

O No O Don't know
O Yes, explain with date and location

____

____

____

Reset

33348

DD FORM 2796, APR 2003

Health Care Provider Only

SERVICE MEMBER'S SOCIAL SECURITY # ☐☐☐ — ☐☐ — ☐☐☐☐

Post-Deployment Health Care Provider Review, Interview, and Assessment

Interview

1. Would you say your health in general is: ○ Excellent ○ Very Good ○ Good ○ Fair ○ Poor
2. Do you have any medical or dental problems that developed during this deployment? ○ Yes ○ No
3. Are you currently on a profile or light duty? ○ Yes ○ No
4. During this deployment have you sought, or do you now intend to seek, counseling or care for your mental health? ○ Yes ○ No
5. Do you have concerns about possible exposures or events during this deployment that you feel may affect your health? ○ Yes ○ No
   Please list concerns: ______________________________
   ____
6. Do you currently have any questions or concerns about your health? ○ Yes ○ No
   Please list concerns: ______________________________
   ____

Health Assessment

After my interview/exam of the service member and review of this form, there is a need for further evaluation as indicated below. (More than one may be noted for patients with multiple problems. Further documentation of the problem evaluation to be placed in the service member's medical record.)

REFERRAL INDICATED FOR:

○ None
○ Cardiac
○ Combat/Operational Stress Reaction
○ Dental
○ Dermatologic
○ ENT
○ Eye
○ Family Problems
○ Fatigue, Malaise, Multisystem complaint
○ Audiology
○ GI
○ GU
○ GYN
○ Mental Health
○ Neurologic
○ Orthopedic
○ Pregnancy
○ Pulmonary
○ Other ______________________________

EXPOSURE CONCERNS (During deployment):

○ Environmental
○ Occupational
○ Combat or mission related
○ None

Comments: ______________________________
____
____

I certify that this review process has been completed.
Provider's signature and stamp:

This visit is coded by V70.5 _ _ 6

Date (dd/mm/yyyy) ☐☐ / ☐☐ / ☐☐☐☐

End of Health Review

33348

Reset

DD FORM 2796, APR 2003 ASD(HA) APPROVED

This form must be completed electronically. Handwritten forms will not be accepted.

POST-DEPLOYMENT HEALTH RE-ASSESSMENT (PDHRA)

PRIVACY ACT STATEMENT

AUTHORITY: 10 U.S.C. 136, 1074f, 3013, 5013, 8013 and E.O. 9397.

PRINCIPAL PURPOSE(S): To assess your state of health after deployment in support of military operations and to assist military healthcare providers in identifying and providing present and future medical care you may need. The information you provide may result in a referral for additional healthcare that may include medical, dental or behavioral healthcare or diverse community support services.

ROUTINE USE(S): In addition to those disclosures generally permitted under 5 U.S.C. 552a(b) of the Privacy Act, to other Federal and State agencies and civilian healthcare providers, as necessary, in order to provide necessary medical care and treatment.

DISCLOSURE: Voluntary. If not provided, healthcare WILL BE furnished, but comprehensive care may not be possible.

INSTRUCTIONS: Please read each question completely and carefully before entering your response or marking your selection. **YOU ARE ENCOURAGED TO ANSWER EACH QUESTION.** Withholding or providing inaccurate information may impair a healthcare provider's ability to identify health problems and refer you to appropriate sources for additional evaluation or treatment. If you do not understand a question, please ask for help. Please respond based on your **MOST RECENT DEPLOYMENT**.

DEMOGRAPHICS

Last Name ____________ **First Name** ____________ **Middle Initial** ______

Social Security Number ____________ **Date of Birth** *(dd/mmm/yyyy)* ____________ **Today's Date** *(dd/mmm/yyyy)* ____________

Date arrived theater *(dd/mmm/yyyy)* ____________ **Date departed theater** *(dd/mmm/yyyy)* ____________

Gender
- O Male
- O Female

Marital Status
- O Never Married
- O Married
- O Separated
- O Divorced
- O Widowed

Service Branch
- O Air Force
- O Army
- O Navy
- O Marine Corps
- O Coast Guard
- O Civilian Employee
- O Other

Status Prior to Deployment
- O Active Duty
- O Selected Reserves - Reserve - Unit
- O Selected Reserves - Reserve - AGR
- O Selected Reserves - Reserve - IMA
- O Selected Reserves - National Guard - Unit
- O Selected Reserves - National Guard - AGR
- O Ready Reserves - IRR
- O Ready Reserves - ING
- O Civilian Government Employee
- O Other

Pay Grade

O E1	O O1	O W1
O E2	O O2	O W2
O E3	O O3	O W3
O E4	O O4	O W4
O E5	O O5	O W5
O E6	O O6	
O E7	O O7	O Other
O E8	O O8	
O E9	O O9	
	O O10	

Location of Operation
To what areas were you mainly deployed *(land-based operations more than 30 days)*? Please mark all that apply, including the number of months spent at each location.
- O Country 1 ____________ Months ____
- O Country 2 ____________ Months ____
- O Country 3 ____________ Months ____
- O Country 4 ____________ Months ____
- O Country 5 ____________ Months ____

Since return from deployment I have:
- O Maintained/returned to previous status
- O Transitioned to Selected Reserves
- O Transitioned to IRR
- O Transitioned to ING
- O Retired from Military Service
- O Separated from Military Service

Current Contact Information:
Phone: ____________
Cell: ____________
DSN: ____________
Email: ____________
Address: ____________

Total Deployments in Past 5 Years:

OIF	OEF	Other
O 1	O 1	O 1
O 2	O 2	O 2
O 3	O 3	O 3
O 4	O 4	O 4
O 5 or more	O 5 or more	O 5 or more

Current Unit of Assignment ____________

Current Assignment Location ____________

Point of Contact who can always reach you:
Name: ____________
Phone: ____________
Email: ____________
Mailing Address: ____________

DD FORM 2900, JAN 2008 PREVIOUS EDITION IS OBSOLETE. Page 1 of 5 Pages Adobe Professional 7.0

This form must be completed electronically. Handwritten forms will not be accepted.

Service Member's Social Security Number:

1. Overall, how would you rate your health during the PAST MONTH?

- O Excellent
- O Very Good
- O Good
- O Fair
- O Poor

2. Compared to before your most recent deployment, how would you rate your health in general now?

- O Much better now than before I deployed
- O Somewhat better now than before I deployed
- O About the same as before I deployed
- O Somewhat worse now than before I deployed
- O Much worse now than before I deployed

3. During the past 4 weeks, how difficult have physical health problems *(illness or injury)* **made it for you to do your work or other regular daily activities?**

- O Not difficult at all
- O Very difficult
- O Somewhat difficult
- O Extremely difficult

4. During the past 4 weeks, how difficult have emotional problems *(such as feeling depressed or anxious)* **made it for you to do your work, take care of things at home, or get along with other people?**

- O Not difficult at all
- O Very difficult
- O Somewhat difficult
- O Extremely difficult

5. Since you returned from deployment, about how many times have you seen a healthcare provider for any reason, such as in sick call, emergency room, primary care, family doctor, or mental health provider?

O No visits O 1 visit O 2-3 visits O 4-5 visits O 6 or more

6. Since you returned from deployment, have you been hospitalized? O Yes O No

7. During your deployment, were you wounded, injured, assaulted or otherwise physically hurt? O Yes O No

If **NO**, skip to Question 8.

7a. If **YES**, are you still having problems related to this wound, assault, or injury? O Yes O No O Unsure

8. In addition to wounds or injuries you listed in question 7., do you currently have a health concern or condition that you feel is related to your deployment? O Yes O No O Unsure

If **NO**, skip to Question 9.

8a. If **YES**, please mark the item(s) that best describe your deployment-related condition or concern:

O Fever	O Dimming of vision, like the lights were going out
O Cough lasting more than 3 weeks	O Chest pain or pressure
O Trouble breathing	O Dizzy, light headed, passed out
O Bad headaches	O Diarrhea, vomiting, or frequent indigestion/heartburn
O Generally feeling weak	O Problems sleeping or still feeling tired after sleeping
O Muscle aches	O Trouble concentrating, easily distracted
O Swollen, stiff or painful joints	O Forgetful or trouble remembering things
O Back pain	O Hard to make up your mind or make decisions
O Numbness or tingling in hands or feet	O Increased irritability
O Trouble hearing	O Taking more risks such as driving faster
O Ringing in the ears	O Skin diseases or rashes
O Watery, red eyes	O Other *(please list)*: ________

9a. During this deployment, did you experience any of the following events? *(Mark all that apply)*

	Yes	No
(1) Blast or explosion *(IED, RPG, land mine, grenade, etc.)*	O	O
(2) Vehicular accident/crash *(any vehicle, including aircraft)*	O	O
(3) Fragment wound or bullet wound above your shoulders	O	O
(4) Fall	O	O
(5) Other event *(for example, a sports injury to your head)*. Describe: ________	O	O

9b. Did any of the following happen to you, or were you told happened to you, IMMEDIATELY after any of the event(s) you just noted in question 9a.? *(Mark all that apply)*

	Yes	No
(1) Lost consciousness or got "knocked out"	O	O
(2) Felt dazed, confused, or "saw stars"	O	O
(3) Didn't remember the event	O	O
(4) Had a concussion	O	O
(5) Had a head injury	O	O

c. Did any of the following problems begin or get worse after the event(s) you noted in question 9a.? *(Mark all that apply)*

	Yes	No
(1) Memory problems or lapses	O	O
(2) Balance problems or dizziness	O	O
(3) Ringing in the ears	O	O
(4) Sensitivity to bright light	O	O
(5) Irritability	O	O
(6) Headaches	O	O
(7) Sleep problems	O	O

d. In the past week, have you had any of the symptoms you indicated in 9c.? *(Mark all that apply)*

	Yes	No
(1) Memory problems or lapses	O	O
(2) Balance problems or dizziness	O	O
(3) Ringing in the ears	O	O
(4) Sensitivity to bright light	O	O
(5) Irritability	O	O
(6) Headaches	O	O
(7) Sleep problems	O	O

DD FORM 2900, JAN 2008 Page 2 of 5 Pages

This form must be completed electronically. Handwritten forms will not be accepted.

Service Member's Social Security Number:

10. Do you have any persistent major concerns regarding the health effects of something you believe you may have been exposed to or encountered while deployed? O Yes O No
If **NO**, skip to question 11.

10a. If **YES,** please mark the item(s) that best describe your concern:

O Animal bites	O Loud noises
O Animal bodies *(dead)*	O Paints
O Chlorine gas	O Pesticides
O Depleted uranium *(If yes, explain)* ____	O Radar/Microwaves
O Excessive vibration	O Sand/dust
O Fog oils (smoke screen	O Smoke from burning trash or feces
O Garbage	O Smoke from oil fire
O Human blood, body fluids, body parts, or dead bodies	O Solvents
O Industrial pollution	O Tent heater smoke
O Insect bites	O Vehicle or truck exhaust fumes
O Ionizing radiation	O Other exposures to toxic chemicals or materials, such as ammonia, nitric acid, etc.: *(If yes, explain)* ____
O JP8 or other fuels	
O Lasers	

11. Since return from your deployment, have you had serious conflicts with your spouse, family members, close friends, or at work that continue to cause you worry or concern? O Yes O No O Unsure

12. Have you ever had any experience that was so frightening, horrible, or upsetting that, IN THE PAST MONTH, you ....

a. Have had nightmares about it or thought about it when you did not want to? O Yes O No

b. Tried hard not to think about it or went out of your way to avoid situations that remind you of it? O Yes O No

c. Were constantly on guard, watchful, or easily startled? O Yes O No

d. Felt numb or detached from others, activities, or your surroundings? O Yes O No

13a. In the PAST MONTH, Did you use alcohol more than you meant to? O Yes O No

b. In the PAST MONTH, have you felt that you wanted to or needed to cut down on your drinking? O Yes O No

c. How often do you have a drink containing alcohol?
O Never O Monthly or less O 2 to 4 times a month O 2 to 3 times a week O 4 or more times a week

d. How many drinks containing alcohol do you have on a typical day when you are drinking?
O 1 or 2 O 3 or 4 O 5 or 6 O 7 to 9 O 10 or more

e. How often do you have six or more drinks on one occasion?
O Never O Less than monthly O Monthly O Weekly O Daily

14. Over the PAST MONTH, have you been bothered by the following problems?	Not at all	Few or several days	More than half the days	Nearly every day
a. Little interest or pleasure in doing things	O	O	O	O
b. Feeling down, depressed, or hopeless	O	O	O	O

15. Would you like to schedule a visit with a healthcare provider to further discuss your health concern(s)? O Yes O No

16. Are you currently interested in receiving information or assistance for a stress, emotional or alcohol concern? O Yes O No

17. Are you currently interested in receiving assistance for a family or relationship concern? O Yes O No

18. Would you like to schedule a visit with a chaplain or a community support counselor? O Yes O No

DD FORM 2900, JAN 2008 Page 3 of 5 Pages

This form must be completed electronically. Handwritten forms will not be accepted.

Service Member's Social Security Number: **Date** *(dd/mmm/yyyy)*:

Health Care Provider Only

Provider Review and Interview

1. Review symptoms and deployment concerns identified on form:

- ○ Confirmed screening results as reported
- ○ Screening results modified, amended, clarified during interview:

2. Ask behavioral risk questions. Conduct risk assessment.

a. Over the PAST MONTH, have you been bothered by thoughts that you would be better off dead or of hurting yourself in some way? ○ Yes ○ No

IF YES, about how often have you been bothered by these thoughts? ○ Very few days ○ More than half of the time ○ Nearly every day

b. Since return from your deployment, have you had thoughts or concerns that you might hurt or lose control with someone? ○ Yes ○ No ○ Unsure

3. If member reports positive or unsure response to 2a. or 2b., conduct risk assessment.

a. Does member pose a current risk for harm to self or others? ○ No, not a current risk ○ Yes, poses a current risk ○ Unsure

b. Outcome of assessment ○ Immediate referral ○ Routine follow-up referral ○ Referral not indicated

4. Alcohol screening result

- ○ No evidence of alcohol-related problems.
- ○ Potential alcohol problem (positive response to either question 13a. or 13b. and/or AUDIT-C (questions 13c.-e.) score of 4 or more for men or 3 or more for women).
  Refer to PCM for evaluation. ○ Yes ○ No

5. Traumatic Brain Injury (TBI) risk assessment

- ○ No evidence of risk based on responses to questions 9.a. - d.
- ○ Potential TBI with persistent symptoms, based on responses to question 9d.
  Refer for additional evaluation. ○ Yes ○ No

6. Record additional questions or concerns identified by patient during interview:

DD FORM 2900, JAN 2008 Page 4 of 5 Pages

This form must be completed electronically. Handwritten forms will not be accepted.

Service Member's Social Security Number: **Date** *(dd/mmm/yyyy)*:

Assessment and Referral: After my interview with the service member and review of this form, there is a need for further evaluation and follow-up as indicated below. (More than one may be noted for patients with multiple concerns.)

7. Identified Concerns	Minor Concern	Major Concern	Already Under Care: Yes	Already Under Care: No
O Physical Symptom(s)	O	O	O	O
O Exposure Symptom(s)	O	O	O	O
O Depression symptoms	O	O	O	O
O PTSD symptoms	O	O	O	O
O Anger/Aggression	O	O	O	O
O Suicidal Ideation	O	O	O	O
O Social/Family Conflict	O	O	O	O
O Alcohol Use	O	O	O	O
O Other: ______	O	O	O	O

8. Referral Information	Within 24 hours	Within 7 days	Within 30 days
a. Primary Care, Family Practice	O	O	O
b. Behavioral Health in Primary Care	O	O	O
c. Mental Health Specialty Care	O	O	O
d. Other specialty care:			
Audiology	O	O	O
Cardiology	O	O	O
Dentistry	O	O	O
Dermatology	O	O	O
ENT	O	O	O
GI	O	O	O
Internal Medicine	O	O	O
Neurology	O	O	O
OB/GYN	O	O	O
Ophthalmology	O	O	O
Optometry	O	O	O
Orthopedics	O	O	O
Pulmonology	O	O	O
Urology	O	O	O
e. Case Manager, Care Manager	O	O	O
f. Substance Abuse Program	O	O	O
g. Health Promotion, Health Education	O	O	O
h. Chaplain	O	O	O
i. Family Support, Community Service	O	O	O
j. Military OneSource	O	O	O
k. Other: ______	O	O	O
l. No referral made O			

9. Comments:

______

I certify that this review process has been completed.
10. Provider's signature and stamp:

ICD-9 Code for this visit: V70.5 _ F

SAMPLE

Ancillary Staff/Administrative Section

11. Member was provided the following:	12. Referral was made to the following healthcare or support system:
O Health Education and Information	O Military Treatment Facility
O Health Care Benefits and Resources Information	O Division/Line-based medical resource
O Appointment Assistance	O VA Medical Center or Community Clinic
O Service member declined to complete form	O Vet Center
O Service member declined to complete interview/assessment	O TRICARE Provider
O Service member declined referral for services	O Contract Support: ______
O LOD	O Community Service: ______
O Other: ______	O Other: ______
______	O None

DD FORM 2900, JAN 2008 Page 5 of 5 Pages

Chapter 19

TREATMENT OF DEPLOYMENT-RELATED POSTTRAUMATIC STRESS DISORDER

JOSEF I. RUZEK, PhD*; JEFFREY S. YARVIS, PhD†; and STEVEN LINDLEY, MD, PhD‡

*Director, Dissemination and Training Division, National Center for Posttraumatic Stress Disorder, Veterans Affairs Palo Alto Health Care System, 795 Willow Road, Menlo Park, California 94025

†Lieutenant Colonel, Medical Service Corps, US Army; Chief, Behavioral Health, Department of Psychiatry, Borden Pavilion, Walter Reed Army Medical Center, 6900 Georgia Avenue NW, Washington DC 20307; formerly, Director of Social Work, Uniformed Services University of the Health Sciences, Bethesda, Maryland

‡Director of Outpatient Mental Health, Department of Veterans Affairs Palo Alto Health Care System, 795 Willow Road, 116R/MHC, Menlo Park, California 94025; and Associate Professor, Department of Psychiatry, Stanford University, Palo Alto, California

INTRODUCTION

Posttraumatic stress disorder (PTSD) is the most common and conspicuous psychiatric problem associated with the stress experienced by soldiers in combat. By definition, diagnosis of PTSD requires exposure to a traumatic event that involves experiencing, witnessing, or being confronted by death or serious injury to self or others; a response of intense fear, helplessness, or horror; and development of a set of symptoms that persist for at least a month and cause significant impairment of functioning.[1] Some factor analytic studies have demonstrated four basic dimensions of PTSD symptoms[2]—(1) reexperiencing (nightmares, flashbacks), (2) avoidance (efforts to avoid thinking about the trauma), (3) numbing of general responsiveness (restricted range of affect), and (4) hyperarousal (exaggerated startle response)—but some suggest other complex relationships between symptoms.[3]

Most individuals who develop chronic PTSD experience immediate distress that then persists over time.[4] However, a small, but significant, number of individuals report increases in PTSD symptoms over time (delayed onset PTSD[5]). In retrospective studies of the course of PTSD, three different patterns have been identified: (1) high levels of symptoms after the war followed by recovery, (2) chronic symptoms persisting until the time of the assessment, or (3) relapsing-remitting symptoms.[6] Heterogeneity, of course, was also observed in a longitudinal study of a large community sample of Vietnam veterans. Koenen et al[7] found that only 5.3% of veterans met PTSD criteria in both 1984 and 1998, whereas 6.5% and 5.2% met criteria in 1984 and 1998, respectively.

Current data suggest that approximately 5% to 20% of armed forces personnel deployed for combat, peacekeeping, or humanitarian disaster relief will develop PTSD following their tour of duty.[8–12] Among Vietnam veterans, as reported in the National Vietnam Veteran Readjustment Study,[13] the lifetime prevalence for full PTSD was 30.9% for male veterans and 26% for female veterans. At the time of that study, 15.2% were currently suffering from PTSD. Reanalysis of the survey data, applying criteria revised to reflect changes in diagnostic criteria, indicates that 18.7% of the veterans had developed war-related PTSD during their lifetimes and 9.1% were currently suffering from PTSD 11 to 12 years after the war.[9] Despite the impact of methodology and deployment experiences on exact estimates of symptomatology, these findings represent significant rates of distress that often persist over long periods of time[14] and reflect a significant public health problem.

In considering the problem of PTSD, it should also be acknowledged that problematic reactions to trauma are not limited to full-blown disorder. A considerable percentage (ie, 10%–25%) of those not meeting threshold diagnostic criteria for PTSD experience significant subsyndromal symptoms[15] that may require treatment. Subthreshold, or partial, PTSD is associated with significant levels of impairment of social, occupational, and family functioning,[15–19] often similar to those reported in individuals with full PTSD. (Yarvis et al[18] conservatively defined subthreshold PTSD as having met the *Diagnostic and Statistical Manual*, 4th edition, criteria for the re-experiencing cluster *and* at least one other symptom cluster). Subthreshold presentations of PTSD are also associated with rates of help-seeking behaviors similar to those found with individuals who meet all the diagnostic criteria.[16,20,21] These findings raise questions about the clinical significance of subthreshold PTSD and the diagnostic cutoffs. Those being diagnosed with PTSD may fall on the upper end of a stress-response continuum instead of representing a discrete clinical syndrome.[22]

Individuals diagnosed with PTSD almost always experience additional concurrent mental health disorders, such as substance use disorder, other anxiety disorders, and major depressive disorder.[13,23–25] In the National Comorbidity Survey,[25] 88% of men and 79% of women with a lifetime history of PTSD met criteria for at least one other disorder. PTSD is also associated with significant levels of functional impairment and disability in civilian and veteran populations.[10,11,20,26–37] The extent and number of symptoms can often predict physical and mental health problems.[38] The persistence of PTSD as much as 30 years after trauma exposure is associated with continuing family problems and reduced happiness and life satisfaction.[39]

Risk factors for development of PTSD include characteristics of the traumatic event itself, pretrauma factors, and posttrauma factors. Event characteristics that increase the risk for chronic PTSD include type of trauma, greater amount of exposure, injury, involvement in atrocities, and perceived life threat.[13,40–43] Degree of exposure to potentially traumatic combat events during deployment is strongly associated with development of PTSD.[44] Military sexual trauma is more strongly associated with PTSD than premilitary or postmilitary sexual trauma[45] or other traumas.[46] In a sample of female veterans seeking treatment for stress disorders, sexual stress was found to be almost four times as influential in the development of PTSD as duty-related stress.[47] In veterans, predisposing factors have included non-Caucasian ethnicity, lower intelligence or education, younger age at exposure, lower socioeconomic status, family problems in childhood, pretrauma psychopathology, and childhood behavior problems.[13,40,41,48] Postevent factors that predict chronic PTSD in veterans include low levels of social support, negative homecoming experiences, poor coping, and adverse life events posttrauma.[40,41,48,49] Although many risk factors exert a similar effect in military and civilian populations, trauma severity and posttrauma social support may be more important in military than in civilian samples.[50]

PSYCHOLOGICAL THEORIES OF POSTTRAUMATIC STRESS DISORDER AND TREATMENT

Conceptions of the etiology of PTSD, both psychosocial and biological, have implications for the understanding of treatment. Many theories have focused on the intense fear often experienced during traumatic events and the impact of fear on conditioned emotional reactions and encoding of traumatic memories. According to emotional processing theory as applied to PTSD,[51] impaired "emotional processing" of traumatic experiences can result in creation of memories of the trauma ("pathological fear structures") that are disruptively intense, contain unrealistic elements (in which harmless stimuli are associated with escape or avoidance responses), and include erroneous evaluations or interpretations (eg, "anxiety will persist until escape" or "fear will cause harm"). The Ehlers and Clark[52] Cognitive Theory of PTSD is similar to emotion-processing theory in drawing attention to the nature of trauma memories (and their links to other memories), to appraisals of the trauma and its sequelae, and to the behavioral and cognitive responses that prevent cognitive change and therefore maintain the disorder.[52]

Foa and Kozak[51] suggest that there are two conditions for change in these problematic fear-related memories once they have been created: (1) the fear structure must be activated, and (2) there must be an incorporation of new information into the memory. Memory activation alone is insufficient for change. In fact, trauma memories are frequently activated by nightmares, conversations, or trauma reminders without benefit to the survivor. These experiences often increase fear for the person, or prompt maladaptive escape or avoidance behaviors. Dual representation theory argues that activation of memories can lead not only to recovery but also to chronic emotional processing (permanent preoccupation with consequences of trauma and intrusive memories), or to premature inhibition of processing that results from avoidance and is associated with continued phobic avoidance, somatization, and vulnerability to reactivation later in life.[53] When PTSD symptoms become chronic, this is thought to reflect a failure to engage in successful emotional processing of the traumatic experience, because avoidance limits activation of the memory and access to new, corrective information.[54]

Following this thinking, it is the job of the treating provider to encourage conditions for change and reduce emotional avoidance. Deliberate therapeutic activation of traumatic memories is most directly attempted in exposure therapies that require the individual to repetitively talk about the trauma in detail and approach previously avoided trauma-related stimuli. During effective treatment, therefore, avoidance is limited and new information of many kinds is purposefully incorporated into the memory. The individual learns that it is not dangerous to remember the trauma and experience strong emotions, that events can be remembered deliberately with a feeling of personal control and manageable physical reactions, that the trauma memory may not be completely accurate and must be updated, and that some beliefs or judgments about the experience can be challenged and changed.

Although most theories of PTSD emphasize the relationship of fear to the development of PTSD, combat and other deployment-related traumas often activate other intense emotions—including sadness, anger, and guilt—that can be connected to the development of PTSD and other posttrauma problems. In Operation Iraqi Freedom (OIF), for example, substantial percentages of US Army and US Marine Corps personnel reported potentially traumatic experiences that included not only events likely to be associated with fear ("being attacked or ambushed"), but also those related to loss ("knowing someone seriously injured or killed"), moral conflict ("being responsible for the death of a noncombatant"), horror ("handling or uncovering human remains"), or helplessness ("seeing ill or injured women or children whom you were unable to help").[44] These types of experiences are associated with a range of intense emotions that can continue to trouble trauma survivors. Some of these emotions are fueled by negative interpretations or appraisals (of personal behavior during the trauma, or the effects of the trauma); thus it may be important to supplement exposure interventions with those explicitly designed to modify appraisals. The cognitive theory of PTSD emphasizes "idiosyncratic negative appraisals of the traumatic event and/or its sequelae that have the common effect of creating a sense of serious current threat"[52(p320)] and thus serve to maintain acute stress reactions.

Generally, cognitive-behavioral psychological theories and treatment of PTSD instruct that the trauma memory needs to be actively confronted, elaborated, and integrated into the context of the individual's preceding and subsequent experience; problematic appraisals that maintain sense of threat and other negative emotions need to be modified; and dysfunctional coping strategies that prevent emotional processing of the trauma, and thus recovery, need to be reduced.

TREATMENT OF DEPLOYMENT-RELATED POSTTRAUMATIC STRESS DISORDER

Treatment of PTSD depends upon a careful assessment of the individual. Treatment plan formulation should be based on judgments of factors that may have caused problems for that particular person, those that maintain them, co-occurring problems of the person, and priorities for intervention. Regardless of specific interventions, treatment of individuals with PTSD can be conceptualized as a temporal process that starts with client engagement, alliance building, and education about the nature of trauma, posttraumatic stress reactions, and the recovery process. This is followed by coping skills training or trauma-focused interventions or both—aspects of treatment that require greater involvement and commitment by the client. Finally, as treatment intensity is decreased, attention is focused on relapse prevention and maintenance of treatment gains.

Active Engagement and Alliance Building

In order for treatment of PTSD to commence, individuals with PTSD must present for care. However, many are reluctant to seek mental health treatment. Those experiencing higher levels of symptoms may be even less likely to seek help and report more barriers to help-seeking.[55] For example, four US combat infantry units were administered an anonymous survey 3 to 4 months after their return from combat duty in Iraq or Afghanistan.[44] Only 38% to 45% of the soldiers whose responses met criteria for a mental health disorder indicated an interest in receiving help, and only 23% to 40% reported having received professional help in the past year. Those screening positive for disorder were twice as likely to report concern about being stigmatized, as well as other barriers to seeking mental health services. In this study, barriers to seeking help included concern about being seen as weak, feelings of embarrassment, and concern about reactions from leadership. For some, another barrier to seeking treatment for PTSD within a Veterans Healthcare Administration (VHA) or Department of Defense (DoD) setting is fear that documentation of PTSD-related problems in the medical record might have an adverse effect on advancement in a military career or later employment in some civilian occupations (eg, police).

Screening programs can increase rates of identification of PTSD and rates of referral.[56] These screenings should occur at multiple points in time, given that soldiers have been found to report more mental health concerns 3 to 6 months following return than in the first month.[57,58] In some screening environments, however, there may be significant disincentives to give positive responses. Factors that may lead to underreporting of early postdeployment distress in military personnel include positive mood at the time of return, misattributions about existing symptomatology, and reluctance to endorse distress because of perceived stigma.[43] Although many who screen positive will not seek care, many individuals may nonetheless ask for help—35% of Iraq war veterans accessed mental health services in the year after returning home.[59]

Relatively little is known about the determinants of help-seeking in those with PTSD. Treatment seeking in Canadian veterans with lifetime PTSD was predicted by cumulative lifetime trauma exposure, traumatic event type, PTSD symptom interference, and comorbid major depressive disorder.[21] Those with comorbid depressive disorder were 3.75 times more likely to have sought treatment than veterans without concurrent depression. Multiple deployments are associated with greater levels of PTSD symptoms,[38] so that soldiers with more than one deployment should be monitored. In research with veterans, the failure of veterans with PTSD to seek VHA mental healthcare was found to be affected by personal obligations that prevented clinic attendance, inconvenient clinic hours, and current receipt of mental health treatment from a non-VHA provider.[60] Another study suggested that veterans' pursuit of mental health services appears to be driven more by their guilt, and the weakening of their religious faith, than by the severity of their PTSD symptoms or their deficits in social functioning.[61]

Outreach interventions can be investigated empirically. In a study of veterans who were service-connected for PTSD but not receiving PTSD treatment, half received an outreach intervention, and the other half were assigned to a control group.[60] The intervention group received a mailing that included a brochure describing VHA PTSD treatment and a letter telling them how to access care. These individuals were also telephoned and encouraged to enroll in treatment. Results indicated that those receiving the intervention were significantly more likely to schedule an intake appointment, attend the intake, and enroll in treatment.

Initial presentation for help does not necessarily result in active involvement in the treatment process. The importance of this issue is highlighted by clinical experience with OIF veterans 1 and 2 years after their return to the United States. In VHA settings, many veterans come to one or two treatment sessions but do not begin active participation in counseling services. In fact, once an individual presents for help, clinicians must take steps to maintain attendance and achieve active engagement in the treatment process. It is important to assess for obstacles to participation and make efforts to ensure that treatment makes sense to these individuals and is perceived as relevant to their needs.

Ongoing Assessment and Monitoring of Treatment Effectiveness

Initial engagement in treatment can be expected to be affected by the assessment process. Assessment provides practitioners with an opportunity to inquire about perceived needs and to describe treatment in terms that make clear its relevance to those needs. This suggests that assessment must include not only attention to symptoms and problems, but also perceived areas of importance to the help-seeker (eg, partner and family conflict, sexual functioning, work functioning and satisfaction, and parenting experiences). The assessment interaction communicates interest in, and understanding of, the individual, as well as expertise on the part of the provider.

Assessment of military-related PTSD requires a multimethod approach in which multiple measures are used to assess different domains of functioning, both to improve diagnostic confidence and to identify multiple targets for intervention.[62] A few key issues can be identified. First, it is important for the provider to gather information about the individual's experiences during deployment. Use of self-report questionnaires, such as the Deployment Risk and Resilience Inventory, can make this process more complete and efficient for provider and patient.[63] Second, findings of high rates of lifetime physical and sexual victimization among veterans in treatment for chronic PTSD support the need for routine assessment of history of trauma exposure.[64] Adverse childhood experiences are strongly associated with mental health symptoms[65] and predict the presence of PTSD and depression among active duty soldiers seeking mental health services.[66] Third, it is important that clinicians engage in ongoing assessment and monitoring of treatment impact. Although this is not currently routine practice in many treatment settings, it is important to help provider and survivor evaluate the effectiveness of their work together, and make changes when necessary. The clinical practice guideline for PTSD, jointly developed by the VHA and the DoD, recommends routine use of validated self-administered checklists (and interviews as appropriate) at intake and to monitor follow-up status (at least every 3 months).[67]

Ongoing Interactive Education

Patient education comprises a basic component of most forms of psychotherapy for PTSD, and should be introduced early and continued throughout all stages of the treatment process. To this end, traumatic stress education classes are often included as part of a first phase of comprehensive treatment programs. Traumatic stress education includes a number of components: (*a*) information about how traumatic experiences can affect individuals; (*b*) information about common reactions to trauma; (*c*) "normalization" of reactions; (*d*) emotional support and reassurance; (*e*) presentation of a rationale for, and description of, what happens in treatment and what the individual will be asked to do; and (*f*) a description of how recovery can happen. Education for the family is also important. Although education alone is unlikely to result in remission of PTSD, it is important to building commitment to treatment participation and helping the survivor more clearly understand the traumatic experience and how to actively participate in treatment.[68]

Coping Skills Training

There is a great difference between knowing what to do versus knowing how to do it. Skills training methods are designed to help individuals learn and practice what to do to cope more effectively with the various kinds of situations that challenge them. Skills training methods are commonly used to help those suffering with PTSD to increase their ability to reduce anxiety, communicate with loved ones, manage anger, and respond assertively (not aggressively) to conflict situations. Through a cycle of instruction, demonstration, rehearsal/practice, feedback/coaching, and more practice, survivors learn skills in treatment sessions and practice them in the natural environment. They keep written records of their attempts to apply the skills, which help them learn and provide practitioner and survivor with real-world experiences to review. Clinical experience indicates that survivors are typically attracted to the idea of learning skills ("tools") for coping. The methods of skills training help to actively involve the survivor in treatment, provide a greater sense of control (and responsibility for active participation in treatment), and strengthen the transfer of what is learned in treatment to the natural environment of the client. For example, stress inoculation training (SIT)[69] focuses on teaching the survivor skills for managing anxiety symptoms, and includes education, muscular relaxation training, breathing retraining (slow abdominal breathing), assertiveness training, covert (imaginal) modeling, role playing, thought stopping, and positive thinking and self-talk. SIT has been found to significantly reduce PTSD symptoms in some treatment research,[70] and is "strongly recommended" in the VA/DoD clinical practice guideline.

Deliberate, Planned Confrontation of Trauma Memories and Reminders

The core element of PTSD treatment is active discussion and exploration of traumatic experiences and their implications. The treatments that focus explicitly on traumatic memories and meanings—prolonged exposure (PE),[71] cognitive therapy (CT), and eye movement desensitization and reprocessing (EMDR)[72]—have received the most empirical support to date, and comprise three of the four "strongly recommended" treatments in the VA/DoD clinical practice guideline.

Methods of therapeutic exposure, such as PE, involve the most direct confrontation of memories and reminders. Imaginal exposure involves a repeated retelling of the trauma story with emotional activation. In vivo exposure adds real-world exposure to stimuli associated with the trauma via confrontation of avoided trauma-related stimuli in the natural environment. These procedures involve multiple repetitions achieved by listening to a cassette recording of the trauma narrative, writing about the experience, or approaching real-world trauma reminders systematically in between-session tasks. A combination of imaginal and in vivo exposure is thought to be more effective than either procedure alone. According to Foa and Jaycox,[73] PE treatment assists the individual to incorporate new information into the memory by reducing cognitive avoidance of trauma-related feelings, demonstrating that remembering the experience is not dangerous and that anxiety will diminish via habituation, fostering discrimination between the trauma and similar nontraumatic situations, strengthening ability to tolerate memories and thereby challenging perceptions of personal incompetence, and reviewing details of the experience that provide evidence against disabling beliefs about danger and incompetence.

Exposure to trauma memories is an element of a number of treatments other than PE that are supported in the research literature. For example, individuals being treated with cognitive processing therapy (CPT)[74] are asked to write out the details of their traumatic experience and to read the account on a regular basis. EMDR includes an exposure component that involves bringing to mind an image of a traumatic event while visually tracking a therapist's finger as it moves back and forth in front of the patient's visual field (or tracking a light moving back and forth, or listening to tones alternating from one ear to the other).

Challenging Negative Trauma-Related Thoughts

CT is a systematic approach that includes education about the role of beliefs in causing distress; identification of distressing beliefs held by the individual; discussion and a review of evidence for and against the beliefs; testing of beliefs; generation of alternative beliefs; and rehearsal of new, more adaptive beliefs. Thoughts that create significant distress (eg, trauma-related guilt, exaggerated thoughts about danger) are replaced with more realistic and self-supportive thoughts. For example, if an individual has the thought "I will never be safe again, the world is a very dangerous place," CT might focus on helping the individual to consider evidence for and against the belief and move toward a more realistic appraisal (eg, "I am safe in most situations and the chances of harm coming to me are quite small in the civilian world"). It is often important that trauma-related guilt be made a formal target of PTSD treatment, and some interventions with a strong CT component, such as CPT[74] and CT for guilt,[75] target guilt explicitly. Instruments designed to assess guilt (eg, Trauma-Related Guilt Inventory[76]) and other trauma-related beliefs (eg, Post-Traumatic Cognitions Inventory[77]) are available.

Negative thoughts can be challenged through direct review of the belief and consideration of alternatives, and through encouraging real-world experiences that can help to disconfirm them. For example, having a successful experience in disclosing personal information to another person can help challenge the belief that "other people cannot be trusted." Successful implementation of PE can also result in modification of distressing trauma-related cognitions by disconfirming beliefs ("anxiety stays forever" or "I will go crazy") and helping the survivor differentiate the trauma from similar but safe events (disconfirming "the world is extremely dangerous"). PTSD symptoms themselves may begin to be associated with mastery rather than incompetence (disconfirming "I am incompetent").

Pharmacotherapy

Medication is an important treatment option that should be considered for almost all patients with significant symptoms of PTSD. The use of a medication in these patients may be directed at PTSD symptoms generally, specific symptoms, common co-occurring symptoms, or comorbid conditions (eg, depression). Initiating a medication trial may occur at different phases in treatment, depending on patient-specific factors. As mentioned earlier, those patients with high levels of symptoms may be the most reluctant to seek psychotherapy care. A medication initiated within the primary care setting may reduce symptoms to a level such that this reluctance can be overcome. However, many military patients may be concerned about the potential side effects of a medication or the stigma of taking a "psych drug" and will need to build trust with their mental health provider before starting a medication can become an option.

Despite the wide use of a variety of medications for the treatment of PTSD, there is a relative lack of definitive evidence for their efficacy.[78] The most thoroughly investigated agents are the selective serotonin reuptake inhibitors (SSRIs). SSRIs have demonstrated superiority over placebo in large randomized controlled trials (RCTs) as well as in a number of smaller investigations, and they are now considered the first-line pharmacological treatment option for PTSD.[79] Sertraline and paroxetine have been subjected to large industry-sponsored trials for the acute treatment of symptoms and have received US Food and Drug Administration approval for treating PTSD.[80–82] Fluoxetine, escitalopram, and citalopram have shown efficacy in smaller randomized or open trials.[83,84] In these trials, SSRIs improved all three clusters of symptoms in PTSD, as well as quality of life and functional impairments. They appear effective in preventing the relapse of symptoms once a patient has responded to treatment.[81,85,86] But the data on SSRIs in the treatment on PTSD in certain populations, including combat veterans, are still limited.[78]

SSRIs have proven effectiveness for many other anxiety and depressive disorders that are highly comorbid with PTSD. PTSD and major depression overlap to a considerable degree; both share sleep disturbances, social withdrawal and isolation, decreased pleasure and enjoyment, and impaired concentration. Major depression is the most common comorbid disorder in patients with PTSD, with close to 50% of PTSD subjects having a history of major depression.[25] Although SSRIs improve both PTSD and depression, SSRIs are efficacious for both PTSD patients with and without depression.[82] Panic disorder and generalized anxiety are also responsive to SSRI treatment and also often co-occur with PTSD.[87]

As with most other disorders treated with antidepressants, a full therapeutic response to SSRIs in PTSD takes 4 to 6 weeks. Although better tolerated than older antidepressants, SSRIs are not without side effects that can include nausea and gastrointestinal distress, insomnia, akathesia, and sexual dysfunction. Many of these side effects are time-limited but still result in relatively high rates of medication discontinuation.[88] Education and support by all members of the treatment team are vital to prevent early discontinuation.

Other antidepressants have less empirical support for the treatment of PTSD than do SSRIs, but available evidence suggests similar efficacy. Therefore, non-SSRI antidepressants should be considered as second-line medication treatment options for PTSD. Antidepressants with RCT data supporting their use in PTSD include venlafaxine,[89] mirtazapine,[90] and nefazodone.[91] Clinically, the choice of an antidepressant is often based on comorbid symptoms and conditions. Venlafaxine, as well as duloxatine, are efficacious in some chronic pain conditions[92] and may be useful in PTSD patients with diabetic neuropathy, fibromyalgia, or certain other pain disorders. Mirtazapine is generally sedating and may be useful in targeting insomnia in PTSD, but weight gain can be a problem. Although the efficacy of bupropion in PTSD is uncertain,[93] it is an option for patients with PTSD who are also attempting to stop smoking.[94] There is limited RCT data to support the efficacy of tricyclic antidepressants and monoamine oxidase inhibitors. Furthermore, their clinical use is limited by their higher rate of side effects, from common dry mouth and constipation to more serious cardiac conduction delays and a lower safety index in overdose. Noradrenergic reuptake inhibiting tricyclic antidepressants, such as nortriptyline, are efficacious for chronic pain conditions[92] and may also be used in PTSD patients with these conditions. Trazodone is widely used at lower dose as a hypnotic in PTSD due to lack of addiction potential.

If antidepressant treatment fails to produce a sufficient treatment response, other psychopharmacological treatment options are available, but with even less empirical support. After antidepressants, the atypical antipsychotics have the most RCT data supporting their efficacy in the treatment of PTSD. Data support their use either as an augmentation therapy to SSRI treatment[95–98] or as a single agent therapy,[99] although not all studies have been positive[100] and the studies conducted to date have been limited in size. In addition to targeting core PTSD symptoms, atypical antipsychotics are often used to treat comorbid psychotic symptoms[96] or as mood stabilizers to treat symptoms related to bipolar disorder or symptoms associated with borderline personality disorder. Another class of mood stabilizers, the third-generation anticonvulsants, had shown promising findings in early clinical case reports and open-label investigations, but small RCT investigations of valproate,[101] topiramate[102] and tiagabine[103] have all failed to demonstrate statistically significant efficacy in PTSD. Therefore, their use should be limited to treating refractory cases or comorbid mood disorders.

Agents targeting noradrenergic neurotransmission have been proposed as possible treatments for PTSD, based in part on the role noradrenergic neurons play in the biological response to stress.[104] Due in part to their ability to decrease central and peripheral noradrenergic activity, the α-2 adrenergic receptor agonists clonidine and guanfacine had been suggested as treatments for PTSD. But RCT investigations of guanfacine have failed to demonstrate efficacy in patients with chronic PTSD.[101,105] Centrally active β-adrenergic receptor antagonists, such as propranolol, may influence how stressful memories are stored[106] and have been efficacious in some,[107] but not all,[108] preliminary studies in preventing the development of PTSD in traumatized individuals. There are also limited data indicating that the α-1 adrenergic agonist prazosin has efficacy in treating nightmares and sleep disturbances in PTSD patients.[109,110] Both propranolol and prazosin are currently under investigation in larger RCT trials.

Benzodiazepines are effective in treating time-limited anxiety, but have significant dependence and abuse potential and are associated with adverse effects, including short-term memory impairment. Small RCTs have failed to demonstrate efficacy for benzodiazepines in the treatment of PTSD[111,112] or in preventing the development of PTSD in trauma survivors.[113] If benzodiazepines are prescribed, they should be used in a time-limited manner and with great caution in patients with PTSD due to the high rates of substance use disorders.[114]

A possible problem with prescription of medications (as with nonpharmacological interventions) is nonadherence to appropriate use. Indeed, many trauma survivors discontinue their medications without discussion with their provider. It can often be important to explore the meaning of medication for the person. When survivors interpret their need for medication as a sign of personal weakness or inability to cope, a judgment of failure in psychotherapy, evidence of the clinician's lack of personal interest, or avoidance of dealing with the "real" problem, they may be less likely to adhere to appropriate use.

In summary, medications, particularly antidepressants, may reduce the overall severity of PTSD symptoms and serve as useful tools in the treatment of PTSD. Psychotropic medications may also be used to treat associated features or comorbid conditions or both. But the practitioner and the patient must be aware that, with the exception of antidepressants, their use is off label. Drug treatments for PTSD should not be used as a routine first-line treatment in preference to a trauma-focused psychological therapy. Individuals with PTSD should be offered a course of trauma-focused cognitive-behavioral therapy or EMDR, regardless of time since trauma.[115] If the PTSD sufferer reports little or no improvement after one of these psychological treatments, an alternative trauma-focused treatment, and then augmentation with pharmacological treatment, can be considered. It is important to consider the least restrictive or intrusive treatment model and choose efficacious treatments.[116] Medications may be warranted, particularly when symptoms are significant and daily functioning is severely impaired, the person has severe insomnia, an additional psychiatric condition (eg, depression) is present, or if significant symptoms are still present following psychological treatment. Polypharmacy can occur in patients with PTSD in the absence of empirical support[117] and should be avoided.

Maintenance and Relapse Prevention

Relatively little is known about rates and processes of relapse after treatment for PTSD. Studies in the civilian sector suggest that improvements resulting from use of evidence-based treatments can be maintained for significant periods of time.[118] Some evidence suggests that patients discharging from residential PTSD treatment and referred for outpatient aftercare are more likely to make an outpatient visit within 1 month of discharge if they receive biweekly telephone calls after discharge.[119] Research also suggests that long-term treatment of PTSD with SSRIs maintains treatment response and quality-of-life improvements, and that discontinuation of SSRI treatment after 12 weeks results in a greater relapse risk, compared with extended treatment.[120]

ASSOCIATED PROBLEMS IN POSTTRAUMATIC STRESS DISORDER TREATMENT

As noted above, approximately 80% of those diagnosed with PTSD experience concurrent additional mental health disorders.[25] They also experience a range of problems in living that are often addressed in treatment. PTSD symptoms are associated with reduced quality of life before treatment. Evidence suggests that positive change in PTSD is significantly associated with positive change in quality of life.[121] Most PTSD outcomes research has focused on reduction of PTSD symptoms; the impact of treatment on the wider range of quality of life and functional outcomes is less well investigated. Successful treatment should be accompanied not only by a reduction in PTSD symptoms but also by an improvement in quality of life.[122] To address the many problems for which those with PTSD seek help, it will often be important to supplement PTSD symptom-focused interventions with adjunctive treatment components targeted at other clinically significant problems identified in the assessment process, especially if these problems do not remit once PTSD-focused interventions have been provided.

Substance Abuse and Addictive Behaviors

Co-occurrence of PTSD and substance abuse (SA) problems is well documented in populations of civilians and veterans.[123,124] For example, Kulka et al[13] reported that 73% of Vietnam veterans with PTSD met criteria for lifetime alcohol abuse or dependence. It is likely that untreated alcohol and drug problems will impede treatment of PTSD; continuing PTSD symptoms may make sobriety more difficult to achieve. Some research suggests that veterans with PTSD who also abuse substances will benefit more from SA treatment if they also address PTSD. Patients who received PTSD treatment in the first 3 months following discharge from SA treatment were more likely to be in remission from substance use disorders at follow-up than those who did not receive PTSD treatment.[123] The interconnectedness of these disorders has generated increased development of integrated PTSD/SA treatments.[125] However, the widespread organization of PTSD and SA care in separate clinics, and the lack of cross-training of professionals in these areas, are among the impediments to delivery of integrated care.

Evidence also suggests that PTSD is associated with increased risk of smoking[26] and that unremitted PTSD is a risk factor for late-onset smoking among individuals who were nonsmokers prior to developing PTSD.[126] In an RCT, McFall et al[127] demonstrated that smoking cessation intervention incorporated into routine mental health care for PTSD is more effective than treatment delivered separately by a specialized smoking-cessation clinic.

Other addictive behaviors may also be associated with PTSD. In civilians seeking treatment for pathological gambling, frequency of PTSD symptoms has been found to predict greater lifetime gambling severity.[128] A study of Australian PTSD treatment-seeking veterans found that the veterans were likely to be problem gamblers, but that PTSD was unrelated to the behavior.[129] However, because all subjects had PTSD, the study was not optimally designed to detect a relationship.

Depression and Suicidality

PTSD is strongly comorbid with depression.[18,23,25,38,130,131] For example, Vietnam veterans with PTSD have higher levels of depression than veterans without PTSD.[13] In retrospective studies, most individuals with both disorders report that PTSD developed first.[25] A 2-year prospective study of the temporal relationship between PTSD and depression symptomatology in Gulf War veterans indicated a bidirectional relationship in which initial PTSD symptoms predicted increases in depression symptoms and initial depression symptoms predicted PTSD, although initial PTSD symptoms were more strongly predictive of later depression.[132] Breslau et al found greatly increased risk for major depression in persons with PTSD,[23] but not in exposed persons without PTSD, suggesting that exposure to traumatic events does not increase the risk for major depression independent of its effects on PTSD.

Presence of PTSD is associated with increased risk of suicide. Sareen et al used data from the nationally representative National Comorbidity Survey to investigate the relationships between anxiety disorders and suicidal ideation and attempts.[133] PTSD was significantly associated with suicidal ideation and suicide attempts; none of the other anxiety disorders showed such an association. Generally, PTSD in US Army veterans is associated with mortality from external causes, including homicide, suicide, drug overdoses, and unintended injury.[134] Clinicians treating PTSD should therefore routinely screen for suicidality and remain alert to the need to monitor suicidal ideation and provide preventive interventions.

Anxiety

PTSD, itself classified as an anxiety disorder, is highly comorbid with other anxiety disorders, including panic disorder, generalized anxiety disorder, social anxiety disorder, obsessive-compulsive disorder, and phobias. Among veterans receiving medical care in primary care clinics, those with PTSD have greater rates of social anxiety disorder (22%) than those without PTSD (1.1%).[135] Development of obsessive-compulsive disorder can be precipitated by trauma in combat.[136] Little research has examined the impact of PTSD treatment on co-occurring anxiety problems, but a treatment for individuals with PTSD who also experience panic attacks has been developed.[137]

Anger and Violence

Anger and irritability comprise one of the symptoms of PTSD. Intense anger is commonly part of the presentation of those with PTSD[138] and is more significant among those whose traumas were experienced during military service.[139] Vietnam veterans with PTSD have higher levels of anger than veterans without PTSD,[13] and high levels of anger have been reported among Iraq and Afghanistan War veterans.[140] Compared to veterans without PTSD, those with it take less time to feel anger, have greater mean heart rate and diastolic blood pressure responses during relived anger, and report greater anger and anxiety during a laboratory task in which they are asked to relive a self-chosen anger memory.[141]

The volatile anger reactions of their patients can present treatment providers with challenges in establishing therapeutic relationships and in delivering treatment itself. In a study of Australian veterans, anger at intake was the most potent predictor of failure to show symptom change.[142] Anger might interfere with the confrontation with, and processing of, traumatic memories that can be important in recovery from the disorder.[71] A high level of anger at the beginning of PE treatment interferes with response to treatment.[143] Anger reduction should often be made an explicit goal of treatment; individuals can be taught skills (eg, time out/cool down, anger self-monitoring, identifying anger situations, relaxation/breathing, anger discrimination, self-talk, assertion training) to reduce their anger or modify its expression.

Anger problems may also require the provider to assist the veteran in reducing risk of violence. Research has indicated that veterans receiving inpatient treatment for PTSD are more violent than male psychiatric inpatients without PTSD and community Vietnam veterans with PTSD not undergoing inpatient treatment.[144] Domestic violence may be an accompanying problem,[145,146] and experiencing PTSD symptoms increases risk for perpetrating intimate partner violence.[147] Moreover, veterans with PTSD often have ready access to weapons and engage in potentially dangerous firearm-related behaviors.[148] Thus, clinicians should routinely address gun storage and safety issues as part of the treatment process.

Complicated or Traumatic Bereavement

Many of those deployed to a war zone will be exposed to significant personal losses, and these deaths will often be encountered in traumatic circumstances. Traumatic bereavement can lead to anhedonia and depression; grief about fallen friends can make social interaction and activity seem pointless. Loss of close comrades and friends in battle is associated with postwar distress and social dysfunction.[149,150] Pivar and Field found that grief-specific symptoms can be distinguished from other war trauma-related symptoms in combat veterans with PTSD. In their sample, veterans' mean scores on grief measures 30 years after their losses were higher than those found in studies of midlife individuals whose spouses had died within the previous 6 months.[151] The authors argued that unresolved grief will endure over time for many individuals if not addressed by clinical intervention. Indeed, treating symptoms of unresolved grief may be as important as treating fear-based symptoms associated with PTSD. Unfortunately, treatment for traumatic or complicated grief has received relatively little formal evaluation. However, most treatments include education about grief, restructuring of cognitive distortions about events, restoration of positive memories of the deceased, acknowledgment of caring feelings toward those lost, retelling the story of the death, and help in tolerating painful feelings.[152] Elements of treatment for PTSD can be adapted for treatment of complicated grief.[153]

Physical Health Problems

PTSD is associated with poorer perceived health status, greater somatic complaints, greater number of chronic health problems, and increased levels of healthcare utilization.[13,18,154–156] Overall, studies suggest that PTSD mediates the relationship between war zone exposure and physical health for both men and women.[155] The majority of veterans seeking PTSD treatment do not engage in preventive health behaviors (eg, exercise and medical screening) at levels consistent with healthcare guidelines.[157] These issues should be assessed and, if necessary, addressed in treatment.

Attention to management of health problems in veterans with PTSD is especially important in light of the "graying" of the veteran population. Veterans with PTSD report greater increases in psychological and physical symptoms during retirement than other veterans.[158] Some research suggests that the challenges of aging may be associated with exacerbation of PTSD symptoms.[159,160] Davison and colleagues, for example, described a phenomenon observed in aging combat veterans that they labeled late-onset stress symptomatology, or "LOSS." For many veterans who experienced highly stressful combat events in early adulthood, and then managed to function successfully throughout their lives without chronic stress-related disorders, the changes of aging are associated with increased combat-related thoughts, memories, and symptoms.[159] The strong relationships between PTSD and health outcomes also extend to OIF returnees.[161] For this latter population, early severity of physical injury is strongly associated with development of later PTSD or depression.[162] Such findings support the need for increasing integration of mental health screening and services in primary care and other medical settings.

Traumatic Brain Injury

The high rate of co-occurring traumatic brain injury (TBI) and PTSD in those returning from deployment to Iraq and Afghanistan poses clinical challenges that are ill understood at present. Evidence suggests that PTSD can develop following both mild and severe TBI, even in individuals who have lost consciousness during the event or display posttraumatic amnesia.[163] In one study of military personnel deployed to Iraq, mild TBI (ie, concussion) was found to be strongly correlated with PTSD and physical health problems 3 to 4 months after return to the United States. The relationship between mild TBI and health was largely mediated by PTSD and depression.[164] Thus, PTSD treatment for those with TBI may need to include modifications that address difficulties that may be associated with injury, including difficulty in retrieving the traumatic memory, comprehending and remembering treatment recommendations, and reporting on symptoms and experience. Bryant et al demonstrated that civilians diagnosed with mild TBI and acute stress disorder could be effectively treated with a brief cognitive-behavioral therapy protocol designed to prevent development of PTSD.[165]

AREAS OF IMPAIRED FUNCTIONING

Family

The anger, emotional numbing, and social withdrawal often associated with PTSD can isolate veterans from their families. PTSD veterans and their partners report more problems in their relationships and more difficulties with intimacy (and have taken more steps toward separation and divorce) than veterans without PTSD and their partners. The degree of relationship distress is correlated with the severity of veterans' PTSD symptoms, particularly symptoms of emotional numbing.[34] Emotional numbing symptoms are also correlated with perceived relationship quality with children.[166] Higher levels of PTSD symptoms (avoidance and emotional numbing symptoms in particular) may lower parent–child relationship satisfaction.[167] Men reporting combat as their worst trauma are more likely to be divorced and physically abusive to their spouses than men reporting other traumas as their worst experience.[168]

Partners of those with PTSD are significantly affected by the symptoms of their loved one and experience burdens associated with care giving.[169] Compared to partners of Dutch peacekeepers without PTSD symptoms, partners of peacekeepers with PTSD symptoms reported more sleep and somatic problems, more negative social support, and poorer marital relationships.[170] PTSD symptomatology places veterans at increased risk for perpetrating relationship aggression against their partners.[171] Such findings suggest that more attention should be paid to supporting partners. Treatment goals should include reduction of problems for the partner and family.

A treatment focus on improvement of family functioning would suggest that steps should be taken to more systematically involve spouses or partners in care.[172,173] Significant others can be included in the assessment process, in the setting of treatment goals, and in treatment itself. Although couples' interventions require systematic development, early work suggests that they can reduce survivors' self-reported levels of anxiety and depression.[174] However, combining family therapy with exposure is not more effective than exposure alone in reducing symptoms of PTSD.[175]

Social Connections

Military-related PTSD is often associated with withdrawal from participation in social activities, limited friendships, and reduced emotional intimacy.[34,176,177] As noted above, some research suggests that veterans with PTSD have greater rates of social anxiety disorder. Poor social support predicts development of PTSD and a more chronic course of the disorder. Veterans with PTSD who are more involved in the community are more likely to show remission in PTSD symptoms than those with less community involvement[7] and adjustment to peacekeeping stressors is significantly related to self-disclosure, especially to supportive significant others.[178] Overcoming problems in social functioning and promoting social participation may require active, sustained intervention. When indicated, improvements in social functioning should be established as a formal treatment goal.

Workplace

Evidence indicates that PTSD impairs work performance and reduces work productivity.[179] Savoca and Rosenheck found that, on average, veterans with a lifetime diagnosis of PTSD were less likely to be currently working than veterans who did not meet diagnostic criteria.[180] Among those who were employed, veterans with PTSD earned less per hour. Veterans with more severe symptoms were more likely to work part-time or not at all. Men reporting combat as their worst trauma are more likely to be unemployed, or fired, compared to men reporting other traumas as their worst experience.[168] It has been suggested that even modest reductions in PTSD symptoms may lead to employment gains, even if the overall symptom levels remain severe.[181]

No interventions to date have targeted the workplace functioning of individuals with PTSD. It would, however, seem useful for clinicians to assist employed patients to apply stress and anger management skills on the job. Patients could also be taught to use problem-solving skills in difficult situations. These strategies would help reduce the impact of traumatic stress reactions on this important domain of patient functioning.

TREATMENT OUTCOME RESEARCH

Reviews of the impact of PTSD interventions have generally concluded that PTSD treatment can be efficacious.[182] In their meta-analysis of PTSD outcome studies, Bradley and colleagues[183] reported that 40% to 70% of trauma survivors included in controlled research trials showed substantial reduction in symptoms or were no longer diagnosable with PTSD posttreatment. To what extent these gains are sustained beyond 6 to 12 months following completion of treatment is relatively unknown. Although there is little empirical support for group-administered treatments at present,[184,185] research suggests that several kinds of individually administered psychological interventions, including exposure-based interventions (eg, PE), EMDR, CPT, and SIT, are effective in reducing PTSD symptomatology.

CPT and PE were compared in treating a sample of chronically distressed rape victims with PTSD.[186] Compared to a group of victims receiving only minimal attention and assessment, both treatments were effective in reducing PTSD and depression symptoms. CPT was superior to PE in reducing some kinds of guilt cognition. Some research has suggested that adding CT to PE appears not to improve PTSD outcomes,[187,188] but findings are mixed.[186,189] It should be noted that although CT and exposure have been separated for research purposes, they are usually combined in clinical practice. For example, PE treatment includes extensive processing of trauma memories that assists in modification of trauma-related cognition. CPT combines repeated writing about the trauma memory with a systematic approach to challenging negative beliefs or meanings associated with the trauma.

The few studies that have compared CT and imaginal (not in vivo) exposure have found no significant differences between the two approaches at the end of treatment.[190] However, a long-term, 5-year follow-up of patients who had taken part in a randomized clinical trial comparing imaginal exposure and CT showed a clear superiority of CT,[191] although there had been no difference at 12 months posttreatment. Those receiving CT showed significantly fewer PTSD symptoms and were less likely to meet criteria for PTSD. Indeed, no patients who received CT were diagnosed with full PTSD, compared to 29% of those who received imaginal exposure. These results cannot be generalized to exposure treatments, however, because imaginal exposure should be combined with in vivo exposure for best effects.

There is little research comparing cognitive-behavioral or other psychological interventions to medications or examining the combination of these approaches for treating PTSD. Individuals with PTSD were randomly assigned by van der Kolk et al to eight sessions of EMDR, 8 weeks of fluoxetine, or placebo. Immediately following treatment, there were no differences among the three groups. At 6-month follow-up, the EMDR group was more likely to show reductions in PTSD symptom severity and remission and depression symptoms than the other two groups.[192] For individuals showing only a partial response to sertraline, PE treatment has been found to further reduce PTSD severity following 10 weeks of medication treatment.[193] More research is needed before recommendations regarding the relative and combined effectiveness of medications and psychosocial interventions can be made with confidence.

Research With Veterans and Active Duty Military Personnel

Several studies have examined various trauma-focused interventions with veterans who have combat-related PTSD. Individually administered imaginal (without in vivo) exposure has been associated with modest but significantly improved PTSD symptom outcomes compared to other treatment as usual.[194–196] Glynn et al found that a combination of imaginal exposure plus cognitive restructuring was more effective than a wait-list control condition.[175] These studies also suggested that in veterans with chronic PTSD, avoidance and emotional numbing symptoms may respond less well to treatment than symptoms of reexperiencing and hyperarousal.

Schnurr et al compared two treatments for male veterans with chronic PTSD: (1) trauma-focused group psychotherapy, and (2) a present-centered comparison treatment that avoided detailed discussion of the military trauma.[197] Weekly group treatment was provided for 30 weeks (followed by 5 monthly "booster" sessions). Follow-up assessments were conducted at the end of treatment (7 months) and at the end of the booster sessions (12 months). A subset of participants was also followed up at 18 and 24 months. Both treatments resulted in modest but significant improvements in PTSD symptoms and other outcomes, but no differences between the two interventions were observed.

In a trial of CPT, significant improvements were reported in PTSD and comorbid symptoms in those receiving CPT compared with a wait-list control group.[198] Forty percent of the intention-to-treat sample receiving CPT did not meet criteria for a PTSD diagnosis at posttreatment, and 50% had a reliable change in their PTSD symptoms.[198] The positive effects of CPT extended beyond PTSD symptoms to include improvements in frequently co-occurring symptoms of depression and general anxiety, affective functioning, guilt, and social adjustment. This trial provides some of the most encouraging results to date related to treatment of male veterans with chronic PTSD.

Positive results have also been obtained with female veterans with chronic PTSD. Schnurr et al compared two types of individually administered cognitive-behavioral therapy—PE and present-centered therapy (a supportive intervention)—for female veterans with PTSD in an RCT. PE treatment was associated with greater reduction of PTSD symptoms, decreased likelihood of meeting PTSD diagnostic criteria, and greater total remission (15.2% vs 6.9%) posttreatment and at follow-up.[199] This study is especially significant in that it demonstrated increased impact of PE when compared with a well-designed alternative treatment, and when delivered by practitioners in the VHA and DoD health care systems.

Studies have also investigated the effectiveness of EMDR as a treatment for veterans with PTSD. A number of studies have produced positive findings with veterans,[200,201] but there is some reason for concern that changes may not be maintained over time. For example, Devilly and colleagues found that Australian veterans treated with EMDR were initially more likely to display reliable posttreatment improvement in trauma symptomatology than those in a control group, but that at 6-month follow-up, reductions in symptomatology were not maintained and there were no differences between groups.[202] A 5-year follow-up evaluation of 13 US combat veterans of the Vietnam War with chronic PTSD who participated in a study of EMDR found that the moderate therapeutic benefits that were obtained immediately were lost at 5-year follow-up. Furthermore, there was an overall worsening of PTSD symptomatology over the 5-year follow-up period in both EMDR-treated subjects and nontreated control subjects.[203]

Some research with veterans has targeted the sleep disturbance associated with PTSD. In a placebo-controlled, blinded study of veterans of multiple conflicts, prazosin was found to be significantly more effective than placebo in reducing trauma nightmares, improving sleep quality, and improving the general clinical condition of the treated patients.[204] Prazosin has also been effective with OIF returnees.[205] In an uncontrolled investigation, Forbes et al offered preliminary evidence for the impact of imagery rehearsal therapy in veterans with PTSD.[206] The treatment reduced nightmare frequency and intensity and overall PTSD, depression, and anxiety symptomatology. Changes were maintained at 12-month follow-up. Some research has suggested that imagery rehearsal therapy can reduce nightmares and improve sleep quality in civilians with PTSD.[207]

In a comprehensive review of PTSD treatment effectiveness, the Institute of Medicine Committee on Treatment of Posttraumatic Stress Disorder applied conservative methodological criteria and found that the research evidence is sufficient to conclude that exposure therapies are efficacious in the treatment of PTSD.[208] The Institute of Medicine found that the evidence for other psychopharmacological treatments and psychosocial interventions is inadequate to reach clear conclusions. It was also judged that the evidence supporting PE was less consistent for veteran populations, especially male veterans with chronic PTSD. Generally, treatment outcomes in veteran samples have been less robust than those obtained with civilian groups.[183] The reasons for this are not well understood, but may include a number of factors. Those who seek treatment at VHA hospitals may have more severe pathology than some civilian samples. Veteran samples have typically been characterized by PTSD that has existed for many years. Veterans seeking care for chronic PTSD may represent a treatment-refractory subgroup of the more general PTSD veteran population. Veterans whose problems were more malleable may have already recovered and thus be underrepresented in the treatment system. The PTSD disorder commonly observed in veterans may also differ in various ways from PTSD among other groups. Or, the compensation system for PTSD may cause some veterans to be reluctant to report symptom improvement.

Posttraumatic Stress Disorder Program Evaluation

Some uncontrolled studies have evaluated individual treatment programs for veterans.[209,210] Johnson et al analyzed the outcome of a 4-month intensive inpatient program for combat-related PTSD among Vietnam veterans.[209,210] Comprehensive measures of PTSD and psychiatric symptoms, as well as social functioning, were assessed at admission, discharge, and 6, 12, and 18 months after discharge from the intervention program. The study showed an increase in symptoms from admission to follow-up, but a decrease in violent actions, thoughts, and legal problems. Family and interpersonal relationships and overall morale were improved at discharge but then returned to pretreatment levels at 18 months.

Johnson et al conducted a long-term follow-up of the program at 18 months and 6 years later because previous studies had shown that program impact on course of illness had been negligible.[211] The sample of 51 veterans showed an extremely high mortality rate of 17% over 6 years. Nearly three-fourths of the sample had experienced an inpatient hospitalization. Self-ratings showed significant improvement in all areas of functioning except employment, and a positive view of the effects of the program. The majority had experienced some improvement in their ability to cope with their chronic illness and decreased their use of violence and substance abuse. Nevertheless, most continued to experience high levels of symptomatology with worsening of hyperarousal symptoms and social isolation.

Bolton et al studied veterans with PTSD who participated in a series of groups focusing on understanding PTSD (education), stress management, and anger management.[212] Although the impact on PTSD symptoms was small, there were moderate impacts on depression and overall life satisfaction, and strong declines in reports of recent violent behavior and improvements in self-reported physical health. Ready et al[185] evaluated a VHA specialized PTSD outpatient program that delivered a three-phase treatment that included group-based exposure therapy. At posttreatment and at 6-month follow-up, veteran patients showed significant reductions in PTSD symptoms.[185]

Findings of evaluations of individual PTSD programs are difficult to generalize to the larger population of treatment programs. However, larger scale evaluations of PTSD treatment are available. Creamer et al reported on the effectiveness of hospital-based programs for Australian veterans with PTSD.[213] These group-based programs deliver a set of cognitive-behavioral interventions, including psychoeducation about PTSD and its treatment; symptom management for anxiety and depression; anger management; interpersonal, problem-solving, and communication skills training; attention to substance abuse, physical health and lifestyle issues; and relapse prevention. Trauma focus work (or direct therapeutic exposure) is delivered in group or individual formats or both. Individual counseling is provided throughout the 12 weeks, in addition to regular medication reviews. Education and support are provided for veterans' partners, often in the form of a weekly group. Overall, individuals in these programs showed significant improvements in core PTSD symptoms, anxiety, depression, alcohol abuse, social dysfunction, and anger. Changes occurred most frequently between admission and 3 months posttreatment, and were maintained at 9 months. Patients and partners reported perceived improvement and strong satisfaction with treatment. Nevertheless, treatment gains were variable and, for most veterans, considerable pathology remained following the program. Creamer et al reported 2-year follow-up outcomes for 1,508 Australian veterans receiving care in the same treatment system. Self-report measures of PTSD,[214] anxiety, depression, anger, alcohol use, and general functioning showed significant improvements at 6 months (with smaller gains continuing through to the 24-month assessment) for PTSD (effect size = 0.8), anxiety (0.5), and depression (0.5). These results suggest that specialized treatment programs for combat-related PTSD can be effective and that improvements are maintained over time.

As noted earlier, existing treatments are often not as effective for veterans as they are for civilian populations with PTSD. Studies of individual programs attest to the difficulty of treating PTSD in veterans whose problems have lasted many years. Veterans themselves report greater satisfaction with participation in specialized PTSD programs than nonspecialized psychiatry programs[215] and high absolute levels of satisfaction.[216] National program evaluation in VHA PTSD residential rehabilitation programs shows significant decreases in PTSD symptoms, alcohol and drug abuse, and violence,[216] but the magnitude of changes in PTSD is modest. Increasingly, PTSD is treated in outpatient settings. Therefore, future research should compare the impact of various forms of intensive outpatient treatment on the full range of outcomes related to traumatization.

TOWARD IMPROVEMENT OF POSTTRAUMATIC STRESS DISORDER SERVICES

Despite the existence of a VHA-DoD clinical practice guideline for PTSD that spells out recommended practices derived from clinical consensus and research findings (available online at www.QMO.amedd.army.mil or www.oqp.med.va.gov/cpg/cpg.htm), there is wide variation in treatment of deployment-related PTSD within VHA[217] and DoD healthcare systems and in the civilian community. Programs vary along many dimensions, including the nature of interventions, intensity of treatment, balance of group or individual therapy, and relative reliance on psychosocial interventions versus medication. This variation reflects the fact that there are many ways of structuring care for PTSD and many treatment options that may in principle be concordant with treatment guidelines. However, variation in treatment practices illustrates the challenge of ensuring that key elements of practice guidelines are implemented in routine care. Central to service improvement is the dissemination of evidence-based treatments.[218] Consistent with reviews of the general PTSD treatment outcome literature, the VA/DoD clinical practice guideline endorses four interventions most strongly: (1) exposure therapy, (2) CT, (3) SIT, and (4) EMDR. In the past, empirically supported treatments for PTSD have not been widely available in most treatment settings, including military mental health settings and the VHA.[219] Some treatments, such as PE, have occasionally been seen as difficult or risky to administer, despite the fact that the evidence does not support the validity of these perceptions.[187,220] In the civilian community, Becker et al found that two major barriers to clinician use of exposure therapy in treatment of PTSD are (1) lack of sufficient training, and (2) concern about the safety of exposure therapy.[221] Findings from research evaluating whether more patients drop out from PE than other treatments for PTSD and whether PE causes symptom worsening have not supported such concerns.[222] Dissemination initiatives are now underway to ensure that PE and CPT are accessible to veterans and active duty personnel with PTSD.

In addition to implementation of evidence-based interventions, another important way to use evidence to enhance treatment delivery is to establish routine monitoring of outcomes in PTSD services. For the individual clinician, it is important to monitor changes in key indicators throughout treatment, to evaluate the impact of intervention, and to inform ongoing redesign of treatment. At the level of the treatment program, outcomes-based program evaluation can assist teams with redesign of services to ensure program improvement over time. Ongoing administration of validated questionnaires as measures of change has not been standard practice in PTSD treatment or in mental health treatment generally. With the use of computerized self-administration of measures, this situation can be expected to change, thereby leading to more rapid improvement of treatment.

In many settings, including the VHA, PTSD treatment is commonly delivered through programs that combine delivery of focal PTSD treatment with other intervention components designed to address concurrent disorders and difficulties.[223] Treatment of PTSD in such programs commonly involves participating in both individual and group activities that includes individual assessment, PTSD education classes, problem-targeted groups (eg, anger management groups, communication skills groups), trauma-focused interventions (eg, PE), case management, and pharmacotherapy. Treatment programs are often delivered in phases, with a beginning, middle, and end of active treatment, followed by lower-intensity maintenance support as needed. Little is known about the best way to organize these structures of care. More research into the types of services that are being provided and the real-world effectiveness of such services is required. Establishment of systematic outcome monitoring of treatment programs can facilitate research and enable comparison of treatment structure.

In fact, there are many treatments for PTSD and co-occurring problems,[224] and new treatments are being developed at an increasing rate. The increasing complexity of the field means that, especially in large-scale treatment systems like the DoD and VHA, it will be important to develop more effective ways to "manage knowledge" within the field of PTSD.[225] It will also be important to help providers upgrade their information, acquire new skills, and learn new interventions, as well as to assist providers and program managers in sharing experiences and learning from one another's efforts.

SUMMARY

Management of deployment-related PTSD has been changing rapidly. Screening for PTSD is widespread, returning personnel are informed about the disorder, and the VHA and DoD have collaborated to establish clinical practice guidelines for responding to the specific needs of those with PTSD. As treatment systems evolve, it is critical that more and better quality evaluation of treatment effectiveness be undertaken. More treatment outcome research is needed, and program evaluative outcomes monitoring, if extended routinely to active duty and veteran treatment systems, can inform all aspects of care and enable more rapid and effective improvement of services. Because PTSD is associated with a wide array of co-occurring disorders and associated problems in living, assessment and program evaluation must be expanded beyond PTSD symptomatology. And because PTSD and other posttraumatic problems affect the whole family, their needs, too, should receive consideration when evaluating and providing services. More systematic monitoring of the effectiveness of PTSD services, along with increasing systemic and public knowledge of PTSD, will inform discussions on disability, fitness for military service, and, most importantly, what constitutes satisfactory support following deployment. As approaches to treatment of deployment-related PTSD continue to develop, the authors anticipate that use of evidence-based practices will increase, routine evaluation of outcomes will become standard practice, and care decisions will become increasingly guided by empirical data.

REFERENCES

1. American Psychiatric Association. *Diagnostic and Statistical Manual of Mental Health Disorders*. 4th-TR ed. Washington, DC: APA; 2005.

2. King D, Leskin G, King L, Weathers FW. Confirmatory factor analysis of the clinician-administered PTSD scale: evidence for the dimensionality of posttraumatic stress disorder. *Psychol Assess*. 1998;10:90–96.

3. McWilliams LA, Cox BJ, Asmundson GJ. Symptom structure of posttraumatic stress disorder in a nationally representative sample. *J Anxiety Disord*. 2005;19(6):626–641.

4. Buckley T, Blanchard E, Hickling E. A prospective examination of delayed onset PTSD secondary to motor vehicle accidents. *J Abnorm Psychol*. 1996;105:617–625.

5. Gray MJ, Bolton EE, Litz BT. A longitudinal analysis of PTSD symptom course: delayed-onset PTSD in Somalia peacekeepers. *J Consult Clin Psychol*. 2004;72(5):909–913.

6. Zeiss RA, Dickman HR. PTSD 40 years later: incidence and person-situation correlates in former POWs. *J Clin Psychol*. 1989;45(1):80–87.

7. Koenen KC, Stellman JM, Stellman SD, Sommer JF Jr. Risk factors for course of posttraumatic stress disorder among Vietnam veterans: a 14-year follow-up of American Legionnaires. *J Consult Clin Psychol*. 2003;71(6):980–986.

8. Bramsen I, Dirkzwager A, van der Ploeg H. Predeployment personality traits and exposure to trauma as predictors of posttraumatic stress symptoms: a prospective study of former peacekeepers. *Am J Psychiatry*. 2000;157:1115–1119.

9. Dohrenwend B, Turner J, Turse N, Adams B, Koenen K, Marshall R. The psychological risks of Vietnam for US veterans: a revisit with new data and methods. *Science*. 2006;313:979–982.

10. Litz BT, Orsillo SM, Friedman M, Ehlich P, Batres A. Posttraumatic stress disorder associated with peacekeeping duty in Somalia for US military personnel. *Am J Psychiatry*. 1997;154(2):178–184.

11. Mehlum L, Weisaeth L. Predictors of posttraumatic stress reactions in Norwegian UN peacekeepers 7 years after service. *J Trauma Stress*. 2002;15(1):17–26.

12. Ramchand R, Karney B, Osilla K, Burns R, Caldarone L. Prevalence of PTSD, depression, and TBI among returning service members. In: Tanielian T, Jaycox LH, eds. *Invisible Wounds of War: Psychological and Cognitive Injuries, Their Consequences, and Services to Assist Recovery*. Santa Monica, Calif: RAND; 2008: 35–85.

13. Kulka RA, Schlenger WE, Fairbank JA, et al. *Trauma and the Vietnam War Generation: Report of the Findings From the National Vietnam Veterans Readjustment Study*. New York, NY: Bruner/Mazel; 1990.

14. Roy-Byrne P, Arguelles L, Vitek ME, et al. Persistence and change of PTSD symptomatology—a longitudinal co-twin control analysis of the Vietnam Era Twin Registry. *Soc Psychiatry Psychiatr Epidemiol*. 2004;39(9):681–685.

15. Schlenger WE, Fairbank JA, Jordan BK. Combat-related posttraumatic stress disorder: prevalence, risk factors and comorbidity. In: Saigh PA, Bremner JD, eds. *Posttraumatic Stress Disorder: A Comprehensive Text*. Boston, Mass: Allyn and Bacon; 1999: 69–91.

16. Stein MB, Walker JR, Hazen AL, Forde DR. Full and partial posttraumatic stress disorder: findings from a community survey. *Am J Psychiatry*. 1997;154(8):1114–1119.

17. Weiss DS, Marmar CR, Schlenger WE, Fairbank JA, Jordan BK, Hough RL. The prevalence of lifetime and partial posttraumatic stress disorder in Vietnam theater veterans. *J Trauma Stress*. 1992;5(3):365–376.

18. Yarvis J, Bordnick P, Spivey C, Pedlar D. Subthreshold PTSD: a comparison of alcohol, depression, and health problems in Canadian peacekeepers with different levels of traumatic stress. *Stress Trauma Crisis*. 2005;8:195–213.

19. Zlotnick C, Franklin CL, Zimmerman M. Does "subthreshold" posttraumatic stress disorder have any clinical relevance? *Compr Psychiatry*. 2002;43(6):413–419.

20. Asmundson G, Stein M, McCreary D. PTSD symptoms influence health status of deployed peacekeepers and nondeployed personnel. *J Nerv Ment Dis*. 2002;180:807–815.

21. Fikretoglu D, Brunet A, Guay S, Pedlar D. Mental health treatment seeking by military members with posttraumatic stress disorder: findings on rates, characteristics, and predictors from a nationally representative Canadian military sample. *Can J Psychiatry*. 2007;52(2):49–55.

22. Ruscio AM, Ruscio J, Keane TM. The latent structure of posttraumatic stress disorder: a taxometric investigation of reactions to extreme stress. *J Abnorm Psychol*. 2002;111(2):290–301.

23. Breslau N, Davis GC, Peterson EL, Schultz LR. A second look at comorbidity in victims of trauma: the posttraumatic stress disorder–major depression connection. *Biol Psychiatry*. 2000;48:902–909.

24. Helzer JE, Robins LN, McEvoy L. Posttraumatic stress disorder in the general population. Findings of the epidemiologic catchment area survey. *N Engl J Med*. 1987;317(26):1630–1634.

25. Kessler RC, Sonnega A, Bromet E, Hughes M, Nelson CB. Posttraumatic stress disorder in the National Comorbidity Survey. *Arch Gen Psychiatry*. 1995;52(12):1048–1060.

26. Beckham J, Kirby A, Feldman M. Prevalence and correlates of heavy smoking in Vietnam veterans with chronic posttraumatic stress disorder. *Addict Behav*. 1997;22:637–647.

27. Beckham JC, Moore SD, Feldman ME, Herzberg MA, Kirby AC, Fairbank JA. Health status, somatization and severity of posttraumatic stress disorder in Vietnam combat veterans with posttraumatic stress disorder. *Am J Psychiatry*. 1998;155:1565–1569.

28. Brown P, Wolfe J. Substance abuse and posttraumatic stress disorder comorbidity. *Drug Alcohol Dependency*. 1994;35:51–59.

29. Clum G, Calhoun K, Kimerling R. Associations among symptoms of depression and posttraumatic stress disorder and self-reported health in sexually assaulted women. *J Nerv Ment Dis*. 2000;188:671–678.

30. Ferrada-Noli M, Asberg M, Ormstad K, Lundin T, Sundbom E. Suicidal behavior after severe trauma, part 1: PTSD diagnoses, psychiatric comorbidity, and assessments of suicidal behavior. *J Trauma Stress*. 1998;11:103–122.

31. Kang HK, Natelson BH, Mahan CM, Lee KY, Murphy FM. Posttraumatic stress disorder and chronic fatigue syndrome-like illness among Gulf War veterans: a population-based survey of 30,000 veterans. *Am J Epidemiol*. 2003;157(2):141–148.

32. Marshall RD, Olfson M, Hellman F, Blanco C, Guardino M, Struening EL. Comorbidity, impairment, and suicidality in subthreshold PTSD. *Am J Psychiatry*. 2001;158(9):1467–1473.

33. Neal LA, Hill N, Hughes J, Middleton A, Busuttil W. Convergent validity of measures of PTSD in an elderly population of former prisoners of war. *Int J Geriatr Psychiatry*. 1995;10:617–622.

34. Riggs DS, Byrne CA, Weathers FW, Litz BT. The quality of the intimate relationships of male Vietnam veterans: problems associated with posttraumatic stress disorder. *J Trauma Stress*. 1998;11(1):87–101.

35. Sharp TJ, Harvey AG. Chronic pain and posttraumatic stress disorder: mutual maintenance? *Clin Psychol Rev*. 2001;21(6):857–877.

36. Wagner AW, Wolfe J, Rotnitsky A, Proctor SP, Erickson DJ. An investigation of the impact of posttraumatic stress disorder on physical health. *J Trauma Stress*. 2000;13(1):41–55.

37. Westerink J, Giarratano L. The impact of posttraumatic stress disorder on partners and children of Australian Vietnam veterans. *Aust N Z J Psychiatry*. 1999;33(6):841–847.

38. Yarvis J, Schiess L. Subthreshold PTSD as a predictor of depression, alcohol use, and health problems in veterans. *J Workplace Behav Hlth*. 2008;23:4.

39. Koenen KC, Stellman SD, Sommer JF Jr, Stellman JM. Persisting posttraumatic stress disorder symptoms and their relationship to functioning in Vietnam veterans: a 14-year follow-up. *J Trauma Stress*. 2008;21(1):49–57.

40. Engdahl B, Dikel TN, Eberly R, Blank A. Posttraumatic stress disorder in a community group of former prisoners of war: a normative response to severe trauma. *Am J Psychiatry*. 1997;154(11):1576–1581.

41. Green BL, Lindy JD, Grace MC, Leonard AC. Chronic posttraumatic stress disorder and diagnostic comorbidity in a disaster sample. *J Nerv Ment Dis*. 1992;180(12):760–766.

42. King DW, King LA, Foy DW, Gudanowski DM. Prewar factors in combat-related posttraumatic stress disorder: structural equation modeling with a national sample of female and male Vietnam veterans. *J Consult Clin Psychol*. 1996;64(3):520–531.

43. Wolfe J, Erickson DJ, Sharkansky EJ, King DW, King LA. Course and predictors of posttraumatic stress disorder among Gulf War veterans: a prospective analysis. *J Consult Clin Psychol*. 1999;67(4):520–528.

44. Hoge CW, Castro CA, Messer SC, McGurk D, Cotting DI, Koffman RL. Combat duty in Iraq and Afghanistan, mental health problems, and barriers to care. *N Engl J Med*. 2004;351(1):13–22.

45. Himmelfarb N, Yaeger D, Mintz J. Posttraumatic stress disorder in female veterans with military and civilian sexual trauma. *J Trauma Stress*. 2006;19(6):837–846.

46. Yaeger D, Himmelfarb N, Cammack A, Mintz J. DSM-IV diagnosed posttraumatic stress disorder in women veterans with and without military sexual trauma. *J Gen Intern Med*. 2006;21(Suppl 3):S65–S69.

47. Fontana A, Rosenheck R. Duty-related and sexual stress in the etiology of PTSD among women veterans who seek treatment. *Psychiatric Serv*. 1998;49:658–662.

48. King LA, King DW, Fairbank JA, Keane TM, Adams GA. Resilience-recovery factors in posttraumatic stress disorder among female and male Vietnam veterans: hardiness, postwar social support, and additional stressful life events. *J Pers Soc Psychol*. 1998;74(2):420–434.

49. Boscarino J. Posttraumatic stress and associated disorders among Vietnam veterans: the significance of combat exposure and social support. *J Trauma Stress*. 1995;8:317–336.

50. Brewin CR, Andrews B, Valentine JD. Meta-analysis of risk factors for posttraumatic stress disorder in trauma-exposed adults. *J Consult Clin Psychol*. 2000;68:748–766.

51. Foa E, Kozak M. Emotional processing of fear: exposure to corrective information. *Psychol Bull*. 1986;99:20–35.

52. Ehlers A, Clark D. A cognitive model of posttraumatic stress disorder. *Behav Res Ther*. 2000;38:319–345.

53. Brewin C, Dalgleish T, Joseph S. A dual representation theory of posttraumatic stress disorder. *Psychol Rev*. 1996;103:670–686.

54. Foa E, Cahill S. Psychological therapies: emotional processing. In: Smelser N, Bates P, eds. *International Encyclopedia of the Social and Behavioral Sciences*. Oxford, UK: Elsevier, 2001; 12363–12369.

55. Maguen S, Litz BT. Predictors of barriers to mental health treatment for Kosovo and Bosnia peacekeepers: a preliminary report. *Mil Med*. 2006;171(5):454–458.

56. Kimerling R, Trafton JA, Nguyen B. Validation of a brief screen for posttraumatic stress disorder with substance use disorder patients. *Addict Behav*. 2006;31(11):2074–2079.

57. Bliese P, Wright K, Adler A. Timing of postcombat mental health assessments. *Psychol Serv*. 2007;4:141–148.

58. Milliken CS, Auchterlonie JL, Hoge CW. Longitudinal assessment of mental health problems among active and reserve component soldiers returning from the Iraq war. *JAMA*. 2007;298(18):2141–2148.

59. Hoge CW, Auchterlonie JL, Milliken CS. Mental health problems, use of mental health services, and attrition from military service after returning from deployment to Iraq or Afghanistan. *JAMA*. 2006;295(9):1023–1032.

60. McFall M, Malte C, Fontana A, Rosenheck RA. Effects of an outreach intervention on use of mental health services by veterans with posttraumatic stress disorder. *Psychiatr Serv*. 2000;51(3):369–374.

61. Fontana A, Rosenheck R. Trauma, change in strength of religious faith, and mental health service use among veterans treated for PTSD. *J Nerv Ment Dis*. 2004;192:579–584.

62. Keane T, Street A, Stafford J. The assessment of military-related PTSD. In: Wilson J, Keane T, eds. *Assessing Psychological Trauma and PTSD*. New York, NY: Guilford Press; 2004: 262–285.

63. King LA, King DW, Vogt DS, Knight J, Samper RE. Deployment Risk and Resilience Inventory: a collection of measures for studying deployment-related experiences of military personnel and veterans. *Mil Psychol*. 2006;18:89–120.

64. Lapp KG, Bosworth HB, Strauss JL, et al. Lifetime sexual and physical victimization among male veterans with combat-related posttraumatic stress disorder. *Mil Med*. 2005;170(9):787–790.

65. Cabrera O, Hoge C, Bliese P. Childhood adversity and combat as predictors of depression and post-traumatic stress in deployed troops. *Am J Prev Med*. 2007;33:77–82.

66. Gahm GA, Lucenko BA. Screening soldiers in outpatient care for mental health concerns. *Mil Med*. 2008;173(1):17–24.

67. Department of Veterans Affairs/Department of Defense (VA/DoD). *Clinical Practice Guideline for the Management of Posttraumatic Stress*. Washington, DC: VA/DoD Clinical Practice Guideline Working Group, Veterans Health Administration, Department of Veterans Affairs and Health Affairs, Department of Defense. 2004.

68. Gray MJ, Elhai JD, Frueh BC. Enhancing patient satisfaction and increasing treatment compliance: patient education as a fundamental component of PTSD treatment. *Psychiatr Q*. 2004;75(4):321–332.

69. Meichenbaum D. *Stress Inoculation Training*. New York, NY: Pergamon; 1985.

70. Foa E, Dancu C, Hembree E. A comparison of exposure therapy, stress inoculation training, and their combination for reducing posttraumatic stress disorder in female assault victims. *J Consult Clin Psychol*. 1999;67:194–200.

71. Foa E, Rothbaum B. *Treating the Trauma of Rape: Cognitive-Behavioral Therapy for PTSD*. New York, NY: Guilford Press; 1998.

72. Shapiro F. *Eye Movement Desensitization and Reprocessing: Basic Principles, Protocols, and Procedures*. New York, NY: Guilford Press; 2001.

73. Foa E, Jaycox L. Cognitive-behavioral theory and treatment of posttraumatic stress disorder. In: Spiegel D, ed. *Efficacy and Cost-Effectiveness of Psychotherapy*. Washington, DC: American Psychiatric Press; 1999: 23–61.

74. Resick PA, Schnicke MK. Cognitive processing therapy for sexual assault victims. *J Consult Clin Psychol*. 1992;60(5):748–756.

75. Kubany ES. Cognitive therapy for trauma-related guilt. In: Follette V, Ruzek JI, Abueg F, eds. *Cognitive-Behavioral Therapies for Trauma*. New York, NY: Guilford Press; 1998: 124–161.

76. Kubany ES, Abueg FR, Kilauano WL, Manke FP, Kaplan AS. Development and validation of the sources of trauma-related guilt survey-war-zone version. *J Trauma Stress*. 1997;10(2):235–258.

77. Foa E, Ehlers A, Clark D. The Post-Traumatic Cognitions Inventory (PTCI): development and validation. *Psychol Assess*. 1999;11:303–314.

78. The Committee on Treatment of Posttraumatic Stress Disorder. *Treatment of Posttraumatic Stress Disorder: An Assessment of the Evidence*. Washington, DC: Institute of Medicine; 2007.

79. Ballenger JC, Davidson JR, Lecrubier Y, et al. Consensus statement update on posttraumatic stress disorder from the international consensus group on depression and anxiety. *J Clin Psychiatry*. 2004;65(Suppl 1):55–62.

80. Brady K, Pearlstein T, Asnis G, et al. Efficacy and safety of sertraline treatment of posttraumatic stress disorder: a randomized controlled trial. *JAMA*. 2000;283:1837–1844.

81. Davidson J, Pearlstein T, Londborg P, et al. Efficacy of sertraline in preventing relapse of posttraumatic stress disorder: results of a 28-week double-blind, placebo-controlled study. *Am J Psychol*. 2001;158:1974–1981.

82. Stein DJ, Davidson J, Seedat S, Beebe K. Paroxetine in the treatment of posttraumatic stress disorder: pooled analysis of placebo-controlled studies. *Expert Opin Pharmacother*. 2003;4(10):1829–1838.

83. Robert S, Hamner MB, Ulmer HG, Lorberbaum JP, Durkalski VL. Open-label trial of escitalopram in the treatment of posttraumatic stress disorder. *J Clin Psychiatry*. 2006;67(10):1522–1526.

84. Seedat S, Stein DJ, Emsley RA. Open trial of citalopram in adults with posttraumatic stress disorder. *Int J Neuropsychopharmacol*. 2000;3(2):135–140.

85. Martenyi F, Brown EB, Zhang H, Koke SC, Prakash A. Fluoxetine versus placebo in prevention of relapse in post-traumatic stress disorder. *Br J Psychiatry*. 2002;181:315–320.

86. Martenyi F, Brown EB, Zhang H, Prakash A, Koke SC. Fluoxetine versus placebo in posttraumatic stress disorder. *J Clin Psychiatry*. 2002;63(3):199–206.

87. Stein MB, McQuaid JR, Pedrelli P, Lenox R, McCahill ME. Posttraumatic stress disorder in the primary care medical setting. *Gen Hosp Psychiatry*. 2000;22(4):261–269.

88. Mullins CD, Shaya FT, Meng F, Wang J, Harrison D. Persistence, switching, and discontinuation rates among patients receiving sertraline, paroxetine, and citalopram. *Pharmacother*. 2005;25(5):660–667.

89. Davidson J, Rothbaum B, Tucker P, Asnis G, Benattia I, Musgnung J. Venlafaxine extended release in posttraumatic stress disorder: a sertraline- and placebo-controlled study. *J Clin Psychopharmacol*. 2006;26:259–267.

90. Davidson J, Weisler R, Butterfield M, et al. Mirtazapine vs placebo in posttraumatic stress disorder: a pilot trial. *Biol Psychiatry*. 2003;53:188–191.

91. Davis LL, Jewell ME, Ambrose S, et al. A placebo-controlled study of nefazodone for the treatment of chronic posttraumatic stress disorder: a preliminary study. *J Clin Psychopharmacol*. 2004;24(3):291–297.

92. Briley M. Clinical experience with dual action antidepressants in different chronic pain syndromes. *Hum Psychopharmacol*. 2004;19(Suppl 1):S21–S25.

93. Becker M, Hertzberg M, Moore S, Dennis M, Bukenya D, Beckham J. A placebo-controlled trial of bupropion SR in the treatment of chronic posttraumatic stress disorder. *J Clin Psychopharmacol*. 2007;27:193–197.

94. Hertzberg MA, Moore SD, Feldman ME, Beckham JC. A preliminary study of bupropion sustained-release for smoking cessation in patients with chronic posttraumatic stress disorder. *J Clin Psychopharmacol*. 2001;21(1):94–98.

95. Bartzokis G, Lu PH, Turner J, Mintz J, Saunders CS. Adjunctive risperidone in the treatment of chronic combat-related posttraumatic stress disorder. *Biol Psychiatry*. 2005;57:474–479.

96. Hamner MB, Faldowski RA, Ulmer HG, Frueh BC, Huber MG, Arana GW. Adjunctive risperidone treatment in posttraumatic stress disorder: a preliminary controlled trial of effects on comorbid psychotic symptoms. *Int Clin Psychopharmacol*. 2003;18(1):1–8.

97. Monnelly EP, Ciraulo DA, Knapp C, Keane T. Low-dose risperidone as adjunctive therapy for irritable aggression in posttraumatic stress disorder. *J Clin Psychopharmacol*. 2003;23(2):193–196.

98. Padala PR, Madison J, Monnahan M, et al. Risperidone monotherapy for posttraumatic stress disorder related to sexual assault and domestic abuse in women. *Int Clin Psychopharmacol*. 2006;21(5):275–280.

99. Stein MB, Kline NA, Matloff JL. Adjunctive olanzapine for SSRI-resistant combat-related PTSD: a double-blind, placebo-controlled study. *Am J Psychiatry*. 2002;159(10):1777–1779.

100. Rothbaum BO, Killeen TK, Davidson JR, Brady KT, Connor KM, Heekin MH. Placebo-controlled trial of risperidone augmentation for selective serotonin reuptake inhibitor-resistant civilian posttraumatic stress disorder. *J Clin Psychiatry*. 2008;69(4):520–525.

101. Davis LL, Ward C, Rasmusson A, Newell JM, Frazier E, Southwick SM. A placebo-controlled trial of guanfacine for the treatment of posttraumatic stress disorder in veterans. *Psychopharmacol Bull*. 2008;41:8–18.

102. Lindley SE, Carlson EB, Hill K. A randomized, double-blind, placebo-controlled trial of augmentation topiramate for chronic combat-related posttraumatic stress disorder. *J Clin Psychopharmacol*. 2007;27(6):677–681.

103. Davidson J, Brady K, Mellman T, Stein M, Pollack M. The efficacy and tolerability of tiagabine in adult patients with posttraumatic stress disorder. *J Clin Psychopharmacol*. 2007;27:85–88.

104. Southwick SM, Bremner JD, Rasmusson A, Morgan CA 3rd, Arnsten A, Charney DS. Role of norepinephrine in the pathophysiology and treatment of posttraumatic stress disorder. *Biol Psychiatry*. 1999;46(9):1192–1204.

105. Neylan TC, Lenoci M, Samuelson KW, et al. No improvement of posttraumatic stress disorder symptoms with guanfacine treatment. *Am J Psychiatry*. 2006;163(12):2186–2188.

106. Reist C, Duffy JG, Fujimoto K, Cahill L. β-Adrenergic blockade and emotional memory in PTSD. *Int J Neuropsychopharmacol*. 2001;4(4):377–383.

107. Pitman RK, Sanders KM, Zusman RM, et al. Pilot study of secondary prevention of posttraumatic stress disorder with propranolol. *Biol Psychiatry*. 2002;51(2):189–192.

108. Stein MB, Kerridge C, Dimsdale JE, Hoyt DB. Pharmacotherapy to prevent PTSD: results from a randomized controlled proof-of-concept trial in physically injured patients. *J Trauma Stress*. 2007;20(6):923–932.

109. Raskind MA, Peskind ER, Hoff DJ, et al. A parallel group placebo controlled study of prazosin for trauma nightmares and sleep disturbance in combat veterans with posttraumatic stress disorder. *Biol Psychiatry*. 2007;61(8):928–934.

110. Raskind MA, Peskind ER, Kanter ED, et al. Reduction of nightmares and other PTSD symptoms in combat veterans by prazosin: a placebo-controlled study. *Am J Psychiatry*. 2003;160(2):371–373.

111. Braun P, Greenberg D, Dasberg H, Lerer B. Core symptoms of posttraumatic stress disorder unimproved by alprazolam treatment. *J Clin Psychiatry*. 1990;51:236–238.

112. Cates M, Bishop M, Davis L, Lowe J, Woolley T. Clonazepam for treatment of sleep disturbances associated with combat-related posttraumatic stress disorder. *Ann Pharmacother*. 2004;38:1395–1399.

113. Gelpin E, Bonne O, Peri T, Brandes D, Shalev AY. Treatment of recent trauma survivors with benzodiazepines: a prospective study. *J Clin Psychiatry*. 1996;57(9):390–394.

114. Hermos JA, Young MM, Lawler EV, Rosenbloom D, Fiore LD. Long-term, high-dose benzodiazepine prescriptions in veteran patients with PTSD: influence of preexisting alcoholism and drug-abuse diagnoses. *J Trauma Stress*. 2007;20(5):909–914.

115. Bisson J. Pharmacological treatment of posttraumatic stress disorder. *Adv Psychiatr Treatment*. 2007;13:119–126.

116. NICE: National Institute for Health and Clinical Excellence Report. Birmingham, UK: National Institute for Health and Clinical Excellence, 2005. Available at: http://www.nice.org.uk/nicemedia/pdf/CG026NICEguideline.pdf. Accessed February 18, 2009.

117. Mellman TA, Clark RE, Peacock WJ. Prescribing patterns for patients with posttraumatic stress disorder. *Psychiatr Serv*. 2003;54(12):1618–1621.

118. Resick PA, Williams L, Orazem R, Gutner C. Can we cure PTSD? Five-year follow-up of a clinical trial comparing cognitive processing therapy and prolonged exposure. Paper presented at: The Association for Behavioral and Cognitive Therapies; 2005; Washington, DC.

119. Rosen CS, DiLandro C, Corwin KN, Drescher KD, Cooney JH, Gusman F. Telephone monitoring and support for veterans with chronic posttraumatic stress disorder: a pilot study. *Community Ment Health J*. 2006;42(5):501–508.

120. Davis LL, Frazier EC, Williford RB, Newell JM. Long-term pharmacotherapy for posttraumatic stress disorder. *CNS Drugs*. 2006;20(6):465–476.

121. Schnurr PP, Hayes AF, Lunney CA, McFall M, Uddo M. Longitudinal analysis of the relationship between symptoms and quality of life in veterans treated for posttraumatic stress disorder. *J Consult Clin Psychol*. 2006;74(4):707–713.

122. Gladis MM, Gosch EA, Dishuk NM, Crits-Christoph P. Quality of life: expanding the scope of clinical significance. *J Consult Clin Psychol*. 1999;67(3):320–331.

123. Ouimette P, Moos RH, Finney JW. PTSD treatment and 5-year remission among patients with substance use and posttraumatic stress disorders. *J Consult Clin Psychol*. 2003;71(2):410–414.

124. Ruzek JI. Concurrent posttraumatic stress disorder and substance use disorder among veterans: evidence and treatment issues. In: Ouimette P, Brown P, eds. *Trauma and Substance Abuse: Causes, Consequences, and Treatment of Comorbid Disorders*. Washington, DC: American Psychological Association; 2002: 191–207.

125. Najavits LM. *Seeking Safety: A Treatment Manual for PTSD and Substance Abuse*. New York, NY: Guilford Press; 2002.

126. Koenen KC, Hitsman B, Lyons MJ, et al. Posttraumatic stress disorder and late-onset smoking in the Vietnam era twin registry. *J Consult Clin Psychol*. 2006;74(1):186–190.

127. McFall M, Saxon AJ, Thompson CE, et al. Improving the rates of quitting smoking for veterans with posttraumatic stress disorder. *Am J Psychiatry*. 2005;162(7):1311–1319.

128. Ledgerwood DM, Petry NM. Posttraumatic stress disorder symptoms in treatment-seeking pathological gamblers. *J Trauma Stress*. 2006;19(3):411–416.

129. Biddle D, Hawthorne G, Forbes D, Coman G. Problem gambling in Australian PTSD treatment-seeking veterans. *J Trauma Stress*. 2005;18:759–767.

130. Blanchard E, Buckley T, Hickling E, Taylor A. Posttraumatic stress disorder and comorbid depression: is the correlation an illusion? *J Anxiety Dis*. 1998;12:21–37.

131. Shalev AY, Freedman S, Peri T, et al. Prospective study of posttraumatic stress disorder and depression following trauma. *Am J Psychiatry*. 1998;155(5):630–637.

132. Erickson D, Wolfe J, King DW, King LA, Sharkansky EJ. Posttraumatic stress disorder and depression symptomatology in a sample of Gulf War veterans: a prospective analysis. *J Consult Clin Psychol*. 2001;69:41–49.

133. Sareen J, Houlahan T, Cox BJ, Asmundson GJ. Anxiety disorders associated with suicidal ideation and suicide attempts in the National Comorbidity Survey. *J Nerv Ment Dis*. 2005;193(7):450–454.

134. Boscarino J. External-cause mortality after psychologic trauma: the effects of stress exposure and predisposition. *Compr Psychiatry*. 2006;47:503–514.

135. Kashdan TB, Frueh BC, Knapp RG, Hebert R, Magruder KM. Social anxiety disorder in Veterans Affairs primary care clinics. *Behav Res Ther*. 2006;44(2):233–247.

136. Sasson Y, Dekel S, Nacasch N, et al. Posttraumatic obsessive-compulsive disorder: a case series. *Psychiatry Res*. 2005;135(2):145–152.

137. Falsetti S, Davis J. Multiple channel exposure therapy: combining cognitive-behavioral therapies for the treatment of posttraumatic stress disorder with panic attacks. *Behav Modif*. 2005;29:70–94.

138. Novaco RW, Chemtob CM. Anger and combat-related posttraumatic stress disorder. *J Trauma Stress*. 2002;15(2):123–132.

139. Orth U, Wieland E. Anger, hostility, and posttraumatic stress disorder in trauma-exposed adults: a meta-analysis. *J Consult Clin Psychol*. 2006;74(4):698–706.

140. Jakupcak M, Conybeare D, Phelps L, et al. Anger, hostility, and aggression among Iraq and Afghanistan war veterans reporting PTSD and subthreshold PTSD. *J Trauma Stress*. 2007;20(6):945–954.

141. Beckham J, Vrana S, Barefoot J, Feldman M, Fairbank J, Moore S. Magnitude and duration of cardiovascular response to anger in Vietnam veterans with and without posttraumatic stress disorder. *J Consult Clin Psychol*. 2002;70:228–234.

142. Forbes D, Creamer M, Hawthorne G. Comorbidity as a predictor of symptom change after treatment in combat-related posttraumatic stress disorder. *J Nerv Ment Dis*. 2003;191:93–99.

143. Foa E, Riggs D, Massie E, Yarczower M. The impact of fear activation and anger on the efficacy of exposure treatment for posttraumatic stress disorder. *Behav Ther*. 1995;26:487–499.

144. McFall M, Fontana A, Raskind M, Rosenheck R. Analysis of violent behavior in Vietnam combat veteran psychiatric inpatients with posttraumatic stress disorder. *J Trauma Stress*. 1999;12(3):501–517.

145. Sherman MD, Sautter F, Jackson MH, Lyons JA, Han X. Domestic violence in veterans with posttraumatic stress disorder who seek couples therapy. *J Marital Fam Ther*. 2006;32(4):479–490.

146. Taft CT, Pless AP, Stalans LJ, Koenen KC, King LA, King DW. Risk factors for partner violence among a national sample of combat veterans. *J Consult Clin Psychol*. 2005;73(1):151–159.

147. Orcutt HK, King LA, King DW. Male-perpetrated violence among Vietnam veteran couples: relationships with veteran's early life characteristics, trauma history, and PTSD symptomatology. *J Trauma Stress*. 2003;16(4):381–390.

148. Freeman T, Roca V, Kimbrell T. A survey of gun collection and use among three groups of veteran patients admitted to Veterans Affairs hospital treatment programs. *South Med J*. 2003;96:240–243.

149. Holman EA, Silver RC. Getting "stuck" in the past: temporal orientation and coping with trauma. *J Pers Soc Psychol*. 1998;74(5):1146–1163.

150. Neria Y. Coping with tangible and intangible traumatic losses in prisoners of war. *Isr J Psychiatry Relat Sci*. 2001;38(3–4):216–225.

151. Pivar IL, Field NP. Unresolved grief in combat veterans with PTSD. *J Anxiety Disord*. 2004;18(6):745–755.

152. Shear K, Frank E. Treatment of complicated grief: integrating cognitive-behavioral methods with other treatment approaches. In: Follette V, Ruzek JI, eds. *Cognitive-Behavioral Therapies for Trauma*. 2nd ed. New York, NY: Guilford Press; 2006: 290–320.

153. Ehlers A. Understanding and treating complicated grief: what can we learn from posttraumatic stress disorder? *Clin Psychol Sci Pract*. 2006;13:135–140.

154. Richardson JD, Elhai JD, Pedlar DJ. Association of PTSD and depression with medical and specialist care utilization in modern peacekeeping veterans in Canada with health-related disabilities. *J Clin Psychiatry*. 2006;67(8):1240–1245.

155. Schnurr PP, Green BL. Understanding relationships among trauma, posttraumatic stress disorder, and health outcomes. *Adv Mind-Body Med*. 2004;20:18–29.

156. Stapleton JA, Asmundson GJ, Woods M, Taylor S, Stein MB. Health care utilization by United Nations peacekeeping veterans with co-occurring, self-reported, posttraumatic stress disorder and depression symptoms versus those without. *Mil Med*. 2006;171(6):562–566.

157. Buckley TC, Mozley SL, Bedard MA, Dewulf AC, Greif J. Preventive health behaviors, health-risk behaviors, physical morbidity, and health-related role functioning impairment in veterans with posttraumatic stress disorder. *Mil Med*. 2004;169:536–540.

158. Schnurr PP, Lunney CA, Sengupta A, Spiro A III. A longitudinal study of retirement in older male veterans. *J Consult Clin Psychol*. 2005;73(3):561–566.

159. Davison E, Pless A, Gugliucci M, et al. Late-life emergence of early life trauma: the phenomenon of late-onset stress symptomatology among aging combat veterans. *Res Aging*. 2006(28):84–114.

160. Solomon Z, Mikulincer M. Trajectories of PTSD: a 20-year longitudinal study. *Am J Psychiatry*. 2006;163(4):659–666.

161. Hoge CW, Terhakopian A, Castro CA, Messer SC, Engel CC. Association of posttraumatic stress disorder with somatic symptoms, health care visits, and absenteeism among Iraq war veterans. *Am J Psychiatry*. 2007;164(1):150–153.

162. Grieger TA, Cozza SJ, Ursano RJ, et al. Posttraumatic stress disorder and depression in battle-injured soldiers. *Am J Psychiatry*. 2006;163(10):1777–1783.

163. McMillan TM, Williams WH, Bryant R. Posttraumatic stress disorder and traumatic brain injury: a review of causal mechanisms, assessment, and treatment. *Neuropsychol Rehab*. 2003;13:149–164.

164. Hoge CW, McGurk D, Thomas JL, Cox AL, Engel CC, Castro CA. Mild traumatic brain injury in US soldiers returning from Iraq. *N Engl J Med*. 2008;358(5):453–463.

165. Bryant R, Moulds M, Guthrie R. Treating acute stress disorder following mild traumatic brain injury. *Am J Psychiatry*. 2003;160:585–587.

166. Ruscio AM, Weathers FW, King LA, King DW. Male war-zone veterans' perceived relationships with their children: the importance of emotional numbing. *J Trauma Stress*. 2002;15(5):351–357.

167. Samper RE, Taft CT, King DW, King LA. Posttraumatic stress disorder symptoms and parenting satisfaction among a national sample of male Vietnam veterans. *J Trauma Stress*. 2004;17(4):311–315.

168. Prigerson HG, Maciejewski PK, Rosenheck RA. Combat trauma: trauma with highest risk of delayed onset and unresolved posttraumatic stress disorder symptoms, unemployment, and abuse among men. *J Nerv Ment Dis*. 2001;189(2):99–108.

169. Calhoun P, Beckham J, Bosworth H. Caregiver burden and psychological distress in partners of veterans with chronic posttraumatic stress disorder. *J Trauma Stress*. 2002;15:205–212.

170. Dirkzwager A, Bramsen I, Adèr H. Secondary traumatization in partners and parents of Dutch peacekeeping soldiers. *J Fam Psychol*. 2005;19:217–226.

171. Byrne C, Riggs D. The cycle of trauma: relationship aggression in male Vietnam veterans with symptoms of posttraumatic stress disorder. *Violence Vict*. 1996;11:213–225.

172. Devilly GJ. The psychological effects of a lifestyle management course on war veterans and their spouses. *J Clin Psychol*. 2002;58:1119–1134.

173. Sautter F, Lyons JA, Manguno-Mire G, et al. Predictors of partner engagement in PTSD treatment. *J Psychopathol Behav Assess*. 2006;28:123–130.

174. Monson CM, Schnurr PP, Stevens SP, Guthrie KA. Cognitive-behavioral couple's treatment for posttraumatic stress disorder: initial findings. *J Trauma Stress*. 2004;17(4):341–344.

175. Glynn SM, Eth S, Randolph ET, et al. A test of behavioral family therapy to augment exposure for combat-related posttraumatic stress disorder. *J Consult Clin Psychol*. 1999;67(2):243–251.

176. Frueh BC, Turner SM, Beidel DC, Cahill S. Assessment of social functioning in combat veterans with PTSD. *Aggression Violent Behav*. 2001;6:79–90.

177. Jordan BK, Marmar CR, Fairbank JA, et al. Problems in families of male Vietnam veterans with posttraumatic stress disorder. *J Consult Clin Psychol*. 1992;60(6):916–926.

178. Bolton E, Glenn D, Orsillo S, Roemer L, Litz B. The relationship between self-disclosure and symptoms of posttraumatic stress disorder in peacekeepers deployed to Somalia. *J Trauma Stress*. 2003;10:203–210.

179. Kessler RC, Frank RG. The impact of psychiatric disorders on work loss days. *Psychol Med*. 1997;27(4):861–873.

180. Savoca E, Rosenheck R. The civilian labor market experiences of Vietnam-era veterans: the influence of psychiatric disorders. *J Ment Health Policy Econ*. 2000;3(4):199–207.

181. Smith MW, Schnurr PP, Rosenheck RA. Employment outcomes and PTSD symptom severity. *Ment Health Serv Res*. 2005;7(2):89–101.

182. Foa E, Keane T, Friedman M, Cohen J. *Effective Treatments for PTSD. Practice Guidelines From the International Society for Traumatic Stress Studies.* 2nd ed. New York, NY: Guilford Press; 2008.

183. Bradley R, Greene J, Russ E, Dutra L, Western D. A multidimensional meta-analysis of psychotherapy for PTSD. *Am J Psychiatry*. 2005;162:214–227.

184. Foy D, Glynn S, Schnurr P, et al. Group therapy. In: Foa E, Keane T, Friedman M, Cohen J, eds. *Effective Treatments for PTSD: Practice Guidelines From the International Society for Traumatic Stress Studies.* New York, NY: Guilford Press; 2000: 155–175.

185. Ready DJ, Thomas KR, Worley V, et al. A field test of group based exposure therapy with 102 veterans with war-related posttraumatic stress disorder. *J Trauma Stress*. 2008;21(2):150–157.

186. Resick PA, Nishith P, Weaver TL, Astin MC, Feuer CA. A comparison of cognitive-processing therapy with prolonged exposure and a waiting condition for the treatment of chronic posttraumatic stress disorder in female rape victims. *J Consult Clin Psychol*. 2002;70(4):867–879.

187. Foa EB, Zoellner LA, Feeny NC, Hembree EA, Alvarez-Conrad J. Does imaginal exposure exacerbate PTSD symptoms? *J Consult Clin Psychol*. 2002;70:1022–1028.

188. Paunovic N, Ost LG. Cognitive-behavior therapy vs exposure therapy in the treatment of PTSD in refugees. *Behav Res Ther*. 2001;39(10):1183–1197.

189. Bryant R, Moulds M, Guthrie R. Imaginal exposure alone and imaginal exposure with cognitive restructuring in treatment of posttraumatic stress disorder. *J Consult Clin Psychol*. 2003;71:706–712.

190. Tarrier N, Pilgrim H, Sommerfield C, et al. A randomized trial of cognitive therapy and imaginal exposure in the treatment of chronic posttraumatic stress disorder. *J Consult Clin Psychol*. 1999;67(1):13–18.

191. Tarrier N, Sommerfield C. Treatment of chronic PTSD by cognitive therapy and exposure: 5-year follow-up. *Behav Ther*. 2004;35:231–246.

192. van der Kolk BA, Spinazzola J, Blaustein ME, et al. A randomized clinical trial of eye movement desensitization and reprocessing (EMDR), fluoxetine, and pill placebo in the treatment of posttraumatic stress disorder: treatment effects and long-term maintenance. *J Clin Psychiatry*. 2007;68(1):37–46.

193. Rothbaum BO, Cahill SP, Foa EB, et al. Augmentation of sertraline with prolonged exposure in the treatment of posttraumatic stress disorder. *J Trauma Stress*. 2006;19(5):625–638.

194. Boudewyns P, Hyer L, Woods M, Harrison W, McCranie E. PTSD among Vietnam veterans: an early look at treatment outcome using direct therapeutic exposure. *J Trauma Stress*. 1990;3:359–368.

195. Cooper N, Clum G. Imaginal flooding as a supplementary treatment for PTSD in combat veterans: a controlled study. *Behav Ther*. 1989;20:381–391.

196. Keane T, Fairbank JA, Caddell J, Zimering R. Implosive (flooding) therapy reduces symptoms of PTSD in Vietnam combat veterans. *Behav Ther*. 1989;20:245–260.

197. Schnurr PP, Friedman MJ, Foy DW, et al. Randomized trial of trauma-focused group therapy for posttraumatic stress disorder: results from a Department of Veterans Affairs cooperative study. *Arch Gen Psychiatry*. 2003;60(5):481–489.

198. Monson CM, Schnurr PP, Resick PA, Friedman MJ, Young-Xu Y, Stevens SP. Cognitive processing therapy for veterans with military-related posttraumatic stress disorder. *J Consult Clin Psychol*. 2006;74(5):898–907.

199. Schnurr PP, Friedman MJ, Engel CC, et al. Cognitive behavioral therapy for posttraumatic stress disorder in women: a randomized controlled trial. *JAMA*. 2007;297(8):820–830.

200. Boudewyns P, Hyer L. Eye movement desensitization and reprocessing (EMDR) as a treatment for posttraumatic stress disorder. *Clin Psychol Psychother*. 1996;3:185–195.

201. Carlson JG, Chemtob CM, Rusnack K, Hedlund NL, Muraoka MY. Eye movement desensitization and reprocessing (EDMR) treatment for combat-related posttraumatic stress disorder. *J Trauma Stress*. 1998;11:3–24.

202. Devilly G, Spence S, Rapee R. Statistical and reliable change with eye movement desensitization and reprocessing: treating trauma within a veteran population. *Behav Ther*. 1998;29:435–455.

203. Macklin ML, Metzger LJ, Lasko NB, Berry NJ, Orr SP, Pitman RK. Five-year follow-up study of eye movement desensitization and reprocessing therapy for combat-related posttraumatic stress disorder. *Compr Psychiatry*. 2000;41(1):24–27.

204. Raskind MA, Peskind ER, Kanter ED, et al. *Prazosin for Treating Noncombat Trauma Post-Traumatic Stress Disorder*. Bethesda, Md: National Institute of Mental Health; 2007. Clinical Trial #NCT00183430.

205. Daly C, Doyle M, Raskind M, Raskind E, Daniels C. Clinical case series: the use of prazosin for combat-related recurrent nightmares among Operation Iraqi Freedom combat veterans. *Mil Med*. 2005;170:513–515.

206. Forbes D, Phelps A, McHugh A, Debenham P, Hopwood M, Creamer M. Imagery rehearsal in the treatment of posttraumatic nightmares in Australian veterans with chronic combat-related PTSD: 12-month follow-up data. *J Trauma Stress*. 2003;16:509–513.

207. Krakow B, Hollifield M, Schrader R, et al. A controlled study of imagery rehearsal for chronic nightmares in sexual assault survivors with PTSD: a preliminary report. *J Trauma Stress*. 2000;13(4):589–609.

208. Institute of Medicine Committee on Treatment of Posttraumatic Stress Disorder. *Treatment of Posttraumatic Stress Disorder: An Assessment of the Evidence*. Washington, DC: The National Academies Press; 2008.

209. Frueh BC, Turner SM, Beidel DC, Mirabella RF, Jones WJ. Trauma management therapy: a preliminary evaluation of a multicomponent behavioral treatment for chronic combat-related PTSD. *Behav Res Ther*. 1996;34(7):533–543.

210. Johnson DR, Rosenheck R, Fontana A, Lubin H, Charney D, Southwick S. Outcome of intensive inpatient treatment for combat-related posttraumatic stress disorder. *Am J Psychiatry*. 1996;153(6):771–777.

211. Johnson DR, Fontana A, Lubin H, Corn B, Rosenheck R. Long-term course of treatment-seeking Vietnam veterans with posttraumatic stress disorder: mortality, clinical condition, and life satisfaction. *J Nerv Ment Dis*. 2004;192(1):35–41.

212. Bolton EE, Lambert JF, Wolf EJ, Raja S, Varra AA, Fisher LM. Evaluating a cognitive-behavioral group treatment program for veterans with posttraumatic stress disorder. *Psychol Serv*. 2004;1:140–146.

213. Creamer M, Morris P, Biddle D, Elliott P. Treatment outcome in Australian veterans with combat-related posttraumatic stress disorder: a cause for cautious optimism? *J Trauma Stress*. 1999;12:545–558.

214. Creamer M, Elliott P, Forbes D, Biddle D, Hawthorne G. Treatment for combat-related posttraumatic stress disorder: two-year follow-up. *J Trauma Stress*. 2006;19:675–685.

215. Fontana A, Rosenheck R. *An Evaluation of the Inpatient Treatment of Posttraumatic Stress Disorder in Specialized PTSD Programs*. West Haven, Conn: Northeast Program Evaluation Center, Department of Veterans Affairs; 1996.

216. Fontana A, Rosenheck R, Spencer H, Gray S. *The Long Journey Home XVI: Treatment of Posttraumatic Stress Disorder in the Department of Veterans Affairs: Fiscal Year 2006 Service Delivery and Performance*. West Haven, Conn: Department of Veterans Affairs, Northeast Program Evaluation Center; 2007.

217. Dieperink M, Erbes C, Leskela J, et al. Comparison of treatment for posttraumatic stress disorder among three Department of Veterans Affairs medical centers. *Mil Med*. 2005;170:305–308.

218. Tanielian TL, Jaycox LH. *Invisible Wounds of War: Psychological and Cognitive Injuries, Their Consequences, and Services to Assist Recovery*. Santa Monica, Calif: RAND; 2008.

219. Rosen CS, Chow HC, Finney JF, et al. VA practice patterns and practice guidelines for treating posttraumatic stress disorder. *J Trauma Stress*. 2004;17(3):213–222.

220. Hembree EA, Foa EB, Dorfan NM, Street GP, Kowalski J, Tu X. Do patients drop out prematurely from exposure therapy for PTSD? *J Trauma Stress*. 2003;16(6):555–562.

221. Becker CB, Zayfert C, Anderson E. A survey of psychologists' attitudes towards and utilization of exposure therapy for PTSD. *Behav Res Ther*. 2004;42:277–292.

222. Riggs DS, Cahill SP, Foa EB. Prolonged exposure treatment of PTSD. In: Follette V, Ruzek JI, eds. *Cognitive-Behavioral Therapies for Trauma*. 2nd ed. New York, NY: Guilford Press; 2006: 65–95.

223. Turner SM, Beidel DC, Frueh BC. Multicomponent behavioral treatment for chronic combat-related posttraumatic stress disorder: trauma management therapy. *Behav Modif.* 2005;29(1):39–69.

224. Follette V, Ruzek JI. *Cognitive-Behavioral Therapies for Trauma*. 2nd ed. New York, NY: Guilford Press; 2006.

225. Ruzek JI, Friedman MJ, Murray S. Towards a PTSD knowledge management system in veterans health care. *Psychiatr Ann*. 2005;35:911–920.

Chapter 20

THE CONTINUUM OF CARE FOR NEW COMBAT VETERANS AND THEIR FAMILIES: A PUBLIC HEALTH APPROACH

HAROLD KUDLER, MD*; ALFONSO R. BATRES, PhD[†]; CHARLES M. FLORA, MSW[‡]; TERRY C. WASHAM, MSSA, LISW[§]; MARSHALL J. GOBY, PhD[¥]; and LAURENT S. LEHMANN, MD[¶]

*Associate Clinical Professor, Department of Psychiatry, Duke University Medical Center, Durham North Carolina; Associate Director, Mental Illness Research, Education and Clinical Center, Mid-Atlantic Veterans Integrated Service Network (VISN 6), VA Medical Center, 508 Fulton Street, #166A, Durham, North Carolina 27705

[†]Chief Officer and Director, Readjustment Counseling Service, Department of Veterans Affairs, 810 Vermont Avenue NW, Washington, DC 20420

[‡]Associate Director, Readjustment Counseling Service, Department of Veterans Affairs, 810 Vermont Avenue NW, Washington, DC 20420

[§]Colonel, Medical Service Corps, US Army Reserve; Military Liaison Coordinator, Office of Seamless Transition, Department of Veterans Affairs, VA Medical Center, 10000 Brecksville Road, Brecksville, Ohio 44141

[¥]Colonel, US Army (Retired); Team Leader/Supervisory Psychologist, Veterans Affairs Readjustment Counseling Service, Palm Beach Veterans Center, 2311 10th Avenue North, #13, Lake Worth, Florida 33461; formerly, Reserve Psychology Consultant, Office of The Surgeon General, US Army, Falls Church, Virginia

[¶]Associate Chief Consultant in Mental Health, Office of Mental Health Services, Department of Veterans Affairs, 810 Vermont Avenue NW, Room 966, Washington, DC 20420

INTRODUCTION

On October 16, 2003, the US House of Representatives Committee on Veterans' Affairs held a hearing on healthcare for veterans, later published as *Handoff or Fumble? Do DoD and VA Provide Seamless Health Care Coverage to Transitioning Veterans?*[1] Testimony summarized developments to that date, including the push for systematic, standardized posttraumatic stress disorder (PTSD) screening and triage for all patients seen in Department of Defense (DoD) and Department of Veterans Affairs (VA) primary care and mental health settings; the release of the DoD/VA Clinical Practice Guideline for Management of Post-Traumatic Stress[2]; the placement of VA liaisons in major military medical treatment facilities (MTFs); the importance of coordination between medical personnel and chaplains in identifying and reaching out to veterans and their families; and the need for new information technologies capable of integrating best practices into DoD and VA computerized medical record systems.

A key observation made in this hearing was that

> the VA is the world leader in the care of post-traumatic stress disorder, but its clinical and research programs have primarily been directed towards veterans who suffer from chronic PTSD from Vietnam, Korea, and World War II. Starting with the first Gulf War and gaining momentum with [the attacks of] September 11 [2001 and] the conflicts in Afghanistan and Iraq, the VA is learning to tackle PTSD proactively.[2(p40)]

Furthermore, it was noted that

> real grunts see post-traumatic stress disorders, not as a reaction of a normal person exposed to a very abnormal situation, but rather, as a failure of training, of leadership, strength, or, perhaps, character. This is a stigma and it's the single greatest impediment to effective intervention and continuity of care.[2(p41)]

This observation was subsequently validated by Hoge et al in their seminal report, "Combat Duty in Iraq and Afghanistan, Mental Health Problems, and Barriers to Care," that appeared in the *New England Journal of Medicine* in July 2004.[3] These considerations helped set the stage for the ongoing efforts to strengthen and integrate the continuum of care for combat veterans and their families across DoD, VA, state, and community settings described in this chapter.

A BRIEF OVERVIEW OF THE DEPARTMENT OF VETERANS AFFAIRS

Although the VA is well known nationally and internationally, it may still be helpful to provide a brief description of what the VA is and who it serves. The following information is primarily derived from the VA Web site, www.va.gov.[4] Established as a cabinet-level agency in 1989 succeeding the Veterans Administration, the department is responsible for providing federal benefits to veterans and their families. Its mission is inspired by the words of Abraham Lincoln's second inaugural address, delivered in the final days of the Civil War: "to care for him who shall have borne the battle and for his widow and his orphan." Headed by the Secretary of Veterans Affairs, the VA is the second largest of the 15 cabinet departments. The VA operates nationwide programs for healthcare (the Veterans Health Administration [VHA]), financial assistance (the Veterans Benefits Administration [VBA]), and burial benefits (the National Cemetery Administration). In fiscal year 2007, the VA's spending totaled over $80 billion, including $34.9 billion for healthcare and $41.5 billion for benefits.

Of the 24 million American veterans currently alive, nearly three quarters served during a war or an official period of conflict. About a quarter of the nation's population, approximately 74.5 million, are potentially eligible for VA benefits and services because they are either veterans, family members of veterans, or survivors of veterans. The VHA provided healthcare to almost 5.5 million people in 2006, a 29% increase since 2001. By the end of fiscal year 2006, 78% of all disabled and low-income veterans had enrolled for VA healthcare, and 65% of these had received care from the VA. The VA provides care at over 1,400 sites, including 155 VA medical centers, 872 community-based outpatient clinics, and 209 community-based Vet Centers. Expansion plans will bring the number of Vet Centers to 232. Facilities are located in all 50 states and in the District of Columbia, Puerto Rico, Guam, and the Philippines. VA services also extend over time: as of December 2007, VA was providing benefits to three children of Civil War veterans and 232 children and widows of Spanish–American War veterans. The VA also provides medical backup to DoD at times of national emergency or disaster.

The VA is the nation's largest provider of graduate medical education and a major contributor to medical and scientific research. Each year about 90,000 health professionals train in VA medical centers, and more than half of the physicians practicing in the United States received some part of their professional education through the VA. The quality of VA medical care significantly exceeds that of the Medicare fee-for-service program across a wide range of objective performance measures.[5]

Readjustment Counseling Service: The Vet Centers

The Readjustment Counseling Service (RCS), also known as the Vet Center system, plays a unique and pivotal role in the DoD/VA/state/community continuum of care. RCS was established by Congress in 1979 because of the recognition that many Vietnam veterans still struggled with readjustment problems years after that war's end.[6] Vet Centers are community-based and staffed by small multidisciplinary teams of dedicated providers, many of whom are combat veterans. Services are available to any veteran who served in the military in a combat theater or anywhere during a period of armed hostilities. Family members are also eligible for Vet Center services, such as support for the families of veterans coping with deployment-related stress and bereavement counseling services to surviving parents, spouses, children, and siblings of service members (including federally activated reserve and National Guard personnel) who die of any cause while on active duty.

To better respond to the needs of the newest generation of US combat veterans, Congress authorized RCS to hire and train 100 veterans of Operation Enduring Freedom (OEF) or Operation Iraqi Freedom (OIF) as global war on terror (GWOT) outreach workers. These counselors provide briefings on readjustment and VA services to active and reserve component service members after deployment and help enroll new veterans in RCS and VA programs once they become eligible for services. Their shared military experience promotes rapport between GWOT outreach workers and their fellow OEF/OIF veterans, which helps greatly to reduce the stigma associated with discussing postdeployment problems.

Vet Centers seek to increase the resilience of new combat veterans and their families through early intervention. The ultimate aim of these efforts is to prevent the development of more chronic postwar problems including occupational, marital/family, social, financial, or psychological problems. There is never a fee or co-pay for RCS services, and veterans do not have to be enrolled in VA healthcare to access them. Following a tradition of providing "help without hassles," Vet Centers are designed to decrease the stigma that veterans and their families often associate with talking about deployment-related issues in traditional healthcare settings by providing a veteran- and family-centered approach emphasizing access and understanding. These characteristics of RCS have recently been featured (and sensitively portrayed) in Gary Trudeau's *Doonesbury* cartoon series, which depicts the readjustment struggles of a newly returned OIF veteran as he works with his Vet Center counselor (himself a Vietnam veteran).[7]

In addition to psychological counseling for combat-related trauma, RCS services include community outreach, case management and referral, supportive social services, and counseling for veterans who were sexually assaulted or harassed while on active duty. Vet Centers play an important role in connecting veterans with appropriate VA services. Since the first Vet Center opened, more than 2 million veterans have been served. Each year, RCS serves more than 130,000 veterans and provides more than 1 million visits to veterans and family members.[4] From the beginning of the conflicts in Afghanistan and Iraq through the second quarter of fiscal year 2007, Vet Centers had contact with over 227,000 OEF/OIF veterans (this represents over one quarter of discharged OEF/OIF veterans to date). Over 54,000 of these new veterans presented directly to Vet Centers, and the remainder have been contacted at Post-Deployment Health Re-Assessment (PDHRA) programs and through outreach efforts conducted primarily at active duty and reserve component demobilization sites.

Seamless Transition, Care Management, and Social Work

In August 2003, to ensure that returning OEF and OIF combat veterans have timely access to VA care following discharge from military service, then-VA Secretary for Veterans Affairs Anthony Principi and Dr Michael J Kussman, deputy chief in the Office for Patient Care Services, undertook an unprecedented shift in VA policy. Dr Kussman, a retired Army general who had previously commanded Walter Reed Army Medical Center (WRAMC), arranged for VA social workers to work side-by-side with Army medical staff to facilitate the seamless transition of wounded veterans to VA medical care.[8] From the beginning of OIF, the VBA had stationed VA benefits counselors in DoD MTFs to inform wounded service members about VA services and help them begin the claims process. These benefits counselors could not, however, enroll service members for VA healthcare or transfer them to VA facilities. A new clinical system was needed that would involve VHA staff with the clinical experience needed to triage new veterans to the right level and location of care. In Dr Kussman's words: "We just cut through the paperwork and got this going."[8(p17)]

Within a month, a VA social worker from the Washington, DC, VA medical center was detailed to the new VA Seamless Transition Office at WRAMC. In rounding with the Army treatment teams, she and the VA social workers who took up the same efforts at Brooke, Eisenhower, and Madigan Army medical centers overcame the lack of a common computer record system (or even a shared set of paper forms) to develop innovative ways to help new veterans access needed VA services. One of their findings was that when a veteran was to be discharged from the MTF into care at a VA facility, it was often difficult to identify the person at the receiving facility responsible for ensuring follow-up. Within weeks, VA established a list of seamless transition points of contact for administrative issues and seamless transition care managers (usually social workers) for clinical issues at every VA medical facility and VBA regional office nationwide. Seamless transition workers at each VA medical center subsequently enlarged their scope of service to become the point of contact for all new combat veterans presenting to the VA. The success and value of this effort led the VA to develop what is intended to stand as a permanent policy[8(p19)] on DoD/VA care coordination. In January 2005, the VA established the Office of Seamless Transition to assist in working with the DoD on strengthening transition efforts.

These transition efforts have continued to expand. The VA now has social workers and benefits counselors attached to 11 MTFs and the newly created "Center for the Intrepid" rehabilitation facility in San Antonio, Texas. The US Army surgeon general assigned an Army Medical Department soldier to each of the four VA polytrauma rehabilitation centers in March 2005 to assist all active duty service members and their families with transition issues. The VA has posted Army Wounded Warrior (AW2) soldier–family management specialists to VA medical centers across the nation. The VA also detailed a certified rehabilitation registered nurse to WRAMC to assist in the transition of soldiers to VA care. In 2006 the VA established a polytrauma call center operating 24 hours a day, 7 days a week, to help seriously injured service members and their families connect with needed care and benefits. The VA has formed a partnership with the National Guard Bureau that provides for 54 transition assistance advisors, one stationed in each state and territory, to assist with transition issues among National Guard members. The VA is working with the Army Manpower and Reserve Affairs program on the Army Physical Disability Evaluation System improvement initiative. These and other efforts, including a 2007 VA conference, "Evolving Paradigms: Providing Health Care to Transitioning Combat Veterans," attended by 250 DoD and 1,000 VA participants, have further extended the integration of healthcare services and benefits provided by the DoD and VA.

In March 2007, the Secretary of Veterans Affairs authorized a number of additional positions at VA medical centers and outpatient clinics to provide expanded support for OEF/OIF veterans and their families. Each VA medical center has a full-time nurse or social worker who serves as an OEF/OIF program manager. These program managers are the primary coordinators for VA liaisons stationed at MTFs. They work with, and manage the activities of, the VA facility case managers and points of contact to assure seamless transition for all OEF/OIF service members and veterans. Program managers oversee facility outreach efforts including PDHRA events to OEF/OIF veterans including National Guard and reserve members. They work closely with VBA regional offices to track claims, and they also assign case managers for all severely injured or ill OEF/OIF veterans and others who may need or want case management.

Additionally, 100 transition patient advocates have been strategically distributed throughout the 21 veteran integrated service networks to function as ombudsmen for severely injured or ill OEF/OIF veterans and their families as they exit the military and enter the VA. The transition patient advocate, assigned to these service members while they are still at the MTF, arranges for the patients and their families to meet (virtually) with the treatment team at the receiving VA medical center and assists them with transition to the new medical center (escorting them when needed) and into the VA benefits system.[9] These programs are now organized under VA's Care Management and Social Work Service.

Much of the success of this integration is built upon VHA Directive 2002-049.[10] Enacted September 11, 2002, it ensured that hospital care, medical services, and nursing-home care were made available to recent combat veterans for 2 years beginning on the date of the veteran's discharge from military service. In January 2008, the period of service was extended to 5 years. During this 5-year period, these veterans are accorded high priority for VA care and are never charged a fee or co-pay for treatment of any illness that, in the clinician's opinion, is attributable to military service. Veterans are encouraged to begin the application process for any appropriate service connection so that military-related medical problems can be identified and rated for VA care to continue after the initial 5 years have elapsed. The provisions of VHA Directive 2002-049 ensure that recently discharged service members have expedited and unambiguous access to VA services.

In October 2007, the VA and DoD partnered to establish the Joint VA/DoD Federal Recovery Coordination Program to further integrate medical and nonmedical care and services. This program will focus on recovery, rehabilitation, and community reintegration to extend the close care coordination between the DoD and VA and across the lifetime continuum of care for severely injured service members, veterans, and their families.

SERVICES FOR VETERANS OF AFGHANISTAN AND IRAQ

As of February 2008, the DoD reported that 837,458 OEF/OIF veterans had become eligible for VA services. The VA tracks their care through its Environmental Epidemiology Service.[11] Of these new veterans, 39% (324,846) have already registered with the VHA for medical services (notably, the total number of OEF/OIF veterans who have presented for VA healthcare at the time of this writing represents only about 6% of the VA's current caseload).

Among the OEF/OIF veterans who have presented to VA medical facilities, the three most common health problems are (1) musculoskeletal injuries (including serious wounds and injuries but primarily joint and back problems commonly associated with deployment to the rocky terrains of Afghanistan and Iraq); (2) mental health problems; and (3) symptoms, signs, and ill-defined conditions. This third category is a diagnostic placeholder that designates a condition still in the process of evaluation.

Mental health issues reported by OEF/OIF veterans who have so far presented for VA care are represented in Table 20-1 (note that these numbers reflect only OEF/OIF veterans who have presented to VA medical centers and registered for care through the VHA). Over 11,000 other OEF/OIF veterans with a possible diagnosis of PTSD have presented to Vet Centers but not to VA medical facilities. It must be emphasized that the table lists provisional diagnoses. In many cases, the categories simply represent the results of positive screens for mental health diagnoses. Although positive screens are strongly suggestive of a diagnosis, they are not the same as a diagnosis. The VA has developed a "pop-up" clinical reminder within its computerized medical record[12] that prompts clinicians to screen OEF/OIF veterans for a number of mental health problems including PTSD, major depression, alcohol abuse or dependence, and traumatic brain injury. The range and number of mental health diagnoses can be expected to shift over time as clinical evaluations progress.

Diagnoses may also shift as some health issues improve and others develop. The Walter Reed Army Institute of Research (WRAIR) has reported that the majority of soldiers diagnosed with PTSD or depression at 7 months postdeployment did not meet criteria for either condition during the first month after deployment.[13] Given the stigma associated with mental health problems in general, and with postdeployment mental health problems in particular,[3] veterans with such problems may be hesitant to discuss them when they first present for care. Over time, as a clinician–patient trust develops and family or social pressure to seek help mounts, veterans and their family members may become more willing to report such problems. Kang and Hyams[14] have shown that although the rate at which medical problems are reported among OEF/OIF veterans in the VA is fairly constant, the rate at which mental health problems are reported increases with time.

The VA findings summarized in Table 20-1 demonstrate the broad range of mental health diagnoses to consider, including about as many cases of mood disorder and substance abuse or dependence as of PTSD. A similar ratio was observed in New York City in the wake of the September 11, 2001, attack on the World Trade Center.[15] Hoge et al[3] noted a significant increase in major depression and generalized anxiety disorder, as well as in PTSD, among recently deployed soldiers and marines. Postdeployment mental health cannot be about just PTSD anymore.

TABLE 20-1

PROVISIONAL MENTAL HEALTH DIAGNOSES AMONG OEF/OIF VETERANS PRESENTING FOR VA MEDICAL CARE

Diagnosis	Number
Posttraumatic stress disorder	67,525*
Acute reaction to stress	4,070
Nondependent abuse of drugs†	54,415
Depressive disorder	45,155
Affective psychoses	25,399
Neurotic disorders‡	35,605
Alcohol dependence	11,245
Drug dependence	5,062

*21% of total

†Excessive tobacco use accounts for a large portion of those identified as involved in nondependent abuse of drugs.

‡This category includes a number of anxiety disorders such as generalized anxiety disorder and panic disorder.

OEF: Operation Enduring Freedom

OIF: Operation Iraqi Freedom

VA: Department of Veterans Affairs

NEW PROGRAMS FOR COMBAT VETERANS AND THEIR FAMILIES

As noted above, Hoge and colleagues at WRAIR demonstrated that the stigma associated with reporting postdeployment mental health problems may be the single greatest obstacle to accessing care.[3] Their 2004 study reported findings from over 3,600 active duty soldiers and marines 3 to 4 months after their return from service in Afghanistan or Iraq. For example, they found that when asked whether they had concerns about their decision to receive mental healthcare, 65% of these combat veterans were concerned that "I would be seen as weak," 63% were concerned that "my leadership might treat me differently," and 59% were concerned that "members of my unit might have less confidence in me."[3]

The Joint Conference on Postdeployment Mental Health

Hoge and colleagues' 2004 findings[3] and strong interagency desire to optimize mental healthcare across the DoD/VA continuum inspired plans for a joint DoD/VA conference on postdeployment mental health. Held in Alexandria, Virginia, on March 8–10, 2005, this conference was cochaired by Colonel Elspeth Ritchie, psychiatry consultant to the Army surgeon general, and Harold Kudler, MD, then cochair of the VA Under Secretary for Health's Special Committee on PTSD. Among the over 50 participants were the assistant secretary of defense for health affairs; the deputy secretary for veterans affairs; the surgeons general of the Army, Navy, and Air Force; mental health experts from across the DoD and VA, other representatives of Army, Navy, Marine Corps, Air Force, Coast Guard, National Guard, and reserve forces; and leading researchers and health systems planners from across the DoD and VA. Given the composition of its membership and the agenda set, the meeting might have been expected to result in the definition of a medical model for assessing and treating PTSD, depression, substance abuse, and other mental health diagnoses. Instead, the participants concluded this historic conference by defining a public health model for deployment mental health that has set the tone for DoD/VA efforts ever since.

The Public Health Model for Deployment Mental Health

The public health model sprang from the observation that most warfighters or veterans will not develop a mental illness, but that all warfighters or veterans and their families face important readjustment issues. These problems in living may be painful and at times disabling, but they are, nonetheless, normal responses to extreme stress rather than medical illnesses. Within the public health model, the focus is less on making diagnoses than on helping individuals and families retain or regain a healthy balance despite the multiple stressors associated with the deployment cycle. This approach incorporates the recovery model and other principles of the President's New Freedom Commission on Mental Health,[16] including the importance of fostering resiliency and independence.

The term "recovery" is generally associated with the reduction or remission of symptoms and signs specific to a given disease. Recovery also refers to the process by which people become progressively more able to live, learn, work, love, and fulfill a valuable and satisfying role within their families and their communities despite an ongoing medical problem. Thus, "recovery" may not be the same thing as "cure." As Parsons has shown,[17] disease is a biomedical process, but illness is largely a social process in which a person who has a disease accepts the sick role and its implicit and explicit limitations. Not everyone who has a disease lives within the sick role; there is a difference between having a significant problem (even a significant medical problem) and being disabled. Even when the signs and symptoms of disease are clearly disabling, recovery can be understood as the ability to live a fulfilling and productive life despite medical limitations. Recovery might also be understood as a life in which hope succeeds in sustaining the individual and the family even when medical efforts have failed.

"Resilience" refers to the qualities of an individual, a family, or a community that enable it to cope and rebound despite extreme stress. Resilience likely has psychological, biological, and social underpinnings with a different configuration in every person, family, and society. Resilient people retain or regain a sense of mastery, competence, and hope in response to adversity. Jerome Frank, who served as an Army psychiatrist during World War II, and went on to study how people cope with and recover from illness and stress in diverse cultures,[18] suggested that the restoration of morale was the common element in all successful forms of therapy.[19]

A public health model, while medically informed, is quite different than a traditional medical model. It coordinates the efforts of traditional medical programs but also extends into nonmedical settings. In a public health model based on recovery and resilience, the question is less "How do you feel?" than "How are you doing?" New combat veterans usually experience the first question as insensitive and difficult to answer. The latter question places the focus on function and readjustment and will, therefore, engage the veteran in a more useful conversation.[20]

Hoge et als' findings,[3] and the VA utilization statistics provided above, demonstrate that it is not sufficient to announce that effective mental health treatment exists within the DoD and VA. Although many will appreciate the offer of care, only a minority will access it; the stigma associated with needing help is simply too powerful. The public health model circumvents the stigma associated with traditional mental health services by reaching directly into primary care settings and into the larger community. The primary care clinic is the de facto mental health system for a significant portion of the population. In times of trouble, people trust their primary care providers more than any other authority in their community.[21] Web sites and public service announcements help get the word out, but for the message to take hold and access to be maximized, it is necessary to partner with allies in the greater community. Among the most important of these is the veteran's family, because family members often decide when and where the veteran will seek help. Furthermore, resilient, supportive families significantly increase the resiliency of their members.[22,23]

Other allies include DoD and VA chaplains, DoD's family support programs for active and reserve component members, military medical boards, VBA, local health providers (including TRICARE providers), community mental health centers, public schools, local colleges (where many new combat veterans study), employers, local congregations, military unit associations, and veterans' service organizations. Military OneSource, a telephone and Web-based service available free of charge to service members and their families through a contract with DoD,[24] is a confidential and highly accessible outreach tool, but its service is most effective in coordination with the full range of public health resources available to veterans.

The highly successful Vet Center program was founded on public health principles and serves as a model for current efforts. RCS was specifically engineered to meet the needs of those Vietnam veterans who had reservations about seeking care at VA medical centers. RCS Vet Centers are neither hospitals nor mental health centers; they are community-based "storefront" operations. As its name clearly implies, RCS is about readjustment, not about mental illness. RCS freely involves family members and encourages them to share their concerns and express their own needs. RCS has proven effective in overcoming the stigma that kept many combat veterans from presenting to military or VA medical centers. Current public health efforts to reach a new generation of combat veterans and their families build upon the success of the RCS model.

Because the needs of OEF/OIF veterans and their families change over time (as does their access to different services), the public health approach requires a progressively engaging, phase-appropriate integration of services across the DoD/VA continuum. This program must (*a*) be driven by the needs of the veterans and their families rather than by existing organizational structures and processes; (*b*) meet prospective users where they live rather than wait for them to find their way to the right mix of services; and (*c*) better articulate the transition between DoD and VA. Shared computerized medical record systems, and standardized, longitudinal follow-up of mutually agreed upon baseline assessment measures may in time significantly strengthen the DoD/VA continuum of care. There is also an opportunity to optimize the interplay between the DoD medical board and the VBA service connection processes to accelerate the rate at which new veterans and their families can access the constellation of services designed to meet their needs.

Post-Deployment Health Re-Assessment: A New Level of Service Integration

In recognition that physical health, mental health, or other readjustment problems may not be immediately apparent or may take time to develop,[3] DoD developed the PDHRA as a follow-up to the postdeployment health assessment performed at the time of return from a contingency operation. PDHRA is performed 3 to 6 months postdeployment to ensure timely outreach, education, training, screening, assessment, triage, treatment, and follow-up. This intervention incorporates a nonpathologizing public health approach framed within a global health initiative.

Screening utilizes a standardized tool, the DD Form 2900. Service members fill out the self-report section of the form within the context of a special education and training session, focused on common deployment-related health concerns, that provides information on the range of responses and benefits available to meet their needs. Each service member's responses are reviewed with a healthcare provider to clarify issues, gather any needed clinical information, and ensure appropriate connection to services ranging from community-based support and preclinical counseling to referral for treatment in primary care, mental healthcare, other specialty care, or rehabilitative care as appropriate.

PDHRA is medically informed to effectively identify clinical problems and facilitate access to care, but, in line with the public health model, the intervention emphasizes readjustment opportunities rather than pathology and disability. Vet Center and VA Seamless Transition staff and veterans' benefits counselors are on hand at PDHRA events to assist service members entering veteran status. To improve access to mental healthcare, military and VA medical systems are both in the process of increasing its integration into primary care settings. Efforts are underway to allow sharing of DD Form 2900 findings between DoD and VA clinicians to assure continuity of care across systems.

Battlemind Training

Hoge and colleagues[3] demonstrated that the stigma surrounding postdeployment readjustment stress is a significant barrier to new combat veterans receiving appropriate care. To get around this stigma, Hoge and his team at WRAIR developed and tested a new outreach approach to engage OEF/OIF combat veterans: Battlemind training.[25] Battlemind training has now been incorporated into the PDHRA intervention for the Army. (The US Marine Corps' Warrior Transition Program[26] addresses similar issues but is adapted to meet the unique needs of marines.)

"Battlemind" is an acronym for:

Buddies vs withdrawal
Accountability vs control
Targeted vs inappropriate aggression
Tactical awareness vs hypervigilance
Lethally armed vs unarmed
Emotional control vs anger or detachment
Mission and operational security vs secretiveness
Individual responsibility vs guilt
Nondefensive (combat) driving vs aggressive driving
Discipline and ordering vs conflict

Each element of Battlemind training speaks to an important aspect of postdeployment readjustment, and each is illustrated and explained in the video presentation (viewable at https://www.battlemind.army.mil/) that forms the centerpiece of training. Consonant with the public health model, Battlemind emphasizes resiliency rather than pathology, and engages service members through training rather than direct offers of treatment. Further interventions up to and including appropriate clinical assessment and treatment are more likely to be accepted if this initial outreach is accepted.

Battlemind training is designed to be highly acceptable to new combat veterans. Its key message is that combat skills and battle mindset sustained the warfighter's survival in the war zone. Battlemind is defined as the service member's inner strength to face fear and adversity in combat with courage. If, on returning home, service members find that they still "sleep with one eye open," are constantly on alert for signs of danger, and respond reflexively with aggression, this is evidence that they have adapted to the war zone. This explanation is quite different than telling new combat veterans that they may be expressing symptoms of a mental disorder such as PTSD. The clear implication is a positive one: if you were able to adapt to life in a war zone, you should be able to adapt again to life at home. In short, Battlemind training tells new combat veterans that their responses are the normal responses of good warfighters, but it also stresses that Battlemind may be hazardous to social and behavioral health on the home front if it is not transitioned: in other words, "don't try this at home." Battlemind training has been expanded to include spouse Battlemind training for both predeployment and postdeployment use. During 2006, qualified instructors from WRAIR trained all Vet Center staff members in Battlemind principles.

Extending and Strengthening the Continuum of Care

As this review demonstrates, DoD and VA have worked steadily since the start of operations in Afghanistan and Iraq to mesh the gears of their respective agencies through the development of joint clinical practice guidelines, the Joint VA/DoD Federal Recovery Coordination Program, PDHRA, and Battlemind training to extend and enhance the continuum of care for OEF/OIF veterans and their families. These steps can be understood as practical applications of a public health model particularly suited to this newest generation of combat veterans.

In 2005 the VA implemented a new program founded on these same principles, which was subsequently named Services for Returning Veterans-Mental Health (SeRV-MH). Rather than diagnosing specific disorders or limiting services to highly specialized interventions for PTSD, depression, or substance abuse, the goals of SeRV-MH are engagement, health promotion, recovery, and rehabilitation. Triage to primary care, general mental health services, and subspecialty services are available through SeRV-MH teams. SeRV-MH teams actively engage other VHA, VBA, and Vet Center programs; DoD active duty and reserve components; and other federal, state, and community agencies and programs in support of new combat veterans and their families.

Although outreach was initially identified as a core

SeRV-MH function, that role is, as noted above, the purview of Vet Centers, so SeRV-MH outreach is carried out in collaboration with Vet Center initiatives. SeRV-MH teams are distinguished by their unique "in-reach" function, which includes services in primary care settings designed to enhance access to behavioral health services while reducing the stigma that veterans and their families often associate with formal mental health settings. SeRV-MH staff members also support facility polytrauma services, including those for veterans with traumatic brain injury. Service delivery innovations to meet the needs of returning veterans who go to work or school include the establishment of weekend and evening SeRV-MH clinic hours.

SeRV-MH teams are agents of change within the various programs, promoting a view of mental health as an essential part of overall health and function. They help other VA clinical, administrative, and support staff to become aware of the special characteristics of OEF/OIF veterans and their families and develop new methods of intervention. They embody and disseminate the public health model. More than 80 SeRV-MH teams are now distributed across the nation (at least one per state), and nationally coordinated training (developed by a multidisciplinary DoD/VA team) is being rolled out. This training includes information on the Army Battlemind approach and education on topics not addressed in more traditional curricula on war stress disorders, such as improving closeness among family members and addressing traumatic grief.

The VA has also launched a Mental Illness Research, Education, and Clinic Center (MIRECC) dedicated to postdeployment mental health.[27] MIRECCs were established by Congress in 1997 as translational research centers. Ten MIRECCs exist nationwide and each is dedicated to a specific area of mental illness, such as schizophrenia, substance abuse, or dementia. Their stated mission is

> to generate new knowledge about the causes and treatments of mental disorders, apply new findings to model clinical programs, and widely disseminate new findings through education to improve the quality of veterans' lives and their daily functioning in their recovering from mental illness.[28]

The postdeployment MIRECC works with clinicians and researchers across the DoD/VA continuum to identify, develop, and disseminate best clinical practices in the service of new combat veterans and their families. Some of this work stems from MIRECC laboratory, health services, and epidemiological research, while other efforts apply and test new clinical models and educate other health workers, the general public, and OEF/OIF veterans and their families.

BEYOND THE DEPARTMENT OF DEFENSE/VETERANS AFFAIRS CONTINUUM

Ideally, the postdeployment readjustment and mental health problems of OEF/OIF veterans would be identified and addressed somewhere within the DoD/VA continuum of care, but this may not be a realistic expectation. Hoge et al[29] conducted a population-based descriptive study of all soldiers and marines who returned from deployment to OEF (n = 16,318), OIF (n = 222,620), and other locations (n = 64,967) between May 1, 2003, and April 30, 2004. They found that the prevalence of reporting a mental health problem was 19.1% among service members returning from Iraq, 11.3% after returning from Afghanistan, and 8.5% (close to the base rate in the military) after returning from other locations ($P < 0.001$). Although 35% of all OIF veterans accessed mental health services at least once within a year after their return home, 60% of those who screened positive for PTSD, major depression, or generalized anxiety (substance abuse was not addressed in this study) failed to present for any mental health service. These DoD findings closely parallel those in the VA that (as noted above) show that, as of February 2008, only 39% of all OEF/OIF veterans eligible for VA care have come to the VA for health services. Where are the other 61% of OEF/OIF veterans, and what are their mental health needs?

Another parallel exists between this information and the findings of the National Vietnam Veterans Readjustment Study,[30] which found that only 20% of Vietnam veterans who fulfilled diagnostic criteria for PTSD at the time of the study (conducted in the late 1980s) had ever gone to the VA for mental healthcare.[30(p228)] The same study found that 62% of all Vietnam veterans with PTSD had sought mental healthcare somewhere at some point in time. In other words, among Vietnam veterans with PTSD at the time of the study who ever sought mental healthcare, only 32% came to the VA for that care, while 68% went elsewhere for care.

These findings suggest that a "silent majority" of OEF/OIF veterans with postdeployment readjustment or mental health issues may not seek help within the DoD/VA continuum of care. Stigma may be the key reason for this. But if a silent majority does exist, several important questions face DoD and VA planners and clinicians:

- Who among these veterans should be reached?
- What are the best ways to reach them?

- At what point should they be reached?
- What interventions would be most appropriate once they have been reached?
- What about their families?

Work with the families is particularly important because the level of postdeployment social support received by combat veterans strongly predicts their resilience.[22,23] In addition, if new combat veterans are going to get needed help, family members will likely be instrumental in their getting it. Finally, families have needs of their own that, if left unmet, could have serious consequences for the families and their communities. To reach new combat veterans and their families, it is necessary for the DoD and VA to look beyond their own continuum of care towards partnerships at the state and community levels.

State and Community Partnerships

The DoD and VA realize a number of advantages in partnering at the state and community levels. Such partnerships enhance access for service members, veterans, and family members who are concerned about seeking help within the DoD/VA continuum. Partnerships may also enhance the quality of services new combat veterans and their family members receive in the community through joint training and improved interagency cooperation.

Because National Guard programs are organized at the state level, it makes sense for DoD and VA to develop state-level partnerships. Furthermore, each state has its own veterans' service program. Veterans' service officers in each county or region of the state work with veterans and their families to connect them with federal, state, and local programs that significantly improve their access to care, benefits, and reliable information. Finally, partnerships among the DoD, VA, states, and local communities help build new systems of interagency communication and coordination that may serve well at times of local or regional disaster. A number of DoD, VA, state, and community partnerships already exist in areas such as upstate New York, Washington state, Ohio, North Carolina, Virginia, Alabama, Vermont, and Rhode Island. Because each state has a different array of military bases, reserve units, VA facilities, and veteran populations, each faces unique challenges and opportunities.

One recent example of the DoD, VA, state, and community partnership was introduced on February 12, 2007, when the VA announced a national roll out of a partnership with state veterans' service officers through the National Association of State Directors of Veterans Affairs. This program links VA staff based at 10 DoD MTFs around the country with state veterans' service officers in all 50 states. The program helps identify injured military members who are being transferred to VA care so that state veterans' officers can more efficiently identify, locate, and link them and their family members to appropriate state benefits and services.[31]

Partnerships can and should extend well beyond the traditional scope of mental health and substance abuse services to include local primary care providers, pediatricians, ministers and congregations, teachers and school guidance counselors, campus-based veterans' benefits specialists, veterans' service organizations, mental health associations and advocacy organizations, employers and supervisors, law enforcement agents, judges, and others in order to make diverse members of the community more aware of the problems faced by OEF/OIF veterans and their families and of the resources available to assist them.

These partnerships often begin with a state-level summit meeting of potential partners including state-based DoD and VA elements. These conferences generally open with a presentation of the "boots on the ground" experiences of new combat veterans and the deployment cycle experiences of their families. The presence of top leadership, including the governor, the state secretary for health and human services, the adjutant general of the state National Guard, senior leadership from state-based DoD military programs and medical facilities, and VA network leadership, provides a strong and positive message to participants about the importance of the effort and the will of each respective partner to pursue it.

Representatives to the summit meeting exchange key information about their respective agencies' assets and goals to identify strategic partnerships in service for new combat veterans and their families. Attendees work to articulate an integrated continuum of care that emphasizes access, quality, effectiveness, efficiency, and compassion. Services are centered on service members or veterans and their families. Principles of resilience, prevention, and recovery are emphasized. Attendees agree to work together to optimize access to information, support, and, when necessary, clinical services across systems as part of a balanced public health approach. The product envisioned is a network of informational, supportive, clinical, and administrative services through which citizens of the state will have ready access to postdeployment readjustment assistance. The DoD, VA, state, and community partnership may begin with a single high-profile meeting as described above, but if the process is to be successful, it must be sustained. This calls for ongoing meetings of working subgroups, continued support within each partnering entity, and a clear and practical joint plan with scheduled deliverables and clear lines of responsibility.

Key Elements Replicable in Every State

Some states are home to major military bases embedded within strong military-friendly communities. In such settings, postdeployment issues are often well recognized by local leaders, health professionals, teachers, guidance counselors, school principals, and local clergy. Many community support mechanisms may already be in place. Other states have few, if any, major bases, but have large numbers of reserve or National Guard members. Because these citizen soldiers tend to be scattered across communities (and relatively invisible within them), local leaders, health professionals, school personnel, and religious leaders may be less aware of deployment-related issues and less knowledgeable about how to access resources once a need is identified. Nonetheless, there are certain core elements of the DoD, VA, state, and community partnerships that can be successfully replicated in every community and state.

The first element is effective outreach. One basic mechanism is development of a governor's letter to new combat veterans and their families. Because each state director of veterans' services receives a list of the names and mailing addresses of every OEF/OIF veteran living within the state, it is possible for the governor's office to reach out to every affected household. The North Carolina Governor's Focus on Returning Combat Veterans and Their Families recommended in its final report[32] that such a letter be sent to all service members and their families, thanking them on behalf of the entire state. The letter also invites recipients to make use of local resources as they readjust. In North Carolina, the letter provides a toll-free telephone number that combat veterans or family members can call for information and guidance to appropriate resources. As a key step toward enhancing resilience, the governor can conclude the letter by recognizing the strength, skills, and willingness to sacrifice demonstrated by veterans and their families.

The toll-free number used in North Carolina is an application of a preexisting "care line" system established by the state Department of Health and Human Services. It is staffed by information-and-referral specialists trained about a wide variety of human service programs across the state.[33] Care line services are provided in English and in Spanish and as a TTY (text telephone) service for the hearing-impaired (an important consideration among combat veterans). Until recently, these specialists did not routinely inquire whether a caller was a service member, a veteran, or someone calling about a service member or a veteran or in relation to postdeployment issues. These specialists have now undergone training on deployment mental health issues and have begun applying a simple algorithm when fielding calls. They ask about the caller's service in Iraq or Afghanistan, military branch, current military status (active duty or reserve component), date separated from service, date of return from last deployment, and zip code or county of residence.

With this information in hand, a range of services can quickly be identified and located in proximity to the caller's residence. The list of potential access points resides on an electronic database of over 10,000 agencies and programs across the state. The referral specialist can identify the caller's local Vet Center (and its GWOT outreach worker if one exists); the county veterans' services officer; the seamless transition case manager at the local VA medical center; any service-appropriate family program (such as the Guard Family Readiness Group); and the nearest regional VBA. The specialist can also put the caller in touch with Military OneSource or TRICARE services as appropriate to the caller's needs. This information can also be obtained at the care line Web site (http://www.nccareline.org).

Joint training efforts are required to build strong bridges between the DoD, VA, state, and community programs. These should include leaders and clinicians working in local mental health, primary care, and family support programs, as well as professional organizations and other state and community groups. Area Health Education Centers (AHECs), developed by Congress in 1971 to recruit, train, and retain a health professions workforce committed to underserved populations,[34] exist in almost every state. AHECs can play an important role in disseminating best practices and developing a common language and approach among federal, state, and community systems.

One strategy that can be employed with relative ease is to develop an AHEC educational program based on Battlemind training. Trainers can be recruited from local DoD and VA sites. Battlemind training videos and supporting materials are available in the public domain. Although Battlemind is an Army program and the Warrior Transition Program is a Marine Corps program, both incorporate principles that speak to universal issues of the deployment cycle and can be adapted to different audiences while still respecting distinct cultural differences among the military branches.

Local PDHRA events also offer important opportunities for the DoD, VA, state, and community cooperation. DoD and VA staffs routinely meet with local military units (and often with their family members) during PDHRA. State and community representatives could be invited to attend to help reinforce transition back to the community and inform service members and their families about readjustment resources such as medical, vocational, and benefits programs. At the same time, participating state and community representatives have the opportunity to learn more about the challenges faced by new combat veterans and their families, which can then inform further efforts on their behalf. Partnerships should coordinate DoD, VA, state, and community efforts with those of local providers who contract with TRICARE and Military OneSource to assure full and ready access to well-trained clinicians for service members, new veterans, and their families. AHECs can disseminate needed clinical training and can also provide information about working with TRICARE (which could lead to more providers choosing to become TRICARE providers).

Many service members, veterans, and family members prefer to bring readjustment issues to their chaplain or local religious leader rather than to a medical provider. DoD, VA, state, and community partnerships offer a unique opportunity for interchange between military and VA chaplains and local clergy and their faith communities. These partnerships can substantially increase social support for returning combat veterans and their families. Clinical pastoral education programs are ideally suited to develop outreach and educational activities that promote readjustment, resilience, and recovery. Again, Army Battlemind training and the Marine Corps Warrior Transition Program can provide core content for instruction that can be adapted for specific faith communities. The strategies and tactics presented here are not meant to serve as an exhaustive list but rather as a jumping-off point for new ideas. It is essential that each community explore and develop partnerships specific to its own unique needs and assets.

SUMMARY

The VA has long-standing readjustment services stemming from Vietnam-era initiatives such as the Vet Center program; however, new programs have arisen in response to studies finding these efforts inadequate. The DoD and VA have established joint efforts built on a public health model, including partnerships with state and community resources. These partnerships are designed to enhance support and outreach, improve referral systems, reduce stigma, and promote better health outcomes for new combat veterans and their families. The goals of all these programs are to provide a seamless continuum of care that will support increased resilience, decreased military attrition, and decreased disability, as well as increased satisfaction among consumers and providers. Experience to date indicates that these ambitious goals are attainable. The ultimate goal is to transform the postdeployment health system: there should be no wrong door to which OEF/OIF veterans or their families can come for help. The DoD and VA have made significant progress in providing seamless healthcare coverage to transitioning veterans and their families since the start of military operations in Afghanistan and Iraq. The public health model and the DoD, VA, state, and community partnerships help mark the path for future progress.

Acknowledgment

The authors gratefully acknowledge the careful review and suggestions made by Dr Kristy Straits-Tröster of the VA Mid-Atlantic Health Care Network's Mental Illness Research, Education, and Clinical Center in the course of developing this chapter.

REFERENCES

1. *Handoff or Fumble? Do DoD and VA Provide Seamless Health Care Coverage to Transitioning Veterans? Hearing before the Committee on Veterans' Affairs, House of Representatives, One Hundred Eighth Congress, First Session, October 16, 2003.* Washington, DC: US Government Printing Office; 2004: No. 108-26.

2. *VA/DoD Clinical Practice Guideline for the Management of Post-Traumatic Stress.* Washington, DC: VA/DoD Clinical Practice Guideline Working Group, Veterans Health Administration, Department of Veterans Affairs and Health Affairs, Department of Defense; December 2003. Office of Quality and Performance publication 10Q-CPG/PTSD-04. Available at: http://www.guideline.gov/summary/summary.aspx?ss=15&doc_id=5187. Accessed December 16, 2009.

3. Hoge CW, Castro CA, Messer SC, McGurk D, Cotting DI, Koffman RL. Combat duty in Iraq and Afghanistan, mental health problems, and barriers to care. *N Engl J Med*. 2004;351:13–22.

4. US Department of Veterans Affairs. *Fact Sheet: Facts About the Department of Veterans Affairs*. Washington, DC: VA; 2009. Available at: http://www1.va.gov/opa/fact/docs/vafacts.doc. Accessed December 16, 2009.

5. Jha AK, Perlin JB, Kizer KW, Dudley RA. Effect of the transformation of the Veterans Affairs Health Care System on the quality of care. *N Engl J Med*. 2003;348:2218–2227.

6. US Department of Veterans Affairs. Vet Center: Who we are. VA Web site. Available at: http://www.vetcenter.va.gov/About_US.asp. Accessed December 16, 2009.

7. Trudeau GB. *The War Within*. Kansas City, Mo: Andrews McMeel Publishing, LLC; 2006.

8. Bristol M. Mission status: not business as usual. *Vanguard*. 2004;L:16–19.

9. US Department of Veterans Affairs. *Transition Assistance and Case Management of Operation Enduring Freedom (OEF) and Operation Iraqi Freedom (OIF) Veterans*. Washington, DC: VA; 2007. VHA Handbook 1010.01.

10. US Department of Veterans Affairs. *Combat Veterans Are Eligible for Medical Services for 2 Years After Separation From Military Service Notwithstanding Lack of Evidence for Service Connection*. Washington, DC: VA; 2002. VHA Directive 2002-049. Available at: http://www1.va.gov/environagents/docs/VHADirective2002-049_Sept_11_2002.pdf. Accessed December 16, 2009.

11. US Department of Veterans Affairs. Environmental Epidemiology Service. VA Web site. Available at: http://www.vethealth.cio.med.va.gov/Epidemiology.htm. Accessed December 16, 2009.

12. US Department of Veterans Affairs. *Iraq & Afghan Post-Deployment Screen Reminder Setup Guide*. Washington, DC: VA; 2004. Available at: http://www.va.gov/vdl/documents/Clinical/CPRS-Clinical_Reminders/pxrm_1_5_21_setup.pdf. Accessed December 16, 2009.

13. Grieger TA, Cozza, SJ, Ursano RJ, et al. Posttraumatic stress disorder and depression in battle-injured soldiers. *Am J Psychiatry*. 2006;163:1777–1783.

14. Kang HK, Hyams KC. Mental health care needs among recent war veterans. *N Engl J Med*. 2005;352:1280–1289.

15. Adams RE, Boscarino JA, Galea S. Alcohol use, mental health status and psychological well-being 2 years after the World Trade Center attacks in New York City. *Am J Drug Alcohol Abuse*. 2006;32:203–224.

16. President's New Freedom Commission on Mental Health. *Achieving the Promise: Transforming Mental Health Care in America. Final Report*. Rockville, Md: President's New Freedom Commission on Mental Health; 2003. DHHS Pub. No. SMA-03-3832. Available at: http://www.mentalhealthcommission.gov/reports/FinalReport/toc.html. Accessed December 16, 2009.

17. Parsons T. *The Social System*. London; England: Routledge and Kegan Paul Ltd; 1951.

18. Frank JD, Frank JB. *Persuasion and Healing: A Comparative Study of Psychotherapy*. Baltimore, Md: Johns Hopkins University Press; 1991.

19. Frank JD. Psychotherapy: the restoration of morale. *Am J Psychiatry*. 1974;131:271–274.

20. US Department of Veterans Affairs. *2005 Report of the Under Secretary's Special Committee on PTSD*. Washington, DC: VA; 2005.

21. Heldring M, Kudler H. The primary health care system as a core resource in the response to terrorism. *J Aggression Maltreatment Trauma*. 2005;10:541–552.

22. King LA, King DW, Fairbank JA, Keane TM, Adams GA. Resilience-recovery factors in post-traumatic stress disorder among female and male Vietnam veterans: hardiness, postwar social support, and additional stressful life events. *J Pers Soc Psychol*. 1998;74:420–434.

23. Vogt DVS, Tanner LR. Risk and resilience factors for posttraumatic stress symptomatology in Gulf War I veterans. *J Trauma Stress*. 2007;20:27–38.

24. US Department of Defense, Ceridian Corporation. Military OneSource Web site. Available at: http://www.military-onesource.com. Accessed December 16, 2009.

25. US Army Battlemind soldier support Web site. Available at: https://www.battlemind.army.mil/. Accessed December 16, 2009.

26. US Marine Corps. Marine Corps combat operational control (COSC) program Web site. Available at: http://www.marines.mil/news/messages/Pages/2007/MARINE%20CORPS%20COMBAT%20OPERATIONAL%20STRESS%20%20CONTROL%20(COSC)%20PROGRAM.aspx. Accessed December 16, 2009.

27. US Department of Veterans Affairs. MIRECC centers home. VA Web site. Available at: http://www.mirecc.va.gov/. Accessed December 16, 2009.

28. US Department of Veterans Affairs. MIRECC centers: MIRECC program overview. VA Web site. Available at: http://www.mirecc.va.gov/national-mirecc-overview.asp. Accessed December 16, 2009.

29. Hoge CW, Auchterlonie JL, Milliken CS. Mental health problems, use of mental health services, and attrition from military service after returning from deployment to Iraq or Afghanistan. *JAMA*. 2006;295:1023–1032.

30. Kulka RA, Schlenger WE, Fairbank JA, et al. *Trauma and the Vietnam War Generation: Report of Findings From the National Vietnam Veterans Readjustment Study*. New York, NY: Brunner/Mazel; 1990.

31. VA partnering with states to help injured veterans [press release]. Washington, DC: US Department of Veterans Affairs; February 12, 2007. Available at: www1.va.gov/opa/pressrel/docs/State_Outreach.doc. Accessed December 16, 2009.

32. The governor's focus on returning combat veterans and their families: substance abuse and mental health services. North Carolina Governor's Focus on Returning Combat Veterans and Their Families Web site. Available at: http://veteransfocus.org/. Accessed December 16, 2009.

33. North Caroline Department of Health and Human Services. Care-line Web site. Available at: www.dhhs.state.nc.us/ocs/careline.htm. Accessed December 16, 2009.

34. National Area Health Education Center Organization Web site. Available at: http://www.nationalahec.org/About/AboutUs.asp. Accessed December 16, 2009.

Chapter 21

PAIN MANAGEMENT

FREDERICK J. STODDARD, JR, MD*; ROBERT L. SHERIDAN, MD†; JEEVENDRA MARTYN, MD‡; JAMES E. CZARNIK, MD§; AND VIRGIL T. DEAL, MD¥

*Associate Clinical Professor, Department of Psychiatry, Harvard Medical School at the Massachusetts General Hospital; and Chief of Psychiatry, Shriners Burn Hospital, 51 Blossom Street, Boston, Massachusetts 02114; Formerly, Senior Surgeon, US Public Health Service

†Associate Professor, Department of Surgery, Harvard Medical School at the Massachusetts General Hospital; and Assistant Chief of Staff, Shriners Burn Hospital, 51 Blossom Street, Boston, Massachusetts 02114; formerly, Lieutenant Colonel, Medical Corps, US Army; US Army Institute of Surgical Research, Brooke Army Medical Center, San Antonio, Texas

‡Professor/Chief, Department of Anesthesiology and Critical Care, Harvard Medical School/Shriners Hospital for Children, 51 Blossom Street, Room 206, Boston, Massachusetts 02114

§Colonel, Medical Corps, US Army; Command Surgeon, Joint Special Operations Command, PO Box 70239, Fort Bragg, North Carolina 28307-5000; formerly, Deputy Command Surgeon, US Army Special Operations Command, Fort Bragg, North Carolina

¥Colonel, Medical Corps, US Army; United States Special Operations Command, 7701 Tampa Point Boulevard, MacDill Air Force Base, Florida 33621-5323; formerly, Commander, Walter Reed Health Care System, Washington, DC

INTRODUCTION

How should acute or chronic pain from combat and noncombat wounds and injuries be managed? What are the psychiatric implications of the control or elimination of the pain of injuries?[1] Which wounds cause the worst pain? Do the manifestations of pain in (or treatment strategies for) civilians differ from those for soldiers? Which emerging treatments can help? Are analgesic requirements met, or are they underestimated as in the past?[2,3] Is drug-seeking behavior a contraindication to use of analgesics, or not? It is important to differentiate, with the patient's help, pain resulting from injury, surgery, dressings, amputation, and physical therapy, as well as other types of pain associated with injury, illness, and emotional suffering. Pain caused by combat wounds and noncombat injuries in military personnel and in affected civilians are significant in the current context and may cause subsequent psychopathology.[4–7] Consistent with the medical team approach, collaboration of surgeons, psychiatrists, anesthesiologists, and allied personnel is key to optimal management of pain due to wounds and injuries.

A primary task of medical personnel caring for the wounded, second only to assuring the safety of the patient and staff, is to relieve pain. Prompt, accurate diagnosis of mental disorders is key to the effective and safe relief of pain. Diagnosis of delirium,[8] preexisting brain injury, substance abuse, psychosis, posttraumatic stress disorder (PTSD), Axis II disorder, or depression will affect measurement of pain, diagnostic procedures, precautions, and choice of analgesia. Failure to observe the lack of a pain response in a patient with a history of serious past trauma, or in a chemically paralyzed patient with the inability to communicate a pain response, or not diagnosing delirium, risk of violence, or high alcohol or drug levels, may cause preventable suffering or even death.

Finding solutions to managing pain leads to central clinical and research questions in the care of injuries to patients of all ages. The answers have been modified or discovered in the last 25 years. Previous publications by the authors of this chapter have addressed posttraumatic psychological and neurobiological aspects of injury pain at different stages in the life cycle, and different stages postinjury.[9–12] Pain is an essential focus of the requirements of the Joint Commission (formerly the Joint Commission on Accreditation of Healthcare Organizations), practice guidelines, treatment protocols, and continuing education. Prevention and relief of acute or chronic pain is more achievable as a result of treatment initiated at the scene of injury and continued throughout care. Pain relief for adults and children has a primary place in life-saving surgical care. Furthermore, it is important from a metabolic point of view because it decreases the stress response that activates the release of the catabolic hormones, catecholamines, and cortisol. Treatment to control metabolic and stress responses in burns, for example, has been tested to confirm a reduction in subsequent stress as outlined below.

Which wounds cause the worst pain? The patient is the judge of this, and will answer with self-report if asked, but may not volunteer this information, especially if stoical in temperament. Orthopaedic injuries including amputation may cause patients to rate pain "25" on a 0-to-10 scale, and the pain may rapidly recur with a delay in administering a dose of morphine. Burn patients frequently report their most severe pain being caused by dressing changes or from the donor sites for skin grafts. Although any bodily location—including internal organs—can be the site of severe pain, areas that are highly innervated, and thus most likely to be painful after wounds, are common locations of the most severe pain. These include parts of the face, scalp and neck, arms and hands, genitals and perianal area, and legs. Unexplained behavioral symptoms including confusion, combativeness, anger, emotional withdrawal, or anxiety may be secondary to an unrecognized wound, or a wound causing unrecognized pain.

There is growing evidence to indicate that successful pain relief appears to lessen posttraumatic stress, anxiety, and depression, although in one study, the *N*-methyl-D-aspartic acid (NMDA) antagonist ketamine, which is widely used in burn care, was shown to increase PTSD symptoms while protecting against posttraumatic reduction of hippocampal volume.[13] That study is of 30 burned adults, 15 with and 15 without PTSD, and provides "evidence that smaller hippocampal size in trauma-exposed individuals is a result of traumatic stress."[13(p2194)] Pain continues to be the subject of extensive research, and in hospital settings ongoing pain monitoring and team consultations for complex cases is the standard of care. Such teams include nurses, surgeons, anesthesiologists, psychiatrists, neurologists, pharmacists, physical therapists, ethicists, and others. Pain in those with injuries is the subject of great clinical attention, systematic evaluation, focused research, and a broad and growing range of pharmacological and psychological treatment options. Converging research in both genomics and neurobiology promises to offer new options to improve pain management for the injured patient in the future.

There is a well-established knowledge base with

which to design plans to manage and eliminate pain in injured children and adults.[14,15] Making appropriate use of this knowledge is important for everyone caring for those in pain. The evaluation of children's pain requires understanding their ways of communicating, stage of development, their mental impairments, and the emotional, as well as physical, effects of pain in selecting the appropriate treatments. Similarly, evaluation of adults' pain requires listening to their complaints of pain and recognizing the unique needs of special populations, such as intensive care patients, those with mental or physical disability, substance abusers, and the elderly.

Although psychological elements of treatment, such as preparation for painful procedures and hypnosis, are less likely to be covered by protocols than pharmacological approaches, they enable patients to lessen their own pain and are effective components of care.[1,16–18] Psychological methods of pain relief do not have the risks of drug side effects, toxicity, or dependence but may be less effective than drugs. Systematic pharmacological research with severely injured patients has established the benefits of acute management with high-dose morphine and possibly benzodiazepines (although some literature indicates lorazepam may worsen outcomes),[19] other analgesics, and adjuvants, utilizing intravenous and other routes of administration, mainly in ventilated patients. Further advances in management of injury pain are continuing.

A large contribution to pain control for military wounded has been in the field of regional pain control. It is now possible for casualties of bullet or blast injuries to have at least one extremity rendered pain free by the ultrasound-guided placement of a nerve-block catheter and administration of appropriate anesthetic. These catheters may be maintained in place and connected to infusion pumps. This may allow the casualty to remain pain free during the first surgical interventions in theater, through the evacuation to Europe, and through washout and further debridement at Landstuhl Army Regional Hospital in Germany and across the Atlantic to military hospitals in the United States. It is anticipated that this will prove to be another contribution to a lower incidence of narcotic addiction and complex regional pain syndromes in casualties of the global war on terror.

The two temporal components of pain due to acute injuries include acute and chronic pain, which are further classified. Acute pain, the principal subject of this chapter, includes both background pain and procedural pain. Acute pain may be worsened by anxiety, depression, sleep deprivation, and "regeneration of nerve endings (possible neuroma formation, known as postburn neuralgia)."[20(p319)] Chronic pain is usually present for months to years and may not be easily relieved. It may result from scarring, contractures, and injury to a bone or joint; from bone formation in soft tissues (heterotopic ossification)[21,22]; or injury to the peripheral nerves (neuropathic pain). Although this chapter is not comprehensive, it provides scientific background, case illustrations, clinical approaches, and pertinent references to assist in developing an optimal multidisciplinary plan for pain management of patients suffering from combat and noncombat injuries.

ANATOMY OF INJURY-RELATED PAIN

The anatomic location of pain is a sign of tissue injury, underlying infection, or systemic illness. The sensory detection of pain (nociception) and pain are not the same. Nociception is, according to Sherrington,[23] the sensory detection of a noxious event of potentially harmful environmental stimulus. Pain, in contrast, involves sensory and cognitive components, and is defined by the International Association for the Study of Pain as "an unpleasant sensory and emotional experience associated with actual or potential tissue damage."[24] The anatomy of pain involves both central and peripheral nervous systems.[25] Patients with larger injuries generally suffer more pain. Due to the involvement of both central and peripheral nervous systems, and afferent and efferent pathways, approaches to pain management are needed to address both central brain and spinal cord receptors and peripheral nerve receptors.

Injury-Related Pain Cases

Case Study 21-1: A 26-year-old Afghani civilian male was injured by enemy rocket fire, sustaining a gaping penetrating injury to his left knee. The patient was dragged by his comrades to an austere casualty collection point inside a secure bunker. He presented screaming and clutching his left knee. Primary survey revealed normal mentation and respiratory status. A rapid secondary survey revealed no other injuries.

The patient was clearly stirred by the visual appearance of his knee. He was given an 800-µg fentanyl transmucosal lozenge to suck on while his knee was rapidly immobilized and dressed and he was comforted by one of his battle buddies. By the time intravenous access was obtained (less than 5 min), his pain response had significantly improved. The simple act of immobilizing and dressing (and thereby concealing) his injury was the essential treatment for his pain. Thirty minutes after his initial assessment, he was titrated with small boluses of intravenous ketamine (0.25 mg/

kg) to a comfortably dissociated state, whereupon a gross decontamination of his wound with copious irrigation could be performed.

The patient's pain was subsequently controlled with immobilization and intermittent use of self-administered transmucosal fentanyl during the next 8 hours until transport could be arranged. The profound effect of covering and immobilizing his wound significantly decreased his pain response.

Case Study 21-2: A 55-year-old Iraqi male sustained direct-fire injury to his left foot, ankle, and tibia. He was treated with a tourniquet for hemorrhage control in the field and was rapidly transported to a surgical element. He was otherwise uninjured and remained alert through his transport. The associated direct-fire injury to several key nerves limited his immediate pain response; pain control was achieved initially through immobilization and intermittent small doses of intravenous morphine.

The surgeon's assessment was that the patient's best option for a functional recovery in the current environment was through a below-the-knee amputation allowing for maximum stump length. As the patient was counseled (through an interpreter) as to the surgical options of either attempts at limb salvage (with tremendous potential for follow-up infection, difficult rehabilitation, and fusion with limited range of motion) or amputation, the patient's "pain" became acutely worse.

After confirming that there had been no change in the status of his injured extremity to account for the surprising increase in pain, the interpreter was asked to inquire from the patient what would alleviate his new increase in "pain." Upon questioning, he made clear the overwhelming angst he felt at the recommendation to amputate his leg. His answer routinely was "Insha'Allah" (English translation "God willing" or "If it is God's will"). The surgeon required a decision from the patient, but the patient was unable to make the decision.

It became apparent that to treat the patient's pain and to continue with any treatment regimen, the patient's psychological pain needed to be addressed. Through the continued verbal analgesic work and religious discourse of the Muslim interpreter, the patient eventually became much less distraught and his pain improved markedly. The patient was subsequently able to make a decision.

This case demonstrates the multifactorial components of pain generation, even in relatively acute traumatic denervation, and how these factors can precipitate a clinically severe pain syndrome, which may be relieved by a culturally appropriate intervention in the patient's own language.

Case Study 21-3: A 4-year-old girl was caught in a burning house, sustaining a 55% full-thickness flame burn and an inhalation injury. Immediately after rescue, she was intubated at the scene by responding medics because of respiratory distress. To facilitate intubation and ventilation during transport, she was chemically paralyzed with cisatracurium and sedated with approximately 0.05 mg/kg of midazolam and 0.05 mg/kg of morphine sulfate as single bolus doses. As a result of witnessing her injuries, her parents were severely traumatized, but reassured that she was receiving optimal care.

On arrival to the burn unit she was placed on continuous infusions of these same drugs, at 0.05 mg/kg/h each, and muscle relaxation was stopped to allow a more accurate assessment of comfort. Assessment after spontaneous reversal of neuromuscular blockade revealed a grimacing, writhing child in need of further analgesia and sedation. The morphine sulfate and midazolam infusions were increased, titrating to a Richmond Agitation-Sedation Score of -2.[3] Over the following 2 weeks, until she was extubated, background infusions of these agents were gradually increased, as tolerance developed, in response to continuous monitoring of the status of her comfort. During this time she needed several skin grafting operations, which are associated with substantial postoperative pain. At maximum, doses required to maintain appropriate comfort were 0.50 mg/kg/h of morphine sulfate and 0.40 mg/kg/h of midazolam.

Procedural pain and anticipatory anxiety were important issues for her because she required at least daily bedside procedures during this period of intubation. Sedation for these interventions (dressing changes, intravenous line placement, wound debridement) was provided by the addition of ketamine intravenous boluses at 1 mg/kg, repeated every 20 minutes as needed. When she was awake, the continuous presence of her parents, their verbal explanations and reassurance, and their touching her also facilitated her coping with pain, fear, and hospitalization.

Donor site and skin graft healing were complete by 2 weeks, coincident in improvement of the child's inhalation injury. After extubation, the need for sedation was lessened by removal of the endotracheal tube and for analgesia by healing of wounds. Intravenous background infusions were reduced by 10% per day, alternating drug reductions every 12 hours (eg, 0600 hours reduction in morphine and 1800 hours reduction in midazolam). During this period, as her pain and anxiety lessened, her parents became less stressed and more effective in supporting her and participating in dressing changes.[26]

Case Study 21-4: An 18-year-old man was involved in a high-speed truck accident and trapped in the wreck, which then caught fire. He suffered fractures and deep burns to both legs, a 65% mixed second- and third-degree surface area burn, and a comminuted closed fracture of the right humerus. After extrication and transport, he was intubated and mechanically ventilated for 4 weeks. His comfort management plan included escalating infusions of morphine sulfate and midazolam, supplemented by intravenous boluses of propofol (2–3 mg/kg) for procedures. At day 10 he underwent tracheotomy, which reduced his requirement for intravenous sedation. He underwent excision and grafting of his wounds, but required bilateral below-the-knee amputations. On weaning his sedation he was transiently delirious, and then manifested intrusive recall of the accident contributing to flashbacks and insomnia, which were relieved by lorazepam. He was initially depressed in response to his massive injuries, but this lessened with supportive psychotherapy, acceptance by his friends, and messages of family support. In his recovery phase, he developed severe neuropathic phantom leg pain that interfered with his rehabilitation. This improved with gabapentin, allowing him to be successfully fitted with prosthetics. After 6 months he was able to discontinue the gabapentin.[27]

BIOLOGY OF PAIN

There are several important concepts relevant to pain mechanisms to consider: (*a*) pain receptors in the skin (nociceptors), (*b*) the opioid system, (*c*) increased pain sensitivity (hyperalgesia), and (*d*) the emerging role of the nonopiate pain adjuncts including inhibitors of the enzyme cyclooxygenase-2 (COX-2) and gabapentin.

Pain associated with trauma including burn or other tissue injury is transmitted by peripheral nociceptors—the peripheral endings of primary sensory neurons whose cell bodies are in the dorsal root of the spinal cord and trigeminal ganglia. Unlike other sensory receptors in the skin, nociceptors are without specialized transducing structures and essentially exist as free nerve endings. Different classes of nociceptive fibers can be involved in the experience of pain. Thermal or mechanical nociceptors convey stimuli rapidly (up to 30 m/sec) via thinly myelinated, small-diameter fibers classified as "A" or "A delta." Polymodal nociceptors are also activated by hot stimuli, but transmit impulses more slowly (up to 2 m/sec) along small-diameter unmyelinated "C" fibers. Both A delta and C fibers are widely distributed in skin and in deep tissues.[12] Nociceptive fibers, both A and C, enter the dorsal horn of the spinal cord and split into ascending and descending branches. The fibers terminate primarily in lamina I and in lamina II, although some A-fiber afferents may terminate more deeply in lamina V. Within lamina I, different projection neurons process the incoming stimuli. "Nociceptive-specific" neurons are only excited by nociceptors, but "wide-dynamic-range" neurons receive their input from both nociceptors and other mechanoreceptors.

Several ascending pathways convey afferent stimuli to the brain. The spinothalamic tract originates in lamina I and laminae V–VII and is the major ascending pathway for nociceptive input. The nociceptive-specific and wide-dynamic-range projection neurons in this tract terminate in the contralateral thalamus, particularly ventrobasal and posterior thalamic nuclei. The spinoreticular tract originates in laminae VII and VIII and sends both ipsilateral and contralateral projections to the reticular formation and thalamus. The spinomesencephalic tract originates in laminae I and V, where it projects to the contralateral mesencephalic reticular formation, the periaqueductal gray, and other sites within the midbrain. The spinocervical tract, and even the dorsal column of the spinal cord, also can convey nociceptive stimuli. In addition, in the dorsal horn, A-B fibers conveying sensations such as vibration and light touch are involved in the modification of pain transmission via inhibitory interneurons.

There are multiple projections from thalamic nuclei to the cortex, primarily somatic sensory and association cortex. Although at least two classes of somatosensory cortical neurons can be identified with respect to their receptive fields and source of thalamic input, nociceptive inputs do not map to the cortex as do tactile inputs. Further, lesions to the somatosensory cortex do not result in loss of pain, suggesting that parallel or distributed processing of nociception in the cortex is likely.[28,29] Studies examining cortical activation following painful stimuli highlight the multiplicity of regions involved, including the contralateral prefrontal cortex, as well as the middle and inferior frontal gyrus (Brodmann areas 6, 8, 9, 44, and 45).[30,31]

The intense barrage of incoming pain stimuli associated with a trauma results in a decrease in thresholds for subsequent excitation of spinal neurons, as well as a greater response to subsequent stimuli and an expansion of receptive fields.[32]All of these adaptive changes likely underlie the increased pain sensitivity, or hyperalgesia, that typically follows a significant burn or multiple traumas. Hyperalgesia has long been characterized as "primary" if limited to the area of injury or "secondary" if it extends to areas adjacent to the site of damage.[33] Primary hyperalgesia appears to require sensitization of both peripheral nociceptors and spinal neurons, whereas secondary hyperalgesia seems to depend on sensitization of spinal neurons alone.[34,35] Both types of increased pain sensitivity can occur immediately following injury, but secondary hyperalgesia may take hours before reaching its peak and is likely to resolve before primary hyperalgesia.[30] Interestingly, experimental data suggest that chemosensitive nociceptors can be recruited to become mechanosensitive receptors following injury.[31] This ability to recruit otherwise "silent" nociceptors may play a role in primary hyperalgesia following injury or inflammation.

Any form of major trauma, including burn injury, results in a local and systemic response that includes fever, anorexia, and pain in the injured (primary hyperalgesia) and uninjured areas. Until recently, as indicated in the previous paragraph, this sensation was thought to occur by transmission of nerve impulses from the injured region to the spinal cord and the brain.[36] Other mechanisms, in addition to nerves, may play a role.[37] Drugs that silence sensory nerves work well to relieve acute pain. When inflammation occurs, drugs for acute pain are less effective. Local inflammation at the site of injury (eg, burn) causes a rapid and long-lasting increase in the proinflammatory-signaling molecule in the brain, especially interleukin-1β in the cerebral spinal fluid. Blockers of interleukin 1β (eg, COX-2 inhibitors) strongly inhibit the hypersensitivity to pain.[36,37] Increased levels of interleukin-1β cause increased expression of COX-2 and prostaglandin E synthase, with a resultant increase in prostaglandin E_2. Thus the use of COX-2 inhibitors currently available will not only have antiinflammatory and antipyretic effects but also have antihyperalgesic effects by acting at local and central sites. Among those available are celecoxib (Celebrex [Pfizer Inc, New York, NY), nimesulide (Mesulid [various manufacturers], and meloxicam (Mobic [Abbott Laboratories, Abbott Park, Ill]). Additionally, trauma/inflammation-induced upregulation of protein kinase Cδ (PKCδ) and NMDA in the spinal neurons may also play a role in the hyperalgesia and mechanical allodynic.[38] A growing body of evidence supports the notion that the upregulation of protein kinase Cα (PKCα) and NMDA are implicated in the mechanisms of chronic nociception.[38] Hence the rationale for use of drugs such as ketamine, an NMDA antagonist.

PRINCIPLES OF PAIN THERAPY

Laboratory research is clarifying the synthetic and degradative pathways by which the levels of endogenous opioids are maintained in the body.[39,40] In addition to the clarification of the dynorphin gene, the neural systems involved in pain and anxiety have been located. The three classes of endogenous opioid peptides are: (1) endorphin, (2) met-leu-enkephalin, and (3) dynorphin. Additional transmitters modulating pain include the monoamine (dopamine, norepinephrine, and serotonin) systems, substance P, and the γ-aminobutyric acid system—each with its own specific brain receptor sites. Clinically, opioids are the first-line drug used to treat pain associated with injury. Selection of analgesics such as nonsteroidal antiinflammatory drugs (NSAIDs), COX-2 inhibitors, benzodiazepines, anticonvulsants, and adjuvants (eg, stimulants, tricyclic or serotonergic antidepressants, neuroleptics) may be made to modulate and potentiate the effects of narcotics. However, the analgesic effects of opioids are unpredictable, particularly under chronic pain conditions. This is partly due to downregulation of opioid receptors,[37] and to the development of a condition called opioid-induced hyperalgesia (OIH).

Recent observations suggest that chronic administration of opioids leads to OIH. Thus, treatment with opioids is a double-edged sword; the treatment of pain may lead to a hyperalgesic state. OIH can occur during maintenance therapy, withdrawal, or both. OIH has been studied in three different clinical settings: (1) in former opioid addicts on methadone therapy, (2) in patients treated with opioids, and (3) in human volunteers. OIH can occur following both low-dose and high-dose opiate therapy.[41–43] Mechanisms involved in OIH include sensitization of peripheral nerve endings, enhanced facilitation of the nociceptive signal transduction, altered kinetics of nociceptive transmitters, and increased sensitization of the second-order neurons to neurotransmitters.[41,43] Excitatory amino acids (glutamate), NMDA receptors, and PKC seem to play a role in the development of OIH. The greater the opioid therapy, the greater the OIH will be.

Tolerance to opioids can also occur acutely[44]; this emphasizes the importance of alternative or adjunct therapy with opioids for treatment of pain. Strategies to treat tolerance and OIH can include rotation from phenanthrene (morphine) to a piperidine (fentanyl) opioid derivative. The administration of NMDA antagonists (ketamine) prevents opioid-induced hyperalgesia and also overcomes tolerance.[45] Dexmedetomidine, an α_2 agonist more potent than clonidine, has analgesic/sedative effects, particularly in combination with other drugs, and may reduce the incidence of delirium and other complications of withdrawal from opiates.[46–49]

Experience gained from treating other pain-associated conditions such as cancer, herpes, diabetic neuropathy, and degenerative diseases can also be applied to posttraumatic pain syndromes.[50] The available therapies shown to be effective include anticonvulsant drugs, tricyclic and other antidepressants (duloxetine, venlafaxine), topical lidocaine, and tramadol. Of great recent interest is gabapentin. The mechanism of its action is unclear, but its effects on the $\alpha_2\delta$ calcium-channel subunit may result in decreased release of the neurotransmitter and suppression of central sensitization.[51] The combination therapy of gabapentin with morphine resulted in greater reduction of pain than did either drug alone or placebo. The combination also had beneficial effects on pain-related interference with daily activities, mood, and quality of life.[51] Combination therapies have the potential to simultaneously alleviate pain, insomnia, and mood instability or depression. Tolerance will most likely develop to this combination based on previous reports on receptor behavior and neuroplasticity.

ADVERSE EFFECTS OF PAIN

Many factors contribute adverse physiological, behavioral, and psychological effects to the experience of pain and injuries.[52] It is often difficult to differentiate the specific contribution of pain to the range of psychological problems that develop following injury. The injury itself may or may not be unexpected and normally initiates an ongoing experience of severe pain. Shortly after the injury, these patients often find themselves in an emergency setting where they may undergo application of wound dressings and possibly extensive surgery. Hospitalization involves separation from the military component and friends, who themselves may have been injured or killed. Treatment usually includes painful dressing changes and support for adjustment to permanent and emotionally traumatic changes in their bodies' appearance and function. The traumatic nature of severe injuries is compounded by the fact that some are inflicted in battle, while others are due to mistakes, accidents, or intoxication, or are intentionally inflicted or self-inflicted. Injured patients frequently manifest severe psychological reactions such as nightmares, flashbacks, acute sadness and grief, irritability or anger, and behavioral regression.[11,53] For example, the psychological intensity of burn trauma, and particularly the relentless stress of extended hospital treatment for a burn, has been compared to "inescapable shock" or "learned helplessness,"[54] both of which are models for PTSD.[55,56]

About one third to one half of injured people eventually develop PTSD, and over half display significant posttraumatic stress symptoms.[57] PTSD and posttraumatic stress symptoms are reactions to diverse traumatic events related to combat and civilian injuries, assaults, witnessing violence, disasters, medical illness, physical and sexual abuse, and other psychological traumas not involving injury.[58,59] Symptoms of this disorder include increased intrusive recollections, numbing and avoidance, and hyperarousal.[60] The manifestation of these symptoms is triggered by environmental factors, such as exposure to objects, people, or situations reminiscent of the trauma. PTSD occurs when symptoms are experienced for most days and interfere in either a social or occupational setting. PTSD causes significant difficulties for a person's social, educational, occupational, biological, and life-cycle development. Children with PTSD are often so preoccupied with intrusive recollections or are so hyperaroused that they have difficulty processing social information.[61,62]

The intrusion of trauma-related memories and extreme levels of arousal that traumatized individuals experience interfere with job performance and learning at school. Traumatized people often avoid social situations secondary to fear and anxiety that memories will reoccur. Patients with injuries also develop mood (especially depressive), anxiety, sleep, sexual, behavioral, elimination, and attentional problems. PTSD symptoms cause tremendous morbidity and may persist for many years. Evidence indicates that once posttraumatic symptoms become persistent, they are refractory to treatment.[63] Accordingly, it is important in each case of a person sustaining an injury to seek interventions that may prevent or ameliorate the development of PTSD. Evidence is slowly accumulating suggesting that the early postinjury preventive or therapeutic administration of cognitive behavior therapy, or of drugs (eg, morphine, propranolol, serotonin reuptake inhibitors, or tricyclic antidepressants) can block the emergence of PTSD symptoms in some cases, including combat injuries.[64–68]

GENETICS

This section briefly outlines the genetics of pain, the genetics of opiate drug responses, and the important genetic determinants of racial differences in response to pain or its treatment. The human genome project has revealed data on genomic variations that may influence pathologic states, and are certain to influence treatment advances in the future. Nevertheless, the molecular biology and genetics of pain has lagged behind the research in diseases such as hereditary, cardiovascular, and oncologic disorders. Reports continue to emanate, however, on the genetic factors influencing nociceptive sensitivity and responses to drugs. Genes involved in pain perception, pain processing, and pain management include opioid receptors, transporters, NMDA receptors, α_{2A} adrenoceptors, and more recently discovered, guanine triphosphate cyclohydrolase—the rate-limiting enzyme for tetrahydrobiopterin synthesis, a key modulator of peripheral neuropathic and inflammatory pain.[69,70]

Pain is a complex trait with interaction of multiple genes, each with varying effect, that together with environmental and cultural factors, play a role in sensation of pain. Altered sensitivity to pain can be due to hereditary disorders; usually these are due to homozygous disorders. For example, a mutation in nerve growth factor has been found and in this instance there was complete absence of pain.[71] Recently, a "pain protective haplotype," the guanine triphosphate gene, has been identified with allelic frequency of 15%.[72] This haplotype was associated with decreased pain sensitivity in low-back-pain patients following herniated disc surgery and in volunteers undergoing experimental pain.[70] The degree of activity or inactivity of enzymes that metabolize drugs may also influence drug efficacy. It is well established that polymorphisms of the cytochrome P-450 (CYP2D6) enzymes influence analgesic efficacy of codeine, tramadol, and tricyclic antidepressants.[69] Similarly, blood levels of some NSAIDS are dependent on CYP2C9 activity.

Catechol-o-methyltransferase is a key regulator of pain perception, cognitive function, and affective mood. Polymorphisms in this enzyme and μ-opioid receptors are known modulators of pain sensitivity and opioid efficacy.[73,74] In addition to endogenous factors that alter pain sensitivity, exogenously administered small molecules (peptides) that can alter gene activity have been shown to influence pain response. Progress in molecular biology has enabled gene expression modulation (in animal models) using "knock outs" or antisense ribonucleic acid (RNAi) and small RNA molecules (sRNA). Gene therapy for patients with chronic pain shows encouraging results. Additional studies that have been performed on candidate genes transmitting pain include opioid receptors, transporters, and other targets of pharmacotherapy. Future studies should also elucidate the side-effect profiles of these gene manipulations. The challenge is to deliver this RNAi or sRNAs to target tissues such as the central nervous system. Genes can also affect signaling pathways related to pain sensitivity and clinical response.[7,74] Future studies could characterize the roles of different genes and metabolizing enzymes along with demographic and clinical variables that may influence treatment of pain both in acute and chronic situations.[75]

Few studies of pain in humans have described the ethnic or racial background of their subjects. In spite of this limitation, findings from any given study are then generalized to other ethnic and social groups, although there is no evidence base for such generalization of the results of these studies. Therefore, genetic studies of varying ethnic and social groups are indicated. The importance of genetic factors controlling drug disposition and response has received increased attention.[76] For example, the variability of a single drug, midazolam, was 11-fold.[77] Selective sequencing of CYP3A4 and CYP3A5 genes revealed 18 single-nucleotide polymorphisms (SNPs), including eight novel CYP3A4 SNPs. These differences may or may not account for such variability. Thus, the so-called standard doses of a drug may have toxic effects in some but fail to produce expected effect in others. Racial and ethnic differences have been described for a range of drugs and reflect genetic, environmental (cultural and dietary), and pathogenetic causes. Polymorphism of drug-metabolizing enzymes (eg, CYP2D6 of the cytochrome P-450 system) is well recognized and can affect drug therapy, such that lower or higher drug doses should be used. Thus, differences in response to pain treatment can be due to pharmacokinetic, pharmacodynamic, or pharmacogenetic factors. The identification of such genetic differences will result in better therapeutics. The role of pharmacogenetics can also be confounded by injury-induced alterations in drug metabolism.[78]

METHODS OF PAIN ASSESSMENT

The perception of pain is subjective and poses unique challenges for its objective assessment. The measurement of pain has developed to assess both the self-report of pain experience and behavioral observations. Behavioral measurements can lead to data correlating behaviors to subjective reports of pain. Self-report measures are used for patients over 4 years of age, and require sufficient cognitive and language abilities. Psychiatric disorders may indicate an increased requirement for analgesia. For example, a severely injured woman with borderline personality disorder who complained constantly of pain was later shown to have had negligible levels of endorphins. Alternatively, patients with Axis II psychiatric disorders may exaggerate their needs for analgesia and need psychiatric or substance abuse evaluation, especially in later stages of care when their wounds are largely healed. Other patients, such as those suffering depression or bipolar disorder, once treated with antidepressants or mood stabilizers may have significantly reduced pain. Patients with factitious disorders may use pain or self-inflicted injuries to obtain opiates. Patients with a brain injury, delirium, or limited cognitive and language skills may not be able to accurately complete self-report measures of pain.

Various methods assess pain in children.[79] Surveys of pediatric anesthesiologists have reported that the infant's respiratory rate is commonly used as an indicator of pain.[80] Other useful behavioral indices in young children include facial expression,[81] body movement (particularly limb withdrawal to painful signals[82]), and crying. Psychophysiological indices include blood pressure, pulse, respiratory rate, and neurochemical activity.[82] There are combined behavioral and psychophysiological indices (eg, the COMFORT scale,[83] which is composed of six behavioral dimensions [alertness, calmness, muscle tone, movement, facial tension, and respiratory response] and two physiological dimensions [heart rate and mean arterial pressure]) to assess postoperative pain. Using this scale, it was found that the most accurate variables for measuring pain were behavioral activity, mean arterial pressure, and heart rate.[84] Methods in older patients take advantage of the ability to self-report symptoms and experiences. The Poker Chip Tool[85] allows children ages 4 to 8 to describe their pain as "pieces of hurt," using one to four poker chips. The Faces Scale[86] asks children to choose a picture of a face with expressions of various gradations of pain, rated 0 to 5, from "no pain" to "the worst pain."

The most practical and standard pain assessment tools in adolescents and adults are verbal or visual (or both) analogue scales, asking patients to rate their pain on a continuum of intensity along a line using numerical anchors, commonly from 0 to 10, from "no pain" to "the worst pain."[87] Visual analogue scales, the most commonly used instruments, have good psychometric properties and are easily administered. The numerical anchors have been enhanced in the visual analogue instruments by adding colors to the intensity ratings.[75] Pain diaries are also useful, and require the repeated numerical rating of pain over the course of time along with other relevant information such as activities, stressors, or alleviation with medications.

Comfort management will have different priorities depending on the locale of care: prehospital, inpatient, and outpatient. In the prehospital setting, the priority must be safe and efficient care. The airway must be secured. The patient must cooperate with evaluation and transport. Medication policies should be simple and follow trained protocols. These protocols generally rely on intravenous opiate and benzodiazepine dosing, and may include drugs to facilitate endotracheal intubation, including neuromuscular blocking agents.[88]

In the inpatient setting, the focus is on continuous evaluation and titration of sedatives and analgesics. Inpatient protocols may be more complex, and importantly include regular objective evaluations of pain and anxiety using one or more of several available scales.[89,90] Inpatients may also benefit from patient-controlled analgesia devices, which have been shown to be associated with reduced total opiate requirements.[91] Peripheral nerve blocks[92] or continuous epidural anesthesia are an excellent adjunct in some patients, particularly in the management of short-term or postoperative lower body pain.[93]

In the outpatient setting, where monitoring is less feasible, patient safety is an added important consideration. A differentiation should be made between neuropathic pain (eg, phantom pain) and more standard pain (eg, open wounds). The former is ideally addressed with nonopiate medication or alternative therapies to avoid the specter of opiate dependence.[94]

METHODS OF PAIN MANAGEMENT: OVERVIEW

Until 20 years ago, pain management for acutely injured patients was relatively neglected due to concerns about respiratory depression and its effect on survival. Pain became recognized as critically undertreated, increasing physiological stress and adversely affecting outcomes. Improved pain relief became a priority and was successfully addressed by increased use of opiates, benzodiazepines, other analgesics, and anxiolytics. Today, in managing the pain of severely injured patients with intractable pain and anxiety, combinations of agents are commonly used, with close monitoring of vital signs and symptoms. Among these agents are high-dose opiates and benzodiazepines, NSAIDs, and the judicious use of both atypical and typical antipsychotics, antiepileptic drugs, and antidepressants. Signs of physiological dependence such as increased pulse, blood pressure, or insomnia are common upon tapering sedatives after prolonged administration but do not indicate psychological addiction; these signs are managed by adjusting the weaning regimen.

Pharmacological approaches are the first-line treatment in management of pain due to combat or noncombat injuries. In addition, psychological methods are essential in conjunction with drugs, and their effectiveness is also well established. These include psychoeducation, psychological preparation for procedures, relaxation techniques, hypnosis and self-hypnosis, guided imagery, and therapeutic touch. Psychological approaches enhance trust and communication with the patient, facilitating hope, positive coping, and optimal recovery despite potentially stigmatizing disfigurement and functional losses.

PHARMACOLOGICAL MANAGEMENT OF ACUTE PAIN

Two key principles in acute management of pain include frequent reassessment and dose titration. It is not possible to predict with accuracy the medication requirements of an individual patient. These will vary with pain intensity, anxiety state, personality characteristics, and distractions. Frequent reassessment of the efficacy of pain and anxiety control is essential. Ideally, these findings are documented so that pain and anxiety control can smoothly transition between shifts of caregivers. There are several acceptable scales that are validated for this purpose.[95] Analgesic and anxiolytic doses will need to be titrated to the findings from these reassessments.

Ideally, every patient care unit will have specific written guidelines describing the preferred methods of pharmacological pain management. These guidelines should have a limited formulary to facilitate development of a working knowledge of drugs used by all staff, and allow for bedside dose-ranging depending on the findings at regular reassessment.

There are a limited number of drug classes used in acute comfort management. The cornerstones are opiates and benzodiazepines. Opiates are potent analgesics with some sedative properties. Although they are very effective, side effects are common and include respiratory depression and ileus. Benzodiazepines are potent anxiolytics. The synergy between these two classes of drugs is strong.[96] Other drugs useful in this setting are propofol (a short-acting intravenous anesthetic), ketamine (an intravenous dissociative agent), haloperidol (an intravenous antipsychotic), and dexmedetomidine (a centrally acting α_2 agonist). A complete program of pain and anxiety management in the intensive care unit is beyond the scope of this chapter, but the reader is referred to many excellent reviews.[97] The important point is that acute pain and anxiety management will have an important effect on subsequent incidence and severity of acute and posttraumatic stress symptoms.[65] Frequent pain and anxiety assessment should be a regular part of care of all acutely injured patients.

PSYCHOLOGICAL MANAGEMENT OF PAIN AND GRIEF

Psychological strategies are quite effective for pain[1] and for associated anxiety and grief. Reassurance, supportive interventions, increasing structure, and a variety of psychosocial interventions geared to the patient's interests can be extraordinarily helpful in relieving pain, anxiety, and the sense of helplessness. Videos, television, hypnosis,[18] guided imagery, relaxation, virtual-reality methods, and therapeutic touch may also effectively relieve pain and discomfort. They should be individualized, because some methods are more acceptable for one individual than for another; they are well established as key interventions for pain relief, with a very low risk of adverse or toxic effects. Psychological management of the patient and interventions also include assessment for safety, empathic listening, modifying cognitive distortions through cognitive behavior therapy, providing hope, and facilitating a positive long-term attitude toward recovery.

Regarding pain-associated sadness and grief, psychotherapeutic approaches should respond to the phase of grief (including grieving their injury) the patients are in, and their phase of recovery from injury. Such grief exacerbates pain, and may be triggered by loss of a close buddy, seeing children die, mass casualties, or terrorist attacks. Some bereaved patients will have prolonged grief disorder, newly proposed for DSM-V.[98] Prolonged grief disorder is distinguished from bereavement by causing impairment for at least 6 months with one of these three symptoms in criterion B, which is called "separation distress":

1. intrusive thoughts related to the deceased,
2. intense pangs of separation distress, and
3. distressingly strong yearnings for that which was lost.

These symptoms must occur daily or to an intense or disruptive degree. In addition, five of the following nine symptoms of criterion C, "cognitive, emotional, and behavioral symptoms," must be present daily or to an intense or disruptive degree:

1. confusion about one's role in life or diminished sense of self;
2. difficulty accepting the loss;
3. avoidance of reminders of the reality of the loss;
4. inability to trust others since the loss;
5. bitterness or anger related to the loss;
6. difficulty moving on with life;
7. numbness (absence of emotion) since the loss;
8. feeling that life is unfulfilling, empty, and meaningless since the loss; and
9. feeling stunned, dazed or shocked by the loss.

The duration must be at least 6 months from the onset of separation distress; it must cause clinically significant distress or impairment in social, occupational or other important areas of functioning; and lastly, it cannot be due to a substance, general medical condition, or other disorder. When present, family support is key to relieving pain, anxiety, and grief. Family understanding, coping, resilience, and capacity to support need to be assessed and reinforced. Provision of supports, including counseling and psychotropic medications where indicated, facilitates the capacity to care for the patient.

SPECIAL PROBLEMS

Ventilated Patient

Analgesia and sedation in the mechanically ventilated patient has the added factor of maintaining airway security and patient safety. The agitated patient will not only suffer emotionally, but may die if the endotracheal tube or vascular access devices are dislodged.[99] A "lightly asleep but arousable" state, or a Richmond Agitation-Sedation Score of -2, is a common objective when caring for intubated patients in the intensive care unit.

Burns and Multiple Traumas

Patients with burns and multiple traumas will have very large amounts of noxious stimulation associated with wounds and their management. The level of analgesic required can have adverse effects on respiratory and hemodynamic status. At times, these adverse effects must be accepted and managed (via mechanical ventilatory or vasopressor support or both) to ensure adequate patient comfort and safety. It is important that other potential causes of these problems (most commonly sepsis) be excluded.

Amputation Pain

Amputated limbs are a common cause of acute and chronic pain syndromes. It is important to distinguish acute surgical pain (eg, bone and soft-tissue pain) from neuropathic pain (eg, phantom pain), as pharmacological and nonpharmacological management strategies differ.[100]

Weaning

Most pain and anxiety medications stimulate receptor changes that mandate weaning if consequences of abrupt withdrawal are to be avoided.[101] Opiate withdrawal will cause tremulousness, autonomic hyperactivity, diarrhea, and emesis. Benzodiazepine withdrawal can result in seizures. Gradual weaning is well tolerated, with low rates of withdrawal symptoms or drug dependence, even when very high drug doses are used acutely.[102]

Pediatric Pain

Pain in children is treated according to similar principles to those outlined in this chapter, but with specific changes adapted to the pediatric population for body weight, any pediatric illnesses, developmental status, and dependency on parents and family.[10] Dosages are calculated on a milligram per kilogram basis, and treatment is modified if there is concomitant pediatric illness. The developmental status of the child—infant, toddler, school age, and adolescent—requires adaptation to the physical, mental, emotional, and relationship characteristics of those stages.

Psychiatric Risk Factors

The principal risk factors for pain complications include inadequate analgesia, delirium, unrecognized infection or injury, sleep disorders, preexisting psychopathology, self-inflicted injuries, prior addiction, PTSD or other anxiety disorder, emergent depression, somatoform disorders, and factitious disorder. Diagnosis and specific treatment of these conditions or disorders is essential to effectively manage the associated pain. Not all apparently psychological contributions to pain are that, and further diagnostic investigation is often warranted.

Pain Management and the Issue of Addiction

Prior addiction to or abuse of alcohol or other substances is very commonly associated with noncombat injuries, as is withdrawal from the drug of abuse, especially alcohol, during acute treatment of the injuries. As a result, treatment of all injuries should include a careful history of substance abuse, toxicology screening, ongoing evaluation of possible withdrawal, treatment of withdrawal symptoms, and interventions to reduce the risk of continuing addictive behavior posttreatment.[103]

THE ETHICS OF PAIN CONTROL

Pain control may become complicated. As noted above, inadequate relief of pain results in increased risk for adverse psychiatric sequelae and poorer outcomes. There is therefore an ethical obligation to relieve pain to reduce the likelihood of harm. Acutely, treatment of serious pain is occasionally complicated by excess sedation, respiratory depression, or hypotension. Over the longer term with chronic pain management, drug dependency can occur, particularly in patients who have been substance abusers. If, in the management of chronic pain, overuse of pain medication occurs or is perceived, serious medical complications may arise and could result in challenging medicolegal consequences. It is an ethical imperative that such risks, as well as those of undertreatment, are acknowledged, considered, and appropriately managed in formulating a sound treatment plan for the injured patient.[104–106]

SUMMARY

The objective of this chapter is to aid in improving management of acute or chronic pain from combat and noncombat wounds. It addresses the psychiatric implications of the control or elimination of injury pain, the wounds causing the worst pain, and differences in treating soldiers from civilians. Four case examples (of patients aged 4, 18, 26, and 55) that were presented with combat and noncombat injuries provide practical illustrations of the range of approaches to pain problems needing evaluation and treatment. Biological factors are presented that affect pain, including anatomic, genetic, and pharmacological considerations. A range of established and emerging treatments is described, and ways to assess whether or not analgesic requirements are met, underestimated, or exceeded are detailed. The problem of addictive behavior in the military must be considered both acutely, and later in care, but is not a contraindication to providing adequate pain relief. Approaches to pain from injury, surgery, dressings, amputation, and emotional causes are discussed. Pain caused by wounds and other injuries in military personnel and civilians is significant, and may trigger subsequent PTSD, depression, or behaviors associated with disability, especially in vulnerable individuals. Consistent with the medical team approach, as well as the authorship of this chapter, multidisciplinary collaboration of psychiatrists, surgeons, anesthesiologists, and allied personnel is key to optimal pain management.

REFERENCES

1. Wain HJ, Grammer GG, Stasinos J, DeBoer CM. Psychiatric intervention for medical and surgical patients following traumatic injuries. In: Ritchie EC, Friedman MJ, Watson PJ, eds. *Interventions Following Mass Violence and Disasters: Strategies for Mental Health Practice*. New York, NY: Guilford Press; 2006: 278–299.

2. Perry SW. Undermedication for pain on a burn unit. *Gen Hosp Psychiatry*. 1984;6:308–316.

3. Ely EW, Truman B, Shintani A, et al. Monitoring sedation status over time in ICU patients: reliability and validity of the Richmond Agitation-Sedation Scale (RASS). *JAMA*. 2003;289(22):2983–2991.

4. Stoddard FJ, Norman DK, Murphy JM. A diagnostic outcome study of children and adolescents with severe burns. *J Trauma*. 1989;29:471–477.

5. Schreiber S, Galai-Gat T. Uncontrolled pain following physical injury as the core-trauma in post-traumatic stress disorder. *Pain*. 1993;54:107–110.

6. Koren D, Hemel D, Klein E. Injury increases the risk for PTSD: an examination of potential neurobiological and psychological mediators. *CNS Spectr*. 2006;11(8):616–624.

7. Koren D, Norman D, Cohen A, Berman J, Klein EM. Increased PTSD risk with combat-related injury: a matched comparison study of injured and uninjured soldiers experiencing the same combat events. *Am J Psychiatry*. 2005;162:276–282.

8. Cassem NH, Murray GB, Lafayette JM, Stern TA. Delirious patients. In: Stern TA, Fricchione GL, Cassem NH, Jellinek MS, Rosenbaum JF, eds. *Massachusetts General Hospital Handbook of General Hospital Psychiatry*. 5th ed. Philadelphia, Penn: Mosby; 2004: 119–134.

9. Stoddard FJ, Martyn J, Sheridan R. Psychiatric issues in pain of burn injury. *Curr Rev Pain*. 1997;1(2):130–136.

10. Stoddard FJ, Sheridan RL, Saxe GN, et al. Treatment of pain in acutely burned children. *J Burn Care Rehabil*. 2002;23(2):135–156.

11. Stoddard FJ. Care of infants, children and adolescents with burn injuries. In: Lewis M, ed. *Child and Adolescent Psychiatry: A Comprehensive Textbook*. 3rd ed. Philadelphia, Penn: Lippincott Williams & Wilkins; 2002: 1188–1208.

12. Stoddard FJ, Levine JB, Lund K. Burn injuries. In: Blumenfield M, Strain JJ, eds. *Psychosomatic Medicine*. Philadelphia, Penn: Lippincott Williams & Wilkins; 2006: 309–336.

13. Winter H, Irle E. Hippocampal volume in adult burn patients with and without posttraumatic stress disorder. *Am J Psychiatry*. 2004;161:2194–2200.

14. Schechter N, Berde CB, Yaster M, eds. *Pain in Infants, Children and Adolescents*. 2nd ed. Philadelphia, Penn: Lippincott Williams & Wilkins; 2003.

15. Wall PD, Melzack R, eds. *Textbook of Pain*. 3rd ed. New York, NY: Churchill Livingstone; 1994.

16. Rasnake L, Linscheid TR. Anxiety reduction in children receiving medical care: developmental considerations. *J Dev Behav Pediatr*. 1989;10:169–175.

17. Kuttner L, Solomon R. Hypnotherapy and imagery for managing children's pain. In: Schechter NL, Berde CB, Yaster M, eds. *Pain in Infants, Children and Adolescents*. 2nd ed. Philadelphia, Penn: Lippincott Williams & Wilkins; 2003: 317–328.

18. Spiegel H, Spiegel D. *Trance and Treatment: Clinical Uses of Hypnosis*. 2nd ed. Washington, DC: American Psychiatric Press Inc; 2004.

19. Pandharipande P, Shintani A, Peterson J, et al. Lorazepam is an independent risk factor for transitioning to delirium in intensive care unit patients. *Anesthesiology*. 2006;104(1):21–26.

20. Abdi S, McPeek B. Pain in burn patients. In: Ballantyne JC, ed. *The Massachusetts General Hospital Handbook of Pain Management*. 3rd ed. Philadelphia, Penn: Lippincott Williams & Wilkins; 2006: 317–322.

21. Balboni TA, Gobezie R, Mamon HJ. Heterotopic ossification: pathophysiology, clinical features, and the role of radiotherapy for prophylaxis. *Int J Radiat Oncol Biol Physics*. 2006;65(5):1289–1299.

22. Esselman PC, Thombs BD, Magyar-Russell G, Fauerbach JR. Burn rehabilitation: state of the science. *Am J Phys Med Rehabil*. 2006;85(4):383–413.

23. Sherrington CS. *The Integrative Action of the Nervous System*. New York, NY: Scribner; 1906.

24. International Association for the Study of Pain. IASP pain terminology page. Available at: http://www.iasp-pain.org/AM/Template.cfm?Section=Pain_Definitions&Template=/CM/HTMLDisplay.cfm&ContentID=1728. Accessed September 26, 2008.

25. Hyman SE, Cassem NH: Pain. In: Rubenstein E, Federman DD, eds. *Scientific American Medicine, Current Topics in Medicine*. New York, NY: Scientific American; 1989: 1–17.

26. Stoddard FJ, Ronfeldt H, Kagan J, et al. Young burned children: the course of acute stress and physiological and behavioral responses. *Am J Psychiatry*. 2006;163:1084–1090.

27. Wain HJ, Cozza SJ, Grammer GG, et al. Treating the traumatized amputee. In: *Caring for the Clinicians Who Care for Traumatically Injured Patients: Iraq War Clinician Guide*. 2nd ed. Washington, DC: National Center for Posttraumatic Stress Disorder; 2004: Chap 8. Available at: http://www.ptsd.va.gov/professional/manuals/iraq-war-clinician-guide.asp. Accessed January 5, 2010.

28. Jessell TM, Kelly DD. Pain and analgesia. In: Kandel ER, Schwartz JH, Jessell TM, eds. *Principles of Neural Science*. Norwalk, Conn: Appleton and Lange; 1991: 385–399.

29. Baron R, Baron Y, Disbrow E, Roberts TP. Brain processing of capsaicin-induced secondary hyperalgesia: a functional MRI study. *Neurology*. 1999;53:548–557.

30. Lundell JC, Silverman DG, Brull SJ, et al. Reduction of postburn hyperalgesia after local injection of ketorolac in healthy volunteers. *Anesthesiology*. 1996;84:502–509.

31. Hardy JD, Wolff HG, Goodell H. Experimental evidence on the nature of cutaneous hyperalgesia. *J Clin Invest.*1950;29:115–140.

32. Warncke T, Stubhaug A, Jorum E. Preinjury treatment with morphine or ketamine inhibits the development of experimentally induced secondary hyperalgesia in man. *Pain*. 2000;86:293–303.

33. Treede RD, Magerl W. Multiple mechanisms of secondary hyperalgesia. *Prog Brain Res*. 2000;129:331–341.

34. Holthusen H, Irsfeld S, Lipfert P. Effect of pre- or post-traumatically applied i.v. lidocaine on primary and secondary hyperalgesia after experimental heat trauma in humans. *Pain*. 2000;88:295–302.

35. Pedersen JL, Kehlet H. Hyperalgesia in a human model of acute inflammatory pain: a methodological study. *Pain*. 1998;74(2–3):139–151.

36. Bartfai T. Immunology. Telling the brain about pain. *Nature*. 2001;410:425,427.

37. Samad TA, Moore KA, Sapirstein A, et al. Interleukin-1beta-mediated induction of Cox-2 in the CNS contributes to inflammatory pain hypersensitivity. *Nature*. 2001;410:471–475.

38. Wang S, Lim G, Yang L, et al. A rat model of unilateral hindpaw burn injury: slowly developing rightwards shift of the morphine dose-response curve. *Pain*. 2005;116:87–95.

39. Borsook D, Falkowski O, Rosen H, Comb M, Hyman SE. Opioids modulate stress-induced proenkephalin in the hypothalamus of transgenic mice: a model of endogenous opioid gene regulation by exogenous opioids. *J Neurosci.* 1994;14:7261–7271.

40. Hyman SE, Nestler EJ. Initiation and adaptation: a paradigm for understanding psychotropic drug action. *Am J Psychiatry*. 1996;153:151–162.

41. Angst MS, Clark JD. Opioid-induced hyperalgesia: a qualitative systematic review. *Anesthesiology*. 2006;104:570–587.

42. Eisenach JC. Preemptive hyperalgesia, not analgesia? *Anesthesiology*. 2000;92:308–309.

43. Liang DY, Liao G, Lighthall GK, Peltz G, Clark DJ. Genetic variants of the P-glycoprotein gene Abcb1b modulate opioid-induced hyperalgesia, tolerance and dependence. *Pharmacogenet Genomics*. 2006;16(11):825–835.

44. Vinik HR, Kissin I. Rapid development of tolerance to analgesia during remifentanil infusion in humans. *Anesth Analg*. 1998;86:1307–1311.

45. Shimoyama N, Shimoyama M, Inturrisi CE, Elliott KJ. Ketamine attenuates and reverses morphine tolerance in rodents. *Anesthesiology*. 1996;85:1357–1366.

46. Pandharipande PP, Pun BT, Herr DL, et al. Effect of sedation with dexmedetomidine vs lorazepam on acute brain dysfunction in mechanically ventilated patients: the MENDS randomized controlled trial. *JAMA*. 2007;298(22):2644–2653.

47. Dasta JF, Jacobi J, Sesti AM, McLaughlin TP. Addition of dexmedetomidine to standard sedation regimens after cardiac surgery: an outcomes analysis. *Pharmacotherapy*. 2006:26(6):798–805.

48. Chrysostomou C, Di Filippo S, Manrique AM, et al. Use of dexmedetomidine in children in cardiac and thoracic surgery. *Pediatr Crit Care Med*. 2006;7(2):126–131.

49. Petroz GC, Sikich N, James M, et al. A phase I, two-center study of the pharmacokinetics and pharmacodynamics of dexmedetomidine in children. *Anesthesiology*. 2006;105(6):1098–1110.

50. Gilron I, Bailey JM, Tu D, Holden RR, Weaver DF, Houlden RL. Morphine, gabapentin, or their combination for neuropathic pain. *N Engl J Med*. 2005;352:1324–1334.

51. Raja SN, Haythornthwaite JA. Combination therapy for neuropathic pain—which drugs, which combination, which patients? *N Engl J Med*. 2005;352:1373–1375.

52. Stoddard FJ, Saxe G. Ten-year research review of physical injuries. *J Am Acad Child Adolesc Psychiatry*. 2001;40(10):1128–1145.

53. Zatzick DF, Rivara FP, Nathens AB, et al. A nationwide US study of post-traumatic stress after hospitalization for physical injury. *Psychol Med*. 2007;37(10):1469–1480.

54. Kavanagh CK, Lasoff E, Eide Y, et al. Learned helplessness and the pediatric burn patient: dressing change behavior and serum cortisol and beta-endorphin. *Adv Pediatr*. 1991;38:335–363.

55. Charney DS, Deutch AY, Krystal JH, Southwick SM, Davis M. Psychobiologic mechanisms of posttraumatic stress disorder. *Arch Gen Psychiatry*. 1993;50:295–305.

56. van der Kolk BA. The body keeps the score: memory and the evolving psychobiology of posttraumatic stress. *Harv Rev Psychiatry*. 1994;1:253–265.

57. Thombs BD, Fauerbach JA, McCann UD. Stress disorders following traumatic injury: assessment and treatment considerations. *Primary Psychiatry*. 2005;12(3):51–55. Available at: http://www.primarypsychiatry.com/aspx/articledetail.aspx?articleid=319. Accessed September 29, 2008.

58. Saigh PA, Yasik AE, Sack WH, et al. Child-adolescent posttraumatic stress disorder: prevalence, risk factors, and comorbidity. In: Saigh PA, Brenner JD, eds. *Posttraumatic Stress Disorder: A Comprehensive Text*. Needham Heights, Mass: Allyn and Bacon; 1999: 18–43.

59. Davidson JR, Stein DJ, Shalev AY, Yehuda R. Posttraumatic stress disorder: acquisition, recognition, course, and treatment. *J Neuropsychiatry Clin Neurosci*. 2004;16:135–147.

60. American Psychiatric Association. *Diagnostic and Statistical Manual of Mental Disorders, Text Revision*. 4th ed. Washington, DC: APA Press; 2000.

61. Pynoos RS. Traumatic stress and developmental psychopathology in children and adolescents. In: Oldham JM, Riba MB, Tasman A, eds. *American Psychiatric Press Review of Psychiatry*. Vol 12. Washington, DC: American Psychiatric Publishing; 1993: 205–238.

62. Grieger TA, Cozza SJ, Ursano RJ, et al. Posttraumatic stress disorder and depression in battle-injured soldiers. *Am J Psychiatry*. 2006;163:1777–1783.

63. Shalev AY, Bonne O, Eth S. Treatment of posttraumatic stress disorder: a review. *Psychosom Med*. 1996;58:165–182.

64. Bisson JI, Shepherd JP, Joy D, Probert R, Newcombe RG. Early cognitive-behavioural therapy for post-traumatic stress symptoms after physical injury. Randomised controlled trial. *Br J Psychiatry*. 2004;184:63–69.

65. Saxe G, Stoddard F, Courtney D, et al. Relationship between acute morphine and the course of PTSD in children with burns. *J Am Acad Child Adolesc Psychiatry*. 2001;40:915–921.

66. Stoddard FJ Jr, Sorrentino EA, Ceranoglu TA, et al. Preliminary evidence for the effects of morphine on posttraumatic stress disorder symptoms in one- to four-year olds with burns. *J Burn Care Res*. 2009;30(5)836–843.

67. Pitman RK, Delahanty DL. Conceptually driven pharmacologic approaches to acute trauma. *CNS Spectr*. 2005;10(2):99–106.

68. Holbrook TL, Galarneau MS, Dye JL, Quinn K, Dougherty AL. Morphine use after combat injury in Iraq and post-traumatic stress disorder. *N Engl J Med*. 2010;362:110–117.

69. Stamer U, Bayerer B, Stüber F. Genetics, pain and analgesia [Review. German]. *Anaesthesist*. 2006;55:746–752.

70. Tegeder I, Costigan M, Griffin RS, et al. GTP cyclohydrolase and tetrahydrobiopterin regulate pain sensitivity and persistence. *Nat Med*. 2006;12:1269–1277.

71. Minde JK. Norrbottnian congenital insensitivity to pain. *Acta Orthop Suppl*. 2006;77:2–32.

72. Pasternak GW, Inturrisi CE. Feeling pain? Who's your daddy. . . . *Nat Med*. 2006;12(11):1243–1244.

73. Reyes-Gibby CC, Shete S, Rakvåg T, et al. Exploring joint effects of genes and the clinical efficacy of morphine for cancer pain: OPRM1 and COMT gene. *Pain*. 2007;130(1–2):25–30.

74. Nackley AG, Tan KS, Fecho K, Flood P, Diatchenko L, Maixner W. Catechol-O-methyltransferase inhibition increases pain sensitivity through activation of both beta2- and beta3-adrenergic receptors. *Pain*. 2007;128(3):199–208.

75. McGrath PA, Brigham MC. The assessment of pain in children and adolescents. In: Turk DC, Melzack R, eds. *Handbook of Pain Assessment*. New York, NY: Guilford Press; 1992: 295–314.

76. Wood AJ. Racial differences in the response to drugs—pointers to genetic differences. *N Engl J Med*. 2001;344:1394–1396.

77. Court MH, Hao Q, Krishnaswamy S, et al. UDP-glucuronosyltansferase (UGT) 2B15 pharmacogenetics: UGT2B15 D85Y genotype and gender are major determinants of oxazepam glucuronidation by human liver. *J Pharmacol Exp Ther*. 2004;310:656–665.

78. Martyn J. Clinical pharmacology and drug therapy in the burned patient. *Anesthesiology*. 1986;65:67–75.

79. Gaffney A, McGrath PJ, Dick B. Measuring pain in children: developmental and instrument issues. In: Schechter NL, Berde CB, Yaster M, eds. *Pain in Infants, Children, and Adolescents*. 2nd ed. Philadelphia, Penn: Lippincott Williams & Wilkins; 2003: 128–141.

80. Purcell-Jones G, Dormon F, Sumner E. Paediatric anaesthetists' perceptions of neonatal and infant pain. *Pain*. 1988;33:181–187.

81. Ekman P, Rosenberg EL, eds. *What the Face Reveals: Basic and Applied Studies of Spontaneous Expression Using the Facial Action Coding System* (FACS). New York, NY: Oxford University Press; 1997.

82. Fitzgerald M, Millard C, McIntosh N. Cutaneous hypersensitivity following peripheral tissue damage in newborn infants and its reversal with topical anesthesia. *Pain*. 1989;39:31–36.

83. Ambuel B, Hamlett KW, Marx CM, Blumer JL. Assessing distress in pediatric intensive-care environments: the COMFORT Scale. *J Pediatr Psychol*. 1992;17(1):95–109.

84. van Dijk M, de Boer JB, Koot HM, Tibboel D, Passchier J, Duivenvoorden HJ. The reliability and validity of the COMFORT scale as a postoperative pain instrument in 0 to 3-year-old infants. *Pain*. 2000;84:367–377.

85. Hester NO, Foster RL, Kristensen K. Measurement of pain in children: generalizability and validity of the pain ladder and the poker chip tool. In: Tyler DC, Krane EJ, eds. *Advances in Pain Research and Therapy. Pediatric Pain*. New York, NY: Raven Press; 1990: 79–84.

86. Bieri D, Reeve RA, Champion GD, Addicoat L, Ziegler JB. The Faces Pain Scale for the self-assessment of the severity of pain experienced by children: development, initial validation, and preliminary investigation for ratio scale properties. *Pain*. 1990;41:139–150.

87. Wallenstein SL. Scaling clinical pain and pain relief. In: Bromm B, ed. *Pain Measurement in Man: Neurophysiological Correlates of Pain*. New York, NY: Elsevier Science Publishers; 1984: 389–394.

88. Klemen P, Grmec S. Effect of pre-hospital advanced life support with rapid sequence intubation on outcome of severe traumatic brain injury. *Acta Anaesthesiol Scand*. 2006;50(10):1250–1254.

89. Sessler CN. Sedation scales in the ICU. *Chest*. 2004;126(6):1727–1730.

90. Sheridan RL, Hinson M, Nackel A, et al. Development of a pediatric burn pain and anxiety management program. *J Burn Care Rehabil*. 1997;18(5):455–459.

91. Grass JA. Patient-controlled analgesia. *Anesth Analg*. 2005;101(5 Suppl):S44–S61.

92. Grossi P, Urmey WF. Peripheral nerve blocks for anaesthesia and postoperative analgesia. *Curr Opin Anaesthesiol*. 2003;16(5):493–501.

93. Schug SA, Saunders D, Kurowski I, Paech MJ. Neuraxial drug administration: a review of treatment options for anaesthesia and analgesia. *CNS Drugs*. 2006;20(11):917–933.

94. Roganovic Z, Mandic-Gajic G. Pain syndromes after missile-caused peripheral nerve lesions: part 2—treatment. *Neurosurgery*. 2006;59(6):1238–1249.

95. Kwekkeboom KL, Herr K. Assessment of pain in the critically ill. *Crit Care Nurs Clin North Am*. 2001;13(2):181–194.

96. Hogarth DK, Hall J. Management of sedation in mechanically ventilated patients. *Curr Opin Crit Care*. 2004;10(1):40–46.

97. Adam C, Rosser D, Manji M. Impact of introducing a sedation management guideline in intensive care. *Anaesthesia*. 2006;61(3):260–263.

98. Zhang B, El-Jawahri A, Prigerson HG. Update on bereavement research: evidence-based guidelines of the diagnosis and treatment of complicated bereavement. *J Palliat Med*. 2006;9(5):1188–1203.

99. Krinsley JS, Barone JE. The drive to survive: unplanned extubation in the ICU. *Chest*. 2005;128(2):560–566.

100. Bosmans JC, Suurmeijer TP, Hulsink M, van der Schans CP, Geertzen JH, Dijkstra PU. Amputation, phantom pain and subjective well-being: a qualitative study. *Int J Rehabil Res*. 2007;30(1):1–8.

101. Cammarano WB, Pittet JF, Weitz S, Schlobohm RM, Marks JD. Acute withdrawal syndrome related to the administration of analgesic and sedative medications in adult intensive care unit patients. *Crit Care Med*. 1998;26(4):676–684.

102. Zapantis A, Leung S. Tolerance and withdrawal issues with sedation. *Crit Care Nurs Clin North Am*. 2005;17(3):211–223.

103. Findley JK, Park L. Psychiatric issues in trauma. In: Sheridan RL, ed. *The Trauma Handbook of the Massachusetts General Hospital*. Philadelphia, Penn: Lippincott Williams & Wilkins; 2004: 662–681.

104. Ballantyne JC. Opioids for chronic nonterminal pain. *South Med J*. 2006;99(11):1245–1255.

105. Magnusson RS. The devil's choice: re-thinking law, ethics, and symptom relief in palliative care. *J Law Med Ethics*. 2006;34(3):559–569, 481.

106. Green C, Todd KH, Lebovits A, Francis M. American Academy of Pain Medicine Council on Ethics. Disparities in pain: ethical issues. *Pain Med*. 2006;7(6):530–533.

Chapter 22

US ARMY OCCUPATIONAL THERAPY: PROMOTING OPTIMAL PERFORMANCE

MARY W. ERICKSON, MAOL, OTR/L*; TERESA L.BRININGER, PhD, CHT, OTR/L†; SHARON M. NEWTON, OTR/L, MHS‡; AMY M. MATTILA, MS, MBA§; AND JAMES P. BURNS, OTR/L, MOT¥

*Colonel, Individual Mobilization Augmentee, US Army Reserve; Chief, Occupational Therapy, Reintegration Branch Chief for the Proponency Office for Rehabilitation and Reintegration, Office of The Surgeon General, Falls Church, Virginia

†Lieutenant Colonel, Medical Specialist Corps, US Army; Deputy for Rehabilitation and Reintegration, Telemedicine and Advanced Technology Research Center, Medical Research and Materiel Command, 504 Scott Street, Building 722, Room 30, Fort Detrick, Maryland 21702

‡Lieutenant Colonel, Medical Specialist Corps, US Army; Command Inspector General, 30th Medical Command, CMR 442, APO AE 09042; formerly Theater Consultant for Combat and Operational Stress Control, Iraq

§Captain, Medical Specialist Corps, US Army; Chief, Department of Occupational Therapy, Reynolds Army Community Hospital, 4301 Wilson Street, Fort Sill, Oklahoma 73503; formerly, Chief, Occupational Therapy, 254th Medical Detachment (Combat Operational Stress Control), Germany

¥Major, Medical Specialist Corps, US Army; Occupational Therapist, Department of Orthopaedics and Rehabilitation, Building 2, Room 3J04, Walter Reed Army Medical Center, 6900 Georgia Avenue NW, Washington, DC 20307-5001; formerly, Chief Occupational Therapist, Department of Surgery, Fort Jackson, South Carolina

INTRODUCTION

Occupational therapy (OT) utilizes engagement in meaningful occupation (purposeful everyday tasks and activities that "occupy" one's time) to facilitate function and achieve a healthy and balanced lifestyle.[1,2] Early history records the use of activity, music, and games to assist with the recovery of mental health. In 172 CE, Galan wrote: "Employment is nature's best physician and is essential to human happiness."[3] The profession grew out of the moral treatment movement of the early 19th century, with a focus on compassion and occupation using manual labor such as agriculture, sewing, and tailoring to treat the insane.[4] The founders of OT in the United States came from a variety of backgrounds including psychiatry, social work, and architecture. Adolf Meyer, a psychiatrist, observed human behavior and habit in relation to the environment, writing

> the whole of human organization has its shape in a kind of rhythm...work and play and rest and sleep, which our organism must be able to balance even under difficulty. The only way to attain actual balance in all of this is actual doing, actual practice, a program of wholesome living as the basis of wholesome feeling and thinking and fancy of interests.[5]

During the 20th century, OT became closely aligned with treating wounded soldiers and sailors in response to the two world wars.[6(p158),7] Then, as now, the profession's foundation is the belief that occupation, or purposeful activity, is vital to regaining or maintaining the health of the entire person. This purposeful activity is graded according to the individual's ability. Furthermore, the philosophies of OT and treating service members with combat or operational stress reactions go hand-in-hand.[6]

The use of OT in the US military dates to World War I, when the US Civil Service Commission (precursor to the Office of Personnel Management) called for individuals trained in OT and other professions such as teachers and artists to serve as reconstruction aides in military hospitals. Early in 1918, the Surgeon General's Office began recruiting reconstruction aides to work with and treat service members who were wounded or suffered from battle neurosis to return to the battlefield. In February of that year, the Army's first trial of OT, occurring at Walter Reed Hospital, demonstrated its value in treating both the mind and the body of the wounded service member using occupation in the form of treatment: physically, to improve upper extremity function; and psychologically, to help prevent depression, control attention, and calm the wounded.[3(pp159–160)] By June 1918 the first OTs arrived at Base Hospital 117 in France, serving as civilians in the American Expeditionary Forces.[3]

During World War I, OT was established in Army hospitals for the reconditioning of convalescent soldiers by the Division of Physical Reconstruction within the Office of The Surgeon General, established in January 1918. Its intent was "through the use of mental and manual work, to restore to complete or maximum possible function, any military person disabled in line of duty."[7(p70)] The overall goal of the reconditioning program was to return soldiers to military duty in the highest state of physical and mental fitness in the shortest possible time. If disqualified for further military service, the aim of reconditioning was to return the soldier to civilian life in the best possible physical condition, "well oriented in the responsibilities of citizenship and prepared to adjust successfully to social and vocational pursuits."[8(p329)] The mission was accomplished by a coordinated program of educational reconditioning, physical reconditioning, and occupational therapy.

OCCUPATIONAL THERAPY IN WORLD WAR II

During World War II, OT grew in breadth and scope of practice in both physical medicine and neuropsychiatry. Programs developed to treat the physical and psychological injuries incorporated educational reconditioning, activity-based workshops, industrial therapy, and recreational therapy. OT carried out within physical medicine addressed "the restoration of physical function to impaired joints and muscles...seeking (1) improvement of the general physical condition, (2) the development of work tolerance through graded activity, and (3) stimulation of mental acuity through interesting occupation."[8(p344)] Occupational therapists' observations of behavior, attitude, and reactions of patients were extremely valuable to the medical team and were reported during interdisciplinary staff conferences. These regularly scheduled meetings helped staff to plan and adjust the overall treatment program as needed.

OT in the neuropsychiatric section was placed under the immediate direction of the psychiatrist. The goals of OT within neuropsychiatry were "(1) to guide mental attitudes into healthy channels, (2) to promote a desire to get well, (3) to restore self-confidence and a sense of security, (4) to substitute encouragement for discouragement, (5) to establish and maintain good work habits and (6) to afford opportunity for socialization."[8(p348)] General treatment principles used with neuropsychiatric patients included (*a*) quiet, soothing work to help calm patients; (*b*) noisy, active work to discharge tension; (*c*) responsible work to promote self-confidence; (*d*) simple, easily completed tasks for encouragement; (*e*) interesting, colorful work for stimulation; (*f*) absorbing, detailed tasks for improving concentration; and (*g*) group work for socialization.

OT's role in educational reconditioning included identifying the service members' goals and interests and providing valuable information for the establishment of individualized treatment programs. Essential components of the educational reconditioning program included OT laboratory shops that provided practical experience for patients following the completion of academic courses sponsored by the educational reconditioning program in fields such as photography, radio, electricity, and motor mechanics. The "noisy" shop was used for patients who needed to discharge tensions through work. Activities in the noisy shop included carpentry, metalworking, work with plastics, and printing. The "quiet" shop was used for patients who were easily distracted or disturbed by noise and included activities such as weaving, leatherworking, ceramics, and art. Patients confined to the ward participated in OT through the use of small handicrafts carried out under close supervision.

An industrial therapy program also emerged during World War II, in which occupational therapists organized therapeutic "industrial" assignments involving hospital maintenance. The program included identifying available job assignments by gathering information on each job title, duties required, physical and mental requirements, and work standards. The program successfully provided participants a balanced work program, helped maintenance personnel complete daily tasks, and provided therapeutic activity for a large number of patients while requiring few trained supervisors. It was designed as a transitional program to meet the work requirements of patients who had progressed beyond the need for specific therapy but could not yet return to full duty. The work activities improved

> general physical ability including muscle tone, strength, and joint motion, to combat the effects of prolonged hospitalization, to increase work tolerance, to re-establish work habits counteracting the effect of periods of mental and physical idleness and to stimulate mental alertness.[8(p352)]

Job task analysis was an essential component in the World War II reconditioning program. Occupational therapists analyzed jobs from both a physical and a psychological perspective, and subsequently identified a variety of job opportunities. Work areas utilized for reconditioning included the utility shop, motor pool, warehouse, post office, laundry, mess hall, supply department, administrative office, medical laboratory, photographic laboratory, orthopaedic shop, messenger service, drafting, landscaping, and gardening. The patients' clinical appointments and medical consultations took precedence over industrial work assignments, and high standards were maintained: work projects were not allowed to deteriorate into a source of "cheap labor," and the therapists ensured that the job task was appropriate for the soldiers' physical and mental capabilities.

Another OT effort was a recreational (or "diversional") program used "to divert the patient's mind from thinking of himself constantly, to provide for the constructive use of leisure time, to furnish opportunity for self-expression, to stimulate interests and sustain morale, to conserve initiative and maintain good work habits, to promote socialization by group activities and to improve general physical fitness by stimulating the appetite and the circulation."[8(pp353–354)] The Arts and Skills Corps, composed of craftspeople recruited and organized by the Red Cross; the "Gray Ladies," a group of volunteers assigned to hospital OT departments; and Women's Army Corps assistants expanded the reach of OT to include minor crafts such as model making, art, wood and soap carving, plastics, leatherwork, ceramics, fly-tying, and weaving. Shop programs included photography, radio and electrical work, motor mechanics, and the use of power equipment.[8(p355)] In 1947, the Army established the Women's Medical Specialist Corps under Public Law 36, 80th Congress, giving OTs a permanent military status. In 1955 the name was changed to the Army Medical Specialists Corps under Public Law 294, 84th Congress, reflecting the inclusion of men in the corps.[7(pp5,402)] Current Army OT policies and practices are built on the foundations established in World War II.

ARMY OCCUPATIONAL THERAPY IN THE 21ST CENTURY

Serving throughout the world in times of war and peace, Army occupational therapists (OTs, military occupational specialty [MOS] 65A) and military occupational therapy assistants (OTAs, MOS 68WN3) currently number over 200 in strength. The mission of OT in today's Army is to promote soldier readiness, healthy living, and optimal performance among all Department of Defense (DoD) beneficiaries using OT principles and practices (Exhibit 22-1). Army OTs incorporate best clinical practices and strive to deliver them in a timely and cost-efficient manner.[9]

Today, Army OT practitioners function as human performance experts whose innovative programs and services help to optimize soldier performance and readiness in both field and garrison settings. OTs treat a wide range of conditions with many soldiers impacted by both physical and psychological injuries. In addition to the behavioral health role of OT in combat and operational stress control (COSC) efforts, OTs provide neuromusculoskeletal evaluation and rehabilitation with an emphasis on the upper extremity; inpatient and outpatient rehabilitation, including specialty areas such as cognitive rehabilitation, community reintegration, driving rehabilitation, and burn care; neurology and orthopaedics; ergonomics, including the development of strategies to prevent injuries and decrease human and economic costs of injuries in the DoD; peak performance training; use of assistive

EXHIBIT 22-1

US ARMY OCCUPATIONAL THERAPY SCOPE OF PRACTICE

The unique role of occupational therapy (OT) emphasizes the enhancing of each individual's performance in his or her various life roles (ie, soldier, worker, parent, student, and retiree). Occupational therapy's services are designed to respond to soldier, patient, family, and military organizational needs and expectations. Army OT helps prevent dysfunction, promotes and develops healthy lifestyles, and facilitates adaptation and recovery. Army OT helps the wounded, injured, or ill adapt daily occupations and routines in the areas of self-care, home management, community participation, education, work, and/or leisure activities. New Army OT initiatives include standardization of a military-specific Functional Capacity Evaluation, driving rehabilitation including the use of driving simulation, animal-assisted therapy, warrior goal-setting training, and use of a toolkit to evaluate and treat concussion/mild traumatic brain injury.

Occupational therapy's scope in the provision of services encompasses the following:

- **Military readiness.** All services provided to the soldier population target optimized effective performance, prevention, and expeditious return to duty following medical or psychological conditions.
- **Priority of care** is directed to the soldier to assist in maintaining his or her highest level of performance and ensure fitness to fight.
- **Prevention and wellness.** Includes screening and health promotion interventions to maintain and promote effective performance of soldiers and Department of Defense beneficiaries.
- **Combat stress prevention and intervention** in the combat environment and in stability and support operations.
- **Unit consultation** to promote psychosocial well-being, including ergonomic evaluation, training, and work-site analysis; identification of and ergonomic intervention for conditions where the etiology is physical or stress-related.
- **Support of humanitarian missions** in the primary care role for upper extremity neuromuscular screening or stress prevention and intervention.
- **Direct patient care** may include but is not limited to basic and advanced self-care (activities of daily living) evaluation and training. Training emphasizes regaining and sustaining functional performance while developing and improving diverse, complex skills including problem-solving and decision-making capabilities.
- **Psychosocial treatment** with emphasis on functional performance in various life roles through insight development, skill acquisition, education, and treatment programs.
- **Work reintegration,** including ergonomic analysis, fit-for-duty programs, and injury prevention and training that keep workers on the job, reduce costs, and improve productivity. Programs that promote work behaviors for improved physical and psychological performance include stress, coping, and life skills education programs.
- **Evaluation and treatment of upper extremity conditions**, including upper extremity neuromusculoskeletal evaluations in support of the orthopaedic physician.
- **Orthotic (splint) fabrication**. Adaptive technology evaluation and recommendations for, or fabrication of, equipment.
- **Developmental pediatric evaluation and treatment** (at specified treatment facilities).

technology; and work reintegration programs within warrior transition units (WTUs). Recognizing the psychological as well as functional value of early return to wearing the uniform following injury, OTs helped develop the Army's Wounded Warrior Clothing Support Program in 2008, which authorizes the wear of uniforms with adaptations/modifications prescribed by OTs or other rehabilitation specialists. Additionally, Army OTs serve in dedicated research positions as well as academic appointments.

Emerging OT practice areas include pilot programs in brigade combat teams to treat individuals with traumatic brain injury, animal-assisted therapy and animal-assisted activities in COSC units, and service-dog training programs. Creative partnerships with 501(c)(3) (nonprofit) organizations have produced successful service-dog training programs. For instance, initial service-dog training may be conducted within a civilian prison with specialized service-dog skills training conducted as part of a WTU work therapy program to prepare future service dogs to meet the unique needs of wounded soldiers. OTs are involved in a growing use of therapeutic riding programs as well. An integrated process team consisting of OTs, veterinarians, and behavioral health specialists is addressing principles and standards, and updating policies related to the human-animal bond.

Army Occupational Therapy Credentials and Training

Army OT practitioners, who serve in command and executive positions throughout the Army Medical Department, must be versatile, competent leaders to successfully operate and manage clinic operations in both deployed and garrison environments. Army OTs are credentialed healthcare providers and, as commissioned officers, they require National Board for Certification in Occupational Therapy (NBCOT) registration and a current, active, valid, and unrestricted OT license from a US state or jurisdiction. Currently, OT recruits entering the Army with a master's degree in OT will be able to earn a doctorate of science in occupational therapy (DSCOT). The DSCOT program and the enlisted 68WN3 OTA program are taught at the Army Medical Department Center and School at Fort Sam Houston in San Antonio, Texas. As of 2010, Army OTAs are required to obtain NBCOT national certification and state licensure. Civilian OTs working within a military setting must be registered by NBCOT and licensed according to the regulatory requirements of the state in which they are practicing.[9] Civilian OTAs are required to take the NBCOT examination and be credentialed as a certified occupational therapy assistant (COTA) with licensure according to the regulatory requirements of the state in which they are practicing.

Role of Occupational Therapy Assistants

OTAs are specialists who bring the perspective of the enlisted soldier to the therapeutic process by assisting the supervising OT in evaluating a service member's occupational performance; conducting initial occupational performance history interviews and mental status evaluations; using observation to gather data as part of task-performance skill assessments; and implementing OT interventions under the supervision of a credentialed OT. OTAs coordinate, set up, and oversee work hardening sites; lead OT groups; and monitor, facilitate, and supervise therapeutic activities. The OTA supervises combat and operational stress reaction casualties, provides status updates for these casualties, and conducts classes on selected stress-related topics. OTAs assist in all COSC functional areas including unit needs assessments and traumatic event management in the deployed environment.

Overview of Occupational Therapy Services in Combat and Operational Stress Control

The role of the OT practitioner in Army COSC is to evaluate occupational performance and implement interventions to enhance that performance.[6] OT's unique core skills are aimed at keeping soldiers able to perform their mission and include

- analysis of jobs and job tasks for underlying requisites (required subtasks, performance standards, equipment used, the social and physical work environment, occupational hazards);
- assessment of occupational performance (functional abilities) relating to specific tasks and jobs;
- configuration of a therapeutic, structured environment in which skills can be developed;
- analysis, selection, and application of occupations (activities) as therapeutic media; and
- the ability to match the individual to tasks he or she can successfully perform.[2(p22),6,7]

Army OTs evaluate soldier performance across the spectrum of occupational areas including activities of daily living, work, education, leisure, and social participation. The OT, or a COSC team member under the guidance of the OT, selects therapeutic occupations (purposeful activities) based on the soldier's current functional ability that support maintaining the soldier's military identity, enhances the soldier's sense of competence, and restores confidence. OTs perform task analysis and functional assessments, structure a therapeutic environment, provide occupation-based treatment, and match soldiers' abilities to the tasks or jobs they can perform. OTs also identify and evaluate mental and physical stressors, stress reactions, and cognitive function. They subsequently develop a treatment plan, which often includes teaching prevention, adaptive coping, and psychosocial skills. Additionally, they utilize therapeutic media and therapeutic use of self within individual and group settings to enhance environmental adaptation and maximize treatment.[10(pp3–8)] Army OTs integrate their diverse training in upper extremity orthopaedics, rehabilitation, ergonomics, and COSC techniques to identify areas of need for both individual soldiers and organizational units. Functional assessments include analysis of skills required by the soldier's MOS, identification of tasks the soldier can perform, and synthesis of therapeutic occupations. Interventions such as "work hardening for Warriors" involve occupation-based treatment that matches the soldier's functional ability with therapeutic occupations that he or she can perform.

OT groups engage in work activities, cognitive and sensorimotor activities, activities that parallel task-performance skills, cooperative activities, expressive arts, and exercise. Psychoeducational training may include selected common and collective soldier tasks or life skills such as stress management, relaxation skills, sleep hygiene, anger management, communication skills, problem solving, assertiveness training, and time management. Therapeutic activities of daily living may include personal hygiene and uniform maintenance; work/productive activities may include military-relevant tasks such as vehicle or site maintenance; and social and leisure activities may include cooperative or competitive sports, games, ceremonies, or celebrations. Therapeutic occupations are graded to offer challenges that are "just right" for each individual, leading to successful performance that instills competence and confidence. The soldier then gradually improves his or her functional capacity and ability to return to duty.[10(pp10–12)]

OT personnel also provide services as members of fitness teams and preventive teams in the delivery of behavioral health services in a deployed setting. The OT's role in a preventive team is the same as the other team members: providing outreach services through establishing rapport with supported units and leaders, assessing unit needs, and making regular contacts with supported units. An OT approaches these tasks from a unique perspective of assessing and addressing functional performance. The OT evaluates a soldier's current level of functional performance in a deployed environment. OTs also assess how psychological and cognitive function impacts task performance. They draw from a battery of standardized assessments that can help identify the presence of a combat and operational stress reaction, behavioral health problem, or traumatic brain injury. Collaborating with the rest of the team, the OT assimilates this information in determining the appropriate interventions, referrals, or other necessary action. For example, the OT may find that the best intervention is to restructure the soldier's job or environment to ensure successful completion of a task. Interventions often involve educating both the soldiers and their leaders.

Observation is one of the tools the OT uses to assess function. Observation can be especially valuable while conducting outreach visits. While performing "walk-abouts" within the area of operation, OTs work alongside soldiers and use their expertise to help them retain the functional ability to perform their mission. By working alongside soldiers, OTs can observe how each soldier is functioning and assess the mental or physical demands required to complete a particular job. Using this knowledge, the OT can begin to identify potential problems in task performance and intervene before problems escalate. For example, during Operation Iraqi Freedom (OIF) I (2003), an OT on the preventive team helped prepare and serve a meal in a mobile kitchen trailer. The OT talked casually with soldiers preparing the meal, getting a better idea of how they were dealing with the stress of operations. Additional stressors quickly presented themselves: working in a hot, crowded kitchen and dealing with large numbers of flies. Even the manner in which the food on the serving line was placed created physical stress. The OT provided suggestions for a more efficient and safer order of food trays, and adjusted the height of a work surface for one of the soldiers so she could more easily reach it. An added bonus was getting a glimpse into the basic cognitive function and general mood of hundreds of soldiers as they filed past the serving line.

The OT's observation skills are helpful when performing a unit needs assessment through evaluating the occupational performance needs of individuals in the unit. OTs identify component factors that are essential to successful performance. They may also assess the behavioral health training needs of soldiers, leaders, the unit ministry team, and other medical personnel within the unit. This may lead to additional interventions to enhance occupational performance and the development of plans to meet the future COSC needs of soldiers and units based on prevention and early intervention.

To enhance the provision of COSC services, Army OT practitioners utilize their background and training in upper extremity orthopaedics, rehabilitation, and ergonomics in both garrison and theater. Since the early 1980s, OTs have proposed and participated in programs designed to promote the soldier's job performance in garrison.[6(p56)] Occupational therapists have been included in missions to Bosnia-Herzegovina, Peru, and Russia, to name a few. The global war on terror continues to provide opportunities for OTs to utilize their unique skills to promote the health and welfare of service members. OTs have deployed to Afghanistan and Guantanamo Bay in support of Operation Enduring Freedom. In the Iraq and Afghanistan theaters of operations, they offer OT services to US and Coalition military members, national security forces and civilians, and the detainee population. OT practitioners within WTUs help meet the needs of injured, ill, and wounded soldiers through a focus on life skills training and work reintegration. OT personnel were also involved in the development of regional Army Reserve COSC programs on the home front.

AN INTEGRATED ARMY RESERVE REGIONAL COMBAT AND OPERATIONAL STRESS CONTROL PROGRAM

Identifying the need for home-front support as large numbers of Army Reserve soldiers began to deploy in 2003, the commanding general from the 88th Regional Readiness Command (RRC) initiated a COSC program for Army Reserve soldiers and their families within a six-state region in the upper Midwest (Minnesota, Wisconsin, Ohio, Michigan, Indiana, and Illinois). Two COSC officers from the 785th Medical Company (Combat Stress Control) were mobilized (an OT and a social work officer) to initiate a deployment cycle support program. From the inception of the program, the team used an interdisciplinary psychoeducational approach to help build resiliency and coping skills in soldiers and their families (Figure 22-1; Table 22-1). When available, Reserve component behavioral health specialists within the region augmented the team to provide local support. In 2005, a psychiatric nurse was mobilized to enhance the capabilities of the 88th RRC COSC team.

The COSC team established a strong working relationship with the other RRC elements that had direct roles in preparing and supporting deploying soldiers and their families. Program staff brought together representatives from family readiness groups; the chaplain's, public affairs, and casualty affairs offices; and the RRC leadership to establish an integrated approach to meet the comprehensive needs of soldiers and families. A multilevel needs assessment was conducted to identify capabilities, needs, and resources for soldiers, leaders, and families throughout the region. The implementation of an integrated operational stress management program was seen as an essential element in producing secure and resilient soldiers with families prepared to withstand the rigors of military separation, combat operations, and the more routine stressors common to the military lifestyle. The COSC team explained to unit leaders that its mission is to keep their soldiers with them, doing their jobs through programs designed to promote resiliency in the workplace, the family, and the community.

Through a series of meetings and site visits a plan of operation emerged. The plan included the provision of information to leaders, soldiers, and family members as well as other regional military and civilian organizations. The team's goal was rapid response: to provide soldiers and their families with educational, spiritual, and psychological resources to strengthen the basic bonds essential to high morale and good order. The expected outcomes included mission-capable soldiers and self-reliant families who were stress resilient, confident, secure, supported, and healthy (physically,

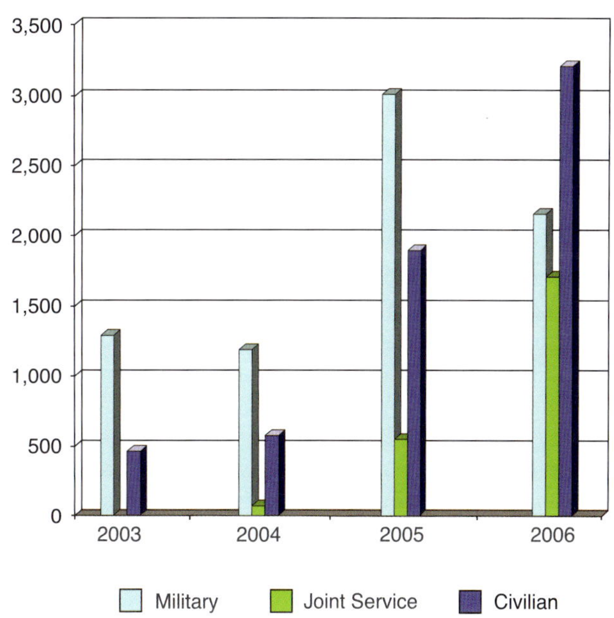

Figure 22-1. 88th Regional Readiness Command educational stress briefings, numbers of participants, 2003–2007.

TABLE 22-1

88TH REGIONAL READINESS COMMAND COMBAT AND OPERATIONAL STRESS CONTROL PROGRAM: ACTIVITY SUMMARY, APRIL 2003–DECEMBER 2006

COSC Briefings*		Individual Counseling	
Mobilization (soldiers/families)	13,398	Soldier/family and stress/PTSD issues	2,363
Midcycle (families)	4,826	Bereavement support (ie, funeral, follow-up, etc)	496
Homecoming (families/friends)	13,839	Well-being (acupuncture and therapeutic massage)	1,901
Reconstitution support (first postdeployment drill)	8,541	PREP couples' support†	934
SRP training	28,247	Marriage/relationship‡	228
Educational stress briefings			
Community groups	6,045		
Military groups	7,548		
Other military (NG, Navy, etc)	2,258		

*Number of participants
†Marriage retreat. No program participation in 2006
‡Single soldier retreat
COSC: combat and operational stress control
NG: National Guard
PREP: Prevention and Relationship Enhancement Program
PTSD: posttraumatic stress disorder
SRP: Soldier Readiness Program

emotionally, psychologically, and spiritually). Soldiers departing for extended missions would have confidence that their families were prepared and supported, and would be more likely to resist the debilitating effects of long-term operational stress. Families who knew their soldiers had a solid base of preparation and training would feel more secure sending them out to serve and would be more likely to support a soldier's decision to make the Army a career. Outcome measures were based on assessments of physical, social, and environmental factors with direct and indirect feedback from soldiers, family members, and leaders. Metrics included the number of training sessions conducted, attendees at each, individual consultations and follow-up referrals, and requests for further information and training sessions, as well as feedback on the effectiveness of the educational material including handouts, presentations, and resources provided.

Training (including informational briefings), command consultation and support, and referral were core features of the program. Crisis intervention, sexual assault prevention and advocacy programs, suicide prevention training and briefings, and grief-counseling support were also incorporated. Family stress support services included community outreach programs and collaborative programs with other branches of the military. For instance, Army Reserve family readiness groups (FRGs) "adopted" family members of service members from other components of the military who were living within their local area.

Training for leaders and soldiers included prevention, identification, and management of combat and high-intensity training stressors and battle-fatigue–related injuries (Exhibit 22-2). The training covered stress reduction techniques, predeployment "hardening," anger management, suicide prevention, sexual assault prevention training, first responder (unit level) training in combat stress control, and buddy aid. The team provided briefings for soldiers and family members, addressing predeployment stressors and coping techniques, midcycle issues related to rest and recuperation visits by soldiers halfway through their deployment, redeployment (reunification) stressors and coping techniques, and reconstitution issues including reestablishing family roles and relationships, anger management, operational stress reactions, traumatic brain injury, and posttraumatic stress disorder. Family stress support services included direct and indirect (consultation support) services to help families develop stress coping skills, address couple dynamics, deal with children's issues, and prepare for reunification. The team worked closely with FRGs following the loss or severe injury of unit members. Linking FRGs with Reserve combat stress control assets and other military, veteran, and community-based resources was a significant part of the COSC team's role.

A well-being program was established at the RRC Headquarters to provide a variety of self-care services teaching leaders, soldiers, and contract personnel ways to build personal coping skills and resiliency. Inte-

EXHIBIT 22-2

88TH REGIONAL READINESS COMMAND COMBAT AND OPERATIONAL STRESS CONTROL TEAM FIRST RESPONDER TRAINING

1. **MISSION**. The Combat Operational Stress Control Team (COSC) of the 88th Regional Readiness Command Surgeon's office will conduct **Operational Stress Control First Responder Training** for Command-designated representatives from subordinate units in support of Department of Defense Directive 6490.5 (Combat Stress Control [CSC] Programs) JP-1-02, Force Protection.
2. **EXECUTION**.

   a. **Intent**: Prepare Soldiers / leaders within the USAR in basic principles of Combat Operational Stress Control to enhance force protection and improve Soldier readiness in support of Contingency Operations. Embedding Soldiers and FRG representatives knowledgeable in COSC into each unit will enhance early recognition, intervention / referral with stress issues that often result in problems that may affect unit efficiency and degrade the quality of life of soldiers and their families. It is assumed that this trained group of first responders will maintain contact with a COSC team and their commands on a regular and as-needed basis.

   b. **Concept of Training**. Conduct 2½-day course with training consisting of Power Point slide presentations, video, handouts and role-playing to familiarize non-medical Soldiers with concepts of operational stress and battle fatigue. A team consisting of operational stress control personnel and chaplains will conduct the training. Both a pre- and a post-test will be administered in order to evaluate the effectiveness of the training. (Training Annex W)
3. **CONCEPT OF OPERATIONS**. To train the participants in the following topics.

   a. Basic combat operational stress principles

   b. Emotional cycles of deployment

   c. Identifying and responding to individuals with suicidal and homicidal behaviors

   d. Recognizing and responding to:
   - aggression
   - domestic violence
   - depression
   - posttraumatic stress disorder
   - combat stress reactions and battle fatigue
   - methods of deescalating potentially dangerous situations
   - sexual assault prevention and identifying sexual harassment

   e. Available military, VA, civilian and other resources—how to access and use them

COSC: combat and operational stress control
USAR: US Army Reserves
VA: Department of Veterans Affairs
Data source: 88th Regional Readiness Command Headquarters, Surgeon's Office, Fort Snelling, Minnesota.

grative healthcare providers from the civilian sector volunteered their services to provide a variety of self-care techniques including seated chair massage, acupuncture, guided imagery, healing touch, reflexology, Reiki, aroma therapy, and relaxation skills training. Information on a variety of stress management topics was provided in the form of brochures, handouts, computer disks, and posters. Topics included but were not limited to information on stress and anger management, sleep hygiene, communication skills, parenting, transitioning, suicide prevention, brain injury, and posttraumatic stress, with resources from Military OneSource, the Brain Injury Association, Veterans Affairs (VA), chaplains, and the Public Health Command (Provisional), formerly the US Army's Center for Health Promotion and Preventive Medicine. Personnel who participated in the program reported decreased pain and stress levels and increased awareness of stress management techniques.

The 88th RRC sustained the highest number of Army Reserve soldiers killed in action during the early part of the war. The COSC team worked closely with chaplains, public affairs staff, and casualty affairs personnel to establish strong support networks for grieving families, units, and communities. The team addressed the topic of grief and loss at the leadership, FRG, and soldier level. Frequently accompanying the chaplain, public affairs office, and the funeral honors team, the COSC officer provided support to the family, unit leadership, and other unit members and their families, as well as the honors team. In specific instances, COSC team members met with FRGs to provide bereavement support and education on ways to deal with loss. For instance, while five sisters anxiously awaited the beginning of their brother's memorial service, the OT taught them some simple relaxation skills for self-calming. The family reported later how much those simple techniques helped them get through that difficult time. During a funeral, one of the honors team members was having a hard time standing still for his 20-minute rotation. A few minutes spent helping him refocus and practice some simple breathing techniques allowed him to successfully manage the task. In another case, the COSC team provided bereavement support for family members during an FRG meeting following the battlefield death of one of the soldiers. They discussed factors involved in grief and loss including the associated fear of having a loved one still in harm's way, taught self-care techniques for adults and children, and explained how to locate resources for additional support. Following the educational part of the meeting, families shared a potluck meal, local massage therapists provided "pro bono" seated chair massage, and families participated in structured leisure activities while socially engaging with one another within a safe environment. The COSC team provided one-on-one consultation support during this time. Throughout the remainder of the unit's deployment the team provided periodic support to the FRG.

Located in a predominately civilian region, outreach to civilian organizations within the 88th RRC was vital to help the community understand the unique and changing culture of the citizen soldier (the next-door neighbor, coworker, or church member serving as a Reservist). A concerted effort was launched in partnership with the National Guard, VA, and veterans' service organizations to address the reintegration of soldiers into the workplace and community following their return home. Briefings were prepared to meet the individual needs of employers, community groups, and faith-based groups. For instance, OT staff developed briefing material to alert leaders, units, and care providers about the impact of traumatic brain injury, combat stress reactions, and posttraumatic stress disorder.

Community outreach presentations on a regional, state, and national level also provided training and workshops for civilian healthcare workers. Law enforcement training was provided through interagency partnerships. State-based postdeployment healthcare collaborations were supported by the COSC teams in Wisconsin, Ohio (Ohio Cares), and Minnesota (postdeployment collaboration with the VA, DoD, and community health professionals). The team provided training for both Minnesota and North Dakota county veterans' service officers, helping the officers to understand the changing culture and needs of redeployed soldiers and refer them to the appropriate level of services.

College and university presentations focused on the needs of returning combat veterans in the classroom, the needs of families and friends of a combat veterans, and resources available to returning veterans. The state of Minnesota allocated funds for the state college and university consortium to establish campus-based veterans' transition centers. Veterans were encouraged to utilize the services of these centers to identify "battle buddies" as they returned to college living and to focus on formation of attitudes and behaviors to promote success in their college experience. A county library donated thousands of books for deploying troops at Soldier Readiness Processing centers as well as their families to provide constructive diversion from deployment cycle stress. Exhibit 22-3 describes the types of soldier and family briefings provided throughout the deployment cycle.

OCCUPATIONAL THERAPY IN SUPPORT OF OPERATION IRAQI FREEDOM DETAINEE HEALTHCARE

US Army combat support hospitals are responsible for providing quality healthcare with dignity and respect to Iraqi civilians as well as detained insurgents. Individuals with acute injuries can be admitted day and night in an intensive combat environment. Patients on detained status are required to live in the theater internment facility while they receive medical treatment. A dynamic and multifaceted rehabilitation program is necessary not only for the improvement of patients' performance in all areas of occupation, but also to enhance their functional outcomes. The goal is for the patient to achieve a functional level sufficient for discharge in a facility with a rapid turnover rate.

Patients admitted to a combat support hospital have often sustained polytrauma, which can include

EXHIBIT 22-3

88TH REGIONAL READINESS COMMAND COMBAT AND OPERATIONAL STRESS CONTROL TEAM DEPLOYMENT CYCLE SUPPORT BRIEFINGS

Deployment cycle support briefings are the single most important mechanism for establishing rapport with soldiers and family members. Through these briefings, soldiers and family members learn about the effects of chronic stress on the body and on performance. A significant element in all the presentations is improving communication skills: a factual presentation of the negative results of poor communication is given, followed by suggestions for developing positive communication skills. Effects of the deployment cycle on children and significant others are also presented.

Soldier readiness processing briefings consist of 30-minute slide presentation that alerts soldiers to the need to prepare themselves and their families for deployment. Briefings discuss preparation in terms of Preventative Maintenance Checks and Services (PMCS; a routine personal self-care program to maintain mission capability) and stress the need to start working on communication skills and problems before the soldier is mobilized.

Premobilization briefings consist of a 45-minute slide presentation describing the ramp-up to deployment and the effect this process has on soldiers, their spouses and significant others, and the children. Handouts are used to reinforce the briefings.

Mid-cycle briefings are presented to members of a family readiness group. The loosely structured briefings are used to answer questions and allay fears that have become burdens to family members and children, and may include one-on-one talks with individuals with specific questions. Most of the issues revolve around communication. Handouts are used to reinforce the briefings.

Demobilization briefings are ideally presented to family members and interested others 2 to 4 weeks before the soldiers return home; however, they are usually presented the same day the soldiers return. The slide presentations used at homecoming try to cover a range of issues from readjustment of roles to intimacy issues. Handouts are used to reinforce the material.

Reconstitution briefings are directed sessions of teaching followed by small group and one-on-one discussions on issues that have come up since the soldiers' return. Issues include operational stress reactions, posttraumatic stress reactions, and marital and parenting problems. A slide presentation can be used to present issues, but often this briefing takes the form of a more relaxed and unstructured conversation. Handouts are used to reinforce the material.

Data source: 88th Regional Readiness Command Headquarters, Surgeon's Office, Fort Snelling, Minnesota.

many orthopaedic or neurological deficits. OT staff members critically observe and analyze patients to determine a baseline performance for motor, cognitive, and communication skills. OTs and OTAs then work with patients to reconcile the changes to their bodies by empowering them to establish new habits, routines, and roles to maximize performance during daily activities. The model of human occupation frame of reference provides theoretical guidance to OT staff working with detainees, aimed at enabling inpatients to make order out of the disorder that they are experiencing.[11] Active involvement in improving health and learned wellness are two key constructs of the model that are directly applied to detainee healthcare. Detainees may not readily expect to take an active approach in their own recovery process; therefore, adding a patient education piece to other aspects of healthcare service delivery is an important aspect of recovery. Patients must cope with the transition from the status of "detained patient" to an ordinary "detainee" upon discharge. Detainees are expected to perform the activities of daily living requirements independently in the internment facility.

Cultural differences bring particular challenges to detainee care. Many detained patients do not speak English, necessitating interpreters. In addition, gender roles within the Muslim culture are significantly different than Americans are accustomed to; for example, the expectation of taking direction from primarily female nurses can pose difficulty for male patients raised in a male-dominated society. If a detainee is having difficulty complying with medical instructions from staff, the OT may become involved. The therapist would work with the detainee to facilitate understanding of the benefits of inpatient care using the *listen, learn, and comply* approach: the OT explains that it is the patient's responsibility to listen to directives put forth by the staff to maximize the benefit of multidisciplinary healthcare. For patients to take responsibility for the personal management of their own health, patient education about the injury or illness is imperative. Patient compliance is necessary because the staff must meet the needs of the other patients in a timely manner.

PEAK PERFORMANCE TRAINING IN OCCUPATIONAL THERAPY

The concept of peak performance, developed originally at the US Military Academy's Center for Enhanced Performance and currently used by Army OTs, is derived from "mental toughness training to develop the Army pentathlete."[12] It is based on the principle that Army leaders must be self-aware, mentally agile, and adaptive. Peak performance has been described as "sports psychology taken to the battlefield" in that the core components rely on human performance and behavior, but the thought–performance interaction is essential in successfully completing warrior tasks. A mental imagery research study found that mental imagery (imagining squeezing an immobilized hand without performing any movement) might be of benefit in preventing strength loss during immobilization.[13] OTs have successfully utilized peak performance training with Operation Iraqi Freedom/Enduring Freedom patients, specifically in combat stress casualties or those diagnosed with posttraumatic stress disorder. Peak performance techniques decrease recovery time and prepare individuals for success both physically and mentally in returning to their respective areas of expertise. The OT uses peak performance concepts to help maximize soldiers' physical, mental, and emotional performance during periods of temporary or permanent life changes following illness or injury. Through their knowledge of human factors, occupational performance, and occupational adaptation, OTs help soldiers build their performance capabilities in overcoming physical, cognitive, and emotional challenges posed by illness or injury.

The five core foundations of peak performance are (1) a cognitive foundation, (2) attention control, (3) goal setting, (4) stress and energy management, and (5) visualization and imagery. Improving skills related to each of the five components ultimately leads to optimizing mental agility and performance. An example of an effective therapeutic intervention derived from peak performance training is the use of guided imagery and relaxation. Guided imagery involves using a series of thoughts or suggestions to direct a person's mental focus toward a more relaxed state. Nightingale[14] suggested various ways that imagery could be used for counseling, such as motivation by imagining a positive future, insight through exploration of possibilities, and problem solving. In warrior training and rehabilitation programs, OT services are conducted by an OT and an OTA. The OTA conducts the group program and implements orthopaedic treatments, while the OT completes individual evaluations and treatment sessions.

Peak performance training has been implemented in the form of group intervention, 1 hour per week for 6 weeks. The OT staff facilitates a group addressing the following six topics: (1) goal setting, (2) stress and energy management, (3) visualization and imagery, (4) confidence, (5) attention control, and (6) anger management. To foster esprit de corps, the soldiers in the program develop a unit creed while participating. Group interventions focus on enhancing the thought–performance interaction to maximize performance outcomes. For example, one group might focus on recognizing physiological changes such as skin temperature, heart rate, and muscle tension while experiencing both physical and mental stressors to allow participants to experience physical manifestations of stress. Participants would then implement steps to enhance performance in this stressful environment. Both negative and positive self-fulfilling prophecies can ultimately affect performance on any given event, not only during the training but also in many settings throughout soldiers' lives. These core areas are essential to enhancing soldier performance and can ultimately be applied to either battlefield or garrison environments.

Individual peak performance training augments group topics to develop the skills necessary for successful performance. Soldiers can choose goal setting and/or stress management for their care plan. During goal setting, the soldier develops personal goals ranging from graduating from the Warrior Training and Rehabilitation Program (WTRP) to military retirement. In the goal-setting session, soldiers identify the reasons for participating in any given event, what they want to accomplish, and most importantly, how they will achieve their goals. The end result is energy, persistence, and a prime selection of strategies for achieving each person's goals.[12] Ultimately a personalized "goal sheet" is developed and kept with participants at all times. The stress management option involves the use of Freeze Framer, a computerized biofeedback program, or a relaxation plan. Individual peak performance intervention can either be self-referred or command-referred if the soldier is not adapting well to WTRP.

The stress and energy management model in peak performance is based on a concept called "grip and gravity,"[12] based on identifying things individuals cannot control (gravity), and redirecting focus to things individuals have the ability to control (grip). In a setting where many injured soldiers feel out of control, future plans, current situations, attitudes, and perceptions will always be within their "grip" forces. Once the soldier has grasped the concept of taking control over his or her own life, biofeedback and relaxation techniques can be introduced into the treatment plan.

Biofeedback tools are used to teach soldiers how to recognize physiological changes (such as heart rate and breathing patterns) that occur with stress and make the necessary changes to reduce the magnitude of the stress response. By using biofeedback instruments, the soldier gains increased awareness and sensitivity to internal stress responses. The ultimate goal of this treatment is for the soldiers to recognize internal cues of stress without the aid of the instrument, and implement the steps to regain control. This reemphasizes the thought–performance interaction concept discussed during the group intervention. Equipment required for this program includes a computerized biofeedback instrument for treatment sessions and a relaxation chamber, which allows for optimal relaxation positioning and control of environmental stimuli during the intervention. The biofeedback equipment has been shown to improve overall physical speed and accuracy, enhance problem-focused coping skills, sustain concentration, and manage stress and anger.[12]

Using the peak performance model and its inherent mental agility intervention can improve soldiers' satisfaction with themselves, their careers, and their families. With dedicated work and intervention, it can facilitate patients' return to the unit without removal from theater or return to garrison duty. When utilized in the garrison setting, peak performance training at WTRP enabled soldiers' return to duty earlier when compared to programs that do not incorporate peak performance concepts. Soldiers also reported increased satisfaction in their own outcomes as well as a decrease in negative thoughts. Overall, the peak performance program integrates psychological, cognitive, and physiological concepts to enhance performance and promote positive attitudes among soldiers both in theater and in garrison.

Case Study 22-1: SGT JS, an infantryman, was initially seen by OT for an upper extremity injury following his return from Operation Iraqi Freedom. The therapist noticed that JS was having difficulty dealing with issues related to his deployment, specifically with anger and depression. He was referred to a community mental health social worker and a posttraumatic stress disorder group, which met once a week for 6 weeks. He decided immediately that his goal was to work on anger management, specifically when it came to his relationship with his wife. In a group-learning environment, he acquired many of the skills of the peak performance model, including energy management and goal setting. SGT JS also attended OT for one-on-one intervention for 8 weeks, incorporating a biofeedback heart rate program, guided imagery, and progressive muscle relaxation to gain control and composure when dealing with stressful situations. SGT JS reported an increase in confidence, increased satisfaction with his marriage since his return, and an overall increase in well being after attending the group and one-on-one sessions.

OCCUPATIONAL THERAPY IN THE WARRIOR TRANSITION UNIT

Since World War I, OT's philosophy of matching interventions to the soldier's ability has been an integral part of the effort to help those wounded in combat return to work. It was thought that wounded soldiers should be "restored to trades appropriate to their abilities, interest, and background."[3(p152)] Contributions did not end with direct care. Early OTs were also instrumental in setting national policy, contributing to the passage of the Soldiers Rehabilitation Act in June 1918.[3(p158)] Similar involvement continues today, with OT personnel instrumental in the formation of the Army's Proponency Office for Rehabilitation and Reintegration in May 2007, the development of the Comprehensive Transition Plan, and the development of the role of OT within WTUs.

The goal of a WTU is to promote soldiers' abilities to return to the force or transition to a productive civilian life. OT helps individuals regain, develop, or master everyday skills to live independent, productive, and satisfying lives.[15] Within the WTU, OT's primary role is to address life-skills needs and coordinate work reintegration, thus assisting soldiers to return to productive living. Work includes activities needed for engaging in paid employment or volunteer activities.[16(p341)] Occupation refers to the everyday activities of life that are named, organized, and given value and meaning by individuals and a culture. "Occupation is everything people do to occupy themselves including looking after themselves, enjoying life and contributing to the social and economic fabric of their communities."[17(p34)] Work reintegration is defined as a program that provides a structured environment with participation in vocationally related activities. The participant must be medically stable and have a goal of competitive employment.[18]

The Comprehensive Transition Plan

The desired outcome is for each participant to be a successful soldier or successful veteran, physically and mentally strengthened, vocationally enabled, with a life-care plan established, able to maintain relationships, and proud of his or her military service.[19] Each soldier's comprehensive transition plan is an individualized, multiphased process with overlapping boundaries. The reception phase is generally 1 week in duration. Upon arrival at the WTU, soldiers are greeted with a unit welcome and orientation that delineates the expectation that they will actively participate in their own healing process. They are educated on the overall mission statement that will be inculcated into their daily life within the WTU:

> I am a warrior in transition. My job is to heal as I transition back to duty or continue serving the nation as a veteran in my community. This is not a status, but a mission. I will succeed in this mission because I AM A WARRIOR AND I AM ARMY STRONG.

The soldier is issued a "Warrior Toolkit" that includes the soldier mission statement, orientation materials, and life-skills material designed to encourage self-empowerment in the healing process.

Next comes the assessment and goal-setting phase, which generally lasts a month. During this initial period, soldiers undergo assessments for behavioral health risk; pain, sleep, and safety (including cognitive awareness, mobility, vision, and hearing tests); and requirements for housing assistance, medical supplies, family needs, and nutrition management. The staff members also appraise the soldier's level of function, vocational goals, skills, abilities, health maintenance and lifestyle, and the initiation/sustainment of rehabilitation. At the same time, the soldier's goal-setting phase begins with a focus on the development of positive life skills and habits. The soldier works with the nurse case manager, primary care manager (a physician or physician's assistant), squad leader, OT personnel, social work, and unit ministry teams to develop goals for improvement in body, mind, and spirit. OTs have a leadership role in warrior goal-setting training. Functional independence and mobility goals are established, including accessing transportation resources. Vocational, educational, social, leisure, and recreation goals are also established during this phase. Intrapersonal goals are identified to enhance self-esteem, responsibility to self, interpersonal relationships, and community responsibility.

Next, during the active rehabilitation phase, the soldier works toward attaining specific goals. This phase is divided into four tiers based on the soldier's abilities, and a training calendar is established to help reset the soldier. Tier assignment levels include tier A (medical recovery/rest) for soldiers who are placed on quarters. Soldiers in tier A are generally unable to participate in any physical, mental, relationship, or spiritual strengthening programs. Tier B (basic reset) consists of soldiers who spend their training day in rehabilitation basics. These soldiers are actively engaged in medical appointments; group or individual therapy to improve strength, range of motion, or endurance; programs and classes in nutrition or weight management; classes in life skills; or classes and workshops on relationships. Tier B includes programs that every warrior in transition needs to build basic skills and strengths as well as individualized programs to address unique circumstances.

Tier C (advanced reset) follows completion of the basic skills program. These soldiers spend part of their duty day in vocational or educational activities, but still require significant time for activities specifically designed to rehabilitate their body, mind, and spirit. Tier C generally involves interventions targeted at addressing a specific goal. Tier D (life reset) is focused on vocational, educational, family, and community pursuits. Soldiers in this tier must have completed tier B basics. They spend the majority of their duty day in vocational or educational activities, but still require ongoing medical treatment or rehabilitation. Throughout the active rehabilitation phase, a mandatory review of progress and reassessment occurs on a regular basis, with the soldier actively participating in multidisciplinary team meetings coordinated by the nurse case manager.

The final transition preparation phase, which may last up to 90 days, occurs once each individual's disposition decision has been made. During this phase, the soldier undergoes final preparation for the expected disposition. Details regarding return to home, family, and community living as well as ongoing vocational or educational pursuits after they leave the WTU are addressed and coordinated to assure a smooth transition.

Work Reintegration Programs

The objectives of a work reintegration program involve returning the soldier to the role of worker either in a military or civilian capacity. This is done through promoting, improving, conserving, and restoring the skills, abilities, and aptitudes of soldiers through both vocational and avocational reintegration services. A soldier-centered work reintegration program pursues these goals for the soldier in transition. The program focuses on the behavioral, psychosocial, vocational, avocational, and educational needs of the soldier using techniques to facilitate independence and empowerment. The work reintegration program involves collaboration with military and civilian communities to set up safe work sites that promote quality work performance and enhance the quality of the service member's everyday life. The soldier actively participates in the work reintegration program, developing an understanding of how the services provided can positively impact his or her ability to function in a work environment.

The program also incorporates collaboration with appropriate professionals and community members to minimize impairment, maximize independent function, and enhance the quality of life of the service member in transition. Through the use of performance indicators, the work reintegration program measures the effectiveness of services provided along the continuum of care. OTs assist service members to develop and attain realistic short-term and long-term goals that reflect their interests in vocational and avocational pursuits. Service members benefit from this program by increasing the likelihood of attaining their personal goals, while the community benefits by reacquiring responsible and competent workers.

Occupational Therapy's Focus in Work Reintegration

The director of the work reintegration program is a registered and licensed OT who is qualified in both OT and work reintegration. Certified OTAs provide support in areas including screening, programming, life skills training, work-site development and coordination, and networking with internal and external resources to assure a well-balanced program aimed at returning soldiers to productive living. OT personnel work closely with other WTU staff to develop and implement the work reintegration program, which the OT is then responsible for overseeing. OTs are located in proximity to the WTU to facilitate communication with the cadre and increase interactions with participants. The OT and COTAs should be allocated appropriate space to develop and conduct a successful work reintegration program. Responsibilities of the OT assigned to the WTU include but are not limited to:

- working closely with OTs at the medical treatment facility to ensure continuity of care;
- developing and implementing standard operating procedures that support the overall goals and objectives of the work reintegration program;
- assessing limitations that prevent or delay return to work and providing recommendations for modifications and equipment needs;
- working closely with case mangers in coordinating vocational training, job skills training, and work placement;
- conducting visits to work sites to ensure job appropriateness and verifying that the participant is performing the agreed-upon job tasks;
- developing collaborations within the community to determine resources and to prevent duplication of services;
- working closely with other WTU staff to ensure continuity of care and accountability;
- establishing specific quantifiable standards to measure the work reintegration program success; and
- supervising the COTA personnel assigned to the WTU.

All soldiers assigned to the WTU undergo a comprehensive evaluation by the OT to determine eligibility and placement in the work reintegration program. Tools used by the OT may include a vocational interest survey, vocational aptitude assessment, career assessment tests, life skills assessments, cognitive skills assessments, occupational performance assessments, functional capacity evaluations, a driving evaluation in a simulator, and an evaluation of firearm performance in a simulator. All soldiers in transition also should be evaluated by the OT within 1 to 2 weeks of in-processing to determine if they are eligible to participate in the work reintegration program. Soldiers eligible for the program will be assigned a meaningful job within the limits of their physical profile and commensurate with their grade. Work internships are being developed in collaboration with the VA and 501(c)(3) (nonprofit) organizations to provide work experiences in areas of potential career fields. Each work reintegration program should maintain a file on each work site including a job description with work hours, dress code (if civilian), point of contact, memorandum of agreement, and the physical, cognitive, and psychosocial requirements of the job.

OTs collaborate with unit training personnel to help develop a structured daily schedule for each participant consisting of life skills development, work preparation, education, training, and structured duty assignments to prepare soldiers for return to functional living. Activities are matched to the individual's needs and abilities and may include (*a*) stress management, (*b*) anger management, (*c*) assertiveness/communication skills training, (*d*) functional activities, (*e*) soldier basic skill training, (*f*) MOS training, (*g*) problem-solving and goal-setting skills training, (*h*) financial management skills training, (*i*) time management skills training, and (*j*) work readiness skills—work habits, values, interests, skills, and vocational exploration.

The supervisor at each work reintegration site provides weekly progress reports to the OT. In addition, the OT conducts at least bimonthly follow-ups to reassess each participant for continuance of the current work placement. The OT also decides what type of follow-up is needed when participants leave the unit. By the day of discharge/transition, written recommendations are given to providers in the continuum of care and other stakeholders as appropriate. Depending on the needs of the soldier, the written recommendations address:

- medical issues relevant to job placement;
- functional issues relevant to job performance;
- psychological issues relevant to job placement;
- significant abilities, relevant aptitude scores;
- areas for growth;
- identification of additional training if needed; and
- available community integration services, including local, regional, provincial, or national consumer organizations.

The work reintegration program includes a data collection system for performance indicators—collected initially and reevaluated over time—to measure the effectiveness of services provided across the continuum, including the number of WTU soldiers who were discharged from the military, who returned to duty, who received a permanent job placement, and who enrolled in school. Program staff also record satisfaction of the job site from the participant and family members.

OCCUPATIONAL THERAPY ON THE HOME FRONT

The emotional cycle of deployment affects not only soldiers, but also their families, employers, coworkers, schools, and the surrounding community.[20] The role of OT on the home front involves building skills to withstand the stress of deployment separation as well as focusing on habit training to assist soldiers and their families in the reintegration process. Incorporating rituals and traditions that can carry over throughout the deployment may provide a sense of consistency and order during a chaotic time. A psychoeducational approach using a resiliency model to enhance life skills in predeploying soldiers and their families may act as a protective measure in preparing them to overcome the hardships of deployment separation.

Returning combat troops and their families frequently report increased levels of anxiety and risk-taking behaviors when the soldier resumes driving at home.[21] This may be due to the retention of automatic combat driving behaviors that were overlearned to help the soldier survive in a hostile environment. Although appropriate on the battlefield, automatic combat driving behaviors do not mesh well with local traffic laws at home. OT personnel assess the physical, cognitive, and behavioral components of driving to help soldiers safely perform this daily living skill. Awareness training and specific interventions are useful in managing maladaptive postcombat driving behaviors. Using a consultative approach, occupational therapists collaborated with Military OneSource to develop a handout for service members and their families, providing awareness of and tips for managing postcombat driving behaviors. An article published in a national newsletter for traffic court judges also helped to increase the judges' awareness of these issues when returning soldiers have pending legal action in the traffic court system.[21,22]

A collaborative relationship between an academic institution and an Army OT resulted in the development of postdeployment driving reintegration tools. Research conducted by OT faculty and students at the University of Minnesota described postcombat soldier driving responses and identified specific interventions that effectively enhance driving safety. In consultation with the Proponency Office for Rehabilitation and Reintegration, the student/faculty team incorporated survey results, focus groups, and one-to-one interviews to develop informational brochures for soldiers and family members. The brochures address postcombat driving on the American road and include suggestions to help returning soldiers drive safely at home. In addition, the OT academic researcher developed clinician training for OTs working in military settings to help standardize the use of driving simulation.

SUMMARY

Army OTs are human performance experts and dedicated leaders whose innovative programs and services help optimize soldier performance and readiness in theater and garrison. Providing a functional approach to healing through doing, OTs match the individual's interests, skills, and abilities with activities that have meaning and purpose, along with a "just right" challenge. A focus on occupational performance helps to restore soldier confidence and competence. Life skills components of OT promote functional independence, which enhances future quality of life and productivity. Participation in work and productive activities promotes a sense of mastery, a positive self-identity, and a responsibility to take control over one's future. Bridging the gap between medical care and military performance training, OTs help unit leaders retain their soldiers through assessing physical, social, and environmental factors and recommending interventions to enhance unit climate and living conditions.

The practice of OT has been essential in the rehabilitation of military personnel since World War I. OTs use a variety of strategies to enhance occupational performance, a key factor in retention of the soldier who has sustained a physical or psychological injury. They also assess the soldier's performance and help the service member gain the skills and resilience to remain functional whether returning to the battlefield or transitioning to the civilian community. OTs provide a vital link to practical living and a more satisfactory life through occupational engagement and enhancement of physical, psychological, cognitive, and social aspects of performance.

REFERENCES

1. American Occupational Therapy Association. Occupational therapy practice model: domain and process. *Am J Occup Ther.* 2002;56:609–639.

2. Gerardi S, Newton S. The role of the occupational therapist in CSC [combat stress control] operations. *US Army Med Dep J.* 2004;Jul–Sep:20–27. Available at: http://www.dtic.mil/cgi-bin/GetTRDoc?Location=U@&doc=GetTRDoc.pdf&AD=ADA493056. Accessed October 7, 2010.

3. Quiroga VAM. *Occupational Therapy: The First 30 Years, 1900 to 1930.* Bethesda, Md: American Occupational Therapy Association; 1995.

4. Crepeau EB, Cohn DS, Shell BB, eds. *Willard and Spackman's Occupational Therapy.* 11th ed. Philadelphia, Penn: Lippincott-Raven Publishers; 2008.

5. Creek J, ed. *Occupational Therapy and Mental Health.* 3rd ed. New York, NY: Churchill Livingstone; 2002: 8.

6. Newton SM. The growth of the profession of occupational therapy. *US Army Med Dep J.* 2007;Jan–Mar:51–58.

7. Department of the Army. *Army Medical Specialist Corps.* Washington, DC: Office of The Surgeon General; 1968.

8. Neistadt ME, Crepeau EB, eds. *Willard and Spackman's Occupational Therapy.* 9th ed. Philadelphia, Penn: Lippincott-Raven Publishers; 1998.

9. US Department of the Army. *Clinical Quality Management.* Washington, DC: DA; 2004. Army Regulation 40-68.

10. US Department of the Army. *Combat and Operational Stress Control.* Washington, DC: DA; 2006. Field Manual 4-02.51.

11. Kielhofner G. *Model of Human Occupation: Theory and Application.* 4th ed. Baltimore, Md: Lippincott Williams & Wilkins; 2008.

12. Corbari G. Performance enhancement program at the Center for Enhanced Performance. Paper presented at: Peak Performance Training Conference; November 2005; West Point, New York.

13. Newsom J, Knight P, Balnave R. Use of mental imagery to limit strength after immobilization. *Sport Rehabil.* 2003;12:249–258.

14. Nightingale L. What is interactive guided imagery? [1998]. Available at: http://www.nightingalecenter.com/guided.html. Accessed October 25, 2010.

15. American Occupational Therapy Association. For prospective students. Available at: http://www.aota.org/Students/Prospective. Accessed October 25, 2010.

16. Mosey AC. *Applied Scientific Inquiry in the Health Professions: An Epistemological Orientation.* 2nd ed. Bethesda, Md: American Occupational Therapy Association; 1996.

17. Law M, Polatajko H, Baptiste W, Townsend E. Core concepts of occupational therapy. In: Townsend E, ed. *Enabling Occupation: An Occupational Therapy Perspective.* Ottawa, Ont: Canadian Association of Occupational Therapists; 1997.

18. US Department of Veterans Affairs. Compensated work therapy. Available at: http://www.cwt.va.gov/. Accessed October 25, 2010.

19. Department of the Army. *MEDCOM Warrior in Transition Comprehensive Care Plan Policy.* Washington, DC: DA; January 2008.

20. Pincus SH, House J, Christenson J, Adler LE. The emotional cycle of deployment: a military family perspective. Available at: http://hooah4health.com/deployment/familymatters/emotionalcycle.htm. Accessed October 25, 2010.

21. Stern E. Driving behaviors of returning combat troops [unpublished survey results]. Minneapolis, Minn: University of Minnesota; 2008.

22. Stern EB, Erickson M. Readjustment to civilian life doesn't stop at the garage door: driving infractions of post deployment citizen soldiers. *Experience.* 2008;18(2):22–24. [Published earlier under same title in *Highway to Justice.* 2007;Spring:2–6.]

Chapter 23

PROVIDER FATIGUE AND PROVIDER RESILIENCY TRAINING

MARY ANN PECHACEK, PsyD, LMFT*; GRAEME C. BICKNELL, PhD, LISW†; and LISA LANDRY, PhD‡

*Psychologist and Instructor/Writer, Department of Behavioral Health Sciences, Special Subjects Branch, Army Medical Department Center and School, 3151 Scott Road, Building 2840, Fort Sam Houston, Texas 78234

†Lieutenant Colonel, Medical Service Corps, US Army; Deputy Chief, Behavioral Health Division, US Medical Command, 2050 Worth Road, Building 2792, Fort Sam Houston, San Antonio, Texas 78234-6010s

‡Instructor/Writer, Department of Behavioral Health Sciences, Army Medical Department Center and School, 3151 Scott Road, Building 2840, Office #32, Fort Sam Houston, Texas 78234

INTRODUCTION

The effects of caring for traumatized individuals have been characterized in numerous ways and given different names over time during many traumatic events. Although each of these concepts was originally developed in a specific context with individual nuances, they have also been used interchangeably in connection with the phenomenon of secondary trauma—the reaction of caregivers to the traumatic events experienced by those they serve. Current military behavioral healthcare providers have built on the efforts of their predecessors, who have attempted to capture and understand the effects of trauma through the years. Providers are resilient by nature and military providers are especially so, as seen in their focusing, building, and reinforcing the resilience in achievable balanced health.

All members of the Department of Defense—soldiers, sailors, airmen, marines, and civilians—have been affected by the global war on terror. The US military has developed many programs and services to aid military personnel and their families, addressing psychological, spiritual, and physical recovery; however, only a few programs are directed toward caregivers. One such program is Provider Resiliency Training (PRT), created and implemented by the Soldier and Family Support Branch at the Army Medical Department (AMEDD) Center and School at Fort Sam Houston, Texas.

PRT has three phases. During the first phase of training, all care providers throughout the medical command (MEDCOM) watch a video on PRT and take the Professional Quality of Life (Pro-QOL) Scale (discussed in detail in this chapter). This phase takes approximately 30 minutes to complete. The second phase of PRT involves the development of initial self-care plans by all MEDCOM medical treatment facilities' staff, and takes about 2 hours to complete. The third phase—annual maintenance of the plan—is completed during the care provider's birth month and is used to readminister the Pro-QOL screening tool completed during the first phase. This allows trainers to review those results with individual participants. This third and final phase takes about 1 hour to complete.

PRT is a comprehensive course in definitions, concepts, models, and methods for dealing with provider fatigue. This training is designed for audiences at all levels of care provision. The first half of the introduction to PRT defines and clarifies the challenge of compassion fatigue/provider fatigue and the "cost of caring," as well as principles of practical holistic renewal. The second half is focused on strength and resiliency: How do individuals stay strong? Where does resiliency come from? How might resiliency be encouraged in self, colleagues, systems, and soldiers?

Like a mental gymnasium geared toward the overall fitness of caregivers and the development of their resiliency in the face of challenges, PRT aims to help providers find the inner strength to face fear and adversity with courage. Furthermore, PRT is focused on military providers who care for those who have experienced suffering and trauma. The stress of contemporary combat and operational environments is unlike that experienced by physicians, nurses, or chaplains in the civilian sector.

TERMS AND DEFINITIONS

A number of terms have been used to capture secondary reactions to trauma, including "burnout,"[1] "secondary victimization,"[2] "secondary traumatic stress disorder,"[3–7] "secondary survivor,"[8] "vicarious traumatization,"[9,10] "traumatic countertransference,"[11] and "compassion fatigue." A similar concept, "emotional contagion," is defined as an affective process in which "an individual observing another person experiences emotional responses parallel to that person's actual or anticipated emotions."[12(p338)] Furthermore, "rape-related family crisis"[13,14] and "proximity effects" on female partners of war veterans[15] are related concepts. The generational effects of trauma[16,17] and the need for family "detoxification" from war-related traumatic stress[18] have been noted. Finally, difficulties with client problems have been considered as simple countertransference and discussed within the context of posttraumatic stress disorder (PTSD) treatment.[2,11,19,20] However, the concept is difficult to measure or to separate from other factors of client-therapist transactions.

Historically, compassion fatigue, compassion stress, vicarious traumatization, secondary PTSD, and the current military concept of provider fatigue all involve the empathic connection with people experiencing the emotions of trauma, resulting in the provider experiencing the same emotions. Provider fatigue is related to the other concepts, primarily compassion fatigue, previously the latest in an evolving concept known in the field of traumatology as "secondary traumatic stress." Most often this phenomenon is associated with the "cost of caring"[3] for others in emotional pain.

The term "provider fatigue" was first used in 1992 by Joinson,[21] who described nurses worn down by daily hospital emergencies. The same year, in his book *Compassionate Therapy*, Kottler[22] emphasized the importance of compassion in dealing with extremely difficult and resistant patients. However, neither publication adequately defined "compassion." Most past research emphasized only why practitioners lose compassion as a result of working with the suffering. On the other hand, some people, including military care providers, may feel that it is wrong for a practitioner to have deep feelings of sympathy and sorrow for a client's suffering. And practitioners certainly must understand their limitations in helping to alleviate the pain suffered by patients.

The American Psychiatric Association's *Diagnostic and Statistical Manual of Mental Disorders* (4th ed)[23] notes that PTSD is possible when one is traumatized either directly (in harm's way) or indirectly, for example, as a parent witnessing a child's injury. Those involved in both types of incidents may experience trauma, although through different social pathways. The latter pathway is called "secondary traumatic stress." Few reports of the incidence and prevalence of this type of stress reaction exist; however, based on secondary data and theory analysis, it is possible that burnout, countertransference, worker dissatisfaction, and other related concepts may have masked this common problem.[2] Vicarious traumatization, for example, refers to a transformation in the therapist's inner experience resulting from empathic engagement with clients' trauma material. These effects are cumulative and permanent, and evident in both a therapist's professional and personal life.[10] Compassion or provider fatigue is a more user-friendly term for secondary traumatic stress disorder, which is nearly identical to PTSD except that it affects those emotionally affected by the trauma of another (usually a client or a family member). Terms as used in this chapter are defined as follows:

- **Primary traumatic stress** results from stressors inherent in an extreme event—what was immediately experienced or witnessed, especially things that contributed most to a traumatic response. For example, the military healthcare provider may be in danger of direct fire while assisting fellow soldiers.
- **Compassion stress** is the residue of emotional energy from the empathic response to the client, as well as the ongoing demand for action to relieve the client's suffering. It flows from having an empathic, caring response. Together with other factors it can contribute to provider fatigue unless the provider acts to manage the stress.
- **Compassion or provider fatigue** is the emotional residue or strain of exposure from working with those suffering the consequences of traumatic events. A form of secondary traumatic stress—compassion or provider fatigue—is the result of a healthcare provider engaging in the treatment of individuals exposed to various traumas. It is natural and normal for providers to experience compassion fatigue; if a provider is doing a job well, it is normal to feel fatigued, similar to an athlete feeling fatigued after a good workout. Provider fatigue should be expected, mitigated, and processed by every professional caregiver.
- **Burnout** is a cumulative process marked by emotional exhaustion and withdrawal associated with increased workload and institutional stress. Burnout is not necessarily trauma-related; it can occur in any job with an ongoing overwhelming workload. Burnout occurs when a person loses the ability to care.
- **Resiliency** is the ability to recover rapidly from illness, change, or misfortune. (In objects, it is the ability to regain the original shape after being bent, stretched, or compressed.) Resiliency occurs on a continuum (it is not an either/or proposition) and relates to a person's overall growth and development. Resiliency is about who the person is, while stress management is about what that person is doing; however, a provider's level of resiliency is evident in how he or she responds to stressors. Resiliency grows through healthy responses to stressors.

FIGLEY'S COMPASSION FATIGUE MODEL

In 1995, Charles Figley, a former Marine and leader in the field of traumatology, created a model of compassion fatigue delineating how exposure to suffering and an empathic response can lead to compassion stress and compassion fatigue.[24] The same experiences can be seen in the area of provider fatigue, and will be further discussed in the next section. Elements in the model include the following:

- **Emotional contagion** is experiencing the feelings of the sufferer as a function of exposure to the sufferer.
- **Empathic concern** is the motivation to respond to people in need.

- **Empathic ability** is the aptitude for noticing the pain of others.
- **Empathic response** is the extent to which the helper makes an effort to reduce the suffering of the sufferer.
- **Disengagement** is the extent to which helpers can distance themselves from the ongoing misery of the traumatized person.
- **Sense of achievement** is the extent to which helpers are satisfied with their efforts to help the client/sufferer.
- **Compassion stress** is the compulsive demand for action to relieve the suffering of others.
- **Prolonged exposure** is the ongoing sense of responsibility for the care of the suffering, over a protracted period of time.
- **Traumatic recollections** are memories that trigger the symptoms of PTSD and associated reactions, such as depression and generalized anxiety.
- **Life disruption** is the unexpected change in schedule, routine, and managing life responsibilities caused by experiences that demand attention (eg, changes in health, lifestyle, social status, or professional or personal circumstances).
- **Compassion fatigue** is the state of tension and preoccupation with the traumatized by (*a*) reexperiencing the traumatic events; (*b*) avoidance/numbing of reminders, and (*c*) persistent arousal. It is a natural consequence of behaviors and emotions resulting from knowing about a traumatizing event experienced by another.
- **Compassion trap** is the inability to let go of the thoughts, feelings, and emotions useful in helping another, long after they are useful.[24]

It is thought that "other-centered" people, who are good at providing care, are vulnerable to compassion fatigue. Those without as much compassion suffer these effects less dramatically. The first author of this chapter conceptualizes this as follows: "the caregivers' gift is their burden." Being a compassionate person is helpful in the healing process, but that compassion may become a challenge if it is not balanced by resiliency.

Providers who are strongly empathetic may be most at risk of provider fatigue. No provider witnesses trauma in the abstract; for those who are strongly empathic it can be, and is, personal. The actual experience is felt vicariously as pain, with a consequential psychological impact. Often providers do not see self-care as a priority, which places them in jeopardy of burning out.

Another factor that puts the provider at risk for secondary traumatization is a personal history of trauma. When providers have experienced a significant loss in their own lives, the experiences and images of trauma may trigger those memories and stimulate fresh grief. Many providers are secondary witnesses to trauma on a regular basis. As witnesses and providers, they are vulnerable to the emotional pain of victims. Providers picture bits and pieces of the trauma in their minds and may experience intense feelings in their bodies.

Many military providers are both participants in the trauma (eg, being shot at) and caregivers of others affected. Figley summarized these experiences by noting that helping the traumatized can itself be quite traumatizing. An Army chaplain related the story of being part of a convoy in which a vehicle in front of him was blown up. He was in imminent danger himself. As he participated in helping his comrades through the trauma and debriefing that followed it, he found himself alone, wondering who would help him. He turned to his God and returned to camp. The next day was Sunday and his job took him to the pulpit, where he delivered an inspiring sermon to the soldiers he served.[25] The point made is that one may be in the face of danger, help those in danger, be alone in danger, and then rise the next day to serve those in danger. This situation occurs in the life of the military care provider on a regular basis.

FACTORS CONTRIBUTING TO COMPASSION STRESS

Empathic responses in the provider occur when the ability and desire to help others converges with exposure to suffering. Compassion stress flows from having an empathic, caring response to the work or to those who suffer. It is how providers feel (physically and/or emotionally) the trauma of the patients with whom they are working. For example, hearing of terrible abuse stirs within the provider a feeling of disgust and gastrointestinal upset. The level of stress is determined by how much the provider relates to or identifies with another's suffering and trauma. The following characteristics, based on Figley's model, often propel people to become healthcare providers, yet also predispose them to experience compassion stress: (*a*) the ability to be empathic, (*b*) the desire to help, and (*c*) the level of exposure to suffering. The chances of experiencing compassion fatigue are reduced to the degree that these features are lacking.[2,24]

- **Empathic ability** is the aptitude of the provider for noticing the pain of others. Figley's model suggests that without empathy, providers experience little if any compassion stress and no compassion fatigue. However, without empathy they feel little if any empathic response to suffering clients. Thus, the ability to empathize is key both to helping others and being vulnerable to the costs of caring.
- **Empathic concern** is the motivation to respond to people in need. The ability to be empathic is insufficient unless motivation exists to help others who require the services of a concerned psychotherapist. With sufficient concern, the empathic provider draws upon his or her talent, training, and knowledge to deliver the highest quality of services possible to those who seek it.
- **Exposure to the client** is experiencing the emotional energy of client's suffering through direct exposure. Mental health professionals directly employed in human services may decide to become supervisors, administrators, or teachers because of the costs of direct exposure to clients (of course, determining individual motivation is difficult, and some make the shift from direct practice because of additional pay, improved working conditions, and higher status).[24]
- **Empathic response** is the extent to which the provider makes an effort to reduce the suffering of the client through empathic understanding. This insight into feelings, thoughts, and behaviors of the client is achieved by projecting one's self into the perspective of the client. In doing so, the provider might experience the client's hurt, fear, anger, or other emotions. Therein lie both the benefits and the costs of such a powerful therapeutic response. The benefits are immediately obvious to every provider who practices his or her skills with another. The benefit for the provider is that a sense of bonding and understanding with the hurting person may emerge. This may be demonstrated by the latter feeling understood and having the pain/trauma be normalized by the provider's expression of empathy. The costs, rarely discussed, must be experienced for the provider to guard against or mitigate the effects.
- **Compassion stress,** the residue of emotional energy from the empathic response, is experienced as an ongoing demand for action to relieve the client's suffering. As with any stress, compassion stress with sufficient intensity can have a negative effect on the immune system and quality of life. Together with other factors, this stress can contribute to compassion fatigue unless the psychotherapist acts to control it. Two major types of coping actions appear to help control compassion stress:
    - A **sense of achievement,** the extent to which providers are satisfied with their efforts to help the client, can lower or prevent compassion stress. Having a sense of achievement involves a conscious, rational effort to recognize where the provider's responsibility ends and the client's begins.
    - **Detachment,** the extent to which providers can distance themselves from the ongoing misery of the client between treatment sessions, can lower or prevent compassion stress. The ability to disengage also requires a conscious, rational effort to recognize that to live their own lives providers must "let go" of the thoughts, feelings, and sensations associated with clients. Disengagement is the recognition of importance of self-care.[24]

Compassion stress can also be mitigated by both individual and unit management of stressors. If there is a sense of achievement, an ability to disengage, and the stress is well managed, the stress will be maintained at normal levels. If these are insufficient or not present, then the level of stress will rise. If compassion stress is permitted to build, despite the provider's effort at disengagement and a sense of work satisfaction, the provider is at a greater risk of compassion fatigue. Three other factors play a role in increasing compassion/provider fatigue:

1. **Prolonged exposure** is the ongoing sense of responsibility for the care of the suffering, over a protracted period of time (eg, multiple sessions with one individual or multiple contacts from large-scale disasters such as the 2004 tsunami in Asia). To prevent prolonged exposure, providers should have regular breaks from client appointments, lasting from a day off to a week's vacation.
2. **Traumatic recollections** are memories that trigger symptoms of PTSD and associated reactions, such as depression and anxiety. These memories may be from the provider's experiences with either demanding or threat-

ening clients, clients who were especially sad or suffering, or clients with experiences that have a connection to traumatic events experienced by the provider.

3. **Life disruptions** are unexpected changes in schedule, routine, and managing life responsibilities that demand attention (eg, personal home-front concerns while at war; illness; or changes in lifestyle, social status, or professional or personal responsibilities). Normally such disruptions would cause a certain but tolerable level of distress. However, when combined with the other factors, these disruptions can increase the chances of the provider developing compassion fatigue.[24]

SYNERGISTIC EFFECTS OF PROVIDER FATIGUE

For the military healthcare provider, numerous sources of stress may come together to bring about provider fatigue. Although the primary ingredient of provider fatigue is unmanaged compassion stress, operational stress also contributes to the provider fatigue of military healthcare providers, as well as chaplains, support staff, and family members. Unresolved primary traumatic stress, secondary traumatic stress, and burnout, when added to unmanaged compassion stress, directly affect the overall level of provider fatigue. For example, providers may experience burnout from a continuously heavy workload (unrelated to trauma); secondary trauma from repeated exposure to the suffering of coworkers or family members; or primary trauma in the form of direct or indirect fire in a war zone, or the sights, smells, and sounds of providing direct humanitarian care. The interactive effect of different types of stressors can shape the overall development of provider fatigue. Military healthcare providers are at increased risk of provider fatigue because of both exposure to others' suffering and the risk of personal injury or death.

For many military providers, symptoms of secondary traumatization have a delayed onset. Many providers also have prior traumatic experiences that may cause no symptoms until associated with the stressors of working with traumatic material presented by patients. Some may develop clinical PTSD-like symptoms associated with their previously "benign" historical experiences. It is often necessary to resolve primary traumatic stress before addressing any issues of secondary stress or burnout.

Primary stress, secondary stress, operational stress, and burnout symptoms have a synergistic or interactive effect with compassion stress (Figure 23-1). Experiencing symptoms from any one of these sources appears to diminish resiliency and lower thresholds for the adverse impact of the stressors, which can in turn lead to a rapid onset of severe symptoms that can become debilitating to the provider within a very short period of time. The experiences of military providers differ from those of civilian providers because of danger while delivering service, multiple deployments, working with detainees, cultural differences, and lack of time for reprieve. Military-specific operational stress includes

- lack of reprieves, breaks, and exits during operations;
- experience of primary trauma while helping others;
- a cumulative effect of the provider's and clients' repeated deployments;
- isolation and relational issues;
- ethical issues, such as determining who the client is; and
- competing demands for treatment of the client versus the provider.

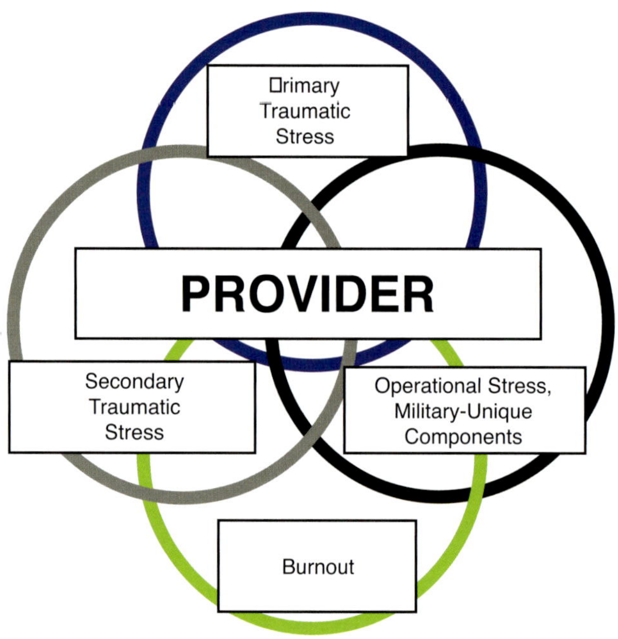

Figure 23-1. Synergistic effects of primary, secondary, and operational stress, combined with burnout symptoms, on providers.

WAYS TO IDENTIFY PROVIDER FATIGUE

Symptoms of provider fatigue may include withdrawal from family and friends; emotional numbing; loss of interest in things usually enjoyed; persistent thoughts and images related to the problems of others; physical symptoms such as headaches, gastrointestinal disturbances, and muscle tightness; sleep disturbance; and jumpiness.

Markers

Healthcare providers must monitor themselves and coworkers for the following markers. The more markers observed or felt, the greater the risk of provider fatigue. The markers fall into the categories of cognitive, emotional, behavioral, spiritual, somatic, and social.[2]

Cognitive Markers

- Intrusive thoughts and disturbing memories
- Preoccupation with trauma
- Lowered concentration
- Disorientation
- Thoughts of self-harm or harm to others
- Reduced sense of safety

Emotional Markers

- Powerlessness
- Anxiety or fear
- Anger
- Survivor's guilt
- Numbness or inability to feel emotions
- Sadness
- Emotional roller coaster
- Feelings of depletion, being run down, or out of steam
- Irritability
- Decreased self-esteem

Behavioral Markers

- Impatience
- Being snappy or short tempered with others
- Poor sleep
- Nightmares
- Appetite changes, eating more or less than normal
- Being jumpy or on edge; startling easily
- Being accident prone
- Losing things
- Being rigid or inflexible, wanting to do everything the same way
- Using ineffective or harmful self-care practices

Spiritual Markers

- Loss of hope
- Loss of purpose
- Anger at God
- Questioning prior religious beliefs
- Skepticism toward religion
- Reduced joy and sense of purpose with career
- Loss of compassion

Somatic Markers

- Shock
- Rapid heartbeat and sweating
- Breathing difficulties
- Aches and pains
- Dizziness
- Impaired immune system; being more prone to illness
- Exhaustion
- Gastrointestinal problems and headaches

Social Markers

- Decreased interest in emotional intimacy
- Mistrust and isolation
- Being overprotective as a parent or as a leader; not allowing others to have normal activities
- Loneliness
- Increased interpersonal conflicts
- Trouble separating work from personal life

Behavior Changes After Exposure to Trauma

Numerous problems including absenteeism have been documented after exposure to trauma. This is a real phenomenon that can affect military healthcare providers and their ability to do their jobs. In a mixed method study by Regehr, Goldberg, and Hughes,[26] emergency workers routinely exposed to pain and suffering were examined to better understand factors leading to higher levels of distress within the theoretical framework of emotional and cognitive empathy. Researchers found a significant increase in alcohol-related problems, an increase in mental health stress leave, and an increase in use of psychiatric medications after these providers were exposed to a traumatic event. The study concluded that paramedics, who are exposed to many events outside the everyday experiences of the average person, have for the most part learned to deal with the events and take them in stride. A coping technique commonly used by paramedics is to deal with the events cognitively and technically while maintaining an emotional distance. At times, however, certain circumstances lead workers to develop an emotional connection with events based on their awareness of other aspects of the patient's experience. Aspects that can trigger this connection include the victim's alienation from others, profound loss, or the abuse of an innocent child. When this connection occurs, paramedics report increased symptoms of traumatic stress.[26]

Provider fatigue can be recognized on the job by its effects on work performance, morale, behavior, and relationships.[2]

Effects on Work Performance

- Decreased quality
- Decreased quantity
- Low motivation
- Avoidance of tasks
- Increased mistakes
- Setting perfectionist standards
- Obsession about details

Effects on Morale

- Decrease in confidence
- Loss of interest
- Dissatisfaction
- Negative attitude
- Apathy
- Demoralization
- Lack of appreciation
- Detachment
- Feelings of incompleteness

Effects on Behavior

- Absenteeism
- Exhaustion
- Faulty judgment
- Irritability
- Tardiness
- Irresponsibility
- Frequent job changes
- Overwork

Effects on Interpersonal Relationships

- Withdrawal from colleagues
- Impatience
- Decrease in quality of relationship
- Poor communication
- Subsuming own needs
- Staff conflicts

In addition to direct observation, compassion can be indirectly identified through self-administered survey instruments.

US Medical Command Use of the Professional Quality of Life Scale

The ProQOL[27] scale is the current version of the old Compassion Fatigue Self Test[2] and has been widely used in assessing compassion fatigue. The ProQOL is a 30-item survey instrument that consists of three subscales: (1) compassion fatigue, also known as secondary trauma scale; (2) burnout; and (3) compassion satisfaction. In keeping with the tone of this chapter, the discussion will focus specifically on issues related to compassion fatigue. The compassion fatigue variable is measured with 10 questions, and each response option ranges from 0 (never) through 5 (very often). Stamm[28] reported updated descriptive statistics for the ProQOL to include compassion fatigue. Based on a comprehensive reanalysis of existing published research, she found the compassion fatigue mean score to be 12, with a standard deviation of 6.9 and a Cronbach's alpha reliability score of .80. Throughout the remainder of this discussion, Stamm's new results and the research it was based on will be referred to as ProQOL data. Additionally, because the ProQOL attempts to identify persons who are "compassion fatigued," the instrument uses quartile scores as cutoff scores. In the ProQOL data the top quartile score is 17, meaning that respondents scoring 17 or above on the compassion fatigue scale are considered compassion fatigued.

Compassion fatigue is described as "your work-related, secondary exposure to extremely stressful events."[27] The list below contains the 10 items on the Trauma/Compassion Fatigue Scale taken directly from the ProQOL:

- I am preoccupied with more than one person I help.
- I jump or am startled by unexpected sounds.
- I find it difficult to separate my personal life from my life as a helper.
- I think that I might have been "infected" by the traumatic stress of those I help.
- Because of my helping, I have felt "on edge" about various things.

- I feel depressed as a result of my work as a helper.
- I feel as though I am experiencing the trauma of someone I have helped.
- I avoid certain activities or situations because they remind me of frightening experiences of the people I help.
- As a result of my helping, I have intrusive, frightening thoughts.
- I can't recall important parts of my work with trauma victims.[27]

In 2008 the Surgeon General of the US Army, Lieutenant General Schoomaker, required all Army MEDCOM personnel to complete the ProQOL. This requirement met the intent to assess MEDCOM personnel on compassion fatigue, burnout, and compassion satisfaction. MEDCOM personnel accessed the ProQOL scale through a secure Army Web site. Respondents were assured that "[t]he information on the ProQOL is protected. Scores on the assessment are for use in helping individuals to develop a self-care plan. Employees are not required to share the information with their supervisors."[29]

The de-identified database was analyzed by personnel assigned to the Soldier Family Support Branch of the AMEDD Center and School, using SPSS (Version 16, SPSS Inc, Chicago, Illinois) statistical software. To meet the Surgeon General's intent of assessing the levels of compassion fatigue in MEDCOM personnel, the analysis started with descriptive statistics for MEDCOM population demographics and population scores. As the name implies, MEDCOM is a medical organization that has about 27,000 soldiers and 28,000 civilian employees[30] assigned across 35 medical treatment facilities. For parity's sake, demographic description is limited to respondent medical specialty. Figure 23-2 illustrates the percentage of MEDCOM personnel by medical specialty.

Using inferential statistics, the data were then analyzed to see whether MEDCOM scores differed from ProQOL data scores in a statistically significant way. A P value of < .001 was considered statistically significant. Analysis then focused on establishing descriptive statistics specific to MEDCOM compassion fatigue scores. With valid N = 50,478, the MEDCOM mean score for compassion fatigue was 9.8823 (minimum = 0.00, maximum = 50.00, ST = 6.71681, variance = 45.116).

A one-sample t test is an appropriate statistical test to compare a sample score to a known population score.[31] In this case, MEDCOM is considered a sample of the greater population represented by the ProQOL data scores. A one-sample t test was conducted to compare the MEDCOM compassion fatigue mean score of 9.88 to the ProQOL data compassion fatigue mean score of 12. The MEDCOM compassion fatigue mean score was lower than the ProQOL data score and the difference was statistically significant with a 2-tailed test (t_{12} = -70.835, P < .001, df = 50,477). The mean difference was -2.11768 (95% CI, -2.1763 to -2.0591).

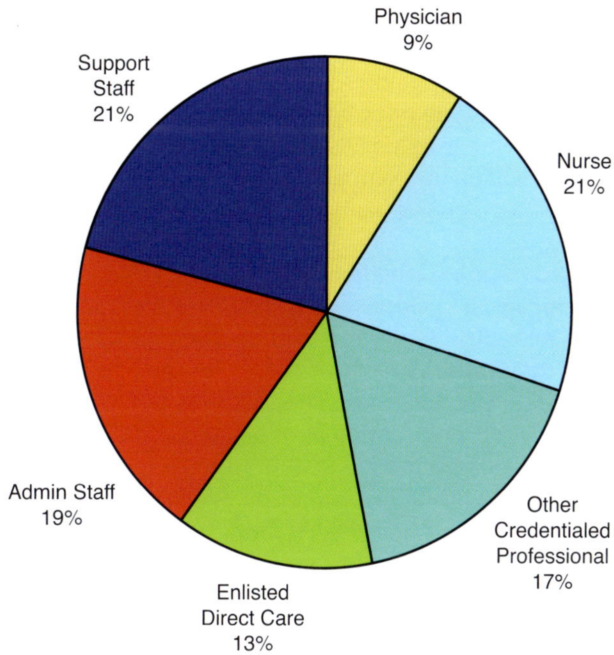

Figure 23-2. Percentage of US Army Medical Command personnel, by specialty, who completed the ProQOL survey in 2008. N=50,478.

TABLE 23-1

PERCENTAGE OF MEDICAL COMMAND PERSONNEL WHO MEET COMPASSION FATIGUE CUT SCORE

	Frequency	Percent	Valid Percent	Cumulative Percent
Not Compassion Fatigued	43,595	86.4	86.4	86.4
Compassion Fatigued	6,883	13.6	13.6	100.0
Total	50,478	100.0	100.0	

Another question of interest is how the percentage of MEDCOM personnel with compassion fatigue differs from the percentage of personnel with compassion fatigue in the ProQOL data. Stamm's establishment of a compassion fatigue cut score of 17, representing 25% of the ProQOL data population, allows this comparison. The percentage of MEDCOM personnel that scored at or above 17 on the compassion fatigue score was 13.6% (Table 23-1). This is further graphically represented in Figure 23-3.

To determine whether this difference is statistically significant, a goodness-of-fit test was conducted. A goodness-of-fit test is appropriate when the data score is nonparametric,[31] which is true in this case using quartile-based cut scores. The goodness-of-fit test compares the observed number of personnel (MEDCOM) that meet or exceed the cutoff score to the expected percentage (ProQOL data) of personnel that meet or exceed the cutoff score (Table 23-2). The difference was found to be statistically significant with a chi-square of 3,477.4 ($df = 1$, P value < .001).

This study focused on assessing the level of compassion fatigue among MEDCOM personnel and then comparing it to levels of compassion fatigue in the ProQOL data that represent the greater population. The findings establish that MEDCOM personnel report less compassion fatigue overall and MEDCOM has a lower percentage of personnel who meet criteria for compassion fatigue when compared to the cumulative samples in published research. Though important, speculations about the reasons for this difference are beyond the scope of this discussion; further research is warranted.

TABLE 23-2

MEDICAL COMMAND OBSERVED COMPASSION FATIGUE CUT SCORE FREQUENCIES COMPARED TO EXPECTED FREQUENCIES BASED ON ProQOL DATA*

	Observed N	Expected N	Residual
Not Compassion Fatigued	43,595	37,858.0	5,737.0
Compassion Fatigued	6,883	12,620.0	-5,737.0
Total	50,478		

*No cells (.0%) have expected frequencies less than 5. The minimum expected cell frequency is 12,620.0.
ProQOL: Professional Quality of Life scale

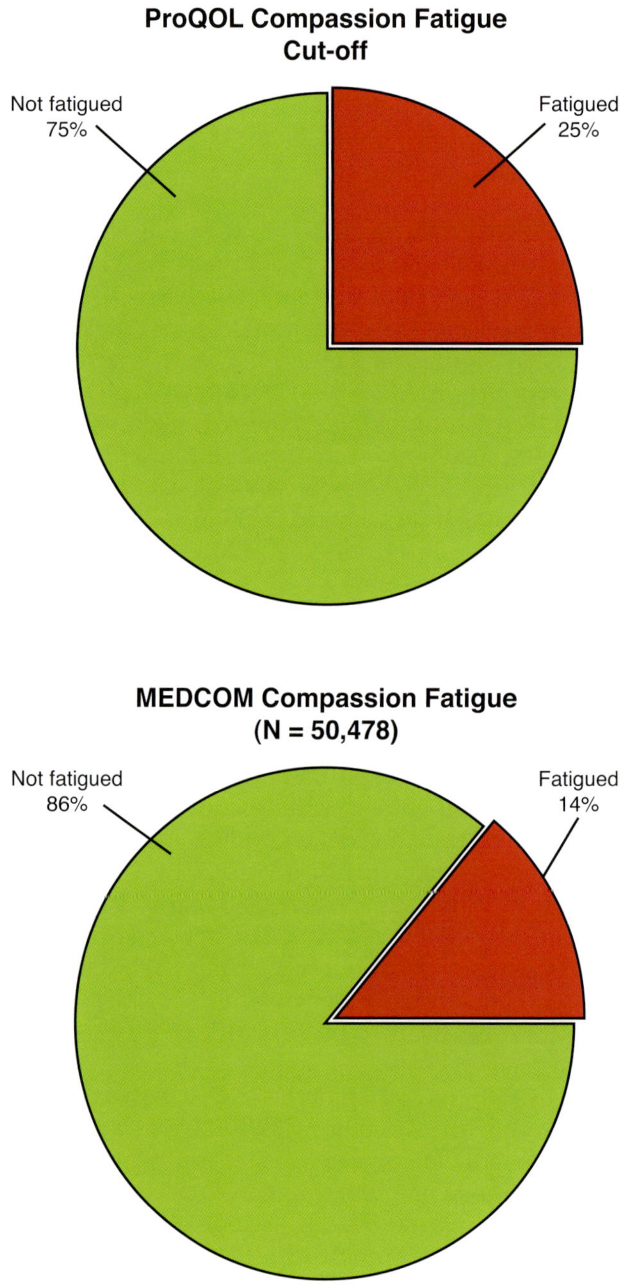

Figure 23-3. Percentage of ProQOL respondents with compassion fatigue compared to US Army Medical Command personnel with compassion fatigue.
MEDCOM: US Army Medical Command ProQOL: Professional Quality of Life scale

WAYS TO COMBAT PROVIDER FATIGUE

The EAT Model

The EAT model was created by Pechacek as a teaching tool for the AMEDD Center and School. The model offers a simple, easy-to-remember way for leaders, providers, wounded individuals, and anyone in the helping profession to articulate a way to manage provider fatigue and / or burnout. One way to combat provider fatigue is using the "EAT" action plan (Figure 23-4): **E**ducate yourself; **A**ssess your level of provider fatigue; and **T**ake action to build resiliency, create a self-care plan, and seek professional help if needed. Figure 23-5 is a visual reminder that focus on the provider is essential to combating provider fatigue. Providers are involved with many relationships, including those with a patient, soldier, and client, as well as those with a colleague who shares stories of trauma. The work environment may include many cases of trauma, and its resources may be stressed in the attempt to provide services to providers and others. Providers are also affected by war, disaster, or other traumatic event. The level of provider fatigue may be assessed with the markers and effects listed above through self and buddy observation and discussion, as well as through self-tests such as Figley's Secondary Trauma Scale[2] and the Professional Quality of Life: Compassion Satisfaction and Fatigue Subscales–III.[32]

Building Resiliency

Resiliency training focuses on strength rather than on pathology. For providers, it is important to have a resiliency model and to know where resilient strength comes from. Providers should identify a resilient role model: Who has the qualities that you as a provider would like to have? Have any of the people you work with inspired you? Resiliency, like the "Battlemind" concept (see Chapter 4, Combat and Operational Stress Control, in this volume), is a person's inner ability to face fear and adversity with courage, and the will to persevere and overcome adversity.

To build resiliency, providers must accomplish two difficult tasks simultaneously in a stressful situation: "self-soothing" and "self-confronting."[33] Self-soothing

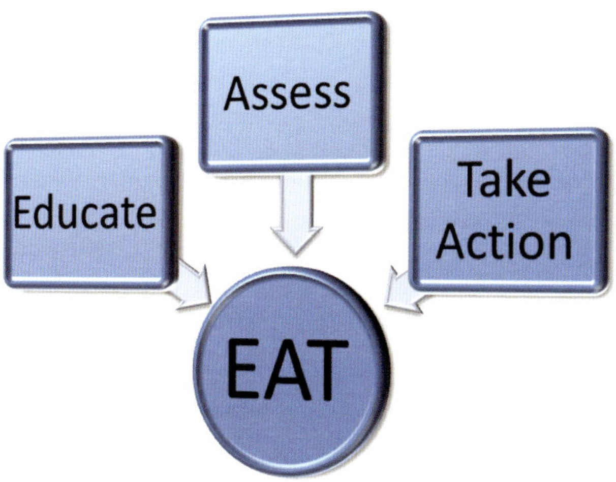

Figure 23-4. "EAT" to combat provider fatigue.
- **E**ducate yourself:
  - Who is affected?
  - What is provider fatigue?
  - What is resiliency?
- **A**ssess your level of provider fatigue:
  - What is the provider fatigue severity level?
  - What is the resiliency level?
  - How might resiliency be increased?
- **T**ake action:
  - Build up your resiliency
  - Create a self-care plan
  - Seek professional help if needed

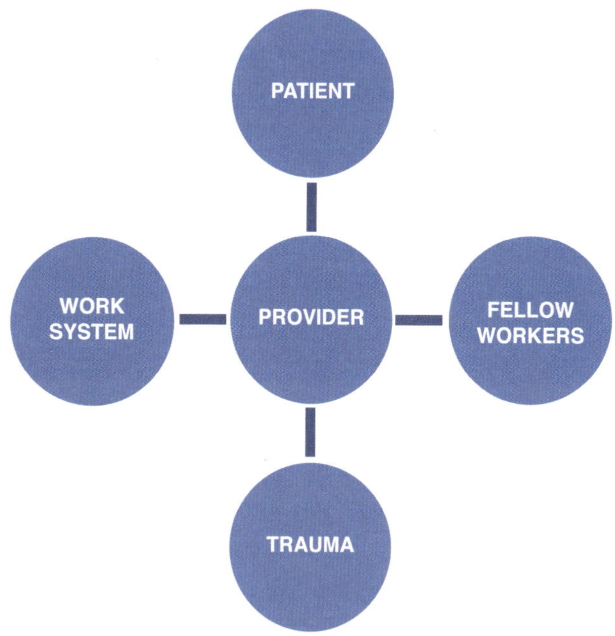

Figure 23-5. Focus on the provider is essential to combating provider fatigue. Providers are affected by their many relationships with patients and clients as well as colleagues, in a work environment with exposure to various types of trauma.

is the ability to deliberately relax while facing a stressful situation. Examples of self-soothing activities include working out, running, taking a bubble bath, hiking, diving, dancing, or just breathing deeply. The purpose of self-soothing is to enable the second step, self-confronting. Self-confronting is the process of assessing one's own anxiety and examining what might be learned from the situation. Providers should ask themselves questions such as:

- Why am I anxious?
- What am I trying to prove?
- Who am I trying to impress?
- What am I trying to fix?
- Am I depending on someone else to validate my sense of self-worth?
- What is the growth potential in this situation?

Self-soothing without self-confronting leads to avoidance, such as withdrawing, being demanding or driven by emotions, overeating, or substance abuse. Self-confronting without self-soothing leads to the risk of negativity without the willingness to step back and look for growth opportunities.

A Holistic Approach to Renewal

A provider can work to combat provider fatigue and build resiliency in five ways: (1) physically, (2) mentally, (3) emotionally, (4) spiritually, and (5) socially.

Physical Renewal

Nutrition is the first consideration in physical renewal. Under stress, some providers use food for comfort, and some refrain from eating. Maintaining good nutrition while avoiding fast food provides the best results. Furthermore, drinking the appropriate amount of water is important to fighting stress. Secondly, rest and relaxation are important for physical renewal, including sleep at night, breaks at work, and vacation time away from trauma.

Other means of physical renewal are exercise and laughter. Exertion through exercise releases pent-up frustrations and renews energy. Studies have shown that consistent exercise is associated with improved depression scores in patients with depression, cancer, and cardiac disease, and even in healthy subjects.[33] Other studies[34] have shown that laughter can reduce or prevent hypertension. Laughter may initially cause blood pressure to increase, but it then decreases and breathing becomes deeper, sending oxygen-enriched blood and nutrients throughout the body. This increase in blood flow and oxygenation of blood can actually assist in healing. Not conducive to physical renewal are forms of avoidance such as substance abuse, gambling, or other addictions.

Mental Renewal

Fear is normal for providers, who may worry about how well they are taking care of patients or accomplishing other duties. Fear can also lead to feelings of shame and guilt. Like physical renewal, mental renewal results from relaxation, through activities like reading books, listening to music, or learning relaxation techniques from tapes or seminars. When the sympathetic nervous system is calmed and quieted by relaxation, muscle tension decreases, the heart rate slows, and a feeling of well-being occurs.

Emotional Renewal

Emotional renewal means accepting and normalizing experience. Internalized anger, fear, depression, anxiety or other negative emotions can produce biochemical changes that have been shown to adversely affect the mind and body. The experiences of providing military medical care may cause troubling dreams or recurring thoughts. This is normal. Before providers can act to change their emotions, they must accept their situation. Emotional resiliency grows by thinking through daily events, sorting through emotions, talking with trusted friends, keeping a journal, and even laughing. Laughter can activate and strengthen the immune system by reducing four neuroendocrine hormones associated with the stress responses: epinephrine, cortisol, dopamine, and growth hormones.

Spiritual Renewal

Spiritual renewal is important to numerous military providers. Many have claimed that the sense of belonging to God or a higher power has assisted them in coping with anxiety and trauma. For many people, praise and worship with groups of people is uplifting and rejuvenating, listening to inspirational music or reading devotional books may be therapeutic, and taking time out to refocus attention on a greater "problem solver" reduces pressure when working in traumatic circumstances. Meditation can also be a source of provider resiliency; the ability to sit back, observe the mind, and direct attention to the present moment allows people to face challenges with renewed strength and flexibility. And for many, spiritual resiliency and renewal comes from forgiveness. Forgiveness is a way to avoid bitterness and recover from burnout; failing to forgive oneself and others often turns anger inward, resulting in bitterness, depression, and burnout.

For many military healthcare providers, spirituality is a deep sense of comfort, support, and daily inspiration. Studies have demonstrated that religion and spirituality are associated with reduced risk of medical morbidity and mortality and lower rates of divorce, criminal behavior, suicide, and drug abuse.[33] For some individuals, spirituality without a formal religion is their source of resiliency; however, according to a Gallup poll,[34] religion plays a huge role in the lives of others:

- for 70% of Americans, religion is a "very important" part of life;
- over 60% of Americans believe in angels; and
- 82% of Americans express interest in spiritual growth.

Social Renewal

Humans are social creatures. Military providers need to be with and relate to others for growth and development. Making time for others increases positive mental health and builds resilience. Having a social network increases coping strategies, a key ingredient for building resiliency both on the job and in all aspects of life. Providers have often asked, "How do I keep from getting depressed, listening to people's problems day after day?" The answer lies in the basic philosophy of looking for and emphasizing strengths rather than pathology in other people. Maddi[35] studied hardiness and wrote extensively about how people obtain hardiness and thrive under adverse conditions. He has found that people who thrive under stress maintain three key beliefs that help turn adversity into advantage: (1) commitment: striving to become involved in ongoing events rather than feeling isolated; (2) control: trying to influence outcomes rather than lapsing into passivity; and (3) challenge: viewing stressful situations as opportunities for new learning.[35]

Leadership

Like all complex systems, the military is greatly affected by its leadership. It is imperative that leaders at all levels be familiar with the concepts discussed in this chapter and encourage their soldiers to practice them. Colonel Joseph Pecko, former chief of the Soldier and Family Support Branch of the AMEDD Center and School, commented on the role of leadership and its place in striving for resiliency: "Leadership may have many meanings, but leadership practices in regard to provider fatigue are very important." Following the suggestions of PRT ensures strong leadership skills and the best results for all. Colonel Pecko encourages leaders to promote provider resiliency in the following ways:

- Place the care of the military care providers as the highest priority.
- Give credit and reward a job well done.
- Foster an environment of dignity and respect.
- Be available to talk with subordinates; spend time with them. Embrace an open door as well as anonymous "back door" policy. Allow providers to talk about their experiences and feelings. Let providers know that you are aware of their situation and offer help. Often, providers cannot take action on their own because they are too close to the situation, so the suggestions and attitude from leadership can be helpful.
- Keep your staff informed. Clearly express your policies and views on all matters. Allow subordinates to seek clarification on your policies without becoming defensive or seeing subordinates as disloyal. Try not to take subordinates' actions personally.
- Allow providers sufficient time to recover from duties, physically and mentally. Give them private time to do different work or catch up on tasks. Assist with the provider's everyday tasks when possible.
- Establish a climate where subordinate leaders can acknowledge stress and the desire to seek assistance. Teach leaders that seeking help takes courage. Encourage leaders to seek out and identify their most vulnerable and at-risk people.
- Take care of yourself as a leader and set a good example of self-care. Maintain a positive attitude during periods of adversity and challenge. The resiliency and mental toughness of the leader will shine through to others. Leaders setting an example in self-care and speaking the language of resiliency can bring about dramatic positive results in the work environment.

SUMMARY

In the 21st century, military care providers must understand provider fatigue and how it affects their care for those suffering from the effects of trauma. This chapter has defined types of fatigue related to the military healthcare provider and unit ministry teams, discussed Figley's model of compassion fatigue, identified the symptoms and markers of provider fatigue, and listed methods of preventing provider fatigue as well as ways to promote renewal and resiliency for the provider, including the role of leaders. Promoting resiliency for the provider, like the broader mission of providing healthcare for all service members, depends on teamwork. At every level, leaders and providers must begin with self-care before promoting resiliency in their colleagues and subordinates.

REFERENCES

1. Mental Health Advisory Team (MHAT-II). *Operation Iraqi Freedom (OIF-II). Report.* The US Army Surgeon General. January 30, 2005. Available at: www.armymedicine.army.mil/reports/mhat/mhat_ii/mhat.cfm. Accessed November 30, 2010.
2. Figley C. *Compassion Fatigue: Coping With Secondary Traumatic Stress Disorder in Those Who Treat the Traumatized.* New York, NY: Brunner/Mazel; 1995.
3. Figley C. Traumatization and comfort: close relationships may be hazardous to your health. Keynote presentation at: Families and Close Relationships: Individuals in Social Interaction; Texas Tech University, February 1982; Lubbock, Texas.
4. Figley C. Catastrophes: an overview of family reactions. In: Figley CR, McCubbin HI, eds. *Coping With Catastrophe.* Vol 2. In: *Stress and the Family*. New York, NY: Brunner/Mazel; 1983: 3–22.
5. Figley C. The family as victim: mental health implications. *Psychiatry.* 1985;6:283–291.
6. Figley C. *Helping Traumatized Families.* San Francisco, Calif: Jossey-Bass; 1989.
7. Stamm BH. *Secondary Traumatic Stress: Self-Care Issues for Clinicians, Researchers, and Educators.* Lutherville, Md: Sidan Press; 1995.
8. Remer R, Elliott J. Characteristics of secondary victims of sexual assault. *Int J Fam Psychiatry*. 1988;9(4):373–387.
9. McCann IL, Pearlman LA. Vicarious traumatization: a framework for understanding the psychological effects of working with victims. *J Trauma Stress.* 1990;3(2):131–149.
10. Pearlman LA, Saakvitne KW. Treating therapists with vicarious traumatization and secondary traumatic stress disorders. In: Figley CR, ed. *Compassion Fatigue: Coping With Secondary Traumatic Stress Disorder in Those Who Treat the Traumatized.* New York, NY: Brunner/Mazel; 1995: 150–177.
11. Herman JL. *Trauma and Recovery: The Aftermath of Violence—From Domestic Abuse to Political Terror.* New York, NY: Basic Books; 1992.
12. Miller KI, Stiff JB, Ellis BH. Communication and empathy as precursors to burnout among human service workers. *Commun Monographs.* 1988;55(9):336–341.
13. Erickson CA. Rape in the family. In: Figley C. *Treating Stress in Families*. New York, NY: Brunner/Mazel; 1989: 257–290.
14. White PN, Rollins JC. Rape: a family crisis. *Fam Relations.* 1981;30(1):103–109.
15. Verbosky SJ, Ryan DA. Female partners of Vietnam Veterans: stress by proximity. *Issues Ment Health Nurs.* 1988;9(1):95–104.
16. Danieli Y. Treating survivors and children of survivors of the Nazi Holocaust. In: Ochberg F, ed. *Post-Traumatic Therapy and Victims of Violence*. New York, NY: Brunner/Mazel; 1988: 278–294.
17. McCubbin HI, Dahl BB, Lester G, Ross B. The returned prisoner of war and his children: evidence for the origin of second generational effects of captivity. *Intl J Sociol Fam*. 1977;7:25–36.

18. Rosenheck R, Thomson J. Detoxification of Vietnam war trauma: a combined family-individual approach. *Fam Process.* 1986;25(4):559–570.

19. Danieli Y. The treatment and prevention of long-term effects and intergenerational transmission of victimization: a lesson from Holocaust survivors and their children. In: Figley C, ed. *Trauma and its Wake*. New York, NY: Brunner/Mazel; 1988: 295–313.

20. Wilson JP, Lindy JD. *Countertransference in the Treatment of PTSD.* New York, NY: Gilford; 1994.

21. Joinson C. Coping with compassion fatigue. *Nursing*. 1992;22(4):116,118–119,121.

22. Kottler JA. *Compassionate Therapy: Working With Difficult Clients.* San Francisco, Calif: Jossey-Bass; 1992.

23. American Psychiatric Association. *Diagnostic and Statistical Manual of Mental Disorders.* 4th ed. Washington, DC: APA; 1994.

24. Figley CR, ed. *Treating Compassion Fatigue.* New York, NY: Brunner-Rutledge; 2002.

25. Chaplain Wayne Garcia, AMEDD Center and School, PRT Class for Chaplain Training; 2008.

26. Regehr C, Goldberg G, Hughes J. Exposure to human tragedy, empathy, and trauma in ambulance paramedics. *Am J Orthopsychiatry*. 2002;72(4):505–513.

27. Stamm BH. *The ProQOL Manual. The Professional Quality of Life Scale: Compassion Satisfaction, Burnout and Compassion Fatigue/Secondary Trauma Scales*. Baltimore, Md: Sidran; 2005. Available at: http://www.proqol.org/ProQOl_Test_Manuals.html. Accessed December 10, 2010.

28. Stamm BH. Personal communication. June 9, 2009.

29. US Department of the Army. Provider Resiliency Training. Available at: http://www.behavioralhealth.army.mil/prt/index.html. Accessed December 10, 2010.

30. US Department of the Army. Introduction to the US Army Medical Department. Available at: http://www.armymedicine.army.mil/about/introduction.html. Accessed December 10, 2010.

31. Rubin A. *Statistics for Evidence-Based Practice and Evaluation*. Belmont, Calif: Thomas Higher Education; 2007.

32. Stamm BH. *The Professional Quality of Life: Compassion Satisfaction and Fatigue Subscales–III.* Baltimore, Md: Sidran; 1995–2002.

33. Funk JR. *Balancing the Burdens of Caregiving: Avoiding Compassion Fatigue*. Healthcare Chaplains Ministry Association; 2002.

34. Seibert A. *The Survivor Personality: Why Some People Are Stronger, Smarter, and More Skillful at Handling Life's Difficulties… and How You Can Be, Too.* New York, NY: Practical Psychology Press; 1993.

35. Smallwood B. Do you have compassion fatigue? Available at: http://hodu.com/compassion.shtml. Accessed December 10, 2010.

COMBAT AND OPERATIONAL BEHAVIORAL HEALTH

Section V: Surveillance and Intervention

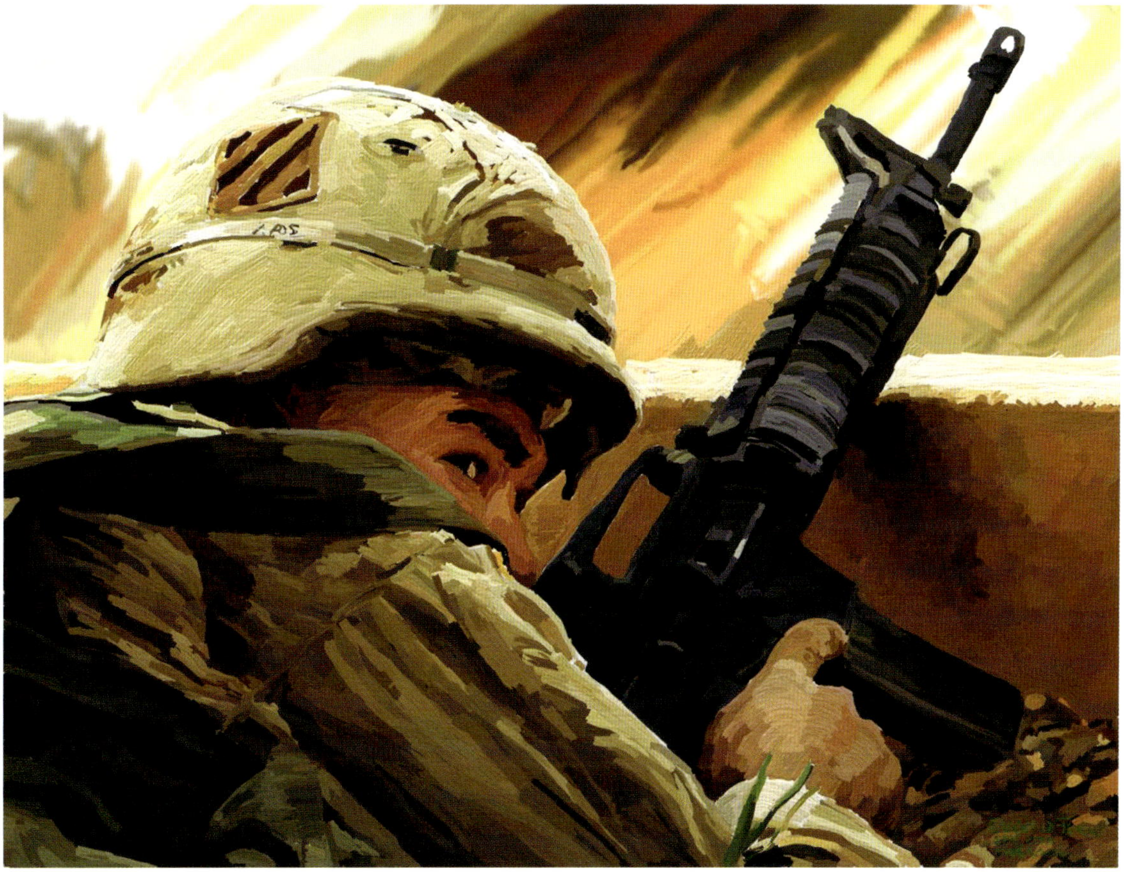

Under Fire, by Darrold Peters, Digital Oils/ArtRage 2.0, 2006.

Art: Courtesy of the US Army Center of Military History.

Chapter 24

ARMY SUICIDE SURVEILLANCE: A PREREQUISITE TO SUICIDE PREVENTION

GREGORY A. GAHM, PhD,* AND MARK A. REGER, PhD†

*Colonel, Medical Service Corps, US Army; Chief, Department of Psychology, Madigan Army Medical Center, 9933C West Hays Street, Fort Lewis, Washington 98431-1100

†Research Psychologist, Department of Psychology, Madigan Army Medical Center, 9933C West Hays Street, Fort Lewis, Washington 98431-1100; Affiliate Assistant Professor, Department of Psychiatry and Behavioral Sciences, University of Washington School of Medicine, 1925 NE Pacific Street, Seattle, Washington 98195-6340

INTRODUCTION

"Mental health specialists are now able to predict and prevent many suicides." At first glance, this statement (and those similar to it) appears to be a reasonable expectation of behavioral health providers. Suicidal ideation is a common presenting problem in outpatient settings,[1,2] and when suicides do occur, they inflict a tremendous emotional toll on family, friends, coworkers, and the broader community. Caring for the psychological needs of individuals requires providers to make suicide risk assessment and prevention a high priority. A general awareness of the significant amount of research that has been conducted to inform clinical decisions about suicidal patients may also suggest that clinicians can predict and prevent many suicides. Hundreds of studies have added to the body of knowledge about suicide, and there are a number of well-respected peer-reviewed journals dedicated solely to suicide research. Furthermore, there is a general recognition that behavioral health providers have specialized training in suicide intervention. Behavioral health providers are often viewed as experts in suicide assessment and prevention, and psychologists are regularly consulted about acute suicide potential in specific individuals, both within the military and in the civilian sector.

However, a closer analysis of the literature supporting the quoted statement suggests that more caution may be indicated. What does it mean to predict suicide? What does current research demonstrate about clinicians' abilities to predict suicide? How does prediction relate to prevention, and what does it mean to prevent suicide? This chapter will review some of the current literature on suicide prediction, suggesting that population surveillance studies provide an important tool to improve knowledge about suicidal behaviors in the military. It will describe an ongoing epidemiological surveillance project in the US Army, and propose future directions that will maximize the benefits of the program.

SUICIDE PREDICTION DEFINED

What does it mean to predict suicide? Prediction requires an individual to "foretell on the basis of observation, experience, or scientific reason."[3] Thus, suicide prediction implies an ability to anticipate future behavior. Obviously, truly knowing the future is not possible, but case law suggests that defendants in legal cases should have intervened when results were "reasonably foreseeable."[4] Certainly, clinical providers are tasked with predicting "reasonably foreseeable" suicide behaviors. Patients often present to providers with questions about their own safety. In addition, US Army commanders frequently consult psychologists for assistance in determining whether suicide is a "reasonably foreseeable" outcome for one of their soldiers. Providers are not only asked to assess *if* a patient will attempt or complete suicide, but *when*. A patient with a high risk of an imminent suicidal behavior requires a different intervention than an individual with chronic risk factors but no imminent risk of self-harm.

A key question, therefore, relates to the definition of "reasonably foreseeable." What research is available to help clinicians predict suicidal behaviors? How well can trained mental health experts currently foresee suicidal behaviors? The next section reviews some of the current research on suicide prediction in an attempt to inform future research priorities.

RESEARCH ON THE PREDICTABILITY OF SUICIDAL BEHAVIORS

Can providers currently predict suicidal behavior? Extensive research has been conducted to identify factors that might help in suicide prediction. Many variables have been studied, including demographic factors, specific risk factors, periods of elevated risk, psychopathology, psychiatric comorbidity, medical disorders, substance use, personality disorders, and personality traits. This body of work has produced some helpful information. For example, individuals who complete suicide are more likely to be white male adolescents or older adults.[5–7] Chronic or recurrent depression,[8] especially with comorbid alcoholism,[9] also increases the risk of suicide. In addition, hopelessness, relationship problems, living alone, chronic medical problems, and a family history of suicidal behaviors appear related to suicide completion.[10,11] Most individuals who complete suicide were seen in primary care within a month of their death,[12] but were less likely to be under the care of a behavioral health provider.[13] Individuals who complete suicide use methods more likely to be fatal, and therefore often die on their first attempt.[14] At the same time, there is strong evidence that a prior suicidal behavior increases the risk of a future suicide attempt[15] or completion.[16]

A variety of other risk and protective factors have varying degrees of support.[10,11] Unfortunately, many of these are based on a single study, or on contradictory evidence.[17] Although a significant body of research exists on the topic of suicide, few well-designed studies are available to answer some of the most basic questions in the field. Suicide research is extremely complex because of the low base rate of completions; ethical problems associated with studying high-risk individuals; biases in retrospective data; the cost of conducting well-designed studies; and differences in suicide rates by gender, age, and ethnicity.

The literature supporting the risk factors reviewed above suggests that even when all the known risk factors are considered together, they may only account for a small proportion of the variance in suicidal behaviors. That is, the known risk factors do not provide clinicians with sufficient information to predict suicide. This assertion is strongly supported by studies that have attempted to predict future suicides using many of the known risk factors described above. In one study at a psychiatric hospital, 1,906 inpatients with affective disorders were linked to their manner of death during a 2- to 14-year follow-up period. Using suicide risk factors judged to have the most robust evidence, researchers attempted to predict which patients would later complete suicide. In the follow-up period, 46 patients completed suicide. None were correctly predicted by the researchers.

In a similar study, 4,800 psychiatric inpatients were prospectively followed for 4 to 6 years.[18] Using a variety of risk factors, the researchers explored several approaches to predicting future suicides. Like the study described above, they characterized their own results as wholly "unsuccessful," even when alternative statistical approaches were employed in later studies.[19] Other studies[20,21] have reported similar results.

Unfortunately, failure to prospectively identify appropriate numbers of suicide completions is only one of the problems related to suicide prediction. A second problem relates to the high false-positive rate of current suicide prediction models. That is, the probability that a person will complete suicide when known risk factors are positive is low.[17] The implications of this problem are magnified exponentially by the fact that suicide is a very rare behavior. This problem is not simply a matter of statistical trivia, but has significant implications for the use of provider time and costs of treatment.

To illustrate the point, the following is an adaptation of an example provided by Gaynes et al.[22] Assume that a provider could predict suicidal behaviors with 80% sensitivity and 70% specificity (rates similar to depression screening). A provider who saw 10,000 patients over a number of years, 10 of whom truly attempt suicide, would correctly predict 8 suicide attempts while committing 2,997 false-positive errors. Thus, even if clinicians could predict suicide with this level of sensitivity and specificity, they would still miss 20% of the suicides, and the low base rate of suicide behaviors would result in significant costs related to false-positive errors.

In summary, behavioral health providers do not currently have the information they need to predict suicidal behaviors with any significant degree of accuracy. This conclusion is shared by many in the field. At the end of one of the prediction studies reviewed above, Pokorny stated, "Identification of particular persons who will (complete) suicide is not currently feasible."[18(p249)] After reviewing the literature on suicide prediction, Paris stated that "it is not possible to predict suicide with any degree of accuracy."[23(p235)] Bryan and Rudd stated that there is an "inability to predict suicidal behavior reliably."[24(p186)]

Although many of the studies reviewed above were based on actuarial prediction models, conclusions about the accuracy of clinical judgment do not differ from those summarized for statistical prediction models. Gaynes et al stated, "Despite the public health import of suicide and the Surgeon General's call to action, evidence to guide the primary care clinician's assessment and management of suicide risk is extremely limited."[22(p831)] Goldstein et al made the sobering statement that beyond identifying individuals with multiple risk factors, "it appears unrealistic for the general public or the legal system to expect that health professionals be able to predict suicide in specific patients based on our present knowledge."[25(p422)] Many clinicians and researchers prefer to define the clinician's role in terms of a "risk assessment process,"[24] suggesting a general recognition that providers are not capable of predicting suicide.

IMPORTANCE OF SUICIDE PREDICTION

Is suicide prediction important? Because current research to support suicide prediction is immature, and well-designed suicide research is extremely difficult and costly to conduct, it may be worth considering whether prediction is actually an important goal. Unfortunately, an analysis of the question results in the inescapable conclusion that without a reasonable ability to predict suicide, prevention efforts are extremely ineffective and costly.

Prediction is in many ways a prerequisite of prevention. In order to prevent a condition, prevention programs must generally be able to predict, with some degree of accuracy, who will benefit from a preventive effort. Without any predictive information, preventive actions can still be conducted, but high-risk individuals cannot be targeted, the effective components cannot be evaluated, and the costs are significant. Options for population-targeted prevention programs include conducting preventive activities with no one, with random individuals (or those with the most financial resources), or with groups who are *believed* to be at greater risk. These options are usually unacceptable. Clearly, when there is reason to believe that effective preventive efforts are available, failure to conduct any such activities is far from ideal. Performing preventive efforts among only those with sufficient economic resources devalues human life. However, applying preventive efforts to an entire population requires significant financial resources and exposes everyone in the group to any risks that are associated with the prevention efforts. Predictive information is essential for helping clinicians and patients balance the costs and benefits of specific preventive efforts.

An example from the field of dementia illustrates the latter point. Results from a number of studies suggest that high-dose treatment with the antioxidant vitamin E may slow disease progression and reduce the incidence of dementia.[26–29] Recently, however, new safety concerns related to high-dose vitamin E treatments have emerged.[30,31] Although prophylactic vitamin E supplementation may not be indicated for all older adults, some patients with known risk factors for Alzheimer's disease (eg, genetic vulnerabilities) may determine, after weighing the risks and potential benefits with their provider, that the risk–benefit ratio supports their use of vitamin E treatment. Advances in predicting dementia inform decisions related to preventive practices that may be associated with risks.

Similarly, suicide prevention efforts are not without risk. Although biological risks of suicide prevention may not apply, specific interventions to prevent suicide in a high-risk individual may violate confidentiality, harm the therapeutic relationship, increase stigma associated with treatment, decrease the probability of forthright conversations about suicidal ideation in the future, and increase the probability of treatment drop-out. In addition, population-based prevention efforts targeted at those for whom they are not appropriate may, at a minimum, reduce the effectiveness of the program, because messages can be "washed out" for everyone receiving nonspecific prevention efforts and training.

Based on the low base rate of suicide behaviors and the current accuracy of suicide prediction, well-intentioned interventions are surely targeting many for whom the intervention is not needed. It may be argued that as long as the negative impact on nonsuicidal individuals is low and the intervention is palatable to the community, the effort is justified. However, when individuals are targeted for intervention efforts, clinicians are committing numerous false-positive errors. Many individuals who are not "truly suicidal" may be targeted with intrusive interventions and suffer adverse effects because of the inability to predict suicide.

This discussion is not arguing that efforts aimed at prevention should be ended; rather, it is emphasizing the importance of efforts to improve the ability to predict suicide behaviors. In fact, efforts aimed at prediction can contribute significantly to prevention efforts, because progress in prediction often illuminates keys for prevention programs. The following is another example from the literature on Alzheimer's disease. Genetic research has now shown that mutations in three genes cause many of the early onset (before age 65) Alzheimer's disease cases and that these genetic mutations result in a build-up of a toxic protein fragment called amyloid beta, which may eventually lead to the death of nerve cells. This information has been helpful, not only for genetic counseling and predicting which family members will develop the disease, but also for defining new treatment approaches. The genetic data has informed exciting new approaches to treatment and prevention that attempt to "normalize" amyloid beta levels. Significant discoveries about suicide prediction would likely suggest information about the etiology of suicide that could potentially be leveraged by prevention programs. Although the road from prediction to prevention may be less direct for suicide, findings of significant predictive value would, at a minimum, suggest a narrower population in which to focus prevention efforts.

EPIDEMIOLOGICAL SURVEILLANCE STUDIES

Although research has demonstrated that clinicians are currently unable to predict which individuals will complete suicide with any degree of accuracy, suicide reduction is an extremely important health goal, and suicide prediction is in many ways a prerequisite to suicide prevention. This section reviews the use of epidemiological surveillance studies as an important tool for improving suicide prediction.

Suicide is not alone in the prediction challenges it presents due to its low incidence. A key challenge in many areas of medical and psychiatric research is the rarity of the disease or condition of interest. Improving the medical community's ability to predict these rare events requires research methods that are effective for studying low base-rate behaviors or diseases. Epidemiological surveillance studies offer just such a methodology.

Epidemiological methodologies are not composed of a single research design or statistical analysis. Rather, they comprise the body of methods that examine the occurrence of health-related conditions or events in defined populations.[32] Included among these are randomized controlled trials (RCTs), cohort studies, and case-control designs. In RCTs, subjects are randomly assigned to one of several exposures and prospectively followed to determine the effect on outcomes. Cohort studies are observational, in the sense that the researcher does not control which subjects are exposed to specific variables. A group of participants (a "cohort") is instead identified and then classified based on its natural exposure to the variables of interest, and followed over time to measure outcomes. This approach allows for the study of some topics that cannot be studied through RCTs, but cohort studies are inefficient for rare outcomes because a huge sample size is required to identify a sufficient number of infrequent positive outcomes on which to base conclusions. In contrast, a case-control study identifies individuals who are positive for a specific outcome and compares them to controls who are negative for the outcome.

Models for Suicide Research

Consideration of these basic methodologies indicates that RCTs obviously cannot be conducted to determine the effect of numerous exposure variables (eg, child abuse, combat exposure) on suicide. Large cohort studies have clear advantages, but they are extremely costly and inefficient for rare events with delayed outcomes such as suicide. Case-control studies offer an efficient, ethical approach to improving suicide prediction. A case-control surveillance system can efficiently identify individuals with suicidal behaviors and compare them to control subjects.

An Army Suicide Surveillance System

Although a number of suicide surveillance studies have been conducted in the United States and Europe (eg, the National Center for Injury Prevention, the World Health Organization Regional Office for Europe [WHO-EURO] Multicentre Study on Parasuicide), their results may not generalize to the US Army population. Soldiers represent a demographically distinct population that faces unique work-related stressors. The Army cohort is a younger, more ethnically diverse, and disproportionately male group compared to the broader US population.[33] Many soldiers are exposed to unique experiences and stressors, and as the Army mission changes over time, these work-related stressors can shift. Therefore, civilian suicide surveillance efforts may be of limited relevance.

An Army surveillance program offers a number of specific advantages. First, such efforts allow the Army to track trends over time as the military mission changes. Second, unique Army risk factors, such as deployments, combat exposure, training assignments, repeated geographic relocation, and others can be studied. Third, recommendations for refining the Army's suicide prevention efforts can be generated. Finally, a suicide surveillance program may provide opportunities to evaluate the effectiveness of suicide prevention programs and policies.

Additional research on suicide in both the military and civilian sectors is clearly needed. Epidemiological surveillance studies represent one of the more efficient approaches to improving suicide prediction. The Army has recently established a long-term suicide surveillance program to supplement its other risk-tracking efforts.

THE SUICIDE RISK MANAGEMENT AND SURVEILLANCE OFFICE

History of the Office

To effectively execute the suicide surveillance mission, the US Army established the Suicide Risk Management and Surveillance Office (SRMSO), a Medical Command office based at Fort Lewis, Washington. In 2002 and 2003, questions for an epidemiological data collection tool called the Army Suicide Event Report (ASER) were fielded, and content was clarified and revised. The ASER evolved from a scannable, paper-based data capture and processing approach, to an electronic Microsoft Word form, to a Web form submitted on a secure site. On February 4, 2004, Army Suicide Event Reporting Implementation Guidance was signed by Major General Kenneth Farmer, Jr, Deputy Surgeon General. This was followed by a widely circulated memorandum signed by Major General Joseph Webb, Jr, Deputy Surgeon General, stating that "the behavioral health leadership at each medical treatment facility will complete the ASER in accordance with the Implementation Guidance." The ASER requirement is also specifically addressed in the revised Army Regulation 600-63, *Army Health Promotion*.[34]

Army Suicide Event Report Data Collection Process

The ASER is a data collection form intended to standardize the data collected on all suicidal behaviors among Army soldiers. Submission of an ASER is required for all suicide-related behaviors that result in death, hospitalization, or evacuation from theater. To support this requirement, SRMSO has worked with each medical treatment facility (MTF) to identify both a command and an ASER point of contact (POC). The command POC is generally the MTF commander who is responsible for ensuring regional compliance with ASER requirements. The command POC also appoints a provider to serve as the ASER POC, who is responsible for either personally completing the MTF's ASERs, or ensuring that a qualified provider completes the requirements.

For suicide completions, the data collection process generally begins when SRMSO receives notification from the Armed Forces Medical Examiner's Office at the Armed Forces Institute of Pathology that a soldier's death has been confirmed as a suicide (Figure 24-1). Upon such notification, the ASER and command POC for the MTF are notified and requested to complete an ASER within 60 days. Alternatively, ASERs are commonly submitted after a suicide completion is identified locally; SRMSO then confirms this determination with the medical examiner's office.

For suicidal behaviors resulting in hospitalization or evacuation, the data-collection process requires ASER POCs to submit monthly reports for each MTF. This reporting generally involves coordination with inpatient psychiatric personnel and outpatient behavioral health clinic personnel. Because no central system formally tracks nonfatal suicide behaviors, these reports are currently used to determine how many ASERs are required for each MTF. ASER POCs are notified when expected ASERs are past due (30 days).

Army Suicide Event Report Questions

Development of the current ASER content evolved from a structured review of the past versions and data, and a systematic review of the literature. The results of the review were assessed for evidence-based predictors of suicide risk, and additional identified questions were combined into the update of the ASER.

For theoretically meaningful presentation of relevant risk factors for suicide and suicidal behavior, risk variables were organized into four categories using a prototype successfully implemented in the violence

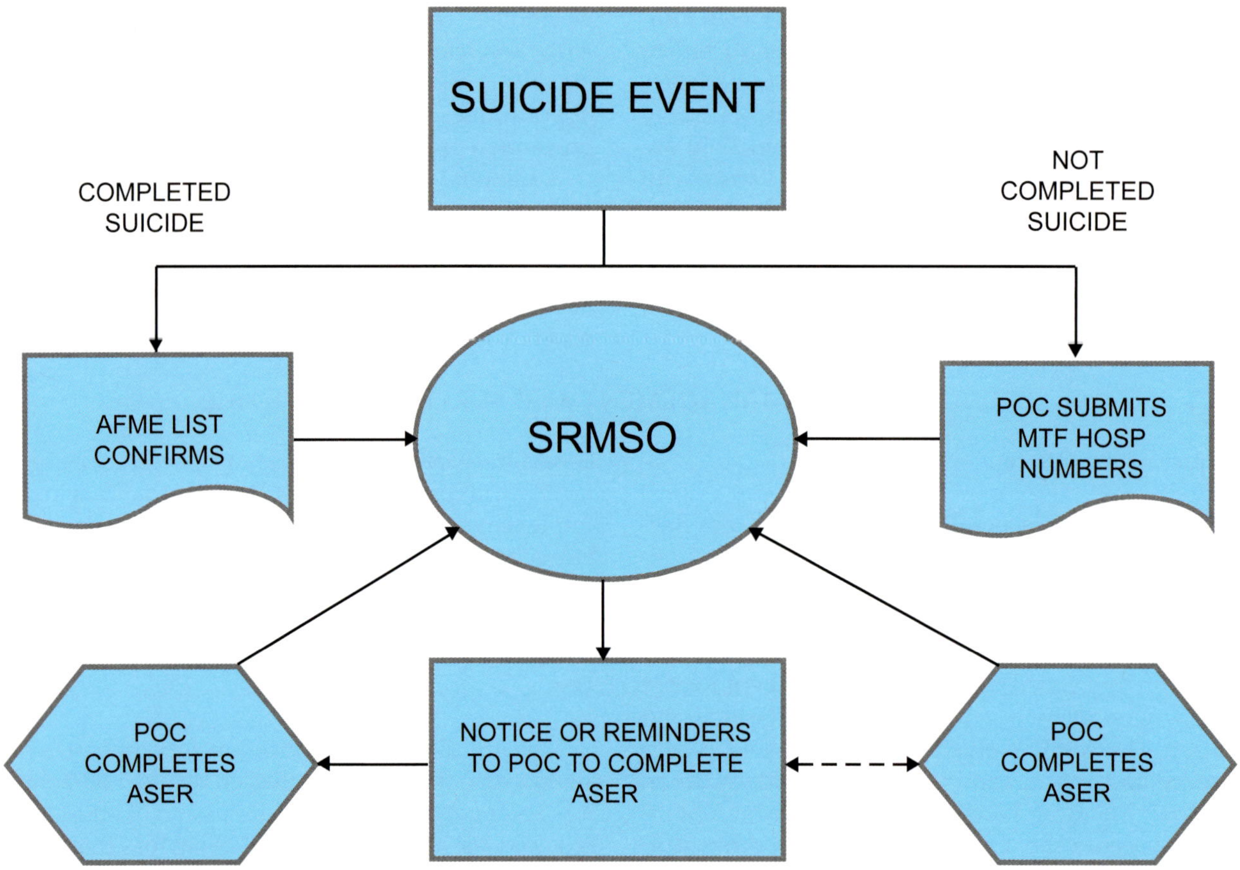

Figure 24-1. Army Suicide Event Report data collection.
AFME: Armed Forces Medical Examiner's Office
ASER: Army Suicide Event Report
HOSP: hospital
MTF: medical treatment facility
POC: point of contact
SRMSO: Suicide Risk Management and Surveillance Office

risk assessment literature[35]: (1) dispositional or personal factors (eg, demographics); (2) historical or developmental factors (eg, family history, prior suicidal behaviors, life events); (3) contextual or situational factors (eg, access to firearms, place of residence); and (4) clinical or symptom factors (eg, posttraumatic stress disorder, other psychiatric disorders or symptoms). This categorical banding of risks is intended to help organize the complex and multifaceted factors that contribute to suicidal behaviors. These factors were combined with a comprehensive set of questions related to the event (eg, method, location, injuries) to form the current ASER.

Required Source Information

Completion of an ASER requires a review of all relevant and available records. In addition, interviews may be needed in some cases, especially when suicidal behaviors resulted in hospitalization or evacuation. These data sources are described in Table 24-1.

Suicide Risk Management and Surveillance Office Reports

SRMSO drafts regular reports of suicide findings and also responds to requests from senior leaders for specific analyses. SRMSO generates quarterly and annual reports that are provided to the behavioral health consultants to the Surgeon General, the Army Suicide Prevention Program (G-1), and all ASER POCs and command POCs.

TABLE 24-1

SOURCE INFORMATION REQUIRED TO COMPLETE AN ARMY SUICIDE EVENT REPORT

Event	Required Data Sources
Completed suicide	Review of medical and behavioral health records
	Personnel and counseling records
	Investigative agency records (eg, Criminal Investigation Division)
	Records related to manner of death (casualty reports, toxicology, autopsy, suicide notes)
	Interview of coworkers and supervisors as needed and appropriate
	Interview of responsible investigative agency officer, as needed and appropriate
	Interview of other involved professionals and family members when appropriate
Attempted suicide	Interview of patient
	Review of medical and behavioral health records
	Interview of coworkers and supervisors as needed

Future Directions

Current SRMSO efforts are focused on improving data quality and accessibility for senior leaders. First, SRMSO is pursuing approaches to populating the ASER database from existing Army and Department of Defense data sources. As described above, the ASER POC must collect all relevant documents and data, extract the information that applies to specific ASER questions, and enter the data manually without errors. Populating the ASER database from existing databases with data quality assurances eliminates many opportunities for error. Significant conclusions and recommendations are drawn from ASER data, and the importance of this data is growing. For example, the Office of The Surgeon General has funded a new Suicide Prevention Office that is charged, in part, with facilitating new Army-wide prevention efforts based on empirical evidence derived from ASER research, the only Army-wide source of information on most aspects of Army suicide. Improving the reliability of ASER data provides Army leadership and the Suicide Prevention Office an improved capacity to make sound conclusions and recommendations.

Second, SRMSO is exploring options to improve the accessibility of ASER data for senior leaders. Currently ASER data are available in an Oracle database at the Fort Lewis, Washington, SRMSO office. Qualified requesters must submit a request for a report to SRMSO. A researcher at SRMSO must then query the database and analyze the results. SRMSO then checks and rechecks the results to assure that they are accurate and will answer the questions asked. Finally, the SRMSO research team must determine the most meaningful graphical representation, create the graphs, and return the results to the requestor. Although SRMSO has a solid track record of timeliness and efficiency, this process is less than ideal, especially given the importance of suicide and the short suspense that Department of Defense leaders often face.

SRMSO is exploring options for a user-friendly data reporting tool that can be configured to rapidly extract information from data sets and provide reports using predetermined statistical analyses and intuitive visual output. The Web-based Injury Statistics Query and Reporting System on the Centers for Disease Control and Prevention Web site provides a good example of such a tool.[6] The user is prompted to select types of data and appropriate categorical grouping variables. The graphical interface is not only informative but also interactive, allowing the user to drill down to get more specific information within a given domain. ASER data reported via a similar output generator would be delivered as an intuitive, interactive graphical output, rapidly generated to support the mission of senior leadership and healthcare providers.

A number of additional future directions are in the planning stages. One goal is to provide behavioral health clinicians access to relevant local ASERs to improve clinical care and safety planning. In addition, SRMSO is pursuing software functionality for command and ASER POCs to view regional ASER data over time. Efforts are also underway to improve the size and quality of control samples to compare to Army data. A large control sample drawn from the Army at large would be of significant value. Finally, SRMSO is focusing on developing a longitudinal data set. Even with a population as large as the Army, some topics cannot be studied because of the low base rate of suicide completions (eg, many questions related to suicides in Iraq). Longitudinal data over several years will allow for richer analysis.

SUMMARY

This chapter reviewed the issues and expectations associated with the prediction of suicides. A generally pessimistic conclusion was drawn regarding the ability to predict suicides with the current level of knowledge. After reviewing methods that may improve prediction of suicide risk, the authors recommended a surveillance model. Finally, the surveillance process within the Army was reviewed in detail, outlining its process, challenges, and goals.

REFERENCES

1. Kessler RC, Berglund P, Borges G, Nock M, Wang PS. Trends in suicide ideation, plans, gestures, and attempts in the United States, 1990–1992 to 2001–2003. *JAMA*. 2005;293(20):2487–2495.
2. Boudreaux ED, Cagande C, Kilgannon H, Kumar A, Camargo CA. A prospective study of depression among adult patients in an urban emergency department. *Prim Care Companion J Clin Psychiatry*. 2006;8(2):66–70.
3. Merriam-Webster Online. Available at: www.m-w.com. Accessed February 28, 2007.
4. Simon RI. Imminent suicide: the illusion of short-term prediction. *Suicide Life Threat Behav*. 2006;36(3):296–301.
5. Beautrais AL. Suicides and serious suicide attempts: two populations or one? *Psychol Med*. 2001;31(5):837–845.
6. National Center for Injury Prevention and Control. Web-based Injury Statistic Query and Reporting System (WISQARS). Available at: http://webappa.cdc.gov/sasweb/ncipc/mortrate.html. Accessed February 28, 2007.
7. National Institute of Mental Health. Suicide in the US: statistics and prevention. Available at: www.nimh.nih.gov/publicat/harmsway.cfm. Accessed February 28, 2007.
8. Sokero TP, Melartin TK, Rytsala HJ, Leskela US, Lestela-Mielonen PS, Isometsa ET. Prospective study of risk factors for attempted suicide among patients with DSM-IV major depressive disorder. *Br J Psychiatry*. 2005;186:314–318.
9. Maser JD, Akiskal HS, Schettler P, et al. Can temperament identify affectively ill patients who engage in lethal or near-lethal suicidal behavior? A 14-year prospective study. *Suicide Life Threat Behav*. 2002;32(1):10–32.
10. Hirschfeld RM, Russell JM. Assessment and treatment of suicidal patients. *N Engl J Med*. 1997;337(13):910–915.
11. Mann JJ. A current perspective of suicide and attempted suicide. *Ann Intern Med*. 2002;136(4):302–311.
12. Andersen UA, Andersen M, Rosholm JU, Gram LF. Contacts to the health care system prior to suicide: a comprehensive analysis using registers for general and psychiatric hospital admissions, contacts to general practitioners and practising specialists and drug prescriptions. *Acta Psychiatr Scand*. 2000;102(2):126–134.
13. Lesage AD, Boyer R, Grunberg F, et al. Suicide and mental disorders: a case-control study of young men. *Am J Psychiatry*. 1994;151(7):1063–1068.

14. Maris RW, Lazerwitz B. *Pathways to Suicide: A Survey of Self-Destructive Behaviors*. Baltimore, Md: Johns Hopkins University Press; 1981.

15. Leon AC, Keller MB, Warshaw MG, et al. Prospective study of fluoxetine treatment and suicidal behavior in affectively ill subjects. *Am J Psychiatry*. 1999;156(2):195–201.

16. Schneider B, Philipp M, Muller MJ. Psychopathological predictors of suicide in patients with major depression during a 5-year follow-up. *Eur Psychiatry*. 2001;16(5):283–288.

17. Oquendo MA, Currier D, Mann JJ. Prospective studies of suicidal behavior in major depressive and bipolar disorders: what is the evidence for predictive risk factors? *Acta Psychiatr Scand*. 2006;114(3):151–158.

18. Pokorny AD. Prediction of suicide in psychiatric patients. Report of a prospective study. *Arch Gen Psychiatry*. 1983;40(3):249–257.

19. Pokorny AD. Suicide prediction revisited. *Suicide Life Threat Behav*. 1993;23(1):1–10.

20. Thomas CB, Greenstreet RL. Psychobiological characteristics in youth as predictors of five disease states: suicide, mental illness, hypertension, coronary heart disease and tumor. *Johns Hopkins Med J*. 1973;132(1):16–43.

21. Motto JA, Heilbron DC, Juster RP. Development of a clinical instrument to estimate suicide risk. *Am J Psychiatry*. 1985;142(6):680–686.

22. Gaynes BN, West SL, Ford CA, Frame P, Klein J, Lohr KN. Screening for suicide risk in adults: a summary of the evidence for the US Preventive Services Task Force. *Ann Intern Med*. 2004;140(10):822–835.

23. Paris J. Predicting and preventing suicide: do we know enough to do either? *Harv Rev Psychiatry*. 2006;14(5):233–240.

24. Bryan CJ, Rudd MD. Advances in the assessment of suicide risk. *J Clin Psychol*. 2006;62(2):185–200.

25. Goldstein RB, Black DW, Nasrallah A, Winokur G. The prediction of suicide. Sensitivity, specificity, and predictive value of a multivariate model applied to suicide among 1906 patients with affective disorders. *Arch Gen Psychiatry*. 1991;48(5):418–422.

26. Sano M, Ernesto C, Thomas RG, et al. A controlled trial of selegiline, alpha-tocopherol, or both as treatment for Alzheimer's disease. The Alzheimer's Disease Cooperative Study. *N Engl J Med*. 1997;336(17):1216–1222.

27. Masaki KH, Losonczy KG, Izmirlian G, et al. Association of vitamin E and C supplement use with cognitive function and dementia in elderly men. *Neurology*. 2000;54(6):1265–1272.

28. Morris MC, Beckett LA, Scherr PA, et al. Vitamin E and vitamin C supplement use and risk of incident Alzheimer disease. *Alzheimer Dis Assoc Disord*. 1998;12(3):121–126.

29. Engelhart MJ, Geerlings MI, Ruitenberg A, et al. Dietary intake of antioxidants and risk of Alzheimer disease. *JAMA*. 2002;287(24):3223–3229.

30. Miller ER 3rd, Pastor-Barriuso R, Dalal D, Riemersma RA, Appel LJ, Guallar E. Meta-analysis: high-dosage vitamin E supplementation may increase all-cause mortality. *Ann Intern Med*. 2005;142(1):37–46.

31. Lonn E, Bosch J, Yusuf S, et al. Effects of long-term vitamin E supplementation on cardiovascular events and cancer: a randomized controlled trial. *JAMA*. 2005;293(11):1338–1347.

32. Last JM. *A Dictionary of Epidemiology*. 4th ed. New York, NY: Oxford University Press; 2001.

33. Office of Army Demographics. *Army Profile FY-05*. Washington, DC: Department of the Army; 2005.

34. US Department of the Army. *Army Health Promotion*. Washington, DC: DA; 2007. Army Regulation 600-63.

35. Steadman HJ, Silver E, Monahan J, et al. A classification tree approach to the development of actuarial violence risk assessment tools. *Law Hum Behav*. 2000;24(1):83–100.

Chapter 25

SUICIDE PREVENTION IN THE US ARMY: LESSONS LEARNED AND FUTURE DIRECTIONS

ELSPETH CAMERON RITCHIE, MD, MPH*; WALTER MORALES, MSA†; MICHAEL RUSSELL, PhD‡; BRUCE CROW, PsyD§; WAYNE BOYD, MDiv¥; KELLY FORYS, PhD¶; and STEVEN BREWSTER, MD, MPH**

*Colonel, US Army (Retired); formerly, Psychiatry Consultant to The Surgeon General, US Army, and Director, Behavioral Health Proponency, Office of The Surgeon General, Falls Church, Virginia; currently, Chief Clinical Officer, District of Columbia Department of Mental Health, 64 New York Avenue NE, 4th Floor, Washington, DC 20002

†Sergeant Major, US Army (Retired); Program Manager, Army Suicide Prevention Program, Army G-1, Headquarters, Department of the Army, 300 Army Pentagon, ATTN: Army G-1 (DAPE-HR), Washington, DC 20310-0300

‡Lieutenant Colonel, Medical Service Corps, US Army; Army Medical Department Neuropsychology Consultant, Warrior Resiliency Program, Lincoln Center, Suite 300, 7800 Interstate 10 West, San Antonio, Texas 78230

§Colonel, Medical Service Corps, US Army; Clinical Psychology Consultant to the Surgeon General, US Army, and Director, Warrior Resiliency Program, Southern Regional Medical Command, Brooke Army Medical Center, San Antonio, Texas 78234

¥Colonel, Chaplain Corps, US Army; Staff Officer, Comprehensive Soldier Fitness, Headquarters, Department of the Army, Zachary Taylor Building (NC3), 2530 Crystal Drive, Room 512B, Arlington, Virginia 22202; formerly, Program Manager, Directorate of Health Promotion and Wellness, US Army Center for Health Promotion and Preventive Medicine, Aberdeen Proving Ground, Maryland

¶Psychologist, Department of Outpatient Behavioral Health, Landstuhl Regional Medical Center, CMR 402, Box 1045, APO AE 09180; formerly, Psychologist, US Army Center for Health Promotion and Preventive Medicine, Aberdeen Proving Ground, Maryland

**Colonel, Medical Corps, US Army; Commander, US Army Medical Activity–Bavaria, Vilseck, Germany, Unit 28038, APO AE 09112 formerly, Directorate of Epidemiology and Disease Surveillance, US Army Center for Health Promotion and Preventive Medicine, Aberdeen Proving Ground, Maryland

INTRODUCTION

The goal of all the military services is to provide the serving men and women the best available support to assist them in overcoming the stressors that military service entails. The services utilize training and education, counseling, intervention, and postvention measures to help them find alternative and appropriate ways of dealing with stress and minimize the risk of suicide.

The spectrum of suicide behaviors (which ranges from gestures to serious attempts to completed suicides) and stress from the high operational tempo continue to have an effect on readiness and mission accomplishment. The Army Suicide Prevention Program's mission is to preserve readiness for soldiers, families, and Department of the Army civilians by continuing to develop policies and procedures that are designed to minimize suicidal behavior. Unfortunately, the Army-wide suicide rate has been trending upward every year since 2004. The total Army suicide rate in 2009 was 21.7 per 100,000, an increase from the rate of 9.8 per 100,000 observed at the beginning of hostilities in 2001.[1]

This chapter first describes the history of suicide prevention in the Army, then delineates current initiatives and some recent results of the Epidemiological Consultation Teams, and provides a theater update. This chapter is focused mainly on the Army because the authors are all affiliated with that service. However, all the military services have robust suicide prevention programs and the suicide prevention managers meet regularly. For example, there is a regular Suicide Prevention and Risk Reduction Committee meeting, formerly hosted by Health Affairs and more recently by the Defense Center of Excellence. Likewise, there is an annual Suicide Prevention Conference, which in recent years has included the Department of Veterans Affairs.

HISTORY OF SUICIDE PREVENTION IN THE US ARMY

Psychological characteristics and ideas that can lead a soldier to engage in a heroic disregard of personal safety on the battlefield can also lead to self-destructive behaviors when not at war. In 1897, Emile Durkheim advanced the first theories of suicide in the military. He defined suicide as those cases of death that resulted either indirectly or directly from something that the victim had done, knowing that death would result from this action.[2] Of note were those individuals who were not sufficiently bound to social groups, alienated, and who were said to engage in *egoistic suicide*. At the opposite end of the psychological spectrum, Durkheim proposed the idea of *altruistic suicide*, said to be a result of excessive integration, in which individuals become so immersed into social groups that they lose sight of individuality and are willing to sacrifice themselves to the group's interests, even at the cost of their own lives. Not surprisingly, the most common cases of altruistic suicide were said to occur among members of the military.[3]

The idea that at least some suicides were preventable evolved slowly throughout the 20th century. In the 1930s, Karl Menninger, a psychiatrist, wrote the influential book *Man Against Himself*,[4] which extended Freud's concept of the death instinct. In the 1950s, two psychologists, Norman L Farberow and Edwin S Schneidman, introduced several key concepts in suicide research and prevention. These concepts led to the opening of the Los Angeles Suicide Prevention Center, which provided a model for immediate consultation, guidance, and assistance to the suicidal person.[5]

This activity spurred the Los Angeles County coroner to first engage mental health professionals in determining cause of death via a "psychological autopsy,"[6] which is a methodology for determining not just how a person died, but why. It is a diligent process that requires gathering information from all available records as well as extensive interviews with those who knew the deceased.[7] The US Army relied on psychological autopsies during the 1990s, but that process has now been replaced by the Army Suicide Event Report,[8] which will be covered in more detail in this chapter. Currently, psychological autopsies are principally used to help determine the manner of death in equivocal cases, that is, when there is a question as to whether it was an accident, suicide, or homicide.

The American Association of Suicidology (AAS), founded in 1968, was the first national organization aimed at understanding suicide and its prevention.[9] Coincident with this national presence, publications dealing with the problem in the military began to appear, although no formal suicide prevention program was yet established.[10]

Army research psychologists and psychiatrists at the Walter Reed Army Institute of Research (WRAIR) in Washington, DC, became interested in the causes of suicide among Army personnel and began several influential reviews of suicide deaths.[11] In 1988, Colonel Nicholas Rock published an influential 10-year review of suicide and suicide attempts in the Army.[12] A number of articles by Dr Joseph Rothberg and others followed.[13–20]

The 1980s were a time of increased interest and dramatic progress in military suicide prevention efforts. On November 1, 1985, the Department of the Army (DA) published DA Pamphlet (PAM) 600–70, *Guide to the Prevention of Suicide and Self-Destructive Behavior*,[21] which discussed many of the myths of suicide and suggested a strategy to prevent self-destructive behavior. This was followed on September 30, 1988, by DA PAM 600–24, *Suicide Prevention and Psychological Autopsy*,[22] which detailed many of the principles of suicide prevention first suggested by Farberow and Schneidman, and later the AAS. This pamphlet set forth policy and procedures for establishing the Army Suicide Prevention Program (ASPP) and conducting psychological autopsies. It provided guidance for all suicide-prevention activities of the Army and it also provided the rationale, circumstances of use, and guidance for reporting psychological autopsies.

In 1999, the Army contracted with the AAS to produce *Suicide Prevention: A Resource Manual for the United States Army*,[9] which used principles of community mental health to establish prevention programming "intended to save lives and reduce the impact of self-harm behaviors using a three-tiered approach to achieve the best-coordinated prevention possible."[9(p3)] In general, the first level—primary prevention—consisted of those command programs designed to anticipate critical junctures in a person's career and make these less stressful. The next level—secondary prevention—included those command programs of special support and crisis counseling needed when persons encounter times of crisis and may be helped by a caring professional. The final level—tertiary prevention—was designed to provide immediate care for a potentially life-threatening crisis, and required care by a mental health professional. These common suicide prevention strategies are still in use today.

In December 1999, the chief of staff, US Army, directed a review of the ASPP. In 2000, the Army G-1 (formerly the Army Deputy Chief of Staff for Personnel), in collaboration with the Office of The Surgeon General (OTSG) and the Office of Chief of Chaplains, completed a review and determined that the program was basically sound, but needed to emphasize leadership involvement and offer more advanced training. In 2001, the Army implemented the Suicide Prevention Campaign Plan, which emphasizes preventive and intervention measures, directs commanders to take ownership of the program, and synchronizes and integrates resources at installation level. More recent efforts by the Army Suicide Prevention Task Force have built upon these actions. Despite these efforts, the rate of suicide in the Army has continued to rise (Figure 25-1).

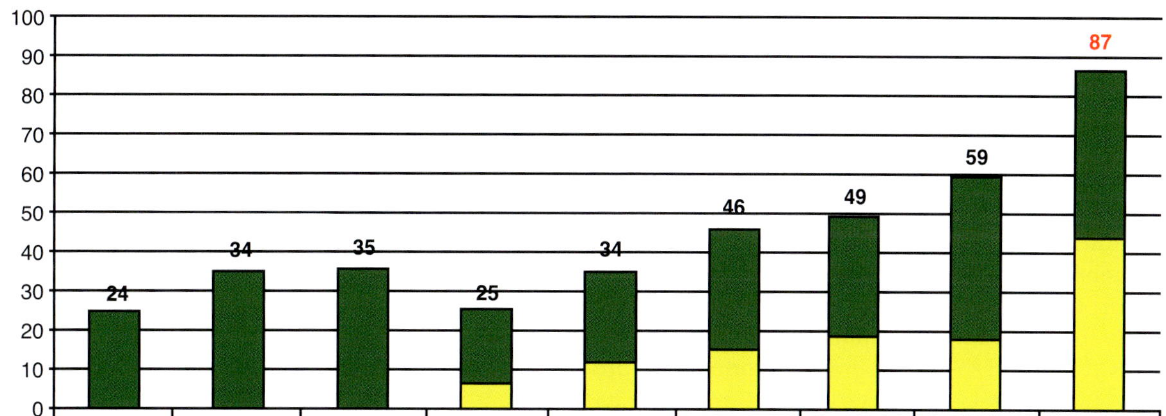

	CY01	CY02	CY03	CY04	CY05	CY06	CY07	CY08	CY09
Confirmed	24	34	35	19	22	31	30	41	44
Pending	0	0	0	6	12	15	19	18	43

Figure 25-1. Active duty suicides in the US Army January 1, 2001, through June 15, 2009. Data includes active duty, Army Reserve, and Army National Guard. "Pending" data not available for 2001 through 2003.
CY: calendar year
Data source: US Army G-1, Human Resources Policy Directorate.

ARMY SUICIDE PREVENTION PROGRAM

Initiatives and Efforts to Minimize Suicidal Behavior

Army G-1

The Army G-1 is the Army's proponent for the ASPP and collects demographic data on completed suicides. These data assist the Army G-1, commanders, program managers at the installation level, and "gatekeepers" Army-wide in the identification of trends and the development of new initiatives, tailored and targeted training, and policies to minimize suicidal behavior. The ASPP, as detailed in DA PAM 600-24,[22] also established a Suicide Prevention Task Force at each installation. In 2006, the Army G-1 formed an "Integrated Product Team" to integrate and synchronize efforts at the Headquarters, Department of the Army level. The team met regularly to identify ongoing initiatives, gaps in resources, and trends. Of main concern was the implementation of tailored and targeted training for soldiers and leaders.

Army programs have focused on training the gatekeepers—leaders, chaplains, behavioral health officers, and others. In the October 26, 2005, issue of the *Journal of the American Medical Association,* Mann and colleagues noted:

> Where the roles of gatekeepers are formalized and pathways to treatment are readily available, such as in the military, educating gatekeepers helps reduce suicidal behavior. Demonstration projects for other gatekeepers with intermediate outcome measures, such as referral rates and psychiatric treatment rates, should be conducted.[23]

To educate gatekeepers, the Army G-1 has contracted with outside organizations like Living Works Education and the QPR (Question, Persuade, Refer) Institute from Spokane, Washington, to provide suicide awareness training.

For several years, the mainstay of Army suicide intervention was the "Applied Suicide Intervention Skills Training" (ASIST) program,[24] a commercial product of LivingWorks, Calgary, Alberta, Canada. In 2002, the Army funded service-wide ASIST workshops[25] with accompanying computer interactive-training software. In 2005, the Army G-1 funded QPR workshops[26] Army-wide to provide additional resources in suicide-prevention awareness training, prevention, intervention skills, and risk identification to installations throughout the Army. Organizations have the option to use the training resource that best meets their needs; many continue to use Living Works Education, which has certified over 700 "gatekeepers" in suicide prevention and intervention,[25] as their primary training resource. In addition, QPR Institute has certified hundreds of trainers in suicide prevention.[26]

The G-1 also conducts many other training activities, to include:

- Ensuring suicide-prevention training is provided to all deployed soldiers as part of the deployment cycle support process.
- Revitalizing the Installation Suicide Prevention Committee/Task Force to adopt Army key strategies for suicide prevention and actively coordinate with efforts of major subordinate units.
- Developing and distributing suicide awareness cards that focus on buddy care, warning signs/risk factors, and resources (the card is a graphic training aid [GTA #12-001-01] that can be ordered through the installation and community Training Audiovisual Support Center).

The Medical Command and The Surgeon General

The OTSG and the US Army Medical Command (MEDCOM) support the ASPP by providing medical care, research and data analysis, and assessment of medical support systems. In 2007, OTSG established a dedicated Suicide Prevention Office within MEDCOM to ensure greater visibility of programs, obtain data, identify trends, and provide timely information to leaders. This office sought to standardize methods and procedures for future epidemiological consultation (EPICON) teams, improve behavioral health surveillance methods for postmortem review, and continue Department of Defense Suicide Event Reports (DoDSER) for suicide attempts and/or completions, which are reported to the installation suicide prevention program manager. However, currently its functions were subsumed under a new suicide surveillance cell managed by the former US Army Center for Health Promotion and Preventive Medicine (CHPPM), recently renamed Public Health Command (Provisional) or PHC(P). In the subsequent discussion, CHPPM will be used for past efforts and PHC(P) for current and future efforts.

CHPPM also supported the ASPP by focusing on continuous research and the development of awareness and training resources. For example, during calendar year 2006, CHPPM's main effort was to distribute 2,000 suicide awareness training kits to chaplains. Topics in this training program include suicide awareness, warning signs of suicidal thinking and behavior, and intervention skills development.

These suicide prevention activities are part of an ongoing effort, which includes suicide awareness briefings tailored for populations, tip cards, and warning signs and risk factors cards for distribution during training. CHPPM developed the acronym ACE — "Ask," "Care," and "Escort" — to serve as the intervention centerpiece idea to assist buddies who may be suicidal (Figure 25-2). "Ask" centers around the idea of asking the buddy about state of mind and whether the buddy is suicidal (ie, "Are you thinking about suicide?"). "Care" focuses on employing active listening skills and understanding the situations to provide the right mix of resources or help. "Escort" involves not leaving the buddy alone, but rather either escorting or finding someone to take this soldier to a professional for help.

Awareness is a key piece of the ASPP. CHPPM took the lead in promoting awareness by the development of posters for dissemination throughout the Regular Army, the Army National Guard (ARNG), and the US Army Reserves (USAR). In 2007, CHPPM finalized and initiated distribution of suicide awareness briefing content, via chaplains' channels, to enhance soldiers' skills in identifying personnel at risk, to assist interventions with the individual, and to provide guidance for referring or escorting the soldier to professional help. Chaplains and other facilitators can obtain all supporting materials (ie, tip cards, brochures, posters, briefings) through CHPPM's suicide prevention Army Knowledge Online (AKO) Web site (https://www.us.army.mil/suite/page/334798) and their Health Information Operations Web site (http://chppm-www.apgea.army.mil/hio_public/orders.aspx).

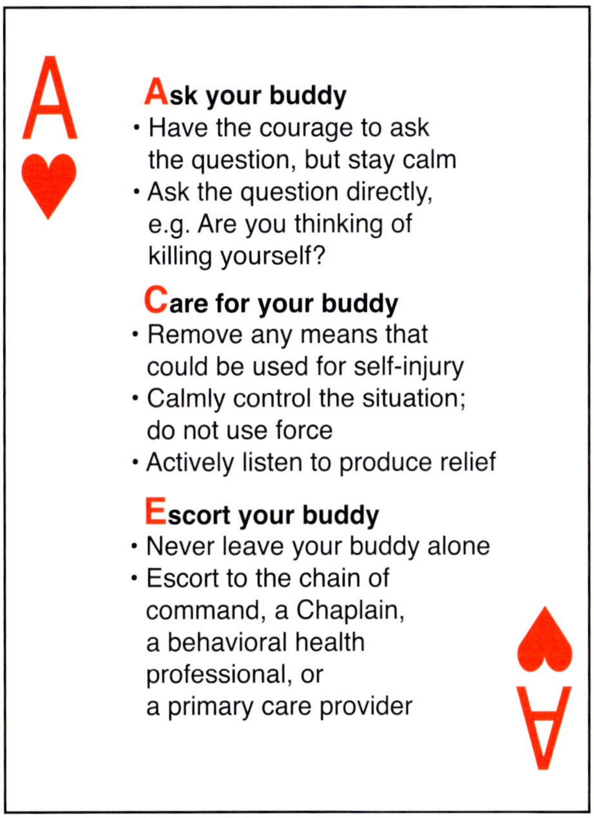

Figure 25-2. "ACE" card developed by US Army Center for Health Promotion and Preventive Medicine.

MEDCOM's Suicide Risk Management and Surveillance Office (SRMSO) managed the primary tool for surveillance of Army suicide, the DoDSER, which is a reporting and tracking mechanism for completed suicides and nonlethal events that result in hospitalization and/or evacuation. The original Army Suicide Event Report (ASER) was developed, with initial validation conducted by the US Army Medical Research Unit, Europe, as a means to track in near, real-time, suicides and suicidal behaviors of Army personnel within the US Army, Europe.[27]

Following the recommendation of the Mental Health Advisory Team (MHAT) I,[28] MEDCOM issued a policy directing that the ASER be used throughout the Iraqi Theater of Operations. The SRMSO, located at Fort Lewis, Washington, had operational oversight of the ASER, and conducted routine data analyses and published reports of these findings. In 2008, all the services began using this report form, which became the DoDSER. The SRMSO also has responsibility for updating changes to the DoDSER.

The SRMSO has directed that the DoDSER should be completed for all fatalities, hospitalizations, and evacuations where the injury or injurious intent is self-directed. It is not meant to replace the psychological autopsy, which is limited to fatalities in which the manner of death is equivocal, (eg, it is unclear whether it is an accident, suicide, or homicide). The DoDSER is available at: https://dodser.t2.health.mil/dodser/. (Chapter 24 in this volume discusses suicide surveillance programs.) CHPPM (now PHC [P])assumed operational control of the Army suicide surveillance program in 2009.

Chief of Chaplains

The Army Chaplaincy continues its "Strong Bonds" program (enriching and developing lasting relationships for both married and single personnel through the use of relationship-building seminars and workshops) Army-wide through the efforts of its 1,500 active duty chaplains and 1,200 reserve component chaplains. Suicide prevention awareness and intervention training continues to be its main effort in support of the ASPP. The Chaplaincy provides extensive counseling to soldiers and family members, some of whom may need to see a mental health professional. The Office of the Chief of Chaplains has worked very closely with CHPPM to develop a standardized suicide prevention awareness briefing for all chaplains and leaders. This training support package was completed in 2007, and is now available to all Army chaplains. Furthermore, the ACE (Peer) Suicide Intervention Program for soldiers and junior leaders is now being taught at the Chaplain Annual Sustainment Training course. Approximately 200 chaplains received this training in 2008.

Installation Management Command

Garrison commanders provide support to tenant units at the installation level. As such, they are charged with coordinating suicide prevention activities at the installation level. The Installation Management Command (IMCOM) has established the garrison director of human resources as responsible for ASPP execution at the installation levels. One of the initiatives is to eliminate confusion about the roles and responsibilities in support of the ASPP. Senior leaders throughout IMCOM support the program by engaging the leadership at the region and installation levels. An additional support to the Army's ASPP is the establishment of community health promotion councils (CHPCs) on every Army installation. The Army, via Army Regulation (AR) 600-63, *Army Health Promotion*,[29] has directed each Army installation to create a CHPC. The CHPC will ensure a proactive, coordinated, and synchronized local program. It will be the responsibility of each CHPC to ensure that suicide prevention activities are carried out in accordance with guidance from the Army's ASPP plan.

Army National Guard

The ARNG coordinates extensively with the active Army for training and policy development, workshops, conferences, and marketing. The ARNG Suicide Prevention Program reflects the active Army's program, with several differences due to the nature of the ARNG. The main differences and challenges involve data collection and availability of resources.

Like the active Army, the ARNG program takes a holistic approach that addresses suicide prevention, intervention, and postvention. Leaders and program managers initiate proactive measures to prevent suicide within their states by enhancing life skills in areas such as alcohol and drug abuse prevention, stress and anger management, communication, and conflict resolution training. In addition, personnel receive training in suicide risk identification and learn procedures for crisis intervention and referral. And finally, considering the devastating impact a suicide has on those who knew the deceased, the ARNG suicide prevention program includes postvention, which is also known as "prevention for the next generation."

In April 2007, the ARNG directed that all states appoint a suicide prevention program manager (SPPM) at each Joint Forces Headquarters. Having a program manager at the state level will allow a greater degree of suicide surveillance for states, as well as more accurate national oversight. The SPPM administers a statewide ARNG Suicide Prevention Program for both military and civilian leaders, managers, supervisors, soldiers, and family members. Administering a program of this magnitude requires coordination with commanders, surgeons, chaplains, personnel officers, mental health staff, health promotion staff, and public affairs personnel throughout the state, as well as local agencies and helping services, local law enforcement, civilian coroners, and hospitals. The SPPMs receive suicide intervention training and conduct suicide prevention, intervention, and postvention training and awareness activities throughout their respective states.

The ARNG goal is to provide intervention skills training to at least one soldier per company-sized unit. All soldiers will receive annual suicide awareness training. To maximize valuable resources, the ARNG SPPM has compiled a directory of all ASIST-trained National Guardsmen to share with active Army and USAR. The services often collaborate to provide training to the different components. The state SPPM tracks and reports all attempted and completed suicides to its state's Joint Forces Headquarters and to the National Guard Bureau SPPM. The state SPPM identifies trends and provides decision support when possible factors lead to an increase of suicides.

The challenges inherent in collecting accurate data about the suspected suicide of a soldier serving in a traditional status ("M Day," or one weekend a month) lie in the fact that the details of the suicide are contingent upon reports by family members, medical authorities, and local law enforcement investigations. Most ARNG soldiers who died by suicide had been in a traditional drilling status, rather than on active duty in a Title 10 status. Although AR 600-63, *Army Health Promotion*, requires a review to be conducted by a mental health officer for any active or reserve component soldier on active duty whose death meets specific criteria for suicide or suspected suicide,[29(chap5, para5-8)] there is no such requirement for ARNG soldiers not on active duty.

In addition to tracking and reporting, the ARNG

differs from the active Army in terms of resources available. Whereas active duty soldiers deploy from and return to a post where all resources for support are usually available without charge, easily identifiable, and in a designated geographic area, the ARNG deploys from and returns to communities across the state. Resources available to each ARNG member are dependent on what the local community provides, and therefore vary from member to member. Because the state SPPMs are from the local community, they will be familiar with these local resources. They will ensure soldiers and families are aware of these resources and are able to identify problems and refer personnel in crisis to an appropriate source of help. This information is included in annual suicide prevention briefings and published in Army suicide prevention policies and guidelines.

An increasing number of benefits have become available to all ARNG soldiers. The TRICARE Transitional Assistance Membership Program is available for 6 months to ARNG soldiers returning from deployment, with the option to buy in to the TRICARE program for a length of time determined by the amount of time the soldier was deployed. In addition, all soldiers, regardless of whether they were ever deployed, can take advantage of Military OneSource (available at www.MilitaryOneSource.com), which will contract with a local mental healthcare professional to provide six counseling sessions at no cost to the soldier.

The ARNG SPPM has created two suicide-prevention Web sites for soldiers and families. One is public and can be found at http://www.virtualarmory.com/WellBeing/suicide. The other site is restricted to members of the ARNG who have a Guard Knowledge Online (GKO) account and password and is located at https://gkoportal.ngb.army.mil/C15/C5/SuicidePreventionProgram.

Army Reserves

The USAR faces all of the challenges described by the ARNG. Furthermore, their regions are large, and soldiers are often "cross-leveled" from one area of the country into another. Thus gathering accurate data is an enormous challenge. Recent initiatives in the USAR have included: (*a*) implementing suicide-awareness training into family programs, (*b*) appointing ASPP managers at major subordinate commands, (*c*) forming community health promotion councils, (*d*) developing policy guidance for referral of soldiers to mental health, and (*e*) directing chaplains to develop reporting requirements for suicide prevention training.

Recent Initiatives

The Army Campaign Plan for Health Promotion, Risk Reduction, and Suicide Prevention

The vice chief of staff for the Army established the Army Suicide Prevention Task Force (ASPTF) in March 2009 in response to the Army's increasing suicide rate. The ASPTF's effort has resulted in approximately 250 tasks throughout the Army that are currently being executed. The resultant effort of the ASPTF has been published as the "Army Campaign Plan for Health Promotion, Risk Reduction, and Suicide Prevention," which is directly monitored by the vice chief of staff for the Army; the tasks identified will substantially change the way the Army provides care to its extended family. This campaign plan reaffirms the Army's commitment to care for its greatest strategic assets—soldiers, families, and civilians.

Behavioral and Social Health Outcomes Program

The Army has established an epidemiological surveillance program that will utilize the public health process approach to developing a behavioral health and social outcomes capability. The mission of the PHC(P) Behavioral and Social Health Outcomes Program is to protect combat readiness and soldier health by addressing psychological and social threats through surveillance and in-depth analysis of behavioral health and disease outcomes; tracking rates and changes in trends in deployed and nondeployed populations; and projecting BH epidemiology. In addition, working with the Army G-1, a specialized suicide analysis cell was funded to conduct suicide-specific analysis and surveillance in support of the ASPP.

In 2008, the Army contracted with the National Institute of Mental Health to assist the Army in a comprehensive research effort that will lead to better prevention strategies and fewer suicides. This memorandum of agreement spans over 5 years and represents an Army investment of $50 million. The Behavioral and Social Health Outcomes Program and National Institute of Mental Health are collaborating to provide and analyze these data.

OPERATION IRAQI FREEDOM THEATER SUICIDE ASSESSMENT

The previous MHATs have reviewed the status of the Operation Iraqi Freedom (OIF) theater's suicide prevention and surveillance program, including an analysis of completed suicides (see Exhibit 25-1 for

EXHIBIT 25-1

OPERATION IRAQI FREEDOM AND SUICIDE PREVENTION

In 2003, the Office of The Surgeon General (OTSG) deployed a Mental Health Advisory Team (MHAT) to Kuwait and Iraq to assess soldiers' mental health issues. Every year since then, an MHAT team has visited the theater of operations and produced a comprehensive report. MHAT II and V included Afghanistan. The full reports are available on the www.armymedicine.mil Web site. Recommendations that are especially relevant to suicide prevention include:

1. Establishing a behavioral health consultant position in theater that will synchronize and coordinate behavioral health resources needed across the area of operations.
2. Establishing a modified theater suicide prevention program based on both current installation-based strategies and lessons learned from epidemiological consultations and MHAT visits to the theater of operations. These strategies include:
   a. Designating proponents to manage the suicide prevention program. (The proponent for the Operation Iraqi Freedom theater of operations was appointed in June 2006.)
   b. Establishing a command climate that encourages help-seeking behavior.
   c. Maintaining vigilance by leaders and soldier-peers (buddy care).
   d. Conducting continuous training throughout the deployment cycle.
   e. Implementing the surveillance of completed suicides/suicide attempts using the Army Suicide Event Report .

Nonetheless, military suicide continues to be a significant problem in Iraq. Theater rates of suicide have trended upward since 2004, and remain elevated compared to both the total Army rate and rates observed in the civilian population.

a discussion of the first MHAT). The MHAT V conducted a similar review of Multi-National Force-Iraq's prevention and surveillance program and a detailed analysis of completed suicides.

A team was requested by the Multi-National Corps-Iraq (MNC-I) commander to do a theater assessment in the fall of 2007. The team worked in parallel with MHAT V and with information from the Criminal Investigations Division (CID) and a review by SRMSO. A detailed "Summary of Theater Suicides" for 2007 was presented by the forensic investigator, MNC-I CID, on October 2, 2007.[30] A similar review, limited to Army personnel, was performed by the SRMSO at Fort Lewis, Washington, 2 weeks later, with a focus on soldiers in Iraq and Iraq suicides. The results of all studies are similar, and thus will be examined together.

As has been consistently true for reviews going back as far as 20 years,[12] military suicide is most often precipitated by the loss of a relationship—either a spouse or other intimate partner. The SRMSO study reflected that 68% of Iraq suicides had had an intimate relationship failure, compared to 56% of the suicides in the non-Iraq population. This highlights the importance of the "Dear John" letter or e-mail, or other messages communicating the end of a relationship, as an implicated factor in the deployed setting.

A second major cause implicated in suicide is loss of career, usually through the Uniform Code of Military Justice (UCMJ) or other criminal charges. Approximately 35% of Army suicide cases in the Iraqi theater of operations had recent UCMJ charges—higher than the suicides in the continental United States. The CID review for all services found a 24% incidence of UCMJ charges.[30] These two factors alone—loss of relationship and loss of career—appear to account for the majority of the suicides seen in the Iraqi theater of operations.

The Iraq CID review suggests that 60% of the 2007 suicides showed behavioral changes or signs of depression prior to their suicides. The SRSMO review of DoD-SER data also suggests that a substantial percentage of Army personnel who commit suicide sought help: 50% of all suicides presented to a medical treatment facility (MTF) for care within 30 days of the event. This supports research literature, which suggests that although people considering suicide may not be able to accurately identify their problems as emotional in nature, or marshal the right resources to help them, they manifest an awareness that something is wrong and may seek out primary care.[31–35] This highlights the importance of suicide prevention and awareness in the primary care and pastoral settings.

Discussion

The US Public Health Service considers suicide risk and prevention in terms of relative *risk factors* and *protective factors* for suicide.[36,37] These factors have been adopted by the Centers for Disease Control and Prevention (CDC) and are used to frame the discussion of suicide in Iraq.

Risk Factors

Risk Factors most relevant to Army suicide in Iraq include:

1. *Loss (relational, social, work, or financial).* This has consistently been the key variable associated with suicide. It appears that long tour duration, in itself, does not increase rate of suicide, but rather serves as a secondary factor in provoking marital disruption and in kindling the loss of relationships.
2. *Isolation, a feeling of being cut off from other people.* The Soldier Survey assesses this directly by asking whether soldiers are "feeling distant or cut off from people." Results note that 51.8% of all soldiers surveyed have experienced these feelings of isolation. Morale, Welfare and Recreation efforts to deliver mail and enhance Internet and phones, have probably helped, but this variable should continue to be monitored over time, and efforts to keep soldiers feeling engaged in what is going on "back home" should be encouraged.
3. *Barriers to accessing behavioral health treatment.* As the troop footprint in Iraq surged, the supply of behavioral healthcare providers in theater expanded less robustly in 2006 and 2007.
4. *Easy access to lethal methods.* It has been proposed that the ready availability of weapons is a contributory factor for the elevated suicide rate in theater. Although firearms do increase the lethality of suicide attempts, epidemiological studies do not clearly support a finding that either gun ownership, in general, or living in a country that bans firearms result in a lower population suicide rate. Furthermore, the troops that have been deployed in Iraq since 2003 have had weapons readily available. Any rise in this rate cannot solely be attributed to weapons availability.
5. *Unwillingness to seek help because of the stigma attached to mental healthcare.* Stigma continues to be a major issue in the willingness of service members to seek care. Soldier and leader interviews indicate first-line supervisors are the primary barriers to seeking care. This is fueled by a perception that seeking behavioral healthcare is "shamming" or attempting to avoid duty. A need for further efforts to educate these first-line supervisors is indicated (Exhibit 25-2).

EXHIBIT 25-2

STIGMA ASSOCIATED WITH SEEKING BEHAVIORAL HEALTHCARE

Four types of stigma are generally seen: (1) career, (2) leadership, (3) peer-to-peer, and (4) personal. Stigma was reported differently across rank groups; lower enlisted were more concerned about peer and self-perceptions, senior enlisted were most concerned about their careers and perceived leadership abilities.

Career

- On permanent record, affects future promotion and employment
- End career, lose retirement
- Lose security clearance
- "Boarded out" rather than rehabilitated

Leadership

- Some "old school," senior NCOs, and early promoted NCOs create/maintain stigma
- More stigma for senior enlisted, others think they can't lead, fear of affecting retirement
- Many squad/platoon leaders don't support
- Treated differently; doubt "warrior" abilities; ridicule those with a profile

Peer-to-Peer

- Peer stigma is the worst
- More stigma if never deployed
- Treated differently, ridiculed
- Gossiped about/perceived as faking

Personal

- Weak, isolated, embarrassed
- Profile makes them feel worthless
- Pride/denial
- Don't want to be viewed as a "bad" soldier

Protective Factors

Protective factors for suicide buffer individuals from suicidal thoughts and behavior. To date, protective factors have not been studied as extensively or rigorously as risk factors. Identifying and understanding protective factors is, however, equally as important as researching risk factors. Protective factors that act to reduce suicide probability in Iraq include:

1. *Lack of intoxicants*. Alcohol is a known risk factor for both civilian and military suicides. The relative lack of availability of intoxicants in the theater of operations should therefore act to lower the rate of suicide. It has long been known that intoxicants make the act of suicide more likely through disinhibition effects. (The National Violent Death Reporting System examined toxicology tests of those who committed suicide in 13 states, and 33.3% tested positive for alcohol; 16.4% for opiates; 9.4% for cocaine; 7.7% for marijuana; and 3.9% for amphetamines.[38])
2. *Effective clinical care for mental, physical, and substance abuse disorders*. Certain units within the theater of operations deployed with a comprehensive plan for deployment cycle support, and a number of best practices for effective soldier support, which appear to have produced a significant decrease in aberrant behaviors, including suicide, after the program was implemented.[39] These results suggest wider adoption of the deployment cycle support model for the brigade combat team.
3. *Easy access to a variety of clinical interventions and support for help seeking*. Recent redistribution of troops in the battle space calls for equally agile shifts in behavioral health support, which is a strong argument for locating the theater mental health consultant at the MNC-I level. This also calls for increased efforts to destigmatize the act of seeking mental healthcare services.
4. *Family and community support*. Efforts to strengthen family and unit bonds should be encouraged, and the definition needs to be broadened to include significant others regardless of marital status.
5. *Skills in problem solving and conflict resolution*. Relationship enrichment and training, at both the soldier and the family readiness group level, designed to improve communication will assist in reintegration and strengthening relationships. All available evidence supports stabilizing relationships as the single most effective suicide prevention intervention.
6. *Cultural and religious beliefs that discourage suicide and support instincts for self-preservation*. There have long been observed differences in suicide rates across gender, as well as racial and cultural lines.[40] This illustrates the powerful basis of cultural beliefs for acceptable and socially appropriate behavior. For example, certain cultural beliefs support the idea of suicide in response to dishonor. Similar idea threads permeate the military culture (ie, death before dishonor, respect for the Samurai as portrayed in the media, popularity of movies in which suicide or death is seen as a logical approach to failure.) This opens up the possibility of "suicide-proofing" the military culture with carefully crafted messages against soldier suicide (ie, "Don't let the enemy win," "Don't let your buddies down," "Make it home alive").

Summary of Theater Suicide Assessment

The Multi-National Force-Iraq has an active suicide prevention committee, chaired by the chief of clinical operations for the command surgeon. This has recently been augmented by the MNC-I Suicide Prevention Board, which is chaired by the corps chief of staff. The current suicide training program is being completely reconfigured into a much more robust program, which, once established, will require further review to gauge effectiveness.

The DoDSER is being widely used in the theater by behavioral healthcare providers, but only for suicides or suicidal gestures by Army personnel. Although numerous service-specific mental health tracking systems exist, a single, joint tracking system capable of monitoring suicides, mental health evacuations, and use of mental health/combat stress control services in a combat environment does not exist.

PSYCHIATRIC EPIDEMIOLOGICAL CONSULTATIONS IN THE US ARMY

Description and Background

Sending a behavioral health EPICON team to investigate an apparent suicide cluster is an emerging strategy in the US Army (Table 25-1). An epidemiological consultation is analogous to any other medical consultation in that the existence of a problem is verified through history and examination/investigation of the

TABLE 25-1

COMMON BEHAVIORAL HEALTH EPIDEMIOLOGICAL CONSULTATION THEMES

Theme	Ft Leonard Wood 2001 (suicide)	Ft Bragg 2002 (homicide)	Ft Riley 2005 (suicide)	Ft Hood 2006 (suicide)	Ft Campbell 2008 (suicide)	Ft Carson 2009 (homicide)
Individual Risk Factors						
Deployment: length, multiple, unpredictability		✓	✓	✓	✓	
Combat intensity						✓
Family separation, relationship stress, lack of support		✓	✓	✓	✓	✓
Increased violence against persons including spouse / family		✓	✓	✓	✓	✓
Increased use of alcohol and drugs, and related offenses			✓	✓	✓	✓
Previous gestures / attempts / BH contact	✓	✓	✓	✓	✓	✓
Manipulating, malingering	✓		✓		✓	✓
Legal and financial issues		✓	✓	✓	✓	✓
History of misconduct						✓
Systems Issues						
Stigma: personal, leadership, career		✓	✓	✓	✓	✓
Poor service delivery for dependents		✓	✓	✓		
Transition, reintegration (one size fits all)		✓	✓	✓	✓	✓
Problems with BH services, FAP, ASAP	✓	✓	✓	✓	✓	✓
Lack of standardized screening, tracking, intervention, data collection	✓	✓	✓	✓	✓	✓
Leadership / management climate	✓	✓	✓	✓	✓	✓

ASAP: Army Substance Abuse Program
BH: behavioral health
FAP: Family Advocacy Program
Data source: US Army Center for Health Promotion and Preventive Medicine.

problem, a differential list of potential causes may be established, and data analysis is used to generate recommendations for remedy and prevention. EPICONs are public health investigations of clusters, outbreaks, or epidemics of symptoms or illnesses. They are modeled after the CDC's "EPIAID," which is a service that CDC provides to state and local health departments. The concepts behind an EPICON are drawn from the public health literature and are adapted to behavioral health. The EPICON mission was originally established at the WRAIR in 1969 and transferred to CHPPM in 1994. In the Army, EPICONs were originally limited exclusively to infectious diseases and environmental exposures. However, this mechanism was expanded to include clusters of behavioral health problems after an outbreak of suicidal behaviors at Fort Leonard Wood, Missouri, in 2000.

Every suicide case in the US Army receives a thorough investigation, with participation from multiple organizational entities on an installation, to collect data to determine if current factors or conditions exist that may be mitigated to prevent future suicides (Figure 25-3 and Figure 25-4). It is occasionally necessary to replicate this process using the population-based approaches of an EPICON to look at communities and organizations in a similar manner. The authors and others have participated in the five EPICONS that have been performed since 2000: (1) Fort Leonard

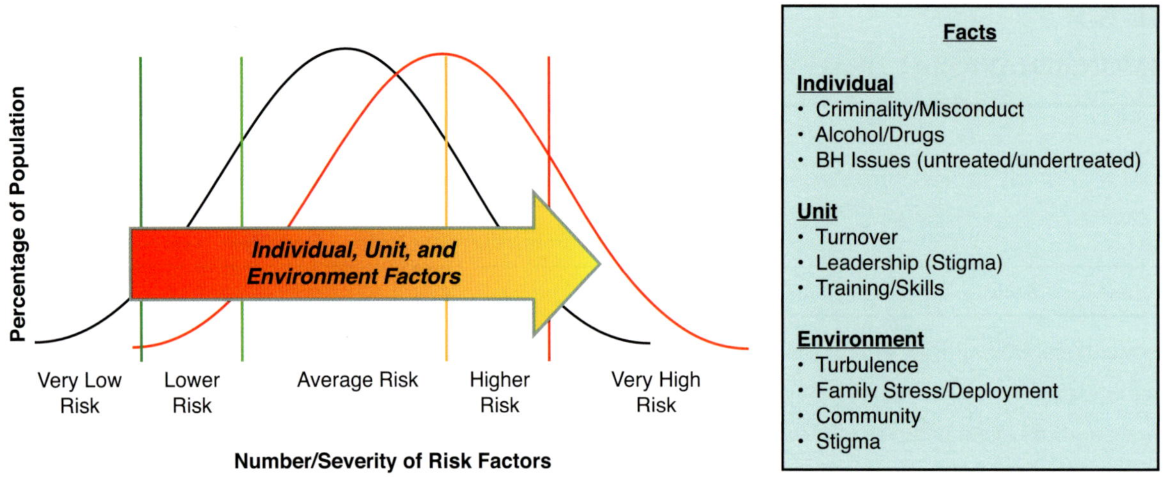

Figure 25-3. Causal factors. Multiple individual, unit, and community factors appear to have converged to shift the population risk to the right. This would put more soldiers in the "very high risk" category, making clustering more likely.
BH: behavioral health

Wood, Missouri, in 2000, following the deaths of two recruits by suicide; (2) Fort Bragg, North Carolina, in 2003 following two murders and two murder-suicides; (3) Fort Riley, Kansas in 2005, following six suicides in 14 months; (4) Fort Hood, Texas, which had 22 suicides between 2003 and 2005, and (5) Fort Campbell, Kentucky, with 14 soldier suicides between 2006 and 2007. There was an EPICON at Fort Carson, Colorado, in 2008, which focused on homicides, but included other violent crimes and suicides. At the time of this writing, there is another EPICON to examine suicides and accidental deaths in the warrior transition units.

An EPICON may become necessary when the requirements for epidemiological expertise or even simple personnel exceed the resources of a theater or regional medical command. EPICON teams hold the benefit of bringing in new resources capable of focusing solely on the issue at hand, free of the distractions and demands inherent to supporting a community or organization. Additionally, the higher level of tasking

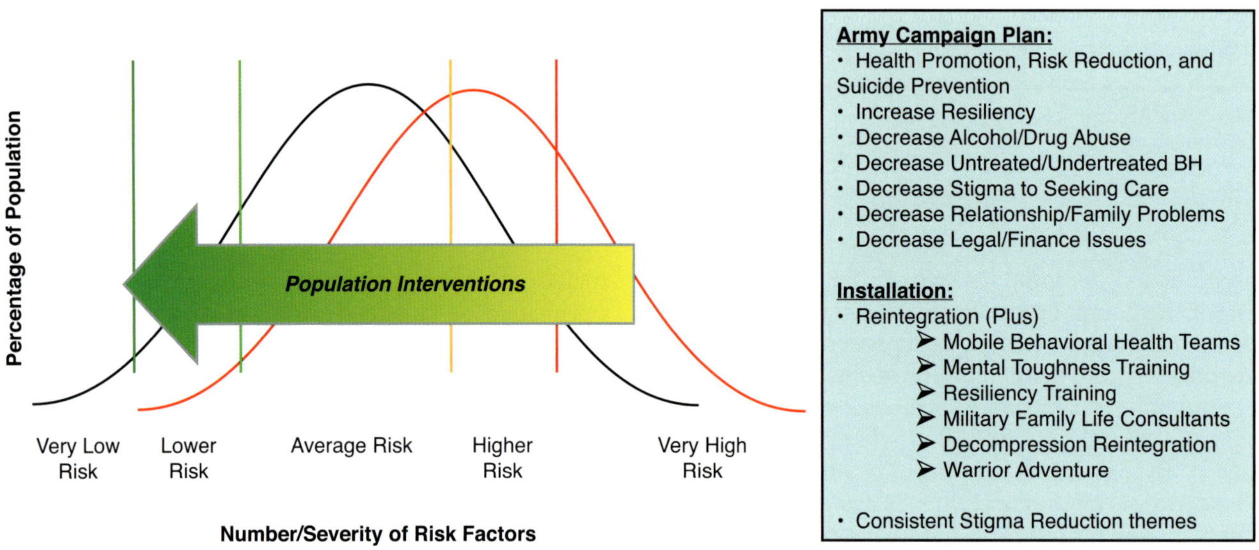

Figure 25-4. Suicide factors to consider. Although it is important to identify and help individual soldiers, the biggest impact will come from programs that shift the overall population risk back to the left. Effective medical treatment can prevent individuals from increasing in risk or decrease their risk, but it cannot shift overall population risk very much.
BH: behavioral health

authority associated with EPICONs may open doors to data sources and collaboration that are difficult to achieve when such investigations are conducted with a local approach. It is important to note that EPICONs are not staff assistance visits or inspections, nor are they research endeavors. EPICONs provide a mechanism to investigate a disease cluster on an urgent/emergent basis. They can be conducted as a public health initiative without a research protocol. The perception that there is a problem (eg, increased numbers of suicide behaviors, homicides, etc) can lead to request for an EPICON.

Initiation of an Epidemiological Consultation and Operational Support

The request for an EPICON usually originates from local leadership (eg, hospital, brigade, or installation commander). Implementing an EPICON requires extensive coordination and approval, particularly from the local leadership of the installation that is involved, as well as OTSG, MEDCOM, and other stakeholders. Both AR 40-5, *Preventive Medicine,*[41] and DA PAM 40-11, *Preventive Medicine,*[42] task the commander, PHC(P), with the responsibility to provide EPICON support worldwide. PHC(P) responds to such taskings from MEDCOM and OTSG through the Proponency Office for Behavioral Health and the Proponency Office for Preventive Medicine. PHC(P) is readily able to assemble a team of experts (often pulling resources from throughout the Army) to deploy on short notice. All tasking should come through OTSG/MEDCOM for purposes of validation, command visibility, and resourcing approval. The process of validation is one that should take place between the theater or regional medical command and MEDCOM/OTSG.

It may be necessary to draw on resources from the Armed Forces Health Surveillance Center and PHC(P) to analyze data in this process. Command interest, political pressure, and media attention may all influence the validation of an EPICON. The PHC(P) operational support section is capable of facilitating country clearances, travel orders, funding citations, travel reservations, hotel accommodations, and even work environment requirements such as computer connections, meeting room reservations, and rental cars. In preparing for an EPICON, it is a great help to prearrange for a meeting room that can accommodate the entire EPICON team during evenings and on weekends. This working space should have computer connections and the ability to accommodate screen projection of computer documents.

A team leader will be selected, usually a senior officer. EPICONs have had teams of varying sizes from 4 to 14 people, composed of individuals from OTSG, PHC(P), the regional medical centers, installation, and subject matter experts from throughout the Army. The challenge is balancing the need to include all of the stakeholders, but not overwhelm the local environment. Appropriate agency representatives may include behavioral health, chaplains, installation management activity, and the G-1. The local behavioral health leadership should be included as much as possible, as they will need to contribute to the analysis and implementation of recommendations.

The following representatives should be considered as members of any behavioral health EPICON team:

- team leader: senior preventive medicine officer or behavioral health specialist;
- local senior behavioral health clinician (social work, psychology, psychiatry);
- epidemiologist with appropriate database development support;
- chaplain;
- Army Substance Abuse Program representative;
- safety officer representative with knowledge of Army risk reduction data;
- health risk communication specialist;
- G-1 representative; and
- unique representation depending on the target population (such as senior noncommissioned officers, unit behavioral health specialist, division surgeon, local civilian resources, and unit/installation public affairs officer).

Once a team has been established, it is essential to formulate a schedule from which all of the team members can work. This timeline will establish the necessary planning meetings, the dates of deployment, and deadlines for work to be done in preparation for the EPICON, as well as documentation requirements. All members must understand the importance of meeting the timelines established by the EPICON leader. Scheduling the time for the team to visit is always a challenge. Most assessments have taken 1 to 2 weeks, and may require repeated visits. An inbrief and outbrief must be arranged with the local installation command, and often the hospital command. Other important agencies with whom to communicate include behavioral health, chaplains, CID, and Army Community Services, including Family Advocacy, Risk Reduction Program, and the Army Substance Abuse Program. Clinical records, including medical, behavioral health, family advocacy, and substance abuse, should be reviewed on the index cases. Much of this work can be done in advance of the actual

EPICON visit by the installation and local MTF in the interest of efficiency and to maximize use of time on the ground once the team arrives. It would be helpful for all established EPICON team members to review previous copies of installation-level EPICONs conducted in the past. Such EPICONs are available through the PHC(P) Directorate of Epidemiology and Disease Surveillance.

The content of the inbrief to be presented to the installation and MTF commands should be completed in advance of the EPICON deployment. The inbrief should clearly reflect the team's understanding of the command's intent for the EPICON. This will often include an initial hypotheses held by those who are at the installation. (Note that initial hypotheses are often wrong, but it is critical to recognize both the concerns and the questions asked by leadership as a starting point.) The inbrief should include a description of the team composition, a schedule (to include the outbrief date), a plan of action, and realistic requirements for support. It is important to establish a senior unit or installation leader to serve as a point of contact in advance of the EPICON's deployment. Discussions prior to the visit with the point of contact and relevant staff will help to reduce any misunderstandings or communication shortfalls in advance of the prebrief to senior leadership, which is most often a general officer.

Epidemiological Consultation Activities on the Ground and Data Sources

As previous team members have performed this mission, they have learned many lessons, both in the science and practical application of this consultative service. Whenever possible, the EPICON team should arrive at its destination on the same day. It is important to have a team meeting immediately after arrival to review the overall plan, schedule, and ground rules. No overt activity or interviews should be conducted before the command has received its prebrief and has given the team permission to proceed. Engaging the command staff early and frequently throughout the EPICON process can be very beneficial.

Outbreaks of completed suicides are hard to study because they are very rare and present challenges for epidemiological analysis. As of 2008, the rate in the US Army was 20/100,000/year. This compares to the demographically matched population of 20/100,000/year. Even more rare in the Army are homicides paired with suicides. However, similar psychological dynamics may lead to both suicides and suicide-homicides. These dynamics are usually in the context of broken intimate relationships, with accompanying fears of humiliation, rejection, and loss. In general the motives for suicide and methods of suicide are reflective of the historical Army findings. The top apparent motivations for suicide in soldiers were found to be relationship failures, followed by legal and occupational difficulties and financial problems. Severe mental illness leading to suicide is rare in the military population but may occur. Among soldiers, impulsivity and substance abuse are more often than not contributing factors. Chronic pain, medical disability, and individual perceptions of general health all merit further analysis as risk factors for suicide in the military. Deaths by firearm, hanging, and jumping are the most common methods. All of the findings above mirror historical trends and substantiate the importance of looking across the spectrum of medical and social data on an installation during an EPICON.

The following data sources have proven helpful in evaluating individual suicides in the military:

- medical and behavioral health records,
- ASERs,
- CID files,
- AR 15-6 (commander's inquiry reports),
- RCA reports,
- Post-Deployment Health Assessment/Post-Deployment Health Re-Assessment records,
- deployment data (date arriving and departing, location, days in theater),
- enlistment medical waiver data,
- Army Substance Abuse Program records,
- Family Advocacy Program data,
- line-of-duty reports, and
- Armed Forces Institute of Pathology data.

The most useful individual suicide data sources have proven to be DoDSERS, RCA reports, and CID reports. It is important to get the installation commander's support to gain access to all of these data sources. Although the above data are useful for looking at the index cases on an installation (see following section on epidemiological methods), it is also useful to evaluate population data from the community. Population-based data from an installation or theater can reveal important information on trends related to leadership, morale, operations tempo, mental health support, alcohol-related events, domestic violence, and so forth. All of these are important indicators of the behavioral health of a community and may offer insight in the generation of hypotheses or reveal associations in the course of epidemiological analysis that lead to recommendations.

The following are useful sources of population data on Army installations:

- installation population size and demographics (denominator data),
- installation deployment cycle and impact on population calculations,
- behavioral health utilization and workload,
- behavioral health staffing,
- Army risk reduction data,
- Military OneSource reports,
- Army Substance Abuse Program data, and
- installation-level Family Assistance Program data.

Additionally, it may be helpful to conduct interviews and focus groups to explore concerns of the soldiers (junior enlisted and junior noncommissioned officers), military leadership, MTF staff, community-based agencies and installation support staff, and military family members or familiy readiness groups. Such sessions, when conducted by experienced health risk communications specialists, can reveal important information on prevailing perceptions, stigma associations, knowledge status, and morale within subpopulations on an installation. When collected early, this information can help guide the course of the EPICON. It also can be useful in targeting intervention strategies at the community level.

Likewise, surveys can be of great assistance when applied to an appropriate number of individuals. In most of the EPICONs that have been completed, staff from WRAIR or PHC(P) performed anonymous soldier surveys. The surveys ask about a wide range of issues, including access to care and command climate. The most recent survey administered by PHC(P) looked for associations with self-reported suicidal ideation. Surveys contribute to the inclusion of quantifiable data into the report. The hardest challenge in working with the command is finding time for their soldiers to take the surveys, especially in a high operations tempo environment. PHC(P) has the ability to generate electronic form surveys, which can greatly reduce data-entry workload and errors in analysis.

During the EPICON visit, it is essential to establish a close working relationship with both the MTF and the installation PAOs. All information released publicly must go through these individuals. Similarly, after the EPICON document summary is drafted, it must go through the local PAOs for review prior to the submission to command or OTSG/MEDCOM.

While working an EPICON, it is necessary to generate daily situation reports, which must be forwarded to PHC(P) Operations and up to OTSG. EPICONs are high visibility missions with tremendous sensitivity to the command. The team should document each day's activities (interviews, meetings, surveys, presentations) to reference in writing the EPICON final document.

Methods in the Epidemiological Consultation

Suicide outbreaks are unique from other types of disease outbreaks because the perception of the outbreak itself may lead to further cases, especially in an adolescent population. This characteristic must be taken into consideration in EPICON activities. Behavioral health assessments may use concepts from infectious diseases epidemiology, such as "exposure" to index cases, "contagion," and "isolation." Epidemiologic methodology in an EPICON should be guided by the services of an experienced epidemiologist on the team. Although the outline presented below is not the focus of this chapter, it is important to briefly discuss epidemiologic methods for understanding behavioral health EPICONS.

During an EPICON, basic epidemiological strategies should be followed, to include:

- defining the questions or current hypotheses (one of these may determine if there is an actual outbreak),
- conducting hypothesis-generating interviews to broaden knowledge of the subject and what should be evaluated more thoroughly,
- establishing a case definition for this public health study,
- conducting an investigation using epidemiological methods,
- completing initial analysis,
- providing initial findings and recommendations to leadership, and
- completing final analysis and write-up.

In general, epidemiologic methods of study include: (*a*) case series (clinical, forensic, etc); (*b*) case-control studies (eg, suicide cases vs controls); (*c*) cross-sectional studies (eg, compare cases with rest of battalion); (*d*) soldier surveys (usually done by WRAIR or PHC(P)); and (*e*) focus-group interviews.

The basic questions are:

- Is there a real outbreak of suicidal behavior?
- Is the rate significantly higher than expected (eg, when compared to like installations or the overall Army)?
- What factors contributed to the outbreak and how can they be compared against one another?
- What recommendations can be made to address the problem?

When defining inclusion criteria for cases, the team must determine an outbreak time frame, the individuals included, and their location. An index case definition must also describe who is not included as a case. An example from the Fort Campbell, Kentucky, index case definition is described below:

> Index cases were defined as all confirmed and pending suicides occurring between January 1, 2006 and October 31, 2007 based on Army G-1 and Armed Forces Institute of Pathology (AFIP) data. There were a total of 14 index cases in this time period. Cases were restricted to active duty soldiers who were assigned to Fort Campbell, Kentucky, at time of death. Family member, civilian, and retiree suicides were not included in this analysis because of limitations to medical and legal data available on non–active-duty deaths.

One useful tool inherent to any EPICON is an "epi-curve." Traditionally, a team shows the time course of an epidemic by drawing a graph of the number of cases by their date of onset. This graph, called an epidemic curve, or "epi-curve," gives a simple visual display of the outbreak's magnitude and time trend.

Suicides and suicide rates on an installation are always sensitive issues. It is critical to keep the command informed of the status of the assessment. The command must be briefed on the results before any information is released outside of the command. It is important to clarify the level of detail (ie, full report or briefing slides) desired by the command.

Writing the report is a laborious and time-consuming process, especially if the team members have been gone for several weeks for the mission. Upon their return, other duties often interfere with report writing. Different sections of the report may be assigned to different people. It is helpful to develop and adhere to a time line, which is set by the senior officer. Another practical suggestion is that plane rides home should be dedicated to report writing; team members should ensure that computer batteries are charged. PHC(P) uses a standardized EPICON report format that may easily be transformed into a publishable document.

Media attention may or may not be present. There was intensive media attention on the Fort Bragg EPICON. The redacted report was eventually put on the Army medicine Web site (www.armymedicine.army.mil). In other cases, media interest is less prominent. However, all team members should be reminded not to discuss their work with the media without appropriate clearances.

Results and Lessons Learned

Each EPICON has led to recommendations based on internal assessments of the particular installation that was evaluated. Although each installation's situation is unique, the overall recommendations will be summarized here, as the reports have had some parallel themes. However, it must be noted that these assessments have been performed on installations where there were apparent suicide clusters, and thus may not be indicative of Army installations as a whole.

The common findings are:

- there is a perceived shortage of behavioral health assets, despite efforts of local commanders to hire more resources,
- there is a stigma involved in seeking help,
- forward-deployed assets are more effective,
- marital therapy should be more available,
- more integration of resources is desirable,
- command is very interested in solving these problems, and
- the effort is essential to maintaining the strength of the fighting force.

Both the local and the overall command have been very interested in these results. In all cases commanders and the medical departments have taken the recommendations seriously. Some examples follow:

- The Fort Leonard Wood, Missouri, report led to the expansion of the "Medical Moment of Truth" at the reception battalion, and to a reexamination of the "unit watch" protocol.
- The Fort Bragg, North Carolina, EPICON spurred development of the Deployment Cycle Support program.
- The Fort Riley, Kansas, EPICON led to an increase in marital therapy resources.
- The Fort Hood, Texas, EPICON reinvigorated the installation-wide risk reduction committees.
- The Fort Campbell, Kentucky, EPICON recommended an improvement in the quality of the "risk reduction" data.

SUMMARY

Suicide prevention is a continuing challenge. The rate continues to increase, despite development and use of educational and training materials. The behavioral health epidemiological consultation process is a useful method of assessing clusters of suicides and suicidal behaviors. The results help to guide both installation and Army-wide efforts to focus on gaps in outreach, education, and treatment.

There are caveats, however. It is notoriously difficult to measure the effectiveness of any suicide prevention program. Because the focus is often on completed suicides, it is not known how many have been prevented via proactive measures by the command and staff. Additionally, the suicide rates are not necessarily a good marker of the mental health of the force. There are other instruments available to assess effectiveness of suicide prevention programs and the quality of services delivered. These include, for example, the DoDSER, unit surveys, and gatekeeper training.

Suicide affects the psychological and physical health of soldiers, units, family members, and friends. The approach to prevention, intervention, and postvention must be an integrated, multifactorial endeavor involving all levels of the command and family resources. The information presented here illustrates the current initiatives, many of which were developed from lessons learned in the past. Building products and strategies based on those lessons should enhance the ability to save lives in the future.

The rate of suicides has doubled in the Army in the last 6 years. Every suicide is a tremendous tragedy, for the soldier, for the family, and for the Army. Risk factors for suicide include a break-up in a relationship and trouble at work. Medical issues, especially chronic pain or disability, may precipitate a suicide attempt. Alcohol abuse can disinhibit someone in many ways and result in self-injury. In recent years, there has been a rise of suicides in senior noncommissioned officers, senior officers, female soldiers, and soldiers in the warrior transition units. Medical soldiers are not immune.

There are numerous educational resources for soldiers and families detailing suicide awareness and intervention for someone in trouble. To take care of fellow soldiers ("Ask, Care, and Escort"), ask about their issues, take care of them, and do not leave them alone. Get them to a chaplain, a medic, combat stress control, or their command. "Shoulder to shoulder: No Soldier stands alone."

REFERENCES

1. Deputy Chief of Staff for Personnel, US Army. The Pentagon, Washington, DC.
2. Durkheim É. *Suicide: A Study in Sociology*, translated by Spaulding JA, Simpson G. 1897. Reprint, Glencoe, Ill: Free Press; 1951.
3. Thompson K. *Emile Durkheim*. London, UK: Tavistock Publications; 1982.
4. Menninger K. *Man Against Himself*. New York, NY: Harcourt, Brace; 1938.
5. Shneidman ES, Farberow NI. *Clues to Suicide*. New York, NY: McGraw-Hill; 1957.
6. Shneidman ES, Leenaars AA. *Lives and Deaths: Selections From the Works of Edwin S. Shneidman*. Philadelphia, Penn: Brunner/Mazel; 1999.
7. Russell S. What is a psychological autopsy? *Author's Den*. 2004. Available at: http://www.authorsden.com/visit/viewarticle.asp?AuthorID=8848&id=14997. Accessed January 28, 2010.
8. Ritchie EC, Gelles M. Psychological autopsies: the current Department of Defense effort to standardize training and quality assurance. *J Forensic Sciences*. 2002;47(6):1370–1372.
9. The American Association of Suicidology and the US Army Center for Health Promotion and Preventive Medicine. Suicide prevention: a resource manual for the United States Army. 1999. Available at: http://www.medtrng.com/suicideprevention/suicide_prevention.htm. Accessed January 28, 2010.
10. Newby JH Jr, Van Der Heide CJ. A review of 139 suicidal gestures: discussion of some psychological implications and treatment techniques. *Mil Med*. 1968;133:629–637.
11. Gaines T Jr, Richmond LH. Assessing suicidal behavior in basic military trainees. *Mil Med*. 1980;145:263–266.
12. Rock NL. Suicide and suicide attempts in the Army: a 10-year review. *Mil Med*. 1988;153:67–69.

13. Rothberg JM, Rock NL, Jones FD. Suicide in United States Army personnel, 1981–1982. *Mil Med.* 1984;149:537–541.

14. Ritchie EC, Keppler W, Rothberg J. Suicidal admissions in the United States military. *Mil Med.* 2003;168(3):177–181.

15. Rothberg JM, Jones FD. Suicide in the US Army: epidemiological and periodic aspects. *Suicide Life Threat Behav.* 1987;17:119–132.

16. Rothberg JM, Ursano RJ, Holloway HC. Suicide in the United States military. *Psychiatric Annals.* 1987;17:545–548.

17. Rothberg JM, Rock NL, Shaw J, Jones FD. Suicide in United States Army personnel, 1983–1984. *Mil Med.* 1988;153:61–64.

18. Rothberg JM, McDowell CP. Suicide in United States Air Force personnel, 1981–1985. *Mil Med.* 1988;153:645–648.

19. Rothberg JM, Bartone PT, Holloway HC, Marlowe DH. Life and death in the US Army: in corpore sano. *JAMA.* 1990;264:2241–2244.

20. Rothberg JM, Fagan J, Shaw J. Suicide in United States Army personnel, 1985–1986. *Mil Med.* 1990;155:452–456

21. US Department of the Army. *Guide to the Prevention of Suicide and Self–Destructive Behavior.* Washington, DC: DA; 1985. DA PAM 600–70.

22. US Department of the Army. *Suicide Prevention and Psychological Autopsy.* Washington, DC: DA; 1988. DA PAM 600-24.

23. Mann JJ, Apter A, Bertolote J, et al. Suicide prevention strategies: a systematic review. *JAMA.* 2005;294:2064–2074. Available at: http://jama.ama-assn.org/cgi/content/full/294/16/2064. Accessed November 27, 2009.

24. *Applied Suicide Intervention Skills Training (ASIST) Manual*, 10th ed. Calgary, Alberta, Canada: Living Works; 2008. Available at: http://www.livingworks.net/LW_Str.php. Accessed November 27, 2009.

25. ASIST workshop: Calgary, Alberta, Canada: Living Works; 2002. Available at: http://www.livingworks.net/AS-T4T.php. Accessed November 27, 2009.

26. Information on the QPR Workshop can be obtained from the QPR Institute, PO Box 2867, Spokane, Washington 99220. Available at: http://www.qprinstitute.com/. Accessed November 27, 2009.

27. Dolan CA, Schroeder ED, Wright KM, Thomas JT, Ness JW. USAREUR suicide surveillance project: data summary and program evaluation. Heidelberg, Germany: US Army Medical Research Unit–Europe; 2003. USAMRU-E Technical Report.

28. Mental Health Advisory Team (MHAT). Operation Iraqi Freedom (OIF). Report. The US Army Surgeon General and HQDA G-1. December 16, 2003. Available at: www.armymedicine.army.mil/reports/mhat.html. Accessed September 4, 2008.

29. US Department of the Army. *Army Health Promotion.* Washington, DC: DA; 2007. Army Regulation 600–63.

30. MNC-I Criminal Investigations Division (CID). October 2, 2007. Personal communication.

31. Nutting PA, Dickinson LM, Rubenstein LV, Keeley RD, Smith JL, Elliott CE. Improving detection of suicidal ideation among depressed patients in primary care. *Ann Fam Med.* 2005;3(6):529–536.

32. Meats P, Solomka B. A perspective on suicides in the '90s. *Psychiatr Bull.* 1995;19:666–669.

33. Vassilas C, Morgan HG. Suicide prevention: service contacts and coordination between primary and secondary care [letter]. *Br J Psychiatry.* 2001;179:271.

34. Vassilas CA, Morgan HG. General practitioners' contact with victims of suicide. *Br Med J.* 1993;307:300–301.

35. Appleby L, Shaw J, Amos T. National confidential inquiry into suicide and homicide by people with mental illness. *Br J Psychiatr.* 1997;170:101–102.

36. Centers for Disease Control and Prevention. Suicide: risk and protective factors. Atlanta, Ga: CDC; 1999. Available at: http://www.cdc.gov/ViolencePrevention/suicide/riskprotectivefactors.html. Accessed January 28, 2010.

37. US Department of Health and Human Services. Office of The Surgeon General. The Surgeon General's call to action to prevent suicide. Washington, DC: OTSG; 1999. Available at: http://www.surgeongeneral.gov/library/calltoaction/default.htm. Accessed January 28, 2010.

38. Karch D, Crosby A, Simon T. Toxicology testing and results for suicide victims–13 states, 2004. *MMWR.* 2006;55:1245–1248.

39. Christopher H Warner, Major, Medical Corps, US Army; Division Psychiatrist, Multi-National Division—Center, Iraq. Personal communication [face-to-face conversation as part of a site visit]; 2007.

40. Centers for Disease Control and Prevention. Web-based Injury Statistics Query and Reporting System (WISQARS). Atlanta, Ga: CDC. Available at: http://www.cdc.gov/injury/wisqars/index.html. Accessed January 28, 2010.

41. US Department of the Army. *Preventive Medicine.* Washington, DC: Headquarters, DA; May 25, 2007 [rapid action revision]. Army Regulation 40-5.

42. US Department of the Army. *Preventive Medicine.* Washington, DC: Headquarters, DA; October 19, 2009 [rapid action revision]. Department of the Army Pamphlet 40-11.

Chapter 26

SUICIDE AND HOMICIDE RISK MANAGEMENT: RATIONALE AND SUGGESTIONS FOR THE USE OF UNIT WATCH IN GARRISON AND DEPLOYED SETTINGS

SAMUEL E. PAYNE, MD*; JEFFREY V. HILL, MD†; AND DAVID E. JOHNSON, MD‡

*Colonel, Medical Corps, US Army; Chief, Outpatient Behavioral Health Services, Dwight D. Eisenhower Army Medical Center, Building 300, Room 13A-15, 300 South Hospital Road Fort Gordon, Georgia 30905

†Lieutenant Colonel, Medical Corps, US Army; Chief, Child and Adolescent Psychiatry, Landstuhl Regional Medical Center, Landstuhl, Germany, CMR 402 Box 1356, APO AE, 09180; formerly, Chief, Outpatient Psychiatry, Landstuhl Regional Medical Center

‡Major, Medical Corps, US Army; Chief, Behavioral Health, US Army MEDDAC Bavaria, IMEU-SFT-DHR, ATTN: OMDC Schweinfurt, Unit 25850, APO AE 09033

An earlier version of this chapter was originally published as: Payne SE, Hill JV, Johnson DE. The use of unit watch or command interest profile in the management of suicide and homicide risk: rationale and guidelines for the military mental health professional. *Mil Med.* 2008;173:25–35.

INTRODUCTION

Unit watch procedures are routinely used in both garrison and operational settings as a tool to enhance the safety of unit personnel when a soldier presents with suicidal or homicidal thoughts. To date, no specific body of literature or US Army publication offers either a rationale or a set of guidelines for their use. This chapter provides both a rationale and a set of suggestions for the use of unit watch based on fundamental military psychiatric principles, review of the relevant literature, and anecdotal experience. Finally, the chapter includes a discussion of the medicolegal issues specific to the use of unit watch.

RATIONALE FOR UNIT WATCH

The management of suicidal and homicidal patients in the military environment is somewhat different from the management of such patients in the civilian sector for several reasons. One reason is that the military community provides additional resources, such as the chain of command and fellow soldiers, to assist the military clinician in addressing suicide and homicide risk. Another important reason is the necessity of managing suicide and homicide risk in a deployed or geographically isolated setting. Finally, management of suicide and homicide risk in the military requires addressing the challenge of heightened access to firearms in many settings. Unit watch has evolved within these circumstances as a practical and effective means to enhance the safety of the soldier and others and has gained some legitimacy in the psychiatric community.[1–3] Unit watches have been used in many environments from the battlefield to the garrison, primarily in cases involving a level of risk that is concerning but does not necessarily warrant hospitalization.

Psychiatric hospitalization, although often necessary for patients at high risk for attempting suicide or homicide, is not always the best option for managing suicide or homicide risk in a military setting for several reasons.[1] Hospitalization necessitates removal of the soldier from the unit and in some cases (notably those involving low to moderate risk of suicide) may delay recovery, especially when the symptoms are precipitated by battle fatigue.[4–6] Anecdotally, the authors have observed cases in which hospitalization seemed to exacerbate the symptoms by placing the soldier in the role of a psychiatric patient. Psychiatric hospitalization carries significant stigma in the military as in the general population and may permanently impede the soldier's reintegration into the unit. Fellow soldiers often make comments about hospitalized soldiers being "psycho" or needing to be "locked in a rubber room." Some soldiers lose their sense of self-worth and belonging when they are separated from their units and cannot maintain occupational functioning.

The unit watch (also known as the "command interest profile") is a term describing the use of the military system to limit the suicidal or homicidal soldier's access to people, places, or objects that might increase that soldier's chances of harming self or others. Based on recommendations from the clinician, a variety of interventions are carried out by the command team, which may include searching the soldier's belongings and living quarters for dangerous items, removing such items from the soldier's possession, prohibiting access to alcohol and drugs, minimizing contact with people who may negatively influence the soldier's mental health, continuously observing the soldier, and ensuring that the soldier returns for mental health follow-up.

A unit watch is an excellent example of the military clinician working with the command team to address a soldier's mental health needs in the least restrictive setting possible through application of the time-honored military psychiatric principles of "PIES" (proximity, immediacy, expectancy, and simplicity), or "BICEPS" (brevity, immediacy, centrality, expectancy, proximity, and simplicity).[7,8] Many soldiers with suicidal or homicidal thoughts have been experiencing stressful life circumstances. Sometimes these circumstances are the direct result of the wartime environment and may represent battle fatigue. Suicidal or homicidal thoughts may occur in the absence of a diagnosable mental illness and may respond to simple interventions such as rest, expectation of recovery, command attention, and support from other members of the soldier's unit. Utilization of the PIES doctrine has demonstrated that suicidal or homicidal soldiers often benefit from brief, immediate care and support near their units. The unit watch is one mechanism for enhancing safety while providing this care and support.

A unit watch can reduce the chances of misperception about the soldier's condition because unit members see and interact with the soldier on a daily basis. Soldiers often report that just talking to other unit members proved helpful. Commanding officers and senior noncommissioned officers often provide invaluable support for soldiers on unit watch by listening to the soldier's concerns, sometimes modifying their style of interaction with the soldier based on a heightened sensitivity to the soldier's personal problems, and by providing social support and advice as they perform their roles in "watching" the soldier.

Though often useful, unit watch may not always be the best approach. The treating mental health professional uses clinical judgment to determine the best course of action. One factor to consider is that a unit watch carries some risk of stigmatization by peers. Fellow soldiers may become frustrated with the soldier because of increased workload and potentially increased hazards as they attempt to cover the soldier's battlefield responsibilities or provide personnel to monitor the soldier. This frustration may be exacerbated if the soldiers experiencing suicidal and homicidal thoughts, who often have a limited ability to give and receive social support, have already marginalized themselves. Many soldiers on unit watch have described to healthcare professionals episodes of ridicule and verbal harassment by both peers and leaders in their units. Regardless of the setting, stigma associated with receiving mental healthcare can be significant.[9] Adequate education of the unit leaders, who then train unit members to envision a unit watch as analogous to "helping a family member in distress," may help alleviate some of the stigma.

Leadership, unit cohesion, and group identification play decisive roles in a soldier's ability to cope with peacetime or wartime duties. A unit watch may focus the command team's attention on issues or stressors affecting their soldiers. In addressing these stressors, the command team may provide enhanced support to the soldier and may actually resolve some of the issues that are contributing to the heightened suicide or homicide risk. Ideally, the command team will consistently communicate the expectation that the unit watch is a team effort designed to help one of their own and to enhance both unit cohesion and the soldier's ability to contribute. Such support can reduce the agitation and hopelessness often present in soldiers with suicidal or homicidal thoughts.[4,10] Working with a command to ensure a unit watch environment that builds social support can be extremely helpful for the soldier. Strengthening such social support may play a key role in the soldier's recovery.[11,12]

Although some risk remains, the authors contend that unit watch significantly reduces the risk of a soldier accessing lethal means such as firearms, ropes, medication, or knives. Of these weapons, firearms deserve special mention. In 2004 and 2005, firearms were the most common method of suicide completion within the US Army (62% and 69%, respectively, per year).[13,14] By limiting access to firearms, a unit watch is likely to reduce the soldier's risk of suicide completion early in the course of treatment, thus allowing time for the treatment and supportive interventions by the command to take effect.

Among US Army soldiers attempting or completing suicide in 2005, 57% of attempts and 17% of completions involved alcohol or drug use.[14] Such substance use may impair judgment and lower inhibitions against acting on suicidal or homicidal impulses. A properly executed unit watch ensures that soldiers at risk are not given access to alcohol or drugs, thereby reducing risk. Also, by limiting contact with people who might exacerbate the soldier's condition or become a victim of the soldier's homicidal intent, a unit watch may further reduce risk and prevent adverse outcomes.

Finally, the utilization of a unit watch for a soldier who presents with "military-specific" suicidal or homicidal ideation may be highly effective in reducing secondary gain, a term that describes the tangible advantages and benefits that result from being sick.[15] The terms "military-specific suicidal ideation" and "military-specific homicidal ideation" refer to the verbal expression of suicidal or homicidal thoughts with the implicit (as determined by the clinician) or explicit goal of avoiding a military duty such as a field training exercise or deployment, of receiving a transfer to another unit or occupational specialty, or of obtaining a separation from active duty. In such cases, soldiers essentially imply or state that they may or will kill themselves or a leader in their unit unless they are allowed to achieve the stated goal. Such statements are often accompanied by allegations of harassment against the unit chain of command that may or may not be well founded. In many cases of military-specific suicidal or homicidal ideation, the soldier's threats are directly linked to a desire to get out of the military. Such soldiers may believe that reporting suicidal or homicidal thoughts is an easy way to "get chaptered" (seek honorable administrative discharge) without negative consequences. In the absence of risk factors requiring hospitalization, military-specific suicidal or homicidal ideation is an indication for a unit watch, thus conserving inpatient treatment services for other service members who are more likely to benefit from these services. Additionally, soldiers in the unit rapidly develop an awareness that the mental health system is not there primarily to provide an escape from duties and responsibilities, but to provide supportive treatment, helping them function more effectively in a military environment.

While useful in the management of military-specific suicidal or homicidal ideation in garrison, unit watches in a theater of operations are even more valuable. Military-specific suicidal and homicidal ideation are arguably two of the most common presenting behavioral health symptoms on today's battlefield and could easily develop into an evacuation syndrome if not managed appropriately.[11] A force that is well-versed in unit watches from its garrison experience is much more likely to successfully employ the intervention in wartime or other operations and thus benefit significantly in conserving its fighting, or peacekeeping, strength. However, the system as utilized in garrison requires modification in a deployed setting (discussed later in the chapter).

Two caveats warrant discussion when considering the rationale for the use of unit watch as a tool for enhancing the safety of soldiers at risk for suicide and homicide. The first is that although the unit watch may be beneficial for the soldier, it is only one component of a multifaceted treatment plan. Military mental health clinicians must provide psychological and pharmacologic treatment, as appropriate, to soldiers who present for care, whether or not a unit watch is used to enhance safety. For example, treating symptoms such as anxiety and insomnia is often essential in reducing suicide risk.[1] Treatment of these symptoms should be a priority in soldiers presenting with suicidal thoughts, and treatment should occur independently of the decision to utilize a unit watch.

The second caveat is that essentially no research exists that directly addresses the safety and efficacy of a unit watch as an intervention. The Army Suicide Event Report (ASER) does provide some data that obliquely address the safety of "under command observation" (defined further on the ASER form as "eg, CIP," a reference to command interest profile). In calendar year 2004, ASER data were received for 54 of 70 suicide completions and 259 other suicide events (including both suicide attempts and other events that did not involve a suicide attempt, eg, hospitalization and evacuation for suicidal thoughts). In that year, one soldier who completed suicide (1%) and one (.4%) who attempted suicide were under command observation.[13] In calendar year 2005, 2 of the 723 reported suicide events (.2%) in the active duty Army population occurred while the soldier was under command observation (of the five ASER reports identified as "under command observation," two cases involved ideation only with no attempt, and one was from another branch of service). During the same year, none (0%) of the 71 completed suicides reported to the Suicide Risk Management and Surveillance Office occurred under command observation.[14] (ASERS were not submitted for 12 of the 83 completed suicides that year; therefore, 71 reports were available.) Considering the widespread use of unit watch procedures in the US Army, these data offer some support to the hypothesis that unit watches are safe and may be effective in reducing suicidal behaviors in the short-term while treatment is initiated. Although a controlled study evaluating the safety and efficacy of unit watch procedures may be difficult to design, research about this common practice is certainly warranted. In the meantime, the decision to use unit watch must be based on clinical judgment and experience with consideration of the potential risks and benefits.

SUICIDE RISK ASSESSMENT

Essential to the appropriate use of unit watches is the ability to assess and document the soldier's risk for suicide in a format that clearly explains the clinician's decision-making process. Much has been written about the factors most often associated with completed suicide in both the civilian population and the US military population.[14–17] These factors can be incorporated into a risk assessment that guides the clinician in appropriately choosing a unit watch or hospitalization. Although discussion of a comprehensive suicide risk assessment is beyond the scope of this chapter, a few risk factors are particularly relevant in a military setting.

One of the risk factors most highly correlative with completed suicide is diagnosis. Almost 95% of patients who attempt or commit suicide have a diagnosis of a mood disorder, a psychotic disorder, a substance-abuse disorder, dementia, or delirium. In populations under 30 years of age, the most common diagnoses among suicide completers in one study were antisocial personality disorder and substance-abuse disorders.[18] Based on anecdotal experience, a significant proportion of soldiers presenting with military-specific suicidal thoughts do not meet criteria for these diagnoses. However, the absence of a psychiatric diagnosis must be interpreted with caution in the active duty Army population, because the ASER data from 2005 indicate that only 26% of suicide completers were given a psychiatric diagnosis.

An "unambiguous wish to die" over a "primary wish for change" as well as "communication internalized" (self-blame) versus "communication externalized" have been cited as important factors associated with high suicide risk.[19] The majority of soldiers with military-specific suicidal thoughts are primarily interested in a change (leaving the military, the theater of operations, or their units) and are angry at an external entity (the military or their chains of command), rather than blaming themselves for their dissatisfaction. Additionally, the association of suicide completion with a conflicted romantic relationship or recent divorce has been particularly well described in the military population.[16]

When many or all of the above-described risk factors for suicide completion are absent, this is often an indication that a unit watch is more appropriate than hospitalization. It is important that the clinician clearly document these and other factors in a formal suicide-risk assessment that provides a rationale for the decision to utilize a unit watch. In a military setting, collateral history from the unit commander or from others in the unit is an important source of information in the suicide-risk assessment. Current practice in the field of suicide-risk assessment also emphasizes the ongoing nature of the evaluation. Individuals on unit watch should undergo frequent reassessments by the mental health professional to determine whether the suicide risk has increased to the point that inpatient hospitalization is now indicated. Homicide risk assessment and management is similar to that described for suicide-risk assessment and management, with examination of risk factors and frequent reassessment playing crucial roles in the decision process.

RECOMMENDATIONS FOR UNIT WATCH PROCEDURES

In Garrison

There are many different approaches to the implementation of unit watch in the military system. A model for conceptualizing the role of unit watches in a garrison setting is presented in Table 26-1. Whatever approach is taken by the clinician, the unit watch should be regarded as a "temporary profile," a recommendation to a commander regarding the soldier's temporary duty restrictions that is likely to be helpful in ensuring the soldier's health and welfare. Most Army commanders are familiar with the concept of unit watch and will support such recommendations, especially when notified via a memorandum signed by the mental health professional. The memorandum format ensures that instructions are written and easily understood.

The memorandum is given to the soldier's escort, usually a noncommissioned officer, who signs for its

TABLE 26-1

MANAGING SUICIDE AND HOMICIDE RISK IN GARRISON

	Full Duty	Buddy Watch	24-Hour Watch	Admit to Psychiatric Ward
	Least restrictive ⟵			⟶ Most restrictive
Actions	Return to duty	1. Secure weapons and medication 2. Soldier is under direct observation from first formation until lights out	1. Secure weapons and medications 2. Soldier is under direct observation 24 h/day	Admit to psychiatric ward
Examples	1. SI/HI without plan/intent, few risk factors, contracts for safety	1. Primary indication is "military-specific" SI/HI, no intent, few risk factors 2. SI/HI due to psychiatric disorder but risk level does not warrant 24 h watch or hospitalization 3. Step down from unit watch	1. Primary indication is "military-specific" SI/HI with plan and/or intent but few risk factors 2. SI/HI due to psychiatric disorder but risk level does not warrant hospitalization	1. High suicide or homicide risk requiring psychiatric hospitalization 2. Suicide/homicide risk not diminishing after (no more than) 5 days despite treatment while on 24 h or buddy watch
Advantages	1. RTD 2. No stigma	1. Less stigma than 24 h watch 2. Some safety precautions 3. Lower personnel demands than 24 h watch 4. Reasonable likelihood of RTD	1. High level of safety precautions 2. Reasonable likelihood of RTD	Highest level of safely precautions
Disadvantages	No safety precautions	Fewer safety precautions vs 24 h watch	Stigma, high personnel demands for unit	Low likelihood of RTD, stigma, loss of social and occupational roles that sometimes support recovery

HI: homicidal ideation; RTD: return to duty; SI: suicidal ideation receipt and is instructed to deliver it to the commander or first sergeant. This allows the clinician to release the service member with a recommendation for a unit watch at times when the clinician may not be able to contact the commander immediately. As with all medical profiles, the commander may choose to ignore the clinician's recommendation, but then assume significant responsibility for the outcome of the case.

The garrison system proposed in this chapter consists of two types of unit watches. The first is called a "buddy watch"; it recommends that the soldier be under direct observation only from first formation until lights out, rather than 24 hours a day, for up to 5 days from the initiation of the watch until a reevaluation occurs. This watch is generally for lower-risk individuals, provides more flexibility for use (eg, over a weekend), and is generally better received by the chain of command and the soldier. It is valuable in a

EXHIBIT 26-1

BUDDY WATCH MEMORANDUM

DATE:
MEMORANDUM FOR (COMMANDER, UNIT)

SUBJECT: Buddy Watch for ______________________ (Soldier's name and last 4)

1. The soldier was evaluated at the __________ Behavioral Health Clinic. The results of the evaluation indicate that this Soldier is at some risk for self-harm or harm to others. The risk level at this time does not warrant hospitalization, but a Buddy Watch for both support and safety is recommended.
2. Buddy Watch procedures are as follows:
   a. Command should assign someone to constantly monitor the soldier from first formation until lights out. The Soldier may be allowed to go to the latrine alone if the latrine doorway is monitored by the buddy or NCO assigned to watch the Soldier. During the night, constant monitoring is not required, but the soldier must not sleep in a room alone. Actions that specifically identify a Soldier on a Buddy Watch to large numbers of unit personnel (e.g. having the Soldier wear a road guard vest throughout the day) are not authorized.
   b. Health and welfare inspection of the soldier's room to remove hazardous material (e.g. pills, knives, etc.).
   c. No access to alcohol or dangerous objects such as:
      1) Personal weapons, knives, cigarette lighters, jewelry with sharp edges, blow dryers (silverware other than sharp knives is acceptable).
      2) Pills (medication should be dispensed one dose at the time by medic, PA, NCO, etc).
      3) The Soldier may carry a military-issued firearm if the firing pin or bolt has been removed from the weapon.
   d. It is recommended that the Soldier perform his/her regular (noncombat) duty and PT. Physical exercise often improves behavioral health symptoms.
3. This plan will be in effect from today until it is terminated by the Behavioral Health clinician in agreement with the commander. Continuing a buddy watch after a Behavioral Health clinician has recommended termination is not authorized and may be perceived as harassment.
4. If this Soldier's condition worsens, the Soldier's supervisor should call the Behavioral Health clinic at xxx-xxxx during duty hours or bring the Soldier to the _________ Emergency Room after hours. If phone contact cannot be established with a Behavioral Health clinician during the duty day, escort the Soldier immediately to the Behavioral Health clinic for evaluation.

This Soldier's next appointment at the ______________ Behavioral Health clinic is on____________________(date) at_________________________ (time).

________________________________ ________________________________
Representative from Command Clinician

Adapted from a form developed at the 2nd Infantry Division, initially by Captain Sally Chessani (now Colonel Sally Harvey), licensed clinical psychologist.
NCO: noncommissioned officer; PA: physician's assistant; PT: physical training

variety of situations, including the typical presentation with military-specific suicidal ideation and very few risk factors for suicide completion.

Another scenario in which this watch may be useful is in managing soldiers who are urgently command-referred for verbal expression of suicidal thoughts or self-injurious behavior the previous night when they were intoxicated. On presentation, the service member may have no current suicidal ideation, may claim to have no memory of the statements or self-injurious

EXHIBIT 26-2

24-HOUR WATCH MEMORANDUM

DATE:

MEMORANDUM FOR (COMMANDER, UNIT)

SUBJECT: 24 Hour Watch for ____________________________ (Soldier's name and last 4)

1. The Soldier was evaluated at the ___________ Behavioral Health clinic on __________________ The results of the evaluation indicate that this Soldier is at some risk for self-harm or harm to others. The risk level at this time does not warrant hospitalization , but a 24 Hour Watch for both support and safety is recommended.
2. 24-Hour Watch procedures are as follows:
   a. Continuous monitoring should occur at all times, including accompanying the soldier to the latrine and during meals.
   b. The soldier should sleep in a room with a unit member who is awake at all times or in a dayroom (cleared of dangerous items) near the Staff Duty/CQ area so that the Soldier is constantly monitored throughout the night. Other actions that specifically identify the Soldier on a 24 Hour Watch to large numbers of unit personnel (e.g. having the Soldier wear a road guard vest throughout the day) are not authorized and may be perceived as harassment.
   c. Health and welfare inspection of the soldier's room to remove hazardous materials (e.g., pills, knives, weapons, etc.). Instead of removing the Soldier's weapon, the weapon may be inactivated (e.g., removing the bolt or firing pin from an M-16.
   d. Other than family members, visitors from outside the unit must be cleared by the commander.
   e. No access to alcohol or dangerous objects such as:
      1) Personal weapons, knives, cigarette lighters, jewelry with sharp edges, blow dryers (silverware other than sharp knives is acceptable).
      2) Pills (medication should be dispensed one dose at a time by medic, PA, NCO, etc.).
      3) The Soldier may carry a military-issued firearm if the firing pin or bolt has been removed from the weapon.
3. Soldier should perform his/her regular (noncombat) duty and PT. Physical exercise often improves behavioral health symptoms.
4. This plan will be in effect from today until it is terminated by the Behavioral Health clinician in agreement with the command. Continuing a 24 hour watch after a Behavioral Health clinician has recommended termination is not authorized and may be perceived as harassment.
5. If this Soldier's condition worsens, the Soldier's supervisor should call the Behavioral Health clinic at xxx-xxxx during duty hours or escort the Soldier to the Emergency Room (or TMC in theater) after duty hours. If phone contact cannot be established with a Behavioral Health clinician during the day, bring the Soldier to the Behavioral Health clinic during duty hours for evaluation.
6. This soldier's next appointment at the____________________ Behavioral Health clinic is on_____________________ at ____________________.

________________________________ ________________________________

Representative from Command Clinician

CQ: charge of quarters; NCO: noncommissioned officer; PA: physician's assistant; TMC: troop medical clinic

EXHIBIT 26-3

INFORMATION PAPER FOR COMMANDERS

MCXC-BH

INFORMATION PAPER

SUBJECT: Management of Soldiers with Suicidal or Homicidal Ideation

1. References: FM 4-02.55 COMBAT AND OPERATIONAL STRESS CONTROL, FM 22-51 Leader's Manual for Combat Stress Control
2. Purpose. To provide information to commanders regarding the use of unit watches in the management of Soldiers who express suicidal and homicidal ideation.
3. Overview:

When it is brought to the commander's attention that a Soldier has expressed suicidal ideation, the commander should immediately contact his supporting behavioral health activity to insure that an evaluation of risk is performed. Procedures for this are not within the scope of this information paper. Once the Soldier is evaluated, the behavioral health professional will have examined the risk factors (e.g. the psychiatric diagnosis, any history of previous attempts, family history of attempts, the presence and lethality of a plan for suicide) and will make recommendations to the commander. These recommendations will include one of the following: return to full duty with close monitoring and support for low risk soldiers, Buddy Watch (or Basic Precautions in Operational environments) for low to moderate risk Soldiers, 24 Hour Watch for moderate risk Soldiers, and hospitalization for soldiers at high risk. The value to the soldier and commander of Basic Precautions, Buddy Watch, and 24 Hour Watch as opposed to hospitalization are as follows:

The soldier is able to maintain occupational functioning at some level and maintains social connection in the unit. This helps to prevent feelings of worthlessness and a sense of isolation that sometimes result from psychiatric hospitalization.

The soldier avoids the stigma that is unfortunately commonly associated with psychiatric hospitalization. While there may be some stigma associated with a unit watch, at least the soldiers in the unit see the soldier on a daily basis and are much less likely to develop misperceptions about the Soldier's problem, e.g. that the Soldier is "psycho" and is "locked in a rubber room". These misperceptions are prevalent in our culture and are sometimes very damaging in the Soldier's reintegration to the unit after a psychiatric hospitalization.

The Soldier has the opportunity to address his or her concerns with the chain of command. NCOs often provide significant relief from depressed feelings when they listen to and support a Soldier who has expressed suicidal ideation. In this way, the unit implements the Army's concept of the unit as the Soldier's "family" and provides extra care and support to a unit member in distress.

Soldiers with "military specific" suicidal ideation (e.g. "I will kill myself if you don't let me out of the Army") become aware more rapidly that the behavioral health system does not provide an escape route from their duties and responsibilities, though it does react to help the Soldier adjust to their situation. This message is transmitted to the entire unit and is likely to lessen the number of Soldiers who develop "military specific" suicidal ideation. This MAY ENHANCE RETENTION AND COMBAT READINESS by reducing the number of soldiers that seek out the mental health system as an escape route from the Army.

The unit chain of command gains significant experience in managing Soldiers who express suicidal ideation. This experience and familiarity with unit watches MAY ENHANCE COMBAT READINESS because the unit will most likely need to employ similar procedures in an operational environment. The proficient use of unit watches in a combat setting may prevent an "evacuation syndrome" in which significant numbers of Soldiers who express suicidal thoughts are evacuated from theater because units have not been trained in the management of this problem.

4. Types of Unit Watches:

a. Buddy Watch: A unit member is assigned to constantly monitor the soldier from first formation until lights out. The soldier should not sleep in a room alone but constant monitoring is not required at night. The Soldier will follow up with Behavioral health within 5 days (usually sooner) of the initiation of the watch so that the risk level can

(**Exhibit 26-3** *continues*)

Exhibit 26-3 *continued*

be reassessed. If significant risk remains at that point, the Soldier is often hospitalized so that the unit's combat readiness is not unduly affected by an extended period of observation of the soldier.

b. 24-Hour Watch: A unit member is assigned to constantly monitor the Soldier throughout an entire 24 hour period. Unit commanders often use a Staff Duty NCO or CQ personnel for this purpose. This type of watch is generally only used in "military specific" suicidal ideation where the Soldier is making specific threats related to a wish for release from the Army or a deployment but does not have other risk factors (eg, a depressive disorder, a history of suicide attempts) that would warrant hospitalization. The Soldier will generally be seen back within 24 hours due to the time-intensive nature of this procedure for the unit. At that point, the clinician will again assess the risk and make a determination regarding the appropriate recommendation.

c. Recommendation for Basic Precautions: While a recommendation for Basic Precautions is not technically a unit watch, it is a set of safety precautions used only in an operational environment. The essential elements of Basic Precautions are that the Soldier does not participate in combat (or "off-FOB") duties and that the firing pin or bolt is removed from the Soldier's weapon.

5. The Homicidal Soldier:

Soldiers who express homicidal thoughts should also be referred to Behavioral Health for an evaluation so that the mental health professional can rule out a mental disorder as a cause of the homicidal thoughts, assess the risk, and initiate treatment if there is evidence of a behavioral health disorder. In the absence of a serious behavioral health disorder contributing to the homicidal thoughts, the presence of homicidal thoughts is often not an indication for psychiatric hospitalization. The mental health professional will generally take steps to insure that the commander warns the personnel who are threatened, and may recommend a Buddy Watch or 24 Hour Watch as a method of protecting the threatened individual. If the risk level is very high, the commander has the option of consulting SJA regarding the possibility of placing the Soldier in pretrial confinement if hospitalization is not indicated.

6. Summary:

The use of unit watches is a valuable tool for the commander in supporting Soldiers and enhancing combat readiness. Behavioral Health clinicians will work with you to determine the appropriate management tool and will hospitalize the Soldier if the risk level warrants this intervention. Behavioral Health clinicians can not predict suicide or homicide but are trained to follow clear guidelines about the level of risk that warrants hospitalization. Your supporting Behavioral Health clinicians will insure that your Soldier receives the most appropriate intervention for their level of risk.

______________________________ ______________________________

Representative from Command Clinician

CQ: charge of quarters; FOB: forward operating base; FM: field manual; NCO: noncommissioned officer; SJA: Staff Judge Advocate

act, and may demonstrate minimal risk factors for a suicidal act. However, there is clearly some risk, especially if alcohol use is resumed. The buddy watch significantly minimizes the opportunity for continued alcohol use, and thus may reduce the suicide risk while outpatient treatment, including referral to the Army Substance Abuse Program, is initiated. Other situations in which a buddy watch may be valuable are situations in which "stepping down" from hospitalization or 24-hour watch is prudent. Exhibit 26-1 is an example of specific procedures for buddy watch.

The second type of unit watch is called a "24-hour watch," avoiding another commonly used term, "CQ (charge-of-quarters) watch," for two reasons. Some units do not have a CQ duty and the commander may infer from the term that the unit is being asked to perform a task for which it is not equipped. The commander may also infer from "CQ watch" that the clinician is recommending that the soldier be moved to a central area (eg, dayroom) in the unit where observation is possible by soldiers performing CQ duty. Moving the soldier to a central area is sometimes necessary but should be avoided whenever possible because such a move may enhance the sense of humiliation or stigma. The primary characteristic of a 24-hour watch is that the soldier is under constant observation during a 24-hour period, after which an evaluation by a mental health officer must take place. Specific procedures for

EXHIBIT 26-4

STANDARD OPERATING PROCEDURES FOR BUDDY WATCH AND 24-HOUR WATCH

STANDARD OPERATING PROCEDURES

Buddy and 24-Hour Unit Watch

1. PURPOSE: To establish procedures for the use of Buddy and 24 Hour Unit Watches in the management of Soldiers undergoing evaluation and treatment for suicidal statements or behaviors.

2. SCOPE: All personnel assigned to or working in the Department of Behavioral Health.

3. GENERAL:

a. All patients seen in the clinic who describe a history of current or recent (i.e. within the past two weeks) suicidal ideation, suicide attempt, or homicidal ideation must be seen by a Behavioral Health clinician prior to release of the soldier. (Risk assessments after clinic hours will be performed by Emergency Department staff, in consultation with the on-call Behavioral Health clinician.)

b. The evaluation of potential for harm will include a thorough psychiatric history and examination of risk factors. The suicide risk factors assessed will include at a minimum the following: history of previous attempts, frequency and duration of suicidal ideation/plan/intent, access to lethal means, presence or absence of substance abuse, signs and symptoms of mood and anxiety disorders, current significant stresses, social supports, reality testing, and any family history of completed suicide. The homicide risk factors assessed will include at a minimum the following: history of previous violence, frequency and duration of homicidal ideation/plan/intent, and determination of access to lethal means.

c. The disposition should be appropriate based on the assessment and must address the safety of all involved.

d. Documentation of the assessment will be completed on the day of the evaluation.

4. PROCEDURES:

a. A Buddy Watch may be recommended to the commander if there is some risk for harm to self or others, but the mental health officer clearly documents a risk assessment explaining that the Soldier's risk is not high enough to warrant hospitalization. The Buddy Watch allows for monitoring the Soldier while treatment is initiated, and may have advantages over hospitalization. These are described in Attachment C.

b. A 24-Hour Watch may be recommended for Soldiers who require more constant supervision than provided by a Buddy Watch and is typically implemented for Soldiers who make specific threats to harm themselves or others in order to avoid duty or to force a discharge from service (eg, "I will kill myself if you don't let me out of the Army"). The risk assessment explaining the clinician's conclusion that the Soldier's risk is not high enough to warrant hospitalization must be clearly documented.

c. The procedures for Buddy Watch and 24-Hour Watch are explained in detail in Attachments A and B. The essential difference in these two procedures is that a Soldier on Buddy Watch requires observation only from first formation until lights out, whereas a Soldier on 24 Hour Watch must be observed at all times.

When a Soldier is placed on a watch, the Behavioral Health clinician will make an attempt to contact the commander to discuss the reasons for the watch and other pertinent concerns. The appropriate form will be forwarded to the commander through the Soldier's escort. If the commander requests additional information about unit watch or expresses uncertainty about unit watch, the information paper titled Management of Soldiers With Suicidal or Homicidal Ideation will be forwarded to the commander through the Soldier's escort. A Soldier on a Buddy Watch will be seen for a follow up appointment at least every five working days until the watch is discontinued. A Soldier on a 24-Hour Watch will be seen for re-evaluation within 24 hours. A Behavioral Health clinician will evaluate the Soldier at each return appointment until the watch is discontinued. The decision to recommend discontinuation of a unit watch will be made only by a Behavioral Health clinician. A memorandum recommending discontinuation of the watch will be signed by the Behavioral Health clinician and forwarded to the commander.

Unit watches are recommendations to commanders. Behavioral Health clinicians must discuss their recommendations with the commander and be sensitive to specific command and unit circumstances. In all cases, the safety of the Soldier and others that might be at risk will be the primary concern.

The Buddy Watch or 24-Hour Unit Watch will only be used for soldiers who have been assessed for their level of risk by a clinician at this institution. Unit watches may be utilized by Emergency Department clinician if the on-call mental health care clinician has been consulted by the Emergency Department clinician and they are in agreement regarding the disposition.

EXHIBIT 26-5

UNIT WATCH DISCONTINUATION MEMORANDUM

Date:

MEMORANDUM FOR (Commander, Unit)

SUBJECT: Release from Twenty Four Hour Watch/Buddy Watch for ______________________

SSN: ____

1. The above named service member was recommended for Twenty Four hour Watch/Buddy Watch on _______ .
2. The above named service member was evaluated at ___________ Behavioral Health clinic again on _______ . I currently do not believe that the service member is an imminent risk to self or others and recommend the service member be removed from Twenty-Four Hour Watch/Buddy Watch.
3. Although this service member is not currently at significant risk for dangerousness to self or others, please understand that the service member's risk level may change.
4. If the service member experiences a recurrence of suicidal or homicidal thoughts or demonstrates other behaviors indicating there is risk for harm to self or others, the service member should be escorted to the clinic (duty hours) or to the Emergency Department (after hours) for evaluation.
5. The service member's next scheduled appointment at Outpatient Behavioral Health Services is on _____________ at ___________.
6. Point of contact for this memorandum is the undersigned at xxx-xxxx.

____

Clinician

this watch are outlined in Exhibit 26-2.

The procedures outlined for both types of unit watch are designed to give the commander specific guidance regarding measures to ensure the soldier's safety. This written guidance helps to reduce confusion, which often results if a more vague verbal recommendation for a unit watch is used to communicate with the chain of command. The 24-hour watch is at times useful in the management of a soldier with military-specific suicidal or homicidal ideation who has very few risk factors except for a verbalized threat, such as "I will kill myself (or my squad leader) if I have to go back to my unit." It is often, though not necessarily, used in conjunction with an environmental change, for instance, an agreement with the commander that the service member will be moved to a different platoon, if the threats of suicide or homicide are specific to alleged harassment by a noncommissioned officer in the service member's section, squad, or platoon.

In addition to the memoranda outlining specific recommendations, the authors suggest that a unit watch information paper (Exhibit 26-3) be forwarded to the commander, especially if the commander expresses confusion or skepticism about the recommendation for a unit watch. This document provides education for the command team and may alleviate concerns about the safety and value of a unit watch. Command support of the unit watch is crucial. If not fully informed and educated about the unit watch, unit leaders may feel compelled to intervene further and attempt to force the mental health system to psychiatrically hospitalize the service member.

Exhibit 26-4 is an example of a standard operating procedure for the behavioral health team, providing a general guide for the use of unit watch in a garrison setting. Clinicians' beliefs about the need for psychiatric hospitalization in various situations differ significantly, so no absolute guidelines about which clinical factors require hospitalization over unit watch are included in this chapter. This variation in decisions regarding hospitalization reinforces the critical role of documenting the clinical assessment and decision-making process in each case. Finally, when the clinician decides to recommend discontinuation of the unit watch, it is helpful to forward to the command team a standard document with this recommendation. Commanders may wait for such written notification before discontinuing a watch. Exhibit 26-5 is a sample memorandum.

Deployed Settings

The garrison system for unit watch must be modified to function in a deployed setting for two reasons. The first is a recognition that access to lethal weapons is heightened immeasurably in a deployed setting; thus, the buddy watch must be removed from the range of options. The 24-hour watch is used instead for soldiers at heightened risk who do not require hospitalization. Another option for lower risk soldiers used during the deployment has been dubbed "basic precautions." The essential elements of the basic precautions profile are removal of the firing pin (or bolt) from the soldier's weapon and suspending combat duties until further notice. Exhibit 26-6 shows the basic precautions memorandum that was used to successfully communicate to the commander the necessary precautions by one of the authors (SP) during a 2006–2007 deployment. During this deployment, basic precautions were applied extensively in a variety of situations, including those involving vague suicidal or homicidal thoughts but few other risk factors in soldiers requiring a period of treatment before return to full duty.

The second reason is that, depending on the unit, the clinician may have ready access to a "patient hold" area such as that operated by the medical company in a brigade support battalion. Although traditional combat stress control doctrine has emphasized separation of soldiers presenting with psychiatric issues from those presenting with medical and surgical illness, utilization of the patient hold area for brief management of suicide risk has been effective in deployed settings. Based on these two modifications, a model for conceptualizing the role of unit watches in a deployed setting is presented in Table 26-2. This model was used by one author (SP) to train primary care clinicians and mental health professionals in the management of suicide and homicide risk during the 2006–2007 deployment. The following is an example of a unit watch used in a deployed setting.

Case Study 26-1: A 31-year-old married African-American man deployed to a combat zone came to the mental health clinic after learning that his wife planned to leave him. He stated that if only he was given the chance to go home, he could save his marriage. He reported that he was

EXHIBIT 26-6

BASIC PRECAUTIONS

________ TMC
FOB ____, Iraq

Date ________________
MEMORANDUM FOR Commander,

SUBJECT: Basic Precaution for ____________________________ SSN:______________________

This service member was evaluated at the FOB ______ TMC. Based on this evaluation of the service member's recent behaviors and current mental status, the following precautions are recommended to the commander for the service member's support and safety. The evaluation did not indicate a high enough risk of dangerousness to warrant hospitalization or a unit watch at this time.

2. Precautions:

   a. Remove the firing pin (or bolt) from this service member's weapon.
   b. No combat or "Off-FOB" duties until further notice.
   c. Service member should perform duties not involving combat operations and should participate in PT. PT may help improve the service member's behavioral health symptoms.

3. If this service member's condition worsens, the service member's supervisor should call FOB ________ TMC Behavioral Health at xxx-xxxx or escort the service member to the TMC for evaluation.

This service member's next appointment at FOB _______ TMC is on______________________
at ________________________ with ____.

______________________________ ______________________________
Representative from Command Clinician

FOB: forward operating base; PT: physcial therapy; SSN: social security number; TMC: troop medical clinic

TABLE 26-2

MANAGING SUICIDE AND HOMICIDE RISK DURING DEPLOYMENT

	Full Combat Duty	**Basic Precautions**	**24-Hour Watch** (or admit patient to hold)	**Evacuation to Combat Support Hospital**
	Least restrictive ⟵			⟶ Most restrictive
Actions	Soldier verbally contracts for safety	1. Secure bolt from weapon until further notice 2. No off-FOB duties until further notice	1. Secure weapons and medications 2. Soldier is under direct observation 24 h/day	Enact evacuation procedures
Examples	Suicidal thoughts, few risk factors, able to contract for safety	1. Primary indication is military-specific SI/HI 2. Psychiatric disorder with SI/HI but risk not high enough to warrant unit watch 3. Step down from unit watch	1. Military-specific SI/HI but risk not high enough to warrant hospitalization 2. Psychiatric disorder with SI/HI but risk not high enough to warrant hospitalization	1. Suicide or homicide risk high enough to warrant hospitalization 2. Medically serious suicide attempt (overdose, lacerations requiring sutures) 3. Suicide/homicide risk not diminishing after (no more than) 5 days despite treatment while on unit watch
Advantages	1. RTD 2. No stigma	1. Much less stigma than unit watch 2. Some level of safety precautions	1. High level of safety precautions 2. High likelihood of RTD 3. Consistent with PIES	Highest level of safety precautions
Disadvantages	No safety precautions	Fewer safety precautions vs unit watch	1. Stigma 2. "Sick role" with patient hold	Low likelihood of RTD, stigma, violates PIES unless clearly indicated

FOB: forward operating base; HI: homicidal ideation; PIES: proximity, immediacy, expectancy, and simplicity; RTD: return to duty; SI: suicidal ideation

suicidal and would kill himself if he wasn't allowed to leave. During the initial evaluation, he didn't describe a defined plan for carrying out his suicide and reported never before experiencing suicidal thoughts. He denied any previous mental health history, had no medical illness, and was not using alcohol, street drugs, or medications. A 24-hour watch was recommended to the commander, along with frequent mental health treatment to help him cope with his emotional crisis. On meeting to discuss a safety plan for the soldier, the command team reported that he had recently been serving well in his role as a member of a logistics team. During the meeting the soldier's first sergeant reminded the soldier how proud the battalion commander was of the soldier's proficiency in a recent task. He then expressed how the command team valued the soldier, not just as a "number" but as a person and team member. The command team agreed to provide 24-hour supervision for the soldier in a nonstigmatizing manner by removing the bolt from his weapon and removing his ammunition and knives from his possession, as well as allowing him to remain on base where he would probably not need his weapons. He was allowed to choose the soldiers who would be assigned to monitor him, selecting those with whom he felt the closest connection. He was then returned to duty with mental health follow-up planned in 2 days. He reported that during the day while on 24-hour watch he spent time talking to his escorts about his problems. During this time period, he continued his usual work schedule and came to the clinic every other day for a brief assessment and supportive therapy. Within 2 weeks, he had come to terms with his pending divorce, realizing that his presence at home would probably not have affected his wife's plans. He also noted that his distress over the loss of his marriage wouldn't resolve by throwing away his life or military career. The 24-hour watch was discontinued at that point. His bolt, ammunition, and knives were returned to him and, though his wife did leave him, he was able to continue with the mission and complete the deployment. His emotional state had returned to near baseline approximately 1 month after his initial presentation. After several months of monthly follow-up, he required no further treatment for the remainder of the deployment.

The soldier in this case presented with suicidal ideation in acute emotional crisis after learning of his wife's plan to divorce him. His access to a weapon and his primary stressor of interpersonal loss placed him at significant risk for a suicide attempt. However, he did not have a formulated plan for suicide, a significant medical or mental health history, or a substance-use problem. Thus, his treating clinician decided that the appropriate treatment setting would be to ensure the patient's safety via a 24-hour watch, long enough for his immediate emotional crisis to resolve. An adequate nonstigmatizing safety environment was created for the soldier, and the unit provided emotional support as well as safety. As expected, his emotional crisis resolved within 2 weeks and his symptoms resolved within 1 month as he gained understanding and acceptance of his changing life situation.

In a garrison or deployed setting, the clinician must clearly document the suicide or homicide risk assessment, giving a clear rationale that makes the case for the specific treatment setting (eg, buddy watch, 24-hour watch, basic precautions, patient hold) rather than hospitalization or evacuation. The military unit is a unique and cohesive community that often allows these interventions to effectively reduce suicide or homicide risk. However, because these interventions are relatively unknown in the civilian sector, meticulous documentation of suicide risk factors and the reason that unit watch was considered a safe intervention for the soldier are essential in each case. Documentation of discussions with command, education given to the command, and assurance that the command is capable of carrying out a proper unit watch are also recommended. Finally, the widespread use of the unit watch by military mental health providers, and its inclusion in the American Psychiatric Association practice guidelines, may help establish this as an appropriate, if not yet evidence-based, intervention within the military.[1]

MEDICOLEGAL ISSUES

The legal implications of using a unit watch are of concern to many clinicians. There is no exact equivalent to the unit watch in the civilian sector, although it is loosely analogous to sending a patient home with parents or family members who promise to watch the patient and confiscate weapons or excess pills. Suicide watches in a prison may use similar procedures, despite the obvious differences between a prison environment and an Army barracks. Although the need for collaboration with the legal community on these issues is obvious, no literature specifically addresses this aspect. The following brief summary lays out the basic medicolegal issues involved.

Mental health clinicians in the civilian community have serious concerns about liability when a patient completes a suicide or commits a homicide. Many malpractice lawsuits involve plaintiffs who complete suicide after a psychiatric assessment concluded that hospitalization was not indicated. Factors in finding the mental health clinician liable for damages often include inadequate risk assessment or inadequate response to that risk.[20] Inadequate documentation of the risk assessment is a frequent factor that leads to a verdict against the clinician. Failure to frequently reevaluate the suicide risk may also be a basis for a finding of malpractice. Prison staff and supervisors have been found liable in cases of completed suicides in civilian prisons because of their responsibility for the health and well-being of their wards. Insufficient training of personnel or inadequate adherence to standard operating procedures may result in findings of negligence.

Military commanders and clinicians have a unique protection from liability in the form of the Feres doctrine, which is an exception to the Federal Tort Claims Act. The doctrine stems from *Feres v US*,[21] which consolidated three lawsuits concerning the injury or death of three service members due to possible negligence on the part of the military. Two of the cases involved physician malpractice. The US Supreme Court ruled that there was no cause of action under the Tort Claims Act for wrongful death of or personal injury to a member of the armed forces if the injury or death was "in the course of activity incident to their service in the Armed Forces."[21] Many lawsuits alleging malpractice or seeking consortium for loss of finances have been barred because of the Feres doctrine, including suits in which unit commanders were accused of failure to take appropriate actions when there was direct evidence of a soldier's suicidal intent. Legal action by both active duty members suing through military courts and civilian dependents suing through federal courts have been barred.

The suicide of a soldier while that individual is under unit watch could potentially call into question whether the mental health clinician did not fully appreciate the suicide risk or did not ensure that an adequate intervention was used. The commander could also be questioned concerning the competence of the unit to perform a unit watch. Another issue is that soldiers performing the watch may have little or no experience with the procedures involved in a unit watch, and they may not fully appreciate that serious adverse outcomes might result if the procedures are not strictly followed. Although lawsuits are often barred through the Feres doctrine, the military may nonetheless take disciplinary action against physicians or commanders if an internal investigation uncovers fault or negligence. Monetary payments may be given out for compensable events. Department of

Defense Directive 6025.13 outlines the procedures for investigation of potential provider malpractice.[22] If the surgeon general for the specific military branch makes a determination that an adverse privileging action should be placed against a physician, then that finding will be entered into the National Practitioner Data Bank (NPDB).[22,23(pA-3)] The NPDB is a database that provides information concerning specific areas of a practitioner's licensure, including professional society memberships, medical malpractice payment history, record of clinical privileges, adverse licensure actions, withdrawal of clinical privileges, and other negative actions taken against an individual healthcare practitioner. Such information is provided through legally authorized queries to assist state licensing boards, hospitals, and other healthcare entities in establishing the qualifications of the healthcare practitioners they seek to license, hire, or privilege. These actions are representative of the military's ongoing efforts to ensure that military healthcare is comparable to civilian standards. A survey of all military malpractice cases from 1978 to 1987 revealed that of 14 cases involving attempted or completed suicide, six cases resulted in monetary settlements totaling $754,000.[24]

The use of unit watch for management of homicide risk is perhaps the easier case to make. The landmark *Tarasoff* decision, although binding only within the state of California, gave clinicians the responsibility to take measures to protect the potential victim if the clinician believes there is a probability that the patient will commit murder.[25,26] In the *Tarasoff* case, a patient told his psychiatrist that he planned to kill a female love interest. The murder was carried out, and the psychiatrist was found liable for not taking action such as alerting the victim and committing the patient. Many states now require *Tarasoff*-like duties to protect potential victims, either through case or statutory law. However, there is no federal law regarding this issue (federal law applies to the military). Some states have ruled that psychiatrists are liable for violent acts by their patients even when no specific victim can be identified, when no specific threat was made, or when homicides occur several months after a risk assessment.[27–29]

The military psychiatric community commonly assumes that a duty to protect exists, despite the lack of clear statutory guidance. The Feres doctrine would not exempt a military clinician from potential liability if an active duty patient hurt or killed an individual not on active duty; in such a case, relevant state law would be applicable. Unless one is familiar with the laws of each state, the best practice in the military is to adhere to a *Tarasoff*-like standard of care. The use of unit watch to prevent an individual from carrying out an act of homicide would be an added medicolegal (and ethical) safeguard when a clinician is assessing a soldier's threats.

In the authors' experience, a large proportion of soldiers presenting with homicidal ideation toward their chains of command have diagnoses of adjustment disorder, personality disorder, or, sometimes, alcohol-abuse disorder. In the absence of a severe mental disorder, these service members do not meet criteria for hospitalization, but are often hospitalized because the clinician believes that it is necessary to protect the potential victim. As an alternative measure, unit watch helps protect potential victims by limiting access to lethal means and providing an observer to notify the chain of command or authorities if the potential perpetrator takes any confrontational action. As an adjunct to the unit watch, additional clinical actions in the case of a potential homicide sometimes include a recommendation that the commander move the soldier to another section of the unit (in the case of homicidal ideation toward an immediate supervisor), that the commander warn the potential victim about the homicide threat, and that the commander give both parties a direct order to avoid all contact except as necessary in the performance of their daily duties. In many cases, these interventions may actually be more effective in minimizing risk than simply notifying the local police and the potential victim, in keeping with the civilian standard of care when the patient does not meet commitment criteria because of the lack of evidence of a severe mental disorder.

SUMMARY

Although there are no simple answers in the assessment and management of suicide and homicide risk in any setting, military clinicians practice in a unique community that necessitates a uniquely military approach to the issue. The recommendations and information presented in this chapter may help validate and standardize a military approach, and will hopefully stimulate research in this area. For example, publication of a case series of soldiers successfully managed with unit watch according to the guidelines discussed above would further validate this technique. A retrospective or prospective study comparing various outcome measures for soldiers at a post where unit watch is commonly used with outcomes for a control group of soldiers at a post where unit watch is not commonly used might also be possible. Optimization, validation, and eventually incorporation of this chapter's recommendations into the curricula in military behavioral health training programs, combat operational stress control doctrine, and other military publications will contribute to a wealth of resources available to military mental health professionals to support and guide the successful management of suicide and homicide risk in the active duty population.

Acknowledgment

The authors would like to express their sincere thanks to Colonel Sally Harvey for developing an earlier version of the example unit watch forms used in this paper. These forms have been modified and utilized in two major conflicts, Operation Iraqi Freedom and Operation Enduring Freedom; in peacekeeping operations in the Balkans; and in garrison settings throughout the United States, Europe, and Asia.

REFERENCES

1. American Psychiatric Association. Practice guideline for the assessment and treatment of patients with suicidal behaviors. *Am J Psychiatry*. 2003;160(11 suppl):1–60.

2. Hassinger AD. Mentoring and monitoring: the use of unit watch in the 4th Infantry Division. *Mil Med*. 2003;168(3):234–238.

3. Pincus SH, Benedek DM. Operational stress control in the former Yugoslavia: a joint endeavor. *Mil Med*. 1998;163(6):358–362.

4. Ritchie EC, Owens M. Military issues. *Psychiatr Clin North Am*. 2004;27:459–471.

5. US Department of the Army. *Combat and Operational Stress Control*. Washington, DC: DA; 2006. Field Manual 4-02.51 (formerly Field Manual 8-51).

6. Jones FD. Psychiatric lessons of war. In: Jones FD, Sparacino LR, Wilcox VL, Rothberg JM, Stokes J, eds. *War Psychiatry*. In: Zajtchuk R, Bellamy R, eds. *Textbooks of Military Medicine*. Washington, DC: Office of The Surgeon General, United States Army and Borden Institute; 1995: 9–25.

7. Solomon Z, Benbenishty R. The role of proximity, immediacy, and expectancy in frontline treatment of combat stress reaction among Israelis in the Lebanon War. *Am J Psychiatry*. 1986;143:613–617.

8. Jones DR. US Air Force combat psychiatry. In: Jones FD, Sparacino LR, Wilcox VL, Rothberg JM, Stokes J, eds. *War Psychiatry*. In: Zajtchuk R, Bellamy R, eds. *The Textbooks of Military Medicine*. Washington, DC: Office of The Surgeon General, United States Army and Borden Institute; 1995: 202.

9. Greene-Shortridge TM, Britt TW, Castro CA. The stigma of mental health problems in the military. *Mil Med*. 2007;172(2):157–161.

10. Gal R, Jones FD. A psychiatric model of combat stress. In: Jones FD, Sparacino LR, Wilcox VL, Rothberg JM, Stokes J, eds. *War Psychiatry*. In: Zajtchuk R, Bellamy R, eds. *The Textbooks of Military Medicine*. Washington, DC: Office of The Surgeon General, United States Army and Borden Institute; 1995: 139.

11. Hill JV, Johnson RC, Barton RA. Suicidal and homicidal soldiers in deployment environments. *Mil Med*. 2006;171(3):228–232.

12. Alaimo CJ, Parker BL. Social support: an undervalued and underused clinical resource. *Fed Pract*. 2004;21(6):27–28,31.

13. Gahm GA, Lucenko BA. Suicide Risk Management and Surveillance Office, Army Behavioral Health Technology Office. *Army Suicide Event Report (ASER) Calendar Year 2004*. Tacoma, Wash: Madigan Army Medical Center; 2005: 16–17.

14. Gahm GA, Lucenko BA. Suicide Risk Management and Surveillance Office, Army Behavioral Health Technology Office. *Army Suicide Event Report (ASER) Calendar Year 2005*. Tacoma, Wash: Madigan Army Medical Center; 2006: 11–17.

15. Sadock BJ, Sadock VA. Somatoform disorders. In: Sadock BJ, Sadock VA, eds. *Kaplan & Sadock's Synopsis of Psychiatry: Behavioral Sciences/Clinical Psychiatry.* 10th ed. Philadelphia, Penn: Lippincott, Williams & Wilkins; 2007: 640.

16. Rothberg JM, Jones FD. Suicide in the US Army: epidemiological and periodic aspects. *Suicide Life Threat Behav.* 1987;17(2):119–132.

17. Helmkamp JC. Occupation and suicide among males in the US armed forces. *Ann Epidemiol.* 1996;6(1):83–88.

18. Sadock BJ, Sadock VA. Emergency psychiatric medicine. In: Sadock BJ, Sadock VA, eds. *Kaplan & Sadock's Synopsis of Psychiatry: Behavioral Sciences/Clinical Psychiatry.* 10th ed. Philadelphia, Penn: Lippincott, Williams & Wilkins; 2007: 898.

19. Adam KS. Attempted suicide. *Psychiatr Clin North Am.* 1985;8(2):183–201.

20. Robertson JD. *Psychiatric Malpractice: Liability of Mental Health Professionals.* New York, NY: Wiley Law Publications; 1988.

21. *Feres v United States,* 340 US 135 (1950).

22. US Department of Defense. Medical Quality Assurance (MQA) in the Military Health System (MHS). Washington, DC: DoD; 2004. DoD Directive 6025.13.

23. National Practitioner Data Bank Guidebook. Available at: http://www.npdb-hipdb.hrsa.gov/npdbguidebook.html. Accessed November 2, 2009.

24. Lande RG, Armitage DT, eds. *Principles and Practice of Military Forensic Psychiatry.* Springfield, Ill: Charles C Thomas; 1997: 387.

25. *Tarasoff v Regents of the University of California,* 551 P2d 334, 131 Cal Rpt 14 (1976).

26. Sadock BJ, Sadock VA. Clinical-legal issues in psychiatry. In: Sadock BJ, Sadock VA, eds. *Kaplan & Sadock's Synopsis of Psychiatry: Behavioral Sciences/Clinical Psychiatry.* 10th ed. Philadelphia, Penn: Lippincott, Williams & Wilkins; 2007: 1374.

27. *Lipari v Sears Roebuck,* 497 F Supp 185 (D Neb 1980).

28. *Jablonski v United States,* 712 F2d 391 (1983).

29. *Naidu v Laird,* 539 A2d 1064 (1988).

Chapter 27

SEVERE PSYCHIATRIC ILLNESS IN THE MILITARY HEALTHCARE SYSTEM

GEOFFREY GRAMMER, MD*

*Lieutenant Colonel, Medical Corps, US Army; Chief, Inpatient Psychiatry, Department of Psychiatry, Walter Reed Army Medical Center, 6900 Georgia Avenue NW, Washington, DC 20307

INTRODUCTION

New military recruits with psychiatric illness often will have their first contact with mental health professionals within the military healthcare system. Demographics, personal development, and life circumstances contribute to first-presentation illness that manifests only after active duty entry. Medical standards for enlistment or commission and retention effectively select out service members with recurrent or chronic mental illness. Providers who care for military service members are thus afforded a unique opportunity to set the tone for therapeutic alliances with patients unfamiliar with mental healthcare. Providers must also contend with patients struggling with insight and acceptance of newly diagnosed mental illness.

Several assumptions are made in this discussion of severe psychiatric illness in the military. Diagnoses elaborated in this chapter are based on the 4th edition of the *Diagnostic and Statistical Manual* (DSM-IV-TR) of the American Psychiatric Association. Combat zones are considered to be outside the continental United States. Severe mental illnesses include, but are not limited to, the diagnoses of brief psychotic disorder, schizophreniform disorder, schizophrenia, schizoaffective disorder, delusional disorder, major depressive disorder–severe, and bipolar disorder types I and II. And finally, the use of antidepressants and neuroleptics requires 4 to 6 weeks before efficacy can be fully realized.

Almost 90% of new recruits enlist in the Army before the age of 25, thus falling within the window of the average age of onset for many psychiatric illnesses.[1] Schizophrenia will begin earlier in men than women, but excepting less distinct prodomes, the average age of onset falls well within this window. Bipolar disorder is considered to have a bimodal peak onset, both in early adulthood and again later in life (around age 50), a time when many are ending their military careers. Depression can begin at any age, but the average age of onset is 25, falling well within the new-recruit age range.

Entering into military service is not a decision that most take lightly. It requires geographic separation from friends and family, changes in daily activities, loss of some flexibility enjoyed by civilians, and the potential for hazardous deployments. A decision to join can challenge one's existential and phase-of-life development and presents service members with stressors rarely found in the civilian workforce. Drastic life changes can be accompanied by destabilizing anxiety, a precipitate of psychiatric illness.

Some new recruits enter military service to bring a change of direction to their lives. Although most often this is a personal developmental milestone followed by a successful career, it can sometimes be the result of premilitary failings resulting from subclinical or fully developed mental illnesses. Obligations required of soldiers and the stringent fitness for duty requirements may be unknown to those who see military service as a chance to bring about a change in their lives. At its extreme, recruits may join the military with preexisting severe mental illness, often stopping pharmacologic treatment shortly before entering basic training to facilitate acceptance into service.

The military operates in environments ranging from remote locales with few to no medical facilities through major academic medical centers. Soldiers may find themselves in garrison, peacetime missions, training exercises, or combat zones. Each of these environments presents its own unique challenges to new onset or recurrence of major psychiatric symptoms. Resources at each locale are utilized to control symptoms and agitation until definitive care can be administered, often within the confines of continental United States military medical facilities.

Military mental health professionals provide care within the context of the physical disability system and military regulations. Providers must often comply with the actions of the physical evaluation board (which will determine fitness for duty and potential disability ratings), while simultaneously attempting to maximize clinical improvement. These competing agendas and potential conflicting interests can add an unwelcome complexity to patient management. Patients undergoing fitness-for-duty and disability determination may have a financial or administrative disincentive for improvement or accurate reporting of decline in their clinical status due to varying degrees of conscious and unconscious secondary gain.

BRIEF PSYCHOTIC DISORDER, SCHIZOPHRENIFORM, AND SCHIZOPHRENIA

The spectrum of primary thought disorders described in the DSM-IV-TR may present uniquely in a military community. Though predominately distinguished by length of symptoms, brief psychotic disorder may terminate in non-thought-disorder diagnoses such as adjustment disorders.[2] Differentiating true schizophreniform disorder (as defined by complete resolution of symptoms within 6 months of onset) from first-break schizophrenia (which has the same symptoms as schizophreniform disorder but lasts for a lifetime) may be possible only after clinical observation. Often the clinician will need to wait to see if the symptoms persist over time; it is estimated that 25% of these cases will resolve.[3] Unfortunately for many patients, both brief psychotic disorder and schizophreniform disorder may serve only as place markers in the timeline of new onset schizophrenia, most commonly a chronic and disabling disease.

A detriment to clinical accuracy can occur with such early presentation of primary thought disorders. It is common for psychotic symptoms to not be fully developed leading to ambiguous perceptual disturbances, delusional beliefs, or executive functioning that may make diagnosis more difficult. Premature diagnoses of delusional disorder and psychosis not otherwise specified may underestimate the severity of illness and long-term functional implications if the true disorder is schizophrenia. Military providers should consider this phenomenon when applying diagnoses and determining treatments and disposition management.

Presentation of psychotic illness is different than that seen in the general community. Closer scrutiny and command oversight can result in a greater interpersonal immersion than in the civilian workplace. Command-directed evaluations can require service members to undergo evaluation with a level of dysfunction that may not have reached threshold criteria in a civilian healthcare system. Early referral may be beneficial, as symptoms may be present for shorter periods before presentation to mental healthcare and thus offer an opportunity to positively effect long-term outcome through early treatment.[4,5] Ensuring compliance during initial treatment may enhance outcomes and slow declines in function seen in naturalistic studies.[6] Service members undergoing a medical evaluation board often wait for months, if not more than a year, before adjudication, which offers an opportune time for close monitoring of compliance and subsequent clinical status.

Pharmacologic management of primary thought disorder extends beyond the scope of this chapter. Long-term metabolic and extrapyramidal side effects should be weighed against proven efficacy for positive and negative symptoms and receptor profiles.[7] When psychosis arises in remote locations, choice of an antipsychotic agent is often more dictated by availability than the previously described variables. This may be problematic if efficacy is achieved despite long-term issues of toxicity.

SUBSTANCE-INDUCED PSYCHOSIS

Intentional and unintentional ingestions of supplements, medications, or illicit substances can result in mental status changes that may mimic severe thought disorders. History, physical examination, and laboratory testing sometimes detect a particular agent, but history may be difficult to obtain from an acutely agitated patient. Furthermore, not all substances are readily detected in drug screens or routine laboratory tests, or laboratory testing may not be possible in some field environments.

Illicit substances and novel ways of utilizing items not intended for consumption have their own usage trends in the community. Illicit substance use has its own variations in popularity depending on street costs, accessibility, and cultural acceptance. Knowing which items are "in style" can assist with more rapid diagnosis of sudden changes in mental status. In addition, novel ways of ingesting or inhaling routine items, such as pressurized air, solvents, or even brake fluid, can alter mental status. Familiarity with these substances may allow for more rapid detection of their use and intervention for the potentially life-threatening complications that may develop. Collateral history from fellow service members, barracks health and welfare inspections, and prior substance abuse history may help providers determine if a particular agent is associated with behavioral change.

Withdrawal from substance dependence can not only result in an acute change in mental status indistinguishable from primary mental illness, but it may also be associated with life-threatening complications. Military service with controlled environments—weekend drills, field exercises, combat deployments, and military training schools—can interrupt accessibility to drugs or alcohol for a chronic substance-using service member. Healthcare providers should remain vigilant for, and be prepared to treat, such events.

BIPOLAR DISORDER

Bipolar disorder presents diagnostic and management considerations for service members presenting with current or past histories of mania. With a bimodal onset, it can affect new recruits in their second decade or those getting ready to retire in their fifth decade.[8] Both are associated with significant adjustments, as younger patients will have to contend with management of an indefinite mental illness, and those in mid-life have retirement and generational phase-of-life development potentially derailed with a new-onset mental illness.

Bipolar disorder type I can present with frank psychosis, making diagnosis more difficult. Acutely agitated patients with grandiose delusions may be indistinguishable from those with agitated schizophrenia without collateral history to suggest prior and current mood criteria. Misdiagnosis may be more common in certain ethnic groups and thus caution should be taken when suggesting diagnoses in minority populations.[9]

Bipolar type II can be less dramatic in its presentations with hypomania. A decreased need for sleep, narcissism, and increased goal-directed activity can be adaptive for noncommissioned and commissioned officers. Presentation for care can commonly occur under times of marked duress, such as a combat deployment, when defenses used in a hypomanic state are overwhelmed (leading to decompensation) or during depressed mood episodes. Traditional antidepressant medications can cause destabilization and thus a careful collateral history is needed for any service member presenting with depression, to ensure there have not been prior manic symptoms.

Bipolar disorder has a high likelihood of recurrent mood episodes and providers should give strong consideration for initiation of a medical evaluation board.[10] Environmental changes, lack of access to laboratory monitoring, and sleep-cycle changes can destabilize this condition, and conversely, early treatment, avoidance of illicit drug and alcohol use, and lifestyle management can improve long-term prognosis.[11] Military mental healthcare providers are in a unique position to affect the course of this illness long after patients have separated from the service.

Choice of pharmacologic agents should account for likely indefinite treatment and potential long-term side effects, such as metabolic impact and tolerance. Practice guidelines continue to push the envelope of evidenced-based treatments and extend beyond the scope of this chapter. Providers, however, should seek these resources to remain abreast of agents with the most evidence-based efficacy while mitigating potential side effects.[12]

MAJOR DEPRESSIVE DISORDER

Depression is a common disorder affecting service members of all ages.[13] The effect of this illness on performance can be more variable than seen with primary thought disorders or bipolar disorder, ranging between little to no impact on performance to marked decrement with potential harm to self or others. Remote locales, variable pharmacologic and psychotherapeutic resources, command support, and psychosocial stressors all can affect treatment decisions and disposition.

The DSM-IV-TR does not distinguish between exogenous or endogenous depression. Although many cases have some components of external influences and endogenous predispositions, unique military environments can bring about extraordinary levels of environmental stress that challenge the most resilient of personalities. Geographic separation from friends and family, combat exposure, obligated tours of duty, scrutiny from command, loss of privacy, and physical demands are some of the unique military stressors than can help precipitate a depressed mood. Because service members are often unable to change their occupations or duty assignments and thus avoid an unpleasant stressor, hopelessness may ensue, leading to suicidal and/or homicidal thoughts. Even though meeting criteria for major depressive disorder, many of these service members will have rapid resolution of symptoms if medically removed from the situation, such as through evacuation, more fitting the intent of the diagnosis of adjustment disorder despite being incorrect by criteria.[14]

Whereas overt behavior associated with mania and psychosis will garner the attention of peers and commanders, isolation associated with a worsening depression may go unnoticed. Deployment to areas far from mental health resources, stigma associated with accessing care, and unwarranted fear of career damage if treated may delay entry into care. Ongoing military efforts to raise awareness and ease access cannot completely negate these effects. Unfortunately, ready access to firearms and heavy machinery make self-injurious behavior lethal in a military with a predominately younger male population, which has tended to prefer this mechanism for suicide.

Fortunately, mild to moderate depression can be treated with relative ease using both therapy and psychopharmacology, with medical assets allowing care in almost all austere locations. Providers who choose to use medications in their treatment of mild to moderate depression should consider agents less likely to cause sedation, ataxia, weight gain, or anticholinergic side effects because all of these can impair a soldier's performance. Antidepressants with shorter half-lives and associated withdrawal phenomenon should also be avoided because compliance is not always accommodated by operational tempos.

Severe depression may be associated with marked performance decrement, reality testing impairment, or injurious behavior, and should be managed at fixed facilities removed from active military operations. Diagnostic clarity often requires inpatient observation to rule out a depressive episode of bipolar disorder, or the presence of a primary thought disorder such as schizoaffective disorder, especially if there are comorbid psychotic symptoms. Treatments will likely require antidepressant and antipsychotic administration, with electroconvulsant therapy (ECT) as an option for those refractory to medication, unable to tolerate medication, or those with life-threatening severity, such as imminent suicidality or catatonia. Single episode severe depression with psychosis warrants strong consideration for a medical board.

POSTTRAUMATIC STRESS DISORDER

Combat-related posttraumatic stress disorder (PTSD) may account for up to 20% of inpatient admission to CONUS medical facilities through the aeromedical evacuation system.[15] Often the symptoms of PTSD alone do not lead to inpatient treatment, but rather comorbid psychiatric conditions (with or without illicit substance use) manifest potentially dangerous clinic states that necessitate inpatient psychiatric treatment. With increased awareness of the phenomenon of PTSD and possible financial disability compensation, patients may find PTSD symptoms easier to discuss with providers, thereby masking another major psychiatric illness. Providers should remain vigilant for confounding illness present in patients who arrive with severe disability or safety concerns and insist on a sole diagnosis of PTSD. Further discussion of PTSD is covered elsewhere and readers are referred to those relevant sections of this book.

REMOTE SITE TREATMENT CONSIDERATIONS

Any mental health facility must be prepared to handle agitated and violent patients no matter how remote the location. Treatment teams need to construct contingency plans utilizing whatever resources they have available to secure a violent or agitated patient, including using restraint and emergency pharmacologic management. For smaller teams, other personnel may need to be enlisted to train and potentially assist with a restraint. Potential personnel resources may include medics, other unit members, military police, and battalion aid station staff. Soft-point restraints are a Joint Commission standard, but not always available on site. Providers may have to use locking ties typically reserved for detainees until appropriate restraint can be obtained. Pharmacologic treatment of agitation may require intramuscular injections that do not require refrigeration.

Pharmacologic options may be limited, particularly in immature operational areas. Providers should be aware of what medications are available to them and, when possible, assist with deciding which medications to pack at the start of a mission. Availability of medical supplies and utilizing surrounding medical facilities can help expand medication options.

If troop movements are ongoing, medical facilities may find themselves occupied with tasks of unit relocation and thereby have less capability to provide resource intensive care. The threshold for evacuation will need to change to accommodate operational tempo in these situations. Skill sets of providers may also dictate what is feasible, as does patient availability. Expectations of patients to follow up weekly in an active combat environment may not be appropriate if traveling to and from the medical site is a hazard itself. Attending line unit battle update briefings will help with accurate intelligence acquisition for ongoing operations as well as foster a collaborative relationship with commands.

While awaiting air evacuation, patients should be kept in a quiet room with minimal distractions. Patients who suffer from psychosis can misunderstand the most basic voice inflection, so providers should interact with these patients in a neutral tone and focus on factual information, such as current location, plan for evacuation, dosing of medications, and formal names of the people who are involved in the patient's care. A patient who is psychotic at a combat stress center can be disruptive to soldiers recovering from mood and anxiety conditions. Providers should educate other patients at the facility about differing disease presentations in an effort to minimize pathologic identification for those for whom this would be a concern.

AIR EVACUATION

The international deployment of military forces creates a unique situation where patients may be evacuated across continents at the beginning of their mental healthcare. Although hospitalization alone can be an adjustment, time-zone changes, layover in medical facilities, and long evacuation flights may affect the presentation of patients as they move through the system.[16] Exposing patients to this process is justified by the need to get them to a fixed medical facility for definitive treatment and fitness-for-duty determination.[17] Given the risks of symptom exacerbation and subsequent agitation, a low threshold for pharmacologic treatment and possible physical restraint should be considered.

Another consequence of medical evacuation is evolution of clinical state when service members reach rear-echelon medical facilities. There may be numerous reasons for such an occurrence. Once removed from whatever stressor may have precipitated or aggravated their condition, some service members will reconstitute quickly en route. Other patients may have time to reflect on consequences of admitting to delusional belief systems or to the presence of hallucinatory events, and thus began to recant their stories given the reaction of those to whom they had confided. Some service members may admit to severe psychiatric symptoms with secondary gain as a motivator and, upon seemingly realizing their objective, begin to report a rapid recovery to escape the mental healthcare system. Treatments instituted at the lower echelon of care may have a rapid effect leading to genuine symptom improvement. The end result is that patients diagnosed with severe psychiatric disorders at lower echelons of care may look different and much less ill when arriving at a tertiary treatment facility.

Providers should not dismiss collateral and observed behavior noted downrange. Underestimation of severity of illness can have consequences to both patient care and unit readiness. Upon arrival at the definitive care facility, medical records should be reviewed and collateral contacts made with medical personnel involved in the care of the patient prior to that point. Existence of electronic record systems should facilitate continuity of care, but austere environments may not allow for such a convenience and physical records may not survive extensive evacuation routes. Providers should make concerted efforts at overcoming inherent obstacles to continuity that military operations may create.

Command should be notified of the patient's arrival at each step along an evacuation route. It is not uncommon for patients to be evacuated from an operational area with such efficiency as to outpace command notification. In addition, commands can provide invaluable collateral data on history of presentation, premorbid functioning, known interpersonal and social stressors, environmental exposures, and actions that may be subject to the Uniform Code of Military Justice.

Patients should receive a thorough medical-psychiatric assessment upon arrival at definitive treatment facilities. Lower echelons of care may not have resources available to meet practice guideline recommendations for medical workup of the psychiatric patient. The receiving facility should ensure that psychiatric symptoms do not have a medical or substance-induced cause. Operational environments downrange may also have competing priorities, such as ongoing combat operations, that prevent providers from completing a thorough assessment. In some cases, an expeditious evaluation may have been formed to determine appropriateness for evacuation and initial management. Some patients may require tests, such as a positron emission tomography scan, magnetic resonance imaging, or electroencephalography, that can only be performed at higher echelon facilities. Finally, case load downrange may not lend itself to a thorough psychiatric assessment that can be performed at a major medical facility with subspecialty consultations and graduate medical education programs.

SUMMARY

Severe psychiatric illness represents an important component of military mental healthcare. Unique aspects of military service and operations may impact presentation and disease processes. Military mental health providers should be familiar with the management of severe psychiatric illness and the nuances of its treatment in an operational environment.

REFERENCES

1. Civilian data from Bureau of Labor Statistics Current Population Survey File; 2004. Available at: http://www.defenselink.mil/prhome/poprep2004/enlisted_accessions/age.html. Accessed May 28, 2008.

2. Beighley PS, Brown GR, Thompson JW Jr. DSM-III-R brief reactive psychosis among Air Force recruits. *J Clin Psychiatry*. 1992;53:283–288.

3. Zhang-Wong J, Beiser M, Bean G, Iacono WG. Five-year course of schizophreniform disorder. *Psychiatry Res*. 1995;59(1–2):109–117.

4. Jarskog LF, Lieberman JA. Neuroprotection in schizophrenia. *J Clin Psychiatry*. 2006;67(9):e09.

5. Wyatt RJ, Henter I. Rationale for the study of early intervention. *Schizophr Res*. 2001;51(1):69–76.

6. McGlashan TH. A selective review of recent North American long-term followup studies of schizophrenia. *Schizophr Bull*. 1988;14:515–542.

7. Lieberman JA, Stroup TS, McEvoy JP, et al. Effectiveness of antipsychotic drugs in patients with chronic schizophrenia. *N Engl J Med*. 2005;353(12):1209–1223.

8. Hale RE, Yudofsky SC, eds. *The American Psychiatric Publishing Textbook of Clinical Psychiatry.* 4th ed. Washington, DC: American Psychiatric Publishing; 2003: 490.

9. Mukherjee S, Shukla S, Woodle J, Rosen AM, Olarte S. Misdiagnosis of schizophrenia in bipolar patients: a multiethnic comparison. *Am J Psychiatry.* 1983;140(12):1571–1574.

10. Tohen M, Zarate CA Jr, Hennen J, et al. The McLean-Harvard First-Episode Mania Study: prediction of recovery and first recurrence. *Am J Psychiatry*. 2003;160(12):2099–2107.

11. Post RM. Kindling and sensitization as models for affective episode recurrence, cyclicity, and tolerance phenomena. *Neurosci Biobehav Rev*. 2007;31(6):858–873.

12. Suppes T, Dennehy EB, Hirschfeld RM, et al. The Texas implementation of medication algorithms: update to the algorithms for treatment of bipolar I disorder. *J Clin Psychiatry*. 2005;66(7):870–886.

13. Grammer GG, Cooper M. *National Collaborative Study of Early Psychosis and Suicide: New Onset Psychosis in New Military Service Members*. Bailey K Ashford Research Award. Washington, DC: Walter Reed Army Medical Center; 2001.

14. American Psychiatric Association. *Quick Reference to the Diagnostic Criteria From DSM-IV-TR.* Washington, DC: American Psychiatric Association; 2005.

15. Data on file at Department of Psychiatry, Walter Reed Army Medical Center, Washington, DC; 2004.

16. Ritchie EC. Psychiatric patients. In: Hurd WW, Jernigan JG, eds. *Aeromedical Evacuation: Management of Acute and Stabilized Patients*. New York, NY: Springer-Verlag; 2003: Chap 26.

17. Ritchie EC, Morse JH, Brewer PG. Surviving the "air evac": medical and logistical issues of evacuating psychiatric patients by air from Korea to the United States. *Mil Med.* 1996;161(5):298–302.

Chapter 28

EATING DISORDERS

GAIL H. MANOS, MD*; JANIS CARLTON, MD, PhD†; AND AILEEN KIM, MD‡

*Captain, Medical Corps, US Navy; Navy Psychiatry Specialty Leader and Senior Medical Officer, Director of Mental Health, Naval Medical Center Portsmouth, 620 John Paul Jones Road, Portsmouth, Virginia 23708; formerly, Psychiatry Residency Training Director, Department of Psychiatry, Naval Medical Center Portsmouth, Portsmouth, Virginia

†Commander, Medical Corps, US Navy; Department Head, Psychological Health and Traumatic Brain Injury, Building 7, Room 600, National Naval Medical Center, 8901 Wisconsin Avenue, Bethesda, Maryland 20889; formerly, Department Head, Mental Health, Naval Hospital, Camp Lejeune, North Carolina

‡Lieutenant Commander, Medical Corps, US Navy; Staff Psychiatrist, Department of Behavioral Health, Building 7, 3rd Floor, National Naval Medical Center, 8901 Wisconsin Avenue, Bethesda, Maryland 20889; formerly, Chief Resident, Department of Psychiatry, Naval Medical Center Portsmouth, Portsmouth, Virginia

INTRODUCTION

Over the past decade, the growing obesity epidemic in the United States has received increased attention. Like the general population, the US military is experiencing an increase in those classified as overweight (54%) despite high physical activity levels.[1] Although the majority of Americans are overweight or even obese by Centers for Disease Control and Prevention standards,[2] the ideal body image as portrayed by television, movie, and fashion mediums appears to be underweight. This ideal may drive some individuals to abnormal eating behaviors, such as food restriction or bingeing with compensatory behaviors. Military service members may be particularly at risk because of the expectation that they conform to specific weight standards, with adverse career consequences for those who fail to live up to those standards. Under the stress of deployment to a combat zone, service members with an eating disorder may experience an exacerbation of their illness. Even those without a history of an eating disorder may develop poor eating habits as a reaction to stress, or, ironically, due to the ready availability of fast food in some locations. On the other hand, for some individuals, eating behaviors and overall fitness may improve in the military, with nutritional counseling and time for physical exercise more available.

The rates of eating disorders in the military parallel those reported in high-risk groups such as athletes and dancers, who place an emphasis on thinness.[3,4] Abnormal eating and dieting behaviors are reported in 25% to 76% of female service members, with a significant increase around the time of personal fitness assessments (PFAs).[5] Because deployed service members are not subject to PFAs, they may feel less pressured to engage in the abnormal eating and dieting behaviors. Also, with meals eaten community style and public bathrooms, binge and purge behaviors may be more difficult to enact.

The diagnosis of an established eating disorder does not necessarily preclude deployment if the service member's condition is in remission. For example, a physician deployed several years ago soon became overwhelmed with the stress of her duties and separation from family, leading to repetitive bingeing and intentional vomiting several times a day. She had previously avoided mental health treatment due to concerns about an adverse impact on her career. She was subsequently medically evacuated and treated for her bulimic behaviors and depression by one of the authors. Three years later, both her depressive symptoms and bulimia were in remission, allowing her to successfully deploy to a combat zone. Unlike the outcome in this case, other service members with eating disorders have experienced recurrence of their symptoms under the stress of deployment, resulting in early returns.

This chapter presents information on the identification and recognition of eating disorders, medical complications, treatment, and prognoses. The authors also review available literature on eating disorder behaviors in military populations and potential risks of deploying individuals with an eating disorder.

OVERVIEW OF EATING DISORDERS

Eating disorders consist of a group of increasingly common psychiatric and medical conditions that have been studied extensively in women and in certain groups of men. The risks of both bulimia nervosa (BN) and binge eating disorder (BED) in the general population have increased with successive birth cohorts.[6] Anorexia nervosa (AN) was described in the scientific literature by Sir William Gull (in 1873) as a "mental state [that] destroys the appetite."[7] BN, marked by episodes of bingeing and purging, was first described in 1979.[8] The lifetime prevalence for women in the general population is estimated as 0.5% to 1% for AN and 1% to 3% for BN. Rates for men were previously estimated to be about one tenth as high as those for women.[9] However, in 2007, the National Comorbidity Survey Replication[6] found that the estimated point prevalence of BN in men is significantly higher than previously thought, approximately one fifth that in women. Eating disorder not otherwise specified (EDNOS) is a residual category for conditions that do not meet the full criteria for AN or BN. It is difficult to determine the prevalence of EDNOS, but estimates range from 1% to 30% in men and women.[10] As many as 60% of treated eating disorder cases fall into the EDNOS category.[11] It is estimated that only about one third of individuals with AN and 6% of those with BN receive mental healthcare,[12] although the majority of persons with eating disorders receive treatment for another mental health complaint.[6] Because physicians infrequently assess for eating disorders, and patients rarely spontaneously disclose them, these disorders may be underdiagnosed.[6] Healthcare providers should routinely ask patients about eating disorder symptoms even when these symptoms are not the presenting complaint.

Anorexia Nervosa

AN is a psychiatric disorder characterized by extreme weight loss in the absence of a medical cause, refusal to regain weight, and intense determination to continue or maintain weight loss. Patients with AN may deny that they are underweight and take measures to conceal their emaciation with bulky clothes to avoid being "ordered" to gain weight by family members or doctors. Typically, onset is between the ages of 13 and 20, peaking at 17 to 18 years of age.[10] AN is defined by the *Diagnostic and Statistical Manual of Mental Disorders*, 4th edition (DSM-IV),[9] as including the following conditions:

1. the refusal to maintain body weight at or above a minimally normal weight (approximately 85% of those with the AN are below ideal body weight);
2. an intense fear of gaining weight or becoming fat, even though underweight;
3. a disturbance in the way in which one's body weight or shape is experienced, undue influence of body weight or shape on self-evaluation, or denial of the seriousness of current low body weight; and
4. in postmenarcheal females, amenorrhea (ie, the absence of at least three consecutive menstrual cycles).

AN can be divided into (*a*) the restricting type, in which the individual does not engage regularly in bingeing or purging behaviors, but severely restricts calories intake, and (*b*) the bingeing/purging type, in which the individual meets criteria for AN and engages regularly in binge/purge behaviors such as self-induced vomiting and laxative or diuretic misuse. Exhibit 28-1 lists the warning signs and symptoms of AN.

EXHIBIT 28-1

WARNING SIGNS OF ANOREXIA NERVOSA

- Abnormal weight loss without a medical cause
- Severe restriction of food intake
- Denial of hunger and/or a problem with low weight
- Strict food preferences, such as complete avoidance of foods containing fat or strict vegetarianism
- Intense fear of gaining weight and determination to continue weight loss
- Abnormal reproductive functioning (loss of interest in sex, amenorrhea in females, low testosterone in males)
- Excessive exercise despite fatigue and weakness
- Unusual behaviors or rituals with meal preparation and eating
- Distorted perception of weight or body shape
- Inability to stop losing weight or decrease exercise
- Unrealistically high self-expectations; perfectionism with a sense of ineffectiveness
- Use of dangerous methods to lose weight
- Belief that body weight and shape are extremely important to self-esteem and self-definition
- Psychological symptoms of starvation (eg, depression, difficulty concentrating, social withdrawal)
- Physical signs of starvation (eg, sensitivity to cold, fine hair on the face or body, emaciation)

Bulimia Nervosa

BN is defined according to the DSM-IV[9] as consisting of the following conditions:

1. recurrent episodes of binge eating, with the binge episode characterized by eating within a certain time period more food than most people would eat in the same time period and under the same circumstances, including a sense of lack of control over eating during the episode;
2. recurrent inappropriate compensatory behavior to prevent weight gain;
3. binge eating and inappropriate behaviors occurring at least twice weekly for 3 months;
4. self-evaluation unduly influenced by body shape and weight; and
5. episodes not occurring exclusively during episodes of AN.

BN can be divided into purging and nonpurging types; during the latter, individuals use inappropriate compensatory behaviors such as fasting or excessive exercise rather than engaging regularly in vomiting, laxative use, diuretics, or enemas. Purging-type BN differs from purging-type AN in that patients with the latter are significantly underweight. The onset of BN is usually late adolescence to early adulthood.

Warning signs and symptoms of BN are shown in Exhibit 28-2.

Eating Disorder Not Otherwise Specified

The EDNOS category is considered by some to be overly broad, whereas the criteria for BN or AN may be too rigid. Examples of EDNOS include meeting all the criteria of AN except for amenorrhea or being underweight, meeting criteria for BN except for frequency of episodes, or engaging in purging behaviors without binge episodes. BED, bingeing without compensatory behaviors, is a category proposed in the DSM-IV for further study. Although only 1% of the general population is felt to meet strict DSM-IV diagnostic criteria for BED,[11] the prevalence of binge behaviors is thought to be significantly higher. Night-eating syndrome (NES) is characterized by continual eating during evening hours between dinner and breakfast, accompanied by negative feelings about the eating behavior, insomnia, and nocturnal awakenings followed by food intake. Prevalence for this condition is estimated at 1.5% of the general population.[13] Like BED, the prevalence of NES is significantly higher in overweight and obese individuals. NES is also a category proposed in the DSM-IV for further study.

EXHIBIT 28-2

WARNING SIGNS OF BULIMIA NERVOSA

- Fluctuations in weight, usually within about 15 lb of normal weight
- Fear of gaining weight
- Uncontrollable, secretive episodes of binge eating followed by attempts to purge by vomiting, laxatives, etc
- Excessive exercise for weight control
- Physical problems with the throat, stomach, and colon; swelling of the parotid glands
- Dental problems, tooth decay
- Psychological problems such as depression, mood swings, impulsivity
- Dissatisfaction with body shape and preoccupation with weight loss
- Belief that body weight and shape are extremely important to self-esteem and self-definition
- Unrealistically high self-expectations; perfectionism with a sense of ineffectiveness

Obesity

Increasing media attention has focused on overeating and obesity. According to the World Health Organization, a body mass index (BMI) of 18.5 to 24.9 is normal, a BMI of 25 to 29.9 is overweight, and a BMI greater than 30 is obese. The Centers for Disease Control and Prevention report that 51% of American women are overweight and 34% are obese.[2] Although obesity is not itself considered an eating disorder, up to 50% of obese individuals, particularly those seeking bariatric surgery, have BED or NES.[11,13] A cross-sectional analysis from the US Department of Defense Survey of Health-Related Behaviors found that 10% of active duty men and 4% of active duty women were obese.[14] Based on data from the general population, it is likely that many of these individuals have an eating disorder contributing to their obesity; thus, recognition of eating disorders directly impacts fitness for duty and deployability.

ETIOLOGY

The etiology of eating disorders includes genetic, biological, sociocultural, psychological, familial, developmental, and comorbid factors.[15] Although all eating disorders are characterized by an abnormal relationship with food, and usually a disturbance in body image, the underlying factors vary with the type of eating disorder. Although it is important to understand etiological factors commonly found in the different eating disorders, it is also necessary to remember that each person is an individual with a complex history and a unique set of characteristics.

Biological Factors

Brain serotonin, norepinephrine, dopamine, endogenous opioids, and a variety of neuropeptides (eg, leptin, neuropeptide Y) have been implicated in appetite, food intake, satiety, and the development of eating disorders.[16] Traditionally, the catecholamines, particularly norepinephrine and dopamine, have been associated with appetite or onset of eating. Serotonin has been associated with satiety or cessation of an eating episode as well as specific carbohydrate cravings sometimes associated with binges. Disorders of appetite, satiety, or both, underlie abnormal eating behaviors. This may be relevant to the mechanism of action for medications, particularly antidepressants that modulate brain serotonin and catecholamine activity in the treatment of eating disorders.

Eating disorders co-occur more frequently in

monozygotic twins (50% concordance rate) than in dizygotic twins (10% concordance) and are more likely to occur in first-degree relatives of patients with eating disorders than in the general population. Genetic factors account for 58% to 76% of the variance in AN and for 54% to 83% of the variance in BN, with a 7- to 12-fold increase in prevalence among relatives.[17] Some studies have found a link between the serotonin receptor 5-HT_{2A} gene polymorphism in the promoter region and eating disorders.[18] Enhanced 5-HT_{2A} receptor binding suggestive of serotonergic dysfunction has been found in AN and BN patients.[19] Polymorphism of the 5-HT_{1B} receptor gene has also been linked to minimum lifetime BMI in women with BN.[20] These findings suggest that some individuals are more at risk genetically than others to developing an eating disorder. The increasing incidence of these disorders in society may be the result of the sociocultural importance placed on body image and thinness that has allowed more people with a genetic predisposition for AN or BN to develop an eating disorder.

Although all the complex peripheral and central mechanisms that regulate appetite, food intake, and body weight are not yet understood, most people maintain a body weight around a relatively stable "set point" or "settling point," which changes across the age span in a predictable manner. In individuals with an eating disorder, regulation of appetite—and in many cases body weight—is thrown out of balance. People who engage in periods of excessive food restriction that may be followed by binges ignore the biological signals of hunger and satiation. Binge behaviors may be a natural holdover from a time when humans foraged or hunted for food and needed to eat as much as possible before food was lost to competitors or spoilage.

Sociocultural Factors

Social and cultural factors are important in the development of both AN and BN. Although the stereotype persists that these disorders, particularly AN, are more common in higher socioeconomic groups, most of this evidence is based on small, uncontrolled case series.[7] These eating disorders are most common in Western cultures, where tasty, high-calorie food is abundant. Evidence suggests that, as other cultures have become richer and more Westernized, body dissatisfaction has grown and eating disorders have increased.[21]

Obesity is considered a socioculturally driven eating disorder. Individuals and families dine more often in restaurants, where the food served is often high in fat and in large portions. The media present conflicting signals: on one hand, images show thin, happy families eating at fast food restaurants; on the other hand, magazines present not only the latest fad diet, but also recipes for beautiful, high-calorie dishes. Eating is a social or family event. From an early age, many people learn to see tasty foods as a reward for good behavior or accomplishment. As individuals struggle to lose or maintain weight by severely restricting intake or skipping meals, they may trigger the urge to binge or impulsively overeat, followed by guilt, and in the case of bulimics, purging or using other compensatory behaviors. In an effort to demonstrate control, patients with AN may simply refuse to indulge.

Psychological and Family Factors

Families or first-degree relatives of individuals with eating disorders have a higher rate of eating disorders (approximately 10% vs 1%–3% in the general population). Although these rates may indicate a genetic component, there is also evidence for learning and modeling within the family and from peers.[22] Patients with eating disorders frequently report that their parents or siblings were overly concerned with body weight and external appearances. Often, their first diet was started in response to criticism from a family member or friend.

Families of patients with AN are often described as perfectionistic, with one or both parents described as authoritarian and having high expectations for their children. Psychological factors in the development of AN include a drive to perfection, unrealistic self-expectations, and perhaps a misdirected search for autonomy and self-control through control of food intake and weight. The primary comorbid psychiatric condition associated with AN is depression, although it is not clear if this is a preceding condition or a result of AN.

Families of patients with BN are more often described as chaotic, with a higher rate of mood disorders, substance abuse, and eating disorders. A history of sexual abuse during childhood has been reported in one third to nearly one half of women with BN.[23,24] A review of 53 controlled studies that examined the link between sexual abuse and eating disorders found that childhood sexual abuse was a risk factor for eating disorders, particularly BN, with psychiatric comorbidity.[25] Furthermore, women who had experienced both childhood sexual abuse and rape in adulthood had even higher rates of eating disorder behavior and marked impulsivity.[25] Conditions associated comorbidly with BN—including borderline personality disorder, substance abuse, and mood instability—have also been found to be more prevalent in people with a history of childhood abuse.[26] Childhood sexual abuse may lead to diminished self-esteem, development of maladaptive behaviors (including eating disorders), and placement of individuals at risk for further trauma.

A study of 1,887 female Navy recruits found that 57% had a history of childhood physical or sexual abuse or both, and 35% had been sexually assaulted as adults.[27] In addition, women who were raped as adults were 4.8-fold more likely to have experienced childhood sexual abuse. Trauma may also result in psychobiological changes that increase vulnerability to developing an eating disorder. These findings suggest that healthcare providers should ask about eating patterns, purging behaviors, and body image in female service members with a history of abuse.

CLINICAL FEATURES

Eating disorders are often hidden.[28] The individual may consider these behaviors to be shameful or may lack insight into their pathological nature. Patients with restricting-type AN may move food around on their plates or otherwise disguise their lack of food consumption. Individuals with BN may eat normally but subsequently purge in secret. Those with AN may be easier to identify based on height and weight measurements and their emaciated appearance. A BMI of less than 17.5 in an individual from Western cultures, where food is abundant, should raise suspicion among healthcare workers and prompt further evaluation. It may be more difficult to spot BN or EDNOS among normal-weight individuals.

In an operational environment, service members with BN may find it more difficult to binge and purge because of lack of privacy for these behaviors. One of the authors treated a female service member who carried a plastic bag into which she vomited in secret due to lack of privacy in the latrine area. She would then wait to dispose of the bag into a trash receptacle when no one was looking. On the other hand, excessive exercise as a compensatory behavior may easily be overlooked as adaptive rather than disguising pathological behavior.

Medical Findings

Anorexia Nervosa

In addition to an emaciated appearance with sunken cheeks, prominent bone structure, low body fat, and muscle wasting, patients with AN may have dry skin, hypercarotenemia (manifested by a yellow-orange discoloration of the skin); lanugo (fine, downy hair covering the body to compensate for lower body temperature resulting from loss of body fat); acrocyanosis (digits of the hands and feet become blue and sweaty from decreased circulation); and atrophy of the breasts.[28–30] Symptoms of concomitant hypothyroidism include hair loss, peripheral edema, and sensitivity to cold. Tachypnea and shortness of breath may result from metabolic alkalosis caused by vomiting. Conversely, metabolic acidosis may occur from laxative abuse.[31] Gastrointestinal symptoms include pain, bloating, and severe constipation (from starvation, chronic laxative abuse, or both) that may result in obstruction and megacolon. Exercise-induced disorders (eg, hernias, shin splints, and other injuries) are also common.

Cardiac problems include mitral valve prolapse, prolongation of the corrected QT interval, sinus bradycardia, and arrhythmias from electrolyte imbalance (particularly hypokalemia).[27] Pneumomediastinum induced by vomiting[32] or cardiomyopathy (from ipecac poisoning)[28] may be seen on a radiograph. The heart is often strophic due to chronic hypovolemia.[33] The second leading cause of death in AN is cardiac arrhythmia. Central nervous system changes include nonspecific electroencephalogram changes and generalized reversible atrophy associated with starvation and dehydration.

Osteoporosis occurs in half of women with AN and can lead to compression fractures and kyphosis.[34,35] Patients with AN have a 3-fold higher risk of fracture than those who do not. Bone loss may develop in as short a time as 6 months after onset of the illness and persist even after recovery, leading to a long-term risk of fractures. Fractures were found in 57% of women with AN in the ensuing 20-year period after onset.[36] Although most studies of osteoporosis in AN have focused on women, one study[37] found that 50% of men with eating disorders had lumbar spine and femoral neck bone densities more than two standard deviations below those of age-matched controls. Compared with women with eating disorders, this group of men had more severe bone loss. Andersen, Watson, and Schlechte[37] suggested that the correlation between reduced body weight in men and lowered testosterone led to more bone loss. Given the increased physical demands in an operational environment, those with AN may be at even higher risk for fractures.

Bulimia Nervosa

Patients with BN and other binge/purge conditions usually have normal weight without the concomitant features of starvation. Even patients with bingeing/purging-type AN do not achieve as low a body weight as restrictive-type AN patients. External examination may reveal damage to teeth and gums from acidic vomit. Russell sign is the calloused posterior surface of one or more fingers used to induce vomiting. Physical findings include gastrointestinal disorders (eg, sequelae of laxative abuse, esophageal tearing from excessive vomiting, and complications of electrolyte imbalance, including metabolic alkalosis and cardiac arrhythmias).[28,31]

Laboratory Studies

Serum chemistry may show electrolyte disturbances. Patients who purge may develop hypokalemia, hypochloremia, and elevated serum bicarbonate.[38] Hypokalemia appears to be particularly common, occurring in up to one half of those who purge; however, the ratio of urinary sodium to urinary chloride may be a better predictor of purging behavior than serum hypokalemia.[39] Metabolic acidosis with low serum bicarbonate may occur in laxative abusers.[38] Hyponatremia may result from water intoxication or a syndrome of inappropriate antidiuretic hormone.[28]

Other laboratory abnormalities include anemia; leucopenia, neutropenia, and thrombocytopenia[40]; hypercholesterolemia[41]; and euthyroid sick syndrome with normal thyroid-stimulating hormone and low triiodothyronine and thyroxine.[28,42] Hypercarotenemia has been proposed as a laboratory marker for restricting-type AN, with a sensitivity of 62% and a specificity of 83% when a cutoff marker of 200 μg/mL is used.[30] In one study of patients with AN, high serum creatinine and uric acid levels were associated with a chronic disease course, whereas low serum albumin and low body weight predicted lethality.[38]

DIFFERENTIAL DIAGNOSIS

Medical conditions that must be considered in the differential diagnosis include inflammatory bowel disease, thyroid disease, abdominal malignancy, central nervous system disease or tumor, and new-onset diabetes mellitus. The psychiatric differential includes depression, substance abuse, psychosis, and obsessive-compulsive disorder. Comorbidity with psychiatric conditions (including depression, psychosis, anxiety, personality disorder, and substance abuse) must also be addressed.

COURSE AND PROGNOSIS

Anorexia Nervosa

AN is associated with significant morbidity and mortality. It is usually a chronic, sometimes life-long disease with low full recovery rates. In a review of studies[43] conducted with patients at least 4 years after onset of illness, approximately 24% had what was considered a poor outcome (eg, never reached target weight gain within 15% of normal, had not established regular menses). Another 44% were considered to have a good outcome (eg, achieved and maintained weight within 15% of normal, had regular menses). About 28% had outcomes that fell between poor and good. The mortality rate was 5%. Even among those judged to be recovered based on body weight and menses, two thirds continued to struggle with body image, obsessive preoccupation with weight and appearance, and disordered eating habits.

Crude 10-year mortality rates for patients receiving treatment for AN has been cited at 3.3% to 5.6%.[44,45] Twenty-year mortality rates are 15% to 20%, with suicide and cardiac arrest the leading causes of death.[46–49] The annual mortality rate associated with AN is 12-fold higher than the annual death rate as a result of all causes of death for women in the general population 15 to 24 years of age.[46] AN is associated with social and functional impairments,[41] as well as with medical and psychiatric morbidities.[47]

Bulimia Nervosa

There is limited evidence that some untreated patients with BN have modest rates of improvement or recovery. For patients treated with either psychotherapy or medication, the short-term improvement rates are 50% to 70%; however, relapse rates are high (30%–50% in 6 months to 6 years follow-up).[50,51] Longer-term prognosis may be somewhat better. Patients with milder symptoms and fewer medical and psychiatric comorbidities who do not require hospitalization have a better course and prognosis. The mortality rate for BN has been cited at 0.3% per year.[52] A metaanalysis of standardized mortality rates in BN 5 to 11 years after diagnosis found a 7-fold greater mortality rate than expected.[51]

Eating Disorder Not Otherwise Specified

The only study to date that reported mortality information on EDNOS found that 4 of 28 subjects had died in an 11-year follow-up.[53] The risk of dying may be greater in the first few years after diagnosis of an eating disorder. A review of 10 eating disorder populations found a 2% risk of dying for women in the first year after presentation and a 5% risk of dying for men in the first and second years.[53]

ABNORMAL EATING IN MILITARY POPULATIONS

Research on eating disorders in military populations primarily consists of case reports[54–56] and surveys of military populations within gender or service. These surveys generally rely on self-reporting, which in civilian populations has been shown to underestimate pathological weight-control behaviors.[57] A summary of the published literature assessing eating disorders in military populations is provided in Table 28-1. There are no studies of eating disorders in military populations in combat operational environments.

McNulty[5] surveyed prevalence and contributing factors of abnormal eating behaviors in 3,000 active duty women in the US Army, Navy, Air Force, and Marine Corps. The rate of AN was highest in the Marine Corps, at 4.9%. Rates across the other services were Army, 1.3%; Navy, 1.1%; and Air Force, 0.8%. The rate of BN was again highest among marines at 15.9%. Rates in other services were Army, 4.3%; Navy, 5.2%; and Air Force, 9.3%. Rates of EDNOS were far higher: 62.8% of the total population met the criteria for this diagnosis. Again, the Marine Corps reported a significantly higher rate: 76.7%. The rates for the other services were Army, 57.4%; Navy, 61.2%; and Air Force, 58.6%. Notably, more than 60% of respondents had some type of eating disorder, and nearly every Marine Corps respondent (97.5%) met criteria for an eating disorder. Of those with an eating disorder at the time of the survey, the overwhelming majority had no history of previous eating disorder and negative family histories. Fasting or purging increased during PFA periods, suggesting that the military environment may put women at risk for eating disorders and increased use of unhealthy strategies of weight reduction to meet standards.

In a survey of 423 active duty Army women (officers and enlisted personnel) from medical and field commands, Lauder and colleagues[58] found that 142 women (33.6%) were at risk for abnormal eating behaviors. These at-risk women admitted to abnormal eating or purging behaviors more than once a month for 3 months, or had high scores of body dissatisfaction and a drive for thinness associated with a BMI of less than 21. Of the 142 women deemed at risk by the survey, 108 completed a structured interview with a board-certified psychiatrist. Of this number, 33 were diagnosed with an eating disorder. The other women had specific stressors, such as PFA periods, that prompted their abnormal eating behaviors. Therefore, 8% of the total sample was diagnosed with an eating disorder, and 3.1% met criteria for an eating disorder situational to the military environment. In a follow-up study of this same population, Lauder et al[59] evaluated their subjects for the prevalence of the female athlete triad, defined by the presence of an eating disorder, amenorrhea, and osteoporosis. They found no subjects who met the full triad, although, as they pointed out, the military physical activities that the subjects participated in may have had a protective effect on bone mass density.

McNulty[60] surveyed 1,425 Navy men from medical and line communities. She reported prevalence for AN (2.5%), BN (6.8%), and EDNOS (40.8%) in this population. Purging behaviors increased dramatically (up to 15%) during PFA periods. Fasting during these times occurred in nearly one third of respondents. Stressors of military life significant for AN, BN, or EDNOS included failing to be selected for advanced training schools, fear of being involuntarily separated, mandatory physical fitness, nonsupport of a supervisor, height/weight requirements, and rotating shifts. McNulty further reported that some sailors spoke of anger and discouragement over the PFA and their personal struggles with weight. One soldier even reported past suicidal ideation associated with the issue.

In a similar survey of 1,323 female Navy nurses, McNulty[61] reported the prevalence of AN (1.1%), BN (12.5%), and EDNOS (36%). To lose weight rapidly, these respondents reported skipping meals (44.4%), binge eating (19.2%), exercising excessively (16.9%), using diet pills (8.5%), using laxatives (7.1%), and vomiting (3%). Poor body image and satisfaction were predictors of eating disorders, as were height (in AN) and weight (in BN). Work-related stressors that adversely impacted eating disorder behaviors included working in an undesired area or in the intensive care unit, rotating shifts, and being a staff nurse. It is unclear if the high rates of BN and EDNOS in the survey personnel, compared with the general population, were related to their status as military officers or their occupation as nurses. Other studies of eating behaviors in nursing students have found conflicting results. A study of female medical students and nursing students found abnormal eating behaviors in one fifth of the respondents, with a higher rate in the nursing students.[62] Another study found a similar rate of overall abnormal eating behaviors in nursing, medical, and art students (~20%), but no difference among the three groups.[63]

TABLE 28-1

SUMMARY OF ABNORMAL EATING BEHAVIOR STUDIES IN MILITARY POPULATIONS

Subjects	N	Findings	Study
Army ROTC	310	20% subjects with increased bulimic behaviors, body dissatisfaction, drive for thinness	Lauder TD. Abnormal eating behaviors in female Reserve Officer Training Corps cadets. *Mil Med.* 2001;166:264–268.
Women in the Army, Navy, Air Force, and Marines	3,000	AN (%) / BN (%) / EDNOS (%) Marines 4.9 / 15.9 / 76.7 Navy 1.1 / 5.2 / 61.2 Air Force 0.8 / 9.3 / 58.6 Army 1.3 / 4.3 / 57.4	McNulty P. Prevalence and contributing factors of eating disorder behaviors in active duty service women in the Army, Navy, Air Force, and Marines. *Mil Med.* 2001;166:53–58.
Army women	423	33.6% abnormal eating or purging behaviors and increased body dissatisfaction; 8% diagnosed with eating disorder; 3.1% situational eating disorder	Lauder T, Williams MV, Campbell CS, Davis GD, Sherman RA. Abnormal eating behaviors in military women. *Med Sci Sports Exerc.* 1999;31:1265–1271.
Army women with "at- risk" eating behaviors	108	None with female athlete triad (osteoporosis, amenorrhea, eating disorder)	Lauder T, Williams M, Campbell C, Davis G, Sherman R. The female athlete triad: prevalence in military women. *Mil Med.* 1999;164:630–635.
Navy men Navy women (nurses)	1,425 1,323	AN (%) / BN (%) / EDNOS (%) Men 2.5 / 6.8 / 40.8 Women 1.1 / 12.5 / 36.0	McNulty P. Prevalence and contributing factors of eating disorder behaviors in active duty Navy men. *Mil Med.* 1997;162:753–758. McNulty P. Prevalence and contributing factors of eating disorder behaviors in a population of female Navy nurses. *Mil Med.* 1997;162:703–706.
Air Force weight-management patients + Civilian weight-management patients + Military control population	155	Air Force group: 4 times more purging behaviors than civilian group, 2–5 times more purging behaviors than military control group; great fluctuations in weight	Peterson AL, Talcott GW. Bulimic weight-loss behaviors in military versus civilian weight-management programs. *Mil Med.* 1995;160:616–620.
Israeli Army women diagnosed with anorexia	16	6/1,000 had AN; 16 treated with CBT and clomipramine; 12 returned to full duty; 3 returned to limited duty; 1 discharged	Mark M, Rabinowitz J, Rabinowitz S, Gaoni B, Babur I, Danon Y. Brief treatment of anorexia nervosa in military personnel. *Hosp Community Psychiatry.* 1993;44:69–71.
Male Hungarian military college students Male Hungarian general college students	480 752	No anorexic or bulimic subjects but general college students more likely to have behavioral and psychological characteristics of eating disorders. Body builders in both groups more likely to be perfectionistic	Lukacs L, Muranyi I, Tury F. Eating and body attitudes related to noncompetitive bodybuilding in military and general Hungarian male student populations. *Mil Med.* 2007;172:152–156.
Army women and men in advanced individual training	1,090	40% overweight; 10.8% with prior psychiatric history; 25.4% with history of verbal abuse; 9.8% reported disordered eating. Females, overweight, and those with previous psychiatric treatment and history of verbal abuse most at risk	Warner C, Warner C, Matuszak T, Rachal J, Flynn J, Grieger TA. Disordered eating in entry-level military personnel. *Mil Med.* 2007;172:147–151.

AN: anorexia nervosa
BN: bulimia nervosa
CBT: cognitive-behavioral therapy
EDNOS: eating disorder not otherwise specified
ROTC: Reserve Officer Training Corps

Peterson and colleagues[64] compared the prevalence of bulimic weight-loss behaviors in patients enrolled in an Air Force weight-management program with civilians enrolled in a weight-management program and with normal military controls. The Air Force members in the weight-management program vomited, engaged in strenuous exercise, or used the sauna/steam room four times more often than the civilian group. They were 2- to 5-fold more likely than the military comparison group to engage in bulimic weight-loss behaviors. They also lost more weight than the other two groups: 53% of the Air Force members in the weight-management program, but only 10% of the other two groups, reported a weight loss of more than 10 pounds in 1 month. The Air Force members in the weight-management group also showed more variability, with 41% gaining more than 5 pounds in 1 week, compared with 27% in the civilian group and 14% in the military control group. Fixed-interval reinforcement operant conditioning may have affected the fluctuations in weight and heightened weight-loss behaviors seen in the Air Force weight-management group, because participants were required to weigh in every month on a specified date. Thus, they may have continued with their routine eating habits until just a few days before the weigh-in and made drastic, last-minute attempts to drop weight, similar to the behaviors seen in the 6-month PFA cycles.

Warner et al[65] assessed prevalence and risks factors for disordered eating in a cross-sectional survey of over 1,000 advanced individual training soldiers. Even in this entry-level population, 40% were overweight and 9.8% endorsed disordered eating (7.0% of the men, 29.6 % of the women). Risk factors for abnormal eating behaviors included being a woman, being overweight, having a history of previous psychiatric treatment, and having a history of verbal abuse.

Carlton et al[66] surveyed eating disorders in a mixed military population at a large Navy medical center. A relatively high percentage of respondents were men, officers, or both, which reflected the general makeup of the population studied. The average BMI reported by the respondents—both men and women—would put them in the overweight category. More than 50% of respondents reported a BMI of 25 or greater.

Overall, the findings were consistent with those of other studies on eating and dieting behavior in the military, with high rates of body image dissatisfaction, abnormal patterns of eating and dieting, and a high correlation between these behaviors and the PFA cycle. Nearly 40% of respondents reported bingeing or binge-like behaviors, 18% or more reported some type of purging behavior, and 25% reported fasting. These behaviors were associated with worrying about the PFA and were more likely to occur in those with higher BMI, poor body image, or both. A high percentage of the study population reported dissatisfaction with body appearance and self-esteem dependent on body image. Women scored higher; however, data indicated that a significant proportion of men in the Navy are also dissatisfied with their bodies and engage in abnormal eating behaviors. These unhealthy attitudes and behaviors were common even though the sample was from a medical command; however, other studies in Navy personnel have found lower rates of abnormal eating behaviors in healthcare workers (30%) and medical doctors (6%), compared with the rate in shipboard service members (65%).[60]

Although the data indicate that one third or more of the population sample exhibited abnormal eating and weight-loss behaviors, only 2% had actually been clinically diagnosed.[66] This finding is consistent with other indications that eating disorders are underreported in the military, even at a medical command. It is not surprising that service members are reluctant to come forward. In addition to the stigma, the diagnosis may be grounds for disqualification from many assignments, mandatory enrollment in weight-loss programs, denial of promotion, and involuntary separation from service. McNulty[5] reported that in fiscal year 1995 approximately 5,000 people were discharged from military service for failure to meet weight standards. Military providers may be reluctant to diagnose eating disorders because they are traditionally considered difficult to treat and may end a service member's career.

MEDICAL AND PSYCHIATRIC TREATMENT OF EATING DISORDERS

Anorexia Nervosa

Medical Assessment and Treatment

Patients with AN have poor insight into their conditions. They may perceive their low body weight as an accomplishment and have limited motivation to change their behaviors.[67] The American Psychiatric Association guidelines recommend that patients weighing less than 75% of ideal body weight be treated on an inpatient basis.[68] Other indications for hospitalization are shown in Exhibit 28-3. The hospital utilization rate for individuals with AN is higher than that for any other psychiatric disorder except schizophrenia and organic mental disorders.[69] The cost of treatment is substantial and is estimated to be even higher than

EXHIBIT 28-3

INDICATIONS FOR HOSPITALIZATION IN ANOREXIA NERVOSA*

- Limited motivation to change abnormal eating behaviors
- Intractable (or rapid) weight loss despite treatment
- Refusal to eat
- Prolonged QT interval
- Bradycardia < 40 beats per minute
- Arrhythmia
- Hypothermia
- Symptomatic hypotension
- Less than 75% ideal body weight
- Persistent suicidal ideation
- Need for withdrawal/detoxification from laxatives, diet pills, or diuretics

*This list is not all-inclusive, and a decision to admit a patient to a hospital should always be based on a clinical assessment of the patient's psychiatric and general medical conditions.

that for schizophrenia.[70] Some patients may refuse treatment out of dread of weight gain and limited insight. In these cases, involuntary hospitalization may be necessary. Patients involuntarily committed for AN may show short-term benefit as manifested by weight gain, but have a higher mortality rate than those who undergo treatment voluntarily.[71] With changes in managed care, treatment for AN is increasingly moving toward partial-day programs or outpatient treatment. Hospitalization is often reserved for patients with serious life-threatening medical complications or those who can afford to pay privately.

Once diagnosed with AN, an individual's general medical condition should be assessed. Medical comorbidities, if they exist, must be addressed, although many (such as electrolyte imbalance) may resolve or improve once malnutrition and purging behaviors are rectified. Patients who require hospitalization need careful management because rapid refeeding can lead to gastric bloating, edema, arrhythmia, tachycardia, congestive heart failure, and sudden cardiac death.[33,72] Vitamin supplementation, with calcium at doses of 1,000 to 1,500 mg in addition to a multivitamin, is recommended.[73] Alendronate[74] and etidronate[75] have been found helpful in promoting bone formation in patients with anorexia; however, bone restoration appears to be most determined by weight restoration.

Psychotherapy

There are fewer controlled trials in the psychotherapeutic management of AN compared to BN.[76] Family therapy for adolescent patients may be one of the more effective treatments[77,78]; however, this approach is impractical in the military setting. Although better studied in BN, cognitive-behaviorial therapy (CBT)—in which cognitive distortions of body image and feelings of self-worth are addressed—has been applied with some success to patients with AN.[79]

Mark et al[80] reported on a treatment protocol implemented by the Israeli Defence Forces to treat AN in their armed forces. They surveyed, weighed, and measured all female soldiers over a 6-month period. In this sample, 6 of every 1,000 (0.6%) female soldiers were anorexic. Requirements for enrollment in the treatment program were an identifiable trigger for the disorder, motivation for treatment and military service, a social support system, and self-acknowledgment of the eating disorder. As part of the treatment program, the soldiers were educated on the serious medical nature of AN and instructed that they could be discharged if they failed or refused treatment. Service members were hospitalized for 4 to 6 weeks. During this time, each underwent a thorough medical workup, was placed on a high-calorie diet, and set goals for weekly weight gain. Therapy was based on a CBT model. All patients were initially given clomipramine to decrease obsessional ruminations; this drug was tapered off over several months. Of the 16 patients followed in the study for 1 year after discharge from the program, 12 were returned to full duty, three were returned to limited duty, and one was discharged.

In one study,[81] interpersonal therapy (IPT), CBT, and "nonspecific supportive clinical management"—defined as supportive therapy techniques, education, and nutritional advice—were compared in a randomized trial. Surprisingly, nonspecific supportive clinical management was found superior to both CBT and IPT, with CBT yielding superior results to IPT. Therapists administering the treatments investigated in the study were not eating-disorder specialists. Results of this study have yet to be replicated, but may have implications for the feasibility of treating AN in the military healthcare setting.

In general, the treatment plan for AN patients should involve a multidisciplinary team, including experts in mental health, nutrition, and internal medicine or primary care. The therapeutic approach should be to treat the whole patient. It is often better to focus away from food and toward resolving underlying issues of self-esteem and perfectionism.

Medications

Controlled trials of medications in the treatment of AN are summarized in Exhibit 28-4. Restoring weight and subsequent metabolic stabilization are treatment priorities for patients with AN. Cyproheptadine (32 mg/day) was found to improve weight gain in patients with restricting-type AN but not those with bingeing/purging-type AN.[78] Because zinc deficiency has been linked to AN through inhibition of release of neuropeptide Y,[82] supplementation with this mineral may be beneficial in promoting recovery from AN and improving these patients' levels of anxiety and depression.[83] In a controlled trial of 35 female inpatients with AN, supplementation with zinc promoted a rate of increase of BMI twice that of placebo.[84] Birmingham and Gritzner[85] recommend oral administration of 14 mg daily of elemental zinc for 2 months. A double-blind trial[86] of cisapride (10 mg tid) found reduction in subjective distress during meals in a small group of AN patients, but did not find a difference in gastric emptying or weight gain.

To date, no antidepressant or antipsychotic has been demonstrated to improve the long-term recovery rate from anorexia.[87,88] Tricyclic antidepressants (TCAs) have not only been shown ineffective, but also given their potential lethality, may be risky in this patient population.[89,90] Selective serotonin reuptake inhibitors (SSRIs) have not been found useful in low-weight patients.[91] This may be because of the general state of malnutrition of low-weight patients with AN, resulting in deficiency of tryptophan, the amino acid required for serotonin synthesis.[92] One SSRI, fluoxetine, was shown to be useful at higher doses in preventing relapse in those who have regained weight[93]; however, a larger study reported negative results.[94]

Antipsychotic drugs may have an augmenting role, particularly in patients with AN who have poor insight into their conditions.[95–98] However, not all studies have demonstrated the efficacy of antipsychotics,[99,100] and their use may have serious adverse effects in this population.[73] In a small, randomized trial, olanzapine was superior in reducing ego-syntonic anorexic ruminations compared to chlorpromazine, although there was no difference in weight gain.[101] Theoretically opiate antagonists may be helpful for subgroups of eating-disorder patients who fit an addiction model. Marrazzi et al[102] reported reduction in binge/purge

EXHIBIT 28-4

MEDICATIONS EFFECTIVE* AS MONOTHERAPY IN PLACEBO-CONTROLLED TRIALS FOR ANOREXIA NERVOSA

- Zinc[1]
- Cyproheptadine[2]
- Fluoxetine (after weight restoration, bingeing/purging subtype)[3,4]
- Naltrexone (bulimic subtype)[5]
- Olanzapine[6]

*Defined as fewer days to reach healthy BMI or reduction in binge/purge behavior for bulimia nervosa subtype of anorexia nervosa.

BMI: body mass index

(1) Birmingham CL, Goldner FM, Bakan R. Controlled trial of zinc supplementation in anorexia nervosa. *Int J Eat Disord*. 1994;15:251–255. (2) Halmi KA, Eckert E, LaDu TJ, Cohen J. Anorexia nervosa. Treatment efficacy of cyproheptadine and amitriptyline. *Arch Gen Psychiatry*. 1986;43:177–181. (3) Kaye WH, Nagata T, Weltzin TE, et al. Double-blind placebo-controlled administration of fluoxetine in restricting- and restricting-purging-type anorexia nervosa. *Biol Psychiatry*. 2001;49:644–652. (4) Walsh BT, Kaplan AS, Attia E, et al. Fluoxetine after weight restoration in anorexia nervosa: a randomized controlled trial. *JAMA*. 2006;295:2605–2612. (5) Marrazzi MA, Bacon JP, Kinzie J, Luby ED. Naltrexone use in the treatment of anorexia nervosa and bulimia nervosa. *Int Clin Psychopharmacol*. 1995;10:163–172. (6) Bissada H, Tasca GA, Barber AM, Bradwejn J. Olanzapine in the treatment of low body weight and obsessive thinking in women with anorexia nervosa: a randomized, double-blind, placebo-controlled trial. *Am J Psychiatry*. 2008;165:1281–1288.

EXHIBIT 28-5

INDICATIONS FOR HOSPITALIZATION IN BULIMIA NERVOSA*

- Changes in vital signs (pulse, blood pressure)
- Syncope
- Hypothermia
- Suicide risk
- Alcohol or drug abuse
- Uncontrolled vomiting
- Hematemesis (vomiting of blood)
- Arrhythmia
- Electrolyte imbalance
- Need for withdrawal from laxatives, diet pills, and diuretics

*This list is not all-inclusive, and a decision to admit a patient to the hospital should always be based on a clinical assessment of the patient's psychiatric and general medical conditions.

behaviors in a mixed population of BN and AN (bulimic subtype) patients treated with naltrexone in a randomized trial of 37 patients.

Bulimia Nervosa

Literature to guide treatment of BN is fairly extensive; hospitalization is seldom necessary unless there are medical complications (Exhibit 28-5). Compared to AN, evidence shows that BN can be treated more effectively with medication, although psychotherapy remains the cornerstone of treatment. The most established treatment for BN is CBT; in one study,[103] however, fewer than 10% of patients with bulimia who received psychotherapy were treated with this type of therapy. Guided self-help manuals that use CBT principles have also been found effective.[92,104] Even with CBT, it is estimated that only 50% of patients with BN recover.[105]

Patients with BN who fail to respond to psychotherapeutic techniques may benefit from pharmacotherapy. Medications that have been shown effective in randomized, placebo-controlled trials in the treatment of BN are listed in Exhibit 28-6. Controlled trial data have shown efficacy for TCAs[106–110] and monoamine oxidase inhibitors,[111,112] with the latter demonstrating some superiority.[113] Both TCAs and monoamine oxidase inhibitors may have lethal adverse effects in

EXHIBIT 28-6

MEDICATIONS EFFECTIVE IN PLACEBO-CONTROLLED TRIALS FOR BULIMIA NERVOSA

- Tricyclic antidepressants (desipramine, imipramine)[1–4]
- Monoamine oxidase inhibitors (phenelzine, isocarboxazid)[5,6]
- Fenfluramine[7]
- Fluoxetine[8–11]
- Buproprion*[,12]
- Trazodone[13]
- Naltrexone (high dose)[14]
- Ondansetron[15]
- Topiramate[16,17]
- Flutamide[18]
- Citalopram[19]
- Sertraline[2o]
- Fluvoxamine[11]

*Contraindicated in treatment of bulimia because of increased risk of seizure.

(1) Pope HG Jr, Hudson JI, Jonas JM, Yurgelun-Todd D. Bulimia treated with imipramine: a placebo-controlled, double-blind study. *Am J Psychiatry.* 1983;140:554–558. (2) Agras WS, Dorian B, Kirkley BG, Arnow B, Bachman J. Imipramine in the treatment of bulimia: a double-blind controlled study. *Int J Eat Disord.* 1987;6:29–38. (3) Barlow J, Blouin J, Blouin A, Perez E. Treatment of bulimia with desipramine: a double-blind crossover study. *Can J Psychiatry.* 1988;33:129–133. (4) Hughes PL, Wells LA, Cunningham CJ, Ilstrup DM. Treating bulimia with desipramine. A double-blind, placebo-controlled study. *Arch Gen Psychiatry.* 1986;43:182–186. (5) Walsh BT, Gladis M, Roose SP, Stewart JW, Stetner F, Glassman AH. Phenelzine vs placebo in 50 patients with bulimia. *Arch Gen Psychiatry.* 1988;45:471–475. (6) Kennedy SH, Piran N, Warsh JJ, et al. A trial of isocarboxazid in the treatment of bulimia nervosa. *J Clin Psychopharmacol.* 1988;8:391–396. (7) Blouin AG, Blouin JH, Perez EL, Bushnik T, Zuro C, Mulder E. Treatment of bulimia with fenfluramine and desipramine. *J Clin Psychopharmacol.* 1988;8:261–269. (8) Walsh BT, Agras WS, Devlin MJ, et al. Fluoxetine for bulimia nervosa following poor response to psychotherapy. *Am J Psychiatry.* 2000;157:1332–1334. (9) Fluoxetine Bulimia Nervosa Collaborative Study Group. Fluoxetine in the treatment of bulimia nervosa: a multicenter, placebo-controlled, double-blind trial. *Arch Gen Psychiatry.* 1992;49:139–147. (10) Goldstein DJ, Wilson MG, Thompson VL, Potvin JH, Rampey AH Jr. Fluoxetine Bulimia Nervosa Research Group. Long-term fluoxetine treatment of bulimia nervosa. *Br J Psychiatry.* 1995;166:660–666. (11) Romano SJ, Halmi KA, Sarkar NP, Koke SC, Lee JS. A placebo-controlled study of fluoxetine in continued treatment of bulimia nervosa after successful acute fluoxetine treatment. *Am J Psychiatry.* 2002;159:96–102. (12) Horne RL, Ferguson JM, Pope HG Jr, et al. Treatment of bulimia with bupropion: a multicenter controlled trial. *J Clin Psychiatry.* 1988;49:262–266. (13) Pope HG Jr, Keck PE Jr, McElroy SL, Hudson JI. A placebo-contolled study of trazodone in bulimia nervosa. *J Clin Psychopharmacol.* 1989;9:254–259. (14) Marrazzi MA, Bacon JP, Kinzie J, Luby ED. Naltrexone use in the treatment of anorexia nervosa and bulimia nervosa. *Int Clin Psychopharmacol.* 1995;10:163–172. (15) Faris PL, Kim SW, Meller WH, et al. Effect of decreasing afferent vagal activity with ondansetron on symptoms of bulimia nervosa: a randomised, double-blind trial. *Lancet.* 2000;355:792–797. (16) Hoopes SP, Reimherr FW, Hedges DW, et al. Treatment of bulimia nervosa with topiramate in a randomized, double-blind, placebo-controlled trial, part 1: improvement in binge and purge measures. *J Clin Psychiatry.* 2003;64:1335–1341. (17) Nickel C, Tritt K, Muehlbacher M, et al. Topiramate treatment in bulimia nervosa patients: a randomized, double-blind, placebo-controlled trial. *Int J Eat Disord.* 2005;38:295–300. (18) Sundblad C, Landén M, Eriksson T, Bergman L, Eriksson E. Effects of the androgen antagonist flutamide and the serotonin reuptake inhibitor citalopram in bulimia nervosa: a placebo-controlled pilot study. *J Clin Psychopharmacol.* 2005;25:85–88. (19) Leombruni P, Amianto F, Delsedime N, Gramaglia C, Abbate-Daga G, Fassino S. Citalopram versus fluoxetine for the treatment of patients with bulimia nervosa: a single-blind randomized controlled trial. *Adv Ther.* 2006;23:481–494. (20) Milano W, Petrella C, Sabatino C, Capasso A. Treatment of bulimia nervosa with sertraline: a randomized controlled trial. *Adv Ther.* 2004;21:232–237.

this patient population (potentially made worse by underlying electrolyte imbalance) and are not currently recommended as first-line treatment. Fenfluramine, a serotonergic agonist withdrawn from the market, was shown to be superior to both placebo and desipramine (a TCA).[110] The SSRI antidepressants are, similarly, serotonergic agonists and theoretically may work through a similar mechanism. Fluoxetine at high doses (60 mg/day) was superior to placebo in two 8-week trials[114,115] and one 16-week trial.[116] Fluoxetine's efficacy in BN, as with the TCAs,[117] is not a secondary effect of its antidepressant properties.[118] As many as one third of initial responders may relapse by the end of 1 year despite continued treatment,[119] suggesting that, whereas continued treatment may afford some protective effect, additional treatments may be needed for sustained effectiveness.

Although fluoxetine is the only antidepressant currently approved for BN, other SSRIs may also be effective. In a randomized, placebo-controlled trial, sertraline 100 (mg/d for 12 weeks) was found to be significantly more effective than placebo in reducing binge/purge behaviors in 20 female outpatients.[120] Fluvoxamine has been found effective in preventing relapse in patients with BN who had responded to inpatient behavioral psychotherapy.[121] In a single-blind trial comparing citalopram to fluoxetine, both agents resulted in significant improvement in eating psychopathology. Patients on fluoxetine displayed greater reduction in introjected anger, whereas those on citalopram demonstrated greater improvement in depressive feelings.[122] In comparison, another study found that use of the androgen receptor antagonist flutamide reduced craving and binge behaviors but not purging, whereas citalopram did not separate from placebo on these measures.[123] Among the newer, non-SSRI antidepressants, only bupropion has been studied in a controlled trial. Although bupropion was highly effective in reducing bingeing, there was a 5.8% incidence of seizure among study participants.[124] As a result, this agent is contraindicated in BN. As a class, antidepressants reduce binge eating by 61.4% (remission rate: 22%) and reduce purging by 58.9% (remission rate: 34%).[125] Unfortunately, up to 45% of patients who respond to pharmacotherapy may relapse in the first 6 months.[126]

Topiramate is becoming increasingly popular for treating BN after two randomized, double-blind, placebo-controlled trials established efficacy.[127,128] Other agents that have been found effective in at least one double-blind trial include the 5-HT_3 antagonist ondansetron,[129] the opioid antagonist naltrexone,[102] and trazodone.[130]

Several studies have compared psychotherapy to pharmacotherapy and failed to find any advantage of combining medication with therapy versus therapy alone.[131–133] Results from two metaanalyses found that combination approaches were associated with higher remission rates, although adding medication to therapy increased the dropout rate.[134,135] In summary, the preference is to treat BN with psychotherapy, primarily CBT, or a combination of psychotherapy and medication.

Eating Disorder Not Otherwise Specified

Because EDNOS is a nonspecific diagnostic category, treatment approaches depend on symptoms. The one category of EDNOS for which there appears to be a growing body of literature is BED. In general, the treatment resembles that for BN, with outcome measures defined by reduction in bingeing. The best-studied psychotropic agents used to treat BED and obesity are antidepressants and anticonvulsants. SSRIs have been found effective in double-blind trials for treatment of BED.[136–138] The anticonvulsant topiramate has also been found effective in double-blind trials for BED associated with obesity,[139] and a similar agent, zonisamide, was also associated with significant weight loss in a double-blind trial of obese adults.[140] Alternatively, agents specifically marketed for weight loss (including phentermine, sibutramine, and orlistat)[141,142] have been used to treat weight gain in overweight or obese patients with BED. Although several agents have been found effective for short-term weight loss, there are relatively few data on long-term efficacy with these agents. A review of the Cochrane database system found that, compared with placebo, the number of patients achieving 10% or more weight loss was 12% higher with orlistat and 15% higher with sibutramine in double-blind trials that lasted more than 1 year.[143] However, there was significant attrition in these studies, with an average of 33% of those on orlistat and 43% of those on sibutramine dropping out.

TREATMENT OF EATING DISORDER ISSUES IN THE COMBAT ENVIRONMENT

No formal studies have been conducted of disorders of eating behavior among military personnel in a combat environment. Operation Enduring Freedom and Operation Iraqi Freedom are the first US military actions in which women play a major part in combat; given their higher incidence in this group, eating disorders may become an increasingly important issue. Although significant evidence shows that abnormal eating and weight-loss behaviors are more prevalent in the military than in the general population, the actual rates of eating-disorder diagnoses in the military are at or below the civilian rates. This discrepancy may be due to a variety of reasons, including the pronounced situational component in the military (such as the PFA) producing abnormal eating and dieting patterns, the fear of adverse career actions probably leading to underreporting, and the fact that those with severe eating disorders are screened out prior to enlistment or are discharged when their eating disorders become evident. Additionally, service members with an eating disorder may try to conceal it in order to deploy, because operational and combat experience can be an important step toward promotion.

It is likely that few service members with a recognized eating disorder will be deployed to a combat zone. Individuals who meet criteria for AN clearly should not deploy, and probably should not be on active duty, due to the high rates of morbidity and mortality in AN as well as specialized treatment requirements. Those with a history of BN or EDNOS whose symptoms are well controlled should be considered on a case-by-case basis.

A careful history and evaluation should be conducted prior to the decision allowing affected service members to deploy. Given the chronicity of eating, only those who display good insight, treatment compliance, adequate symptom control, and a general high function should be considered for deployment. Potential side effects and availability of the prescribed medication should be considered. If multiple psychotropic agents, antipsychotics, or anticonvulsants are required for symptom stabilization, the service member should not be deployed. In particular, it should be noted that topiramate is becoming increasingly popular for bulimia but carries a warning for anhidrosis and hyperthermia,[144] which would be particularly problematic in a desert environment. Additional factors to consider include assessment of strengths and weaknesses, support systems, past aggravating factors, comorbidity with substance abuse or depression, motivation for deployment, anticipated job while deployed, the deployment site, and anticipated access to mental healthcare.

It is more likely that a service member with a previously concealed or controlled eating disorder will present in theater when symptoms become obvious to coworkers or impact the individual's ability to perform. Once again a careful assessment is needed to determine if the service member can remain in theater or should be returned. Factors to consider are similar to those above and include the severity of current symptoms, prior history, comorbidity, the individual's job, the location, access to care, and impact on the mission. Metabolic abnormalities and dehydration are of particular concern in strenuous or hot climates; thus, bulimic patients with such abnormalities should be medically evacuated.

Both positive and negative situational factors are associated with deployment, and their effects may vary on an individual basis. During deployment PFAs are suspended, so the pressure of the weigh-in and measurements are removed. In most deployment situations personnel have more time to exercise. Also, a hot climate affects appetite and food intake. Most dining facilities offer a variety of foods so that an individual can make healthy choices; however, some may find that the buffet style (usually including a dessert and ice cream bar) leads to overeating. The communal eating and living environment may make bingeing and purging less likely (although not impossible). Laxatives and diuretics are more difficult to obtain in the combat environment, thus further reducing purging options. Structured meal times can also either decrease the likelihood of overeating or increase the urge to binge. There are clearly fewer environmental cues such as food commercials and restaurants, although many areas have fast food restaurants that are open for extended hours. The separation from home environment and family may have either a positive or negative impact and should be individually assessed for each patient.

AREAS FOR FURTHER RESEARCH

Further research is necessary to improve the understanding of eating disorders in several areas. It is likely that the global war on terror will continue for some time, either as continued combat or with a US operational presence at widespread locations around the world. Given the known high incidence of abnormal eating behaviors in military personnel across services, military medical providers must understand how or if these conditions impact operational readiness and performance. Anecdotally, it appears that most service members who deploy lose weight during the deployment, most likely in healthy ways from increased exercise and decreased food intake. Deployment may somehow be protective for eating disorders due to decreases in certain types of stress. Additionally, a primary symptom in eating disorders is an overconcern about physical appearance and self-esteem tied to appearance. It may be that in a combat zone these issues are less important, and that personal satisfaction and feelings of reward derive from sources other than food or physical appearance. Other valuable research would be measuring the actual amount of weight loss during deployment, identifying any difference in weight loss among those who are and are not overweight prior to deployment, and determining whether the incidence of eating disorder behaviors is increased or decreased with deployment.

Another area of research interest is the potential for comorbid development of posttraumatic stress disorder (PTSD) in patients with eating disorders. Both eating disorders[23–27] and adult PTSD[145,146] have been linked independently to a history of childhood trauma and sexual abuse. It is not known if there is an independent link between eating disorders and the development of PTSD. An additional area for further research is the effect, currently unknown, of combat trauma on the risk of developing an eating disorder.

SUMMARY

Eating disorders are common among service members, and the military environment includes stressors that may contribute to unhealthy behaviors. Healthcare providers must be aware of the signs and symptoms of each disorder, capable of accurate diagnoses, and proactive in offering the available treatments, both medial and psychiatric. Vigilance is especially important with troops preparing for deployment, for these disorders may be exacerbated in theater, with negative consequences for individuals, their units, and their missions. Despite significant long-term morbidity and mortality associated with these conditions, eating disorders are treatable. The military may be an advantageous environment to provide deterrents to unhealthy behaviors, structured support and treatment for affected individuals, and opportunities for further research to increase the understanding of these disorders.

REFERENCES

1. Lindquist CH, Bray RM. Trends in overweight and physical activity among US military personnel, 1995–1998. *Prev Med*. 2001;32:57–65.

2. Centers for Disease Control and Prevention. *Overweight and Obesity: Selected US National Research Findings*. Available at: http://www.cdc.gov/women/natstat/overwght.htm. Accessed March 2, 2010.

3. Byrne S, McLean N. Eating disorders in athletes: a review of the literature. *J Sci Med Sport*. 2001;4:145–159.

4. Marshall JD, Harber VJ. Body dissatisfaction and drive for thinness in high performance field hockey athletes. *Int J Sports Med*. 1996;17:541–544.

5. McNulty PA. Prevalence and contributing factors of eating disorder behaviors in active duty service women in the Army, Navy, Air Force, and Marines. *Mil Med*. 2001;166:53–58.

6. Hudson JI, Hiripi E, Pope HG Jr, Kessler RC. The prevalence and correlates of eating disorders in the National Comorbidity Survey Replication. *Biol Psychiatry*. 2007;61:348–358.

7. Silverman JA. Sir William Gull (1819–1890). Limner of anorexia nervosa and myxoedema. An historical essay and encomium. *Eat Weight Disord*. 1997;2:111–116.

8. Gard MCE, Freeman CP. The dismantling of a myth: a review of eating disorders and socioeconomic status. *Int J Eat Disord*. 1996;20:1–12.

9. American Psychiatric Association. *Diagnostic and Statistical Manual of Mental Disorders*. 4th ed. Washington, DC: APA; 1994.

10. Dorian BJ, Garfinkel PE. The contributions of epidemiologic studies to the etiology and treatment of the eating disorders. *Psychiatric Ann*. 1999;29:187–196.

11. Andersen AE, Bowers WA, Watson T. A slimming program for eating disorders not otherwise specified. Reconceptualizing a confusing, residual diagnostic category. *Psychiatr Clin North Am*. 2001;24:271–280.

12. Hoek HW, van Hoeken D. Review of the prevalence and incidence of eating disorders. *Int J Eat Disord*. 2003;34:383–396.

13. O'Reardon JP, Peshek A, Allison KC. Night eating syndrome: diagnosis, epidemiology and management. *CNS Drugs*. 2005;19:997–1008.

14. Kress AM, Peterson MR, Hartzell MD. Association between obesity and depressive symptoms among US military active duty service personnel, 2002. *J Psychosom Res*. 2006;60(3):263–271.

15. Rodin G. The etiology of eating disorders: lessons from high-risk groups. *Psychiatr Ann*. 1999;29:181–182.

16. Bailer UF, Kaye WH. A review of neuropeptide and neuroendocrine dysregulation in anorexia and bulimia nervosa. *Curr Drug Targets CNS Neurol Disord*. 2003;2:53–59.

17. Klump KL, Kaye WH, Strober M. The evolving genetic foundations of eating disorders. *Psychiatr Clin North Am*. 2001;24:215–225.

18. Nacmias B, Ricca V, Tedde A, Mezzani B, Rotella CM, Sorbi S. 5-HT_A receptor gene polymorphisms in anorexia nervosa and bulimia nervosa. *Neurosci Lett*. 1999;277:134–136.

19. Spigset O, Andersen T, Hägg S, Mjöndal T. Enhanced platelet serotonin 5-HT_{2A} receptor binding in anorexia nervosa and bulimia nervosa. *Eur Neuropsychopharmacol*. 1999;9:469–473.

20. Levitan RD, Kaplan AS, Masellis M, et al. Polymorphism of the serotonin 5-HT_{1B} receptor gene (HTR_{1B}) associated with minimum lifetime body mass index in women with bulimia nervosa. *Biol Psychiatry*. 2001;50:640–643.

21. King M. The epidemiology of eating disorders. *Epidemiol Psichiatr Soc*. 1998;7:32–41.

22. Levine MP, Smolak L, Moodey AF, Shuman MD, Hessen LD. Normative developmental challenges and dieting and eating disturbances in middle school girls. *Int J Eat Disord*. 1994;15:11–20.

23. Connors ME, Morse W. Sexual abuse and eating disorders: a review. *Int J Eat Disord*. 1993;13:1–11.

24. Léonard S, Steiger H, Kao A. Childhood and adulthood abuse in bulimic and nonbulimic women: prevalences and psychological correlates. *Int J Eat Disord*. 2003;33:397–405.

25. Wonderlich SA, Brewerton TD, Jocic Z, Dansky BS, Abbott DW. Relationship of childhood sexual abuse and eating disorders. *J Am Acad Child Adolesc Psychiatry*. 1997;36:1107–1115.

26. Wonderlich SA, Crosby RD, Mitchell JE, et al. Eating disturbance and sexual trauma in childhood and adulthood. *Int J Eat Disord*. 2001;30:401–412.

27. Merrill LL, Newell CE, Thomsen CJ, et al. Childhood abuse and sexual revictimization in a female Navy recruit sample. *J Trauma Stress*. 1999;12:211–225.

28. Becker AE, Grinspoon SK, Klibanski A, Herzog DB. Eating disorders. *N Engl J Med*. 1999;340:1092–1098.

29. Birmingham CL. Hypercarotenemia [letter]. *N Engl J Med*. 2002;347:222–223.

30. Boland B, Beguin C, Zech F, Desager JP, Lambert M. Serum beta-carotene in anorexia nervosa patients: a case-control study. *Int J Eat Disord*. 2001;30:299–305.

31. Mitchell JE, Seim HC, Colon E, Pomeroy C. Medical complications and medical management of bulimia. *Ann Intern Med*. 1987;107:71–77.

32. Karim A, Ahmed S, Rossoff L. Pneumomediastinum simulating a panic attack in a patient with anorexia nervosa. *Int J Eat Disord*. 2003;33:104–107.

33. Casiero D, Frishman WH. Cardiovascular complications of eating disorders. *Cardio Rev.* 2006;14:227–231.

34. Mehler PS. Osteoporosis in anorexia nervosa: prevention and treatment. *Int J Eat Disord.* 2003;33:113–126.

35. Powers PS. Osteoporosis and eating disorders. *J Pediatr Adolesc Gynecol.* 1999;12:51–57.

36. Lucas AR, Melton LJ 3rd, Crowson CS, O'Fallon WM. Long-term fracture risk among women with anorexia nervosa: a population-based cohort study. *Mayo Clin Proc.* 1999;74:972–977.

37. Andersen AE, Watson T, Schlechte J. Osteoporosis and osteopenia in men with eating disorders. *Lancet.* 2000;355:1967–1968.

38. Wolfe BE, Metzger ED, Levine JM, Jimerson DC. Laboratory screening for electrolyte abnormalities and anemia in bulimia nervosa: a controlled study. *Int J Eat Disord.* 2001;30:288–293.

39. Crow SJ, Rosenberg ME, Mitchell JE, Thuras P. Urine electrolytes as markers of bulimia nervosa. *Int J Eat Disord.* 2001;30:279–287.

40. Devuyst O, Lambert M, Rodhain J, Lefebvre C, Coche E. Haematological changes and infectious complications in anorexia nervosa: a case-control study. *Q J Med.* 1993;86:791–799.

41. Pauporte J, Walsh BT. Serum cholesterol in bulimia nervosa. *Int J Eat Disord.* 2001;30:294–298.

42. Pritts SD, Susman J. Diagnosis of eating disorders in primary care. *Am Fam Physician.* 2003;67:297–304.

43. American Psychiatric Association. *Practice Guideline for the Treatment of Patients With Eating Disorders.* 2nd ed. Washington, DC: APA; 2000.

44. Patton GC. Mortality in eating disorders. *Psychol Med.* 1988;18:947–951.

45. Sullivan PF. Mortality in anorexia nervosa. *Am J Psychiatry.* 1995;152:1073–1074.

46. Eckert ED, Halmi KA, Marchi P, Grove W, Crosby R. Ten-year follow-up of anorexia nervosa: clinical course and outcome. *Psychol Med.* 1995;25:143–156.

47. Herzog W, Deter HC, Fiehn W, Petzold E. Medical findings and predictors of long-term physical outcome in anorexia nervosa: a prospective 12-year follow-up study. *Psychol Med.* 1997;27:269–279.

48. Ratnasuriya RH, Eisler I, Szmukler GI, Russell GF. Anorexia nervosa: outcome and prognostic factors after 20 years. *Br J Psychiatry.* 1991;158:495–502.

49. Zipfel S, Löwe B, Reas DL, Deter HC, Herzog W. Long-term prognosis in anorexia nervosa: lessons from a 21-year follow-up study. *Lancet.* 2000;355:721–722.

50. Herzog DB, Nussbaum KM, Marmor AK. Comorbidity and outcome in eating disorders. *Psychiatr Clin North Am.* 1996;19:843–859.

51. Keel PK, Mitchell JE. Outcome in bulimia nervosa. *Am J Psychiatry.* 1997;154:313–321.

52. Nielsen S. Epidemiology and mortality of eating disorders. *Psychiatr Clin North Am.* 2001;24:201–214, vii–viii.

53. Nielsen S, Moller-Madsen S, Isager T, Jorgensen J, Pagsberg K, Theander S. Standardized mortality in eating disorders—a quantitative summary of previously published and new evidence. *J Psychosom Res.* 1998;44:413–434.

54. Davidson DM. Anorexia nervosa in a serviceman: case report. *Mil Med.* 1976;141:617–619.

55. Voge VM, Yacavone D. Bulimia: an uncommon problem in aircrewmen—a case report. *Aviat Space Environ Med.* 1987;58:347–349.

56. Berg JS, Moore JL. A case of "eating disorder NOS": aeromedical implications of DSM-IV diagnostic criteria. *Aviat Space Environ Med.* 1996;67:157–160.

57. Sundgot-Borgen J. Risk and trigger factors for the development of eating disorders in female elite athletes. *Med Sci Sports Exerc.* 1994;26:414–419.

58. Lauder TD, Williams MV, Campbell CS, Davis GD, Sherman RA. Abnormal eating behaviors in military women. *Med Sci Sports Exerc.* 1999;31:1265–1271.

59. Lauder TD, Williams MV, Campbell CS, Davis G, Sherman R, Pulos E. The female athlete triad: prevalence in military women. *Mil Med.* 1999;164:630–635.

60. McNulty PA. Prevalence and contributing factors of eating disorder behaviors in active duty Navy men. *Mil Med.* 1997;162:753–758.

61. McNulty PA. Prevalence and contributing factors of eating disorder behaviors in a population of female Navy nurses. *Mil Med.* 1997;162:703–706.

62. Babar N, Alam M, Ali SS, et al. Anorexic behaviour and attitudes among female medical and nursing students at a private university hospital. *J Pak Med Assoc.* 2002;52:272–276.

63. Szweda S, Thorne P. The prevalence of eating disorders in female health care students. *Occup Med (Lond).* 2002;52:113–119.

64. Peterson AL, Talcott GW, Kelleher WJ, Smith SD. Bulimic weight-loss behaviors in military versus civilian weight-management programs. *Mil Med.* 1995;160:616–620.

65. Warner C, Warner C, Matuszak T, Rachal J, Flynn J, Grieger TA. Disordered eating in entry-level military personnel. *Mil Med.* 2007;172:147–151.

66. Carlton JR, Manos GH, Van Slyke JA. Anxiety and abnormal eating behaviors associated with cyclical readiness testing in a naval hospital active duty population. *Mil Med.* 2005;170:663–667.

67. Vitousek K, Watson S, Wilson GT. Enhancing motivation for change in treatment-resistant eating disorders. *Clin Psychol Rev.* 1998;18:391–420.

68. American Psychiatric Association. Practice Guidelines for the Treatment of Patients with Eating Disorders [revised]. *Am J Psychiatry.* 2000;157(suppl):1.

69. McKenzie JM, Joyce PR. Hospitalization for anorexia nervosa. *Int J Eat Disord.* 1992;11:235–241.

70. Agras WS. The consequences and costs of the eating disorders. *Psychiatr Clin North Am.* 2001;24:371–379.

71. Russell GF. Involuntary treatment in anorexia nervosa. *Psychiatr Clin North Am.* 2001;24:337–349.

72. Rigotti NA. Eating disorders. In: Carlson KJ, Eisenstat SA, eds. *Primary Care of Women.* St Louis, Mo: Mosby-Year Book; 1995: 443–449.

73. Becker AE, Hamburg P, Herzog DB. The role of psychopharmacologic management in the treatment of eating disorders. *Psychiatr Clin North Am.* 1998;5:17–51.

74. Golden NM, Iglesias EA, Jacobson MS, et al. Alendronate for the treatment of osteopenia in anorexia nervosa: a randomized, double-blind, placebo-controlled trial. *J Clin Endocrinol Metab.* 2005;90:3179–3185.

75. Nakahara T, Nagai N, Tanaka M, et al. The effects of bone therapy on tibial bone loss in young women with anorexia nervosa. *Int J Eat Disord.* 2006;39:20–26.

76. Mitchell JE, Peterson CB, Myers T, Wonderlich S. Combining pharmacotherapy and psychotherapy in treatment of patients with eating disorders. *Psychiatr Clin North Am.* 2001;24:315–323.

77. Russell GF, Szmukler GI, Dare C, Eisler I. An evaluation of family therapy in anorexia nervosa and bulimia nervosa. *Arch Gen Psychiatry.* 1987;44:1047–1056.

78. Lock J, le Grange D, Agras WS, Dare C. *Treatment Manual for Anorexia Nervosa: A Family Based Approach.* New York, NY: Guilford Press; 2001.

79. Bowers WA. Basic principles for applying cognitive-behavioral therapy to anorexia nervosa. *Psychiatr Clin North Am.* 2001;24:293–303, x.

80. Mark M, Rabinowitz J, Rabinowitz S, Gaoni B, Babur I, Danon Y. Brief treatment of anorexia nervosa in military personnel. *Hosp Community Psychiatry.* 1993;44:69–71.

81. McIntosh VV, Jordan J, Carter FA, et al. Three psychotherapies for anorexia nervosa: a randomized, controlled trial. *Am J Pscyhiatry.* 2005;162:741–747.

82. Levenson CW. Zinc regulation of food intake: new insights on the role of neuropeptide Y. *Nutr Rev.* 2003;61:247–249.

83. Su JC, Birmingham CL. Zinc supplementation in the treatment of anorexia nervosa. *Eat Weight Disord.* 2002;7:20–22.

84. Birmingham CL, Goldner FM, Bakan R. Controlled trial of zinc supplementation in anorexia nervosa. *Int J Eat Disord.* 1994;15:251–255.

85. Birmingham CL, Gritzner S. How does zinc supplementation benefit anorexia nervosa? *Eat Weight Disord.* 2006;11:e109–e111.

86. Szmukler GI, Young GP, Miller G, Lichenstein M, Binns DS. A controlled trial of cisapride in anorexia nervosa. *Int J Eat Disord.* 1995;17:347–357.

87. Attia E, Schroeder L. Pharmacologic treatment of anorexia nervosa: where do we go from here? *Int J Eat Disord.* 2005;37(suppl):s60–s63.

88. Bulik CM, Berkman ND, Brownley KA, Sedway JA, Lohr KN. Anorexia nervosa treatment: a systematic review of randomized controlled trials. *Int J Eat Disord.* 2007;40:310–320.

89. Halmi KA, Eckert E, LaDu TJ, Cohen J. Anorexia nervosa. Treatment efficacy of cyproheptadine and amitriptyline. *Arch Gen Psychiatry.* 1986;43:177–181.

90. Lacey JH, Crisp AH. Hunger, food intake and weight: the impact of clomipramine on a refeeding anorexia nervosa population. *Postgrad Med J.* 1980;56(suppl 1):79–85.

91. Ruggiero GM, Laini V, Mauri MC, et al. A single blind comparison of amisulpride, fluoxetine and clomipramine in the treatment of restricting anorectics. *Prog Neuropsychopharmacol Biol Psychiatry.* 2001;25:1049–1059.

92. Mitchell JE, Fletcher L, Hanson K, et al. The relative efficacy of fluoxetine and manual-based self-help in the treatment of outpatients with bulimia nervosa. *J Clin Psychopharmacol.* 2001;21:298–304.

93. Kaye WH, Nagata T, Weltzin TE, et al. Double-blind placebo-controlled administration of fluoxetine in restricting- and restricting-purging-type anorexia nervosa. *Biol Psychiatry.* 2001;49:644–652.

94. Anderson IM, Parry-Billings M, Newsholme EA, Fairburn CG, Cowen PJ. Dieting reduces plasma tryptophan and alters brain 5-HT function in women. *Psychol Med.* 1990;20:785–791.

95. Walsh BT, Kaplan AS, Attia E, et al. Fluoxetine after weight restoration in anorexia nervosa: a randomized controlled trial. *JAMA.* 2006;295:2605–2612.

96. Cassano GB, Miniati M, Pini S, et al. Six-month open trial of haloperidol as an adjunctive treatment for anorexia nervosa: a preliminary report. *Int J Eat Disord.* 2003;33:172–177.

97. La Via MC, Gray N, Kaye WH. Case reports of olanzapine treatment of anorexia nervosa. *Int J Eat Disord.* 2000;27:363–366.

98. Hansen L. Olanzapine in the treatment of anorexia nervosa. *Br J Psychiatry.* 1999;175:592.

99. Vandereycken W. Neuroleptics in the short-term treatment of anorexia nervosa. A double-blind placebo-controlled study with sulpiride. *Br J Psychiatry.* 1984;144:288–292.

100. Vandereycken W, Pierloot R. Pimozide combined with behavior therapy in the short-term treatment of anorexia nervosa. A double-blind pacebo-controlled cross-over study. *Acta Psychiatr Scand.* 1982;66:445–450.

101. Mondraty N, Birmingham CL, Touyz S, Sundakov V, Chapman L, Beumont P. Randomized controlled trial of olanzapine in the treatment of cognitions in anorexia nervosa. *Australas Psychiatry.* 2005;13:72–75.

102. Marrazzi MA, Bacon JP, Kinzie J, Luby ED. Naltrexone use in the treatment of anorexia nervosa and bulimia nervosa. *Int Clin Psychopharmacol.* 1995;10:163–172.

103. Crow S, Mussell MP, Peterson C, Knopke A, Mitchell J. Prior treatment received by patients with bulimia nervosa. *Int J Eat Disord.* 1999;25:39–44.

104. Thiels C, Schmidt U, Treasure J, Garthe R, Troop N. Guided self-change for bulimia nervosa incorporating use of a self-care manual. *Am J Psychiatry.* 1998;155:947–953.

105. Agras WS, Crow SJ, Halmi KA, Mitchell JE, Wilson GT, Kraemer HC. Outcome predictors for the cognitive behavior treatment of bulimia nervosa: data from a multisite study. *Am J Psychiatry.* 2000;157:1302–1308.

106. Pope HG Jr, Hudson JI, Jonas JM, Yurgelun-Todd D. Bulimia treated with imipramine: a placebo-controlled, double-blind study. *Am J Psychiatry.* 1983;140:554–558.

107. Agras WS, Dorian B, Kirkley BG, Arnow B, Bachman J. Imipramine in the treatment of bulimia: a double-blind controlled study. *Int J Eat Disord.* 1987;6:29–38.

108. Barlow J, Blouin J, Blouin A, Perez E. Treatment of bulimia with desipramine: a double-blind crossover study. *Can J Psychiatry.* 1988;33:129–133.

109. Hughes PL, Wells LA, Cunningham CJ, Ilstrup DM. Treating bulimia with desipramine. A double-blind, placebo-controlled study. *Arch Gen Psychiatry.* 1986;43:182–186.

110. Blouin AG, Blouin JH, Perez EL, Bushnik T, Zuro C, Mulder E. Treatment of bulimia with fenfluramine and desipramine. *J Clin Psychopharmacol.* 1988;8:261–269.

111. Walsh BT, Gladis M, Roose SP, Stewart JW, Stetner F, Glassman AH. Phenelzine vs placebo in 50 patients with bulimia. *Arch Gen Psychiatry.* 1988;45:471–475.

112. Kennedy SH, Piran N, Warsh JJ, et al. A trial of isocarboxazid in the treatment of bulimia nervosa. *J Clin Psychopharmacol.* 1988;8:391–396.

113. Rothschild R, Quitkin HM, Quitkin FM, et al. A double-blind placebo-controlled comparison of phenelzine and imipramine in the treatment of bulimia in atypical depressives. *Int J Eat Disord.* 1994;15:1–9.

114. Walsh BT, Agras WS, Devlin MJ, et al. Fluoxetine for bulimia nervosa following poor response to psychotherapy. *Am J Psychiatry.* 2000;157:1332–1334.

115. Fluoxetine Bulimia Nervosa Collaborative Study Group. Fluoxetine in the treatment of bulimia nervosa: a multicenter, placebo-controlled, double-blind trial. *Arch Gen Psychiatry.* 1992;49:139–147.

116. Goldstein DJ, Wilson MG, Thompson VL, Potvin JH, Rampey AH Jr. Fluoxetine Bulimia Nervosa Research Group. Long-term fluoxetine treatment of bulimia nervosa. *Br J Psychiatry.* 1995;166:660–666.

117. Blouin J, Blouin A, Perez E, Barlow J. Bulimia: independence of antibulimic and antidepressant properties of desipramine. *Can J Psychiatry.* 1989;34:24–29.

118. Goldstein DJ, Wilson MG, Ascroft RC, al-Banna M. Effectiveness of fluoxetine therapy in bulimia nervosa regardless of comorbid depression. *Int J Eat Disord.* 1999;25:19–27.

119. Romano SJ, Halmi KA, Sarkar NP, Koke SC, Lee JS. A placebo-controlled study of fluoxetine in continued treatment of bulimia nervosa after successful acute fluoxetine treatment. *Am J Psychiatry.* 2002;159:96–102.

120. Milano W, Petrella C, Sabatino C, Capasso A. Treatment of bulimia nervosa with sertraline: a randomized controlled trial. *Adv Ther.* 2004;21:232–237.

121. Fichter MM, Krüger R, Rief W, Holland R, Döhne J. Fluvoxamine in prevention of relapse in bulimia nervosa: effects on eating-specific psychopathology. *J Clin Psychopharmacol.* 1996;16:9–18.

122. Leombruni P, Amianto F, Delsedime N, Gramaglia C, Abbate-Daga G, Fassino S. Citalopram versus fluoxetine for the treatment of patients with bulimia nervosa: a single-blind randomized controlled trial. *Adv Ther.* 2006;23:481–494.

123. Sundblad C, Landén M, Eriksson T, Bergman L, Eriksson E. Effects of the androgen antagonist flutamide and the serotonin reuptake inhibitor citalopram in bulimia nervosa: a placebo-controlled pilot study. *J Clin Psychopharmacol.* 2005;25:85–88.

124. Horne RL, Ferguson JM, Pope HG Jr, et al. Treatment of bulimia with bupropion: a multicenter controlled trial. *J Clin Psychiatry.* 1988;49:262–266.

125. Nathan PE, Gorman JM. *Treatments That Work.* 2nd ed. New York, NY: Oxford University Press; 2002: 560.

126. Walsh BT, Hadigan CM, Devlin MJ, Gladis M, Roose SP. Long-term outcome of antidepressant treatment for bulimia nervosa. *Am J Psychiatry.* 1991;148:1206–1212.

127. Hoopes SP, Reimherr FW, Hedges DW, et al. Treatment of bulimia nervosa with topiramate in a randomized, double-blind, placebo-controlled trial, part 1: improvement in binge and purge measures. *J Clin Psychiatry.* 2003;64:1335–1341.

128. Nickel C, Tritt K, Muehlbacher M, et al. Topiramate treatment in bulimia nervosa patients: a randomized, double-blind, placebo-controlled trial. *Int J Eat Disord.* 2005;38:295–300.

129. Faris PL, Kim SW, Meller WH, et al. Effect of decreasing afferent vagal activity with ondansetron on symptoms of bulimia nervosa: a randomised, double-blind trial. *Lancet.* 2000;355:792–797.

130. Pope HG Jr, Keck PE Jr, McElroy SL, Hudson JI. A placebo-contolled study of trazodone in bulimia nervosa. *J Clin Psychopharmacol.* 1989;9:254–259.

131. Goldbloom DS, Olmsted M, Davis R, et al. A randomized controlled trial of fluoxetine and cognitive behavioral therapy for bulimia nervosa: short-term outcome. *Behav Res Ther.* 1997;35:803–811.

132. Fichter MM, Leibl K, Rief W, Brunner E, Schmidt-Auberger S, Engel RR. Fluoxetine versus placebo: a double-blind study with bulimic inpatients undergoing intensive psychotherapy. *Pharmacopsychiatry.* 1991;24:1–7.

133. Mitchell JE, Pyle RL, Eckert ED, Hatsukami D, Pomeroy C, Zimmerman R. A comparison study of antidepressants and structured intensive group psychotherapy in the treatment of bulimia nervosa. *Arch Gen Psychiatry.* 1990;47:149–157.

134. Bacaltchuk J, Trefiglio RP, de Oliveira IR, Lima MS, Mari JJ. Antidepressants versus psychotherapy for bulimia nervosa: a systematic review. *J Clin Pharm Ther.* 1999;24:23–31.

135. Bacaltchuk J, Trefiglio RP, Oliveira IR, Hay P, Lima MS, Mari JJ. Combination of antidepressants and psychological treatments for bulimia nervosa: a systematic review. *Acta Psychiatr Scand.* 2000;101:256–264.

136. Arnold LM, McElroy SL, Hudson JI, Welge JA, Bennett AJ, Keck PE. A placebo-controlled, randomized trial of fluoxetine in the treatment of binge-eating disorder. *J Clin Psychiatry*. 2002;63:1028–1033.

137. Ricca V, Mannucci E, Mezzani S, et al. Fluoxetine and fluvoxamine combined with individual cognitive-behaviour therapy in binge eating disorder: a one-year follow-up study. *Psychother Psychosom*. 2001;70:298–306.

138. Guerdjikova AI, McElroy SL, Kotwal R, et al. High-dose escitalopram in the treatment of binge-eating disorder with obesity: a placebo-controlled monotherapy trial. *Hum Psychopharmacol*. 2008;23:1–11.

139. McElroy SL, Arnold LM, Shapira NA, et al. Topiramate in the treatment of binge eating disorder associated with obesity: a randomized, placebo-controlled trial. *Am J Psychiatry*. 2003;160:255–261.

140. Gadde KM, Franciscy DM, Wagner HR II, Krishnan KR. Zonisamide for weight loss in obese adults: a randomized controlled trial. *JAMA*. 2003;289:1820–1825.

141. Wilfley DE, Crow SJ, Hudson JI, et al. Efficacy of sibutramine for the treatment of binge eating disorder: a randomized multicenter placebo-controlled double-blind study. *Am J Psychiatry*. 2008;165:51–58. Epub December 3, 2007.

142. Bays H, Dujovne C. Pharmacotherapy of obesity: currently marketed and upcoming agents. *Am J Cardiovasc Drugs*. 2002;2:245–253.

143. Padwal R, Li SK, Lau DC. Long-term pharmacotherapy for obesity and overweight. *Cochrane Database Syst Rev*. 2004;3:CD004094.

144. Hulihan J, Ortho-McNeil Pharmacutical. Important drug warning letter to healthcare professionals, December 18, 2003. http://www.fda.gov/downloads/Safety/MedWatch/SafetyInformation/SafetyAlertsforHumanMedicalProducts/UCM169494.pdf. Accessed March 2, 2010.

145. Clancy CP, Graybeal A, Tompson WP, et al. Lifetime trauma exposure in veterans with military-related posttraumatic stress disorder: association with current symptomatology. *J Clin Psychiatry*. 2006;67:1346–1353.

146. Lapp KG, Bosworth HB, Strauss JL, et al. Lifetime sexual and physical victimization among male veterans with combat-related post-traumatic stress disorder. *Mil Med*. 2005;170:787–790.

Chapter 29

SUBSTANCE USE AND ABUSE IN THE MILITARY

R. GREGORY LANDE, DO*; BARBARA A. MARIN, PHD†; JAMES J. STAUDENMEIER, MD, MPH‡; AND DARYL HAWKINS, PHD§

*Chief, Psychiatry Continuity Service, Department of Psychiatry, Walter Reed Army Medical Center, 6900 Georgia Avenue NW, Building 2, Room 5343, Washington, DC 20307; Clinical Consultant, Walter Reed Army Medical Center Substance Abuse Program, Washington, DC

†Integrated Chief, Department of Addictions Treatment and Clinical Director, Army Substance Abuse Program, Walter Reed Army Medical Center, 6900 Georgia Avenue NW, Washington, DC 20307-5001

‡Colonel, Medical Corps, US Army; Consultant, Army Substance Abuse Program, Department of Psychiatry, USAMEDDAC, 11050 Mount Belvedere Boulevard, BMD (Wilcox), Fort Drum, New York 13602; formerly, Fellow in Geriatric Psychiatry, Walter Reed Army Medical Center, Washington, DC

§Alcohol and Drug Control Officer, Army Substance Abuse Program, Building 6, Room 2066, Walter Reed Army Medical Center, 6900 Georgia Avenue NW, Washington, DC 20307-5001

INTRODUCTION

Through the centuries of armed conflict, soldiers have sought to immunize themselves from the fear and uncertainty of combat. The principle shield that protects these combatants is training. Endless training breeds confidence in military skills and weapons. A strong group milieu firmly centered around camaraderie, mutual support, and confidence further strengthens emotional resilience. These are the positive factors reinforcing a sense of "invulnerability."

The emotional shield protecting soldiers from the stress of combat is further strengthened by training and group cohesion, but weakened by other hidden, pernicious factors. Chief among the factors battering the emotional shield are individually experienced traumas. Although substance use may be perceived by soldiers as a way of reducing the stress of these traumas, the corrosive influence of substance abuse is substantial.

Modern militaries are dominated by complex machinery, precision weaponry, advanced information technologies, and a structural agility necessary for rapid adaptation to a wide range of threats. In a similar fashion, today's soldier is more sophisticated, relying more than ever on "brain over brawn." Nonetheless, physical stamina is important, given the grinding endurance required of combat operations. As a consequence, all military personnel must maintain a level of physical fitness. Despite the obvious importance of physical training, cognitive stamina may be even more important. A successful military career requires persistent honing of the basic cognitive tasks involving information processing and psychomotor skills.

EFFECTS OF ALCOHOL ABUSE ON PERFORMANCE

Cognitive Impairment

The use of alcohol promotes a wide range of biobehavioral impairments, many of which have particular significance to military activities. Alcohol impairs cognitive function in ways both subtle and severe. The nature and intensity of alcohol-related impairments vary according to consumption patterns, physiologic response, social acceptance, and the presence of co-occurring medical or psychiatric problems. Despite these intraindividual variations, at least for the purposes of comparison, the average man weighing 150 pounds can reliably achieve a blood alcohol concentration (BAC) of 0.04% following the consumption of two standard alcohol drinks in 1 hour.[1] Thus, even low levels of alcohol consumption impair cognition. Complex tasks are even more sensitive to the intoxicating influence of alcohol.

Mental activities that require divided attention, such as managing a weapon and scanning the environment, can suffer when blood alcohol levels hover as low as 0.02%.[2] The brain's information processing system attempts to compensate by focusing mental acuity in one area. This can lead to a devastating outcome when mental agility and survival are closely linked. The average man can achieve a BAC of 0.02% with as little as one standard drink in 1 hour, or be on the downward alcohol concentration slope after a bout of heavier drinking.[2]

One psychomotor task with special significance in military operations involves the ability to visually track objects. Whether sighting a weapon or driving a vehicle, the smooth and accurate control of eye motion is critical to mission success. Military personnel can experience impaired visual acuity, mostly in terms of difficulty focusing, with BAC as low as 0.03%.[2]

Clearly, the "blurred" vision associated with alcohol use is common. A less recognized, but potentially more hazardous, consequence of consumption involves a visual–spatial impairment. Visual–spatial exercises require the proper placement of objects in space. To effectively respond to an enemy sniper firing from multiple areas requires recognition of the sniper's relative positions and possible extrapolation to the next location. This sort of analysis relies on accurate perception and the application of abstract thinking.

Alcohol interferes with visual–spatial processing in two broad ways: intoxication makes multitasking more difficult or it simply renders the vision less accurate. The long-term use of alcohol, where duration and quantity are not fully defined, seems to produce a fixed change in cognition. The change is expressed in a loss of mental agility, inhibiting the ability to confront a novel problem with a creative solution. Clues to this condition emerge when an otherwise adequately performing individual is thrust into a new environment and cannot adapt old skills to the current reality.[2]

The greatest degree of impairment in the ability to apply abstract reasoning occurs in the weeks following reduction or cessation of significant alcohol consumption. Military personnel accustomed to substantial levels of alcohol use may be forced into an unwelcome abstinence when deployed, which can be accompanied by the emergence of worrisome symptoms of cognitive decline.

Memory Impairment

Chronic alcohol use disrupts the communication paths between areas of the brain responsible for processing memories, specifically the frontal lobes and the hippocampus.[3] In fact, long-term alcohol use structurally reduces brain volume.[4] The resulting memory deficits profoundly influence the acquisition and retention of knowledge.

A more intriguing and potentially harmful effect of alcohol use arises from acute intoxication. It seems increasingly apparent that alcohol consumption interferes with memory formation. The risk of acute alcohol-related memory impairment correlates closely with quantity consumed and the speed of absorption. Bolus, or binge, drinking among men is defined as five or more drinks in 2 hours. For women, four or more drinks in 2 hours constitutes bolus drinking. A much higher probability of memory impairment exists if bolus drinking occurs on an empty stomach.

Blackouts—the complete failure to transcribe events into memory—are not a rare phenomenon. Indeed, surveys among college students, a cohort closely age-matched with the largest military contingent, would suggest that blackouts are common. Based on these surveys, an estimated 40% to 50% of college students report a prior blackout. Fragmented memory loss is more common than a total blackout.[3] Just a few drinks, ambiguously regarded as "social drinking," can produce lapses in attention and word finding. Neither condition benefits military personnel engaged in fast-paced military operations.

Sleep Impairment

Alcohol's negative impact on cognition and memory is amplified by another side effect of consumption. Even small amounts of alcohol can profoundly affect the sleep cycle.[5] Although alcohol consumption reduces the amount of time necessary to fall asleep, it disturbs the late parts of the sleep cycle. The night is spent with frequent awakenings, many of which occur during rapid eye movement (REM) sleep. Disruption of REM sleep may have particular relevance in exacerbating fatigue, irritability, and the recall of disturbing dreams.

The sleep-inducing benefits of alcohol fade with repeated use, while at the same time the sleep cycle becomes ever more fragmented. It seems natural enough to use alcohol as a soporific during periods of stress and trauma. However, shift work and deployment across time zones may synergistically combine with an alcohol-induced sleep disorder to further impair the individual.

Alcohol withdrawal, perhaps induced by the forced abstinence of rapid mobilization, characteristically produces marked insomnia, disturbing dreams, and even hallucinations.[5] This can be an especially troublesome development when a service member deploys to an area of combat operations. The normal anxiety associated with deployment fuses with the symptoms of withdrawal and may produce substantial incapacitation.

SCREENING FOR ALCOHOL ABUSE

The detection of alcohol abuse begins with an understanding of its prevalence. Epidemiologic studies categorize alcohol use as light, moderate, and heavy.[6] Light drinking consists of three or fewer beverages per week. Light drinking is common. Nearly 43% of Americans meet the consumption criteria for light drinking.

Gender influences the values associated with moderate and heavy drinking. Moderate drinking among women consists of more than three but less than eight drinks per week; for men, no more than 14 drinks per week. Heavy drinking among women consists of more than one daily drink per week; for men it is more than two daily drinks per week. Based on these criteria, 14% of Americans are moderate drinkers and almost 4.5% meet the definition of heavy drinking.[6]

Epidemiologic consumption patterns contributed to the development of a simple screening tool referred to as the "Quantity Frequency Questionnaire."[7] The first set of questions queries quantity by asking, "On average, how many days a week do you drink alcohol?" and "On a typical day when you do drink, how many do you have?" If the multiplied sum of the two responses exceeds 14 for men (or seven for women) this can be considered "at-risk" drinking.

Bolus drinking is another "at-risk" drinking behavior. This pattern of drinking is the other half of the Quantity Frequency Questionnaire. The individual is asked, "What is the maximum number of drinks you had on any given day in the past month?" "At risk" bolus drinking occurs when men exceed four (and women three) drinks at one time. If the person is deemed "at-risk" based on the Quantity Frequency Questionnaire, then the CAGE questions should be asked.[8] The CAGE questionnaire inquires about alcohol use over the past year by asking:

C: Have you ever felt that you should CUT down on your drinking?

A: Have people ANNOYED you by criticizing your drinking?
G: Have you ever felt bad or GUILTY about your drinking?
E: Have you ever tried a drink first thing in the morning? (EYE opener)

If the person answers yes to any of the CAGE questions, this should trigger a more comprehensive assessment of substance use.

Alcohol screening questionnaires can be combined with certain laboratory tests. (Most biochemical markers require a blood sample.) The accuracy of these tests in detecting alcohol use depends on the tests' sensitivity and specificity. By itself, no single test conclusively identifies alcohol use. Multiple tests, combined with an "at risk" history, provide better evidence of problem drinking.[9] Perhaps the best single biochemical marker of alcohol use is gamma glutamyl transferase, or GGT. Elevated GGT occurs in a range of 30% to 50% among problem drinkers.

Problem drinking may also elevate aspartate aminotransferase and mean corpuscular volume, but both are less sensitive than GGT. Carbohydrate deficient transferrin is elevated among heavy drinkers and has sensitivity levels approaching GGT. Ethyl glucuronide can be detected in a urine specimen up to 5 days after heavy alcohol use. Ethyl glucuronide might play a clinically useful role in detecting alcohol use after bolus drinking on weekends.

TOBACCO USE

Although alcohol remains the most commonly used substance, tobacco use is almost as frequent. Approximately 29% of Americans use tobacco, with nearly 24% of that figure accounted for by cigarettes. Another 3% of the population uses smokeless tobacco.[10] Thus, healthcare practitioners should inquire about all forms of tobacco, including smokeless products.

During periods of major upheaval, such as natural or manmade disasters, an increase in the use of tobacco occurs. Several studies explored tobacco use among individuals exposed to the Oklahoma City bombing in 1995, in the aftermath of the 2001 terrorist attack on the twin towers of the World Trade Center in New York, and during other stressful events.[11–13] The findings from these collective studies provide evidence of increased smoking among traumatized individuals. Individuals who increase their smoking during periods of stress subsequently develop the symptoms of posttraumatic stress disorder (PTSD) at rates exceeding nonsmokers. The problem is further compounded when traumatized individuals report an inability to quit smoking. In a more quantifiable way, smoking appears to double the risk of developing PTSD.[14]

Tobacco use appears to play a key role in amplifying anxiety, inhibiting more effective coping strategies, and possibly contributing to heightened irritability. Military planners and healthcare practitioners can monitor tobacco use as a potential risk factor for emotional distress. For example, the predeployment phase begins with official notification of a pending assignment. Some military personnel may respond by initiating or markedly increasing their use of tobacco.

The Fagerström Test for Nicotine Dependence[15] is a screening tool used to assess cigarette use and can be administered at any phase of the deployment cycle, be it pre-, during, or postdeployment, to assess the degree of nicotine use. The test has a total of six questions, covering the following areas for an individual smoker:

1. time of day first cigarette is smoked;
2. whether the subject has difficulty refraining from smoking in places where it is not allowed;
3. time of day it would be most difficult to go without a cigarette;
4. total number of cigarettes smoked each day;
5. time of day, if any, when the subject smokes more frequently; and
6. whether or not the subject smokes even when ill enough to be home in bed.[15]

Points are assigned to the responses, ranging from 0 to 3 points, depending on the particular question. The test has a maximum total of 16 points; any score above 7 points is considered a very high addiction.[15] Military personnel scoring at the higher levels may be at increased risk of emotional deterioration. The increased use of tobacco may be an effort to self-medicate. Healthcare practitioners should take the opportunity to explore this possibility.

OTHER DRUGS OF ABUSE

A sizable minority of the American public regularly skirts potentially severe legal penalties to use, abuse, or sell a wide range of illegal drugs. A person's drug of choice is a complex judgment based on personality dynamics, cost, availability, and the drug's effects. In some situations, such as deployment to foreign locations, the new environment can either restrict options or provide new opportunities.

The National Survey on Drug Use examined patterns among individuals 18 to 25 years old, the age range that correlates well with the majority of the military population. Among this group, the survey reported 16.4% used marijuana, 6% used prescription drugs for recreational purposes, 1.7% used cocaine, and 1.5% used a hallucinogen.[10]

Marijuana is the most commonly used illegal drug, with 5.8% of Americans 12 years and older reporting use in the month proceeding the administration of the National Survey on Drug Use.[16] During the same time period, 2.1% reported the nonmedical use of prescription pain relievers, 0.8% of Americans reported the use of cocaine, and 0.4% used a hallucinogen. "Ecstasy" accounts for half of the reported hallucinogen use.[10]

The nonmedical use of prescription pain-relieving drugs is an area of special concern. The most likely source of these prescription drugs was a friend or family member.

The extent to which military use of illegal drugs bears some similarity to the National Survey on Drug Use is not precisely known. It seems reasonable to conclude that social trends are reflected in the military population. Following this line of reasoning, marijuana, cocaine, and the nonmedical use of prescription drugs would be the most likely problem areas.

The abuse of prescription pain relieving medications is particularly vexing. Traditional medical tests designed to detect opiate use will not identify the most likely offenders. Medications derived naturally from the poppy plant include morphine and codeine. These naturally occurring compounds are referred to as opiates and are included in most standard urine drug screens. Opioids are semisynthetic or fully synthetic opiates. Heroin, hydromorphone, hydrocodone, oxycodone, and fentanyl are examples of opioids. Opioids are not included in most standard medical urine drug tests and must be specifically ordered by name. If a clinician suspects the nonmedical use of oxycodone, for example, then oxycodone must be ordered by name from the testing laboratory. Clinicians should consult their laboratories for guidance.

Military planners and healthcare professionals should recognize the difficulty identifying opioid abuse and the ease in obtaining these medications. Detection of the nonmedical use of prescription drugs begins with an increasing index of suspicion triggered by certain behaviors. Routine screening should be part of every health encounter, which should include several questions aimed at understanding the person's use of addicting medications. Greater concern is occasioned by frequent medical visits rewarded with overlapping prescriptions. Some of the excess medications may be destined for diversion. The truly resourceful individual will seek prescription medications from multiple healthcare providers, both military and civilian, as well as the Internet.

The US government, through the Controlled Substances Act, classifies drugs into five schedules based on abuse potential. Drugs in schedule I or II are considered "illegal drugs" for purposes of prosecution. The Controlled Substances Act applies in all settings, be it a tertiary care medical facility in the United States, a regional military hospital in a foreign country, or mobile medical assets in support of combat operations.

The US military fields a robust drug-testing program. Today's modern drug-testing programs are direct descendants of embryonic military efforts initiated in the 1970s. Roughly a decade later, President Ronald Reagan signed Executive Order 12564,[17] mandating federal drug testing. Federal regulators understood the importance of clinical oversight and by the mid-1980s created the position of a medical review officer (MRO). The MRO plays a critical role in the fair and effective administration of the Federal Drug Testing Program. The US Department of Transportation and the Substance Abuse and Mental Health Services Administration both have extensive print and online documentation outlining the exact responsibilities of the MRO. US Army policies and procedures are found in Medical Command Regulation 40-51.[18]

THE ROLE OF THE MILITARY MEDICAL REVIEW OFFICER

For the sake of brevity, and in light of the changing rules and variances among the services, this chapter will not cover all the responsibilities and regulations pertaining to the military MRO. The official definition of the MRO is "a licensed physician responsible for receiving laboratory results generated by an agency's drug testing program who has knowledge of substance abuse disorders and has appropriate medical training to interpret and evaluate an individual's positive test result together with his or her medical history and any other relevant biomedical information."[19(p5)]

The military treatment commander appoints the MRO (always a physician) specifically to function in that capacity. The MRO must be familiar with laboratory procedures, which include screening immunoassay, gas chromatography, and mass spectrometry. The

AUTHORIZED FOR LOCAL REPRODUCTION

MEDICAL RECORD	CONSULTATION SHEET

REQUEST

TO:	FROM: *(Requesting physician or activity)*	DATE OF REQUEST

REASON FOR REQUEST *(Complaints and findings)*

PROVISIONAL DIAGNOSIS

DOCTOR'S SIGNATURE	APPROVED	PLACE OF CONSULTATION ☐ BEDSIDE ☐ ON CALL	☐ ROUTINE ☐ TODAY ☐ 72 HOURS ☐ EMERGENCY

CONSULTATION REPORT

RECORD REVIEWED ☐ YES ☐ NO PATIENT EXAMINED ☐ YES ☐ NO TELEMEDICINE ☐ YES ☐ NO

(Continue on reverse side)

SIGNATURE AND TITLE	DATE

HOSPITAL OR MEDICAL FACILITY	RECORDS MAINTAINED AT	DEPARTMENT/SERVICE OF PATIENT

RELATION TO SPONSOR	SPONSOR'S NAME *(Last, first, middle)*	SPONSOR'S ID NUMBER *(SSN or Other)*

PATIENT'S IDENTIFICATION *(For typed or written entries, give: Name – last, first, middle; ID no. (SSN or other); Sex; Date of Birth; Rank/Grade)*	REGISTER NO.	WARD NO.

CONSULTATION SHEET
Medical Record

STANDARD FORM 513 (REV. 4-98)
Prescribed by GSA/ICMR FPMR (41 CFR) 101-11.203(b)(10)
USAPA V1.00

Figure 29-1. Standard Form 513, Medical Record Consultation Sheet.

testing procedures are consistent among the services. For purposes of illustration, the Army's procedures are set forth in Army Regulation (AR) 600-85,[20] Chapter 8, which places the responsibility of test result reporting in the hands of the alcohol and drug control officer (ADCO). The ADCO is a member of the garrison or administrative section of Army Substance Abuse Program (ASAP). The installation biochemical testing coordinator (IBTC) works for the ADCO and coordinates the testing and review of the urinalysis. The IBTC and ADCO do not have a direct affiliation with the military treatment facility. The IBTC or ADCO sends the MRO a consult or request (using an SF-513, shown in Figure 29-1) requesting a review of the positive urinalysis. The SF-513 request should include the military person's identifying data, specific drugs in question, and the date the biochemical test was conducted. The MRO should also review DD Form 2624 (Figure 29-2), otherwise known as the Specimen Custody Document: Drug Testing.

The MRO will review the military person's medical records seeking a legitimate medical prescription that would account for the biochemical test result. If such evidence is lacking, the MRO will document this finding on the consult and forward the response to the ADCO or IBTC. The MRO's response triggers one of the important safeguards of the biochemical testing program. Up to this point, the MRO's opinion rested solely on medical documentation. To ensure that a comprehensive medical review occurs before a drug test is deemed "positive," the military person will have the opportunity to meet with the MRO and present medical evidence that might account for the test result. Normally, the ADCO or IBTC will arrange the interview with the MRO.

If the service member agrees to proceed, the MRO reviews the purpose of the interview and reviews the test results. Most importantly, the service member is afforded the opportunity to present evidence, such as a valid prescription, that might account for

SPECIMEN CUSTODY DOCUMENT - DRUG TESTING

1. SUBMITTING UNIT	2. ADDITIONAL SERVICE INFORMATION *(Second Echelon)*	A. LABORATORY CONDUCTING DRUG TESTING
		B. BATCH NUMBER / C. REPORT OF RESULT (DTG/Serial No.)
3. BASE/AREA CODE / 4. UNIT IDENTIFICATION CODE	5. DOCUMENT/ BATCH NUMBER / 6. DATE SPECIMEN COLLECTED YYYY MM DD	D. DRUGS TESTED

7. SPECIMEN NUMBER	8. COMPLETE SSN	9. TEST BASIS	10. TEST INFO	11. PRESCREEN	E. DISC CODE	F. ACCESSION NUMBER	G. RESULT

H. CERTIFICATION. I certify that I am a laboratory certifying official, that the laboratory results indicated on this form were correctly determined by proper laboratory procedures, and that they are correctly annotated.		(3) CERTIFYING OFFICIAL (Printed Name and Title)
(1) SIGNATURE	(2) DATE SIGNED	

DD Form 2624, FEB 1998 — Previous Edition may be used — Reset — Adobe Professional 7.0

Figure 29-2. DD Form 2624, Specimen Custody Document: Drug Testing, page 1. (**Figure 29-2** *continues*)

12. CHAIN OF CUSTODY		LAN	THRU
DATE (YYMMDD) a.	RELEASED BY b.	RECEIVED BY c.	PURPOSE OF CHANGE/ REMARKS d.
(1)	SIGNATURE NAME	SIGNATURE NAME	
(2)	SIGNATURE NAME	SIGNATURE NAME	
(3)	SIGNATURE NAME	SIGNATURE NAME	
(4)	SIGNATURE NAME	SIGNATURE NAME	
(5)	SIGNATURE NAME	SIGNATURE NAME	
(6)	SIGNATURE NAME	SIGNATURE NAME	
(7)	SIGNATURE NAME	SIGNATURE NAME	
(8)	SIGNATURE NAME	SIGNATURE NAME	
(9)	SIGNATURE NAME	SIGNATURE NAME	
(10)	SIGNATURE NAME	SIGNATURE NAME	

INSTRUCTIONS				
BLOCK		USA	USN/MC	USAF
1	SUBMITTING UNIT	Message address of unit submitting urine samples		
2	ADDITIONAL SERVICE INFORMATION (SECOND ECHELON)	Do not use	Message address of second echelon commander to whom submitting unit reports administratively.	Optional. May be used to identify the base POC.
3	BASE / AREA CODE	Service Code Area	Leave blank for future use.	Four-character Base Identification Code (Ex., F123). Comprises the first four characters of the full 10-character Base Identification Number (BIDN).
4	UNIT IDENTIFICATION CODE	Unit Identification Code (UIC or RUC) of unit submitting urine sample.		Do not use
5	DOCUMENT/BATCH NUMBER	Do not use	Enter the locally assigned batch number. Each batch of 12 samples, or portion thereof, shall be assigned a separate number by the submitting unit.	3-digit batch number common to all specimens in the shipment (Ex.,501). Comprises the middle part of the full 10-character BIDN assigned to each specimen.
6	DATE SPECIMEN COLLECTED	Enter the four-digit year, two-digit month, and two-digit day that samples were collected by submitting unit.		
7	SPECIMEN NUMBER	Use number pre-printed on form to itemize bottle.		Enter 3-digit sequential specimen number (last 3 characters of full BIDN).
8	COMPLETE SSN	Full SSN of person from whom sample obtained.		
9	TEST BASIS	Indicate the testing premise to conduct the collection.		
10	TEST INFORMATION	Military: A = E1 - E4; B = E5 - O10; Civilian only: C = TDP Aviation; D = TDP Guard/Police; E = TDP PRP; F = TDP; ADAPCP Staff: G = other TDP; N = other nonmilitary	Leave blank	Entry required only if additional testing is requested: F = Full Panel; S = Steroids; O = Other drugs - Provide clarification in attached message.
11	PRESCREEN	If screened (field tested) prior to submission and found positive, indicate P for positive or N for negative for drug(s) pre-screened. Leave blank if not screened prior to submission to lab.		Not used

12. CHAIN OF CUSTODY (LINE (1)).

a. DATE - Date of collection/shipment
b. RELEASED BY - Signature and printed or typewritten name of the urinalysis coordinator having custody of the samples.
c. RECEIVED BY - Use only if physical change of custody is occuring prior to shipment. Otherwise leave blank.
d. PURPOSE OF CHANGE/REMARKS - Specify the mode of accountable transportation/system utilized to ship specimens to the lab.

NOTE: If/when custody of specimens changes other than for shipment (unless hand carried to lab), each change of custody requires line number signature in the (b) RELEASED BY and (c) RECEIVED BY blocks to document changes in custody with comment in block (d). If a continuation sheet is necessary, it must contain information/signatures of blocks (a) - (d).

13. DAMAGE TO SHIPPING CONTAINER/DISCREPANCIES

DD Form 2624, FEB 1998 (Back)

Reset

Figure 29-2 *continued*. DD Form 2624, Specimen Custody Document: Drug Testing, page 2.

the drug test. If satisfied that the evidence confirms legitimate drug use, the MRO will annotate "legitimate drug use" on the SF-513 and return the form to the ADCO.

THE ARMY SUBSTANCE ABUSE PROGRAM

Biochemical testing is only one of several methods through which referrals are made to the ASAP, or its counterparts in the other military services. Referrals can also be initiated by commanders and supervisors in response to observed changes in occupational performance, interpersonal relations, and physical fitness or health problems suspected to be secondary to substance use. These referrals are made by physicians and other healthcare providers in the context of routine or emergency medical treatment, as a consequence of military or civilian law enforcement investigation or apprehension identifications, or through the individual's voluntary self-identification to the clinic.

In fiscal year 2008, the Army's Drug and Alcohol Management Information System reported that 10,407 soldiers were enrolled in the ASAP Army-wide. An additional 10,310 soldiers were evaluated, though not enrolled. Of those evaluated and subsequently enrolled for outpatient treatment, 22% were referred through biochemical identification, 27% through commander or supervisory intervention, 11% as a result of a driving under the influence/driving while intoxicated arrest, 5% through other investigation or apprehension identification, 10% as medical referrals, 24% as a result of self-identification, and the remainder through a variety of other channels (ie, security clearances, family members).[21]

Regardless of the method of identification, all of the military substance abuse treatment programs function in large measure within the conceptual model of an employee assistance program, focusing on personnel conservation and military readiness. Optimizing the advantages[25] of coercive treatment through effective leveraging of command oversight, the ASAP benefits from a well-articulated team approach in the service of behavior change. The relationship between the ASAP and the command is clearly defined in AR 600-85,[20] with parallel guidance in Air Force Instruction 44-121,[22] and Operational Navy Instruction 5350.4C.[23] AR 600-85 differentiates the responsibilities of the command from that of the clinical staff, placing clinical decision making in the hands of the ASAP's professional staff. All of the clinical staff is required, per AR 40-68,[24] to be licensed to practice independently and to be certified in substance abuse rehabilitation. The clinical consultant, an addictions-trained physician, assists the ASAP staff, providing medical consultation and adjunctive medication management. It is the ASAP clinical staff's responsibility to advise command of all referrals and to secure command input into their assessments.

Although only the clinical staff may define treatment recommendations, unit commanders retain authority for all administrative decisions, ranging from deployments to retention or separation from service, extensions on active duty to permit reenlistment, or bars to reenlistment.[20(p9)] When retention decisions are required, commanders must assess the service members' rehabilitation efforts in the context of their occupational specialties, prior service records, the needs of the military, and their potential for future military service. In general, each of the military services will tend to separate drug- or alcohol-dependent service members who do not respond to treatment.

The Secretary of Defense is required to identify and treat all active duty service members who are drug and alcohol dependent.[25] Regardless of service designation, referral for evaluation is mandatory and early intervention is key. All of the military services have procedures and policies to identify and offer treatment to those active duty members who have drug and alcohol problems. The unique challenges to deployed commanders in managing substance abuse issues are addressed in an information paper produced by the Army Center for Substance Abuse Programs.[26] It provides guidance to deployed unit commanders regarding accessing ASAP services prior to deployment, in theater, and upon return.

Once identified and referred, a comprehensive biopsychosocial and substance use assessment is completed by the ASAP staff. The assessment explores the extent of substance use; intervention is recommended according to the degree of impairment. Such treatment recommendations are based upon careful consideration of the criteria for substance use disorders, per the current *Diagnostic and Statistical Manual of Mental Disorders*.[27] Diagnoses of abuse and dependence generally require enrollment in treatment for periods of 3 months to 1 year. The intensity of response can range from a 12-hour instructional program called ADAPT (Alcohol and other Drug Abuse Prevention Training) to outpatient treatment activities in the ASAP. Referrals to higher levels of care for detoxification, intensive outpatient programs, partial hospitalization programs, or residential treatment are often incorporated into the treatment plan.

Per Health Affairs Policy 9700029,[28] a continuum of substance abuse care must be considered for active duty service members, consistent with the patient placement criteria of the American Society of Addiction Medicine. "These criteria reflect the philosophy of placing patients in the least intensive/restrictive treatment environment, appropriate to their therapeutic needs."[29(p2)] In addition to defining a crosswalk for level-of-care determinations, the American Society of Addiction Medicine posits a multidimensional analysis to enhance treatment decision making. Acute intoxication or withdrawal potential (Dimension 1) and the patient's biomedical conditions and complications (Dimension 2) must receive primary consideration in the stabilization process, after which the patient's emotional, behavioral, and cognitive conditions and complications (Dimension 3); readiness for change (Dimension 4); relapse, continued use, or continued problem potential (Dimension 5); and recovery/living environment (Dimension 6) are considered in the formulation of a dynamic and individualized treatment plan.[30(p4)] Treatment emphasizes motivational enhancement over confrontational drama, supported by a multidisciplinary team approach to facilitate change.

Although the clinical role of the ASAP providers and the administrative domain of the command are clearly differentiated, a collaborative thread is woven between the command and clinical staff through implementation of the "rehabilitation team." The rehabilitation team concept is developed in AR 600-85,[20(p17)] and is a core ingredient of an effective program. With the ASAP clinician serving as chair, the rehabilitation team is composed of the soldier, the unit commander or first sergeant, and others as needed. In its most effective implementation, the rehabilitation team meeting provides the soldier with a positive outlook to start treatment. It offers a forum to clearly define program expectations and to explain the benefits for successful completion, while also articulating the consequences of failure to comply with treatment guidelines. It also offers a setting in which to provide assurances of support to mitigate a soldier's fears, to explain patient rights, and to discredit some of the myths that pervade early beliefs and undermine success. Careers are more often enhanced than lost through the rehabilitation process. Therefore, it is imperative that soldiers experience the ASAP staff and command group as a unified team whose primary mission is to conserve personnel and promote health and well-being. Career retention goals and personnel conservation thus are married to rehabilitation efforts through the close collaboration with command.

SUMMARY

Today's military requires sophisticated knowledge and advanced technical skills to successfully navigate lethal battlefields. Even modest amounts of alcohol can impair crucial decision-making abilities and negatively affect military operations. Military personnel are not immune to the larger social problem of tobacco, illicit drugs, and the misuse of prescription and over-the-counter medications. The military maintains an active biochemical testing program to constantly assess the use of these substances and their impact on military readiness. In addition, each service offers specific administrative rules and clinical support to address the misuse of substances. The best outcome for the individual and the organization results from a collaborative effort involving clinicians, commanders, and a motivated patient to resolve issues of substance abuse.

REFERENCES

1. National Institute on Alcohol Abuse and Alcoholism. Alcohol-related impairment. *Alcohol Alert.* July 1994; No. 25 PH 351. Available at: http://pubs.niaaa.nih.gov/publications/aa25.htm. Accessed September 10, 2008.
2. National Institute on Alcohol Abuse and Alcoholism. Cognitive impairment and recovery from alcoholism. *Alcohol Alert*. July 2001; No. 53. Available at: http://pubs.niaaa.nih.gov/publications/aa53.htm. Accessed September 10, 2008.
3. White AM. What happened? Alcohol, memory blackouts, and the brain. *Alcohol Research Health*. 2004;2:186–196.
4. National Institute on Alcohol Abuse and Alcoholism. Alcohol's damaging effects on the brain. *Alcohol Alert*. October 2004; No. 63. Available at: http://pubs.niaaa.nih.gov/publications/aa63/aa63.htm. Accessed September 10, 2008.
5. National Institute on Alcohol Abuse and Alcoholism. Alcohol and sleep. *Alcohol Alert*. July 1998; No. 41. Available at: http://pubs.niaaa.nih.gov/publications/aa41.htm. Accessed September 10, 2008.
6. National Institute on Alcohol Abuse and Alcoholism of the National Institutes of Health. Percent distribution of current drinking status, drinking levels, and heavy drinking days by sex for persons 18 years of age and older: United States, NHIS, 1997–2006. Available at: http://www.niaaa.nih.gov/Resources/DatabaseResources/QuickFacts/AlcoholConsumption. Accessed September 10, 2008.
7. Cherpitel CJ. Brief screening instruments for alcoholism. *Alcohol Health Res World*. 1997;21(4):348–351.
8. National Institute on Alcohol Abuse and Alcoholism. Screening for alcoholism. *Alcohol Alert*. April 1990; No. 8 PH 285. Available at: http://pubs.niaaa.nih.gov/publications/aa08.htm. Accessed September 10, 2008.
9. Peterson K. Biomarkers for alcohol use and abuse. *Alcohol Res Health*. 2004/2005;28(1):30–37.
10. Results from the 2007 National Survey on Drug Use and Health: National Findings. Department of Health and Human Services. Substance Abuse and Mental Health Services Administration. Available at: http://www.oas.samhsa.gov/nhsda.htm. Accessed April 21, 2009.
11. Pfefferbaum B, Vinekar SS, Trautman RP, et al. The effect of loss and trauma on substance use behavior in individuals seeking support services after the 1995 Oklahoma City bombing. *Ann Clin Psychiatry*. 2002;14(2):89–95.
12. Vlahov D, Galea S, Resnick H, et al. Increased use of cigarettes, alcohol, and marijuana among Manhattan, New York, residents after the September 11th terrorist attacks. *Am J Epidemiol*. 2002;155(11):988–996.
13. Hapke U, Schumann A, Rumpf HJ, John U, Konerding U, Meyer C. Association of smoking and nicotine dependence with trauma and posttraumatic stress disorder in a general population sample. *J Nerv Ment Dis*. 2005;193(12):843–846.

14. Koenen KC, Hitsman B, Lyons MJ, et al. A twin registry study of the relationship between posttraumatic stress disorder and nicotine dependence in men. *Arch Gen Psychiatry*. 2005;62(11):1258–1265.

15. Fagerström K, Schneider NG. Measuring nicotine dependence: a review of the Fagerström Tolerance Questionnaire. *J Behav Med*. 1989;12:159–182.

16. Office of Applied Studies, Substance Abuse and Mental Health Services Administration, Department of Health and Human Services. *Results From the 2005 National Survey on Drug Use and Health: National Findings.* September 2006. Available at: http://oas.samhsa.gov/NSDUH/2k5NSDUH/2k5results.htm. Accessed September 10, 2008.

17. Ronald Reagan, President. *Drug-Free Federal Workplace*. September 15, 1986. Executive Order 12564. Available at: http://www.archives.gov/federal-register/codification/executive-order/12564.html. Accessed December 18, 2008.

18. US Department of the Army, Medical Command. *Medical Review Officers and Positive Urinalysis Drug Testing Results.* Washington, DC: DA; 2005. MEDCOM Regulation 40-51.

19. Shults TF. *Medical Review Officer Handbook*. 8th ed. Research Triangle Park, NC: Quadrangle Research, LLC; 2005.

20. US Department of the Army. *Army Substance Abuse Program.* Washington, DC: HQDA; 2006. Army Regulation 600-85.

21. Army Center for Substance Abuse Programs 2008 data. Available at: https://ssob.acsap.hqda.pentagon.mil/sso/pages/index.jsp. Accessed April 10, 2009.

22. US Department of the Air Force. *Alcohol and Drug Abuse Prevention and Treatment (ADAPT) Program.* Washington, DC: HQUSAF September 26, 2001. Air Force Instruction 44-121. Available at: http://www.e-publishing.af.mil/shared/media/epubs/AFI44-121.pdf. Accessed December 18, 2008.

23. US Department of the Navy. *Drug and Alcohol Abuse Prevention and Control.* Washington, DC: Department of the Navy, Office of the Chief of Naval Operations; October 15, 2003. OPNAV Instruction 5350.4C. Available at: http://www.navyfitrep.com/inst_files/OPNAVINST_5350.4C_-_DAPA.pdf. Accessed December 18, 2008.

24. US Department of the Army. *Clinical Quality Management.* Washington, DC: HQDA; 2004. Army Regulation 40-68. Available at: http://www.army.mil/USAPA/epubs/pdf/r40_68.pdf. Accessed December 18, 2008.

25. Medical and Dental Care, Identifying and Treating Drug and Alcohol Dependence. 10 USC §1090 (2010).

26. Army Center for Substance Abuse Programs. *Army Substance Abuse Program Guidance for Deployed Commanders*. Washington, DC: DA; 2004.

27. American Psychiatric Association. *Diagnostic and Statistical Manual of Mental Disorders.* 4th ed, text rev. (DSM-IV-TR). Washington, DC: APA; 2000.

28. US Department of Defense. *Curbing Alcohol Abuse.* Posted by Casscells SW, August 21, 2008. Health Affairs Policy Memo 9700029. Available at: http://www.health.mil/MHSBlog/Article.aspx?ID=336. Accessed December 18, 2008.

29. American Society of Addiction Medicine. *Patient Placement Criteria.* Available at: http://www.asam.org/PatientPlacementCriteria.html. Accessed December 18, 2008.

30. American Society of Addiction Medicine. *Patient Placement Criteria for the Treatment of Substance-Related Disorders: ASAM PPC-2R.* 2nd rev ed. Chevy Chase, Md: ASAM; 2001.

COMBAT AND OPERATIONAL BEHAVIORAL HEALTH

Section VI: Military Children and Families

Section Editor:

Stephen J. Cozza, MD
Colonel (Retired), Medical Corps, US Army
Associate Director, Center for the Study of Traumatic Stress, Department of Psychiatry, Uniformed Services University of the Health Sciences

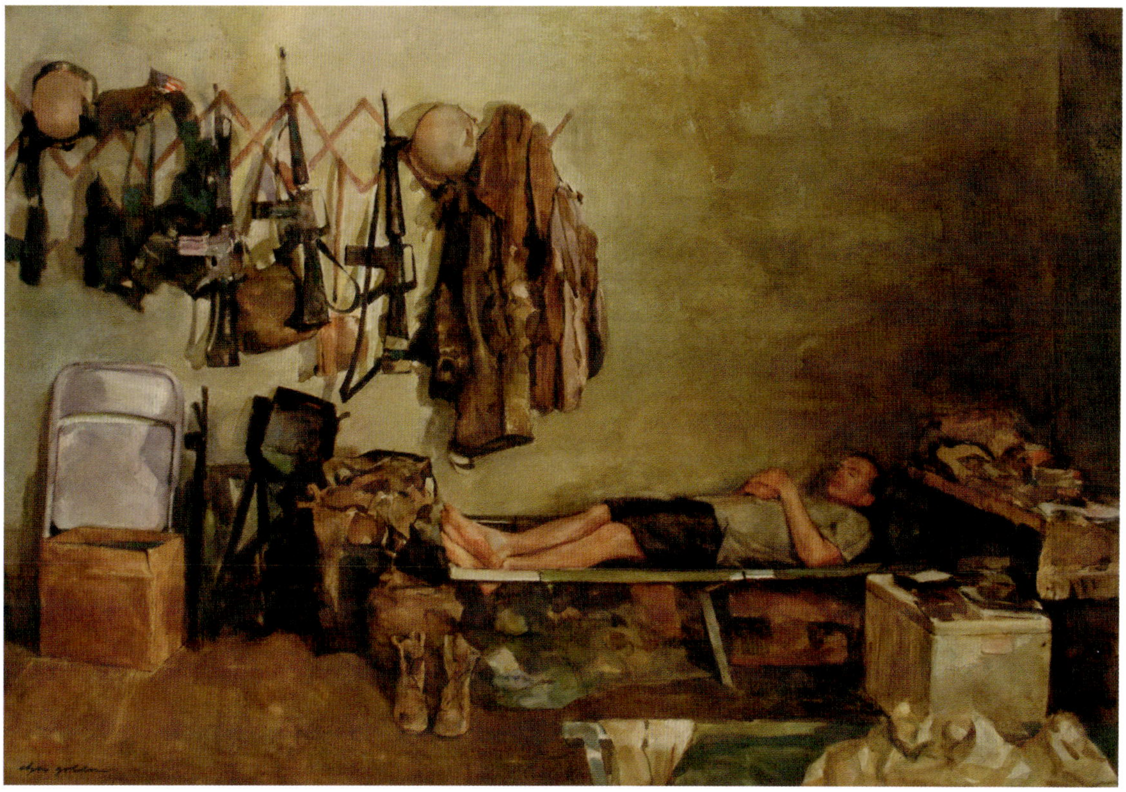

Fallujah, by Elzie Golden, watercolor on paper, 2005.

Art: Courtesy of the Army Art Collection, US Army Center of Military History.

Chapter 30

THE IMPACT OF DEPLOYMENT ON MILITARY FAMILIES AND CHILDREN

SIMON PINCUS, MD*; BARBARA LEINER, MSW, LCSW-C†; NANCY BLACK, MD‡; AND TANGENEARE WARD SINGH, MD§

*Colonel (Retired), US Army; Clinical Director, Department of Mental Health, McChord Medical Clinic, 690 Barnes Boulevard, Joint Base Lewis-McChord (McChord Field), Washington 98438; formerly, Chief, Inpatient Psychiatry, Madigan Army Medical Center, Tacoma, Washington

†Psychiatric Social Worker, Department of Child Psychiatry, Walter Reed Army Medical Center, Borden Pavilion, 6900 Georgia Avenue NW, Washington, DC 20307-5001; formerly, Clinical Case Manager, Department of Child Psychiatry, Kaiser Permanente Mid-Atlantic States, Rockville, Maryland

‡Colonel, Medical Corps, US Army; Training and Program Director, National Capital Consortium of Child and Adolescent Psychiatry Fellowships, Department of Psychiatry, Walter Reed Army Medical Center, Borden Pavilion, 6900 Georgia Avenue NW, Washington, DC 20307-5001

§Major, Medical Corps, US Army; Department of Behavioral Health, Blanchfield Army Community Hospital, 650 Joel Drive, Fort Campbell, Kentucky 42223

INTRODUCTION

"Deployment" is the term used when military personnel leave their usual daily workstations to train for or to perform a mission. Missions vary in length and range from training to humanitarian assistance to combat. Deployment has an effect on the service member, the member's unit, the units that remain to carry on with existing tasks, and the affiliated support systems in the community as well as the member's family. With an increased number of married military service members, deployment affects a growing community of spouses and children, both on and off base. Whether service members are single or married, their parents, siblings, and other relatives are frequently part of an extended family network that is affected by deployment and its outcome. This chapter addresses the complex issues faced by the military family when a service member leaves the home base to perform the mission of war. It also provides a list of resources available to military service members and their families (see Attachment).

In 1994, Peebles-Kleiger and Kleiger[1] wrote about reintegration stress in families with members returning from Operations Desert Shield/Storm (ODS/S). They described two versions of this stress: (1) Logan's seven phases of adjustment and (2) a four-stage version of emotional adjustment based on the Kubler-Ross model of grief.[1(pp176–177)] In a report on the emotional cycle of deployment following the Gulf War and during the rotations to Bosnia and Kosovo, Pincus et al[2] utilized these models to identify five stages: (1) predeployment, (2) deployment, (3) sustainment, (4) late deployment (referred to as "redeployment" in the original online article), and (5) postdeployment. Simon Pincus, MD, is an Army psychiatrist at McChord Medical Clinic (Madigan Army Medical Center) in Tacoma, Washington. He and his colleagues have continued using this approach as they educate families and communities during Operation Enduring Freedom (OEF), Operation Iraqi Freedom (OIF), and Operation Noble Eagle (ONE) engagements. Their goal is to sustain health and function in all family members during the stress of deployment.

In ODS/S (1990–1991), 645,000 troops were deployed to the war zone, including 228,000 National Guard and reserve forces that were brought onto active duty.[3(p273)] OIF and OEF have included an even wider variety and greater number of military service members[4(p233)]: activated reserve and National Guard units and personnel, as well as individual augmentees and ready reserve personnel. During the Balkans engagements service members were occasionally sent on second deployments and multiple tours (some units have had three or four deployments). Longer tours (particularly for the Army) to a combat theater have become common during OIF and OEF. Soldiers who have already endured physical and psychological injuries—including posttraumatic stress disorder (PTSD)—are being returned to combat conditions. The broader involvement of service personnel, who are deployed more frequently and for longer tours of duty, likely increases the impact of the mission on military as well as civilian families and communities.

In many cases during ODS/S, families were less prepared for mobilization and war[5(p442)] than families in today's readiness climate. Many families of ODS/S military personnel were unfamiliar with the larger military system of demands, benefits, and supports that exists for the active duty member and beneficiary. Foreign-born or non-English–speaking spouses, another subset of military families facing unique circumstances, may be less capable or willing to access available resources.[6(p78)]

School enrollment records provide one example of the size of deployment impact on military children. In 2004, Lamberg[7] reported in the *Journal of the American Medical Association* that 191,000 children of soldiers were enrolled in public schools in approximately 35 school districts near military posts around the United States. In addition to this number, the Department of Defense reported approximately 104,000 children enrolled in preschool through 12th grade at DoD schools in seven US states, Guam, and Puerto Rico, and in 13 foreign countries.[7]

To date, national and local community support of troops has been consistently positive in OIF, OEF, and ONE. Although there are differing political views and increasing criticism about the execution of the war in Iraq, the nation as a whole has been able to separate these issues from the role of military service members and to convey support for them and their families. This broad community support creates a positive environment for military families, which in turn results in less isolation and greater overall family resiliency.[8(p1285)]

THE DEPLOYMENT CYCLE

Each stage of deployment involves emotional and organizational elements that affect both individual service members and their families (Figure 30-1). Any impending deployment introduces uncertainty, even for previously deployed and experienced service members. Despite ongoing training, ambiguity likely exists

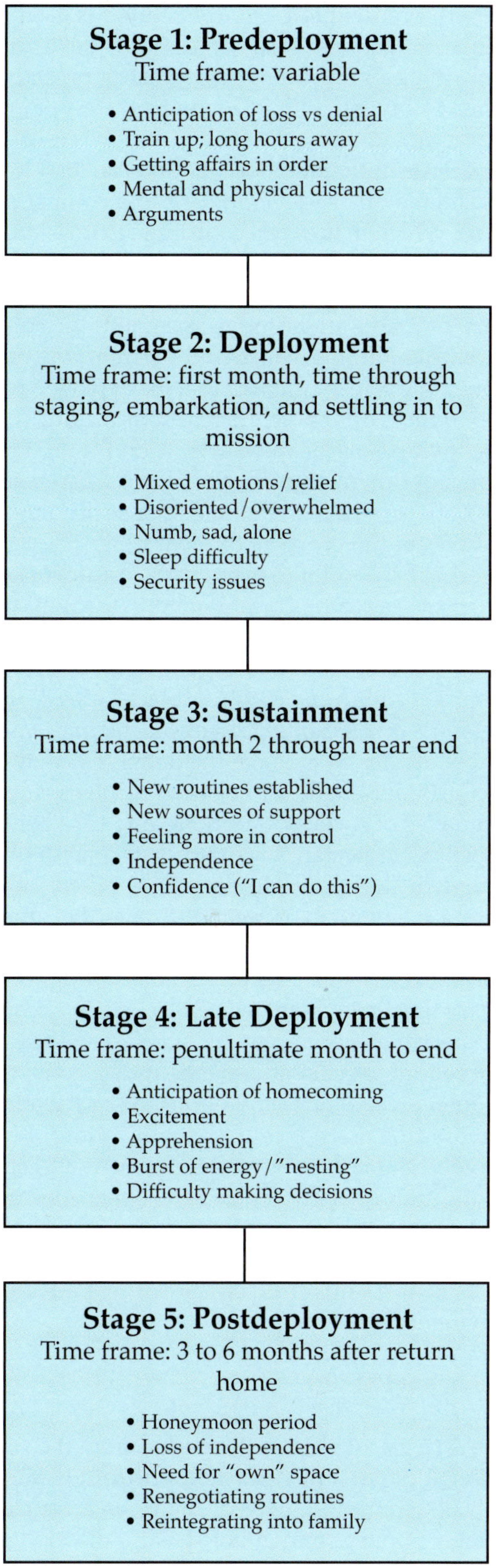

Figure 30-1. Common emotional rections to each stage of deployment.

TABLE 30-1

NEGATIVE EMOTIONAL AND BEHAVIORAL CHANGES IN CHILDREN DURING DEPLOYMENT

Age	Behaviors	Emotions	Remedies
Infants: < 1 y	Refusing to eat	Listlessness	Support from parent, pediatrician
Toddlers: 1–3 y	Crying, tantrums	Irritability, sadness	Increased attention, holding, hugs
Preschoolers: 3–6 y	Potty accidents, clinginess	Irritability, sadness	Increased attention, holding, hugs
School-age children: 6–12 y	Whining, body aches	Irritability, sadness	Spending time, maintaining routines
Teenagers: 12–18 y	Isolating, acting out, using drugs	Anger, apathy	Patience, limit-setting, counseling

about extent of the deployment, associated mission challenges, time commitment, the family's capacity to manage the separation, and the ever-present risk of injury or death.[3(p273),8(p1285)] The stages of military deployment are listed in Table 30-1 and discussed below. The model developed by Pincus, revised to accommodate current deployment cycles during OIF, OEF, and ONE, is the source for the following section.[9]

Predeployment

The *predeployment phase* starts with the alert order for deployment and ends when the service members leave the home station. Its time frame can vary from several weeks to more than a year. The predeployment period often results in both denial and anticipation of separation. For many, the predominant feeling is loss of control.[10(p632)] As the departure date approaches, spouses often ask if the service members really must go. Increased field training, preparation, and long hours away from home mark the beginning of the pending extended separation.

As service members think and talk about the upcoming mission and their unit relationships, bonding with fellow unit members is essential to unit cohesion and safety during the mission, but it can create an increasing sense of emotional and physical distance for military spouses and children.[9,11,12] Because of this psychological distancing, spouses often feel as if their loved ones have already deployed. However, the change in focus from family to unit is a necessary part of the deployment process for active duty service members as they prepare for, and embrace, the mission. It can be especially demanding for the activated National Guard or Reserve service members who are transitioning from civilian to military life. By extension, spouses of National Guard and Reserve service members can have significant adjustment challenges during this transition. These complex issues can increase the individual service member's negative feelings within the context of deployment.[13(p633)]

With deployment pending, families review their personal and family affairs to reorder their lives during the service member's absence. Lists are generated to categorize a variety of expected needs: home repairs, home security, car maintenance, finances, insurance, tax preparation, childcare plans, and wills. Anxiety about financial and bill-paying responsibilities is often significant.[14(p85)] Couples may want increased intimacy and arrange for memorable holidays or anniversaries. Desire for sexual intimacy may be ambivalent, vacillating between wanting and not wanting to be close before the impending separation. Fears about marital fidelity may be raised or may go unspoken. Other frequently voiced concerns include anxiety about children's ability to handle the separation, fears of functioning without the partner, and the survivability of the marriage. Completing the multitude of tasks and fulfilling high expectations before deployment can place tremendous strain on couples and families.

It is not uncommon for military couples to argue before deployment.[3,9] For well-established couples and those familiar with the deployment cycle, arguments may be accepted as part of the rhythm of marital life and adjustment to deployment. For less experienced couples, however, especially those facing an extended separation for the first time, such arguments can lead to fears that the relationship could be over.

In 1980, Valentine cited the work of Evelyn Duvall, who identified "nine ever-changing family developmental tasks that span the life cycle."[15(p350)] These tasks serve to establish and maintain (1) an independent home, (2) satisfactory ways of obtaining and spending money, (3) mutually acceptable patterns in the division of labor, (4) continuity of mutually satisfying sexual relationships, (5) an open system of emotional and intellectual communication, (6) workable relationships with relatives, (7) ways of interacting with associates and the community, (8) competency in bearing and rearing children, and (9) a workable philosophy of life.[15(p350)]

Unresolved family challenges have potentially devastating consequences. To a military commander, a worried, preoccupied service member is easily distracted and unable to focus on essential tasks during critical times. From a psychological perspective, it is easier to be angry than to confront the pain and loss of saying goodbye.[2,16] In the worst-case scenario, unresolved emotional preoccupation can lead to serious accidents or the development of a combat stress disorder, which in turn can contribute to mission ineffectiveness.[17–19] At home, significant spousal distress interferes with completing basic routines, concentrating at work, and attending to the children. This can exacerbate children's fears that the parents are unable to adequately care for them or that the deployed parent will not return. Adverse child reactions include regressive behaviors such as inconsolable crying, apathy, or tantrums. A downward emotional spiral can result in which both service member and spouse become even more upset at the prospect of separating.

Kiser et al[20(p90)] outline seven characteristics of family resiliency: (1) a strong commitment to the family that involves a close bond and stable relationship with at least one person, (2) family organization with shared parental leadership and clear role boundaries, (3) belief in the family and its ability to succeed, (4) implementation of strategies to manage the demands created by stressors, (5) willingness to work to resolve issues, (6) maintenance of social connections, and (7) a coherent and positive understanding of stressors consistent with the family's shared world view.[20(p90)] When military couples are able to explore and discuss their mutual expectations as they prepare for the deployment, they are more likely to successfully adjust throughout the phases of the deployment experience. Healthy couples will expect that nondeploying spouses will exercise their freedom to make independent decisions; maintain contact with same- and opposite-sex friends and neighbors (for assistance and socialization); budget effectively; care for children competently; and stay in touch through letters, care packages, e-mail messaging, and telephone calls. Failure to communicate these and other expectations is frequently a source of misperception, distortion, and hurt feelings during and after the deployment period.

Deployment Phase

The *deployment phase* is the period from the service member's departure from home through the first month of separation. Mixed emotions arise during this stage. Spouses may report feeling disoriented or overwhelmed, or they may feel relieved that they no longer have to appear brave and strong. There may be residual anger about tasks left undone by the deployed spouse. The departure creates a gap that can lead to feelings of numbness, sadness, loneliness, or abandonment. It is common for family members to have difficulty sleeping or coping with everyday challenges. Worries about home security and personal safety may come up again. Other concerns may involve pay problems, sick children, or car repairs. For many, the early part of the deployment stage can be an unpleasant, disorganizing experience.

Although it is often assumed that only wives have such difficulties or concerns, these issues apply to spouses of either gender. Husbands may feel overwhelmed in taking responsibility for childcare, school attendance and homework, meals and shopping, medical and dental care, extracurricular activities, peer groups, friends, and social activities for their children. When new caregivers are brought in to assist families in the absence of the deployed parent, feelings of uncertainty can develop in children as they attempt to integrate another deployment-related change into their lives.

Sustainment Stage

The *sustainment stage* lasts from the end of the first month of the deployment to the month prior to return home. Sustainment is a time of establishing new sources of support and new routines. At home, many Army families rely on the local family readiness group (FRG), a garrison-based function that serves as a close network of community spouses and families. The FRG ideally meets on a regular basis to provide help with problems and disseminate information. The Army's sister services have groups that perform similar functions. In addition, many military spouses are comfortable receiving support from their families, friends, churches, or other cultural, community, ethnic, or religious institutions as their primary means of emotional support. As challenges occur, most spouses find that they are able to cope with crises and make important decisions on their own. They report feeling more confident and in control. During the sustainment stage, most military spouses report that they can do what is needed to keep their families functioning successfully.

Frequency, method, and content of communication between deployed service members and families are important factors at every stage of deployment, but especially during sustainment. The reality that phone contact is unscheduled and initiated by the service member can be frustrating. Spouses can feel tied to the house, not wanting to miss a call. Service members may feel forgotten if they call and no one is home, especially if they waited a long time to get to a phone. When expectations regarding the frequency of calls are unmet, resentment and anger may result. The Defense Satellite Network (DSN) offers time-limited calls home at no cost, depending upon location. Commercial phone lines are an option for some service members, but large phone bills can result, adding to family stress. More recently, some families are able to remain connected through video-teleconference capabilities via the Internet. For most military spouses, reconnecting with their loved ones is a stabilizing experience. For those who have difficult interactions during phone calls, the contact can exacerbate stress in the deployment stage and may result in the need for counseling.[9]

With e-mail now widely available, spouses and service members report feeling more in control; both are able to initiate communication, and they are not limited by the constraints of scheduling phone calls. Another advantage of e-mail is the ability to be more thoughtful about what is said and to monitor intense emotions that may be unnecessarily disturbing. However, e-mail security and restrictions can constrain some communication.

One disadvantage of the improved access to communication (phone calls or e-mail) is the immediacy of, and proximity to, unsettling news from either the family or the service member. It is virtually impossible to disguise negative feelings of hurt, anger, frustration and loss, especially on the phone. Inaccurate and disappointing news may travel quickly by personal cellular phones.

Unsubstantiated rumors can circulate unchecked within the FRG.[9] Rumors involving allegations of infidelity can be particularly damaging. Other troubling rumors may involve innuendo that a particular spouse or service member is handling the deployment poorly, combat accidents or injuries, unexpected changes in the date of return, or disciplinary actions. Rumors can be hurtful to service members, spouses, and the FRG. At its worst, unit cohesion and even mission success can suffer. Limiting the negative effect of rumors is a constant challenge for unit leaders and chaplains. The rapidity of crosscommunication of potentially inaccurate news can undermine the ability of the service member, unit, or family to focus and perform safely.

Late Deployment Stage

The *late deployment stage* is defined as the month before the service member returns home. Deployments occurring during the OIF surge have been marked by unexpected and late announced extensions of combat tours. Deployment extensions typically lead to frustration and anxiety for all involved and can introduce unexpected strain at a time when everyone is looking forward to the service member's return. The late deployment stage is generally one of great anticipation.

As in the deployment stage, there can be a rush of conflicting emotions: excitement that the soldier is coming home, apprehension, concern that spouses may not agree with how things have been managed, worry about whether independence will be lost or how roles will shift, and concern about whether family members will get along. With the separation almost over, there can be renewed difficulty making decisions. A spouse may wonder whether decisions should be deferred until the service member is home to make them. Many spouses also experience a burst of energy during this stage,[9,16] a rush to complete tasks around the home. During late deployment, expectations of service members, spouses, and children all are high.

Postdeployment

Postdeployment begins with the service member's return from theater and arrival home, sometimes first to the clearing station or demobilization station. Like predeployment, the time frame can be variable. The actual homecoming is often ceremonial and can be a joyous occasion. Children rush to the returning parent and the reunited couple embrace. The unit commander calls the unit to attention, praises unit members for their service, and then dismisses them. Weapons and equipment are turned in, and further demobilization tasks (including health evaluations, mental health surveys, and family health surveys) are completed. Finally, the family goes home. Homecoming can also be a frustrating and upsetting experience. The date of return may change, or units may travel home in separate groups over several days. Spouses may be required to attend to other unexpected family obligations, such as sick children.

A "honeymoon" period usually follows the homecoming, during which families reunite; however, they may soon find themselves feeling emotionally distant. Some spouses describe awkwardness in addition to excitement, especially reestablishing intimacy after so many months of separation. Emotional reconnection may require time before sexual intimacy feels comfortable. Eventually, returning service members reassert their role as spouse or parent within the family.[16] This is an essential task that can flow naturally or lead to tension within the family. Service members may feel pressure to make up for lost time and missed milestones. They may want to quickly reestablish the authority they had before. However, some things will have changed in their absence: spouses typically become more autonomous during deployments, children have grown, and individual personal priorities in life may be different. It is not realistic to expect everything to be the same as before the deployment.

During the postdeployment period, spouses may report a lost sense of independence or resentment at having been left on their own. Spouses may consider themselves to be the true heroes, who managed things while service members were away. At least one study[21] suggests that stay-at-home parents are more likely to report distress than the deployed service members. Like their military spouses, nondeployed spouses also have to adapt to changes that result from the homecoming, and may find they are more irritable with their mates around. They may desire to retain a sense of their own space. Basic household chores and routines need to be renegotiated. Roles played by each spouse in the marriage must be reestablished, perhaps in a new form.

Reunions with children can be both joyful and challenging. Youngsters' feelings tend to depend on their age and their understanding of the reason for the service member's absence. Babies less than 1 year old may not know the returned parent and cry when held. Toddlers (1–3 years) may be slow to warm up. Preschoolers (3–6 years) may feel guilty or scared about future separations. School-age children (6–12 years) may want a lot of attention. Teenagers (13–18 years) may be moody and may not appear to care. Children are often loyal to the parent who remained behind and may not respond initially to discipline from the returning service member. Children may also fear the military parent's return if a threat of discipline or consequences has been put forward. Some children may display ongoing anxiety triggered by the real possibility of future deployments. The returned service member may not agree with privileges granted to children by the nondeployed parent. Generally, reunited parents should not make immediate changes, instead taking time to renegotiate family rules and norms. Otherwise, the service member risks invalidating the efforts of the nondeployed parent and alienating the children. Returning service members may feel hurt in response to a perceived ambivalent reception. Clearly, making changes slowly and allowing children to set the pace for reintegration can lead to a successful reunion.

Postdeployment is probably the most critical stage for service member, spouse, and children. Successful reintegration is aided by fostering patient communication, setting reasonable expectations, and taking time for family members to reacquaint.[9,16] Counseling may be required if the soldier is injured, returns with unrelenting psychiatric symptoms, or engages in health-risk behaviors such as excessive alcohol use or physical displays of anger. Nevertheless, the separation experienced during the deployment offers service member and spouse a chance to evaluate changes within themselves and what direction they want their marriage to take. Postdeployment is both a difficult and joyful stage, and many military couples have reported that their relationship is stronger as a result.

EFFECTS OF DEPLOYMENT ON SPOUSES

Soon after the August 1990 announcement that the United States would send troops to the Persian Gulf, Rosen et al[22(p47)] were tasked to study the impact of deployment on service member and family well-being. They studied Army spouses to determine which group had the most difficulty coping during ODS/S. They identified three vulnerable groups: (1) enlisted spouses under 30 years of age, many of whom were Spanish speaking and many married to noncommissioned officers; (2) very young spouses of junior enlisted, especially those living off post; and (3) older, employed spouses who faced their own unique stresses.

In May 2003, Haas et al surveyed[23] pregnant military and civilian women in the antenatal clinic at the Naval Hospital Camp Lejeune to measure stress levels. Almost predictably, women whose partners were deployed and who already had more than one child at home reported higher levels of stress (up to eight times greater than those with no children at home) than their peers who were married to nondeployed military members.[23(p48)]Another study conducted in a southeastern Virginia Navy community looked at families whose service members deployed to the Mediterranean between 1989 and 1991.[24(p103)] The authors found that deployment associated with combat had the strongest effect on spouses, predisposing them to depression.

Not all military families are traditional in constellation; some are single-parent families and some are blended families. Although in past wars most deploying service members were men, this is no longer the case. In 1993, Birgenheier[25] (quoting data from Magnusson and Payne) noted that women comprised more than 10% of the military, and that 14% of them, along with 4% of military service men, were single parents. With the onset of Operation Desert Storm on January 15, 1991, mothers were assigned to combat settings for the first time.[25(p471)]

CHILDREN'S DEVELOPMENTAL RESPONSES DURING DEPLOYMENT

Forty percent of service members have children, approximately one third of whom are less than 5 years of age. Children of varying ages respond differently to deployment stress. Their strengths and vulnerabilities are determined by stages of psychosocial development. Parents or other caring adults must avoid burdening children of any age with matters that are more appropriate to adults.

Some children may have greater difficulty adapting to the stress of a deployed parent. Signs or symptoms indicating an inability to return to normal routines or the presence of more serious problems require a visit to the family doctor or mental health counselor. Despite obstacles, the vast majority of spouses and children successfully negotiate the sustainment stage and look forward to their deployed family member coming home. Table 30-1 provides examples of negative behavioral and emotional changes in children of different ages that require further attention.

Infants

Infants (< 1 year; the Eriksonian psychosocial developmental stage of "trust versus mistrust"[26]) thrive when held and actively nurtured. The infant is at risk when a primary caregiver becomes significantly depressed or otherwise emotionally unavailable. Infantile depression may present with symptoms of apathy, irritability, eating refusal, or weight loss. Early intervention becomes critical to prevent undue harm or neglect. In particular, pediatricians should monitor growth. Personnel in community services, social work, pediatrics, and psychiatry must assist with parental support and treatment, parental skill development, and coordination of appropriate family services.

Toddlers

Toddlers (1–3 years; the Eriksonian psychosocial developmental stage of "autonomy versus shame,"[26]) generally take their emotional and behavioral cues from their primary caregivers. If the home-based parent is coping well, the toddler tends to do well. The opposite is also true. If the primary caregiver is not coping well, then toddlers may become sullen or tearful, throw tantrums, or develop sleep or eating disturbances. Toddlers respond to increased attention such as playing together, hugs, or longer bedtime rituals. Given the challenges of caring for young, active children, home-based parents should balance the demands for caring for children alone with their own needs for time. Parents may also benefit from sharing their day-to-day experiences with other parents facing similar challenges.

Preschoolers

Preschoolers (3–5/6 years; the Eriksonian psychosocial developmental stage of "initiative versus guilt,"[26]) may regress in acquired skills as a result of deployment stress. This regression may manifest itself as loss of toilet training, change in language use, thumb sucking, refusal to sleep alone, or increased neediness. Young children may become more irritable, depressed, or aggressive. They are prone to somatic complaints and can develop more pervasive fears of losing parents or other important adults. Caregivers need to reassure preschoolers with extra attention and physical closeness (hugs, holding hands). Adults should avoid changing family routines; they should support developmental accomplishments, such as encouraging youngsters to continue to sleep in their own bed. Answers to questions about the deployment should be brief, matter-of-fact, and to the point. Consistency of routines and expectations, although important for all age groups, provides greater comfort and security for younger children in particular.

School-Age Children

School-age children (6–12 years; the Eriksonian psychosocial developmental stage of "industry versus inferiority,"[26]) may whine and complain, develop somatic complaints, become aggressive, or otherwise behaviorally demonstrate their feelings. They may focus on the military parent missing a key event such as a birthday, school play, or important game. Depressive symptoms may present as sleep disturbance, loss of interest in school, changes in eating habits, or decreased desire to play with friends. School-age children benefit from talking about their feelings and need more physical attention than usual. Although some reduction in school performance may occur, parental expectations and routines should largely remain the same.

Rosen et al[27] studied children's responses during ODS/S deployments, finding that sadness was fairly widespread in both boys and girls aged 3 to 12 years old. Children's symptoms sometimes varied with birth order. Discipline problems and immature behaviors were more prominent in eldest children (mean age 7.2 +/− 5.4 years). Academic problems and refusing to talk were noted more in second children. Both groups evidenced eating and sleeping problems as well as increased need for adult attention.[27(p466)] Kelley[24] reported that the children of ODS/S combat-deployed service members demonstrated more internalizing and externalizing behaviors that took longer to resolve after the father's return. The frequently quoted study by Jensen et al[28] focused on children's responses to parental separation during ODS/S. In this study, ODS/S combat deployments were related to elevated, but not pathological, depressive and anxiety symptoms for both the nondeployed spouse and the children, as measured by parental reports. Boys and younger children appeared especially vulnerable to deployment effects.[28]

Adolescents

Adolescents (13–18 years; the Eriksonian psychosocial developmental stage of "identity versus role confusion,"[26]) may be irritable or rebellious. Teens might argue or participate in other attention-getting behavior. Huebner and Mancini[29] noted that adolescents face a number of normal developmental stressors, including puberty. These normal stressors combined with the multiple challenges of deployment can push teenagers' coping capacities beyond their limits. With their developing cognitive capacity for abstract thought and more complex emotional lives, adolescents may experience ambivalent feelings, such as anger mixed with pride in the deployed parent. They can also experience a sense of loss and uncertainty about whether they will see the parent again.

Changes in responsibilities and roles during deployment may be challenging, but also provide older children and teens with an opportunity for greater independence and growth. The return of the deployed parent can be more difficult due to the potential loss of these newly earned responsibilities. In Huebner's study, teens were more aware of having become closer to their nondeployed parents (mothers) and struggled to return to their previous roles and relationships at the end of the deployment. These adolescents also reported being aware of more intense family relations and of their own fluctuating emotions.[29(pp3,9,10)]

During parental deployments, adolescents may show a lack of interest in school, peers, and school activities. They are at greater risk for promiscuity, alcohol use, and drug use. Although teens may deny problems and worries, it is extremely important for caregivers to stay engaged and be available to talk about the teens' concerns. Sports and peer or family social activities should be encouraged to give normal structure to teens' lives. Academic tasks can add further order to a teenager's life. Likewise, additional responsibility in the family, commensurate with their emotional maturity, helps teens feel important and needed. Monetary incentives can also contribute positively to the maintenance of grades and chores. Adolescents should not, however, be placed in roles of coparenting or serve as confidantes to the nondeployed spouse. Even the most capable adolescents need to know that competent adults remain in charge and will look after and care for the adolescents' needs.

INTERGENERATIONAL TRANSMISSION OF THE EFFECTS OF WAR AND COMBAT TRAUMA

Newer research has identified elevated rates of PTSD and depression in service members returning from combat deployment in Iraq, with approximately 20% of these personnel evidencing symptoms indicative of a mental disorder.[30] It is essential to consider the impact of these postcombat conditions on families, particularly children. Intergenerational trauma transmission, sometimes referred to as secondary traumatization, is a phenomenon whereby children are affected by their parent's posttraumatic sequelae.[31] A body of literature in this field has emerged since the mid-1960s, when the subject was first considered in work with families of Holocaust survivors.[32] Interest in the subject continued with the 1983 National Vietnam Veterans Readjustment Study (NVVRS), which was established in response to a congressional mandate for an investigation of PTSD and other postwar psychological problems among Vietnam veterans.[33] Numerous studies were conducted with families of Vietnam veterans that examined the psychological, behavioral, and adaptive styles of children of veterans. Additional work in the field of intergenerational trauma studies has focused on the impact of multiple traumas (genocide, political violence, repressive regimes, domestic violence, crime, and life-threatening diseases)[34] on survivor's children. In such cases, the children did not experience the actual traumatic events, but were affected by their parents' traumatic experiences.

The multigenerational repercussions of trauma are well documented in anecdotal data. Children of Holocaust survivors report feeling that they have absorbed their parents' Holocaust experiences as if "through osmosis."[35] Many children of Holocaust survivors describe an unspoken presence of the Holocaust in the home that served as an organizing force underlying family communications and relationships. Many reported that their parents never spoke about the traumas they endured, giving rise to the term "conspiracy of silence."[35] This "conspiracy" refers to an avoidance of discussion within the family as well as within society at large of the horrors experienced by Holocaust survivors. This silence is regarded as a powerful means of transmission of the impact of the parental trauma.

Initial clinical observations in the 1960s noted significant anxiety, depression, and maladaptive behaviors in children of Holocaust survivors.[36] The early literature was generally presumptive of significant psychopathology, given the severity and duration of the traumatic experiences of the parents who had little opportunity to integrate their massive losses and traumatic experiences. Over time, these results were questioned because of methodological weaknesses and lack of reliable data.[37] Questions naturally arose about how to assess the meaning and impact of any parental trauma on a child. New interest developed in considering the strengths that parents confer to their children as a result of their histories of traumatization.[32]

Similarly, studies of children of Vietnam veterans present a range of findings and conclusions. Some reports indicate that children of veterans had difficulties in academic performance, peer relations, and affective coping, with general deficits in psychosocial functioning.[38] The NVVRS determined that on over 100 life-adjustment indices, the majority of Vietnam veterans successfully adjusted to postwar life with few symptoms of psychological disorders.[33] Other studies raised concerns over the adverse impact on children related to their fathers' combat-related PTSD, emotional numbing,[39] or participation in acts of abusive violence during combat.[40] Studies appearing in the literature by the mid-1980s suggested that children of fathers with PTSD were at increased risk for learning disabilities, aggression, depression, and hyperactivity.[41]

A significant factor in the emergence of intergenerational trauma transmission appears to be related to whether the veteran parent had, or did not have, symptoms of PTSD. NVVRS data indicate a relationship between PTSD and family disruption, as well as marital instability and child behavioral problems.[40] Parental feelings of detachment or inability to feel and express emotions were noted to carry over into the parenting relationship, possibly leading to behavioral problems in children. Significantly, affective avoidance and emotional numbing are most highly correlated with behavioral difficulties in children of veterans.[42] The literature also notes that veterans who have participated in abusive violence or atrocities see themselves as social outcasts and have difficulty trusting others. These views can contribute to increased family violence and difficulty with the formation of nurturing parenting bonds.[40]

Intergenerational trauma transmission appears to occur most significantly when second-generation children experience trauma themselves. Vietnam veterans who were sons of World War II veterans and who were diagnosed with PTSD had more severe and persistent symptoms than veterans whose parents had not been exposed to combat. Problems for these Vietnam veterans emerged at the time of homecoming, with clashes in ideology between fathers who fought the "good war" and sons who fought an unpopular war. The lack of support for returning Vietnam veterans may have impeded the resolution of PTSD symptoms and facilitated the intergenerational transmission of combat-related trauma for those with veteran fathers.[43] Similarly, Israeli veterans of the 1982 Lebanon War who were sons of Holocaust survivors were also noted to have especially severe and persistent symptoms of PTSD compared with control groups, suggesting that intergenerational trauma transmission is more pronounced when the offspring experience personal traumas.[44]

A veteran's PTSD can affect children in a number of ways. The parent's reexperiencing of traumatic events can be sudden, intense, and vivid. These intrusions are very frightening to children, who do not understand what is happening. Children may worry about the parent's well-being, or the parent's ability to provide care for them. Parents with emotional numbing and who are "shut down" can seem remote and uninvolved to their children. The parent may seem uncaring, and the child may feel unloved. Symptoms of anxiety, hyperarousal, irritability, and low frustration tolerance can influence a child's sense of safety and can cause the child to question the parent's love.[33]

Children of combat veterans with PTSD have been observed to fall into three general response types: (1) the disengaged child, (2) the overidentified child, and (3) the rescuer child. While the disengaged child may become emotionally detached from family life, the overidentified child tries to become closer to the parent at the expense of age-appropriate activities and peer relationships. This child may experience flashbacks and nightmares that are similar to the veteran parent. The rescuer child, similar to the child of an alcoholic, tends to feel responsible for the parent's problems and guilty when things do not go well. This child takes on parental roles and responsibilities.[38]

Trauma involves a disruption of emotions, beliefs, and cognitions. The parent may return from combat with altered thoughts, feelings, and behaviors in the aftermath of a single traumatic event, or as a result of prolonged exposure to the intensity of the combat experience. There may be change in parents' fundamental sense of themselves as people, and in the way they view themselves within the context of society as well as within their interpersonal relationships. Issues of safety and trust can be deeply affected by trauma, reshaping an individual's beliefs about relationships and about the world at large.[37] Intergenerational transmission of the impact of parental trauma occurs when the parent's disrupted beliefs and assumptions are communicated to a child who has not experienced the trauma but who comes to internalize a set of feelings or beliefs that parallel those of the traumatized parent.

Mechanisms of intergenerational transmission of trauma described by Ancharoff and colleagues[37] include silence, overdisclosure, identification, and reenactment. In an environment of silence, the child experiences the impact of the parent's trauma affectively but in the absence of explanation or reassurance. The family sometimes colludes in avoiding difficult subjects or any trigger to the traumatized parent's symptoms. The child can have frightening fantasies about the parent's unspoken experience and feel anxious about provoking the parent's symptoms. Overdisclosure occurs when the parent reveals frightening or horrific details that the child cannot tolerate and that may cause the child to develop PTSD symptoms. Identification may occur when a child tries to connect emotionally with a parent who is otherwise withdrawn and unavailable. Reenactment occurs when family members are involved in reliving some aspect of a traumatic memory as a result of the parent's difficulty with separating the past from the present.[37]

Not all children develop emotional problems in the aftermath of the parent's combat experience or PTSD symptoms. However, when a child is expressing emotional problems at home or in school, a comprehensive assessment of the child's social and academic status is indicated. This assessment should include an evaluation of overall family functioning and patterns of communication.

Because trauma involves betrayal of trust, all trauma-related work must occur within a safe and trusting therapeutic relationship. Individual treatment may be needed prior to participation in family therapy. The goal of intervention is to help the family recognize its patterns of communication, to develop beliefs and behaviors that distinguish the past from the present, and to have an expanded range of responses.[37] The combat veteran or any survivor of trauma must find a way to integrate past experiences with the present reality in a way that feels meaningful and hopeful. If silence attests to an inability to integrate trauma,[34] then the therapeutic dialogue must skillfully address this silence because it disrupts a sense of continuity of self and experience. The therapist does not seek to elicit detailed descriptions of the parent's traumatic experiences. Rather, assisting the family to develop new interactive patterns through a more informed awareness of family communication patterns is an appropriate goal in addressing the intergenerational transmission of the effects of combat trauma.

The emerging body of anecdotal and empirical literature suggests that interpersonal relationships are affected by the profoundly disruptive nature of trauma. The issues are highly complex; over the past 40 years researchers have sought to identify, qualify, and measure the impact of parental trauma on children. If trauma occurs, how does it occur and how does it affect future generations and manifest in these successive generations? However, over the years since ODS/S, service members and their families have had to adapt to a major shift in US foreign policy and in the role of the US military in extended multinational deployments. The Bosnian experience provided new insight into the different skills needed to minimize familial trauma. Research on ODS/S veterans has further added to knowledge of this subject. However, the multiple and lengthy combat deployments of OEF and OIF have posed new challenges for military service members, their families, and children. It is unclear to what degree the traumatic experiences of service members involved in OEF and OIF will impact their children. Family well-being is not only essential to mission success, but also to the future health of the military in its efforts to retain skilled military service members.[45,46]

SUMMARY

The military, Department of Veterans Affairs, and TRICARE civilian healthcare professionals must be prepared to support service members and their families through the five stages of deployment, and the sequelae that might result from service member combat exposure. Given the established 20% rate of mental illness in returning OIF veterans, the multigenerational effects of combat-related stress and trauma must be considered as a possible health effect of the current conflicts. Public and professional education efforts on these topics are essential for families to cope effectively with the deployment experience and seek help if problems develop. Additional research addressing the impact of deployment on service members and their families will better ensure that US military forces are prepared for the challenges of the next conflict.

REFERENCES

1. Peebles-Kleiger MJ, Kleiger JH. Re-integration stress for Desert Storm families: wartime deployments and family trauma. *J Trauma Stress*. 1994;7(2):173–194.

2. Pincus SH, House R, Christenson J, Adler LE. The emotional cycle of deployment: a military family perspective. Available at: http://www.hooah4health.com/deployment/Familymatters/emotionalcycle.htm. Accessed February 24, 2010.

3. Black WG Jr. Military-induced family separation: a stress reduction intervention. *Soc Work*. 1993;38(3):273–280.

4. Nelson J, Hagedorn ME. Federal Nursing Service Award. Rhythms of war: activation experiences during the Persian Gulf War. *Mil Med*. 1997;162(4):233–239.

5. Rabb DD, Baumer RJ, Wieseler NA. Counseling Army reservists and their families during Operation Desert Shield/Storm. *Community Ment Heath J*. 1993;29(5):441–447.

6. Blount BW, Curry A Jr, Lubin GI. Family separations in the military. *Mil Med*. 1992;157(2):76–80.

7. Lamberg L. When military parents are sent to war, children left behind need ample support. *JAMA*. 2004;292(13):1541–1542.

8. Ursano RJ, Holloway HC, Jones DR, Rodriquez AR, Belenky GL. Psychiatric care in the military community: family and military stressors. *Hosp Community Psychiatry*. 1989;40(12):1284–1289.

9. Pincus SH, Nam TS. Psychological aspects of deployment: the Bosnian experience. *J US Army Med Dep*. 1999;PB8-99-1/2/3:38–44.

10. Wynd CA, Dziedzicki RE. Heightened anxiety in Army Reserve nurses anticipating mobilization during Operation Desert Storm. *Mil Med*. 1992;157(12):630–634.

11. Diedrich J. Deployment overseas can take toll on families. *The Gazette*. October 31,1999:A4.

12. MacIntosh H. Separation problems in military wives. *Am J Psychiatr*. 1968;125(2):260–265.

13. Samler JD. Reserve unit mobilization trauma. *Mil Med*. 1994;159(10):631–635.

14. West L, Mercer SO, Altheimer E. Operation Desert Storm: the response of a social work outreach team. *Soc Work Health Care*. 1993;19(2):81–98.

15. Valentine D. The developmental approach to the study of the family: implications for practice. *Child Welfare*. 1980;59(6):347–355.

16. Logan KL. The emotional cycle of deployment. *US Naval Inst Proc*. 1987;113:43–47.

17. Pincus SH, Benedek DM. Operational stress control in the former Yugoslavia: a joint endeavor. *Mil Med*. 1998;163:358–362.

18. Noy S. Stress and personality as factors in the causality and prognosis of combat reaction. Paper presented at: The Second International Conference on Psychological Stress and Adjustment in Time of War and Peace; June 1978; Jerusalem, Israel.

19. Neumann M, Levy A. A specific military installation for the treatment of combat reactions during the war in Lebanon. *Mil Med*. 1984;149:196–199.

20. Kiser LJ, Ostoja E, Pruitt DB. Dealing with stress and trauma in families. *Child Adolesc Psychiatr Clin N Am*. 1998;7(1):87–103,viii–ix.

21. Zeff KN, Lewis SJ, Hirsch KA. Military family adaptation to United Nations Operations in Somalia. *Mil Med*. 1997;162(6):384–387.

22. Rosen LN, Westhuis DJ, Teitelbaum JM. Patterns of adaptation among Army wives during Operations Desert Shield and Desert Storm. *Mil Med*. 1994;159(1):43–47.

23. Haas DM, Pazdernik LA, Olsen CH. A cross-sectional survey of the relationship between partner deployment and stress in pregnancy during wartime. *Womens Health Issues*. 2005;15(2):48–54.

24. Kelley ML. The effects of military-induced separation on family factors and child behavior. *Am J Orthopsychiatry*. 1994;64(1):103–111.

25. Birgenheier PS. Parents and children, war and separation. *Pediatr Nurs*. 1993;19(5):471–476.

26. Erikson EH. *Childhood and Society*. New York, NY: WW Norton; 1950.

27. Rosen LN, Teitelbaum JM, Westhuis DJ. Children's reactions to the Desert Storm deployment: initial findings from a survey of Army families. *Mil Med*. 1993;158(7):465–469.

28. Jensen PS, Martin D, Watanabe H. Children's response to parental separation during Operation Desert Storm. *J Am Acad Child Adolesc Psychiatry*. 1996;35(4):433–441.

29. Huebner AJ, Mancini JA, Wilcox RM, Grass SR, Grass GA. Parental deployment and youth in military families: exploring uncertainty and ambiguous loss. *Fam Relations*. 2007;56(2):112–122.

30. Hoge CW, Castro CA, Messer SC, McGurk D, Cotting DI, Koffman RL. Combat duty in Iraq and Afghanistan, mental health problems, and barriers to care. *N Engl J Med*. 2004;351(1):13–22.

31. Rosenheck R, Nathan P. Secondary traumatization in children of Vietnam veterans. *Hosp Community Psychiatry*. 1985;36:538–539.

32. Yehuda R, Schmeidler J, Elkin A, et al. Phenomenology and psychobiology of the intergenerational response to trauma. In: Danieli Y, ed. *International Handbook of Multigenerational Legacies of Trauma.* New York, NY: Plenum Press; 1998: 639–656.

33. Price JL. Children of veterans and adults with PTSD. [National Center for PTSD Web site]. Available at: http://ncptsd.va.gov/ncmain/ncdocs/fact_shts/fs_children_veterans.html?opm=1&rr=rr112&srt=d&echorr=true. Accessed February 24, 2010.

34. Danieli Y, ed. *International Handbook of Multigenerational Legacies of Trauma.* New York, NY: Plenum Press; 1998.

35. Danieli Y. The treatment and prevention of long-term effects and intergenerational transmission of victimization: a lesson from Holocaust survivors and their children. In: Figley CR, ed. *Trauma and Its Wake.* New York, NY: Brunner/Mazel; 1985: 295–313.

36. Yehuda R, Schmeidler J, Giller EG Jr, Siever LJ, Binder-Byrnes, K. Relationship between posttraumatic stress disorder characteristics of Holocaust survivors and their adult offspring. *Am J Psychiatry.* 1998;155(6):841–844.

37. Ancharoff MR, Munroe JF, Fisher LM. The legacy of combat trauma: clinical implications of intergenerational transmission. In: Danieli Y, ed. *International Handbook of Multigenerational Legacies of Trauma.* New York, NY: Plenum Press; 1998: 257–276.

38. Harkness L. The effect of combat-related PTSD on children. *Natl Center PTSD Clin Q.* 1991;2(1):12–15. Available at: http://ncptsd.va.gov/ncmain/nc_archives/clnc_qtly/V2N1.pdf?opm=1&rr=rr1046&srt=d&echorr=true. Accessed February 24, 2010.

39. Samper RE, Taft CT, King DW, King LA. Postraumatic stress disorder symptoms and parenting satisfaction among a national sample of male Vietnam veterans. *J Trauma Stress.* 2004;17(4):311–315.

40. Rosenheck R, Fontana A. Transgenerational effects of abusive violence on the children of Vietnam combat veterans. *J Trauma Stress.* 1998;11(4):731–742.

41. Dansby VS, Marinelli RP. Adolescent children of Vietnam combat veteran fathers: a population at risk. *J Adolesc.* 1999;22:329–340.

42. Ruscio AM, Weathers FW, King LA, King DW. Male war-zone veterans' perceived relationships with their children: the importance of emotional numbing. *J Trauma Stress.* 2002;15(5):351–357.

43. Rosenheck R, Fontana A. Warrior fathers and warrior sons. In: Danieli Y, ed. *International Handbook of Multigenerational Legacies of Trauma.* New York, NY: Plenum Press; 1998: 225–242.

44. Solomon Z, Kotler M, Mikulincer M. Combat-related posttraumatic stress disorder among second-generation Holocaust survivors: preliminary findings. *Am J Psychiatry.* 1988;145:865–868.

45. Schneider RJ, Martin JA. Military families and combat readiness. In: Jones FD, Sparacino LR, Wilcox VL, Rothberg JM, eds. *Military Psychiatry: Preparing in Peace for War.* In: Zajtchuk RM, Bellamy RF, eds. *Textbooks of Military Medicine.* Washington, DC: Office of The Surgeon General, US Department of the Army, Borden Institute; 1994: 19–30.

46. van Vranken EW, Jellen LK, Knudson KH, et al. Division of Neuropsychiatry. *The Impact of Deployment Separation on Families.* Washington, DC: Walter Reed Army Institute of Research; 1984. Report NP-84-6.

ATTACHMENT: RESOURCES FOR MILITARY FAMILIES

An important endeavor for military members and their families is navigating through the many resources available to help them through the deployment cycle. Although not an exhaustive list, this attachment includes a number of these resources and a synopsis of their purposes.

Organizations Supporting the Service Member and Military Family

Military OneSource

Military OneSource (available at: http://www.militaryonesource.com) is a service provided by the Department of Defense at no cost to active duty, National Guard, and reserve (regardless of activation status) soldiers and their families. The agency promotes multiple services such as help with childcare, personal finances, emotional support during deployments, relocation information, and resources needed for special circumstances. These services can be accessed by telephone, online, and face to face through private counseling with master's level consultants in the local community.

Information on Helping Military Children

The Department of Defense, in partnership with LIFELines organizations, provide a Web site as the department's official source of education information (available at: www.militarystudent.org). Its purpose is to better enable the children of military personnel, their parents, special needs families, military leaders, and educators deal with the various issues that face the military child by providing each group with access to information, tools, and resources from a central location. Ultimately, the aim is to enhance the educational and social well-being of all military children by increasing the understanding and awareness of how to meet their unique needs.

Educational Resources Available to Aid Bereaved Children and Their Families

The New York University Child Study Center created a Web site (available at: www.aboutourkids.org) dedicated to advancing the field of child mental health through evidence-based practice, science, and education. Using the search engine on the site to look up information on bereavement, users can gain access to a list of books on bereavement, war, terrorism, and tolerance targeted at children of all ages, parents, and professionals.

National Child Traumatic Stress Network Guideline on Managing Childhood Traumatic Grief

The National Child Traumatic Stress Network, a consortium of treatment and research centers across the United States, provides an online guideline (available at: http://www.nctsnet.org/nccts/nav.do?pid=hom_main). The network comprises 70 member centers—45 current grantees and 25 previous grantees —funded by the Center for Mental Health Services, Substance Abuse and Mental Health Services Administration, US Department of Health and Human Services, through a congressional initiative—the Donald J Cohen National Child Traumatic Stress Initiative. This initiative recognizes the profound, destructive, and widespread impact of trauma on American children's lives and seeks to improve the quality, effectiveness, provision, and availability of therapeutic services delivered to all children and adolescents experiencing traumatic events.

Department of Defense Military Assistance Program

The Military Assistance Program (available at: http://dod.mil/mapsite/) aims to provide information and interactive resources for assisting military families with relocation, money management, and job search at a new location.

Operation Special Delivery

Operation Special Delivery (available at: http://www.operationspecialdelivery.com) provides trained volunteer doulas for pregnant women whose husbands or partners have been severely injured or who have lost their lives due to the current war on terror, or who will be deployed at the time they are due to give birth. The doulas are informational, emotional, and physical coaches, not medical providers.

SGT Mom's

SGT Mom's (available at: http://www.family-networks.org/military. cfm) is an interactive Web site created in 1996 and run by a military spouse who handles all e-mails, updates, and additions. It is not an official Department of Defense site and is not related to any official military organization. The Web site contains a communication forum, links to other sites, the latest news about military families, ways to support troops, and a question-and-answer section. SGT Mom's is "military life explained by a military wife."

The National Long Distance Relationship Building Institute (Dads at a Distance)

As stated on the homepage, the Dads at a Distance Web site (available at: http://www.daads.com) was created "to help fathers who are business travelers, military men, non-custodial fathers, airline pilots, travel guides, traveling salesmen, railroad workers, truckers, professional athletes, musicians, entertainers, actors, corporate executives, or any other fathers who have to be away from their children to maintain and strengthen their relationships with their children while they are away." The Web site provides tips for long-distance fathers, links to related Web sites, information on relevant products and books, and stories of long-distance fathering.

The Tragedy Assistance Program for Survivors

The Tragedy Assistance Program for Survivors, or TAPS (Available at: http://www.TAPS.org) was founded after the deaths of eight soldiers aboard an Army National Guard aircraft in November 1992. TAPS provides a support network for the surviving families of those who have died in service to America. To accomplish their mission, TAPS has experienced caseworkers who act as liaisons, assisting the family members in finding solutions to problems. TAPS' small professional staff and a large national volunteer network work hand-in-hand with federal, state, and private agencies in finding solutions to problems of surviving military families.

The Building Strong and Ready Families Program

This is a 2-day program that helps couples develop better communication skills, reinforced by a weekend retreat. Additional information is available at http://www.strongbonds.org/skins/strongbonds/display.aspx.

The PICK (Premarital Interpersonal Choices and Knowledge) a Partner Program

This program helps single soldiers make wise decisions when they choose mates.

Additional Phone Numbers and Web Sites

Army Military Family Research Institute: http://www.mfri.purdue.edu/pages/news/soldier_family_well_being.html
Army OneSource: 1-800-464-8107; http://www.armyonesource.com (User ID: army; Password: onesource)
Department of Veterans Affairs: http://www.va.gov
National Center for PTSD: http://www.ncptsd.org/
Deployment Health Clinical Center: 1-800-796-9699; http://www.pdhealth.mil
HOOAH4HEALTH—Deployment: http://www.hooah4health.com/deployment/default.htm
Institute of Medicine—Health of Veterans and Deployed Forces: http://veterans.iom.edu/
Operations Noble Eagle, Enduring Freedom, and Iraqi Freedom: http://www.odcsper.army.mil/default.asp?pageeid+37
Reserve Affairs—Mobilization and Demobilization: http://www.defenselink.mil/ra/html/mobilization.html
Veterans Benefits Administration: 1-800-827-1000
Veterans Health Administration: 1-800-222-8387

Chapter 31

THE CHILDREN AND FAMILIES OF COMBAT-INJURED SERVICE MEMBERS

STEPHEN J. COZZA, MD*; RYO S. CHUN, MD†; AND CORINA MILLER, MSW‡

*Colonel (Retired), US Army; Associate Director, Center for the Study of Traumatic Stress, and Professor, Department of Psychiatry, Uniformed Services University of the Health Sciences, 4301 Jones Bridge Road, Bethesda, Maryland 20814; formerly, Chief, Department of Psychiatry, Walter Reed Army Medical Center, Washington, DC

†Colonel (Retired), US Army; Clinical Director, Child and Adolescent Psychiatry Service, Department of Psychiatry, Walter Reed Army Medical Center, 6900 Georgia Avenue NW, Washington, DC 20307; formerly, Chief, Child and Adolescent Psychiatry Service, Department of Psychiatry, Walter Reed Army Medical Center, Washington, DC

‡Clinical Social Worker, Department of Psychiatry, Walter Reed Army Medical Center, Building 2, Office #6317, 6900 Georgia Avenue NW, Washington, DC 20307-5001; formerly, Clinical Social Worker, National Naval Medical Center, Bethesda, Maryland

INTRODUCTION

As of July 2008, over 30,000 soldiers, sailors, marines, and airmen have been injured in ongoing operations in Iraq and Afghanistan.[1] A substantial number of these injuries have been serious, resulting in limb amputations, severe soft-tissue and orthopaedic injuries, traumatic brain injuries (TBIs), eye enucleations, and body burns.[2] The effect of these severe injuries on families, parents, and children is not easily ascertained, but will likely be determined by the functional consequences of the injuries. Even when physical recovery is complete, families can be profoundly affected by the injury of a parent. Because 40% of US service members (SMs) have children, averaging about two children per parent,[3] the authors estimate that approximately 24,000 military children have been affected by serious combat-related parental injuries within that same time period. These numbers do not reflect the many other nondependent children whose siblings or other military family members have been injured.

Case reports have described the anecdotal experience of combat-injured families and children.[4,5] The effects appear complex, particularly with children. From the initial distress to the longer-term injury adjustment challenges, children and families face difficult emotional and practical problems. These phenomena have been described and are being addressed in several clinical treatment centers and studied through ongoing research. However, no empirical data have yet been systematically collected examining the effect of combat injury on families. Such investigation is required to inform intervention and treatment planning across the injury-to-recovery timeline. In addition, no family- or parent-focused interventions have been uniformly implemented and no evidence-based treatments developed and evaluated. This chapter describes the clinical experience and insights of mental health practitioners who have been involved with the children and families of the combat injured at Walter Reed Army Medical Center (WRAMC) in Washington, DC, a major military medical center that has been treating injured SMs since the start of global war on terror combat operations.

BACKGROUND LITERATURE

Although no literature exists that systematically examines the effect of parental combat injury on military children, other areas of scientific literature help the understanding of this population. Several types of parental illness have been carefully studied, including parental cancer.[6–9] In these studies, children's emotional and functional responsiveness were affected by their age and gender. A recent study examined the influence of parental multiple sclerosis (MS) on the adjustment of children and adolescents as measured by parental report.[10] The authors found that children of MS parents showed greater difficulty in relating interpersonally and in managing their lives when compared to non-MS children. They also evidenced higher levels of distress, but did not show elevated levels of emotional or behavioral symptoms indicative of psychopathology.

Family function is central to the child's response to parental illness.[11–14] A family's capacity to maintain structure, to provide emotional support, and to diminish distress all appear to help children adjust to parental illness. The level of parental disability is also a principal factor affecting children's responses to parental illness.[15–19] As with many family stresses, children's responses tend to mirror the distress and functional capacity of the important adults in their lives. Whether the seriousness of the illness or resultant parental disability has a greater influence on child functioning and emotional response is less well understood. In either case, these findings highlight the importance of adopting intervention models that improve family and parental functioning when parental health problems exist, to support the health and well-being of children.

Sudden health-altering events, such as combat injury, may have more profound effects on children and families than parental illness. Families have very little time to prepare for the consequences of sudden injuries. The noninjured parents must often make rapid decisions about childcare, or may be so preoccupied by the needs of the injured partner that they are too overwhelmed to address the needs of children.

Of the few studies that have examined the effect of sudden medical events on families, those related to TBI are most instructive.[20–25] TBI often has a profound effect on children and families,[25] with greater difficulty in families with young children, those with lesser social or financial support, or where psychiatric problems are prominent. Elevated levels of emotional and behavioral symptoms in children of TBI patients correlate with compromised parenting in both the injured and noninjured parent, as well as depression in the noninjured parent, suggesting the importance of healthy family and parental functioning to protect children's mental health.[22] Strategies that support such outcomes appear warranted; however, no established family-focused interventions have been empirically studied in TBI populations. In addition, there has been no scientific examination of the psychological effect of parental burns, amputation, or motor vehicle accidents on children that would help in the understanding of the experiences of combat-injured families.

From the initial distress to the longer-term injury adjustment challenges, the children and families of the combat injured face difficult emotional and practical problems. It is likely that the effects of combat parental injury on children are more complicated and potentially more challenging than nonviolent and accident-related injuries. Often immediate information regarding the nature and severity of the injury is limited, and sometimes inaccurate, causing further anxiety. Injuries sustained in combat are likely to result in sudden family distress and a flurry of urgent activity, leading to disruption of family roles, sources of care, and instrumental support. Over time, the consequences of parental injury and required treatment also include changes in the child's residential community, loss of military career by the parent, and changes in parenting capacity. The cascade of events following injury is graphically portrayed in Figure 31-1.

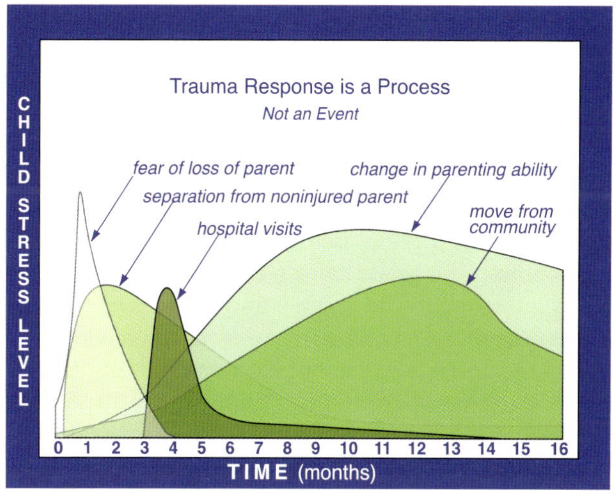

Figure 31-1. Child response to events resulting from combat injury.
Drawing courtesy of: Center for the Study of Traumatic Stress, Uniformed Services University of the Health Sciences, Bethesda, Maryland

Any serious physical injury may result in the development of comorbid psychiatric symptoms,[26] as well as physical injuries. Longitudinal data suggest that combat-injured SMs may develop complicating psychiatric problems, such as posttraumatic stress disorder (PTSD) and depression.[27] Mental health symptoms may present a variable course, resolving or commonly worsening during the first year after hospitalization.[2]

In addition to moderate or severe TBI, researchers have voiced concern about the influence of milder forms of TBI that may not come to medical attention, but can result in serious dysfunction or sense of ill health.[28] When mild TBI is comorbid with other physical injuries, families may contend with the complication of dealing with a parent with psychiatric illness, cognitive or personality alterations, as well as physical injury. When significant changes in parental ability result from injury, parents and children must renegotiate family relationships and integrate the reality of the injury, whether physical, psychological, or both, and its consequences. Continued scientific investigation is required to develop effective preventive interventions that address both short- and long-term effects of these parental injuries.

NOTIFICATION OF INJURY

SM families are faced with multiple challenges, beginning the day the SM receives notification about a combat deployment. These challenges continue through the deployment cycle and can include many changes within the family system resulting from the SM's absence (See Chapter 30, The Impact of Deployment on Military Families and Children). When SMs are injured, facing the threat of permanent bodily changes or reductions in their physical, cognitive, or psychological functions, greater distress is unavoidable.

Family stress begins with notification of the SM's injury. Although there have been improvements in the process of injury notification (eg, when possible, injured SMs may contact a spouse or other family member directly, relieving their loved ones of the worst fear of imminent death), it is not uncommon that initial information pertaining to an injury may be incomplete or inaccurate, leading to even greater worry. Occasionally, information that a member of a military unit has been injured is communicated through informal channels, causing broad confusion and anxiety on the home front. Only when accurate information about the personnel involved and the details of the injury are known is some relief achieved. The manner in which the information of the injury is related to the spouse and family varies significantly from spouse to spouse and unit to unit. Typically, the accuracy and detail of available information, as well as the mode of its communication, reflect the unique circumstances of the injury. Injury notification may be conducted either in person or by telephone.

Several clinical examples help to illustrate. One spouse of an injured SM recalled that she had been visited at home by two rear detachment officers dressed in Army combat uniforms. While the sight of these visitors at her door raised concern about her husband's health, she also noted with great relief that they were not dressed in the formal Class A uniform, indicating that they were not part of a death notification team. Another spouse spoke about how she received telephonic notification of her husband's injury while she was driving. Before relating the news of the injury, the caller made certain that she had pulled off the road, stopped the engine, and was in a safe area, to ensure that she was not in danger of having a motor vehicle accident as a result of receiving the frightening news. Another spouse spoke about having received three separate phone calls from three different offices that related different versions of her husband's injury. Even the simplest inaccuracies can undermine a family's confidence in the care that an SM may receive after an injury, and are often remembered and related by spouses or other family members in the hospital setting. Family members typically describe the most reassuring and trusted information coming from the face-to-face visits of familiar members of their injured SM's unit, rather than from telephone callers who are unknown to them.

Communicating With Children About the Injury

Whether injury notification occurs on the phone or in person, children may be present when news of the injury is shared with adult family members. Children may witness the response of their non-SM parents or other adults, who may become extremely distressed, tearful, or emotionally volatile. When possible, children should be protected from viewing the raw adult emotional response to such news because it can be both confusing and overwhelming. Also, when possible, information should be shared with adults first, so that they can be better emotionally prepared for a discussion with their children that is based on accurate information.

Most adults understand that some information should be shared with children whose parents or close relatives have been injured in combat. It is recommended that all children should be given some explanation to better understand the emotions and behaviors that they see in the adults around them. Depending upon their age and psychological and cognitive abilities, children have different capacities to understand and tolerate sensitive and disturbing news. The amount and type of information that adults share should be based upon the developmental capacity of any given child. Older children and teens are generally capable of understanding and accepting more details, including the cause of the injury, the nature and degree of the physical wounds, the plan for treatment, and the likely effect on the family (eg, expected family separations, visits to the hospital, and changes in childcare arrangements). Adults may be more circumspect about the details that they share with preschoolers or early elementary school children. In some circumstances, facts may be briefly withheld from young children until a parent's immediate survivability is determined. Although infants and toddlers are not cognitively capable of understanding the injury of a SM parent, they will quickly respond to perceived changes in the emotional climate of a household, changes in behavior or availability of any adult childcare providers, or disruptions in their daily schedules or routines. The most important communication to children of any age is that, despite the news of the injury, they will be cared for and that important adults will remain available to them.

It is not recommended that children over the age of 5 or 6 years not be told about an injury for an extended period of time because they are likely to overhear adult conversations or recognize changes in adult behavior that will cause them to worry that something is wrong. Adults should never conduct conversations about the injury within the earshot of children assuming they do not understand. Typically, children will listen and be interested in everything that is discussed. When children ask questions, they should be answered matter-of-factly and with the level of information that seems appropriate and desired by the child. Children should be given permission to ask questions and understand that those questions will be respected and answered truthfully, to the degree that is possible. Sometimes the questions that children ask do not have known answers, in which case adults should say that they do not know. Not uncommonly, children and teenagers may worry that their injured SM parent may die. When an injured SM has stabilized and is not at risk of death, children should be quickly reassured. In situations when health status is precarious, adults should be careful not to unrealistically reassure children. Adults can offer a hopeful message such as, "Dad was hurt very badly, but he is being given the best treatment possible to help him get better."

Often non-SM parents or other adults have trouble gauging what to tell their children. Adults sometimes struggle with their own emotional reactions, which may make it particularly difficult for them to determine what is appropriate to pass on to children. These adults may need help processing and calibrating the amount, content, and timing of the facts that they share. Their description of the injury and its consequences may be based more on their own anxiety than on the needs of the children. Some noninjured parents may choose to share either too much or too little, making it difficult for children to understand the nature or seriousness of the injury and its realistic implications for the injured parent. Knowledgeable professionals should offer parental guidance when needed.

Some adults may choose to withhold important information related to serious injuries from children in an attempt "not to worry them." In such circumstances, clinicians need to challenge the assumption that such "secrets" can realistically be kept from children. The clinician should communicate that even younger children can be given some explanation without causing them to become overly worried, and may help them understand the actions and emotions of the adults they see around them. Just as some parents may provide too little information about the injury, others share more than children are able to tolerate. This may frighten them by unnecessarily bringing up unknown future consequences. The foundation of the clinician's helpful stance toward the families and children of the injured is to increase adult awareness and to help them notice and respond appropriately to children's emotional signals.

All children require some patient adult assistance to better integrate their understanding of serious injuries. Psychologically minded adults implicitly understand this need and may demonstrate tremendous creativity and sensitivity in meeting the needs of young children. As an example, one mother made a thoughtful and developmentally informed decision not to bring her nearly 3-year-old son to visit his seriously injured father until he was no longer intubated, so that the boy could hear his father's voice when first meeting him in the hospital. This sensitive decision enabled the young child to relate with his father in the ways he was accustomed to despite the seriousness of the father's injuries.

Travel to Military Medical Facilities and Family Separations

Once the family has been notified of the injury, a period of intense activity typically follows, often leading to disruptions in the family's schedule or structure. Spouses usually join injured SMs being treated at military hospitals distant from the family home. When necessary, they leave their children under the supervision of other adults either at home or at the homes of other family members or friends in local or distant communities. Sometimes children are uprooted to join parents at the hospital. All these options are likely to be unsettling, particularly for young children, with resultant disruptions of routines and relationships.

Recommendations cannot be broadly made about where children should be cared for when family separations are necessary. When an injury is serious, military spouses might fly alone to join their injured SMs at military medical centers. Spouses must plan for the care of their children and the maintenance of their households while they quickly arrange trips to distant locations, not infrequently overseas. Planning can be complicated as noninjured parents may not know how long they will be away from home. Some spouses make the choice to bring their children with them while others make interim arrangements for childcare with friends or neighbors, or send their children to stay with relatives in distant places for uncertain periods of time. In some cases, families must split the children, due to age, logistical requirements, or because of custody agreements (stepchildren). Siblings may stay with friends, while others move in with relatives. In such circumstances, children are not only separated from their parents, homes, and routines, they are also separated from their siblings, adding distress. Some families are fortunate enough to have their extended families move into their homes with their children, resulting in less disruption. Decisions about childcare and separations are never simple and often can result in parental confusion and guilt as they try to meet competing responsibilities. The following two vignettes provide examples of the complexity of military family situations and the solutions that families found.

Vignette 31-1: Shirlene, the mother of a seriously injured SM, was staying with her son at a military medical center across the country from her home in Washington state. She had been with her injured son since his admission and was torn between staying at the hospital or going home. Her younger daughter, Candace, who was living at home with her stepfather, had requested that Shirlene return home to celebrate the daughter's birthday. Shirlene was hesitant to leave her son's bedside, but was encouraged by the treatment team to visit with her daughter. During the few days that they visited, Candace had the opportunity to talk with her mother about some problems that she was having with friends. She didn't want to burden Shirlene during their phone calls, and she didn't feel comfortable talking with her stepfather about these problems. Shirlene's decision to leave the hospital had been difficult, but upon her return she recognized the importance of this visit and was pleased that she had decided to make it.

Although the decision for children to stay with parents at the hospital can be a helpful way of maintaining the integrity and support of families, many families appropriately choose to have children remain at home. The following example describes how decisions are often complicated and emotionally difficult.

Vignette 31-2: John was injured in an improvised explosive device (IED) blast that resulted in multiple soft-tissue injuries, an upper-extremity amputation, and severe TBI. He and his young wife Miriam were parents of a 10-month-old daughter, Sarah. Miriam had made the decision for Sarah to stay with her parents in Oklahoma during the hospitalization. John's initial prognosis was described as poor and he was not expected to walk or talk again. Miriam, his wife of 2 years, was quite devoted to him and made the decision to remain with him and be there for his ongoing therapies. She received criticism from hospital staff and from some other patients' wives for her decision to leave their young child with her parents. However, she knew that her daughter was in a stable environment with people who loved her. Miriam wanted to provide ongoing support to her husband, something she felt no one else was able to do. The presence of Sarah would have made it hard to give John the care she felt he deserved.

THE HOSPITALIZATION

Duration of hospitalization of combat-injured SMs can vary in length, based upon the type and seriousness of the injury. Critical specialty care services are available at most major military medical centers. Because many war-related injuries are extensive, the care of patients can be time consuming, often requiring months to years of hospital-based treatment and rehabilitative services. Within the hospital setting both formal and informal supports and services are available. Specialty care units, such as the US Army Institute of Surgical Research Burn Unit at Brooke Army Medical Center, San Antonio, Texas, provide specialized care. The course of treatment for the severely injured can be unpredictable, involving multiple surgeries, as well as other treatment procedures and intensive therapies. As a result, treatment plans must be fluid and can change, leading to disappointment in both patients and their families.

Injured patients cannot be effectively treated within the hospital setting without understanding and addressing the needs of families. Loved ones understandably want to spend time with their injured SMs, especially when their health status may be uncertain or when they are undergoing complicated or painful treatments. Some family members may choose to remain in hospital rooms for extended periods of time or even continuously. Although healthcare teams recognize the importance of family member involvement, and work to incorporate families into the overall treatment plan, their presence can also complicate the ability to provide effective care. Family members who have feelings of anger or frustration related to the injury may misdirect those emotions toward the treatment team. Families may also bring preexisting emotional conflicts and challenges or interpersonal difficulties into the hospital setting. It is essential that medical teams recognize and address family conflicts to find resolutions that support effective treatment.

Many military families are nontraditional in their composition. Marital separations and divorces, as well as the young age of many injured SMs, can lead to conflicts between spouses, former spouses, girlfriends, boyfriends, and parents, all of whom may visit the hospital. Due to the stress of the injury, conflict not uncommonly develops along these fracture lines and can lead to interpersonal clashes within the healthcare setting, making treatment more difficult. In young SMs with serious injuries, disagreements can develop between the SMs' mothers, who respond to the regressive needs of their incapacitated sons or daughters, and young spouses who can feel like intruders to the parent–child relationship. Spouses may second guess their commitments to SMs who now are to be permanently altered by the injury. Marital dissolution and divorce are not rare. Sometimes parents, particularly mothers, can unfairly criticize spouses who they believe will abandon their injured children. Legal questions can arise as a result of these conflicts; for example, who in the family will hold medical decision-making capacity or who will be the recipient of insurance or government disability payments?

Marriages are not always healthy or functional prior to the combat deployment or injury. Military family members struggle with many of the same family challenges that all Americans face. Marital conflict, separation, divorce, and infidelity occur. When these problems are present prior to deployment, an injury only compounds them. The case below describes an example.

Case Study 31-1: Peter, a marine, was treated at a military medical center for a left-side below-the-knee amputation. While in Afghanistan he was called by his wife Diane on his birthday, 2 months before his injury. Peter was quite pleased until he heard a voice in the background saying, "Tell him you're engaged and wearing my ring. Tell him the marriage is over." It was in this way he learned that Diane was having an affair. She had also emptied their bank account and sold their home using the power of attorney Peter had provided when he began the deployment. Peter and Diane had a 4-year-old son and 18-month-old daughter. Peter was unable to get in touch with them and didn't know whether they ever learned of his injury. Having been served divorce papers and with no place to return, Peter left the hospital to live on his father's farm in Iowa. He said he would have liked his children to receive counseling to make sure they were handling their new life well but he didn't have the physical ability to pursue this nor did he have the financial ability to fight for custody.

Complicated family situations can affect children as well as adults. When the injured SM is divorced and a child resides with a former spouse with whom the SM sponsor has a conflict-laden relationship, hospital visits or telephone calls with the injured parent become major events to negotiate. When the military parent is remarried, the discussions can become even more difficult because the current spouse, the divorced parent of the children, or other former in-laws may not get along. When families are unable to resolve these differences, clinicians should serve as facilitators to negotiate communication and visitation.

Military family situations can be complex even when relationships are not conflicted. Regulations governing marriage within the military are legally determined and therefore can lack the flexibility that families sometimes wish would be possible. The following case provides an example.

Case Study 31-2: Steven, a transportation driver in the Army, suffered a TBI in Iraq from an IED while he was driving in a convoy. Steven and his wife, Cathy, had divorced prior to his deployment but began working out their differences by e-mail and phone while he was in Iraq and planned to remarry upon his return. They had two children, ages 9 and 12 years. After the injury, Cathy and the children joined Steven at the hospital. However, Steven was listed as "divorced" on all his paperwork and Cathy, unlike other married military spouses, had no rights and was provided no financial compensation for her stay in a hotel close to the hospital. The medical staff members were reluctant to speak with Cathy because she and Steven were divorced. Steven was given written instructions and would lose them. He wanted to pass on information to Cathy but he would forget because of his TBI. Consequently, there were periods of time when he was considered noncompliant, and uninterested and unmotivated in his recovery. During the hospitalization the couple remarried, allowing Cathy and the children access to housing and her greater involvement in the medical care. Prior to the remarriage a well-meaning but misguided administrator counseled Steven that perhaps Cathy only wanted to remarry him because of the money he would be getting from military disability. The family found this to be quite inappropriate and unsupportive.

The following vignette provides another example of a stressful military family situation.

Vignette 31-3: Beth, a divorced mother of three, was injured as a result of crossfire during a small arms firefight. She was hospitalized for sustained injuries to her chest and upper extremities. Beth was injured 9 months into a 12-month deployment with a National Guard unit from the Midwest. Because of her medical treatment, Beth's activation was extended well beyond the original 12-month period. In addition to two biological children, ages 10 and 12, she had a 13-year-old foster daughter. All three children remained with a caregiver in Beth's hometown. Because Beth was the agency-approved foster mother, her ongoing medical care and extended deployment caused the foster daughter to be returned to the agency where another foster home had to be found. This loss was an additional disruption because the foster child had become an important member of the family.

The needs of a family can change dramatically during the course of hospitalization. Attendance to these needs can be extremely supportive to both the SM and family as treatment and rehabilitation progress. Families sometimes require help finding adequate housing, particularly when long-term family stays are required. Questions can arise and practical assistance may be necessary regarding childcare, family health, or educational needs. Familiarity with military regulations and coordination of appropriate paperwork to ensure financial support, adequate housing, and travel arrangements and support are all necessary for military family success during extended combat-injury treatments. Some families are able to demonstrate a tremendous amount of resourcefulness and identify independent ways to meet their own needs. Many others require help through the Family Assistance Center, social work services, or through active case management.

The Psychiatric Consultation Liaison Service (PCLS) at WRAMC has developed a system of care—Preventive Medical Psychiatry (PMP)—that includes ongoing clinical consultation to injured SMs and their families.[29,30] Through PMP, all injured SMs are seen without the need for traditional consultation from the primary treatment team. Patients are told that members of the PCLS routinely see all those who were injured and that PCLS is part of the trauma team. As a result, PMP is met with little patient or family resistance. The major goals of PMP are to place psychological reactions within an appropriate context, to support and encourage healthy defenses, and to monitor for development of psychiatric disorders. Identified posttraumatic symptoms are explained as expected responses to combat and injury, rather than being viewed as necessarily pathological. In addition, PMP serves secondary and tertiary prevention efforts through posthospitalization identification and treatment of at-risk or symptomatic SMs. (For more information see Chapter 16, Psychiatric Intervention for the Battle-Injured Medical-Surgical Patients Following Traumatic Injuries.)

In addition to PMP, PCLS social workers also provide family assistance. Family support services must be individually based, addressing the needs of any particular family in crisis at any given time. Many solutions are met through referral to resources in the surrounding civilian and military communities. Sometimes, effective interventions require more personal professional involvement using creative social work skills, a willingness to get personally involved, and a readiness to "work outside of the box." As examples, WRAMC PCLS social workers have called Operation First Response for portable cribs and have found car seats for spouses who have precipitously flown into town without them. Social workers have arranged for baby items for couples with newborns who were not financially prepared and needed to fully equip a new nursery. Most families are disorganized when they first arrive at the hospital. They may come to the hospital without their automated teller machine (ATM) cards, other bank cards, or their military or other identification cards. Some go months before they can access their pay. Medical treatment centers must expect these problems and attend to them as they would the medical care that is afforded the SMs.

The following vignette is an example of how family needs can arise during hospitalizations.

Vignette 31-4: Enrico, a US Marine from California, was injured by sniper fire to his eye and upper extremity, resulting in eye enucleation and arm amputation. Eventually, 6 months into the hospitalization, Enrico was able to arrange for his fiancée, Maria, to join him from Puerto Rico. They were married shortly thereafter and Maria became pregnant. She precipitously delivered a premature infant at 25-weeks gestation at a local civilian hospital after visiting their emergency room; the infant required a lengthy stay in a neonatal intensive care unit. Maria did not speak English fluently and, therefore, had difficulty communicating the complex healthcare needs of her family to civilian providers. Active military social work assistance was required to coordinate services between Enrico's treatment and the needs of the couple's newborn. Special arrangements were made for vouchers that allowed the couple to travel between the military medical center and the civilian hospital as they were unable to afford these costs. In addition, the social worker coordinated with Army Community Service to ensure that nursery equipment was delivered to Maria's temporary housing unit when their newborn eventually left the hospital.

Other innovative solutions have been developed by PCLS social workers. To help support the family members, a group—Girls Time Out (GTO)—has been meeting weekly since January 2005 at WRAMC. GTO's mission is to provide a forum to support the wives, mothers, sisters, female friends, and fiancées of injured SMs. Group members meet, talk, eat, and learn from one another. They occasionally invite guests who present pertinent information to the group. For the past several years, GTO members have gotten together during the holiday season and made cookies using kitchens available in both Occupational Therapy and Army Community Service. This activity has allowed the women to make and share their favorite seasonal treats while getting away from the hospital setting for a few hours.

Finally, the importance of understanding and attending to family cultural differences cannot be overestimated. Recognizing how different races and ethnicities respond to trauma is quite important. For example, Latinos have been observed to be more "hands on" with their injured loved ones. Very often Latino family members touch injured patients and talk to them regardless of their seeming unresponsiveness. Family members will include the injured in prayers (eg, rosaries, novenas), instruct them, talk to them as they shave them, and give them the latest family news. For non-Latino healthcare providers, these cultural methods may seem foreign. Unfortunately, family members can inadvertently feel demeaned by their sense of the disapproval of the medical staff.

Relationships between family members and the healthcare team can become further complicated when language barriers exist. Some of the Latino family members may believe that their observations are not accepted because they do not speak English. It is as though their comments are tainted by ignorance simply because they are not bilingual. The following vignette provides an example.

Vignette 31-5: Geraldo was wounded by an IED in Iraq and was transported for further medical treatment while in a coma. His mother, Sonia, remained at his bedside and continued to talk to him and to pray out loud. There were times when she felt he was listening to her but was unable to respond. The medical staff continued to tell her not to expect too much and kindly explained that he could not hear her and had no awareness. Although Sonia did not speak English, she understood the looks the medical staff gave her and knew they did not believe her, but this did not deter her and she continued stimulating Geraldo throughout the day and late into the night. She was quite excited on the day after Christmas when she reported that Geraldo had whispered, "Feliz Navidad" on Christmas Eve, but no one believed her. The clinical social worker supported Sonia in her belief that Geraldo had spoken, despite the medical team's skepticism, and encouraged her to continue what she was doing. Ultimately, Geraldo came out of the coma and told his mother he knew she had been with him around the clock. He told her that he had sensed her in his "sleep" and stated that he recognized and was comforted by her perfume, one that she had used throughout his life. Geraldo was also able to relate conversations that had been held in his room while he was in the coma.

CHILDREN IN THE HOSPITAL SETTING

Recognizing and meeting the needs of children within general hospital settings is complex. Most pediatric hospitals have developed effective ways of engaging children and recognizing and meeting them at their developmental levels. Hospitals that provide care to adult populations have been much less effective in planning for the presence of children. Because children are important members of military families, the identification of, and attention to, their unique developmental needs is key if engagement with combat-injured families is to be effective.

When the family of a combat-injured patient arrives at the hospital, the noninjured parent must navigate the medical environment and military system while being available to their injured military service member. Noninjured spouses often are inundated by the requirements they face, and thus the needs of their children can go unmet. When children arrive at the hospital, they can quickly become overwhelmed by the hospital's size and complexity. Young parents may have little understanding of how to best prepare their children for the hospital setting and how to prepare them for the visits with their injured parents.

Family members can have a difficult time with children's activity levels, leading to frustration and unnecessary harshness. Younger children can be loud and boisterous. They may get negative feedback from parents or hospital staff members, leaving them to feel that they are not wanted. Children may also be viewed as obstacles to care. Hospital and nursing personnel typically do not know how to engage younger children. They can benefit from simple recommendations that can make a child's visit much more pleasant. For example, one 4-year-old boy was repeatedly making loud noises and gestures in the hospital that were disturbing other patients and hospital staff members. His parents and grandmother were embarrassed by the behavior and became engaged in a heated and public emotional exchange. After a discussion with Child and Adolescent Psychiatry Service (CAPS) staff, they were helped to recognize that the child had his own ways of expressing worries and needed time to play and unwind outside of the hospital setting.

Children's presence within the hospital should be time limited and structured. Medical centers that provide care to injured service members should ensure that there are appropriate areas for family activities that are "child and family friendly." Specific plans need to be put in place that allow children to be present and involved in their parent's care, while preparing and protecting them from what they are likely to see in the hospital setting. Because of the many injured SMs being treated at military medical centers, children can not only be exposed to their own parent's frightening medical condition, but also the burns, amputations, and serious injuries of those other SMs receiving care. Recommendations for healthcare treatment facilities' support of families of the combat injured are outlined in Exhibit 31-1.

Parents can assist children to prepare for, and comfortably participate in, hospital visits. When possible, it is helpful for parents to settle into the hospital routine alone, before children arrive. If children must accompany parents to the hospital at the first visit, it is best that children remain in the hotel or other living quarters while the noninjured parent gets to know the hospital environment. Parents can help their children understand what they may see or be exposed to. In order to do this, parents must first integrate the experience themselves. The opportunity for parents to describe what the hospital looks like, where it is located, who are the members of the treatment team, the appearance of the hospital room, and the names of individuals with whom the injured parent may share a room, will all help to orient a child to this new setting. When possible, parents can also show children pictures of the hospital, the ward, the hospital room, and their injured SM parent to best prepare them for what they will see when they come.

Preparation for the meeting with the injured parent is a continuation of the discussion that began with injury notification and continues throughout the hospitalization and recovery period. Children typically want to know what is happening and what they can expect when they come to the hospital. Noninjured parents can best accomplish this by gauging the appropriate amount of injury-related information (presence of bandages, casts, amputations, or medical equipment) and mixing the discussion with descriptions of less anxiety-provoking topics, such as the hospital cafeteria, the kind of food that they can eat while in the hospital, or the hotel or living quarters. With proper planning most children will feel comfortable when the time for the visit arrives. It is particularly important to carefully prepare children when dramatic changes in a parent's appearance occur, such as facial wounds or serious burns. The following vignette describes how one couple successfully met their young child's needs.

Vignette 31-6: Teddy was a 3½-year-old boy whose father, Bill, had been deployed to Iraq for 6 months when he was wounded in an IED explosion. The father sustained serious injuries to his face and upper extremities requiring unilateral facial bandaging and resulting in an inability to effectively use his arms and hands. On the day of Teddy's first visit with his father, his mother spent several minutes explaining the nature of the injuries and what he was likely to see upon entering his father's room, to include the presence of facial bandages, as well as his father's hoarse and somewhat unrecognizable voice. Teddy became very excited about the prospect of seeing his father. When they entered the room Teddy became silent and transfixed by his father's appearance. While his mother tried to reassure him, Teddy cautiously approached his father and carefully climbed on Bill's lap when invited. Instinctively, Bill began jostling Teddy between his legs, a game they had played often prior to

EXHIBIT 31-1

TREATMENT FACILITIES' SUPPORT OF FAMILIES OF THE COMBAT INJURED

Recognize the contributions of families as part of treatment and establish appropriate boundaries for involvement

Develop child- and family-friendly treatment environments
- Welcome children and families
- Families don't VISIT, they PARTICIPATE in care
- Develop appropriate areas for family visiting: in room, on ward, off ward, dining area, family lounge
- Develop child-appropriate environments within the hospital
- Ensure adequate available family lodging
- Consider child life worker involvement within the hospital

Protect children from unnecessary exposures
- Educate healthcare providers about child developmental issues and exposure risks
- Develop a systematic methodology to prepare children for hospital visits
- Support parents in parenting role and encourage them to speak with their children about health status

Develop family intervention strategies
- Watch for and address intrafamilial conflicts
- Consider multifamily or spouse group involvement
- Recognize the role of bereavement in family transition
- Actively address expected role changes within the family, especially in TBI and polytrauma victims

Monitor for "at risk" family situations
- Traumatic brain injury
- Polytrauma victims
- Marital or intrafamilial strife/domestic violence
- Substance use problems
- Signs of spousal or parental disengagement

Rally resources to aid
- Practical assistance
- Military Severely Injured Program
- Veterans Administration resources—Seamless Transition
- Military OneSource
- Military treatment facilities/TRICARE
- Self-help and other support organizations

the deployment. The familiarity of this activity eased Teddy, who immediately relaxed and began talking with Bill in a more natural and comfortable way. Recognizing the stress that Teddy faced, his mother limited the amount of time that Teddy stayed in the hospital setting and ensured that he spent considerable time at the hotel pool.

SUPPORT TO COMBAT-INJURED FAMILIES WITH CHILDREN

To better meet the needs of the families and children of injured SMs, the CAPS at WRAMC has established a system of care in which clinicians actively engage families of combat-injured SMs. CAPS staff members are informed of the pending arrival of the families of injured SMs by official notification. Clinicians provide an informational briefing to incoming families during their orientation at the Family Assistance Center, at which time they are given general information about CAPS services and how they can access care for identified problems. Families are also notified that they will be contacted by CAPS providers within the immediate future. This contact is typically made within 1 week of arrival at WRAMC.

Available CAPS services include anticipatory parental guidance to the injured SM and spouse, assistance in preparing children for their visit to the hospital (to include how and what they should be told in anticipation of seeing their wounded parent for the first time), supportive reassurance, anxiety relief, and connection to appropriate resources when required. CAPS staff members work collaboratively with WRAMC PCLS at the hospital bedside. CAPS staff members also provide therapeutic activities to the children living at the Fisher and Malone Houses, where families reside during SM treatment, and at the Military Advanced Training Center, where wounded SMs and their families participate in outpatient occupational and physical rehabilitation. Services are offered in an outreach or "preclinical" format to support healthy family recovery. The goals of the intervention are to assist the reunion of the injured SM family, to promote children's mastery of the complex and stressful injury experience, and to facilitate and promote the rehabilitation process of the injured parent by acknowledging the integral and essential role of parenting in the SM's life. By interacting with families from early in their arrival and developing trusting relationships, CAPS strives to assist families to avert potential difficulties and support their comfort in accepting additional services when indicated. When deemed appropriate, children and families requiring clinical assessment or treatment are referred to the outpatient mental health clinic for formal assessment.

At WRAMC and Brooke Army Medical Center, mental health clinicians have begun using the Parent Guidance Assessment–Combat Injured (PGA–CI) instrument as a mechanism to assist in conducting discussions with injured SMs and their spouses about the needs of their families (especially their children) in response to the combat injury. A copy of the PGA-CI is included in Attachment 1. This semistructured clinical interview is designed to assess family demographics, deployment experience, nature of the combat injury, intrafamilial communication about the injury, and the effect of the event on family members, and to initiate discussion about family expectations and future plans. Often, the PGA-CI interview is the spouses' first opportunity to talk about their personal experiences and to describe the effect of this powerful event on the family. The PGA-CI affords the time to think about their children and to ask questions about how best to meet their children's needs. Ultimately, the PGA-CI was designed to assist healthcare professionals in the formulation of family assistance strategies and plans, with specific interest and emphasis on the positive growth of children.

CHILDREN'S RESPONSES TO COMBAT INJURIES

It is expected that all family members are likely to show some level of distress because of the sudden injury of a military family member. Clinicians have anecdotally observed that although most children do not initially demonstrate symptoms consistent with actual psychiatric disorder, many appear anxious, saddened, or troubled by the news. Parents do not always accurately recognize the emotional effect of the parent's injury on children. Prior studies have shown that parent reports alone are not reliable in the determination of child behavioral and emotional problems and that cross-informant input from others, to include children, is required for accurate assessment.[31] Children who have been exposed to trauma similarly report different and much higher levels of clinical symptoms than their parents, highlighting the importance of direct child assessment for accurate evaluation.[32] No scientific investigation has yet systematically and directly measured the responses of children to parental combat injury. This section provides anecdotal descriptions of children with whom the authors have engaged.

When children first meet their injured parent, their understanding of the injury and the implication of the injuries can be limited. They may experience a broad range of emotional responses that can be confusing both to themselves and to the important adults in their lives. Some children become hesitant and afraid of what they see. They are often distressed and unable to show affection to the injured parent. As a result, some injured SMs express feelings of hurt or disappointment by these reluctant responses. When this occurs, the uninjured parent or another relative may be overly forceful in pushing children, especially young children, to show affection for the injured.

When parents deploy, children are usually told that their parents will safely return home. After the injury, children realize that parents cannot always keep promises that they make. A few children have expressed confusion and anger toward authority, as if they have been wronged. Frequently this anger may be directed toward the caregiver or other adults. Alternatively, children may verbalize fear and ambivalence. They may look to blame others for their parents' injuries or may feel guilty as if somehow they are responsible. After the immediate emotional response, children report feelings of relief and gratitude that the SM parent is alive and safe. However, emotions can fluctuate in character and intensity.

A developmental perspective is helpful when the expected responses of children to parental injury are considered. For example, although infants and toddlers (0–2 years) may be assumed to have little cognitive capacity to appreciate their parents' injuries, they will respond based upon changes in the schedules and routines of their lives, and the physical and emotional availability of important adults, as well as any changes in the emotional tenor (anxiety, interpersonal abruptness, irritability) of these individuals.

Young children (3–6 years) have greater awareness of the actual nature of the injury. However, this understanding is likely to be undeveloped and fragile. Young children use "magical thinking," an immature cognitive process characterized by egocentric thinking, which can lead them to inaccurately take responsibility for events that occur. Young children's cognitive processes become even less reality based at times of high anxiety, as occurs after a parent's injury. For example, one 4-year-old son of an injured SM told his grandparent that he was responsible for his father's injury because he did not remind his dad to be careful when the SM was deploying. The young child needed to be reassured that he did not cause his father's injury.

The immature cognition capacity of young children can lead to an inability to gauge an accurate sense of time. For example, a 3-year-old boy, whose father had multiple injuries and was prescribed extensive bed rest after an amputation, gave his father's wound a kiss and said, "It's all better now, Dad. Let's play." He became confused and frustrated when repeatedly told that his father could not yet play with him. The staff worked with the boy and his parents to establish more circumscribed ways of playing that allowed the father and son to enjoy their time together. Because many serious injuries can result in months, if not years, of medical treatment and rehabilitative services, the patience of young children can rapidly dissipate. Professional intervention that assists parents in understanding the developmental limitations of children and in creating new means of interaction can be invaluable for the future success of the family.

The clinician must recognize how young children perceive and integrate the nature of their parents' injuries. Not uncommonly, young children who see their seriously injured parents become disorganized and extremely anxious. They may wonder "if this powerful and important person in my life can be hurt in this way, what could potentially happen to me?" For example, the mother of two young sons of a seriously injured marine asked to talk with a WRAMC CAPS clinician about their behavior. The boys were becoming increasingly aggressive, impulsive, and active, especially when their father's injury was discussed. While in the room visiting their father, the boys sat quietly and were immobilized, carefully watching him. After leaving the room, they became aggressive with each other and oppositional to their mother.

During the evaluation, each child was asked to "draw a person." They were given no additional directions and were not specifically requested to draw their father. The younger child produced the drawing shown in Figure 31-2. He initiated the drawing as one would expect, completing the face first, but then proceeded to scribble erratically over and around the face. When asked what the picture represented, the young boy stated, "This is a man in an explosion." After completing the drawing, the boy shifted to aggressive play with toy dinosaurs and jungle animals.

The older 5-year-old brother was also asked to produce a drawing of a person. His drawing is shown in Figure 31-3. Unlike his younger brother, he completed the drawing in a very careful and methodical fashion. However, different from his younger brother and the typical approach of other children, the boy started by drawing the figure's feet, which were large and sturdy. He then added extended sections of leg bilaterally. After adding three sections of leg to the drawing, the 5-year-old drew a brace between the two legs to hold them together. The brace was later erased and is not present in the final drawing. This addition betrayed the older son's anxiety about the body's perceived instability that needed to be supported by an armature. He completed the drawing by adding arms, powerful shoulder muscles and a small head. There is no apparent torso and the body is joined at the shoulders.

The children's drawings that appear in these figures give some view into their interior psychological worlds and their drive to process what they had seen and experienced. Their immediate choice to draw injured bodies indicated the psychological challenge that each faced. The younger son was clearly struggling to make

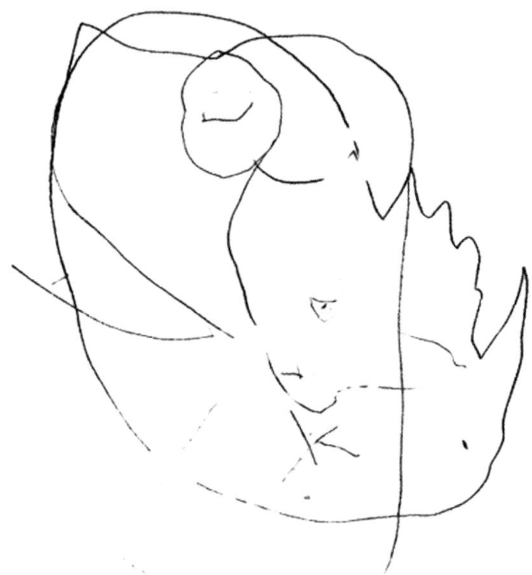

Figure 31-2. Drawing of 3-year-old son of severely injured service member. Image courtesy of Stephen J Cozza, MD.

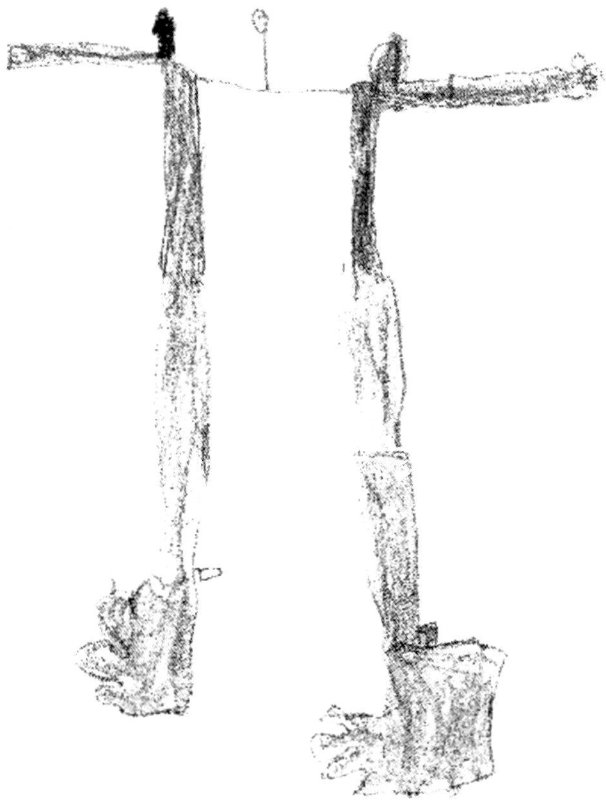

Figure 31-3. Drawing of 5-year-old son of severely injured service member. Image courtesy of Stephen J Cozza, MD.

sense of his father's injury, but was finding difficulty in doing this in any organized way. In comparison, his older brother, while equally preoccupied with his father's injury, demonstrated greater capacity to organize his own thoughts and anxieties and develop his own solutions (as evidenced by the added brace). This greater ability probably indicates the older brother's greater psychological and cognitive capacities. The drawings are not presented as examples of psychopathology, but rather to highlight the challenges that face the young children of combat-injured SMs.

Older children have more mature developmental capacity to meet the stresses of parental injury, both cognitively and emotionally. Nonetheless, the school-aged child may still harbor similar anxieties to those of younger children. Fear, in combination with a sense of guilt and a desire to take responsible action, can complicate the school-aged child's response, as the following two examples illustrate. An 8-year-old boy, whose father had multiple severe injuries and was unconscious as a result of an IED explosion, expressed his reaction to a 4th of July celebration that occurred while he was visiting the hospital. During the celebration he was frightened by both the fireworks and low-flying helicopters. He worried that his family was being targeted by missile attacks from "the bad guys." He imagined another 9/11 terrorist attack near the hospital. He was able to talk with the staff concerning his frequent worries about his and his family's safety. One 10-year-old girl confided that she was sad and missed her two cats that were given to a friend and was sure that she would never see them again. CAPS staff helped her raise these concerns with her parents, who were unaware of the impact of this loss.

Not surprisingly, children can be confused about expectations related to their responses to the injured parent. They may not understand what is or is not appropriate and may feel uneasy bringing up questions. One injured SM expressed concern that her children were reluctant to have physical contact with her. As they had always been affectionate, she could not understand why they no longer wished to be hugged. The mother's apprehension prompted a discussion in which the children described the fear that if they touched her, they might inadvertently add to her ongoing pain. This new understanding allowed the mother to reassure the children and to help them find ways to express their love and care without fear of increasing her pain.

Based upon their developmental stage, teenagers are faced with unique challenges related to parental injury. At a time when they are normally expected to become more independent and less reliant on family, they can be confused by a sudden need to once again be close to, and intensely involved with, their parents and families. Given their near-adult capacity, teenagers may also be asked to shoulder some of the greater demands that result from parental injury, including increased chores, care for younger children, or assistance in the care of the injured parent. Teenagers may be ambivalent and may voice wishes to be with their friends, rather than spend time with their families or injured parent. When visiting the hospital, adolescents have been observed playing electronic games or spending time on computers away from their parents. An adolescent's apparent lack of interest should not be construed as apathy. Clinicians should encourage parents to discuss their teenagers' fears about the injury and their ambivalence about the changed family. Parents may need to be reminded of the importance of remaining involved in their teenagers' lives, especially because this age group is at high risk for engaging in dangerous behaviors. Parents should be encouraged to be clear about their expectations, set appropriate limits on behavior, and consistently administer discipline, when appropriate.

Children and teens can also become activated in healthy ways in response to parental injury. One injured amputee parent proudly shared that his son started a blood drive for a local hospital in appreciation of the care that his father had received. Clearly, this boy was able to redirect the unfortunate experience of his father's injury into altruism and leadership that supported his father's healing. Other children have channeled their energy and desire to help in positive ways within the hospital setting. For example, two preteenage children came to visit their single father who had serious upper extremity injuries as a result of an IED blast. These children cared for their father by bringing food and water and assisting him with some simple and age-appropriate activities of daily living. As a result, the children felt that they were part of their father's treatment and made important contributions to his progress. The clinical staff encouraged the father to include his children in these activities as they requested, while setting limits where developmentally appropriate.

Children whose situations must be closely evaluated are those with preexisting emotional, behavioral, developmental, or medical conditions of their own. For these potentially more vulnerable children, clinicians can expect that the stresses associated with parental injury may lead to greater distress or worsening of their underlying conditions. Healthcare providers should maintain a lower threshold for referral to appropriate clinical resources. At times, families that have children with preexisting conditions may move from their homes to live in the vicinity of the military hospital where the parent is being treated. These parents need to facilitate continuity of care from earlier treatment providers to newly identified clinicians at the military hospital site. Given a family's preoccupation in addressing the medical needs of the injured parent, children's healthcare or educational needs can go unaddressed or inappropriately delayed. Ultimately, children must integrate the realities of the parent's illness over time and adjust to the changes that they face. Exhibit 31-2 highlights the goals of recovery for the children of combat-injured SMs.

EXHIBIT 31-2

GOALS FOR CHILDREN OF INJURED SERVICE MEMBER PARENTS

Develop an age-appropriate understanding of what happened to the parent.

Develop an age-appropriate understanding of the injury and required medical care that can result in

- family separations,
- lengthy hospitalizations,
- multiple procedures, and
- change in family structure/routine.

Accept that they did not create the problems they may now see in their families.

Learn to deal with the sadness, grief, and anxiety related to parental injury.

Accept that the parent who went to war may be "different" than the person who returned, but is still their parent.

Adjust to the "new family" situation by

- staying hopeful,
- having fun,
- being positive about life, and
- maintaining goals for the future.

EFFECT OF THE INJURY ON THE PARENT

In addition to the direct effect of the injury on children, it is important to consider the psychological effect of these injuries on SMs and on their various family roles. Depending upon the nature of the injury, SMs may have resultant physical, psychological, or cognitive changes that affect their abilities to function in virtually all areas of their lives, including parenting. Injuries can alter an SM's capacity to feel comfortable in intimate relationships, may create distance with those to whom they are married or emotionally close, and may undermine their sense of sexual capacity. Because the vast majority of injured SMs are young men, it is important to recognize the potential for narcissistic trauma that negatively affects their sense of competence as men, with resulting effect on spouses and children.

Injured SMs were likely physically active individuals who incorporated these traits in their parenting activities prior to the injury. Physical activities (hiking, backpacking, and camping), hands-on activities (playful wrestling), and athletic activities (ball throwing, skiing, and golfing) were all likely modes of interaction for young military parents with their children. Depending upon the nature of the injury, those modes of interaction either may no longer be possible or may require significant modification to their previous form. In such cases, injured SMs will need to alter their former idealized sense of themselves as parents, mourning any related body change or functional loss. Clinicians should encourage children and parents to explore innovative, mutually developed activities and play that allow parents and children to "try on" fresh ways of relating. The capacity for the parent–child dyad to reestablish enjoyable modes of interaction is critical to future health and happiness. Candid parental discussions can allow injured SM parents to reframe their situations, develop new skills, and achieve greater strength in parenting. Within the hospital setting, occupational therapy and physical therapy services have incorporated children into therapeutic activities with parents in novel and creative ways.

Principles of Caring for Combat-Injured Families

Recognizing that parental combat injury is a life-changing event for SMs, their families, and their children, the Center for the Study of Traumatic Stress at the Uniformed Services University of the Health Sciences convened the Workgroup on Intervention With Combat-Injured Families. This workgroup included expert military and civilian clinicians and academicians from around the country, focusing on the unique needs of this special population. As a result of workgroup meetings, the Center published a fact sheet titled "Principles of Caring for Combat-Injured Families and Their Children" (Attachment 2). These 10 principles can be used by hospital- and community-based professionals in military and civilian settings to support the healthy growth and recovery of this unique population. The principles of caring are summarized in Exhibit 31-3.

Long-Term Rehabilitation and Transitions

Although most of this chapter has addressed the experiences and needs of the families and children of the combat injured during the immediate aftermath of injury, their long-term requirements can vary tremendously and must be planned for. Some data suggest that injured SMs may develop vulnerabilities as they transition back to their homes and communities.[1] When families leave the hospital setting they no longer have the intensive resources that were available. They can lose connection with the families of other injured SMs with whom they may have developed a

EXHIBIT 31-3

PRINCIPLES OF CARING FOR FAMILIES AND CHILDREN OF THE COMBAT INJURED

- Principles of psychological first aid are primary to supporting families of combat-injured service members.
- Medical care for the combat injured must be family focused.
- Service providers should anticipate a range of responses to combat injury.
- Injury communication is an essential component of care of the families of injured service members.
- Programs to assist the families of combat-injured service members must be developmentally sensitive and age appropriate.
- Care of the family of injured service members is longitudinal, extending beyond immediate hospitalization.
- Effective family care requires an interconnected community of care.
- Care must be culturally competent.
- Communities of care should address any barriers to service.
- Families, communities, and service providers must be knowledgeable.

EXHIBIT 31-4

RESOURCES

1. *Resources for Recovery—The Combat Injured Family: Guidelines for Care*. Bethesda, Md: Center for the Study of Traumatic Stress, Uniformed Services University of the Health Sciences. Available at: http://www.centerforthestudyoftraumaticstress.org. Accessed October 14, 2009.
2. Sesame Workshop Talk, Listen, Connect: Deployments, Homecomings, Changes–DVD and print materials. Available through Military OneSource at: http://www.militaryonesource.com, and by online streamed video at: http://www.sesameworkshop.org/tlc. Accessed October 14, 2009.
3. Lee M, Ingram L. *That's My Hope: Featuring a Gallery of Multigenerational Artwork*. Early Light Press, LLC. 2008. Available at: http://www.earlylightpress.com. Accessed September 2, 2009.
4. McCue K, Bonn R. *How to Help Children Through a Parent's Serious Illness*. New York, NY: St. Martin's Press; 1994.
5. Rauch PK, Muriel AC. *Raising an Emotionally Healthy Child When a Parent is Sick*. New York, NY: McGraw-Hill; 2006.
6. Beardslee WR. *Out of the Darkened Room: When a Parent is Depressed.* New York, NY: Little, Brown and Company; 2002.
7. Woodruff L, Woodruff B. *In an Instant: A Family's Journey of Love and Healing*. New York, NY: Random House; 2007.

sense of fellowship and camaraderie. Families may struggle with the realities of being home, having to face responsibilities and routines that no longer seem manageable. Often injured SMs require continuing medical or rehabilitative care. Access to needed services can be problematic or may require the scheduling of appointments at treatment facilities that are at great distance from home, adding more stress to family routines.

With the return of the injured SM, children may expect a return to the lives they remember. They may become disappointed with changes that they experience in the family. Older children and teenagers may have to pick up additional household responsibilities that the injured parent is no longer able to perform. When children are placed in a care-provider role to the injured SM, emotional challenges can be even greater. Teens may be asked to assist with wound care, self-care, or other activities of daily living that require intimate contact with the parent. This contact can be confusing, emotionally upsetting, and lead to resentment and frustration. Such activities should be minimized.

Finally, longer-term consequences of severe combat injury can result in medical retirement from the military service, the loss of a cherished military career, and movement from homes in military communities to other locations or back to families of origin. Although such transitions may increase access to available resources, particularly when the extended family is supportive, these changes are likely to be stressful for both adults and children. Moves from known communities likely mean loss of friends, changes in schools, and possible elimination of enjoyable extracurricular activities. Moves also can cause relocations to communities that have little understanding or appreciation of military culture and the unique challenges that the family has faced. (See Exhibit 31-4 for additional resources available to help families of combat-injured service members.)

SUMMARY

Combat injury can profoundly affect the lives of service members, their families, and their children. Upon injury notification, a cascade of events takes place that can result in distress and interpersonal turmoil for children and adults in the families of the combat injured. Disruptions in parental functioning and family structure are common. The effect on children of serious injury to a parent is likely to be profound, particularly when it leads to long-term or permanent changes in parents, or deterioration in their functioning. Immediately after the injury, noninjured parents are focused on the medical well-being of the injured SMs and may have difficulty recognizing and meeting the needs of their children. Children's developmental and emotional capacities determine their abilities to understand and integrate the experience of parental injury. Parents and healthcare providers benefit from developmentally informed guidance to help children accept the injury, manage their distress, prepare for hospital visits, reengage the injured parent, and effectively communicate their needs. Family and child reactions to combat injury must be understood as a longitudinal process beginning with injury notification and continuing through longer-term rehabilitation and potential transitions to new lives and new communities.

REFERENCES

1. Operation Iraqi Freedom: US Wounded Totals; Operation Enduring Freedom: US Wounded Totals. iCasualities Web site. Available at: www.icasualties.org. Accessed February 8, 2011.

2. Grieger TA, Cozza SJ, Ursano RJ, et al. Posttraumatic stress disorder and depression in battle-injured soldiers. *Am J Psychiatry*. 2006;163:1777–1783.

3. US Department of Defense. *1st Quadrennial Quality of Life Review.* Washington, DC; 2004.

4. Cozza SJ, Chun RS, Polo JA. Military families and children during Operation Iraqi Freedom. *Psychiatr Q*. 2005;76:371–378.

5. Cohen JA, Mannarino AP, Gibson LE, Cozza SJ, Brymer MJ, Murray L. Interventions for children and adolescents. In: Ritchie EC, Friedman MJ, Watson PT, eds. *Mental Health Interventions Following Mass Violence and Disasters*. New York, NY: Guilford; 2006: 227–256.

6. Compas BE, Worsham NL, Epping-Jordan JE, et al. When mom or dad has cancer: markers of psychological distress in cancer patients, spouses, and children. *Health Psychol.* 1994;13:507–515.

7. Compas BE, Worsham NL, Ey S, Howell DC. When mom or dad has cancer: ii. Coping, cognitive appraisals and psychological distress in children of cancer patients. *Health Psychol.* 1996;15:167–175.

8. Huizinga GA, Visser A, van der Graaf WT, Hoekstra HJ, Hoekstra-Weebers JE. The quality of communication between parents and adolescent children in the case of parental cancer. *Ann Oncol.* 2005;16:1956–1961.

9. Visser A, Huizinga GA, Hoekstra HJ, et al. Emotional and behavioral functioning of children of a parent diagnosed with cancer: a cross-informant perspective. *Psychooncology.* 2005;14:746–758.

10. De Judicibus MA, McCabe MP. The impact of parental multiple sclerosis on the adjustment of children and adolescents. *Adolescence.* 2004;39:551–569.

11. Anthony EJ. The mutative impact of serious mental and physical illness of a parent on family life. In: Anthony EJ, Koupernik C, eds. *The Child in His Family*. New York, NY: Wiley-Interscience; 1970: 131–163.

12. Armistead L, Klein K, Forehand R. Parental physical illness and child functioning. *Clin Psychol Rev.* 1995;15:409–422.

13. Finney JW, Miller KM. Children of parents with medical illness. In: Silverman WK, Ollendick TH, eds. *Developmental Issues in the Clinical Treatment of Children.* Needham Heights, Mass: Allyn and Bacon; 1998: 433–442.

14. Korneluk YG, Lee CM. Children's adjustment to parental physical illness. *Clin Child Fam Psychol Rev.* 1998;1:179–193.

15. Power PW. The chronically ill husband and father: his role in the family. *Fam Coordinator.* 1979;28:616–621.

16. Peters LC, Esses LM. Family environment as perceived by children with a chronically ill parent. *J Chronic Diseases.* 1985;38:301–308.

17. LeClere FB, Kowalewski BM. Disability in the family: the effects on children's well-being. *J Marriage Fam.* 1994;56:457–468.

18. Kelley SD, Sikka A. A review of research on parental disability: implications for research and counseling practice. *Rehabil Couns Bull.* 1997;41:105–121.

19. Kotchick BA, Summers P, Forehand R, Steele RG. The role of parental and extrafamilial social support in the psychosocial adjustment of children with a chronically ill father. *Behav Modif.* 1997;21:409–432.

20. Urbach JR. The impact of parental head trauma on families with children. *Psychiatr Med.* 1989;7:17–36.

21. Urbach JR, Culbert JP. Head-injured parents and their children: psychosocial consequences of a traumatic syndrome. *Psychosomatics.* 1991;32:24–33.

22. Pessar LF, Coad ML, Linn RT, Willer BS. The effects of parental traumatic brain injury on the behaviour of parents and children. *Brain Inj.* 1993;7:231–240.

23. Uysal S, Hibbard MR, Robillard D, Pappadopulos E, Jaffe M. The effect of parental traumatic brain injury on parenting and child behavior. *J Head Trauma Rehabil.* 1998;13:57–71.

24. Butera-Prinzi F, Perlesz A. Through children's eyes: children's experience of living with a parent with an acquired brain injury. *Brain Inj.* 2004;18:83–101.

25. Verhaeghe S, Defloor T, Grypdonck M. Stress and coping among families of patients with traumatic brain injury: a review of the literature. *J Clin Nursing.* 2005;14:1004–1012.

26. Zatzick DF, Rivara FP, Nathens AB, et al. A nationwide US study of post-traumatic stress after hospitalization for physical injury. *Psychol Med.* 2007;37:1469–1480.

27. Koren D, Norman D, Cohen A, Berman J, Klein EM. Increased PTSD risk with combat-related injury: a matched comparison study of injured and uninjured soldiers experiencing the same combat events. *Am J Psychiatry*. 2005;162:276–282.

28. Warden D. Military TBI during the Iraq and Afghanistan wars. *J Head Trauma Rehabil*. 2006;21:398–401.

29. Wain HJ, Cozza SJ, Grammer GG, et al. Treating the traumatized amputee. In: Schnurr P, Cozza S, eds. *Iraq War Clinician Guide*. Washington, DC: Department of Veterans Affairs; 2004: 50–57.

30. Wain H, Bradley J, Nam, T, Waldrep D, Cozza S. Psychiatric interventions with returning soldiers at Walter Reed. *Psychiatr Q*. 2005;76:351–360.

31. Achenbach TM, McConaughy SH, Howell CT. Child/adolescent behavioral and emotional problems: implications of cross-informant correlations for situational specificity. *Psychol Bull*. 1987;101:213–232.

32. Meiser-Stedman R, Smith P, Glucksman E, Yule W, Dalgleish T. Parent and child agreement for acute stress disorder, post-traumatic stress disorder and other psychopathology in a prospective study of children and adolescents exposed to single-event trauma. *J Abnorm Child Psychol*. 2007;35:191–201.

ATTACHMENT 1: PARENT GUIDANCE ASSESSMENT—COMBAT INJURY

Center for the Study of Traumatic Stress
Uniformed Services University School of Medicine
Bethesda, MD 20814
www.usuhs.mil/csts/

PARENT GUIDANCE ASSESSMENT – COMBAT INJURY (PGA-CI)

The PGA-CI is a semi-structured clinical interview for collecting preliminary family, child, and parent information from the spouse of recently hospitalized, severely injured service members to guide appropriate child and family interventions. The profound impact on combat injured families necessitates increased support and guidance to sustain parent and family function and child health.

The PGA-CI is a clinical interview to be administered *only* by experienced mental health professionals familiar with the unique issues and challenges of combat-injured soldiers and their families. The PGA-CI provides a selective but sufficiently broad summary portrait of injury-related issues from notification of injury through rehabilitation and recovery as it impacts the wounded service member, his/her children, spouse and other family members. The PGA-CI was developed to assist mental health professionals in the formulation of family assistance strategies and plans.

The PGA-CI is <u>not</u> a self-report questionnaire and therefore should not be used for self-completion by the spouse of combat-injured soldiers. In addition the PGA-CI does not provide prescriptive guidance concerning how the resulting information should be interpreted and utilized.

The PGA-CI is organized thematically and uses both open-ended and response-scale formats. The instrument is not intended to provide an interpretive score. The PGA-CI is not exhaustive in its coverage of these domains. Those who administer this instrument may need additional information to develop and provide appropriate interventions for parents, children and the family.

The PGA-CI is not intended for, but may have applicability, for other families with an injured parent such as might appear in a trauma center after a major motor vehicle accident.

The PGA-CI assesses:

a) Family demographics
b) Family deployment experience
c) Nature of service member's combat injury
d) Injury communication: notification of injury and parent-child injury-related communication
e) Event impact on parent: parent behavioral and emotional responses and concerns
f) Event impact on child(ren): child behavioral and emotional responses and concerns
g) Understanding and preparation for future family needs

FAMILY DEMOGRAPHICS

I would like to begin by asking some basic information about you and your family

Patient Name ______________________________ Age ______ Sex ______

Spouse Name ______________________________ Age ______ Sex ______

Years married ____ Number of Children ________

Child Name ____________________ Age Sex____

Child Name ____________________ Age Sex____

Child Name ____________________ Age Sex____

Child Name ____________________ Age Sex____

Military Branch	Army	Marines	Navy	Air Force	Coast Guard
Active Duty	❒	❒	❒	❒	❒
Reserves	❒	❒	❒	❒	❒
National Guard	❒			❒	

Where do you live? State: __________ City/Town: ___________

Living situation/members – where? ______________________

Do you have access to the military community and services? ❒ Yes ❒ No

Do any members of your extended family live nearby? ❒ Yes ❒ No

Notes

FAMILY DEPLOYMENT EXPERIENCE

I am going to ask you some questions about your spouse's deployment

Dates/scheduled length of deployment ______________________

How many times had your spouse been deployed to combat prior the current deployment ? _____

Current deployment: Location: __________ Date (mm/dd/yy) : / / Duration: ___________

Unit/MOS/Function ____________________

PATIENT IDENTIFIER ____________________ PGA-CI 2

How would you characterize the family impact of your spouse's deployment prior to the injury?

	Minimal Strain		Moderate Strain		Significant Strain
On Children	1	2	3	4	5
On you personally	1	2	3	4	5
On your spouse	1	2	3	4	5

Can you give me some examples?

To what extent did you and your spouse discuss the possibility of combat injury prior to deployment?

No Discussion		Limited Discussion		Significant Discussion
1	2	3	4	5

To what extent did you or your spouse discuss the possibility of parental combat injury with your child prior to deployment?

	No Discussion		Limited Discussion		Significant Discussion
Child Name: ________	1	2	3	4	5
Child Name: ________	1	2	3	4	5
Child Name: ________	1	2	3	4	5
Child Name: ________	1	2	3	4	5

How about any differences in the level of detail you provided different children?

NATURE OF INJURY

Now I am going to ask you some questions about your spouse's injury

Date of injury (mm/dd/yy) ______/________/______

Nature of injury: ❐ TBI ❐ Amputation ❐ Blindness ❐ Multi-trauma ❐ Burn ❐ Other (Describe below)

Describe

PATIENT IDENTIFIER ______________________ PGA-CI 3

How would you rate severity of your spouse's injury?

Minimal Long-Term Impairment		Moderate Long-Term Impairment		Severe Long-Term Impairment
1	2	3	4	5

How difficult has it been for your spouse to relate to you and your children about the injury?

Very Easy		Somewhat Difficult		Very Difficult
1	2	3	4	5

INJURY COMMUNICATION

Notification Process

Next are some questions about how you were told about the injury

How long after the injury were you notified? _____Hours _____Days
Who notified you about the injury? ______________________________

How were you notified injury? ❒ Telephone ❒ In-person ❒ Other _______

Was information passed through informal channels prior to formal channels? ❒ Yes ❒ No

Was the formal notification information accurate? ❒ Yes ❒ No

These next questions concern children about the injury

What have you or anyone else told your child(ren) about the injury? (exact wording)

Child Name ____________ ____

Child Name ____________ ____

Child Name ____________ ____

Child Name ____________ ____

Did you receive any guidance regarding how to share this news with your child(ren)?
❒ No ❒ Yes

From whom?______________________________________

How helpful was this?

Not at All Helpful		Somewhat Helpful		Very Helpful
1	2	3	4	5

PATIENT IDENTIFIER __________________________ PGA-CI 4

How comfortable were you speaking with your children about the injury?

		Very Comfortable		Somewhat Uncomfortable		Very Uncomfortable
Child Name:	________	1	2	3	4	5
Child Name:	________	1	2	3	4	5
Child Name:	________	1	2	3	4	5
Child Name:	________	1	2	3	4	5

How helpful would it have been to have resources or professionals available to help you speak with your child(ren)?

Not Helpful		Somewhat Helpful		Very Helpful
1	2	3	4	5

Comments

FAMILY AND CHILD DISTRESS

Typically after an injury a lot of things happen. May I ask you about that? What things happened to your family immediately after notification?

Clinician please rate the level of organization with which the spouse describes the chain of events after Notification

Very Organized		Variably Organized		Very Disorganized
1	2	3	4	5

What were the 3 most important decisions you had to make immediately after notification?

1 ______________________________

2 ______________________________

3 ______________________________

Did anyone come to be with you or support you and your family following the injury notification?

	Little or No Support		Moderate Support		Significant Support
Family	1	2	3	4	5
Friends	1	2	3	4	5
Neighbors	1	2	3	4	5
Clergy	1	2	3	4	5
Military	1	2	3	4	5

What were the 3 greatest stresses or strains related to this early chain of events?

1 ______________________________

2 ______________________________

3 ______________________________

What 3 three actions by others did you find most helpful to you and your family during this period?

1 ______________________________

2 ______________________________

3 ______________________________

How often have you been separated from your child(ren) in connection with hospital visits related to this injury and for how much time for each period?

		Days	Hours			Days	Hours
Date	/ /			Date	/ /		
Date	/ /			Date	/ /		
Date	/ /			Date	/ /		
Date	/ /			Date	/ /		
Date	/ /			Date	/ /		

To what degree has your spouse's injury disrupted your family/children's lives so far?

	Minimal Disruption		Moderate Disruption		Significant Disruption
Family Routines	1	2	3	4	5
Children's Play Activities	1	2	3	4	5
After School Activities	1	2	3	4	5

Can you give me some examples?

PATIENT IDENTIFIER ______________________ PGA-CI 6

IMPACT ON PARENT

How has this injury impacted on the amount of time you spend with your child?

Minimal Impact		Moderate Impact		Significant Impact
1	2	3	4	5

Can you give me some examples?

To what degree has this injury impacted the way you typically discipline your children?

Significantly More Lenient		About the Same		Significantly More Strict
1	2	3	4	5

Can you give me some examples?

I would be interested in knowing how this injury has impacted you personally

What has been the most challenging part of this injury for you?

What changes have you had to make to your schedule/life (e.g. job, etc)

PATIENT IDENTIFIER ______________________ PGA-CI 7

What has been most helpful to you in dealing with this injury?

Combat injury is a life-changing event that impacts the entire family; at times it may be helpful to talk with a care provider about how your family is coping with your spouse's injury. Would this be helpful for you?
❑ Yes ❑ No

IMPACT ON CHILD AND CHILDREN

Now I'd like to turn to what you think this experience has been like for your child(ren)
Has your child developed any adjustment problems since being informed of your spouse's injury?

(check all that apply)		School Problems	Social Problems	Behavior Problems	Sleeping Problems	Eating Problems
Child Name:	______	❑	❑	❑	❑	❑
Child Name	______	❑	❑	❑	❑	❑
Child Name:	______	❑	❑	❑	❑	❑
Child Name:	______	❑	❑	❑	❑	❑

How difficult has this experience been for your child from an emotional perspective?

		Not al all Difficult		Moderately Difficult		Extremely Difficult
Child Name:	______	1	2	3	4	5
Child Name:	______	1	2	3	4	5
Child Name:	______	1	2	3	4	5
Child Name:	______	1	2	3	4	5

Has your child witnessed any family conflict related to your spouse's injury?

❑ No ❑ Yes

If so, between whom ______

How would you rate the level of conflict?

Little or No Conflict		Moderate Conflict		Significant Conflict
1	2	3	4	5

PATIENT IDENTIFIER ______ PGA-CI 8

Communication support is very important throughout the injured parent's treatment and recovery. Would it be helpful for a care provider to offer guidance on how to communicate with your child(ren) and/or for your child to talk directly with a care provider ?

IMPACT OF HOSPITAL EXPERIENCE ON CHILD/REN

I would like to ask about what it has been like for your child/ren to visit the hospital.

How much preparation did your child receive for his/her first hospital visit?

		Did Not Visit	Minimal Preparation		Moderate Preparation		Significant Preparation
Child Name:		NA	1	2	3	4	5
Child Name:		NA	1	2	3	4	5
Child Name:		NA	1	2	3	4	5
Child Name:		NA	1	2	3	4	5

How distressful was it for your child to visit your spouse in the hospital?

		Did Not Visit	Minimal Distress		Moderate Distress		Significant Distress
Child Name:		NA	1	2	3	4	5
Child Name:		NA	1	2	3	4	5
Child Name:		NA	1	2	3	4	5
Child Name:		NA	1	2	3	4	5

What comments/questions did he/she have about the injury?

Child Name: ________ ____________________

Child Name: ________ ____________________

Child Name: ________ ____________________

Child Name: ________ ____________________

How about your child's exposure to other combat injured soldiers?

		No Other Exposure	Minimal Distress		Moderate Distress		Significant Distress
Child Name		NA	1	2	3	4	5
Child Name:		NA	1	2	3	4	5
Child Name:		NA	1	2	3	4	5
Child Name:		NA	1	2	3	4	5

Has your child participated in his/her injured parent's treatment?

Child Name:	____________	❒ Yes	❒ No
Child Name:	____________	❒ Yes	❒ No
Child Name:	____________	❒ Yes	❒ No
Child Name:	____________	❒ Yes	❒ No

FUTURE PLANS AND ISSUES

Now I'd like to turn to some questions about how you see the future

Have you and your spouse considered long term plans after recovery? ❒ No ❒ Yes

Will he/she be leaving the military? ❒ No ❒ Yes ❒ Unknown

Will you be moving from your current home?

❒ No ❒ Yes ❒ Unknown

If so, where to: ____________________

Do you anticipate any changes in your spouse's role as a parent or partner?

❒ No ❒ Yes ❒ Unknown

If so, what kinds of changes do you anticipate?

How significant do you think these changes will be?

Minimal		Moderate		Profound
1	2	3	4	5

Comments

What impact do you see this injury having over the long-term?:

	Minimal Impact		Moderate Impact		Profound Impact
On you personally	1	2	3	4	5
On your spouse	1	2	3	4	5
On your children	1	2	3	4	5
On your family life	1	2	3	4	5

PATIENT IDENTIFIER ____________________ PGA-CI 10

FAMILY CHALLENDS AND STRENGTHS

As we close I want to ask if there is any other information you would like to share about this experience

What has been the most difficult part of this experience?

What has been the most helpful part of the experience?

What do you wish you had more assistance with?

Of all the choices you have been faced with around this event, what has been the best choice you have made?

Have you developed any new methods of coping based upon this experience (e.g. in what ways have you grown)?

How would you rate your family's need for the following forms of guidance and assistance?

	Little or No Need		Moderate Need		Significant Need
Parenting guidance	1	2	3	4	5
Stress and coping	1	2	3	4	5
Transition planning	1	2	3	4	5
Family communication	1	2	3	4	5
Child counseling	1	2	3	4	5

PATIENT IDENTIFIER ____________ PGA-CI 11

CLINICAL FORMULATION AND CONCLUSIONS

Clinician: List any identified problems, areas of strength/weakness or need for potential referrals.

PATIENT IDENTIFIER ______________________ PGA-CI 12

ATTACHMENT 2:
PRINCIPLES OF CARING FOR COMBAT-INJURED FAMILIES AND THEIR CHILDREN

Principles of Caring for Combat Injured Families and their Children

Combat injury is a life-changing event that impacts a service member, his or her children, as well as other family members and loved ones. Military children are our nation's children, and represent a vulnerable population within the injured family unit. Injury to a parent is a major threat to children of all ages and a challenge for even the most resilient of military families.

Injury to a parent is a major threat to children of all ages and a challenge for even the most resilient of military families.

Parental injury disrupts the family system — its routines, cohesion and sense of safety. Importantly, parental injury can alter the child's view of the wounded parent, and undermine the child's view of his or her own physical integrity. Combat injury also affects existing patterns of parenting, as both injured and uninjured parents experience their own emotional responses and face the complicated reality of medical treatment and rehabilitation over time. Often, adults do not know how to speak to children about the injury, or how much and what kind of information to share.

As a result of parental combat injury, many family members may demonstrate initial distress that is likely to be temporary. Most children will remain healthy in the face of this stress, but some children may sustain life-changing trajectories in their emotional development and/or their interpersonal relationships. The simultaneous use and study of the following principles of care for our combat injured families will foster evidence based approaches that can support their healthy growth and recovery. These principles can be used by hospital and community based professionals in military or civilian settings.

Principles of Caring

- **Principles of *psychological first aid (PFA)* are primary to supporting Injured Families.** Care of injured service members and families should incorporate key elements of PFA: providing safety, comfort, information, practical assistance and connection to appropriate community resources — all serving to support healthy family recovery.
- **Medical care for the combat injured must be *family focused*.** Care of combat injured service members must attend to family needs and specifically should work toward relieving family distress, sustaining parental functioning, and fostering effective injury related parent-child communication.
- **Service providers should anticipate a *range of responses* to combat injury.** Serious injury will challenge our healthiest families. Most service members, their children and families will adjust to the injuries they sustain. But, others may struggle with the changes that they face. Some may even develop problems that require treatment. Service providers should expect this broad range of responses and be prepared to meet family needs as they are identified.
- ***Injury communication* is an essential component of injured family care.** Effective injury communication involves the timely, appropriate and accurate sharing of information with and among family members from the moment of notification of injury throughout treatment and rehabilitation. Communication should be calibrated to address patient and family anxiety and to sustain hope. Because families may be uncertain how to share difficult information with their children, they may benefit from professional guidance on what to say and how to say it.
- **Injured Family programs must be *developmentally sensitive and age appropriate*.** Services and programs must address the unique developmental responses of children of varying age and gender, and recognize that distress, care needs and communication ability will change with children of different ages.
- **Injured Family care is *longitudinal*, extending beyond immediate hospitalization.** Services need to be tailored to the changing needs of the combat injured family throughout the treatment and

Continued

Workgroup on Intervention with Combat Injured Families
Center for the Study of Traumatic Stress, Department of Psychiatry, Uniformed Services University of the Health Sciences

rehabilitation process. Interventions must meet the family where it is within the recovery process, recognizing a family's unique strengths and challenges, as well as anticipate its future needs through transition to a new community or new way-of-life.

- **Effective Injured Family care requires an *interconnected community of care*.** Effective intervention requires collaboration and coordination of services between the family, the health care system, and military and civilian community resources. This collaboration fosters a community of care that reaches across traditional professional boundaries throughout rehabilitation and recovery.
- **Care must be *culturally competent*.** Healthcare and community professionals who interact with combat injured families need to possess the cultural and language competence to engage families that may be traditional or nontraditional in their composition and may be of broad ethnic and religious backgrounds. It is essential that all healthcare and community service providers understand and respect the unique experiences and traditions of military families.
- **Communities of care should address any *barriers to service*.** Barriers to intervention can complicate the healthy recovery of combat injured service and family members. These barriers may include a family's difficulty in accessing health care or community services. In addition, a community's lack of awareness or misunderstanding of the needs of a combat injured family or a family's reluctance to seek assistance (due to stigmatization) can also limit family intervention and recovery
- **Families, communities and service providers must be *knowledgeable*.** Individuals, families, professionals, organizations and communities all have a need for access to quality educational materials to address the challenges that confront combat injured families. Effective education leads to the development of skills in all parties, building empowerment in communities and families. Development of new knowledge is fundamental to better meeting the needs of this unique population.

PLACE LOCAL CONTACT INFORMATION HERE

Center for the Study of Traumatic Stress
Department of Psychiatry
Uniformed Services University of the Health Sciences
4301 Jones Bridge Road
Bethesda, MD 20814-4799
Tel: 301-295-2470 | Fax: 301-319-6965
www.usuhs.mil/csts | www.centerforthestudyoftraumaticstress.org

Chapter 32

FAMILY MALTREATMENT AND MILITARY DEPLOYMENT

RENÉ J. ROBICHAUX, PhD, LCSW,* and JAMES E. McCARROLL, PhD, MPH†

*Colonel, US Army (Retired); Social Work Programs Manager, Behavioral Health Division, US Army Medical Command, 2050 Worth Road, Fort Sam Houston, Texas 78234; formerly, Chief, Department of Social Work, Brooke Army Medical Center, Fort Sam Houston, Texas

†Colonel, US Army (Retired); Psychologist, Center for the Study of Traumatic Stress and Department of Psychiatry, Room B3068, Uniformed Services University of the Health Sciences, 4301 Jones Bridge Road, Bethesda, Maryland 20814; formerly, Psychologist, Walter Reed Army Institute of Research, Silver Spring, Maryland

INTRODUCTION

The relationship between family maltreatment (a term used to describe child abuse and neglect, and domestic violence between married or unmarried partners) and military deployment encompasses a subset of issues related to the effect of war on families—soldiers, spouses, and children. There have been numerous studies describing the effects of deployment on soldiers and families prior to Operation Iraqi Freedom and Operation Enduring Freedom.[1] There are many factors involved in a military deployment, both positive and negative.[2] However, the stresses of the deployment of a service member are timeless. For example, those noted during World War II still occur today: uncertainty, separation, privations, bombing in noncombat areas, isolation, climate, danger, fatigue, differences in status and privilege among ranks and services, the length of the deployment, the degree of security (which may not allow adequate communication with family members or friends), boredom, and interruption of future plans.[3]

In addition to understanding the psychological effect of combat and operational stress on soldiers, the military has begun to more fully appreciate war's impact on family members. Families experience many stressors that affect soldiers along with their own sets of stressors during deployment. Among these are managing physical illnesses of the spouse and children, pregnancy,[4] affective conditions (depression, anger, loneliness), marital adjustment, maintaining the home and car, assuming sole responsibility for family life, playing a dual role as parent, and readjusting following the service member's return from the deployment.[5] Other stressors on families during deployments are the threat of soldiers being killed or injured in combat, parenting responsibilities of families in which the mother deploys,[6] single parents,[7,8] the effects of father absence on children,[9–11] elevated symptoms of depression in parents and in children,[12] and stress-related problems referred to healthcare workers.[13] Finally, for both soldiers and spouses there are the issues of infidelity and marital trust.[2,14]

The ability to communicate under most circumstances is an important morale factor for both spouses and soldiers.[15] During extended conflicts such as World War II, Korea, and Vietnam, communication was limited to letters. More rapid communication during deployment has become possible due to recent technological developments. At the present time, soldiers and families have access to a variety of media depending on their location and mission. The Internet, cellular phones, and e-mail have made virtually instantaneous communication possible, but can also produce emotional turmoil and frustration through system failures and inability to complete conversations.[16]

Army wives who had the most difficulty coping with the absence of their soldier husbands during the 1991 Persian Gulf War were younger women with husbands in the lower ranks.[17] Attempts to reach younger wives in the military community are among the most difficult tasks of Army family assistance workers.

THE ARMY FAMILY ADVOCACY PROGRAM

Since the beginning of military operations in Afghanistan and the subsequent clustering of domestic violence fatalities at Fort Bragg, North Carolina in July, 2002, there has been intense interest in identifying deployment stressors that may contribute to increased domestic violence. The Family Advocacy Program (FAP) is the Army's mechanism for substantiating incidents of maltreatment and caring for victims. The Army FAP was formally established in 1976 following the enactment of the Federal Child Abuse Prevention and Treatment Act of 1974, as amended,[18,19] although less formal programs existed prior to that time.[20] The Army FAP is currently regulated by Department of Defense Directive 6400.1[21] and Army Regulation 608-18.[22] The objectives of the FAP are to prevent abuse, encourage the reporting of all instances of abuse, ensure the prompt assessment and investigation of all abuse cases, protect victims, and treat all family members affected by abuse. The Army is required to investigate all credible reports of family maltreatment.[23]

Incidents of abuse may come to the attention of the FAP from a variety of military and civil sources including law enforcement, medical and dental services, command authorities, and other agencies. When incidents of alleged abuse are reported to an Army installation (regardless of whether the incident occurred on or off the post), a multidisciplinary case review committee at the medical treatment facility on each major Army installation reviews them. Substantiated incidents of child maltreatment may be categorized as one or more of four possible types of maltreatment: (1) deprivation of necessities (neglect), (2) physical abuse, (3) sexual abuse, and (4) emotional abuse. Substantiated domestic violence can be categorized as physical, emotional, or sexual abuse.

If the incident is substantiated, case information is forwarded to the Army Central Registry (ACR), a confidential database of demographic and incident data on all substantiated child and spouse abuse victims and offenders. ACR records are maintained on child victims 17 years of age and younger and on married soldiers and their spouses. Recently the military services expanded their definition of domestic violence to include violence toward a person of the opposite sex who is a current or former spouse, a person with whom the abuser shares a child, or a current or former intimate partner with whom the abuser shares or has shared a common domicile.[24]

MILITARY LIFE AND FAMILY MALTREATMENT

Spouse Maltreatment

Spouse abuse rates in the ACR have steadily declined from 6.3/1,000 in 2001 to 4.4/1,000 in 2007.[25] This decrease is difficult to interpret. Many soldiers have deployed for several tours during this period, thereby decreasing the number of married persons at risk for domestic violence.

It is broadly believed, at least in the media,[26] that the stress of military life contributes to family maltreatment. Is there a difference in military and civilian spouse abuse rates of domestic violence? These populations have not been directly compared, but one study[27] compared a reasonably representative sample of Army couples to previously collected civilian prevalence data of the US national population.[28] The male soldier self-reports of moderate husband-to-wife spousal aggression were not significantly different—11% for the soldiers and 10% for the civilians. However, there was a small, but statistically significant difference in severe aggression in the Army sample (2.5%) compared to the civilian sample (0.7%). The authors concluded that the higher Army rates were mostly due to differences in age and race and not to abuse propensity.

Military deployment has been suggested as a possible cause of domestic violence,[13,25] but little information supports such a claim. Using data from the Heyman and Neidig study,[27] a secondary analysis was performed studying the relationship between the length of deployment and spousal aggression. In this study, using a large-scale database (n = 26,835), with demographic variables controlled, deployment contributed a small, but statistically significant increase in the probability of self-reported severe husband-to-wife violence over a 1-year period.[29] The probability increased from 4% with no deployment to 5% with deployment of 6 to 12 months. The frequency of moderate and severe violence increased with the number of weeks deployed.

Two other studies examined the relationship between deployment and domestic violence. Active duty deployed (n = 313) and nondeployed (n = 712) male soldiers were surveyed after returning from a 6-month peacekeeping deployment to Bosnia.[30] Postdeployment domestic violence by male soldiers was predicted by youthful age and the existence of predeployment domestic violence, but not by deployment. Nonwhite race and off-post residence also contributed to the prediction. The predicted probability of postdeployment domestic violence for a deployed 20-year-old, nonwhite soldier living on the military installation with a history of predeployment domestic violence was 0.20. For the soldier without a history of predeployment domestic violence it was 0.05.[30]

A second study of the relationship between domestic violence and deployment was conducted on wives of male soldiers who deployed to Bosnia.[31] Soldiers in the previous survey[30] and spouses in this survey were not matched because surveys were anonymous; however, both reported their experiences relative to the same deployment. There were 368 wives of soldiers who had been deployed and 528 wives of nondeployed soldiers who retrospectively provided domestic violence data for both the pre- and postdeployment periods. There were no significant differences in the frequency of domestic violence between the deployed and nondeployed groups for pre- or postdeployment time periods. Deployment was not a significant predictor of domestic violence during the first 10 months of the postdeployment period, but younger wives and those who were victims of predeployment domestic violence were more likely to report postdeployment domestic violence than older wives and those who had not been identified as victims during predeployment. Anecdotal reports suggest that abuse is most likely to occur several months after the soldier's return from deployment, but there are no studies to support this observation.

As a result of these latter two studies, it was concluded that prevention and intervention programs for postdeployment domestic violence should target younger families, persons with a domestic violence history, and those who live off post. Increased opportunities for counseling these groups on the risk of postdeployment domestic violence may be helpful. Such programs might emphasize increased awareness of personal risk for domestic violence, self-monitoring, and early help-seeking.

Child Maltreatment

In 1990, prior to the Persian Gulf War (1990–1991), the child victim maltreatment rate was 6.9/1,000 children. After a steady decrease of child maltreatment rates through the 1990s, the rates increased from 5.2/1,000 in 2000 to 6.2/1,000 in 2004, and then decreased to 5.0/1,000 in 2007. Child neglect is the type of maltreatment most affected by the deployments. Neglect rates decreased from a high in 1991 (3.6/1,000) to a low in 2000 (2.7/1,000), an overall decline of 25%. By 2004, however, the rates had increased to 4.5/1,000, which is above the 1991 level. The neglect rates were 3.5/1,000 in 2005, 3.3/1,000 in 2006, and 3.7/1,000 in 2007. Neglect rates were highest for the youngest children and decreased as age increased. The rates of child physical abuse decreased from 3.1/1,000 in 1990 to 1.0/1,000 in 2007.[25]

A study of child maltreatment cases in military families living in Texas between 2000 and 2003 found that both departure to and return from an operational deployment impose stresses on military families and are likely to increase the rate of child maltreatment.[32] For each 1% increase in the percentage of active duty personnel departing to or returning from deployment, there was approximately a 30% increase in the rate of child maltreatment.[32]

A second study found approximately a 40% increased rate of child maltreatment when the soldier parent was deployed.[33] The rates of child neglect were nearly twice as high during deployment. However, the rate of physical abuse was less during deployment. The rate of neglect by female civilian spouses was almost 4 times greater during deployment and the rate of physical abuse was almost twice as great. The authors speculate that the increased risk of child maltreatment may be a function of deployments creating a situation similar to that of single parents in the general population, for whom the research has demonstrated an increased risk for child maltreatment due to limited financial resources and greater levels of physical exhaustion. Finally, a study of trends in child maltreatment cases recorded in the ACR from 1990 to 2004 indicated that child neglect rates increased during the Middle East wars (in the Persian Gulf War [1990–1991] and Operation Iraqi Freedom/Operation Enduring Freedom [2002–2004]).[34]

Earlier research demonstrated little or no relationship between deployment and domestic violence.[29–31] This research, however, was performed during deployments (Bosnia in 1998–1999 and earlier) that were of relatively short duration and did not involve extensive combat operations. These deployments, thus, represent an entirely different scenario for soldiers and families compared to the current conflicts in Iraq and Afghanistan. Recent research has shown a probable effect of lengthy deployment on child maltreatment.[32–34]

EFFECT OF WAR ON FAMILIES

Clinical depression of the nondeployed spouse may contribute substantially to the observed increase in the child neglect rates during combat deployments. The majority of the neglect complaints received by the Army FAP involved both a lack of child supervision and dirty homes, which present a health risk to children. Caretakers who are depressed have little energy to both maintain a house and provide suitable activities for young children. The Army Medical Command (MEDCOM) has published written guidance for its healthcare providers to increase screening for depression in family member spouses. New policy changes encouraging social workers to leave their clinic offices and aggressively reach out to isolated and depressed mothers has underscored the MEDCOM's desire to intervene early and avoid serious negative family outcomes due to depression.

Military spouses have reported their belief that military stress increases the number of divorces.[35,36] If military stress contributes to marital conflict and marital dissolution, deployment should increase both these outcomes. Soldiers have reported that deterioration of a marital or romantic relationship is one of the negative consequences of deployment.[2] Several studies have addressed this point. Spouses of nearly 400 enlisted soldiers who deployed to Somalia in 1992 to 1993 reported that difficulties encountered during the soldier's deployment, such as pregnancy, loneliness, death of a friend or relative, or having problems communicating with the soldier spouse have less impact on marital satisfaction, and are less stressful than is often assumed.[5] A study of over 800 enlisted soldiers who participated in Operations Desert Shield/Storm (1990–1991) found no significant overall change in marital satisfaction.[37]

The "stress hypothesis" is commonly cited to explain the observed increases in divorce rates among military couples and predicts that soldiers who are deployed will experience higher rates of divorce compared to soldiers who do not deploy.[38] Additionally, the hypothesis suggests that longer deployments will be more damaging to marriages than shorter deployments. After correlating deployment histories with personnel records for marital status and controlling for variables such as gender, race, and age at marriage, the opposite outcome was found. For enlisted soldiers, the longer that a service member was deployed while married, the lower the subsequent risk of marital dissolution. The same effect was also observed for soldiers in the Army Reserve and Army National Guard. One of the overall conclusions was that deployment appears to enhance the stability of the marriage. It follows from an analysis of the number of days deployed and its relationship to marital dissolution that the longer the deployment, the greater the benefit to the marriage. However, the effects of military service and deployment in particular on marital stability are complex and are affected by service member factors such as gender, race/ethnicity, age at marriage, and children.[38]

In addition to the stress hypothesis is the selection factor present in service recruitment.[38] Military marriages may be at increased risk for dissolution because the various military services recruit from relatively high-risk populations and provide incentives such as healthcare, housing allowances, separate rations, moving expenses, and survivors' benefits that encourage marriage. Recent challenges to meeting recruiting goals may lead to waivers of some standards for recruitment; these modified standards may lead to a vulnerable group of recruits. In fiscal year 2007, more than 11% of Army recruits were given waivers. Waivers were given to some enlistees for medical problems, drug and alcohol issues, and criminal backgrounds.[39] Although the group with waivers is considered the most vulnerable based on factors associated with impulsivity, anger control, and substance abuse, the remaining 88% are also considered to be vulnerable to marital problems based on age, ethnicity, and potential for career advancement in the civilian labor market.[40] Thus, soldiers marry younger and have children sooner than their civilian counterparts, both of which are associated with increased risk of divorce and marital conflict.[38]

THE ARMY'S RESPONSE TO FAMILY STRESS AND DEPLOYMENT

The Army has responded to its many deployment-related challenges by increasing the number of human service workers to help soldiers and families in the high-tempo environment of repeated deployments to the Middle East. By 2004, the Army had placed 70 clinical social workers at various installations that regularly deployed large numbers of soldiers (power projection platforms) to support soldiers and family members adjusting to the psychological challenges associated with deployment. Additionally, the Department of Defense has provided on contract over 84 military and family life consultants, who arrive at an installation for temporary duty during peak periods of deployment activity, to assist with education and consultation related to deployment stress issues. These contracted master's- and doctoral-level social workers and psychologists have been particularly active in support of Army National Guard and Army Reserve units during their redeployment activities.

Army chaplains have increased their outreach to couples struggling in their marriages against a backdrop of multiple deployments. A program entitled "Strong Bonds" combines elements of marriage preparation and marriage enrichment and is generally delivered in a group setting to both the active and reserve components. Family life chaplains also provide traditional couples' counseling to individual families seeking to improve communication, goal setting, and problem resolution skills.

Funds have recently been set aside to hire approximately 1,000 family readiness support assistants to organize the family support activities centered at the battalion level. Pilot projects have attested to the enormous advantage that can accrue from the networking and outreach efforts provided by the addition of these funded positions. They have succeeded in improving the flow of information between the military unit and the individual family as well as encouraging support between families. Their activities have served to mitigate the feelings of isolation and alienation reported by the wives of young soldiers during the Persian Gulf War (1990–1991).

The FAP is directed by the US Army Family and Morale, Welfare, and Recreation Command. Among the many FAP services provided to families is the New Parent Support Program (NPSP). The NPSP can conduct home visits for high-risk families as well as many educational programs for parents of young children. The FAP currently provides 52 NPSP home visitors and plans to add an additional 100 in support of families who are coping with parenting young children amidst the added stress of multiple deployments.

In July 2006 MEDCOM directed that all parents (both military and civilian spouses) of children born in Army medical treatment facilities and civilian hospitals receive briefings designed to reduce and avoid injuries inflicted in response to children's uncontrolled crying. The Center for Health Promotion and Preventive Medicine has developed materials to educate new parents in understanding the causes of inconsolable crying and offer solutions for them. The Department of Defense, in partnership with the National Center on Shaken Baby Syndrome, has launched a campaign directed at service families to raise awareness while offering sources of help to address this problem.

Drawing from lessons learned from the 2003 and 2004 Fatality Review Board findings, the Army MEDCOM has also directed that when healthcare providers identify high-risk families, their cases be assessed by a team and managed by an identified social worker case manager until the risk is determined to be sufficiently reduced.

Child development centers at various power projection platforms have, since the war's inception, offered hours of free respite care for parents of children while the other parent is deployed. Those installations where this service has been most highly used have seen fewer referrals to the FAP for child neglect.

The programs outlined here represent a broad first effort to manage the psychological stressors associated with high personnel and operational tempo, but more needs to be learned about the effectiveness of these programs. As the Army increases its capacity to address the psychological consequences of deployment for the active force and its relation to family conflict and family maltreatment, a significant benefit would accrue from having trained marriage and family therapists as part of any increased behavioral health workforce. There are about 60 such therapists currently on staff in various hospitals across the Army. They have demonstrated their value in a number of substantive ways. Pre- and postintervention outcome self-report questionnaires indicate clinically significant improvements in distress symptoms. At those installations where marriage and family therapists provided couples' counseling to identified domestic violence cases, the couples were significantly more likely to successfully complete the required treatment. For many soldiers struggling with the need to seek help for depression and posttraumatic stress, family therapy has proven to be extremely efficacious in breaking through denial and rationalizations that may have precluded individual therapy. It is believed that participating as a family in therapy can be helpful to all. War disrupts everyone's lives; therapy with a family can be less threatening than identifying an individual as "damaged" or "broken."

SUMMARY

Deployments place additional stresses on military families. Research conducted prior to the wars in Iraq and Afghanistan showed little or no significant relationship between deployment and domestic violence. More recent research has shown increases in child maltreatment, especially child neglect, during the deployment periods. The Army has responded with many new and expanded efforts to address the many challenges of soldiers and families associated with repeated deployments. The results of some research, such as the effect of deployment on military marriages, have been counterintuitive, showing increased strength of such marriages. However, this finding is not without significant caveats. Much more needs to be learned to address problems encountered in the various phases of deployment: how to prepare soldiers and families for deployment, which services are most helpful to family members while the soldier is deployed, and how to facilitate resumption of post-deployment family life.

REFERENCES

1. McCarroll JE, Hoffman KJ, Grieger TA, Holloway HC. Psychological aspects of deployment and reunion. In: Kelley PW, ed. *Military Preventive Medicine: Mobilization and Deployment.* In: Lounsbury DE, Bellamy RF, eds. *Textbook of Military Medicine.* Washington, DC: Department of the Army, Office of The Surgeon General, Borden Institute; 2005: 1395–1424.

2. Newby JH, McCarroll JE, Ursano RJ, Fan Z, Shigemura J, Tucker-Harris Y. Positive and negative consequences of a military deployment. *Mil Med*. 2005;170:815–819.

3. Menninger WC. *Psychiatry in a Troubled World.* New York, NY: MacMillan; 1948.

4. Haas DM, Pazdernik LA, Olsen CH. A cross-sectional survey of the relationship between partner deployment and stress in pregnancy during wartime. *Women's Health Issues*. 2005;15:48–54.

5. Schumm WR, Bell DB, Knott B, Rice RE. The perceived effect of stressors on marital satisfaction among civilian wives of enlisted soldiers deployed to Somalia for Operation Restore Hope. *Mil Med.* 1996;161:601–606.

6. Kelley ML, Herzog-Simmer PA, Harris MA. Effects of military-induced separation on the parenting stress and family functioning of deploying mothers. *Mil Psychol*. 1994;6:125–138.

7. Bowen GL. Single fathers for the defense. *Soc Casework: J Contemp Soc Work*. 1987;6:339–344.

8. Schumm WR, Rice RE, Bell DB, Perez MMV. Trends in single parenting in the Army. *Psychol Reports*. 1996;78:1311–1328.

9. Jensen PS, Grogan D, Xenakis SN, Bain MW. Father absence: effects on child and maternal psychopathology. *J Am Acad Child Adolesc Psychiatry*. 1989;28:171–175.

10. Jensen PS, Lewis RL, Xenakis SN. The military family in review: context, risk, and prevention. *J Am Acad Child Psychiatry*. 1986;25:225–234.

11. Amen DG, Jellen L, Merves E, Lee RE. Minimizing the impact of deployment separation on military children: stages, current preventive efforts, and system recommendations. *Mil Med*. 1988;153:441–446.

12. Jensen PS, Martin D, Watanabe H. Children's response to parental separation during Operation Desert Storm. *J Am Acad Child Adolesc Psychiatry*. 1996;35;433–441.

13. Blount BW, Curry A Jr, Lubin GI. Family separations in the military. *Mil Med*. 1992;157:76–80.

14. van Vranken EW, Jellen LK, Knudson KH, Marlowe DH, Segal M. *82nd Airborne Division Sinai MFO Deployment Family Health Study I-IV. The Impact of Deployment Separation on Army Families*. Washington, DC: Walter Reed Army Institute of Research; 1983.

15. Schumm WR, Bell DB, Ender MG, Rice RE. Expectations, use, and evaluation of communication media among deployed peacekeepers. *Armed Forces Soc*. 2004;30:649–662.

16. Ross BJ. The emotional impact of e-mail on deployment. *US Naval Institute Proceedings*. 2001;127:85–86.

17. Rosen LR, Westhuis DJ, Teitelbaum JM. Patterns of adaptation among Army wives during Operations Desert Shield and Desert Storm. *Mil Med*. 1994;159:43–47.

18. Child Abuse Prevention and Treatment Act, 42 USC §5101 et seq (1989).

19. Child Abuse Prevention and Treatment Act Amendments of 1996, 42 USC §5116 et seq.

20. Wichlacz CR, Randall DH, Nelson JH, Kempe CH. The characteristics and management of child abuse in the US Army-Europe. *Clin Pediatr (Phila)*. 1975;14:545–548.

21. US Department of Defense. *Family Advocacy Program (FAP)*. Washington, DC: DoD; 2004. DoD Directive 6400.1.

22. US Department of the Army. *The Army Family Advocacy Program*. Washington, DC: HQDA; 2007. Army Regulation 608-18.

23. McCarroll JE, Newby JH, Dooley-Bernard M. Responding to domestic violence in the US Army: the Family Advocacy Program. In: Kendall-Tackett KA, Giacomoni SM, eds. *Intimate Partner Violence*. Kingston, NJ: Civic Research Institute; 2007: Chap 12.

24. US Department of Defense. *Domestic Abuse Involving DoD Military and Certain Affiliated Personnel.* Washington, DC: DoD; 2007. DoD Instruction 6400.06

25. Spouse and child maltreatement rates in the ACR computed from data compiled by James E. McCarroll, Center for the Study of Traumatic Stress, Department of Psychiatry, Uniformed Services University School of Medicine, Bethesda, Md.

26. Thompson M. The living room war. *Time*. 1994;143:48–51.

27. Heyman RE, Neidig PH. A comparison of spousal aggression prevalence rates in US Army and civilian representative samples. *J Consult Clin Psychol*. 1999;67:239–242.

28. Straus MA, Gelles RJ. *Physical Violence in American Families: Risk Factors and Adaptations to Violence in 8,145 Families.* New Brunswick, NJ: Transaction; 1990.

29. McCarroll JE, Ursano RJ, Liu X, et al. Deployment and the probability of spousal aggression by US Army soldiers. *Mil Med*. 2000;165:41–44.

30. McCarroll JE, Ursano RJ, Newby JH, et al. Domestic violence and deployment in US Army soldiers. *J Nerv Ment Dis*. 2003;191:3–9.

31. Newby JH, Ursano RJ, McCarroll JE, Liu X, Fullerton CS, Norwood AE. Postdeployment domestic violence by US Army soldiers. *Mil Med*. 2005;170:643–647.

32. Rentz ED, Marshall SW, Loomis D, Casteel C, Martin SL, Gibbs DA. Effect of deployment on the occurrence of child maltreatment in military and nonmilitary families. *Am J Epidemiol*. 2007;165:1199–1206.

33. Gibbs DA, Martin SL, Kupper LL, Johnson RE. Child maltreatment in enlisted soldiers' families during combat-related deployments. *JAMA*. 2007;298:528–535.

34. McCarroll JE, Fan Z, Newby JH, Ursano RJ. Trends in US Army child maltreatment reports: 1990–2004. *Child Abuse Rev*. 2008;17:108–118.

35. Rosen LN, Durand DB. Coping with the unique demands of military family life. In: Martin JA, Rosen LN, Sparacino LR, eds. *The Military Family: A Practice Guide for Human Service Providers*. Westport, Conn: Praeger; 2000: 55–72.

36. Rosen LN, Durand DB. Marital adjustment following deployment. In: Martin JA, Rosen LN, Sparacino LR, eds. *The Military Family: A Practice Guide for Human Service Providers*. Westport, Conn: Praeger; 2000: 153–165.

37. Schumm WR, Hemesath K, Bell DB, Palmer-Johnson CE, Elig TW. Did Desert Storm reduce marital satisfaction among Army enlisted personnel? *Psychol Reports*. 1996;78:1241–1242.

38. Karney BR, Crown JS. *Families Under Stress: An Assessment of Data, Theory, and Research on Marriage and Divorce in the Military*. Santa Monica, Calif: RAND National Defense Research Institute; 2007. Report No. DRR-4071-OSD.

39. Madhani A. US Army lowers its recruiting standards: more recruits have criminal records, no high school diploma. *Chicago Tribune*. October 11, 2007. Available at: http://archives.chicagotribune.com/2007/oct/11/news/chi-recruit11oct11. Accessed December 17, 2008.

40. Bachman JG, Segal DR, Freedman-Doan P, O'Malley PM. Who chooses military service? Correlates of propensity and enlistment in the US armed forces. *Mil Psychol*. 2000;12:1–30.

Chapter 33

THE FAMILIES AND CHILDREN OF FALLEN MILITARY SERVICE MEMBERS

DOUGLAS H. LEHMAN, MSW, LCSW,* AND STEPHEN J. COZZA, MD†

*Treatment Provider, Department of Behavioral Health and Family Advocacy, Evans Army Community Hospital, 7500 Cochrane Circle, Fort Carson, Colorado 80913

†Colonel, US Army (Retired); Associate Director, Center for the Study of Traumatic Stress, and Professor, Department of Psychiatry, Uniformed Services University of the Health Sciences, 4301 Jones Bridge Road, Bethesda, Maryland 20814; formerly, Chief, Department of Psychiatry, Walter Reed Army Medical Center, Washington, DC

INTRODUCTION

As of October 2007, over 4,000 US service members had died in the line of duty in Iraq and Afghanistan. Forty-four percent of military service members are parents[1] and constitute a relatively young adult population. Families of service members killed in combat are likely to include children of varying ages, one third of whom are under the age of 5. Not infrequently, these young families may include wives who are pregnant at the time of death or newborns who have never met their deceased parents. Deceased service members may have younger siblings, cousins, nieces, or nephews who, while not part of the nuclear military family, are other child mourners. Caring for the family after the loss of a service member requires sensitivity and consistency. This chapter will focus on the needs of the families of the fallen, with special emphasis on the needs of children and the programs in place to meet those needs.

MILITARY RESPONSE TO THE DEATH OF A SERVICE MEMBER

Beginning in 1950, the Army has published an instruction guide to assist survivors of fallen soldiers.[2] *A Guide for the Survivors of Deceased Army Members* describes the notification process and services available to meet the needs of mourning families. Subjects range from discussing the role of the casualty assistance officer (CAO) to funeral and postfuneral procedures. Army Regulation 600-8-1, the *Army Casualty Program*,[3] describes in detail the responsibilities and services provided by the military to families of the deceased, explaining the casualty assistance program and the role and duties of the CAO.

Family notification of combat death has changed in the past century. During World War II, Army families were informed of a service member's death by a telegram from the Army Adjutant General. The telegram, which typically arrived weeks after the death, stated the known factual information about the death and offered a brief statement of regret. A letter offering the military's condolences and outlining survivors' benefits followed the telegram. By the end of the Korean War, the Army sought to improve this process by personalizing notification. Initial notification was still sent by telegram but was followed by the arrival of an Army officer who visited the family's home, verified the death, and provided additional details. The personal visit was meant to convey greater organizational appreciation and respect for the sacrifice of the deceased soldier and the loss to the family.[4]

A substantial change in the notification process occurred during the Vietnam War, when the next of kin was first contacted with the news of death by a "casualty notifier," an officer of equal or higher rank than the deceased. Personal notification was followed by a telegram of confirmation. Only equal ranking officers, senior officers, or noncommissioned officers made the death notification. To minimize the family's shock, death notifications occurred only between 6:00 AM and 10:00 PM. The Vietnam era's expanded casualty assistance program was similar to the current format for notifications and standards.[4] Another significant change occurred in 1970, adding notification of secondary next of kin, identified by the next of kin, such as former spouses, grandparents, or friends. The CAO offered assistance to the family during this difficult time.

Since Vietnam, other changes in notification and family assistance have taken place. After the 1985 airplane crash in Gander, Newfoundland, that killed 248 soldiers and 8 crew members, the CAO's role was expanded to help the immediate family and to support the secondary next of kin in greater depth. These changes included regularly scheduled CAO family briefings, as well as government-funded travel to and from funerals and memorial services for certain family members.[4] Recently, a distinction has been made between the individual (or team) who notifies the family of the soldier's death and the CAO who provides ongoing support to the family. This distinction is recognized as important because of negative associations with the death notification. After the notification, the family is informed of the CAO's role, and the CAO calls on the family to offer assistance and support.[4]

Since 2003, death notification has changed as a result of surveys of Navy families and casualty assistance call officers (CACOs).[5] According to the CACO survey, 95% of the families of deceased Navy military members had a high level of satisfaction with the services they received. Respondents identified the need for more training to increase knowledge of the CACO's duties and responsibilities. The CACOs felt that they should remain engaged with the families for a longer period of time, as well as needing more knowledge about specific benefits. As a result, Navy training has been increased from 1 to 2 days, Web access has been expanded, and personnel services have increased to include operations for survivors available 24 hours a day, 7 days a week. The Navy responds to casualties through its casualty assistance calls program and the assigned program coordinator.

Recent changes to survivor benefits include allowing a surviving spouse and dependents to remain in Army base housing for a full year after the death of a soldier, compared to 6 months, which was the policy before the global war on terror, and an increase in the monetary survivor benefit to $400,000 across the services. Another change requires all death reports to be reviewed by a field-grade or higher-ranking officer. This change was made to ensure the accuracy of the report's details and reduce the likelihood of later changes to the report that could lead to erroneous interpretations of the death.

Since 2006, the National Defense Authorization Act has mandated that all services collect data "regarding the incidence and quality of casualty assistance provided to survivors of military decedents, including surveys of such survivors and military and civilian members assigned casualty duties."[6] In response to the act, the Army's Families First Casualty Call Center created an outreach survey instrument that collects information from outbound calls and mailed questionnaires. The survey was designed to capture feedback and the next of kin's level of satisfaction during the casualty assistance process.

The Army's Casualty and Mortuary Affairs operation center (CMAOC) has been tasked with the collection and analysis of data received from completed surveys. The CMAOC began surveying next of kin in 2005 with 33 questions related to four primary areas: (1) notification, (2) CAO performance, (3) Casualty and Mortuary Affairs activities, and (4) postinterment activities. The survey results below were collected from the families of service members who died between March 2005 and March 2006 (approximately 1,000 identified contacts). The results indicate that families have largely been satisfied with the CMAOC process. A quality-assurance working group has identified key areas where CMAOC scored at least 90% satisfactory from the respondents:

- 97% stated that their CAO displayed/expressed sufficient compassion for their loss;
- 93% stated that their CAO made their family a priority and was responsive to their needs;
- 93% stated that their CAO explained all funeral options and assisted with funeral arrangements;
- 92% stated that the CAO explained all authorized expenses for the funeral; and
- 91% responded that their CAO explained all qualified benefits and entitlements.

The working group also proposed the following procedural changes to address areas of need identified by the survey:

- Command should prioritize predeployment education of benefits, living wills, entitlements, and forms.
- An inventory process should be standardized before deployment, and summary courts-martial officers should determine whether the service member completed an inventory prior to deployment.
- Throughout the CAO assistance process, families should receive continuous updates about survivor benefits.
- CAOs should perform a final review of applicable benefits with the families before ending their assignments (formalized by a check list).
- CAOs should inform survivor families of services available through casualty assistance centers.
- A training module on personal-effect processing should be developed, and CAOs need to be trained in this area.

In addition to these existing tools, the Office of the Secretary of Defense developed a universal survey to assess satisfaction with the casualty assistance process that was disseminated to surviving primary next of kin across all services beginning in the first quarter of 2007.

THE MILITARY CARE TEAM

The care team concept developed from the Spouses' Project at the Army War College, Carlisle Barracks, Pennsylvania.[7] The team typically consists of spouse volunteers from a previously formed family readiness group in the same battalion or company as the deceased service member. Care team training mirrors CAO training, although it has been formalized in different ways at some sites. For example, spouses at Fort Carson, Colorado, have developed and use a "smart book" training manual.[8] In many other places, care team practices have been implemented with less formal procedural development.

The care team offers short-term respite and supportive care to families of the deceased and also helps the families of seriously wounded soldiers. The team is designed as temporary transitional assistance until the survivor's support structure is in place. Each care team consists of an on-site leader as well as other participants. The care team works with the casualty notification team if a surviving family member has agreed to this arrangement. Care team members help activate preestablished plans to assist family members, coordinate more effective use of military and community resources, and develop additional personalized resources to assist surviving family members. Care teams have been successful in personalizing the notification and early assistance support to casualty families. The teams have also reduced stress on spouses of volunteers, relying on team strength rather than overburdening individuals.

GRIEF RESPONSES

Adult Grief Responses

Grief is a reaction people have to loss in their lives. Grief includes a range of responses that vary according to type of loss, its meaning to the individual, and each individual's particular circumstances and experiences. When people grieve, they are coming to terms with life-changing loss. Healthy grieving allows the individual to begin finding new ways of living while coping with the gaps created by the loss. The grief process has no time limit. The phases described in Table 33-1 provide a general timeline that a grieving adult may experience; however, it is not uncommon for individuals to move back and forth between phases or manifest responses from multiple phases simultaneously.

Everyone experiences the grief process physically, emotionally, psychologically, socially, and often spiritually. Physical reactions can include pain, dizziness, shortness of breath, and sleep disturbances (hypersomnia or insomnia). Grieving adults may experience a variety of emotional reactions, including shock, tearfulness, fear, anger, and envy. Adults may sometimes have confusing or contradictory thoughts. They may feel guilty, expect the return of the deceased, or become troubled by disturbed memories or dreams. Socially, a grieving adult is likely to feel lonely or isolated and may find a need to redefine or reestablish relationships. Grieving adults may find spiritual or religious practice to be profoundly helpful and reassuring. Sometimes the death of a loved one can cause adults to question the basis of their religious faith.

Grief symptoms may include an overwhelming sense of loss with strong feelings of yearning or longing for the loved one. Survivors may feel a profound sense of emptiness and a sense that a part of them has died. Grieving survivors often speak of generalized pain or heaviness in their chest. They may feel depressed and hopeless about the future. Things that once were important may no longer seem to matter. Those who suffer traumatic loss may cry easily and lose interest in eating; they may experience stomach upset, headaches, and feelings of restlessness. A commonality among survivors is the desire to preserve the memory of their loved ones and the belief that their loved ones believed in and drew meaning in their military mission. Politi-

TABLE 33-1

ADULT GRIEVING PROCESS TIMELINE

Phase	I	II	III	IV
Description	Responses can result from the initial impact of notification and occur immediately after the notification	Responses comprise withdrawal and confusion	Responses consist of an adjustment to the death	Responses are characterized by reconstruction and reconciliation
Response	"Fight or flight"	Anger, fear, guilt, rage	Positive thoughts begin	Hope
Thought	Numb or disoriented	Ambiguity and uncertainty	Problem solving	Consolidation of problem solving
Direction	Searching for a lost object	Bargaining, detachment, depression	Searching for new objective	Reattachment
Search behavior	Reminiscing	Perplexed and scanning	Focus on exploration	Reality testing
Guidance needed	Accepting feelings	Task orientation and direction	Support and spiritual insights	Breakthrough and reinforced hope

cal, cultural, and economic states are crossed by these dual focuses.[9]

Children's Grief Responses

Children experience a sudden and profound life change when they lose a parent in combat. In all cases, the death of a parent is premature to the age and health of that individual, as well as to the relationship with the child. Since 2001, thousands of children have lost military parents from combat operations in Iraq and Afghanistan. Military deaths have affected countless other children whose service member siblings, cousins, aunts, uncles, and other extended family members have died in the line of duty. These losses can be equally profound.

Similarly to adults, children mourn the deaths of loved ones. Family death affects children of all ages, from infants and toddlers to teenagers (see Exhibit 33-1). Children, like adults, feel a deep sense of loss or sadness when a loved one dies. Many people assume that because children do not understand death in the same way as adults, they have less of an emotional response, but this is not true. Children are likely to be powerfully affected by the deaths of loved ones but may be less able to express confusing thoughts and feelings in words. While many children may express feeling sad, cry, or become more withdrawn, others express their emotions by reverting to earlier childhood behaviors. Infants and toddlers are likely to experience the death through the emotional responses or change in availability of the important adults in their lives, and react to these changes. Very young children can demonstrate changes in sleeping or eating patterns, increasing tantrums, or overactive behavior. School-aged children may express emotional concerns through physical complaints such as stomachaches or headaches. Teenagers often wish to present themselves as independent and not in need of adult help. Their sullenness or seeming disconnectedness should not be mistaken for a lack of emotional response to a death. Behavioral changes in any grieving child are more likely to be an emotional response than a disciplinary problem.

Children who lose military family members during wartime are similar to other grieving children in many ways. However, certain unique aspects characterize military family loss. Service members may be deployed for long periods before a death, and children may have become adjusted to the physical absence of the deceased parent or family member, making it more difficult to accept the permanence of the loss. Because military deaths during wartime are viewed as public events, family privacy during grieving may be diminished. Family members and communities should assist in protecting children from disturbing media exposure or other unwanted intrusions on the grieving process. Bereaved families living on military installations will likely be surrounded by community support and attention. Typically this interest is wanted and appreciated by families, but limits may need to be set by families to ensure that the attention does not become burdensome. Reserve and National Guard families or those living outside of military communities may find their grief is less well understood by well-intentioned civilian families in their neighborhoods. Children who attend schools with few other military children may find themselves isolated in their experiences of loss. Finally, not all military deaths are the same—some children may lose loved ones to combat, but others lose parents as a result of accidents or other causes.

A child's response to parental death is related to the surviving parent's response to the death: "Children appear to be at risk for concurrent and later difficulties primarily in the extent they suffer a higher probability of inadequate parental functioning or other environmental support before as well as after the loss of a parent."[10(p431)] Bivariate and multivariate analyses show that the health of the surviving parent relates directly to how well a child will adjust[11]; however, even a "healthy" parental response does not guarantee a "healthy" child response. Even if a child appears to be transitioning well through the grieving process, it is helpful to notify other adults in the child's life of the death. Teachers, coaches, healthcare providers, and spiritual and religious leaders can often offer support to grieving children within the context of their daily interactions.

Children are extremely aware of the attitudes, behaviors, and emotions of the adults they see around them. Parents and caring adults should help children understand what they are likely to see as people mourn. Children can be reassured when they understand that expressions of emotions, including sorrow, are natural ways of showing how much people cared for the deceased and how much their loved one will be missed. Children will feel more confident when they see adults handling emotionally painful situations without losing control. Tears and sorrow are to be expected. However, adults should protect children from witnessing frightening or uncontrollable displays of emotion. If such a situation occurs, adults should talk to youngsters about what they witness so that the event is more understandable and less frightening.

Very little has been written about children experiencing the loss of a parent in a wartime environment; however, an overwhelming amount of literature explores the issues of grief in children experiencing

EXHIBIT 33-1

CHILDREN'S EMOTIONAL AND BEHAVIORAL RESPONSES TO DEATH

Infants and toddlers:

- crying
- searching for parents/caregivers
- clinging
- changing sleeping and eating habits
- regressing to earlier behavior (eg, bedwetting, thumb sucking)
- repeating play or talk

Preschoolers (age 3–5):

- fearing separation (eg, from parents/loved ones)
- clinging
- throwing tantrums, having irritable outbursts
- fighting
- crying
- withdrawing
- regressing to earlier behavior (eg, bedwetting, thumb sucking)
- sleeping difficulty (eg, nightmares, difficulty sleeping alone)
- increasing occurrence of usual fears (eg, the dark, monsters)
- magical thinking, believing the person will reappear
- acting and talking as if the person is not sick or is still alive

Younger school-age children (ages 6–9):

- reacting in anger, lying, bullying
- denying
- acting irritably
- blaming self
- fluctuating moods
- fearing separation, being alone, or experiencing recurring events
- withdrawing
- regressing to earlier behavior
- having physical complaints (eg, stomachaches, headaches)
- experiencing school problems (eg, avoidance, academic difficulty, difficulty concentrating)

Middle-school children (ages 9–12)

- crying
- longing for someone who has died
- acting aggressively, irritably, bullying
- experiencing resentment
- experiencing sadness, isolation, withdrawal
- having fears, anxiety, pain
- suppressing emotions, denial, avoidance
- blaming self, guilt
- sleeping disturbance
- worrying about physical health and having physical complaints
- declining academic success, discipline, attendance, memory
- thinking and talking repetitively
- expressing "hysterical" concerns and need to help

Early teens and adolescents (ages 13–18):

- experiencing resentment, loss of trust
- feeling guilt, shame
- experiencing depression, having suicidal thoughts
- distancing, withdrawal, panic
- swinging moods, irritability
- experiencing anxiety, panic, dissociation
- experiencing anger
- involving self
- exaggerating euphoria
- acting out (engaging in risky, antisocial, or illegal behavior)
- using substances
- fearing similar events, illness, death, the future
- changing appetite and sleep patterns
- experiencing physical complaints or changes
- declining academics, refusing to go to school

traumatic loss or death of a parent under other circumstances. The distinction is important to understanding how the death and loss of a loved one is further exacerbated by the subsequent social, educational, and financial changes that the military family experiences as isolation from a known life style and disruption of daily routines.[11]

Typically, the family is young; a social change occurs from military family to civilian family; the family moves; and the financial benefits are limited. Family moves likely lead to changes in communities, schools, peer groups, and activities. Thus, the family's changes can limit the children's support systems. Such transitions can be extremely challenging to both children and surviving parents. These transitions can, in some ways, become the most complicating elements of the death for children.

In a briefing for care team training, Chaplain James Ellison of Fort Carson asks the trainees to think about how many times they have experienced the death of an immediate family member and to reflect on the types of life-changing experiences that resulted. He then discusses how children who have experienced the death of a parent have a "life-changing experience" on three levels:

1. the loss of the parent,
2. the loss of the same relationship with the surviving parent, and
3. the loss of a sense of the family system.

Children and Military Funerals

Military traditions and rituals follow the death of a service member from the arrival of the uniformed death notification team through graveside military honors. Family members can decide to what degree they will incorporate military tradition into their mourning process. Many children and families find military ceremonies comforting; others do not. The military funeral tradition is long, rich, and includes activities and rituals that may evoke a variety of reactions. Children may have varying levels of information about the nature of death, and the family funeral may be the child's first exposure to funeral ceremonies. Caskets, military uniforms, the firing of weapons, and the folding of flags can all spark curiosity, interest, and sometimes confusion and fear as well. Helping children prepare for and understand these events also helps them integrate the complex and emotionally charged experience of a military family funeral.

Although funerals are a time of family pain, they are also a time of family gathering. Contact with other family members and close friends before, during, and after the ceremony can be reassuring to children and demonstrate that sadness does not need to be borne alone. Children and family members may choose to express pride for the life of the deceased, reminisce about shared experiences, or say nothing at all. Children particularly value the power of storytelling. Stories evoking positive memories of the deceased can be especially helpful.

It is best to allow children to establish their own levels of comfort and involvement in funeral services. Gentle adult reassurance can be very helpful. However, it is inadvisable to force children to attend viewings or funeral services when they demonstrate significant discomfort in these situations. If the family chooses an open casket viewing, children may or may not want to view the deceased. They should never feel compelled to approach or touch the body, nor should they be forbidden to come near the casket if they wish. When children choose to move closer, adults should monitor younger children, calmly comfort them if necessary, and answer any questions they might have. When properly prepared, most children will feel at ease participating in the funeral service.

Children should be allowed to behave like children. Their participation and activities during the funeral service may vary depending on age. Older children may appear uninterested or bored during the ceremony, but they may actually be trying to observe and integrate what they are experiencing. Some young children may appear to be uninvolved or run around and cause disruptions. Their activity may be the healthy expression of normal childhood behavior or a manifestation of their own anxiety. Disruptive, unruly, and disrespectful behaviors are likely to be signs that children are overwhelmed and would benefit by taking a quiet break away from activities. A funeral is typically not the appropriate time to discipline children.

Traumatic Grief

Death within a family is always a painful experience. Like families of police officers and firefighters, military families are aware of the inherent risks of serving in harm's way. Nevertheless, military deaths are painful and typically sudden and unexpected.

> Combat, combat-related, and training deaths, which are all forms of sudden traumatic death, are especially hard on military (families) widows. These deaths often cause significant damage to the body, often making it non-viewable or non-recoverable.[12(p50)]

Traumatic deaths are distinct from anticipated deaths, and their effect on spouses, families, children, and communities may be profound. The following are general characteristics of traumatic deaths:

- can occur without warning, providing no opportunity to anticipate, prepare, or say goodbye;
- can be untimely, including the death of one's child at any age;
- can occur as the consequence of violence and can result in violent harm to the body;
- can include more than one person; and
- can be the result of the willful misconduct of others, such as carelessness or negligence.

Many individuals experience the sudden traumatic loss of a loved one at some point in their lives. Such losses can be complicated for adults and children to integrate. Communities often share these traumatic losses and experiences.

Traumatic grief symptoms may occur following a sudden traumatic loss. In contrast to normal grief, traumatic grief symptoms may include feelings of horror and anxiety; other feelings may be emotional numbness and a sense of disconnection. Some people cannot remember significant parts of what happened; others are plagued by memories or a sensation that they are reexperiencing or reliving the event through painful flashbacks. Traumatic deaths often cause extreme distress that can interfere significantly with daily functions over an extended period of time.

Those suffering traumatic loss may develop symptoms of posttraumatic stress disorder (PTSD). PTSD is diagnosed when the following three symptom clusters are present: (1) reexperiencing of the traumatic event as indicated by painful, intrusive thoughts or avoidance indicated by marked efforts to stay away from activities, places, or things related to the loved one's death; (2) emotional numbing, as indicated by feeling detached from others; and (3) difficulty sleeping, irritability, difficulty concentrating, and a tendency to become startled easily and detached from others. Even if full criteria for a diagnosis of PTSD are not met, individuals can suffer from symptoms caused by the loss, such as self-blame and guilt. People may imagine ways they could have or should have prevented this loss from occurring or ways they could have rescued the person, and they may experience guilt about events that occurred prior to the death.

Traumatic losses often threaten the survivor's sense of personal safety, security, and ability to trust others. Accepting the reality of the sudden traumatic loss can take a significant amount of time. Survivors may know intellectually that their loved one is dead but may find themselves expecting the loved one to walk through the door or call on the telephone. Parting with a loved one's possessions can be difficult. It may be especially disturbing when a loved one's body is not recovered. Sudden traumatic losses often raise existential and spiritual issues, such an inability to make sense of the loss or a feeling of betrayal by God.[13]

For some children, the extent of emotional response may be similarly extreme, or they may have difficulty grieving in a healthy fashion. Some bereaved military children may reexperience the death through nightmares, troubling memories, or repetitive play. They may avoid being reminded of the person who died or may continue to demonstrate profound sadness or inconsolable anxiety long after the death. In such circumstances a child may demonstrate symptoms of traumatic grief, which requires professional evaluation and treatment. When adults are concerned that a child is struggling to adjust to the death, they should speak with the child's pediatrician and seek referral to a child and adolescent psychiatrist, psychologist, or other mental healthcare provider. Such conditions are treatable but could worsen if left untreated.

Support Services and Organizations

Multiple community and healthcare services are available in military and civilian communities around the country to meet the needs of families that have lost a member during service. Several organizations now exist to provide support to military widows and widowers as well as military children who have lost parents. Gold Star Wives of America is an organization of military widows and widowers whose spouses have died while on active duty or from service-connected disabilities. This organization has been serving war widows and widowers from all conflicts and service-connected disabilities since its founding in 1945.

The Tragedy Assistance Program for Survivors (TAPS) also provides a support network for the surviving families of those who have died in service. TAPS sponsors an annual children's camp in Washington, DC, which provides

> multiple group and individual activities to assist the children in expressing feelings that may not be appreciated by others who cannot relate to their experience. The camp has normal social and outdoors activities to promote peer support and in addition to group sessions that allow the children to do important processing and grieving . . . there is (also) a program enabling the surviving spouses to do similar therapeutic work with other spouses, while the children are engaged in their camp.[13(p273)]

Several other organizations have developed programs to assist military children with the trauma, grief, and loss from their parent's combat death, injury, or illness. More information about the National Military Family Association, Zero to Three's Coming Together Around Military Families program, and the Military Child Education Coalition's Living in the New Normal initiative, as well as other resources are provided in the attachment to this chapter.

Uncomplicated grief is often managed within families, communities, or groups of friends. Widowed spouses and children may find benefit in joining therapeutic or self-help groups that focus on grief. Typically, such groups include other grieving individuals and allow an opportunity for adults and children to interact with others who have had similar experiences. Grief counselors, chaplains, mental health providers, or peer facilitators may lead these groups. For some adults and children, individual grief counseling sessions may be more comfortable. Again, counselors, chaplains, mental health providers, or other professionals may provide these services. Military OneSource is also an important resource for identifying community services for families.

When symptoms of traumatic grief, PTSD, or depression are present, or when health risk behaviors such as increased alcohol use develop, referral to competent mental health treatment is necessary. Psychiatrists, psychologists, social workers, and counselors provide mental healthcare in military medical treatment facilities, through local community mental health services, and by participating TRICARE civilian healthcare professionals. However, the recent Department of Defense Task Force on Mental Health has identified multiple barriers that can block access of bereaved military family members to appropriate care.[14] Widowed spouses and children should be encouraged to advocate for their own needs in finding resources. Primary care providers, chaplains, and community service professionals can all assist in this goal. Health and community professionals can also assist families who avoid mental healthcare because of the associated stigma.

Changes in cultural status of bereaved families can cause them to feel simultaneously disconnected from the military community and not yet comfortable in the civilian community into which they are transitioning. As stated in *Military Widow: A Survival Guide*, bereaved spouses may feel that

> even though you remain a military dependent, your status within the military has changed. You are a dependent without a living spouse. You are no longer affiliated with a particular command or unit. . . . The unspoken lack of acceptance of, or comfort with, widows in the military infrastructure is a key aspect of what contributes to military grief complex.[12(p108)]

Such experiences can complicate the families' ability to connect with needed mental health services.

SPECIAL CIRCUMSTANCES

Death, Illness, or Injury of a Leader

Emotions run high in a unit when a leader is killed. Somehow no one expects the leader to be vulnerable. Because the leader's spouse is usually the one helping others, knowing how to help the spouse is often hard for the unit. Also, the leader's spouse may find accepting help from the unit difficult. When a leader dies, the unit has suddenly lost its direction for the active duty members as well as their family members, creating a significant change in everyone's life. Being aware of this effect can help the unit cope with the loss.

Suicide

For surviving family members dealing with the aftermath of a suicide, the grieving process can be compounded by feelings of failure, shame, and guilt. Public scrutiny and military inquiry into the nature of the death can complicate a family's normal grieving. In such circumstances, families may be uncomfortable about using military or family traditions in honoring the dead. Because adults may be hesitant to share information with children (even information that is appropriate and could be helpful), children may be particularly vulnerable to problems integrating the death. Often children have an awareness of the nature of the death but are met with silence when they ask questions. Being sensitive to the unique nature of the child's loss will better enable a caregiver to provide comfort and support.

Missing in Action and Prisoners of War

Families of service members who are missing in action or prisoners of war are forced to deal with the uncertainty of the status of their loved one. The suffering that might have to be endured for an indefinite period of time exacerbates this highly emotional and painful ordeal. Providing ongoing emotional, spiritual, and logistical support to the families of these service members presents a unique challenge. It should be kept in mind that each family's needs and wants will reflect its particular situation; families should be encouraged to ask for the type and amount of assistance they prefer.

Mass Casualties

Multiple injuries or deaths are certainly one of the most difficult situations a military unit might face. When multiple tragedies occur at the same time, the affected surviving families share a unique bond. After a few days or even weeks, they may be interested in getting connected with each other. Even when tragedies occur at the same time, no two families manage the events exactly the same.

Death of a Spouse or Child

In many instances military units adopt the cohesive characteristics and nurturing tendencies of a family. When trauma occurs within a unit, the potential for impact on many or all members of the "unit family" can be far reaching, especially in the case of the death of an active duty service member's spouse or child. The loss of a spouse or child in any circumstance is traumatic, but when it occurs within the close-knit atmosphere of a military unit, the effects can be compounded. But the same circumstances that make this loss so painful for a unit are the very sources for rallying support, providing comfort, and creating a healing environment for those left behind.

Media

Americans are particularly proud and interested in the lives of their servicemen and women. Today news coverage is instantaneous to audiences throughout the world. Whenever a service member is killed or injured, Americans want to know the "who, what, when, where, and why" of the incident, and the media is eager to report it. Embedded reporters may provide immediate coverage of the spouse's deployed unit, and fatalities may become special reports on the evening news. With the presence of cellular and satellite phones, it is possible for the news of the death of a service member to bypass the normal channels of notification.

In the most stressful hours of coping with trauma in the unit, the media may approach family members for a formal interview, an informal comment, or a gut reaction. Mentoring the affected family members by encouraging them to use the public affairs office for any media interaction is beneficial. Contacting the command whenever the media approaches a unit's family member is also advisable.

SUMMARY

The families and children of service members who die in the line of duty face profound challenges. Most military families are by nature healthy and resilient, and most can be expected to transition through a period of grieving to a new state of health within the civilian communities to which they move. However, all grieving families can benefit from community resources. Professionals need to be mindful of the expected reactions of adults and children as they traverse healthy grieving. As this chapter highlights, impediments to healthy resolution can occur when symptoms of traumatic grief, PTSD, depression, or health-risk behaviors develop. Professionals must also remember that children who lose a parent are at added risk for developing behavioral problems, in comparison to their nongrieving peers. Awareness of developmental differences in children of all ages can be instructive in understanding when children are adjusting well and when they could benefit from additional help.

REFERENCES

1. US Department of Defense. *1st Quadrennial Quality of Life Review.* Washington, DC: DoD; 2004.

2. US Department of the Army. *A Guide for the Survivors of Deceased Army Members*. Washington, DC: DA; 1989. DA Pamphlet 608-4.

3. US Department of the Army. *Army Casualty Program*. Washington, DC: DA; 2007. Army Regulation 600-8-1.

4. Ender MG, Bartone PT, Kolditz TA. Fallen soldiers: death and the US military. In: Bryant CD, ed. *Handbook of Death and Dying.* Thousand Oaks, Calif: Sage; 2003: 544–555.

5. Michael Wardlaw, Casualty Assistance Director, US Navy. *Measuring Customer Satisfaction for Navy Casualty Assistance Calls Program (CACP).* Unpublished research proposal; data are from casualty assistance call officers' surveys, 2003.

6. National Defense Authorization Act. 10 USC §1475. Available at: http://uscode.house.gov/download/pls/10C75.txt. Accessed March 25, 2011.

7. Army War College Spouses' Project. *A Leaders Guide to Trauma in the Unit.* Carlisle Barracks, Penn: Army War College; 2004: 6. Available at: http://www.carlisle.army.mil/usawc/dclm/docs/traumapdf.pdf. Accessed December 12, 2009.

8. Roy C. *Care Team Smart Book* [unpublished manual]. Fort Carson, Colo: Family Readiness Center; 2005.

9. Deb Busch, founder of Helping Unite Gold Star Survivors at Fort Hood, Texas. Personal communication, December 13, 2007.

10. Tremblay GC, Israel AC. Children's adjustment to parental death. *Clin Psychol: Sci Pract.* 1998;5:424–438.

11. Katler N, Lohnes K, Chasin J, et al. The adjustment of parentally bereaved children: factors associated with short-term adjustment. *Omega: J Death Dying.* 2002–2003;46(1):15–34.

12. Steen JM, Asaro MR. *Military Widow: A Survival Guide.* Annapolis, Md: Naval Institute Press; 2006.

13. Hardaway T. Treatment of psychological trauma in children of military families. In: Webb NB, ed. *Mass Trauma and Violence: Helping Families and Children Cope.* New York, NY: Guildford Press; 2004: 259–282.

14. Department of Defense Task Force on Mental Health. *An Achievable Vision: Report of the Department of Defense Task Force on Mental Health.* Falls Church, Va: Defense Health Board; 2007. Available at: http://www.health.mil/dhb/mhtf/MHTF-Report-Final.pdf. Accessed November 5, 2009.

ATTACHMENT: RESOURCES FOR FAMILIES OF DECEASED SERVICE MEMBERS

Organizations and Programs

The Arlington National Cemetery Commemorative Project

In 2009, the Arlington National Cemetery Commemorative Project, in partnership with Rich Clarkson and Associates and the National Geographic Society, produced *For Children of Valor: Arlington National Cemetery*. This volume is a special commemorative gift book for children who since September 11, 2001, have lost close loved ones who were on active duty and are now buried at Arlington National Cemetery. *For Children of Valor* was written to help these children understand and process their grief. The book also includes a resource guide for parents.

Military OneSource

Military OneSource is a service provided by the Department of Defense at no cost to active duty, National Guard, and reserve service members and their families. Military OneSource is available by phone, online, and face-to-face through private counseling sessions in the local community. Its highly qualified consultants provide assistance with childcare, personal finances, emotional support during deployments, relocation information, and resources needed for special circumstances. Assistance includes personalized consultations on specific issues such as education, special needs, and finances, as well as customized research detailing community resources and appropriate military referrals. Available at: http://www.militaryonesource.com. Accessed August 19, 2009.

TRICARE

TRICARE is the healthcare program serving active duty service members, National Guard and reserve members, retirees, their families, and survivors worldwide. As a major component of the military healthcare system, TRICARE brings together the healthcare resources of the uniformed services and supplements them with networks of civilian healthcare professionals, institutions, pharmacies, and suppliers to provide access to high-quality healthcare services while maintaining the capability to support military operations. Available at: http://www.tricare.mil. Accessed August 19, 2009.

Military Homefront

Military life comes with unique challenges, from shopping at the commissary to moving to foreign lands. Having trusted information on how to deal with these challenges can make the difference between stress and success. Military Homefront provides accurate and up-to-date information about Department of Defense programs serving troops and their families. Available at: http://www.militaryhomefront.dod.mil. Accessed August 19, 2009.

The Military Child Education Coalition's Living in the New Normal Initiative

Sparked by concerns about military children dealing with illness, injury, or death of a parent, the Living in the New Normal (LINN): Helping Children Thrive in Good and Challenging Times initiative was developed by the Military Child Education Coalition (MCEC) through collaboration with experts in the fields of trauma and grief, resiliency, healthcare, and child development. LINN encourages families to ensure that their children have the tools to weather life's storms, fosters home-front efforts to support military children, and provides educators and other concerned adults with information to help them support children during times of uncertainty, trauma, and grief. LINN's efforts are predicated on the belief that children are courageous and resilient and that these skills can be strengthened through deliberate encouragement by the adults in their lives. Available at: http://www.militarychild.org/linn.asp. Accessed August 19, 2009.

National Military Family Association

The National Military Family Association is dedicated to providing information to and representing the interests of family members of the uniformed services. Its Web site provides extensive information for military families and support service staff. The association publishes a monthly newsletter as well as a weekly legislative e-mail newsletter, the *Government and You E-News.* Available at: http://www.nmfa.org. Accessed August 19, 2009.

Zero to Three's Coming Together Around Military Families Initiative

The nonprofit Zero to Three organization's Coming Together Around Military Families initiative increases awareness of the impact of trauma, grief, and loss on very young children through specialized training and support for the professionals who are supporting military families in and around military installations with high deployment rates. Of primary focus are the special circumstances of families that experience trauma and loss as a result of a service member's deployment. Available at: http://www.zerotothree.org/military. Accessed August 19, 2009.

Tragedy Assistance Program for Survivors

The Tragedy Assistance Program for Survivors (TAPS) was founded in the wake of a military tragedy in which surviving family members realized that the tragedy they shared, losing a loved one in the line of military duty, was far different from other types of losses. These families shared pride in their spouses' service to America as well as tremendous sadness at the ultimate sacrifice their loved ones made. TAPS has experienced, empathetic caseworkers who act as liaisons with federal, state, and private agencies in helping family members find solutions to problems. Available at: http://www.taps.org. Accessed August 19, 2009.

Gold Star Wives of America

Founded in 1945, Gold Star Wives of America Inc is an organization of military widows and widowers whose spouses died while on active duty or from service-connected disabilities. Gold Star Wives received a federal charter from Congress on December 4, 1980. Available at: http://www.goldstarwives.org. Accessed August 19, 2009.

Uniformed Services University of the Health Sciences Center for the Study of Traumatic Stress

The Center for the Study of Traumatic Stress conducts research, education, consultation, and training on preparing for and responding to the psychological effects and health consequences of traumatic events, including natural (hurricanes, floods, and tsunamis) and human-made disasters (motor vehicle and plane crashes, war, terrorism, and bioterrorism). The center's work spans studies of genetic vulnerability to stress, individual and community responses to terrorism, and policy recommendations to help the nation and its military and civilian populations. Available at: http://www.centerforthestudyoftraumaticstress.org. Accessed August 19, 2009.

The National Child Traumatic Stress Network

Established by Congress in 2000, the National Child Traumatic Stress Network is a unique collaboration of academic and community-based service centers whose mission is to raise the standard of care and increase access to services for traumatized children and their families across the United States. Combining knowledge of child development, expertise in the full range of child traumatic experiences, and attention to cultural perspectives, the network serves as a national resource for developing and disseminating evidence-based interventions, trauma-informed services, and public and professional education. Available at: http://www.nctsn.org. Accessed August 19, 2009.

American Academy of Child and Adolescent Psychiatry

Established in 1953, the American Academy of Child and Adolescent Psychiatry is the leading national professional medical association dedicated to treating and improving the quality of life for children, adolescents, and families affected by mental disorders. The academy is a membership-based organization composed of over 7,500 child and adolescent psychiatrists and other interested physicians. Its members actively research, evaluate, diagnose, and treat psychiatric disorders, giving direction and responding quickly to new developments in addressing the healthcare needs of children and their families. The academy widely distributes information in a effort to promote understanding of mental illnesses and remove the stigma associated with them, advance efforts in prevention of mental illnesses, and assure proper treatment and access to services for children and adolescents. Available at: http://www.aacap.org. Accessed August 19, 2009.

American Academy of Pediatrics

The American Academy of Pediatrics is an organization of 60,000 pediatricians committed to the attainment of optimal physical, mental, and social health and well-being for all infants, children, adolescents, and young adults. Its uniformed services section was founded in 1959 with a mission to improve the health of infants, children, adolescents, and young adults served by medical providers in the US Army, Navy, Air Force, and public health agencies. The section provides unique educational forums to address the global issues of military pediatric providers. Available at: http://www.aap.org. Accessed August 19, 2009.

Suggested Literature and Resources Guide from the Military Child Education Coalition

The MCEC recommends the use of these books by children experiencing and coping with trauma, grief, and loss only with direct parental supervision or guidance and support from other caring adults. This list was compiled by a committee of MCEC advisors representing various perspectives: psychologists, educators, military families, grief specialists, and professional developers, and is reproduced here with permission from the MCEC. The statements included in this list are opinions based on the MCEC perspective and guiding principles and are not intended to be a comprehensive review of the literature, but rather a guide.

Early Elementary Level

- *A Bunch of Balloons,* by Dorothy Ferguson.
  Synopsis: Author discusses loss and grief by introducing a story about a little child who loses a balloon. The author then introduces the topic of death and grief and leads the reader through activities using balloons to capture what is lost and what remains in the grieving child's life. The goal is to help grieving children acknowledge what they have lost and celebrate what they still have left when someone they love has died.

- *I Had a Friend Named Peter: Talking to Children About the Death of a Friend,* by Janice Cohn.
  Synopsis: A young child learns of the sudden death of her school friend, Peter, who was accidentally hit by a car while chasing a ball. Excellent introduction helps adults understand the many questions children pose following the death of a loved one. Addresses dying, funerals, and burial in direct language. Also has a school setting with teacher and classroom. Picture book.
  Teachable moments: Have child talk about memories of the deceased—the likes and dislikes of the person. For sudden death situations, ask children how they would say goodbye to the person.

- *A Good Day,* by Kevin Henkes.
  Synopsis: Four little creatures encounter dilemmas in their day. Using their circumstances, relatable to the young child, this story presents a simple message of reassurance in times of sadness, disappointment and challenge. This book encourages hope and resilience and invites discussion with children regarding their own situations.

- *Ragtail Remembers—A Story That Helps Children Understand Feelings of Guilt,* by Liz Duckworth.
  Synopsis: The death of an old cat who was a playful companion and good friend of the storyteller, a

mouse named Ragtail. The language is clear and direct, which lends to the open discussion of feelings and emotions that are experienced when there is a death and loss. It demonstrates the importance of friends, the help rendered by a wise bluejay that acts as a faithful guide and teacher and becomes a new friend and playmate of the mouse. It is also about honoring and remembering in death.

- *The Fall of Freddie the Leaf,* by Leo Bascaglia.
  Synopsis: Freddie learns about the cycle of life from his fellow leaf friend, Daniel. Freddie comments on his experience regarding his mentor's death and then his own death.
  Caution: ensure child understands that death is not sleeping, but is permanent.
- *The Wall,* by Eve Bunting.
  Synopsis: In this moving picture book, a little boy and his father visit the Vietnam Veterans Memorial ("The Wall") to find the name of the boy's grandfather. They notice details: items left in remembrance, the uniformity of the engraved lettering, a veteran who is an amputee, and more. Together they make a rubbing of the name, which is a popular tradition.
- *When Dinosaurs Die: A Guide to Understanding Death,* by Marc Brown and Laurie Krasney.
  Synopsis: Uses dinosaurs to explain in simple language the feelings people may have regarding death of a loved one and ways to honor the memory of someone who has died. Does not tell a story; addresses fears, curiosity, customs, and acknowledges military death and war.
  Caution: Some may take offense that the death of a pet is represented as equal to the death of a person.
  Teachable moments: Dinosaurs are extinct (this can cause a whole separate discussion). Look closely at the drawings for details related to the children's questions in the book.

Mid-Elementary Level

- *Everett Anderson's Goodbye,* by Lucille Clifton.
  Synopsis: Written in verse and beautifully illustrated with charcoal line drawings, this book features a young African-American boy whose father has died. The theory of stages of grief is presented through the eyes of the young boy and his profound loss. Theories differ in describing grief as stages, phases, or processes. Stages imply a linear progression. Current research emphasizes grief as a process with phases that individuals may experience at different times.
- *Geranium Morning,* by Sandy Powell.
  Synopsis: Two elementary-aged kids, a boy and a girl, each lose a parent, a father and a mother, respectively. The father dies suddenly in an accident and the mother dies from illness. The children help each other deal with their grief; story expresses the value of shared experience as the root of recovery.
  Teachable moments: Talk about the benefit of sharing a new friendship with someone who has had a similar experience.
  Note: This book is out of print, but used copies may be available online.
- *I Don't Have an Uncle Phil Anymore,* by Marjorie Pellegrino.
  Synopsis: When a young boy's uncle dies, he must board a plane and fly to the funeral. He recalls the fun times he had with his Uncle Phil and how he used to play and do special things with his Uncle Phil and his cousin. He worries about his cousin and aunt and who will play with his uncle now. The boy witnesses the support of his uncle's fellow firefighters when the funeral procession passes the firehouse. The boy calls this a sad parade. The boy hugs his cousin Jenny and comforts her when she exclaims while playing blocks, "I don't have a daddy anymore."
- *I Miss You—A First Look at Death,* by Pat Thomas.
  Synopsis: The story uses language that is gentle, simple, clear, and straightforward, directed to a little girl. It explains death as a natural part of life, that after death, the body stops working. It discusses the funeral and provides an excellent discussion of the variation in cultural practices and beliefs regarding death. The question, "What about you?" that appears at the bottom of several pages stimulates discussion of questions a child may have about death, feelings and emotions a child may experience, and the

difficulty of understanding. There are suggestions for how to use the book at the end that are useful and instructive. A list of suggested books and resources is provided; the glossary is rather brief. Caution: On page 23, one line, "the souls of other people who have passed away," is unusual because otherwise very factual and realistic text is used throughout the story.

- *Memory String,* by Eve Bunting.
  Synopsis: A young girl's mother dies and her stepmother helps her remember the love they shared using buttons as mementos. Highlights stepmother relationship as helpful.
  Teachable moments: Gather buttons—including military buttons or insignia—to make a memory string. Discuss the meaning of each button and why it holds that meaning.
- *The Hero in My Pocket,* by Marlene Lee.
  Synopsis: A brother and sister, ages 10 and 7, experience the loss of their father who died serving in the US military. The children progress through the grief process and positive recovery is encouraged.
  Teachable moments: Children can write or draw their part of the story on "Hero Pages" in the book to give voice to their thoughts and feelings. Discuss keepsake memento child may have (or want) of the deceased (95% of children have a keepsake object [transitional linking object] from a deceased parent that they keep in their rooms). Gather "remember letters" or have class write "remember letters."
- *What Does That Mean? A Dictionary of Death, Dying and Grief Terms for Grieving Children and Those Who Love Them,* by Harold Smith and Joy Johnson.
  Synopsis: More of an encyclopedia than a dictionary, the clever format of word, pronunciation, definition and example or quotes, sometimes from known literature, could be a good, objective classroom resource.
- *Owen & Mzee,* by Isabella Hatkoff, Craig Hatkoff, and Paula Kahumbu.
  Synopsis: This is the tale of a baby hippo named Owen and his friend Mzee, a 130-year-old giant tortoise. Owen is a survivor and an orphan as a result of the December 2004 tsunami in Southeast Asia. This profound true story offers a potent reminder that even in the face of tragedy, the power of friendship endures—and that our most important friends are sometimes those we least expect. A true demonstration of resilience and living in a "new normal."
- *Annie Loses Her Leg but Finds Her Way,* by Sandra J Philipson and Robert Takatch.
  Synopsis: Based on an actual incident, this is both a poignant and funny story of a 9-year-old English springer spaniel who loses her front leg to cancer. Two children, Annie and her high-spirited brother, Max, experience her illness and recovery in very different ways. Max is in denial, and Annie is in a state of sad acceptance. This is a book about love, loss, friendship, and optimism.

Elementary and Early Teen Level

- *A Taste of Blackberries,* by Doris Buchanan Smith.
  Synopsis: Two 'tween boys, best friends, "planned to have fun all summer," but one boy dies suddenly. Novel follows range of thoughts, emotions, and actions of surviving best friend.
- *Coping With Death and Grief,* by Marge Eaton Heegaard.
  Synopsis: Eight vignettes about the death of a person and the children affected. Several different kinds of death and relationships are illustrated in easy-to-read format, followed by factual discussion points about grief, changes in relationship, realities of day-to-dayness, and many other aspects. References military funerals, playing "Taps," and much discussion about school settings, including death discussed in the classroom.
  Teachable moments: Discuss the concept of grief as a fact, a normal aspect of the human condition. Discuss how the relationship to someone is a primary factor in one's experience with grief.
- *How It Feels When a Parent Dies,* by Jill Krementz.
  Synopsis: Eighteen kids, boys and girls ages 7 to 16, wrote personal essays about their experiences and feelings about the death of their parent. Different types of loss are represented, as are a range of normal feelings: anguish, guilt, confusion, anger, as well as the children's lives since the death.

Teachable moments: Discuss how book shows that grief reactions and responses are as individual as people. With teenagers, discuss aspects that make it individual (age at time of death, family composition, type of death).

- *Part of Me Died, Too: Stories of Creative Survival Among Bereaved Children and Teenagers,* by Virginia Lynn Fry.
  Synopsis: First-person stories by kids of different ages who experienced loved ones' deaths (father, mother, friend, other relative) from different means (sudden death, lingering illness, and suicide). They describe their reactions and effects. Table of contents lists type of death and ages of kids so reader can go right to the section. In the epilogue the kids reflect on their original writings and talk about how they are now. Also lists follow-on reading suggestions.
  Teachable moments: Discuss how the book shows that grief reactions and responses are as unique as individuals. With teenagers, discuss aspects that make it individual (age at time of death, family composition, type of death).

- *What We Do When Someone Dies,* by Caroline Arnold.
  Synopsis: Fact-based book that explains vocabulary related to someone dying and afterwards (obituaries, funeral service, etc). Ranges from concept that all living things must die to what happens to the body, funeral ceremonies, and afterwards. Acknowledgment of multicultural beliefs and customs. Acknowledges that people die in war. Discusses Memorial Day and Arlington National Cemetery.
  Teachable moments: Discuss military-related traditions ("Taps," veterans' cemeteries, flags, etc). Discuss how having facts helps alleviate some of the fear associated with the difficult topic of death (fear of the unknown, fear of taboo topic, etc). Further discussion on respecting culture and traditions of different religions and nationalities, and allow child to choose topics to discuss further since book is fact-based.

Teen Level

- *Fire in My Heart, Ice in My Veins—A Journal for Teenagers Experiencing Loss,* by Enid Samuel Traisman.
  Synopsis: A workbook that allows teens to describe their feelings and thoughts related to the death of someone they cared about. A brief statement appears at the top of the page, followed by several responses to encourage and focus their expressions in writing or drawings to remember and honor the one who died. The statements are very probing. This process allows teens to be open and candid about their feelings.
  Teachable moment: Provides valuable discussion opportunities between caring adults and teens experiencing loss.

- *The Grieving Teen: A Guide for Teenagers and Their Friends,* by Helen Fitzgerald.
  Synopsis: Written about and for teens, this guidebook covers a wide range of situations and topics—and suggestions—for grieving teens and those who care about them. Teen voices are heard throughout the book. Does not discuss death of service members but it does discuss secondary losses and complicating factors such as dealing with the press and sudden death.
  Teachable moments: Discuss what kind of secondary losses or compounding factors someone may have experienced.

- *The Healing Your Grieving Heart Journal for Teens,* by Alan Wolfelt and Megan Wolfelt.
  Synopsis: Guided journal encourages teens to self-explore through self-expression. Designed as a companion book to *Healing Your Grieving Heart for Teens: 100 Practical Ideas.* Useful weeks, months, or even years following the death of a loved one.

- *When a Friend Dies: A Book for Teens about Grieving and Healing,* by Marilyn Gootman.
  Synopsis: The book is about acceptance and compassion. Focuses on answering teen/preteen questions about death.

- *You Are Not Alone: Teens Talk About Life After the Loss of a Parent,* by Lynne Hughes.
  Synopsis: The author, Lynne Hughes, the founder of the Comfort Zone Camp for grieving children who have lost parents or siblings, personally experienced the death of her parents at an early age. The voices

of teens who have attended the camp provide illustrative insights into ways young people have dealt with loss. As the title suggests, teens are encouraged to seek help and to know that there are others who share feelings of immeasurable loss.

- *Finding My Way: A Teen's Guide to Living With a Parent Who Has Experienced Trauma,* by Michelle D Sherman and DeAnne Sherman.
  Synopsis: An interactive workbook format that offers teens practical tools and information about posttraumatic stress disorder and other responses to trauma. Clearly and concisely written, it encourages teens to address their own emotions and key issues in dealing with a parent who has experienced trauma. The gentle guide, using honest and concise language, offers valuable tools for coping, identifying social support networks, and dealing with friends. An extensive resource list, glossary, and frequently-asked-questions section completes this useful manual.
- *Facing Change: Falling Apart and Coming Together Again in the Teen Years,* by Donna O'Toole.
  Synopsis: Founded on the belief that young adults can make effective choices that can transform pain into resilience, the author provides an abundance of information and coping choices to assist the process. A book about loss, change, and possibilities.

Adults—General

- *Ambiguous Loss: Learning to Live With Unresolved Grief,* by Pauline Boss.
  Synopsis: Offers insight into the meaning and impact of ambiguous loss and suggestions for coping. Author draws from her own research, including interviews with military spouses of service members who are missing in action or prisoners of war. *Ambiguous Loss* is applicable to families of those with traumatic injury or Alzheimer's disease, or who are missing.
- *Helping Children Cope With the Loss of a Loved One: A Guide for Grownups,* by William Kroen.
  Synopsis: Answers questions relative to developmental ages, uses vignettes along with practical and theoretical advice.
- *Life and Loss: A Guide to Help Grieving Children,* by Linda Goldman.
  Synopsis: Tools, ideas, and inventories for educators and other community members to use in helping kids commemorate loss. Discusses different types of childhood losses and avoids clichés. Provides an example of a "community care team" concept to help the grieving child.
- *Raising Our Children to Be Resilient,* by Linda Goldman.
  Synopsis: Resource for adults to understand how children experience traumatic events and empowering them to be resilient.
- *Raising an Emotionally Healthy Child When a Parent Is Sick,* by Paula K Rauch and Anna C Muriel.
  Synopsis: A friendly and accessible guide to communicating with children about illness, death, and dying. Assists parents in understanding unique temperaments of individual children and practical advice and examples of how to establish and organize a family support system.
- *Military Widow,* by Joanne M Steen and Regina Asaro.
  Synopsis: An insider's perspective to understanding and surviving the death of a military service member, as well as implications for surviving dependents. Helpful blend of personal experiences and professional references and research. Addresses the unique aspects and challenges of military widowhood.
- *Authentic Happiness: Using the New Positive Psychology to Realize Your Potential for Lasting Fulfillment,* by Martin EP Seligman.
  Synopsis: "Positive psychology" is a new approach to psychology focusing on mental health rather than mental illness. Readers learn that happiness can be cultivated by identifying and using many of the strengths and traits that they already possess; their signature strengths. By calling upon these strengths in all the critical aspects of life, one develops buffers against misfortune and negative emotion. Break free from learned helplessness to learned optimism resulting in greater resilience.

- *A Parent's Guide to Building Resilience in Children and Teens: Giving Your Child Roots and Wings,* by Kenneth R Ginsburg.
  Synopsis: This practical guide assists parents in showing their children how to be more resilient when facing compounding stressors by developing healthy coping strategies. Dr Ginsburg introduces parents to the seven "crucial Cs": (1) competence, (2) confidence, (3) connection, (4) character, (5) contribution, (6) coping, and (7) control, and how they work together to help kids 18 months to 18 years bounce back from challenges and manage stress.

Adults—Educational Focus

- *Grief Comes to Class: An Educator's Guide,* by Majel Gliko-Brado.
  Synopsis: Short, to-the-point guide, based on results of a study conducted through the College of Education at Montana State University to obtain perceptions and feelings about bereaved children. The views of teachers, parents, and the children are represented in the discussion of the environment, culture, individual personality, and circumstances. Examples of children's experiences are interspersed throughout the text, especially helpful in the section on developmental changes among children of different ages, with special attention on teen grief. The "What You Can Do to Help" section offers sample letters and activities for the classroom, with a teacher/parent/student conference plan that can be modified and personalized.
- *Helping Children Grieve & Grow—A Guide for Those Who Care,* by Donna O'Toole.
  Synopsis: This booklet provides a useful, easily understood synopsis to help children to grieve and to grow. The format is functional in its arrangement of concise information with practical suggestions on understanding reactions and what to do to encourage the children. It speaks of resilience in children and offers resources available both nationally and locally. The language is compassionate and demonstrates that the writer has broad experience in the field.

Adults—Reference

- *25 Things to Do: Activities to Help Children Suffering Loss or Change,* by Laurie A Kanyer.
  Synopsis: Practical and simple activities to engage a child suffering a painful loss or change. A creative, sensitive, "Mr. Rogers"-like reference for parents and caregivers. Encompasses a broad range of loss topics children may encounter in their developmental years; from the loss of a pet, to the divorce of their parents, to the death of a loved one.
- *35 Ways to Help a Grieving Child,* by the Dougy Center: The National Center for Grieving Children and Families.
  Synopsis: Drawn from stories, suggestions, and insight shared by children and their family members at the Dougy Center, this book explores behaviors and reactions of children at different ages and maturity levels; outlets for children to safely express their thoughts and feelings; and ways to be supportive during difficult times, such as a memorial service, anniversary, or holidays.
- *How to Go on Living When Someone You Love Dies,* by Terese A Rando.
  Synopsis: Step-by-step guide for adults to talk about death with children of all ages to help understand what they think, how they feel, and what they comprehend. Directly addresses how adults can help, providing checklists, scripts, and quick reference information.
- *How Do We Tell Children: Helping Children Understand and Cope When Someone Dies,* by Dan Schaefer and Christine Lyons.
  Synopsis: Written by a former funeral home director who dealt with thousands of families, this book helps adults understand how to talk with children openly about death. Covers age range from 2 to teenager. Helpful for adults to understand what children can and cannot grasp at certain developmental stages.
- *Losing Parents to Death in the Early Years,* by Alicia Lieberman.
  Synopsis: Written by one of the most respected professionals in the field of early trauma/loss, the author

explains how vulnerable children can be given their immaturity. Addresses difficult issues that arise as a result of death due to military service or socially-stigmatized causes.

- *Treating Trauma and Traumatic Grief in Children and Adolescents,* by Judith Cohen.
  Synopsis: This book describes the state-of-the-art cognitive-behavioral therapies used in treating children who are exposed to trauma and traumatic death. While it is mainly targeted for therapists and clinicians who work with this population of children, it is also an excellent reference for others who would like to understand the most effective, evidence-based approaches to helping children and adolescents who suffer with trauma-related disorders.

Chapter 34

ESTABLISHING AN INTEGRATED BEHAVIORAL HEALTH SYSTEM OF CARE AT SCHOFIELD BARRACKS

MICHAEL E. FARAN, MD, PhD[*]; ALBERT Y. SAITO, MD[†]; EILEEN U. GODINEZ, PhD[‡]; WENDI M. WAITS, MD[§]; VICTORIA W. OLSON, MBA[¥]; CHRISTINE M. PIPER, APRN, BC[¶]; MARGARET A. McNULTY, DrPH[**]; and CHRISTOPHER G. IVANY, MD[††]

---

*Colonel, US Army (Retired); Director, Child, Adolescent, and Family Behavior Health Proponency, Madigan Army Medical Center, Madigan Annex Building 9913A, Ramp 2, McKinnley Road, Tacoma, Washington 98431; formerly, Director, School Based Mental Health, Child and Adolescent Psychiatry Service, Department of Psychiatry, Tripler Army Medical Center, Honolulu, Hawaii

†Clinical Director, Child and Adolescent Psychiatry Service, Department of Psychiatry, Tripler Army Medical Center, 1 Jarrett White Road, Honolulu, Hawaii 96859-5000; formerly, Staff Psychiatrist, Department of Child Psychiatry, Tripler Army Medical Center, Honolulu, Hawaii

‡Inspector General Chief, Inspections and Outreach Branch, US European Command, CMR 480, Box 1865, APO AE 09128; formerly, Chief, Plans Analysis and Integration Office, US Army Garrison, Hawaii

§Lieutenant Colonel, Medical Corps, US Army; Chief, Inpatient Psychiatry Service, Department of Psychiatry, 1 Jarrett White Road, Room 4B106, Tripler Army Medical Center, Hawaii 96859-5000; formerly, Child and Adolescent Psychiatry Fellow, Tripler Army Medical Center, Honolulu, Hawaii

¥Executive Director, Hawai'i Army Museum Society, Post Office Box 8064, Honolulu, Hawaii 96830-0064

¶Colonel, US Army (Retired); Coaching Trainer/Instructor, LivingWorks, Inc.; formerly, Chief, Soldier and Family Assistance Center, Schofield Barracks, Hawaii

**Captain, US Navy (Retired); Assistant Professor, Department of Nursing, Kapiolani Community College, 4303 Diamond Head Road, Honolulu, Hawaii 96816

††Major, Medical Corps, US Army; Psychiatrist, Department of Behavioral Health, Evans Army Community Hospital, Building 7500, 1650 Cochrane Circle, Fort Carson, Colorado 80913; formerly, Division Psychiatrist, 4th Infantry Division, Fort Hood, Texas

INTRODUCTION

In 2003, members of four US combat infantry units (three Army units and one Marine Corps unit) participated in an anonymous mental health survey taken either before deployment or 3 to 4 months after their return.[1] The percentage of soldiers and marines whose responses met the screening criteria for major depression, generalized anxiety, posttraumatic stress disorder (PTSD), or alcohol misuse was significantly higher after duty in Iraq (15.6%–17.1%) than after duty in Afghanistan (11.2%), particularly with regard to PTSD. The rates of PTSD are similar to those experienced in Vietnam, which led to large numbers of soldiers becoming disabled. Soldiers and marines whose responses were positive for a mental disorder were twice as likely to distrust mental health professionals, viewed seeing mental health practitioners as harmful to their career, and believed that mental healthcare does not work. The stigma of seeking help increased with the presence of mental disorders. Notwithstanding the reported stigma, veterans of Operation Iraqi Freedom (OIF) utilized mental healthcare at a higher rate during the first year postdeployment than veterans of Operation Enduring Freedom (OEF) in Afghanistan or those from other deployments. About one third of the OIF veterans sought mental healthcare during their first year as compared to 22% for OEF and 24% for other regions.[2]

Recent ongoing studies suggest that deployment also significantly increases the risk of mental health problems in military children, family violence, and divorce. Anecdotal reports from the field suggest that soldiers who are worried about their families are not as able to focus on the mission. Family satisfaction and resilience are important factors contributing to soldier readiness and retention, and attrition of soldiers with mental health issues is particularly high. Hoge and colleagues[2] found that attrition for any reason during the first year postdeployment from OIF was 17%, and those who reported a mental health concern were significantly more likely to leave the service. Other studies reported that 47% of all soldiers hospitalized for the first time for any mental disorder were separated from the Army within 6 months.[3] Innovative mental health initiatives are required to meet these and other challenges facing the volunteer Army to conserve the fighting strength and meet the needs of soldiers and their families.

The lineage of community mental healthcare in the military is rich, beginning in earnest during World War II, when clinicians and commanders alike recognized that psychiatric casualties decreased as morale increased.[4] Psychiatrists grasped the importance of treating soldiers within their social structures and strengthening their identification with their units, which led to cohesion with their peers and unit leadership. As clinicians came to recognize the soldier as a part of an interdependent network of social forces, they realized that much of their treatment amounted to intervention in some part of the social structure, and that the psychiatrist was often poorly equipped for these tasks.[5] Individuals in the community—social workers, chaplains, and spouses of active duty members in volunteer positions—encountered less stigma and had greater knowledge of individual units and access to a wider pool of community programs than did hospital-based psychiatrists. As psychiatrists embraced multidisciplinary approaches, treatment moved out of medical centers and became integrated into the military social network, shifting emphasis toward prevention and leading to the community mental healthcare system.

The impetus for extending community mental healthcare to military family members, especially during deployments, rests on the emerging belief that strong social supports enhance the mental well-being of the parent remaining at home, which in turn prevents psychopathology in children. Research has shown that children's behavioral problems increase (especially in young boys) when the nondeployed parent suffers from psychopathology.[6] Practical remedies, such as strong spouse and family support groups; male companionship for young boys (eg, a big brother program or family members); education programs for spouses about separation and reunion; and regular communication with the deployed parent require community-level intervention.[6] Rear detachment units, wives' clubs, schools, childcare groups, and other community organizations can greatly contribute to building resilience in family members. Mental health providers have unique skills for identifying individual problem areas, but their interventions are most effective when integrated with the work of community groups that support families. Likewise, mental health providers working in interdisciplinary clinics located close to military housing areas are better able to implement treatment plans that involve these vital social support systems than those who work in hospital-based programs.

The responsibility for taking care of the physical and emotional needs of soldiers and their families is shared by numerous military, federal, and state agencies. These agencies each have specific portions of the overall caring "pie," but historically have functioned independently. Often agencies staunchly protect their own areas of concern, which unfortunately may result in inefficient and costly duplication of services and staff. It is a significant challenge to integrate agencies in a common goal. Wenger and Synder[7] describe the emerging concept of "communities of practice" and discuss how disparate groups with a shared agenda can come together, learn from each other, and develop strategies that work toward a common goal. Large numbers of corporations and governmental agencies are employing these principles with success; however, many organizations need leadership "buy-in" to facilitate cooperation and collaboration.

The objective of this chapter is to describe the development of a multidisciplinary, integrated system of mental health support and care at Schofield Barracks in Oahu, Hawaii, during the deployment of the 25th Infantry Division Light (25th ID), aimed at promoting resilience and wellness in the Army community. Primary focus will be on the Soldier and Family Assistance Center (SAFAC), followed by a brief discussion of a school mental health initiative,[8] mental health support to family readiness groups (FRGs [composed of Army spouses who support families]), and the Army Community Service (ACS). The discussion of the latter programs will focus on how these efforts came together to provide care for the soldiers and family members in the Schofield catchment area during OIF and OEF. (This chapter will not include detailed discussion of the Family Advocacy Program or the Army Substance Abuse Program [ASAP]. The Family Advocacy Program provides services when domestic violence is identified, and the ASAP delivers a wide range of prevention and treatment services for alcohol and drug abuse.) The overall development of the Schofield community behavioral health system is presented in chronological order to emphasize the importance of the process as it evolved within the entire community.

EARLY EFFORTS

Schofield Barracks, including Wheeler Army Airfield, is located in central Oahu on 167,919 acres of land. It is home to the 25th ID and supports approximately 14,500 active duty soldiers. Additionally, about 9,500 civilian employees and 3,000 contract employees work at Schofield. On post there are three elementary schools and an intermediate school that are part of the Hawaii Department of Education (DoE). Besides the usual stressors for military families, such as frequent moves and transitions, additional stressors of living in Hawaii are the high cost of living, parents' concerns about their children's education, and cultural differences. As with other overseas assignments, most families living in Hawaii are isolated from their extended families and visit their relatives on an infrequent basis because of travel costs. The Army community receives its primary healthcare at Schofield Barracks Health Clinic, except for specialty care, which occurs at Tripler Army Medical Center (TAMC), located 20 miles from Schofield and over an hour's commute during rush hour. Before the establishment of the SAFAC, almost all child, adolescent, and adult mental health services (other than services for active duty personnel) were delivered at TAMC.

In June 2003, the leadership of the 25th ID began preparation for deployment of a brigade combat team (BCT) to Afghanistan. By early fall of that year, the unit rotation schedule had expanded to include deployment of the entire 25th ID at Schofield. The 2nd BCT was slated for deployment to Iraq in January / February 2004, and the 3rd BCT and Division Headquarters were slated for Afghanistan between February and May. At the time, the 25th ID was the only division deploying to two separate theaters of combat operations. The division was also called upon to mobilize the US Army Reserves and Hawaii National Guard as part of the deployment.

Through a combined effort of the 25th ID, Schofield Garrison Command, and TAMC, plans immediately began for soldier and family readiness and assistance during the deployment cycle, which presented significant challenges to these organizations. The 25th ID was deploying over 11,000 soldiers and leaving behind 25,000 family members, including nearly 800 pregnant women. Because of the availability of medical care at TAMC, the division had a higher proportion of families than usual with "exceptional family members," individuals with medical and mental health needs that require specialized care. During the first deployment, 80% of the families of deployed soldiers elected to remain in Hawaii rather than return to their homes on the mainland during the deployment, which increased the need for mental healthcare.

The predeployment preparation for soldiers and families began in earnest in November 2003 with coordination of services among the various on- and off-post agencies. Mental healthcare was already becoming integrated with the involvement of FRGs, schools, and the ACS; for example, since 2001, Child and Adolescent Psychiatry Service (CAPS) at TAMC had already been involved in a school mental health program at Schofield.

During the summer of 2004, it became clear that the OIF and OEF deployments were resulting in significant mental health casualties.[1] The FRGs, CAPS, and ACS began discussing ways to meet the projected increased need for support and mental health services for the entire community, and informed the commander of the 25th ID, Major General Eric Olson, of their concerns. In December 2004, the 25th ID division surgeon returned from Afghanistan to meet with the commander of

Schofield Barracks Health Clinic and leaders in mental health at TAMC. This meeting resulted in a commitment to develop a mental health initiative, which later became the SAFAC.

SOLDIER AND FAMILY ASSISTANCE CENTER

Concept Development, Structural Framework, and Financing

The purpose of the SAFAC was to execute a plan that provides mental health support for returning soldiers and their families. Early in the process, six guiding principles for SAFAC's development emerged:

1. a variety of mental health resources would be developed and integrated under a single umbrella organization to facilitate coordination of services and increase capacity and flexibility in delivery of these services;
2. a single point of entry would be established to make access to care easy and simple;
3. the mental health resources of the 25th ID would be combined with those of the Schofield Barracks Community Mental Health Clinic;
4. the funding of the SAFAC would be shared between Schofield Barracks Health Clinic and the 25th ID;
5. leadership for the newly established clinics could come from either the 25th ID or from Schofield Barracks Health Clinic; and
6. every effort would be made to decrease the stigma in seeking mental health assistance.

Several of these principles were unique to the Army experience, specifically principles 3, 4, and 5. Responsibility and leadership for the SAFAC would be shared so that the 25th ID had a vested interest in the direction and success of the initiative. A process action team, which was established and chaired by the rear division commander of the 25th ID, met monthly to evaluate progress and institute new initiatives or major changes in directions. A work group headed by the commander of Schofield Barracks Health Clinic met weekly to plan the next steps and evaluate progress.

The first task of the work group was to estimate the numbers of various specialty providers that would be required for the SAFAC to adequately meet the needs of the community. This process required estimates of baseline morbidity rates in soldiers and family members during peacetime, as well as rates resulting from deployment. Early estimates for the soldiers deployed to OIF and OEF were based on the research of Hoge et al,[1] and the work group assumed that not all soldiers with difficulties would seek help. Hoge et al[1] reported that rates for PTSD were lower in OEF than OIF. Soldiers of the 25th ID deployed to either OIF or OEF. Rates of PTSD for soldiers were projected to be approximately 8% to 11%. Rates of other anxiety/depression were estimated at 5% to 7%, serious domestic violence at 8%, moderate domestic violence at 22%, divorce at 10%, and children with mental health issues at 25%. Projections of the rates of the mental health problems in the adult family members were based on the rates in soldiers. Because the SAFAC needed to care for not only the current active duty population but also the deployed reserve and National Guard soldiers and their family members, actual numbers for the entire population were not available.

No algorithm was available to estimate the numbers of providers in each specialty needed to serve this population; the Army's system of resource allocation is not based on empirical evidence. To develop an algorithm that later could be tested, several assumptions were necessary. These assumptions were (*a*) the average number of visits per year each individual would make, (*b*) the proportion of individuals who would require medications, (*c*) the numbers of patient visits each specialty provider could reasonably provide in a year, and (*d*) the ratio of patients who could be seen by a nurse practitioner versus a psychiatrist versus another provider. Based on these assumptions and those listed below, algorithms were developed and later refined.

Exhibit 34-1 lists the assumed number of visits per year per specialty provider and the formula for its calculation. For example, it was assumed that an adult psychiatrist would be able to handle 3,290 visits per year based on 7 hours of patient contact a day, two patients per hour, 5 days a week, for 47 weeks each year; each patient visiting the three clinics would require an average of six visits a year; 0.8 of the adults being seen in the Soldier Assistance Center or the Adult Family Member Assistance Center would require medications; and approximately 50% of the patients under 18 years of age seen in the Child and Adolescent Assistance Center would require medications. There would be three psychiatrists to every one nurse practitioner for adults and one child psychiatrist to one nurse practitioner for children and adolescents. The ratio of social workers to psychologists would be 6 to 1. Child psychiatrists, child nurse practitioners, and child psychologists would be in equal proportion. This algorithm could be further refined as actual data were collected, and it could be easily modified to adjust to differences in other clinics or at other installations.

EXHIBIT 34-1

ALGORITHMS FOR CALCULATING PROVIDER NUMBERS

Visits per Practitioner per Year

- Psychiatrist: 3,290*
- Social worker: 1,645†
- Psychologist: 1,645†
- Nurse practitioner: 3,290*
- Child psychiatrist or child nurse practitioner: 2,467‡
- Psychologist: 1,645†

*7 h × 2/h × 5 days/wk × 47 wks = 3,290
†7 h × 1/h × 5 days/wk × 47 wks = 1,645
‡7 h × 1.5/h × 5 days/wk × 47 wks = 2,467

Formulas for Number of Practitioners Required

- Psychiatrists and nurse practitioners: population × 6 visits/patient/year × .8 needing medications ÷ 3,290 visits/psychiatrist/year
- Social workers and psychologists: population × 6 visits/patient ÷ 2,209 visits/provider/year
- Nurse practitioners: population × 6 visits/patient × .8 needing medications ÷ 3290 visits/year
- Child psychiatrists: population × 6 visits/patient × 0.5 needing medications ÷ 2,467 visits per year
- Child nurse practitioners: population × 6 visits/patient × 0.5 needing medications ÷ 1,645 visits/year
- Child psychologists: population × 6 visits/patient ÷ 1,645 visits/year

Proposed Ratios

- Adult psychiatrists to nurse practitioner = 3:1
- Adult social workers to psychologists = 6:1
- Child psychiatrists to child nurse practitioners = 1:1

By January 2005, five areas of care (Exhibit 34-2) were identified and a timeline for implementation of the clinics determined. Table 34-1 lists the projected deployed population and the estimated number of providers required in each of the five areas using the various algorithms. There would be a single point of entry into the mental health system (to be available 24 hours a day), which became known as the Triage Assistance Center. Other areas of care were the establishment of three new clinics and augmentation of the Marriage and Family Assistance Center and the ASAP. The new clinics were called the Soldier Assistance Center (SAC), the Adult Family Member Assistance Center (AFMAC), and the Child and Adolescent Assistance Center (CAAC). The designation "assistance center" was utilized in an attempt to decrease the stigma surrounding mental healthcare.

Funding was approved the same month. Preliminary estimate of the cost of the SAFAC for one year was $5.4 million. The 25th ID agreed to fund approximately 20% of the total, including renovation of a floor in a clinic to house the AFMAC, and hiring three providers to augment drug and alcohol treatment for family members and six social workers to bolster the AFMAC and the Marriage and Family Assistance Center. The remainder of funds came from TAMC. The 25th ID also assumed an active role in the SAFAC's develop-

EXHIBIT 34-2

SOLDIER AND FAMILY ASSISTANCE CENTER FIVE AREAS OF CARE

1. Triage Assistance Center telephone line (24 hours a day/7 days a week)
2. Soldier Assistance Center
3. Adult Family Member Assistance Center
4. Child and Adolescent Assistance Center
5. Marriage and Family Assistance Center

TABLE 34-1

PROJECTED DEMAND OF PROVIDERS BASED ON POPULATION

	Psychiatrists	Psychologists	Nurse Practitioners	Social Workers
Soldier Assistance Center	4.10	1.95	1.37	11.72
Adult Family Member Assistance Center	2.41	1.15	0.80	6.88
Child and Adolescent Assistance Center	1.06	2.13	1.06	0
Marriage and Family Assistance Center	0	0	0	8.07

ment, providing additional leadership and assistance to the assistant division surgeon and technical support through the loan of a division logistics officer.

Recruitment, Advertising, and Implementation

The reorganization of the Community Mental Health Clinic and division mental health services into the SAC occurred immediately, and the SAC opened the second week in January 2005. Demand at the start far outweighed availability, and additional providers were immediately needed. In February, TAMC's chief of psychiatry (Colonel CJ Diebold) and residency program director (Colonel David Orman) provided staff psychiatrists' and residents' time to the SAC as part of the graduate medical education program. This interim solution was essential to maintaining the SAC's function while providers were recruited and hired. Specialty experts at Schofield Barracks Health Clinic or TAMC interviewed prospective candidates and made hiring recommendations. By April 2005, essentially all the positions had been filled.

Although some family members were already being seen in limited numbers in the SAC, the AFMAC and Triage Assistance Center opened on March 15. In April, the division mental health staff returned from OEF and OIF, including the chief, Major Brian Bacon, who was appointed chief of the SAC, and division psychologist Captain Richard Schobitz, who became chief of the AFMAC and CAAC. The opening of the CAAC was delayed a month due to difficulty in recruiting child psychiatrists, but by May 2005 all clinics were operating at or above optimal staffing levels.

Early in the program's development organizers initiated an aggressive campaign to decrease the stigma associated with seeking mental health assistance at the SAFAC, and increase awareness among providers of war-related psychological trauma. Hoge and colleagues[1] found that the greater the likelihood of trauma, the greater the stigma in seeking help. The advertising campaign was initiated in February 2005, promoting the SAFAC and its available resources throughout the community. Ten thousand refrigerator magnets were produced that listed SAFAC's mission and services, as well as the 24-hour triage telephone number. The television channel on post also promoted the new resources and encouraged people in need to seek help. Unit leaders were informed by their chains of command that any soldier having emotional difficulties should be identified and offered the opportunity to visit the SAFAC. Division leaders met regularly before and after redeployment to ensure that soldiers at risk were identified.

The National Center for PTSD was invited to Schofield Barracks to instruct primary care providers in recognizing war-related mental health disorders and to teach behavioral health providers cognitive-behavioral therapy for PTSD. National Center for PTSD staff Matthew Friedman, MD, PhD (the center's director); Frederick Gusman, MSW; Julia Whealin, PhD; and Gregory Leskin, PhD, conducted 3 days of classes for the staff at Schofield Health Clinic and TAMC. Dr Whealin continued to come once a week to colead a soldier PTSD group at the SAC. Efforts by the center increased the knowledge of PTSD and depression among primary care providers and have been very beneficial to the entire Schofield Barracks community. The effectiveness of this campaign in decreasing stigma cannot be known; however, the demand for SAFAC services, particularly during the initial stages, has taxed its resources.

One of the SAFAC's initial efforts was the Soldier Readiness Program (SRP), in which a mental health provider interviewed every soldier prior to and immediately upon redeployment, and those having serious concerns or requesting assistance were immediately referred to a doctoral-level provider. The psychology and psychiatry departments at TAMC supplied additional staff for the SRPs until the SAFAC was fully operational (currently the majority of the staffing of SRPs is done by the SAFAC).

Outcomes and Current Activities

Key to success of the SAFAC team is flexibility. With regular moves of the active duty staff, contracts that require year-to-year negotiation, and deployments, staff flexibility to meet the demand of the current situation is critical. The clinics are organized under an "umbrella" of services, which allows for movement of staff between clinics to meet the changing needs of the population. For example, when some of the soldiers of the 25th ID deployed in summer 2006, staff were shifted from the SAC to the AFMAC, increasing services for family members while the soldiers were deployed. Additionally, two social workers transitioned from the AFMAC to the Marriage and Family Assistance Center in response to increased need. Recently the ASAP had a 2-month backload, which was relieved when the SAC developed a behavioral change group specifically for ASAP clients. In September 2005, the CAAC opened evening hours to see children, facilitating access for parents who work. A new position has been added to conduct outcome studies on the SAFAC's efficacy. Despite minor fluctuations over time in each clinic's staffing, the initial estimates for overall numbers of the various providers have proven to be fairly accurate. Figure 34-1 illustrates the number of client appointments at the three clinics from January 2005 to November 2006.

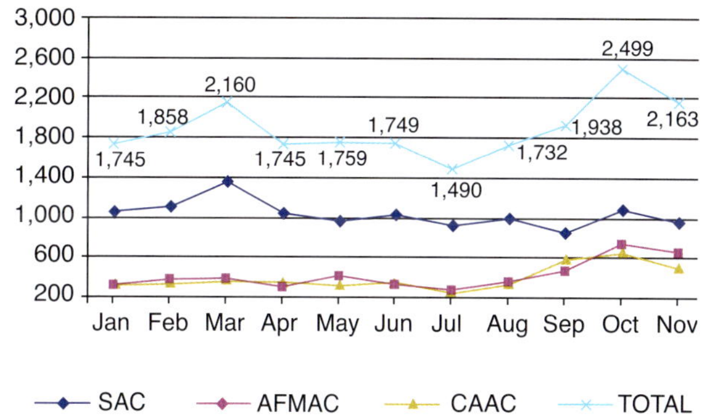

Figure 34-1. Monthly patient or client visits in the three Soldier and Family Assistance Center clinics, January 2005 to November 2006.
AFMAC: Adult Family Member Assistance Center
CAAC: Child and Adolescent Assistance Center
SAC: Soldier Assistance Center

Within the Schofield Barracks community, the SAFAC is involved in a variety of activities. Staff members teach classes and present seminars at ACS. A team composed of an AFMAC child psychologist and an ACS social worker present briefings at district schools on topics relevant to military children, such as "Effects of Deployment on Children," "Children and Redeployment," and "Building Resilience." Every unit that returns from OIF or OEF receives a reintegration briefing from the SAFAC. In addition, a monthly caregiver team meeting is dedicated to improving community outreach, family support, and crisis intervention.

Since the deployments of the Hawaii Army Reserve units and the National Guard, numerous requests have been made for outreach services on other islands in Hawaii, as well as in Alaska, Samoa, Guam, and Saipan. A SAFAC team was appointed to provide services at these geographically remote areas through ongoing visits to each of these locations.

SCHOOL-BASED MENTAL HEALTHCARE

In partnership with Solomon Elementary School in Schofield Barracks, CAPS developed a model for school mental health preventive care, early intervention, evaluation, and treatment of military children. Dr Mark Weist, director of the Center of School Mental Health at the University of Maryland, was consulted during the establishment of the Solomon Wellness Educational Program (SWEP), which began in 2001 with the goal of facilitating easy access to mental healthcare for students.[8] The project initially expanded to four schools. The following discussion only pertains to Solomon Elementary School, because it has the longest history and has received the most evaluation. Although not discussed here, programs at the three other schools are ongoing and highly valued by each school.

Solomon Elementary is a public school administered and funded by the Hawaii DoE. Administrators, teachers, counselors, and support staff are state employees. The school currently has an enrollment of about 830 students, 99% of whom are military dependents. The students come mainly from families of junior enlisted active duty soldiers who are usually assigned to a 3-year tour in Hawaii. Of the students, at least one third transition (move from the area) each year. A large proportion of these families have young children, as reflected by the school's eight kindergarten classes, eight first-grade classes, six second-grade classes, five third-grade classes, four fourth-grade classes, and four fifth-grade classes. Of the children at Solomon, 49% qualify for a reduced-price or free lunch. In addition, seven self-contained special education preschool classes serve 51 young children with severe communication disorders, autistic disorder, global developmental delays, or severe behavioral disorders. An additional 69 special education students are in kindergarten through fifth grade. Three self-contained classrooms are for children with severe behavioral disorders, serving 12 children from 5 years to 11 years of age.

Early History

A formal agreement has existed between Solomon Elementary and the Child Psychiatry Service at TAMC since 1985. Second-year child psychiatry fellows spent one half day per week for 6 months providing consultation services at the school for children referred by school counselors. Fellows mainly provided triage after observing the children and discussing the counselors' concerns. Children in need of services were referred to TAMC or to a civilian provider through TRICARE—the military's health insurance program. In 2000, CAPS decided to offer more services by sending the child psychiatry fellow into the school for a full day each week for the entire school year. The referral process remained the same, but full evaluations were now conducted at the school. These early experiences helped form the vision and goals of a comprehensive, integrated, school mental health program:

Vision: Develop and implement a comprehensive array of school programs and services to support students, family, and community.

Goals:

- Provide a full continuum of mental health promotion and intervention programs and services, including early identification and intervention, prevention, evaluation, and treatment.
- Remove barriers to learning and improve the academic success of students.
- Enhance strengths and protective factors in students, families, and the school community.
- Promote quality of life and wellness in military families.
- Provide training, staff development, and research opportunities to improve children's mental health and education.[8]

Several tenets were developed concurrently to guide program decisions. The first tenet stated that SWEP is a collaborative program responsive to the needs of its stakeholders. An advisory board composed of various stakeholders in the school and community meets on a monthly basis. The board's responsibility is to attend to the mental health of the students, teachers, parents, and the community. For example, to deal with the increased interpersonal difficulties between students at recess, the board developed a program of structured games and contests that resulted in declining referrals to the office during recess. Another example was the regular publication of a newsletter for teachers on mental health topics. During the first OIF deployment of the 25th ID, the advisory board held parent support meetings at the school to help the nondeployed parent and children successfully cope with the situation. The board also established a crisis plan to ensure a coordinated, empathic response to the children and families of soldier parents who were killed or severely injured. The plan called for verification of all information before intervention, followed by a clearly defined, graded approach to meeting families' needs with sensitivity.

The second tenet required that all programs and services for children and families be coordinated. DoE and TAMC policies needed to be integrated, followed by frequent and clear communication. This led to weekly triage meetings following an algorithm for how a child is referred for evaluation and provided care, attended by the treating physicians, counselors, a school behavioral specialist, a student services coordinator, the school principal, and the medical director. After appropriate parental consents are given, information about the child and family is shared, and a coordinated, multidisciplinary treatment plan is devised.

Program Evaluation and Student Demographics

SWEP incorporates ongoing performance improvement to ensure timeliness and quality of services, including a recent review of 133 closed charts of students evaluated from August 2001 to February 2007. Of the 133 children referred to SWEP, nine failed to appear for their initial appointments, for a noncompliance rate of 7%, and 113 of the 124 evaluated were seen within 4 weeks of the date of referral, including over one third of the children who were seen within 10 days of referral. Although 11 children were seen after 4 weeks, three were delayed due to cancellations by the parents and four because of school vacations, particularly during the winter holiday vacation when school was closed for 2 weeks. The majority of the children evaluated were 7 years of age and under (Figure 34-2).

The majority of children had externalizing disorders, with a boy-to-girl ratio of about 4 to 1. Modalities of treatment at the school included individual and group therapy, family therapy, parent guidance, and pharmacotherapy. Of the children treated, only four required a higher level of behavioral intervention, including special education certification. Three of these children were diagnosed with bipolar disorder and the other child (whose parents were both deployed) was

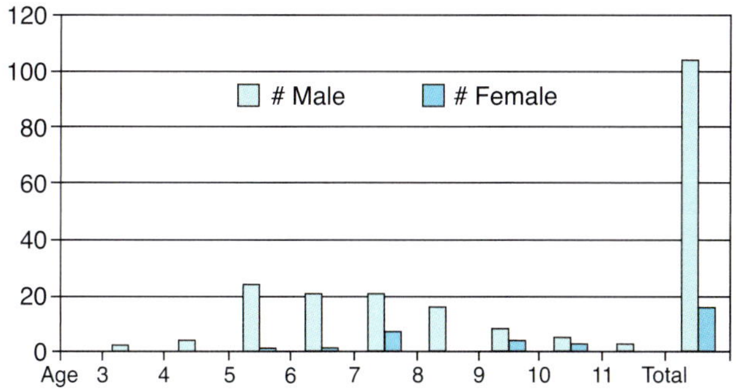

Figure 34-2. Ages and gender of children evaluated at Solomon Elementary School in the Solomon Wellness Educational Program, from August 2001 to February 2007 (total: 133).

diagnosed with severe attention deficit hyperactivity disorder and oppositional defiant disorder.

Other services provided by SWEP included quarterly teachers' workshops and parent workshops on behavioral interventions, as well as a recently initiated bullying awareness and prevention program. For the past 3 years, SWEP physicians have provided weekly consultations to the Primary School Adjustment Program, which screens all younger children and identifies those having trouble adjusting to the school environment. Two paraprofessionals then offer individual and small group services to these children. The child psychiatry fellows have given guidance and instruction on topics such as child development, as well as offering workshops to the parents. Additionally, support groups for children whose parents are separating and divorcing have been initiated.

Along with training opportunities for TAMC child psychiatry fellows, SWEP has expanded to include training of social work students from the University of Hawaii. A formal memorandum of agreement was established whereby master's-level students obtained practicum experience at SWEP under the supervision of the medical director, child fellows, and a DoE school social worker. Practicum students performed intakes and offered individual and family therapy, parent guidance, and group therapy. A similar collaborative agreement was established with the university's Counseling Education Department, whose practicum student performed intakes, provided therapy, and received training in psychological testing.

Future Directions

Efforts are underway to use measurements before and after program participation to document student progress. The Strengths and Difficulties Questionnaire[9] has been administered to teachers and parents before and at selected intervals after to determine the treatment's effect. In addition, patterns of behavioral referrals to counselors or the vice principal are being analyzed before and after treatment to determine if treatment has an impact on disciplinary referrals. Further efforts are planned to identify deployment-related stresses on parents and children, including effects of reunions and postdeployment family readjustment.

BEHAVIORAL HEALTH LIAISON PROJECT

In February 2004, the TAMC psychiatry residency program launched a behavioral health liaison (BHL) project, modeled on a similar program conducted at Letterman Army Medical Center in San Francisco, California (1988–1989), aimed at familiarizing psychiatry residents with operational Army units.[10] Unbeknownst to organizers, it also resembled a program being piloted simultaneously by ACS in the 1st Armored Division using social workers as consultants, which later gained widespread acceptance as the Soldier and Family Life Consultants (or Military Family Life Consultants) program.

The BHL program was different, however, in that residents supported the rear elements of a deployed military force. It included both service and training missions, providing preventive and consultative mental healthcare to rear-detachment units and FRGs, as well as familiarizing residents with these units and their day-to-day activities. The BHL team consisted of 17 TAMC psychiatry residents at various levels of training, along with a supervising attending psychiatrist. Each resident was assigned a 25th ID unit to support; junior residents were given battalions and senior residents were given brigades. Over the course of a 12-month deployment cycle, BHLs provided education on relevant psychosocial issues to rear-detachment commanders and FRG leaders, and facilitated access to mental health resources for soldiers and their family members.

Initial challenges included generating interest among residents while minimizing additional demands on their already burdensome academic schedules. At a minimum, residents were required to contact their assigned unit's FRG leader and offer the group an initial educational briefing. Beyond that, they were encouraged, but not required, to attend their unit's monthly FRG meetings and provide additional education and consultation as requested.

Outcome data later revealed that almost exactly one third of the residents perceived their welcome by the

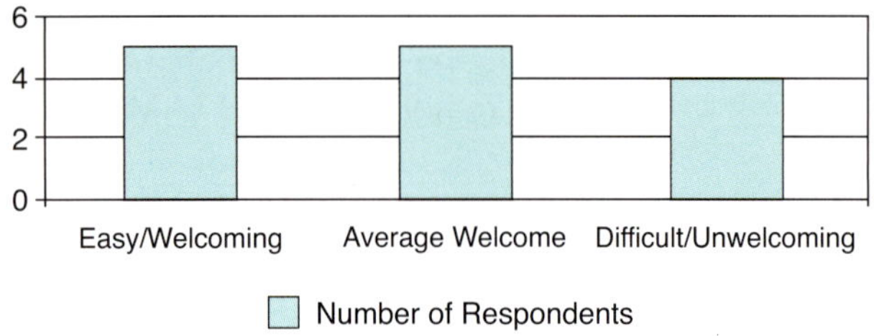

Figure 34-3. Quality of welcome by unit in the behavioral health liaison project.

unit as "easy/welcoming," one third perceived their welcome as "average," and one third perceived their welcome as "difficult/unwelcoming" (Figure 34-3). Although these relationships were not objectively measured, a direct correlation was perceived between the openness with which units welcomed their BHL and the amount of contact the BHLs subsequently had with their assigned units; disinterested units did not receive as many visits or educational briefings as units that proactively reached out for assistance.

Every interested unit received an initial briefing from their BHL on the emotional cycle of deployment, a concept originally described by Pincus and colleagues.[11] Topics covered in subsequent briefings are listed in Exhibit 34-3. Beyond the initial contact, residents had a substantial amount of flexibility in choosing how to work with their FRGs and remained involved with the groups on a variable basis. Some attended FRG meetings every month, kept in close contact with FRG leaders, and attended various unit functions. Others took a more passive role, remaining available to field questions from FRG leaders only when issues arose.

When the program ended, feelings about the program were overwhelmingly positive among FRG leaders, who unanimously felt that the program should be continued following redeployment. The psychiatry residents, however, had a mixed response. Ultimately, the program was discontinued and replaced with a mandatory 2-month senior resident rotation through the SAC, with supervision by either the 25th ID division psychiatrist or an active duty community psychiatrist.

EXHIBIT 34-3

FAMILY READINESS GROUP BRIEFING TOPICS

- Behavioral health liaison introduction
- Emotional cycle of deployment
- Common mental illnesses
- Combat stress/posttraumatic stress disorder
- Children and deployment
- Midtour rest and recuperation
- Loss and grieving
- Reunion and reintegration

Army Community Service Support for 2004–2005 Deployments

The deployment of the 2nd BCT to Iraq in January 2004, followed by the deployment of the 3rd BCT to Afghanistan in March 2004, prompted further community efforts to prepare and support soldiers and families of the 25th ID. ACS took a leadership role in ensuring that 25th ID soldiers and families were trained and ready to handle what became a long and challenging 18 months. ACS concentrated on preparing the families of the 2nd BCT first, followed by the 3rd BCT, and then launched an aggressive sustainment program of continued support to families during the deployment. Finally, ACS developed a robust redeployment program that strategically addressed reintegration issues.

Predeployment Support

ACS developed a four-pronged approach to predeployment support including (1) dissemination of information, (2) training and education, (3) community outreach, and (4) mental health integration. The extensive community outreach element included three deployment information fairs with more than 20 community service organizations participating, such as finance, legal, and housing assistance organizations; TRICARE; child development centers; and SAFAC. Military and civilian organizations were available to answer questions and provide information about making personal deployment decisions for soldiers and families. The fairs were open to the entire community; local sponsors provided door prizes and refreshments. More than 2,500 soldiers, families, and community members attended the three fairs.

A separate job fair was conducted with the community employment assistance program to educate spouses about employment opportunities. Many spouses were undecided about whether to remain in Hawaii or move back to the mainland during deployment. Because employment factored into this decision, ACS partnered with over 30 local businesses and organizations to extend employment opportunities to spouses. More than 250 spouses attended the fair.

Community town hall meetings, beginning several months before deployment, offered the latest information from the division commander about deployment status and myriad community service providers. The division commander and his staff were on hand to answer questions and quell any rumors or misinformation. The town hall meetings continued on a monthly basis throughout the duration of both deployments. Free childcare during the meetings ensured high attendance. Additionally, over 30 school briefings were presented to teachers, school administrators, counselors, and parents, in partnership with CAPS, on deployment-related topics affecting children.

ACS training and education opportunities included:

- preparation and guidance for FRG leaders, either as individuals or in classes, on how to best support families and themselves during deployment;
- education of rear-division commanders (nondeployed) in collaboration with division training resources;
- financial readiness classes for soldiers and families to prepare them for the financial issues of deployment; and
- family wellness classes teamed with various TAMC child and adolescent psychiatrists, SAFAC staff, and chaplains.

The ACS provided over 58 sessions of financial readiness training. Numerous other classes for families covered such topics as "Impact of Deployment on Children," "Helping Children Cope With Stress," and "Dealing With Rumors." Several classes addressed relationship issues for parents and the importance of meaningful communication during separation between spouses. ACS contracted Drs John and Jane Covey to train 27 ACS employees and chaplains for certification in "Seven Habits of Highly Effective Families"; the trainees in turn conducted almost two dozen 1-day sessions for Army couples.

ACS joined with the SRP to offer soldiers a plethora of information, as well as collecting data on soldiers and their families. ACS designed a predeployment information sheet, distributed to all soldiers, asking for information on the soldiers and their families, their needs, potential concerns, and requested assistance. Data were collected for ACS to determine where spouses would be residing during the deployment and any special needs they may have. Single soldiers were asked to provide an address of a parent or friend they wanted to be kept informed during their time deployed. Upon completion of the forms, over 8,500 records were collected and input into a database. Demographics such as spouse or parent addresses, pregnancies, family members with special needs, non–English-speaking spouses, and planned relocations were used to develop specific deployment programs for target audiences. Approximately 22% of spouses moved to the mainland, 9% of married women were pregnant, 13% of spouses did not speak English as their first language, 15% had a special-needs family member, 56% of soldiers were married, and 69% of those married had children. A deployment newsletter was published bimonthly and mailed to over 8,000 spouses, parents, and friends of soldiers, containing information on Army community services available to families and important resource telephone numbers.

Deployment Sustainment

To ensure that quality services were available for spouses, ACS extended its operations to 7 days a week. Classes and training for FRG leaders and family members continued, with frequent seminars on such topics as "Coping With Deployment," "Care for the Care-Giver," and "Taking Care of Me." ACS offered a weekly "spouses night out" every Thursday with pizza and other refreshments provided by sponsors, fun activities, and free childcare (also available for the FRG Wednesday meetings). Guest speakers, craft nights, game nights, support groups, and more were offered during the 52 weekly sessions. In addition, ACS made 20 hours a month of free childcare easily accessible to spouses to provide child-free opportunities for errands or respites. However, 88% of childcare employees were spouses of deployed soldiers, and burnout and stress were common among staff. In hindsight, the free childcare was excessive and created challenges for subsequent deployments when expectations could not be sustained because of decreased funding.

ACS worked directly with the 125th Signal Battalion to connect soldiers and families via video teleconference (VTC) equipment available 7 days a week. Spouses found seeing their deployed spouses and speaking to them face to face to be comforting, but children had mixed experiences with the VTC sessions. Younger children sometimes became visibly upset by seeing mom or dad on the screen, while others used the opportunity to update their parents on school and home activities. In general, the VTC sessions proved to be very valuable to families.

Redeployment and Reintegration

In December 2004, ACS developed a workshop to

prepare spouses and families for reunion after deployment. ACS again invited Drs John and Jane Covey to participate. The workshop included a list of local professionals who offered such classes as "Effects of Combat Stress on Families," "Helping Children Prepare for Reunion," and "Putting the Welcome in Welcome Home." The workshop was in a "round-robin" format, affording spouses the opportunity to attend three of the five sessions provided. Over 150 spouses attended. The workshop was followed by a series of programs with guest speakers offered every 2 weeks in the evenings. Mental healthcare providers, chaplains, and social workers were brought in to present topics on reunion and reintegration.

ACS developed a "Ready 4 Reunion" DVD with three segments that addressed reunion and reintegration, one of which focused on children and deployment and was produced by ACS with the help of local volunteers and a TAMC child psychiatrist. The other two segments were taken from "Operation Ready" material (www.mwrarmyhawaii.com/acs/managing_deployment.asp). Mailed to over 6,000 family members, the DVD had a 3-fold purpose: (1) to reach as many spouses as possible, both those who remained in Hawaii and those who had moved back to the mainland; (2) to provide spouses with reunion information in their own homes; and (3) to generate awareness of the postdeployment reintegration process and encourage spouses to take advantage of the training and services available to them. The DVD was successful in generating interest in reunion training and was later made accessible on the ACS Web site (http://www.mwrarmyhawaii.com/).

To facilitate reintegration, the 25th ID planned to provide comprehensive training to redeploying soldiers and families beginning 90 days before homecoming and ending 30 days after redeployment. The resulting Tropic Lighting University, based on Iron Horse University at Fort Hood, Texas, was a three-phase reunion program designed specifically for intensive reunion training to soldiers and their spouses.

Phase I included intensive reunion training to spouses beginning 90 days prior to homecoming. Phase II, the 3-day deployment cycle support program mandated by the Army, included a series of briefings, mental health screenings, and medical checks. Spouses were invited to attend the briefing portion of this phase. Phase III occurred immediately following the soldier's 30-day leave period and consisted of a series of classes over 2.5 days. Four target audiences were identified for training: (1) single soldiers, (2) single soldiers with children, (3) married soldiers, and (4) married soldiers with children. Unit integrity was maintained throughout the program. Tropic Lighting University trained over 10,000 soldiers. The curriculum included

- stress management (2 hours) for all soldiers,
- anger management (1 hour) for all soldiers,
- money management (1.5 hours) for all soldiers,
- single parent workshop (1.5 hours),
- single soldier workshop (1.5 hours),
- marriage workshop (3 hours),
- communication with children (1 hour), and
- divorce recovery (2 hours) for soldiers going through a divorce.

Lessons Learned

- Partnership with the mental health community was invaluable and should be mirrored on all Army installations.
- Global war on terror funds provided ACS with the needed financial resources to provide extensive deployment services.
- Twenty hours a month of free childcare was excessive and created an unsustainable expectation.
- ACS and childcare staff experienced burnout. Extended hours and additional childcare requirements put a great deal of stress on the staff, many of whom were spouses of deployed soldiers.
- Keeping the community informed and building relationships with schools helped identify potential family issues and at-risk families, and connected families with available resources before issues became elevated. The community served as ACS's eyes and ears.

The responsibility for taking care of the physical and emotional needs of soldiers and their families is shared by numerous military, federal, and state agencies. These agencies each have specific portions of the overall caring "pie," but historically have largely functioned independently. Often agencies staunchly protect their own areas of concern ("defend their turf"), which unfortunately may result in duplication of services and staff, and that is not only inefficient and costly, but also results in barriers to care due to lack of coordination of services and multiple portals of access. It is a significant challenge to integrate agencies in a common goal. Wegner and Synder[10] describe the concept of "Communities of Practice" as being the "organizational frontier" and define how disparate groups that have a "shared agenda" may come together, learn from each other, and develop strategies that work toward a common goal. Large numbers of corporations and governmental agencies are employing the principals embodied in the concept of a "community of practice" with success. However, within many organizations there needs to be a "buy in" from the leadership.

SUMMARY

The rapid development and success of SAFAC is attributable to strong leadership in the 25th ID and TAMC. Likewise, strong leadership from the Schofield Barracks Garrison Command, the National Center for PTSD, and the Hawaii DoE district superintendent facilitated the coming together of the various agencies, schools, and the SAFAC in maximizing resource utilization and cooperation. For example, the SAC, composed of the combined mental health resources of the 25th ID and the Community Mental Health Clinic, greatly increased capacity and access to care for soldiers returning from OIF and OEF. Such collaboration greatly expands the Army's ability to provide mental healthcare for soldiers. Taking mental healthcare to the community is another important principle. School mental healthcare brings services to youth where they spend a large portion of their day. It is often more convenient for parents and has less stigma for children and parents alike than going to a mental health clinic. Outreach in collaboration with ACS educates the community and further decreases stigma. Embedding mental health resources within the FRGs provides direct support to spouses during deployments and makes seeking help easily accessible.

Occasional conflict in Schofield's program had a negative impact on services. Areas that presented difficulties were the direction and control of social work resources and, to a lesser extent, integration of substance abuse resources, particularly for family members. These problems were never fully overcome.

Based on the experience with integrating mental health resources in an Army community like Schofield Barracks, the following is recommended:

- Command and control of mental health resources must be established and made clear under a single umbrella organization. The combination of all mental health resources under a single organization greatly facilitates integration and coordination of services. Failure to integrate such services generates numerous and costly problems even in a peacetime environment. If psychology, psychiatry, and social work need to respond to a crisis as a team, then these agencies should be organized as a team with a leader.
- The current system of accounting for providers' clinical time must be changed to reflect the value of prevention and early identification programs. Under the present accounting system, programs that emphasize prevention and early identification are not counted as patient care and actually count against "productive work." Similarly, community outreach is not quantified as productive workload.
- Army combat units such as the 25th ID should play an integral role in any mental healthcare initiative. Shared responsibility between mental health components and combat units greatly enhances the care of soldiers and their families.

Another important concern is allocation of mental health resources within the Army system. Traditionally, Army staffing guidelines have called for approximately one adult psychiatrist for every 7,000 adults and one child psychiatrist for every 18,000 youths under age 18. The experiences described in this chapter, as well as empirical evidence, suggest that one medication-prescribing practitioner is needed for every 3,000 adults, and one child medication provider for every 3,300 children. This is a greater than 2-fold increase in adult providers and almost a 5-fold increase in child providers. Even so, this staffing level does not take into account the numbers of youth seen in schools or those treated at TAMC. Additionally, these data represent a system that permits ready access to care. Within the SAFAC, nurse practitioners were used as much as possible for prescribing medication in both the adult and child clinics to reduce expenses. The assumptions in the algorithms described in this chapter need further testing; however, the estimated numbers of providers the equations predicted appear to be fairly accurate, and in general do not overestimate the need.

REFERENCES

1. Hoge CW, Castro CA, Messer SC, McGurk D, Cotting DI, Koffman RL. Combat duty in Iraq and Afghanistan, mental health problems, and barriers to care. *N Engl J Med*. 2004;351(1):13–22.

2. Hoge CW, Auchterlonie JL, Milliken CS. Mental health problems, use of mental health services, and attrition from military service after returning from deployment to Iraq or Afghanistan. *JAMA*. 2006;295(9):1023–1032.

3. Hoge CW, Lesikar SE, Guevara R, et al. Mental disorders among US military personnel in the 1990s: association with high levels of health care utilization and early military attrition. *Am J Psychiatry*. 2002;159:1576–1583.

4. Jones FD. From combat to community psychiatry. In: Jones FD, Sparacino LR, Wilcox VL, Rothberg JM, eds. *Military Psychiatry: Preparing in Peace for War*. In: Zajtchuk R, Bellamy RF, eds. *Textbooks of Military Medicine*. Washington, DC: Department of the Army, Office of The Surgeon General, Borden Institute; 1994: 230–235.

5. Satin DG. Allocation of mental health resources in a military setting: a community mental health approach. *Mil Med*. 1967;132:698–703.

6. Jensen PS, Grogan D, Xenakis SN, Bain MW. Father absence: effects on child and maternal psychopathology. *J Am Acad Child Adolesc Psychiatry*. 1989;28:171–175.

7. Wenger E, Snyder WM. Communities of practice: the organizational frontier. *Harvard Bus Rev*. Jan–Feb 2000;139–145.

8. Faran ME, Weist MD, Saito AY, Yoshikami L, Weiser JW, Kaer B. School-based mental health on a United States Army installation. In: Weist M, Evans SW, Lever NA, eds. *Handbook of School Mental Health: Advancing Practice and Research*. New York, NY: Kluwer Academic/Plenum Publishers; 2003: 191–214.

9. Violence Institute of New Jersey at UMDNJ. Strengths and Difficulties Questionnaire. Available at: http://www.sdqinfo.com/. Accessed January 4, 2010.

10. Leamon MH, Sutton LK. Graduate medical educators and infantry commanders: working together to train Army psychiatry residents. *Mil Med*. 1990;155:430–432.

11. Pincus SH, House R, Christenson J, Adler LE. The emotional cycle of deployment: a military family perspective. *US Army Med Depart J*. 2001;PB 8-01-4/5/6:15–23.

COMBAT AND OPERATIONAL BEHAVIORAL HEALTH

Section VII: Operational Behavioral Health

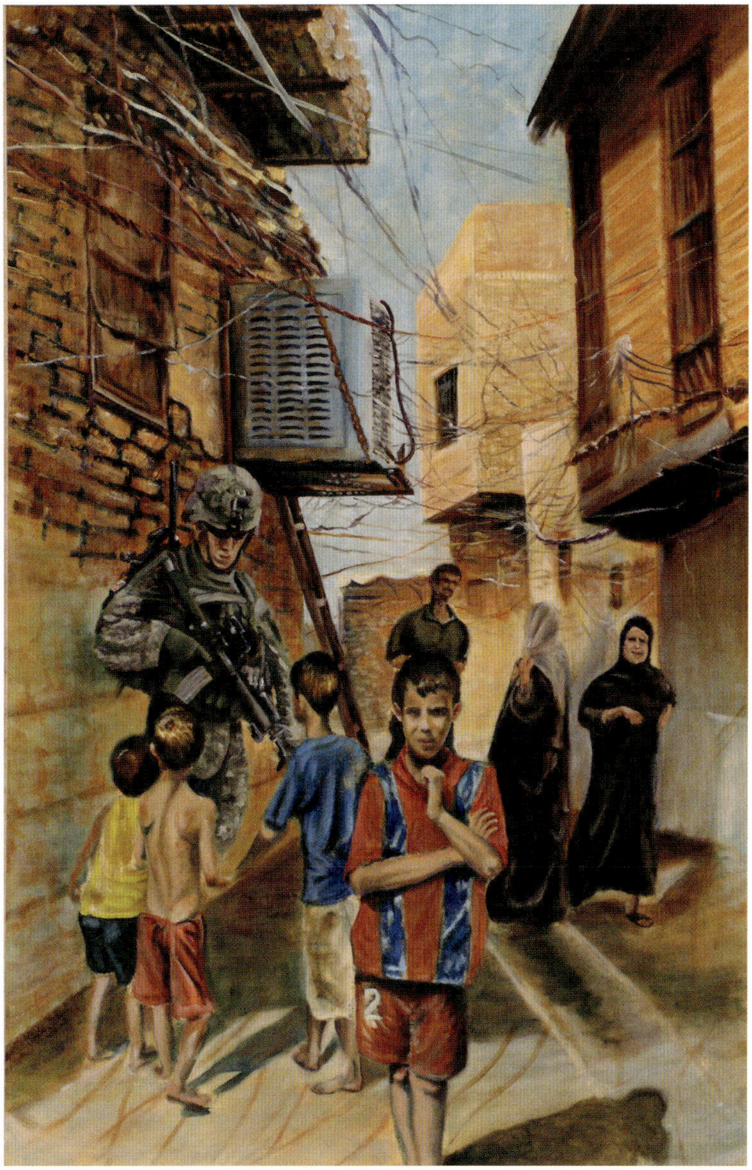

Haifa Street, Bagdad, by Christopher Thiel, oil on canvas, 2008.

Art: Courtesy of the Army Art Collection, US Army Center of Military History.

Chapter 35

DISASTER PSYCHIATRY

ARTIN TERHAKOPIAN, MD, MPH*; DAVID M. BENEDEK, MD†; AND ELSPETH CAMERON RITCHIE, MD, MPH‡

*Major, Medical Corps, US Army; Chief, Inpatient Psychiatry, Department of Behavioral Health, William Beaumont Army Medical Center, 5005 North Piedras Street, El Paso, Texas 79920; formerly, Chief, Behavioral Health, 10th Combat Support Hospital, Baghdad, Iraq

†Colonel, Medical Corps, US Army; Professor and Deputy Chair, Department of Psychiatry, Uniformed Services University of the Health Sciences, 4301 Jones Bridge Road, Bethesda, Maryland 20814

‡Colonel, US Army (Retired); formerly, Psychiatry Consultant to The Surgeon General, US Army, and Director, Behavioral Health Proponency, Office of The Surgeon General, Falls Church, Virginia; currently, Chief Clinical Officer, District of Columbia Department of Mental Health, 64 New York Avenue NE, 4th Floor, Washington, DC 20002

INTRODUCTION

The US military has made significant contributions to medical relief efforts for many devastating civilian events around the world. More recently, military psychiatrists and allied mental healthcare professionals have played major roles in these relief operations. This chapter outlines general principles of disaster psychiatry and illustrates the application of these principles via the response of military psychiatry to recent mass casualty disasters.

The field of disaster psychiatry continues to evolve and inform the conceptualization of disasters and their behavioral health consequences. Knowledge of the proper psychiatric interventions for times of disaster is essential. Although generally well-trained in war or battlefield psychiatry and the application of PIES (proximity, immediacy, expectancy, simplicity) principles, some military psychiatrists, like many of their civilian colleagues, are less familiar with the care of traumatized patients outside the sphere of standard inpatient or office psychiatric settings. Most psychiatrists may be more experienced with the management of conditions such as acute stress disorder or posttraumatic stress disorder (PTSD) in the office than with management of symptoms in the austere and disrupted postdisaster environment. The treatment of disaster-related behavioral health conditions can challenge psychiatric concepts such as those related to intrapsychic determinants of mental disorders[1] and psychiatrist–patient boundaries (eg, cohabiting a tent with a patient).[2] Although knowledge about individually experienced trauma, such as rape and automobile accidents, along with that of war psychiatry, informs the basic principles of disaster psychiatry, psychiatric reactions to disasters where there are often acute, unexpected, and collectively experienced large-scale traumatic events may be different. Much has been learned in recent years as a result of experience following the September 11, 2001, (9/11) attacks, the devastating Indian Ocean tsunami of 2004, and Hurricane Katrina in 2005. The participation of military psychiatrists in relief teams responding to these events has provided a unique opportunity to practice disaster plans, assess the existing framework of disaster psychiatry knowledge, and consider possible modifications for advancement.

This chapter will outline the historical background for the current principles of disaster psychiatry. Descriptions of military psychiatric response to the 9/11 attack on the Pentagon, the Indian Ocean tsunami, and Hurricanes Katrina and Rita will illustrate not only the application of principles of disaster psychiatry but also what military psychiatrists may expect in disaster situations and how they can best assist in relief and recovery. Finally, areas for future research and training emphasis will be identified.

HISTORICAL BACKGROUND

Substantial empirical data regarding medical and surgical needs at times of catastrophe have been accumulated. However, relatively little is known about mental health needs and appropriate psychiatric services. Nonetheless, the nature and extent of mental health needs of populations affected by a disaster and the appropriate psychiatric response has been well articulated in reports regarding a variety of natural and man-made disasters, wars, and public health emergencies.

In disasters, many experience grief and depression, anxiety, and somatic and dissociative reactions.[3–6] Disaster stress reactions may mimic physiological symptoms anticipated by a specific type of disaster event; for example chest tightness and nausea because of anxiety may follow the explosion of a truck carrying chlorine gas. This phenomenon complicates assessment and care of disaster-affected populations and necessitates the collaborative work of psychiatrists with their medical counterparts. Among people with preexisting mental disorders, anxiety and somatic reactions are compounded by fears regarding community disruption, availability of care, and availability of medication supplies.

Psychological reactions to disaster, resulting in presentation for treatment, are well documented in the literature. For example, during the Persian Gulf War (1990–1991) about 40% of Israeli civilians near Scud missile attacks reported symptoms consistent with a chemical weapons' explosion despite the absence of any such exposure.[7] A similar phenomenon was observed in the 1995 sarin gas attack on the Tokyo subway system.[8–10] In a cross-sectional assessment of 182 survivors from the 1995 Oklahoma City bombing 6 months after the disaster, North and colleagues showed elevated rates of PTSD (15% predisaster and 34.3% postdisaster) and depression (12.6% predisaster and 22.5% postdisaster).[11] Five emergency rooms in lower Manhattan near the World Trade Center collapse experienced a surge in patient care in the aftermath of the 9/11 disaster. Of the 950 patients examined during the first 48 hours in these emergency rooms, 14% reported cardiac, neurological, and psychiatric problems.[12] In the months following the World Trade Center destruction, a survey of Connecticut, New Jersey, and New York residents showed nervousness, worry, sleep problems, and increased smoking and alcohol use as a result of the attacks.[13]

The terrorist anthrax attacks in Washington, DC, during November 2001 again demonstrated the need for psychological, emotional, and behavioral healthcare of the affected populations. During the 2 weeks following the anthrax attacks on the Hart Senate Office Building, 1,129 patients with symptoms and concerns of anthrax exposure visited the emergency room of Inova Fairfax Hospital, located in nearby northern Virginia. Of these patients, only two were diagnosed with inhalational anthrax.[14] The reactions of civilians to disasters are fairly similar to those documented among troops as early as World War I.[15] Historically, psychiatric reactions (such as those noted above) have been divided along the time phases of a disaster (predisaster, disaster, and postdisaster), with each phase having its own characteristics with differences essentially determined by the nature and duration of the disaster.[16] Thus, the emotional and behavioral consequences of disasters may cause considerable disruptions in the health and functioning of individuals and societies along a significant timeline. Investigations in the fields of social science, psychology, psychiatry, and public health have provided useful information to enhance resilience, promote effective disaster behaviors, and mitigate mental disorders following traumatic exposures. These have been summarized by Ursano, Fullerton, and Norwood[6]; and Ritchie, Watson, and Friedman.[17] Three broad mental health intervention areas that are informed by the empirical evidence are: (1) community support, (2) education, and (3) definitive care (Table 35-1). These domains of intervention areas are consistent with long-standing

TABLE 35-1

ESSENTIAL DOMAINS OF DISASTER MENTAL HEALTH INTERVENTIONS

Community Support	**Basic Needs:** provide safety, security, water, food, shelter/housing, transportation, contact and/or communication with family and friends
	Psychological First Aid: minimize further harm; reduce psychological arousal and physical pain; mobilize support; maintain families and facilitate their reunion; provide information and education; foster communication about risks; contemplate need for translators
	Needs Assessment: assess current status; know predisaster circumstances; consider silent populations like children and the disabled; think of needs on three levels: (1) populations, (2) groups, and (3) individuals
	Monitoring: listen to those affected; gauge the level of basic needs that are met; measure psychological vital signs like attitudes, hope, expectations, and substance misuse; monitor and dispel rumors
	Fostering Resilience and Recovery: encourage social interaction; allow regular activities such as school and work as far as possible; enhance coping skills; strengthen role system; suggest community action to decrease helplessness and instill hope; build on existing community and organizational fabric; encourage protective community rituals (speeches, memorial services, funerals) to reduce distress and enhance cohesion
Education	**Outreach and Information Dissemination:** ensure wide dissemination of practical information and easy-to-do instruction through media and trusted local leaders; inform the public clearly and repeatedly about recommendations and the rationale behind them; educate about risky behaviors and signs and symptoms of abnormal functioning; be available at common gathering places; make informal services as well as referral to formal services available; use the language of the affected people
	Providing Consultation and Training: transfer needed skills to existing community organizations to improve their ability to meet psychological needs; be available to and educate public officials and religious, civic, and business leaders; encourage local participation in recovery efforts
Definitive Care	**Triage and Clinical Assessment:** stabilize and refer cases of mental disorder or dysfunction; screen highly vulnerable populations; hospitalize to avoid harm
	Treatment: reduce or eliminate symptoms; improve functioning; use psychopharmacy and psychotherapy (individual, family, and group interventions); apply multidisciplinary approach coordinating care with clergy, spiritual healers, counselors, and employers

Adapted from: Ritchie EC, Friedman M, Watson P, Ursano R, Wessely S, Flynn B. Mass violence and early mental health intervention: a proposed application of best practice guidelines to chemical, biological, and radiological attacks. *Mil Med*. 2004;169(8):575–579.

psychiatric conceptualizations of trauma and response such as those of Pierre Janet,[18] Sigmund Freud,[19] and Ivan Petrovich Pavlov.[15]

The appropriate balance of community support, education, and definitive care may enhance individual, group, or community capacity to integrate traumatic experiences, thereby reducing depression, anxiety, somatization, and dissociation. The benefit of interventions along these lines will vary depending on the type of disaster as well as its timing and intensity. Also, many of these efforts (eg, support and education) may be conducted by nontraditional mental healthcare providers, highlighting the importance of liaison among mental healthcare providers and disaster rescue workers including volunteers.

Self-triage and self-soothing can also be enhanced by community support, education, and definitive care. Psychoeducation can help reduce somatization by explaining (and normalizing) the impact of traumatic exposure on personal psychology, spirituality, and physiologic function. Knowledge and understanding of stress reaction may boost the ability of affected individuals to contain their anxiety, curb fear, and mobilize psychological defenses in response to distress by assisting survivors in making sense of the disaster and their emotional responses to it. Support and education may reduce disaster-related chaos by providing instruction and may thus minimize "compensation syndromes" by advocating for postdisaster assistance and community rebuilding programs. Educational and support programs can guide survivors with preexisting mental illness to definitive care centers for medication refills, reevaluation, and hospitalization (or other services as indicated). These mental health interventions, when sustained and tied to surveillance and outreach efforts, may lessen the conversion of minor and short-lived emotional symptoms into more serious and long-lasting mental health problems. Community support, education, and definitive care (when clearly available to those who require it) all serve to enhance community ability to integrate frightening and devastating experiences into cognitive, emotional, and behavioral schemes. From a cognitive and neurobiological perspective, this integration may be viewed as the accumulation of "safety memory," which inhibits the expression of fear memory.[20]

"Project Liberty," a government-funded entity set up after 9/11, illustrates the benefits of the provision of support, education, and definitive care. This program, which provided counseling, education, and outreach services to an estimated 1.2 million individuals during the 27 months following 9/11 in the area around "ground zero" in New York City, is an example of successful community support, education, and definitive care interventions. Project Liberty was particularly effective in facilitating survivors' return to predisaster functioning and guiding those survivors with more serious problems, such as depression and PTSD, to definitive care.[21,22]

An emerging area of concern in disaster psychiatry has been the mental health of disaster workers. Although the evidence is somewhat mixed,[23,24] health problems appear to disproportionately affect disaster workers exposed to psychologically traumatizing exposures.[25–29] Traumatic exposures may have lasting effects on volunteers and rescuers and can diminish their mission effectiveness. Traumatic exposures in military disaster relief and humanitarian assistance operations can include: "a) dead bodies, b) orphaned or abused children, c) uncertainty regarding mission . . . [objectives] and d) unclear chain of command."[30(p63)] Every disaster response plan should include mental health interventions for the affected population and also consider the emotional, behavioral, and mental health needs of rescuers. A psychiatrically informed plan for the support of rescuers can improve mission effectiveness by enhancing worker ability and willingness to report to duty.[31,32] In this era of tremendous advances in medicine, including control of infectious diseases and emergency surgical provisions by disaster workers, and given the recognized health burden of long-term psychiatric illness, the refinement of disaster psychiatric interventions would seem a natural next step in reducing disaster-related morbidity and mortality.

RECENT MISSIONS

Military psychiatrists have supported various disaster relief efforts in the past several years. Among these were the response at the Pentagon following the 9/11 attack, the mission in Southeast Asia following the 2004 tsunami, and the relief operations on the US gulf coast after Hurricanes Katrina and Rita, both in 2005. Military disaster mental health interventions for these catastrophes were tailored to enhance safety and security, mitigate negative long-term psychiatric consequences, ameliorate suffering, and address clinically significant psychiatric reactions. Where possible, research and process improvement procedures were established to gather and document lessons learned. These operations were facilitated greatly by the readiness of military psychiatrists to respond. The extent to which responders were successful depended largely on their military psychiatric training, experience with the practice of caring for war-traumatized soldiers, and access to consultants at national centers of excellence in trauma response and disaster psychiatry such as the Psychiatry Department at the Uniformed Services University of the Health Sciences, located in Bethesda, Maryland.

The September 11, 2001, Attack on the Pentagon

American Airlines Flight 77 crashed into the Pentagon at 9:43 AM EDT on September 11, 2001. It was followed by a rapid, comprehensive, and sustained rescue and recovery response. As part of this response, all military services located near the crash scene dispatched mental healthcare teams to the Pentagon. One rapidly assembled stress management team arrived from Walter Reed Army Medical Center (WRAMC). Other crisis management teams arrived from Andrews, Bolling, and Keesler Air Force bases. A psychiatric intervention team came from the National Naval Medical Center in Bethesda.[33–36] The teams worked with other support personnel, including members of the American Red Cross, Salvation Army personnel, various church volunteers, and Department of Defense (DoD) and fire department chaplains.[34]

Soon after the attack, the DiLorenzo Clinic at the Pentagon was designated as the headquarters for the disaster response. There, on September 12th, more specific plans were developed for the mental health support of personnel at the Pentagon, and the Army was assigned the lead for this mental healthcare effort. Because the Pentagon did not have in-house mental health services for its occupants (beyond a three-person employee assistance program and a single chaplain), Army and Air Force assets were focused on the Pentagon while Navy assets where charged with supporting the Arlington Annex, Marine Corps headquarters,[34] which was a few hundred yards from the crash site.

As observed in other disasters, distressed, sometimes anxious or panicked survivors visited the various organized clinics for assistance and guidance early after the crash. To address the growing need for social and mental health services, a family assistance center was established on September 13th at the Sheraton Crystal City Hotel, which was a short drive from the Pentagon. This facility provided assistance to families of Pentagon personnel as well as families of passengers and crew on Flight 77. Many Air Force mental health personnel, joined by WRAMC mental health team members, supported the mission of this center, including grief counseling, until it was closed 2 weeks after the October 11th memorial service because demand for services had declined.[36]

Consistent with the initial planning, the Air Force established teams that specifically served the personnel falling under the various deputy chiefs of staff in the Pentagon. These teams rotated in the DiLorenzo Clinic generally for 2-week periods until December 10th.[36] The Army divided its charge into an "inside" and an "outside" mission. The "inside" mission included the support of Pentagon personnel while the "outside" mission focused on the large population of first responders encamped on the lawn surrounding the Pentagon. The WRAMC mental health response was based on the accepted premise that most adverse mental health consequences following disasters are "subclinical" (ie, transient and normal responses to trauma).[33] Hence, WRAMC mental health support often took the form of promoting awareness of basic needs such as sleep, food, water, and family contact. It involved modified debriefings through informal conversations and outreach through monitoring of reactions to traumatic exposure among Pentagon employees and responders, particularly high-risk groups such as casualty assistance officers and healthcare workers. This approach allowed for the delivery of support while minimizing the stigma associated with mental health service utilization. When warranted, referral for clinical services was offered for formal evaluation and treatment.[33]

In addition, the WRAMC Psychiatry Consultation Liaison Service (PCLS) team contacted and lent support to attack survivors who were admitted to local civilian hospitals. Using a novel and flexible approach adapted from critical incident stress debriefing models, but with a more targeted emphasis on the observed psychological state of each injured survivor, the WRAMC PCLS team approach helped reduce psychological symptoms, prevent the development of psychopathology, facilitate compliance with medical care, speed recovery, and arrange social support for the 18 attack survivors from the Pentagon who required lengthy hospitalization[37] (Exhibits 35-1, 35-2, and 35-3).

The "therapeutic debriefing" approach advocated mental health contact with all disaster patients and normalization of responses to the disaster with bedside techniques such as cognitive reframing.[37] Here the goal was to help patients integrate their memories in a way that would prevent the disaster experience from "overwhelming" their defenses and that would minimize long-term morbidity.[37] "Therapeutic debriefing" included the use of relaxation breathing, distraction, humor, and creative visualization to speed the return of a sense of agency and mastery to the patient. Addressing the quality of sleep, pain control, and satisfaction with medical treatment was also emphasized.[37] The support provided to the Pentagon was sustained for weeks while psychiatric clinical services and gradu-

EXHIBIT 35-1

GOALS OF PSYCHIATRY CONSULTATION LIAISON SERVICE FOR DISASTER INJURED

- Liaison between medical staff, patients, commands, family, and friends.
- Facilitate medical treatment.
- Reduce psychological-psychiatric morbidity.
- Maintain a flexible evaluation and treatment approach.
- Recognize and reinforce patient's adaptive defense mechanisms.
- Advocate for patient's needs.
- Educate patients and staff.

Adapted from: Wain HJ, Grammer GG, Stasinos JJ, Miller CM. Meeting the patients where they are: consultation-liaison response to trauma victims of the Pentagon attack. *Mil Med.* 2002;167(9 suppl):20.

EXHIBIT 35-2

TREATMENT GOALS OF "THERAPEUTIC DEBRIEFING"

- Establish support.
- Make debriefing a routine preventive measure.
- Emphasize environmental safety.
- Normalize responses and feelings including survivor guilt.
- Reframe loss by recognizing the injured patient's significant sacrifice.
- Help the patient consolidate a narrative of what occurred.
- Console the patient.
- Identify and reinforce healthy coping mechanisms.
- Teach patient mastery techniques using imagery, relaxation, or humor.
- Teach the patient that he or she can be in control.
- Encourage the patient to use social supports.
- Normalize sleep patterns and dietary intake if medical condition permits.
- Clarify patient's medical concerns.
- Educate on the pitfall of self-medication with substance abuse.

Adapted from: Wain HJ, Grammer GG, Stasinos JJ, Miller CM. Meeting the patients where they are: consultation-liaison response to trauma victims of the Pentagon attack. *Mil Med.* 2002;167(9 suppl):20.

ate medical education continued at many of the commands from which the mental health intervention teams came.[33] Psychiatry residents involved in this response reported that their education was enhanced due to their participation in the rescue and recovery operations. The potential benefit of including residents in disaster plans has been echoed by other psychiatry training programs affected by Hurricane Katrina.[38]

Particularly traumatic during the early days of the response to the Pentagon attack were the work of the groups that helped in the recovery of the remains of the dead in the Pentagon.[39] A descriptive report on the effect of recovering human remains on 10 military healthcare workers showed that mental health responses were quite varied and included acute but short-lived—in the order of days—restless sleep, nightmares, and flashbacks. Mission clarity and expectations were cited as ways to enhance coping.[40]

In summary, the military response to the Pentagon attack was rapid; military-specific efforts that were integrated through a series of ongoing planning efforts began immediately after the attack. Sustained mental health outreach efforts helped maximize support for the survivors and rescue workers. The support effort was enhanced by the multidisciplinary composition of the responders, which included psychiatrists, social workers, and chaplains. The "therapeutic debriefing" described by Wain et al[42] stands out as a promising modification of the critical incident stress debriefing model applied in a psychiatry consultation liaison setting. This PCLS approach, which is used with returning injured soldiers at WRAMC, may have contributed to the lower-than-historically observed initial rates of PTSD among battle-injured soldiers and deserves further study in disaster response.[41,42]

Scrutiny of the response to the Pentagon attack points to some weaknesses in terms of coordination and planning of response efforts, as well as mission ambiguity.[33,34,36] Mental healthcare teams that arrived at the Pentagon did not coordinate their initial efforts with the on-scene commander of the disaster response.[34] Each service and each mental health organization came with its own theoretical perspective, response plan, and set of priorities, complicating the response effort. Many have suggested that developing a joint doctrine of disaster response, perhaps along the same lines as the Federal Emergency Management Agency (FEMA) National Incident Management System, and drilling this plan would be a worthy future consideration.[33,34,36,43] Also, the lack of military

EXHIBIT 35-3

PSYCHIATRY CONSULTATION LIAISON SERVICE LESSONS LEARNED IN THE RESPONSE TO THE SEPTEMBER 11, 2001, ATTACKS

- Psychiatric consultation liaison services may need to be exported after a disaster.
- All disaster patients should be seen by mental health providers as a standard protocol.
- Responses of disaster patients should be reframed as normal responses to abnormal events.
- Mental health providers should establish an early therapeutic alliance with other healthcare providers and patients.
- Patient's mature psychological defenses should be supported.
- Mental health resources should remain available to patients irrespective of their current medical status.

Adapted from: Wain HJ, Grammer GG, Stasinos JJ, Miller CM. Meeting the patients where they are: consultation-liaison response to trauma victims of the Pentagon attack. *Mil Med.* 2002;167(9 suppl):21.

administrative support was viewed as contributing to some of the difficulties with coordination.[33] This lack of administrative support may have also contributed to the missed opportunity by military providers to fully integrate the civilian assets into combined plans.[33,34] Inclusion of administrative support for disaster mental health response teams should also be considered.

The December 26, 2004, Southeast Asia Tsunami

A powerful earthquake struck the Indian Ocean basin on December 26, 2004. The aftermath was a tsunami that affected many coastal countries, particularly Indonesia, Thailand, and Sri Lanka. Estimates placed the number of dead and missing at over 250,000 people. The affected people, even if physically unharmed, faced profound grief, loss, and guilt.[44] The US military responded to this disaster by organizing Operation Unified Assistance. The magnitude of the disaster was so great that even highly capable and independent nongovernmental organizations (NGOs) needed the assistance of the US military to reach the devastated areas.[45] The US military mission was subdivided into two groups: one was destined for Sri Lanka and the other to Indonesia. A third group from the Armed Forces Research Institute of Medical Sciences led the assessment of needs in Thailand and coordinated the delivery of assistance in that country.[46]

Soon after the tsunami struck, an advance team was dispatched to the region, which helped coordinate the arrival of US military assets with the respective US embassies and other local and international aid agencies. In addition to military members, the group to Indonesia deliberately included civilian volunteers involved with Project HOPE (Health Opportunities for People Everywhere), an NGO, to enhance the prospects of meeting the mounting needs of the affected people there.[47,48] This group was dispatched to Banda Aceh, Indonesia, on USNS *Mercy* in early 2005, while the other groups were air-lifted to Sri Lanka and Thailand. The group in Sri Lanka eventually worked in the northeastern corner of the island. Once in Thailand, the third group began the task of assessing the damage in Thailand's six coastal provinces affected by the tsunami.

As is established practice with disaster relief and humanitarian assistance operations, relief work entailed providing as much care as possible *in situ* and only bringing back to USNS *Mercy* patients who could not be treated ashore. All operations were in the "spirit of cooperation, collaboration, mutual respect, team-building and team participation, trust, interdependency and consensus-building."[49(p33)] Although only the USNS *Mercy* included mental healthcare providers, all three groups considered the mental health needs of the affected populations as well as the disaster responders. For example, when choosing the housing location for the relief team in Sri Lanka, planners considered the psychological benefits of distance from the major concentration of affected people and physical devastation, allowing team members respite from constant traumatic exposure.[50] Although the team in Sri Lanka provided many interventions that can be considered beneficial to improving mental health, they avoided specific psychological counseling and formal evaluation as it was deemed that these services could not be provided in a culturally relevant manner.[50]

Although the care provided by the team sent to Sri Lanka did not involve formal mental health interventions, the mental healthcare team on USNS *Mercy* specifically planned for and engaged in the provision of mental health services in Banda Aceh, Indonesia. And although the team in Thailand did not directly provide mental health services, its rapid needs assessment alerted Thai officials to the poor preparedness of hospitals for meeting the mental health needs of the affected population. This prompted Thai authorities to organize and deploy mental health teams to the disaster-affected areas and consider changes in their disaster plans that originally did not include mental health elements.[46] The assessment team in Thailand also reported on other facets of disaster response relevant to mental health, such as availability of basic needs, and found them to be well provisioned.[46]

A lesson learned in Operation Unified Assistance was the value of telecommunications. Through data-sharing networks and communication links, the mental health team on the USNS *Mercy* was supported by a virtual group of disaster mental health experts from around the globe. These links enabled the team to assess the needs of the affected population and plan a response. Once it became clear that children were going to be the focus of the team, the same links were invaluable in accessing the latest literature, consulting with experts, and developing an intervention plan.[51,52] With support from consultants, the mental health team aboard USNS *Mercy* was able to implement a program that provided over 80 hours of training in 85 content areas, which reached over 200 child-service staff members and 1,200 teachers in Aceh Province.[53] The data and communication links continue to enhance the effectiveness of the mental health intervention in Aceh Province as they remain in use by mental health providers in the disaster-affected areas.[53]

One study examining rescuers who responded to the tsunami disaster provides some evidence to suggest that certain preventive measures—teaching rescuers about expected traumatic exposures, the range of psychological responses, and appropriate interventions—can reduce the incidence of negative consequences among members of this group. In this study, surveys were used to assess participant health before and 3 months after the mission. Although the small sample size precluded statistically significant conclusions regarding changes from baseline in overall health status, depression, posttraumatic stress disorder, or risk behaviors, responders tended to view favorably and find helpful the mental-health–related briefings and "just-in-time" training they received on the eve of their deployment.[30]

Thus, Operation Unified Assistance rapidly applied validated methods of disaster response. The effort also involved some new components, such as virtual access to global information resources and field experts. This mission illustrated the potential for successful cooperation between military personnel and civilian rescuers. Policies for these types of missions were later enumerated in DoD Directive 3000.05, *Military Support for Stability, Security, Transition, and Reconstruction Operations*.[54] Some areas that require further investigation include those that pertain to clarification of the optimal training for prevention of psychological trauma among disaster workers. One possibility might be the expansion of "just-in-time" training along the same lines as "Battlemind," a training developed for troops before deployment to combat.[55,56]

Hurricanes Katrina and Rita in 2005

Hurricane Katrina struck the coast of Louisiana and Mississippi on Monday, August 29, 2005. As a result of the hurricane's winds, torrential rains, and massive waves, an area the size of the United Kingdom was severely affected. In the aftermath, hundreds of thousands of people remained away from their homes in temporary shelters. Thousands of others less fortunate were stranded in a city that would soon be flooded because of breaches in levees. The contaminated waters pouring into New Orleans flooded hospitals, community mental health centers, pharmacies, and physicians' offices alike, forcing closure of facilities and total displacement of healthcare professionals and patients in the four parishes of Jefferson, Orleans, Plaquemines, and St Bernard.[57–59] Many persons with chronic medical conditions, including those most vulnerable because of psychiatric conditions, were left without care, medication, medical supplies, or support services. Under normal circumstances, Charity Hospital's Crisis Intervention Unit managed about 600 patient encounters each month. These numbers predicted a high post-Katrina demand on mental health services.[60] This potential was identified early on by military disaster psychiatrists and communicated to planners and caregivers.[61,62]

The National Guard mobilized 48 hours before Hurricane Katrina made landfall. The military response, which eventually involved more than 60,000 active duty and National Guard members, accelerated its activities within hours of Hurricane Katrina's landfall despite the presence of half of the Louisiana National Guard in Iraq.[57,63,64] A shelter was established at the Superdome before the hurricane and a medical treatment facility was organized at the convention center 1 day after Katrina made landfall. A field hospital was also established at Louis Armstrong International Airport. By mid-September, Army, Air Force, and Navy medical teams were in and around New Orleans working with the Coast Guard, the US Public Health Service, the Environmental Protection Agency, the Centers for Disease Control and Prevention (CDC), and the Louisiana Department of Health and Hospitals.[57] The first 72 hours following Katrina's landfall were the most hectic. It was during this time that thousands of people were evacuated from the Louis Armstrong International Airport under some of the most distressing conditions.[65]

Health surveillance by the CDC, which commenced

on September 9th (with the assistance of the military), revealed no outbreaks of disease or hazardous environmental exposures as of September 25th. Early surveys noted 42 cases of intentional injuries among the 2,018 cases of injuries reported.[66] The communication of accurate news regarding outbreaks of disease and contamination, as well as education about risks through printed material and the media, were in line with disaster mental healthcare practices that likely calmed public fears of exposure and curbed the propagation of rumors. The rescue of city residents from rooftops kindled hope and strengthened survivors' trust in the arrival of assistance. The hope for outside assistance, at least in terms of augmented medical operations, was realized through the Navy ship USNS *Comfort*. The *Comfort* supported relief efforts at Pascagoula from September 9th through September 20th and at New Orleans from late September to October 8th. Navy medical personnel and volunteers from Project HOPE with experience from the Indian Ocean tsunami helped triage and treat nearly 2,000 patients.[67] However, the confusion regarding the responsibility of recovering human remains and safe travel routes, and the subsequent graphic media coverage, could not have helped allay people's worries and sense of helplessness and abandonment.[57,65]

As the situation in the city stabilized and some degree of order was restored, the mental health burden became more apparent. Hurricane Katrina had caused the deaths of over 1,000 people by early estimates[68]; this would rise to over 1,400 in Louisiana once more accurate counts were available.[69] The dead included two police officers who died by suicide.[70] The news of deaths combined with the realities of scattered families and friends, community destruction, loss of social supports and healthcare, economic devastation, and numerous uncertainties distressed people profoundly, particularly those with existing mental illness. The burden of stress and dysfunction was brought to attention by a CDC survey in October 2005, which showed that 56% of the respondents had a chronically ill family member and only 35% were employed, in contrast to the 73% who were employed before Katrina.[71] Nine hundred New Orleans police officers and about 500 firefighters who completed a CDC survey during October and November 2005 reported mental health problems with symptoms of PTSD and depression, with depression affecting more than a quarter of each group (26% of police officers and 27% of firefighters).[72]

Over half of female caregivers living in FEMA trailers or hotels responding to a February 2006 survey scored at levels consistent with clinically diagnosable depression, anxiety, or other psychiatric disorders.[73] It was not surprising that the New Orleans Coroner's Office reported increased suicide rates from 9 per 100,000 per year to 26 per 100,000 per year in the months from Katrina to the end of 2005.[74] These consequences were exacerbated by the disruption of mental health services at large medical centers like Tulane University and Louisiana State University Health Sciences Center, including problems with methadone clinic patient records.[59,75] Response to Katrina survivors was further complicated by Hurricane Rita, which followed 3 weeks later.

As problems became more evident, programs were organized with the support of local, state, federal, and military organizations. Social workers at Louisiana State University at Baton Rouge arranged for the care of special-needs children displaced by the two hurricanes; Public Health Service staff streamlined credentialing and pharmacy processes for displaced or volunteer physicians.[76] FEMA funding allowed for the start of Project Recovery in Mississippi and supported Louisiana Spirit mental health counselors.[58,70] Project Recovery, which was spearheaded by the Substance Abuse and Mental Health Services Administration (SAMHSA), provided assistance and education to over 1,000,000 people, resulting in more than 10,000 referrals to mental health and substance abuse services. Another SAMHSA program, the Katrina Assistance Project, conducted thousands of counseling sessions.[58] Despite these efforts, the pre-Katrina burden of chronic mental illness in the city, including substance use problems, may have prolonged the "duress" experienced by survivors.[70] Fortunately, psychiatric teaching and treatment programs in New Orleans, borrowing a page from the disaster response literature, were able to return quickly to the city by reestablishing communications, minimizing uncertainty, and applying academic flexibility.[77] Disaster response and recovery in the Gulf Coast still continues, as do efforts to quantify the psychological burden of this disaster and find more effective disaster response paradigms.

SUMMARY

In disaster psychiatry, vast areas of knowledge and practice are by necessity evidence-informed rather than evidence-based. Military psychiatric observation and experience form the basis of much of today's understanding of population response to disaster and mass violence. Considerable knowledge exists with regard to the psychological effects of disasters, but only a smaller body of empirical evidence supports current disaster response practices. Difficulties in the conduct of studies examining relevant questions in this field largely stem from the nature of the traumatizing event; few disasters are clearly anticipated and still fewer are slow to unfold. Further efforts by military and civilian disaster researchers must include rigorous longitudinal studies with baseline predisaster characterization of populations followed by comprehensive health surveillance and ongoing recharacterization of the disaster-affected populations. Measurements of symptoms and functioning before and after mental health interventions with control population comparisons (if ethical) will help quantify the efficacy of intervention programs and help separate cause from effect and modifiers from mediators.

Another area of focus may be the education of disaster psychiatrists. Much is learned and lost in the field of disaster response as a result of the infrequency of large-scale tragedy. Disaster psychiatry training programs may help preserve the gains made in disaster psychiatry and function as institutional memories and resources to be called upon in times of need. Such training programs should emphasize and develop models for cooperation and coordination among the various agencies such as FEMA, the National Center for PTSD, SAMHSA, Uniformed Services University of the Health Sciences, National Institutes of Mental Health, and Project HOPE. Disaster response programs must also strive to more effectively incorporate various professionals (eg, psychiatrists, emergency medical technicians, public health workers, and community politicians) into disaster preparation, response, and recovery efforts.

Specific areas for consideration by the military psychiatric establishment beyond the support of academic centers and research in this area include:

- the development of a common disaster response doctrine, perhaps along the same lines as the National Incident Management System;
- inclusion of disaster psychiatry in psychiatry residency training programs and possible involvement of residents in disaster relief efforts;
- further integration of psychiatry consultation liaison services in the medical care of disaster survivors to reduce stigma and enhance outreach; and
- further development of the concepts of stress inoculation and resilience to find ways to protect disaster workers.

Direct military correlates may be found in the aims of the "Battlemind" program, as discussed in the attachment to Chapter 4, Combat and Operational Stress Control, in this volume.

REFERENCES

1. McCarroll JE, Ursano RJ. Consultation to groups, organizations, and communities. In: Ritchie EC, Watson PJ, Friedman MJ, eds. *Interventions Following Mass Violence and Disasters*. New York, NY: Guilford Press; 2006: 194–195.

2. Croarkin P. Group therapy in a combat zone? *Am J Psychiatry*. 2005;162(8):1504–1505. Available at: http://ajp.psychiatryonline.org/cgi/reprint/162/8/1504.pdf. Accessed July 7, 2010.

3. American Psychiatric Association. Practice guideline for the treatment of patients with acute stress disorder and posttraumatic stress disorder. Available at: http://www.psychiatryonline.com/pracGuide/pracGuideTopic_11.aspx. Accessed May 25, 2010.

4. Fetter JC. Psychosocial response to mass casualty terrorism: guidelines for physicians. *Prim Care Companion J Clin Psychiatry*. 2005;7(2):49–52.

5. Foa EB, Stein DJ, McFarlane AC. Symptomatology and psychopathology of mental health problems after disaster. *J Clin Psychiatry*. 2006;67(suppl 2):15–25.

6. Ursano RJ, Fullerton CS, Norwood AE, eds. *Terrorism and Disaster Individual and Community Mental Health Interventions*. Cambridge, UK: Cambridge University Press; 2003.

7. DiGiovanni C Jr. Domestic terrorism with chemical or biological agents: psychiatric aspects. *Am J Psychiatry*. 1999;156(10):1500–1505.

8. Okumura T, Suzuki K, Fukuda A, et al. The Tokyo subway sarin attack: disaster management, III: national and international responses. *Acad Emerg Med*. 1998;5(6):625–628.

9. Okumura T, Suzuki K, Fukuda A, et al. The Tokyo subway sarin attack: disaster management, II: hospital response. *Acad Emerg Med*. 1998;5(6):618–624.

10. Okumura T, Suzuki K, Fukuda A, et al. The Tokyo subway sarin attack: disaster management, I: community emergency response. *Acad Emerg Med*. 1998;5(6):613–617.

11. North CS, Nixon SJ, Shariat S, et al. Psychiatric disorders among survivors of the Oklahoma City bombing. *JAMA*. 1999;282(8):755–762.

12. Rapid assessment of injuries among survivors of the terrorist attack on the World Trade Center—New York City, September 2001. *MMWR Morb Mortal Wkly Rep*. 2002;51(1):1–5.

13. Psychological and emotional effects of the September 11 attacks on the World Trade Center—Connecticut, New Jersey, and New York, 2001. *MMWR Morb Mortal Wkly Rep*. 2002;51(35):784–786.

14. Howell JM, Mayer TA, Hanfling D, et al. Screening for inhalational anthrax due to bioterrorism: evaluating proposed screening protocols. *Clin Infect Dis*. 2004;39(12):1842–1847.

15. Weisaeth L. The European history of psychotraumatology. *J Trauma Stress*. 2002;15(6):443–452.

16. Jones FD, Harris P, Koshes R, Fong YH. Military psychiatry and disasters. In: Jones FD, Sparacino LR, Wilcox VL, Rothberg JM, eds. *Military Psychiatry: Preparing in Peace for War*. In: Zajtchuk R, Bellamy RF, eds. *Textbooks of Military Medicine*. Washington, DC: Department of the Army, Office of The Surgeon General and Borden Institute; 1994: 239–249.

17. Ritchie EC, Watson PJ, Friedman MJ, eds. *Interventions Following Mass Violence and Disasters*. New York, NY: Guilford Press; 2006.

18. van der Kolk BA, van der Hart O. Pierre Janet and the breakdown of adaptation in psychological trauma. *Am J Psychiatry*. 1989;146(12):1530–1540.

19. Bracken PJ, Giller JE, Summerfield D. Psychological responses to war and atrocity: the limitations of current concepts. *Soc Sci Med*. 1995;40(8):1073–1082.

20. Quirk GJ, Milad MR, Santini E, Lebron K. Learning not to fear: a neural systems approach. In: Kirmayer LJ, Lemelson R, Barad M, eds. *Understanding Trauma Integrating Biological, Clinical and Cultural Perspectives*. Cambridge, UK: Cambridge University Press; 2007: 548.

21. Donahue SA, Jackson CT, Shear KM, Felton CJ, Essock SM. Outcomes of enhanced counseling services provided to adults through Project Liberty. *Psychiatr Serv*. 2006;57(9):1298–1303.

22. Donahue SA, Lanzara CB, Felton CJ, Essock SM, Carpinello S. Project Liberty: New York's crisis counseling program created in the aftermath of September 11, 2001. *Psychiatr Serv*. 2006;57(9):1253–1258.

23. North CS, Tivis L, McMillen JC, et al. Coping, functioning, and adjustment of rescue workers after the Oklahoma City bombing. *J Trauma Stress*. 2002;15(3):171–175.

24. Slottje P, Witteveen AB, Twisk JW, et al. Post-disaster physical symptoms of firefighters and police officers: role of types of exposure and post-traumatic stress symptoms. *Br J Health Psychol*. 2008;13(2):327–342.

25. Galea S. The long-term health consequences of disasters and mass traumas. *CMAJ*. 2007;176(9):1293–1294.

26. Galea S, Nandi A, Vlahov D. The epidemiology of post-traumatic stress disorder after disasters. *Epidemiol Rev*. 2005;27:78–91.

27. Hearns A, Deeny P. The value of support for aid workers in complex emergencies: a phenomenological study. *Disaster Manag Response*. 2007;5(2):28–35.

28. Morren M, Dirkzwager AJ, Kessels FJ, Yzermans CJ. The influence of a disaster on the health of rescue workers: a longitudinal study. *CMAJ*. 2007;176(9):1279–1283.

29. van den Berg B, Grievink L, Yzermans J, Lebret E. Medically unexplained physical symptoms in the aftermath of disasters. *Epidemiol Rev*. 2005;27:92–106.

30. Benedek DM, Ritchie EC. "Just-in-time" mental health training and surveillance for the Project HOPE mission. *Mil Med*. 2006;171(10 suppl 1):63–65.

31. Nickell LA, Crighton EJ, Tracy CS, et al. Psychosocial effects of SARS on hospital staff: survey of a large tertiary care institution. *CMAJ*. 2004;170(5):793–798.

32. Koh D, Lim MK, Chia SE, et al. Risk perception and impact of Severe Acute Respiratory Syndrome (SARS) on work and personal lives of healthcare workers in Singapore: what can we learn? *Med Care*. 2005;43(7):676–682.

33. Cozza SJ, Huleatt WJ, James LC. Walter Reed Army Medical Center's mental health response to the Pentagon attack. *Mil Med*. 2002;167(9 suppl):12–16.

34. Geiling JA. Overview of command and control issues: setting the stage. *Mil Med*. 2002;167(9 suppl):3–5.

35. Grieger TA, Lyszczarz JL. Psychiatric responses by the US Navy to the Pentagon attack. *Mil Med*. 2002;167(9 suppl):24–25.

36. Tarpley AA. A perspective on the Air Force's mental health response to the Pentagon. *Mil Med*. 2002;167(9 suppl):26–30.

37. Wain HJ, Grammer GG, Stasinos JJ, Miller CM. Meeting the patients where they are: consultation-liaison response to trauma victims of the Pentagon attack. *Mil Med*. 2002;167(9 suppl):19–21.

38. McClain TC, Hamilton FC, Clothier J, McGaugh J. Opportunity missed: a lesson learned from evacuating mentally ill patients following Hurricanes Katrina and Rita. *Acad Psychiatry*. 2007;31(3):188–189.

39. Edmondson MW. Professionalism, honor, and respect on September 11th: a historical view of the Initial Response and Recovery Mortuary Team. *Mil Med*. 2002;167(9 suppl):6–7.

40. Keller RT, Bobo WV. Handling human remains following the terrorist attack on the Pentagon: experiences of 10 uniformed health care workers. *Mil Med*. 2002;167(9 suppl):8–11.

41. Grieger TA, Cozza SJ, Ursano RJ, et al. Posttraumatic stress disorder and depression in battle-injured soldiers. *Am J Psychiatry*. 2006;163(10):1777–1783.

42. Wain H, Bradley J, Nam T, Waldrep D, Cozza S. Psychiatric interventions with returning soldiers at Walter Reed. *Psychiatr Q*. 2005;76(4):351–360.

43. Powers R. Help in troubled times: chaplain comments concerning Operation Noble Eagle. *Mil Med*. 2002;167(9 suppl):17–18.

44. Frist WH. Recovering from the tsunami. *N Engl J Med*. 2005;352(5):438.

45. VanRooyen M, Leaning J. After the tsunami—facing the public health challenges. *N Engl J Med*. 2005;352(5):435–438.

46. Guerena-Burgueno F, Jongsakul K, Smith BL, Ittiverakul M, Chiravaratanond O. Rapid assessment of health needs and medical response after the tsunami in Thailand, 2004–2005. *Mil Med*. 2006;171(10 suppl 1):8–11.

47. McCartney SF. Combined Support Force 536: Operation Unified Assistance. *Mil Med*. 2006;171(10 suppl 1):24–26.

48. Peake JB. The Project HOPE and USNS Mercy tsunami "experiment." *Mil Med*. 2006;171(10 suppl 1):27–29.

49. Llewellyn M. Perspectives from MTF USNS Mercy. *Mil Med*. 2006;171(10 suppl 1):30–33.

50. Lane DA. Medical support to Sri Lanka in the wake of tsunamis: planning considerations and lessons learned. *Mil Med*. 2006;171(10 suppl 1):19–23.

51. Center for the Study of Traumatic Stress. Teachers helping students: listening and talking. Available at: http://www.cstsonline.org/csts_items/CSTS_teachers_helping_students.pdf. Accessed May 25, 2010.

52. Lehmann C. APA begins major outreach to tsunami-devastated nations. *Psychiatr News*. February 4, 2005: 1.

53. Reissman DB, Schreiber M, Klomp RW, Hoover M, Kowalski-Trakofler K, Perez J. The virtual network supporting the front lines: addressing emerging behavioral health problems following the tsunami of 2004. *Mil Med*. 2006;171(10 suppl 1):40–43.

54. US Department of Defense. *Military Support for Stability, Security, Transition, and Reconstruction (SSTR) Operations*. Washington, DC: DoD; 2005. DoD Directive 3000.05.

55. Castro C. How to build battlemind: 10 tough facts about combat and what leaders can do to mitigate risk and build resilience. *NCO J*. 2004;14(2):23–24.

56. Munsey C. Armor for the mind. *Monitor on Psychology*. 2007;38(9):45. Available at: http://www.apa.org/monitor/oct07/armor.html. Accessed November 27, 2009.

57. Winslow DL. Wind, rain, flooding, and fear: coordinating military public health in the aftermath of Hurricane Katrina. *Clin Infect Dis*. 2005;41(12):1759–1763.

58. Weisler RH, Barbee JG 4th, Townsend MH. Mental health and recovery in the Gulf Coast after Hurricanes Katrina and Rita. *JAMA*. 2006;296(5):585–588.

59. Osofsky HJ. In the eye of Katrina: surviving the storm and rebuilding an academic department of psychiatry. *Acad Psychiatry*. 2007;31(3):183–187.

60. Townsend MH. Medical student education in psychiatry after Katrina: disaster and renewal. *Acad Psychiatry*. 2007;31(3):205–210.

61. Kaplan A. Helping Katrina survivors: psychiatrists provide insider views. *Psychiatric Times*. November 1, 2005. Available at: http://www.psychiatrictimes.com/display/article/10168/52736?verify=0. Accessed November 27, 2009.

62. Center for the Study of Traumatic Stress. Hurricane Katrina: evacuee mental health and care. Available at: http://www.cstsonline.org/resources/resource-2_hurricane_katrina_evacuee. Accessed May 25, 2010.

63. Miles D. More active, Guard troops join Katrina response. *American Forces Press Service*. September 3, 2005. Available at: http://www.defenselink.mil/news/newsarticle.aspx?id=17417. Accessed November 27, 2009.

64. Miles D. Military response to Katrina intensifies. *American Forces Press Service*. September 7, 2005. Available at: http://www.defenselink.mil/news/newsarticle.aspx?id=17389. Accessed May 25, 2010.

65. Klein KR, Nagel NE. Mass medical evacuation: Hurricane Katrina and nursing experiences at the New Orleans airport. *Disaster Manag Response*. 2007;5(2):56–61.

66. Surveillance for illness and injury after Hurricane Katrina—New Orleans, Louisiana, September 8–25, 2005. *MMWR Morb Mortal Wkly Rep*. 2005;54(40):1018–1021.

67. Military Sealift Command. MSC supports Hurricane Katrina relief efforts. Available at: http://www.msc.navy.mil/comfort/katrina. Accessed May 25, 2010.

68. Cerise FP. Updated number of deceased victims recovered following Hurricane Katrina. Louisiana Department of Health and Hospitals Bureau of Media and Communications News Release. October 21, 2005. Available at: http://www.dhh.louisiana.gov/news.asp?ID=1&Detail=720&Arch=2005. Accessed May 25, 2010.

69. Louisiana Department of Health and Hospitals. Hurricane Katrina reports of missing and deceased. August 2, 2006. Available at: http://www.dhh.louisiana.gov/offices/page.asp?ID=192&Detail=5248&Print=1. Accessed May 25, 2010.

70. Lamberg L. Katrina survivors strive to reclaim their lives. *JAMA*. 2006;296(5):499–502.

71. Assessment of health-related needs after Hurricanes Katrina and Rita—Orleans and Jefferson parishes, New Orleans area, Louisiana, October 17–22, 2005. *MMWR Morb Mortal Wkly Rep*. 2006;55(2):38–41. Available at: http://www.medscape.com/viewarticle/523049. Accessed November 27, 2009.

72. Health hazard evaluation of police officers and firefighters after Hurricane Katrina—New Orleans, Louisiana, October 17–28 and November 30–December 5, 2005. *MMWR Morb Mortal Wkly Rep*. 2006;55(16):456–458. Available at: http://www.cdc.gov/mmWR/preview/mmwrhtml/mm5516a4.htm. Accessed November 27, 2009.

73. The Children's Health Fund. *Responding to an Emerging Humanitarian Crisis in Louisiana and Mississippi: Urgent Need for a Health Care "Marshall Plan."* New York, NY: Columbia University Mailman School of Public Health; April 17, 2006. Available at: http://www.ncdp.mailman.columbia.edu/files/marshall_plan.pdf. Accessed May 25, 2010.

74. Saulny S. A legacy of the storm: depression and suicide. *New York Times*. June 21, 2006. Available at: http://www.nytimes.com/2006/06/21/us/21depress.html. Accessed May 25, 2010.

75. Winstead DK, Legeai C. Lessons learned from Katrina: one department's perspective. *Acad Psychiatry*. 2007;31(3):190–195.

76. Connelly M. IMERT deployment to Baton Rouge, Louisiana in response to Hurricane Katrina, September 2005. *Disaster Manag Response*. 2006;4(1):4–11.

77. Kahn MJ, Markert RJ, Johnson JE, Owens D, Krane NK. Psychiatric issues and answers following Hurricane Katrina. *Acad Psychiatry*. 2007;31(3):200–204.

Chapter 36

TERRORISM AND CHEMICAL, BIOLOGICAL, RADIOLOGICAL, NUCLEAR, AND EXPLOSIVE WEAPONS

ROSS H. PASTEL, PhD,* and ELSPETH CAMERON RITCHIE, MD, MPH†

*Lieutenant Colonel, Medical Service Corps, US Army; Chief, Division of Traumatic Brain Injury, Research Directorate, Defense Centers of Excellence for Psychological Health and Traumatic Brain Injury, 1335 East-West Highway, Suite 900, Silver Spring, Maryland 20910; formerly, Assistant Professor, Department of Medical and Clinical Psychology, Uniformed Services University of the Health Sciences, Bethesda, Maryland

†Colonel, US Army (Retired); formerly, Psychiatry Consultant to The Surgeon General, US Army, and Director, Behavioral Health Proponency, Office of The Surgeon General, Falls Church, Virginia; currently, Chief Clinical Officer, District of Columbia Department of Mental Health, 64 New York Avenue NE, 4th Floor, Washington, DC 20002

INTRODUCTION

Chemical, biological, radiological, nuclear, and explosive (CBRNE) agents have gained increased international attention in the last 20 years. In 1992 Boris Yeltsin, the Russian president, admitted for the first time that the Soviet Union had continued to develop an offensive biological warfare program following the Soviet Union's ratification of the Biological and Toxin Weapon Convention in 1972.[1] In 1995 the world was stunned by two major terrorist attacks. In March the Aum Shinrikyo cult carried out a large-scale sarin attack on the Tokyo subway system. In April two home-grown American terrorists, Timothy McVeigh and Terry Nichols, attacked the Murrah Federal Building in Oklahoma City, Oklahoma, with a large truck bomb. Early in the new millennium on September 11, 2001, the terrorist group al Qaeda attacked the Pentagon and the twin towers of the World Trade Center. Although the anthrax mail attacks followed within the week, they were not recognized until October, when the first victim fell ill. In the midst of these terrorist attacks, an emerging infectious disease outbreak caused by a new contagious disease called severe acute respiratory syndrome (SARS) appeared and caused widespread death and illness around the globe, including in China, Taiwan, Hong Kong, Singapore, Vietnam, and Canada. Although not a terrorist attack, the SARS epidemic resembles what might happen following a terrorist attack with a contagious disease such as smallpox.

CBRNE weapons are no longer weapons only of states; they have become available to terrorists as well. Many experts believe that a large-scale attack with CBRNE weapons is not a matter of if, but of when. Therefore, it is critical that mental healthcare practitioners become aware of the possible psychological consequences following a CBRNE attack.

The psychological effects differ from other medical effects in that personnel do not need to be physically exposed to these agents to exhibit symptoms. Psychological effects can cause symptoms that may mimic the prodromal (or early) symptoms of CBRNE agents. Fortunately, the acute and long-term effects after CBRNE attacks have no apparent unique psychological disorders, but rather seem to exist on a continuum with effects seen after natural disasters or high explosives.[2] Psychophysiologic effects, typically syndromes of medically unexplained symptoms, will likely dominate the long-term picture,[3] and treatment may be difficult because of patient resistance and difficulties with doctor–patient relationships.[4]

This chapter will not be a comprehensive review of the literature; rather, it will introduce the clinician to potential problems resulting from CBRNE attacks. The chapter will briefly cover some unique aspects of such attacks, which can amplify the psychological effects, before reviewing acute and long-term effects.

TERMINOLOGY

Terminology has an important effect on perception. Having a name for something presupposes an understanding. Terminology can be positive, neutral, or negative, depending on the connotations and context. One important collective behavior phenomenon has variously been called mass hysteria, epidemic hysteria, and mass psychogenic illness.[5–7] Unfortunately, these terms have a pejorative connotation. For example, hysteria comes from the Greek word *hystera*, meaning uterus. Thus, when "mass hysteria" is used to describe an event involving medically unexplained physical symptoms, the immediate presupposition is that mostly females are involved. The common connotation for hysteria presupposes an overemotional response to an event, that is, a pejorative connotation. Use of "mass hysteria" by media, medical personnel, or public officials can lead to a negative perception of medical personnel and public officials by people affected by an event and vice versa. Similarly, in "mass psychogenic illness," *psyche* refers to the mind and *genic* refers to genesis or creation. The connotation is that symptoms are "all in the head" and thus not real. A preferred term is "outbreak of multiple unexplained symptoms" (OMUS).[7] Although clumsy, this term is relatively neutral. OMUS is also descriptive—the symptoms are real but unexplained, rather than "all in the head."

Another common term used in CBRNE events is "worried well." This terminology presupposes that the "worried well" are not suffering a real medical effect from a CBRNE exposure, but are simply worried that they might be ill. However, after a CBRNE event, many people with unknown exposures may be symptomatic—distressed and in pain. How can they be "well?" Again, "worried well" is a pejorative term and should be discarded. In the 1950s a more useful term, "disaster fatigue," was used. This term was based on the military experience with combat exhaustion or battle fatigue (now called combat stress reaction). In World War II, battle fatigue was originally called "war neurosis" or "psychoneurosis" (which also had a negative connotation for soldiers).

Panic is another commonly used term, often used in reference to the general public, that is, a "mass panic." In the strict sense, mass panic means an acute fear reaction marked by loss of self-control and followed by nonsocial and unreasoning flight.[8] Flight can be a normal reaction to the presence of an immediate danger. It becomes a mass panic only when large numbers of people stampede without regard to others in an attempt to escape danger. Thus, to describe a panic following the anthrax attacks in 2001 or the New York City outbreak of West Nile virus in 1999 is inaccurate because there was no mass exodus from any city, nor was there an explicit danger from which to escape. A more accurate term would be "mass anxiety."

Terrorism and CBRNE incidents (whether in warfare or in terrorism) are most typically mass casualty events (MCEs). However, MCEs vary widely both in the number and severity of casualties and the ability of the local environment to respond to the event. One group has proposed a useful terminology that categorizes MCEs into emergencies, disasters, and catastrophes based on the demand characteristics (number of people in need of rescue, shelter, or medical treatment) of the event and the locally available response capacity.[9] Disasters are events in which the demands are in excess of the locally available response capacity (eg, the 2001 World Trade Center attack). Although emergencies may have high demand characteristics, they are not disasters because the locally available response capacity can handle the demand (eg, the 2001 attack on the Pentagon). Catastrophes occur when the event not only overwhelms the local response capacity, but also causes substantial damage to the infrastructure supporting the response system (eg, the 1995 Kobe earthquake in Japan).

Persistent idiopathic (medically unexplained) symptoms that drive patients to seek medical care[4] typically fall within syndromes, including chronic fatigue syndrome, fibromyalgia, and multiple chemical sensitivity. These syndromes have overlapping symptom clusters and may be identified more by the specialty of the physician providing treatment than by the patient's symptoms.

RISK COMMUNICATION AND PERCEPTION

Communicating With the Public

In a CBRNE event, it is likely that the extent of the danger will not be known immediately, especially for chemical, biological, radiological, and nuclear (CBRN) weapons. Public health authorities and public officials will attempt to calculate the extent of the threat, and inform the media and the public. New York City Mayor Rudolph Giuliani was extremely effective following the events of September 11, 2001, and demonstrated the value of daily or twice-daily scheduled briefings with the media and the public. Much has been published on principles of health communication, including having a consistent message delivered by a knowledgeable and credible official, listening and responding to the concerns of the public, and avoiding the appearance of defensiveness or concealment.

After any toxic accident or terrorist attack, many people will feel anxious about the potential health effects of a CBRN release. Such anxieties may be multiplied if devastating descriptions of the potential aftermath appear in the media. Following the 2001 events, fears were exacerbated by media suggestions that in an anthrax attack, "your next breath may kill you." Public officials should provide accurate hazard communication and workable measures that can be taken to protect individuals and families. According to one risk communication approach, risk equals hazard plus outrage.[10] Hazard is the scientifically based risk assessment, but outrage is made up of nonquantifiable factors related to the public's concern and perception of the event. Outrage following an attack with weapons of mass destruction will significantly influence both acute and long-term psychological effects.

The US Army Center for Health Promotion and Preventive Medicine has more detailed information and training courses available (see the Center's Web site: http://usachppm.apgea.army.mil/risk/). The Centers for Disease Control and Prevention has developed a course on emergency risk communication training (see the CDC's Web site: http://www.cdc.gov/cdcynergy/emergency/).

Risk Perception

Risk perception is an important driver of the outrage component in risk communication. CBRN weapons involve a number of factors that can increase the perception of risk. Many CBRN weapons are invisible and odorless (radiation, biological agents, and some chemical agents), which leads to uncertainty about both exposure and amount of exposure. In many cases, exposure is not known until the patients become symptomatic. However, these agents may initially induce nonspecific symptoms (eg, fatigue, headache, nausea, dyspnea, dizziness, and muscle and joint ache). Regardless of illness induced, chemical agent and radiation exposures will also increase the fear of the long-term effects of the exposure.

In the risk literature, a number of factors have been

shown to increase the perception of risk, including potentially fatal illness, involuntary exposure (lack of control), a catastrophic event, presence of an unknown perpetrator, delayed detection and reaction by authorities, and potential effect on future generations.[11,12] Fear of radiation, in particular, is prevalent, largely because of ignorance and misinformation. Thoughts and images typically associated with radiation are death, cancer, sterility, and fear for future generations. A number of factors may further amplify risk perception: scapegoating, distrust of governmental and industrial experts, and news media hype and misinformation.

Mass Media

The acute and long-term consequences of terrorism and CBRNE events are certainly shaped by risk perception. Risk perception, at least in part, is shaped by the mass media. Mass media has played an important role in various OMUS situations.[13] Media are an important risk amplifier because they select and frame risk messages to inform the public, and intensive reporting (or media hype) can create continuing waves of news.[13]

The power of the media can be seen in studies that followed both the 1995 Oklahoma City bombing and the events of September 11, 2001. In a study of over 2,000 middle-school children surveyed 7 weeks after the Oklahoma City bombing, both emotional exposure and television exposure were significantly related to posttraumatic stress symptomatology.[14] When children with no direct (felt or heard the explosion) or emotional (knew someone killed or injured) exposure to the bombing were divided into high and low television exposure, children with high television exposure had significantly higher posttraumatic stress scores.[14] A telephone survey study done 3 to 5 days after September 11 found that 44% of the people surveyed had one or more substantial stress symptoms, including sleep difficulties, irritability and anger, difficulty concentrating, and disturbing thoughts, memories, and dreams.[15] The people responding to this survey were not present at the event; therefore, much of what they knew was presumably based on media reporting.

In a contagious disease outbreak, information becomes extremely important. The public is eager for information and needs to know what precautionary measures should be taken. In Hong Kong, most respondents to a survey reported actively seeking SARS information on a daily basis, and relied more on mass media (television, newspapers and radio) than on medical professionals, friends, or the Internet.[16] Substantial misinformation and false beliefs persisted among Hong Kong adults even at an advanced stage of the SARS epidemic, despite constant media and public service announcements.[17] Recommended measures were not practiced uniformly. Many people did not understand transmission routes; only one third of respondents avoided direct contact by touch with contaminated objects (fomites), and less than one half practiced at least five of the seven recommended precautions.

TRIAGE AND ISSUES OF DIFFERENTIAL DIAGNOSIS

An important lesson learned from the Israeli Scud missile experience is the importance of a separate stress center at hospitals, so that psychological casualties can be removed from the emergency room and taken to a less stressful environment. Only recently have neuropsychiatric casualties been included as a triage category.[18] When Israel was attacked with Scud missiles during the Persian Gulf War in 1991, large numbers of people reported to the emergency room for treatment.[19,20] Studies reported that approximately 70% to 80% of the patients in the early attacks had stress-related symptoms.

Psychological Symptoms

Many symptoms commonly seen following a CBRNE incident (fatigue, nausea, vomiting, headaches, and anorexia) are common in combat[21] and can be induced by acute radiation sickness (ARS) and chemical agent exposure, or during the prodromal syndrome of exposure to various biological agents and toxins.[22] Because many CBRN agents are invisible, many soldiers may experience symptoms that they blame on CBRN exposure, regardless of actual exposure or dose of exposure. These patients are not "worried well." They are worried—possibly with good reason—but they are not well if they are in distress and pain.

Some CBRN agents may directly induce psychological effects in addition to medical effects (eg, nerve agents can induce anxiety).[23] In other cases, symptoms may precede signs; that is, patients exposed to pulmonary agents may initially present with respiratory distress without measurable physical signs.[24] Symptomatic ambulatory cases with mild or perceived exposures will present difficulties for CBRN event triage.

Unfortunately, most disaster exercises for CBRNE or other incidents include few psychological casualties. Without proper training based on actual CBRNE accidents, incidents, and attacks, healthcare providers will be unprepared for the sudden onslaught of patients presenting with mild or psychological symptoms who will arrive at the hospital before the severely wounded.

Estimating Psychological Casualties

Based on historical experience in World War II, military medical planners can get a rough estimate of battle fatigue or combat stress casualties, based on the number of wounded in action (WIA) expected from different types of battles.[25,26] In World War II, the ratio of combat stress casualties to WIA was in the range of 1:10 to 1:2.[25,26] The civilian psychological casualty (PC) to WIA ratio for the first Israeli Scud missile attack was 16:1 (if PCs are combined with unjustified atropine injections) or 8:1 (if only the PCs are included). In the 1987 radiological contamination accident in Goiânia, Brazil, where no explosion occurred, the PC to WIA ratio was 500:1 (with WIA defined as anyone contaminated either externally or internally), or 2,500:1 (with WIA defined as those individuals requiring close medical surveillance).

Both examples involve civilians of two foreign nations, so extrapolation to US citizens or military personnel is difficult. The available data suggest that it is unlikely that the PC to WIA ratio following a CBRNE attack or incident will resemble the 1:10 to 1:2 range seen in World War II battles. The low end of the range may resemble World War II statistics, but the high end could go much higher, depending on the characteristics of the CBRNE attack. Most importantly, it is time to ensure that training for disaster and CBRNE incident should involve large numbers of psychological casualties, not the typical token few.

ACUTE EFFECTS

Mass Panic

The common image of behavior during or after a disaster is that of mass panic, described as "highly disorganized flight by hysterical individuals who have stampeded at the sight of actual or potential danger."[27(p68)] During the Cold War, civil defense planners feared that a mass panic would follow a nuclear attack. However, studies of disasters and wars over the last 50 years show that disorganized flight (mass panic) is very rare.[28–30] The few occasions when it did occur were very circumscribed and were characterized by limited escape routes with the possibility of entrapment, a perception of collective powerlessness, and a feeling of individual isolation.[27,29,31] The most frequent historical examples of mass panic are in cases of fires, mine collapses, and sinking ships. Mass anxiety is *not* mass panic.

In the initial use of chlorine gas on the Western front by Germany in 1915, "a full-blown, blind, contagious panic swept portions of the line."[32(p91)] However, no panic occurred farther out on the line where there was little or no gas. In the next six gas attacks over the following 2 months, no mass panics occurred, although protective equipment was rudimentary and not widely available. Only four other gas panics were documented in World War I.

Most victims of the Tokyo sarin subway attack were office workers going to their jobs in central Tokyo. Despite the crowded conditions of the morning rush hour and the limited escape routes, there were no reports of mass panic. One fireman reported a "perplexing silence" at the accident scene—no talking, just the coughing of the victims as they awaited medical assistance.[33]

Distress and Outbreaks of Multiple Unexplained Symptoms

Perceived exposure to a CBRNE agent can result in the appearance of symptoms that may be hard to differentiate from mild symptoms expected from actual exposure. Thus, an OMUS can occur independently or in conjunction with a CBRNE event. However, in a CBRNE event, not all symptomatic casualties have been exposed to a toxic agent.[34] Symptoms of psychological origin can also occur in casualties actually exposed to a CBRNE agent and may make treatment more difficult (victims finding out they have been exposed to a lethal disease such as anthrax or smallpox are unlikely to remain calm). Regardless of the actual exposure, it is important to pay attention to the patient's symptoms of pain and distress while attempting to discern actual exposure.

The US military has experienced several OMUS incidents. In World War I, outbreaks of gas neurosis (gas hysteria) occurred, in which some soldiers experienced symptoms of gas poisoning (eg, dyspnea, coughing, and burning of skin) without clinical exposure to gas.[35] In one incident, 500 battle-tested troops drifted into medical aid stations over a 1-week period following desultory gas shelling. They exhibited chest pain, fatigue, dyspnea, coughing, husky voice, and indefinite eye symptoms, all consistent with chemical exposure.[36] However, the divisional gas officer found no evidence of gas inhalation or burning.

More recently, in 1988, 1,800 male military recruits were evacuated from barracks due to an epidemic of coughing, dyspnea, and chest pain that broke out at a training center.[37] The symptoms were consistent with exposure to a chemical agent or toxin. Recruits and medical personnel suspected an airborne toxin, but none was detected. These examples of OMUS demonstrate that a perceived exposure can induce symptoms resembling an actual exposure.

The Goiânia radiation incident was a dramatic example of a co-occurrence of OMUS and a CBRNE event. Over 125,000 people demanded to be screened for radiological exposure following the news of radiological contamination.[38] Screening identified only 249 persons with any radiological contamination, but 5,000 of the first 60,000 people screened had symptoms consistent with radiation sickness (vomiting, diarrhea, and/or rashes around the face and neck). None of the symptomatic persons were contaminated.

Chemical Warfare Agents

The Israeli experience with 18 Scud missile attacks during the Persian Gulf War involved both the effects of missile explosions and, at least initially, the perception of a possible nerve agent attack. One study of patients arriving in the emergency departments of 11 local hospitals in Israel[19] found that approximately 332 of the 773 casualties (43%) were psychological casualties and an additional 209 (27%) had injected themselves with atropine because they feared the missiles contained nerve agent. After the first Scud attack, there were 365 casualties: 172 psychological casualties (47%), 171 cases of unjustified atropine injections (47%), and only 22 cases of physical injury (6%). Another study[20] looked at patients reporting to the emergency department of a Tel Aviv hospital within 8 hours of a Scud attack. Of the 103 patients admitted, 70 had psychological distress (68%) and 19 had unjustified atropine injections (18%); only 9 had direct injuries (9%). All these findings were among civilians, not soldiers.

After the 1995 sarin attack in the Tokyo subway,[33,39] over 5,500 people visited 280 medical facilities the day of the attack and the following week. Of these, 1,046 were admitted as patients. Saint Luke's International Hospital saw the most patients: 641 patients on the first day and 349 in the following week.[39] Of the 641 patients admitted to the emergency department on the first day, 111 were admitted to the hospital (4 severe cases, 107 moderate cases), and 530 mild cases were observed for 6 hours and then released. The patients with mild cases suffered mainly from eye problems. It is difficult to determine from the literature how many of the mild cases were psychological casualties.

Biological Agents

In 1994 two outbreaks of plague occurred in India: a bubonic plague outbreak in Maharashtra state, followed by a pneumonic plague outbreak 1 month later and 500 km away in Surat.[40] Of the 5,000 suspected cases of plague, there were 167 confirmed cases and 55 deaths.[41] Unfortunately, no data are readily available on psychological reactions or rates of such reactions. However, there were observable effects on behavior. The local media fueled the anxiety with exaggerated reports.[41,42] An estimated 400,000 to 600,000 people fled Surat, including hospital staff, private medical practitioners, and municipal workers.[43,44] In Delhi, 1,200 km from Surat, people fashioned masks from available materials, and many bought and hoarded tetracycline, an antibiotic used to treat plague.[45]

In 2001, after the September 11th attacks and before the first of 23 anthrax cases,[46] the media had already reported increased purchases of gas masks and ciprofloxacin ("cipro," used to treat anthrax). After the anthrax mail attacks, there were increased patient requests for ciprofloxacin and anecdotal reports of increased prescriptions.[47] Hospitals reported their already busy emergency rooms were filled with people anxious about anthrax, many demanding treatment.

The outbreak of SARS, a new and emerging infection, created much fear and anxiety. In Beijing, schools and universities were closed, hundreds of companies closed their doors, and some surrounding villages shut themselves off from contact with others.[48] Rumors of neighborhoods being quarantined led to stockpiling of food.[49] Although officials asked people to avoid travel, thousands of businesspersons, migrant workers, and college students left Beijing. In Taiwan, 160 doctors and nurses quit work at various hospitals, fearing both the disease itself and the inadequacy of infection control measures.[50] SARS patients often spent hours in isolation between contacts with staff and were deprived of family visits, leading to complaints of sadness, anxiety, boredom, loneliness, and nonspecific anger and frustration.[51,52] Fear and anxiety often waxed and waned with fever.[51]

One study measured the psychosocial effects of SARS on hospital staff in a Toronto hospital using questionnaires.[53] Almost two thirds of the respondents reported concerns for their own or their family's health. Factors associated with increased concerns were perception of a greater risk of death from SARS, living with children, personal or family lifestyle affected by SARS outbreak, and being treated differently by other people because of working in a hospital. Emotional distress was found in almost 30% of all responders and in 45% of nurses, who were most at risk for infection. Factors identified for significant association with emotional distress were being a nurse, part-time employment status, lifestyle affected by SARS outbreak, and ability to do one's job affected by precautionary measures.

Radiological Agents

The Three Mile Island (TMI) accident in Pennsylvania in 1979 demonstrated the importance of psychological effects following a CBRNE incident. According to the president's commission that studied the accident, the only medical effect documented was mental distress.[54] There were no cases of ARS, and the estimated exposure doses for people living within 10 miles of TMI were approximately the dose of an average chest radiograph, much lower than the annual background radiation dose.[55] Populations exhibiting the most distress were TMI workers, families with preschool-age children, and those living within 5 miles of TMI. Studies of TMI workers reported no long-term effects, only short-term acute effects. TMI personnel reported nausea, stomach troubles, headaches, diarrhea, sleep disturbances, and loss of appetite in greater frequency than did the control group. These symptoms are also common to the ARS prodrome, but TMI personnel were not exposed to radiation doses that would cause ARS.

Unlike the TMI accident, the 1986 Chernobyl accident in Ukraine did release significant amounts of radiation. Approximately 135,000 people were evacuated from a 30-km zone in the first 2 weeks after the accident. Most of these people had to be permanently relocated. In addition, an estimated 600,000 to 800,000 "liquidators" were brought in to handle the emergency situation and subsequent cleanup operations.[56] Although over 200 cases of ARS were recorded, the primary health effect was widespread psychological distress.[57,58]

In the 1987 Goiânia incident, two scavengers removed a cesium-137 teletherapy unit from an abandoned radiotherapy institute.[59] While dismantling the unit, they accidentally ruptured the source capsule that contained radioactive cesium-137 powder. When the accident became public, the perceived threat of radiation exposure caused over 120,000 people (approximately 10% of the city's population of 1.2 million) to be screened over a 6-month span for possible contamination.[60] Residents and others in the city at that time felt sufficiently at risk that they took time off from work or came on weekends to wait in line to be scanned.[38,61] Approximately 5,000 (8%) of the first 60,000 people screened presented with symptoms that mimicked ARS (eg, rash around neck and upper body, vomiting, diarrhea), but none of these individuals were contaminated.[38] Only 249 people had measurable radiological contamination.

Explosives

Acute psychological effects were reported in 50% of bomb-injured patients in one study.[62] Another study reported that approximately 12% of the casualties presented with emotional distress, with another 6% presenting with medical problems (eg, angina, diabetes, headache, or asthma).[63]

Mental Disorders

Chemical Warfare Agents

Most patients from the Tokyo sarin attack who were admitted to a hospital remained hospitalized for a few days. Some reported sleep disturbances, nightmares, and anxiety. Whether these symptoms were due to acute stress disorder or to exposure to nerve agent is unknown. In studies done 1 month after the event, nearly 60% of casualties reported suffering from postincident symptoms, including fear of using the subway, sleep disturbances, flashbacks, depression, nightmares, irritability, headaches, malaise, physical tension, and emotional lability and irritability.[33,39] Follow-up questionnaires at 3- and 6-month intervals showed little decrease in the percentage reporting symptoms. Unfortunately, it is difficult to determine to what extent these symptoms were psychological effects and to what extent they may have been sequelae to the cholinergic effects of sarin exposure. Because most of the casualties from Saint Luke's International Hospital were mild cases (suffering mainly eye symptoms), it is possible that many of the postincident symptoms were psychological.

Radiological Agents

Most of the 20 hospitalized Goiânia patients suffered from depression and anxiety.[64] The 11 victims most seriously affected were moved to one hospital, where they were kept confined and isolated because of immunosuppression, and the medical personnel treating them wore protective masks. Both measures increased stress in patients. Uncertainty about future health effects also increased stress, as did the lack of information concerning the duration of their treatment and the long-term prognosis.

Nuclear Weapons

Of all CBRNE agents, nuclear weapons have the greatest destructive impact—they are the quintessential weapons of mass destruction. The atomic weapons dropped on Hiroshima and Nagasaki caused incredible devastation, outbreaks of local fires, and large numbers of dead, dying, and injured people.[65] In interviews done after the war, approximately two thirds of survivors described psychological disturbances of intense fear, emotional upset, or depression. However, only a single incident of an apparent mass panic was reported at Hiroshima: a large group of frightened people in a park pressed some victims into a river, and several died.[66]

During the following weeks, survivors continued to witness the sight of severely injured people suffering from burns and blast injuries. In addition, there were outbreaks of ARS. The continued exposures to the devastation and human suffering served as a constant reminder to survivors and reinforced the psychological impact of the original event.[65]

LONG-TERM EFFECTS

Distress and Chronic Outbreaks of Multiple Unexplained Symptoms

Although acute OMUS has been widely studied, the possibility of long-duration and large-scale OMUS syndromes has only lately been suggested.[67] In recent years, a number of different chronic syndromes (eg, chronic fatigue syndrome, environmental somatization syndrome, multiple chemical sensitivity syndrome, and sick building syndrome) have appeared, all characterized by multiple nonspecific symptoms (eg, fatigue, headaches, sleep disturbances, nausea, dizziness, muscle and joint pains, and difficulties with memory and concentration) that are not connected with specific infectious or toxic agents.[68–70] In each of these syndromes, the patient attributes an invisible contaminant or infectious agent as the cause for the symptoms.

Military Experience

The military has seen several chronic OMUS syndromes, including Agent Orange syndrome, atomic veterans syndrome, and Gulf War syndrome.[3] Agent Orange syndrome began when the media publicized an association between exposure of Vietnam veterans to Agent Orange and a reported epidemic of cancer and children born with birth defects. Epidemiological studies done by the Centers for Disease Control and Prevention found no evidence of increased incidence of cancer or birth defects in this population.[71–73] However, an increased prevalence of depression, anxiety, alcohol abuse or dependence, and posttraumatic stress disorder (PTSD) was demonstrated in Vietnam veterans compared with subjects who had not fought in Vietnam.[71] Another study found that symptoms of psychological distress were strongly associated with self-reported herbicide exposure. This group presented with more symptoms than were found in Air Force personnel actively involved in aerial spraying of herbicides.[74] This suggests that Agent Orange syndrome might be more related to a perception of exposure than to actual exposure.

An estimated 200,000 Department of Defense personnel (both military and civilian) observed the early US above-ground nuclear tests.[75] The external doses received by these "atomic veterans" averaged about 0.5 rem, with many receiving no dose and only 1% receiving a dose greater than 5 rem (the maximum annual occupational dose). Several case studies of atomic veterans reported long-term psychological distress.[76,77] Initially, troops at the Desert Rock V test seemed to go through the experience with equanimity,[78] but many years later, an anecdotal study found that veterans reported vivid recollections of an atmosphere of tension and fear at the test sites and thought they had been ill-prepared.[76]

A cluster of functional somatic symptoms was reported in atomic veterans and dubbed the "radiation response syndrome."[77] The syndrome has two components: (1) a core belief that radiation had caused physical harm, and (2) functional somatic symptoms that appeared to be an expression of this belief. The radiation response syndrome belief system included the views "that men were dying, that doctors are of little help, that one doctor may exist who could help, that the government is to blame for their illness, and that people think they are crazy for blaming exposure to ionizing radiation for their illnesses."[77(p128)] Radiation response syndrome resembles delayed-onset PTSD, but rather than reexperiencing the trauma as in PTSD, the veterans are preoccupied with radiation and its effect on their lives.

Chemical Warfare Agents

Three years after World War I, approximately one half of gassed veterans claimed subjective complaints in medical examinations.[79] When there were no objective findings, no compensation or pensions were paid, nor were these complaints included in statistics of permanent disabilities. There were reports of large numbers of men who had recovered from acute gas poisoning and had good physical examinations, but suffered from serious sequelae, most particularly of easy fatigability and difficulty breathing on exertion.[80] This condition was variously known as effort syndrome, disordered action of the heart, and neurocirculatory asthenia. Chronic gas cases often involved acute attacks of breathlessness at night accompanied by nightmares, and patients usually reported insomnia and unrefreshing sleep.[80]

A long-term study of sarin patients who had been hospitalized at Saint Luke's Hospital found that somatic and psychological symptoms continued for 5 years after the incident.[81] A high rate of medically unexplained physical symptoms was reported. Eye symptoms, fatigue, muscle stiffness, and headache were all reported by more than 10% of the study population.

Biological Agents

Puzzling long-term effects were seen in the survivors of the 2001 anthrax attacks. Newspapers reported that survivors continued to exhibit symptoms of fatigue, shortness of breath, chest pains, memory problems, nightmares, and rage 6 to 12 months after their illnesses.[82] Only one of the inhalational anthrax survivors was well enough to return to work at the time of the study. In the one published study of anthrax survivors 1 year after the attack, many of the survivors reported reduced health-related quality of life and psychological distress.[83]

Radiological Agents

No long-term psychological stress in TMI workers has been reported.[84] However, TMI residents, compared to controls, displayed a significant amount of stress on several measures (performance; self-reported measures of anxiety, depression, and somatic complaints; physiological measures of urinary norepinephrine, epinephrine, and cortisol; disturbed sleep; and changes in immune system parameters) for up to 6 years after the accident.[85–87] The TMI symptoms were not the result of exposure to radiation but to perceived radiation threat, demonstrating that fear of exposure to radiation can cause significant distress and stress symptoms that can mimic symptoms of actual radiation exposure.

The large number of people (~10,000) who lived or worked within 300 meters of the contaminated area in Goiânia exhibited fear, psychosomatic reactions, fear about the future, insecurity, and doubt about the effectiveness of government remedial measures.[88] A public opinion poll conducted 6 months after the incident[88] found that two thirds of both affected Goiânia residents and a control group living away from the contamination believed that Goiânia was still contaminated. Research conducted 3 years later showed that stress parameters were still increased and performance decreased both in nonirradiated individuals with perceived exposure (those living within 1 km of the area where contaminated waste from the incident had been stored) and in irradiated individuals from Goiânia.[89]

A variety of psychoneurological syndromes have been reported as sequelae of Chernobyl in the Russian literature.[90–92] These syndromes are characterized by multiple unexplained physical symptoms including fatigue, sleep and mood disturbances, headaches, impaired memory and concentration, and muscle or joint pain. These syndromes were reported in liquidators who both had and had not experienced ARS.[90,92] No significant correlations were found among physical symptoms, radiation dose, and physical examination data.[92]

Nuclear Weapons

Survivors of Hiroshima and Nagasaki were severely stigmatized, especially those with severe burns that resulted in scarring and keloids. Lifton described a "neurasthenic survivor syndrome" characterized by "persistence of symptoms of withdrawal from social life, insomnia, nightmares, chronic depressive and anxiety reactions and far-reaching somatization . . . in addition, fatigue, emotional lability, loss of initiative, and generalized personal, sexual and social maladaptation."[93(p504)] A study of over 7,000 Nagasaki atomic bomb patients done 15 years later showed long-term psychological effects in approximately 7%, with the majority complaining of fatigue, lack of spirit, poor memory, and introversion.[94] These symptoms were twice as common in survivors who had shown ARS symptoms and were related to severity of ARS symptoms.

Mental Disorders

Chemical Warfare Agents

PTSD has been reported in American World War II veterans exposed to mustard agent while participating in field trials and chamber tests.[95] According to follow-up studies of the Tokyo sarin attack, conducted 3 and 5 years after the accident by the National Police Agency and the National Research Institute for Police Science, reporting of somatic complaints—eye strain, weakened eye sight, and easy fatigability—remained relatively stable from the acute stage through both follow-up periods.[33] PTSD symptoms still reported by 14% to 18% of studied survivors included flashbacks, fear of the subway, intense distress at exposure to reminders of the attack, and avoidance of thinking about the attack.

The casualties seen at Saint Luke's were surveyed at 2, 3, and 5 years, using a questionnaire that asked about 14 physical symptoms, 8 eye symptoms, and 11 psychological symptoms (symptoms of avoidance, hyperarousal, and reexperiencing).[81] The most common symptoms across all time periods were eye symptoms: eye strain (33%–39%), dim vision (23%–26%), and difficulties focusing (17%–21%). Physical symptoms (tiredness, fatigue, muscle ache, headache) were also common. Most of the psychological symptoms remained stable over the three time periods, with rates of 10% to 16% still being reported at the 5-year point for memory difficulties, depressed mood, avoidance of accident reminders, flashbacks, and fear in the subway or at the attack site. PTSD frequency, as determined by criteria in the *Diagnostic and Statistical Manual of Mental Disorders, 4th Edition*,[96] remained stable, with 2% to 3% of patients meeting the criteria during the three time points. The incidence of partial PTSD (one symptom from each category) ranged from 7% to 9%. Because of the persistence of physical symptoms, a modified set of PTSD criteria (adding at least one medically unexplained physical symptom to the diagnosis) were developed, and 10% to 14% of patients met these criteria. The physical symptoms were reported to deteriorate following flashbacks and to improve during psychiatric therapy. The victims continued to be stressed by lack of government support, limited resources available for medical follow-ups, and a feeling of stigmatization.

Biological Agents

Several infectious disease outbreaks have been reported to cause both PTSD and a decreased health-related quality of life. For example, the majority of survivors of an outbreak of Legionnaires disease reported fatigue, neurologic symptoms, and neuromuscular symptoms 17 months after diagnosis.[97] Health-related quality of life was impaired in seven of eight dimensions, and 15% of patients experienced PTSD. Similarly, survivors of acute respiratory distress syndrome have also reported PTSD and decreased health-related quality of life.[98,99] Because most category A biological warfare agents cause acute respiratory distress syndrome, similar long-term effects should be expected.

Radiological Agents

A study conducted 8 years after the Chernobyl accident found that 44% of 1,412 Latvian liquidators had mental-psychosomatic disorders: depression (neurotic depression and brief depressive reaction), physiologic malfunction arising from mental factors, or unspecified disorders of the autonomic nervous system.[100] The actual numbers of mental-psychosomatic disorders might have been higher, but anxiety, PTSD, and sleep disturbances were not studied because of the coding scheme used.[101] Two other studies of Chernobyl exposure found PTSD and PTSD symptoms.[102,103]

An epidemiologic study of over 4,700 Estonian liquidators found an increase in suicide, but no increases in cancer, leukemia, or overall mortality.[104] Suicide accounted for almost 20% of mortality in the liquidator cohort. Reasons for the increased suicide rate are not currently known. However, data from Vietnam veterans with PTSD have demonstrated an increased risk for traumatic deaths, including suicide.[105] Other studies demonstrating a variety of mental health disorders in Chernobyl liquidators support the speculation that fear of radiation might cause depression, PTSD, and other disorders associated with increased rates of suicide. The primary toxic agent appears to be fear, rather than radiation.

Explosives

Long-term psychological consequences after terrorist attacks with explosives have been reported. After the Oklahoma City bombing, 45% of the survivors suffered a postdisaster psychiatric disorder, including 34% with PTSD.[106] Another study reported PTSD in 50% of the patients 6 months after a bombing.[107] PTSD patients had a lower mean injury severity score (1.2) than did patients without PTSD (6.6). Nearly one in five civilian survivors of terrorist attacks (18%) in another study suffered from PTSD, while another 13% suffered from major depression.[108] When broken down by severity of injury, PTSD was present in 31% of the severely injured, but in only 11% of the uninjured and 8% of the moderately injured. The adjusted prevalence ratio for PTSD (severely injured / others) was 4.2. Similarly, major depression occurred in 22% of the severely injured, but in only 9% of the moderately injured or uninjured.[108]

SUMMARY

Mass panic is not likely to occur in CBRNE incidents. Although mass panic can occur in situations involving limited escape routes, it will still probably be a rare event. Psychological effects are likely to cause large numbers of casualties following attacks using CBRNE weapons. Initial presentation may resemble combat stress casualties or may include a variety of nonspecific symptoms, such as difficulty breathing, dizziness, fatigue, headache, and sleep disturbances. Triage and differential diagnosis may be challenging in the initial stages. The number of psychological casualties could increase based on possible amplification of risk perception by mass media reporting. Unlike most physical injuries or illnesses caused by CBRNE agents, psychological effects can be contagious. Given the history of postcombat syndromes, long-term effects are also very likely, and will be difficult to diagnose and treat. These chronic OMUS syndromes will also be greatly influenced by risk perception and mass media reporting.

REFERENCES

1. General Accounting Office. *Biological Weapons: Effort to Reduce Former Soviet Threat Offers Benefits, Poses New Risks*. Washington, DC: GAO; 2000. GAO/NSIAD-00-138.

2. Scharf T, Vaught C, Kidd P, et al. Toward a typology of dynamic and hazardous work environments. *Hum Ecol Risk Assessment.* 2001;7(7):1827–1841.

3. Hyams KC, Wignall FS, Roswell R. War syndromes and their evaluation: from the US Civil War to the Persian Gulf War. *Ann Intern Med.* 1996;125(5):398–405.

4. Engel CC Jr, Adkins JA, Cowan DN. Caring for medically unexplained physical symptoms after toxic environmental exposures: effects of contested causation. *Environ Health Perspect.* 2002;110(suppl 4):641–647.

5. Boss LP. Epidemic hysteria: a review of the published literature. *Epidemiol Rev.* 1997;19:233–243.

6. Colligan MJ, Pennebaker JW, Murphy LR. *Mass Psychogenic Illness*. Hillsdale, NJ: Lawrence Erlbaum Associates Publishers; 1983.

7. Pastel RH. Collective behaviors: mass panic and outbreaks of multiple unexplained symptoms. *Mil Med.* 2001;166(suppl 12):44–46.

8. Schultz DP. *Panic Behavior: Discussion and Readings*. New York, NY: Random House; 1964.

9. Glass TA. Emergency, disaster, and catastrophe: a typology with implications for terrorism response. In: Wessely S, Krasnov VN, eds. *Psychological Responses to the New Terrorism: A NATO-Russia Dialogue*. Amsterdam, Netherlands: IOS Press, 2005: 25–36.

10. Sandman PM. Bioterrorism risk communication policy. *J Health Commun.* 2003;8(suppl 1):146–147.

11. Brecher RW, Flynn T. Principles of risk communication: building trust and credibility with the public. In: Haschek WM, Rousseaux CG, Wallig MA, eds. *Handbook of Toxicologic Pathology*. New York, NY: Academic Press; 2002.

12. Covello VT, Peters RG, Wojtecki JG, Hyde RC. Risk communication, the West Nile virus epidemic, and bioterrorism: responding to the communication challenges posed by the intentional or unintentional release of a pathogen in an urban setting. *J Urban Health.* 2001;78(2):382–391.

13. Vasterman P, Yzermans CJ, Dirkzwager AJ. The role of the media and media hypes in the aftermath of disasters. *Epidemiol Rev.* 2005;27:107–114.

14. Pfefferbaum B. Impact of the Oklahoma City bombing on children in the community. *Mil Med.* 2001;166(suppl 2):49–50.

15. Schuster MA, Stein BD, Jaycox L, et al. A national survey of stress reactions after the September 11, 2001, terrorist attacks. *N Engl J Med.* 2001;345(20):1507–1512.

16. Lau JT, Yang X, Tsui H, Kim JH. Monitoring community responses to the SARS epidemic in Hong Kong: from day 10 to day 62. *J Epidemiol Community Health.* 2003;57(11):864–870.

17. Leung GM, Lam TH, Ho LM, et al. The impact of community psychological responses on outbreak control for severe acute respiratory syndrome in Hong Kong. *J Epidemiol Community Health.* 2003;57(11):857–863.

18. Burkle FM. Triage of disaster-related neuropsychiatric casualties. *Emerg Med Clin North Am.* 1991;9(1):87–105.

19. Bleich A, Dycian A, Koslowsky M, Solomon Z, Wiener M. Psychiatric implications of missile attacks on a civilian population. Israeli lessons from the Persian Gulf War. *JAMA.* 1992;268(5):613–615.

20. Rotenberg Z, Noy S, Gabbay U. Israeli ED [emergency department] experience during the Gulf War. *Am J Emerg Med.* 1994;12(1):118–119.

21. Stouffer SA, Lumsdaine AA, Lumsdaine MH, et al. *The American Soldier: Combat and its Aftermath.* Princeton, NJ: Princeton University Press; 1949.

22. Anno GH, Baum SJ, Withers HR, Young RW. Symptomatology of acute radiation effects in humans after exposure to doses of 0.5–30 Gy. *Health Phys.* 1989;56(6):821–838.

23. DiGiovanni C. Domestic terrorism with chemical or biological agents: psychiatric aspects. *Am J Psychiatry.* 1999;156(10):1500–1505.

24. US Army Medical Research Institute of Chemical Defense. Chemical Casualty Care Division. *Medical Management of Chemical Casualties Handbook.* 3rd ed. Aberdeen Proving Ground, Md: USAMRICD; 2000.

25. Levin SG. *Estimating Battle Fatigue Casualties in Tactical Nuclear Combat.* Washington, DC: Defense Nuclear Agency; 1991. DNA-TR-90-114.

26. Vineberg R. *Human Factors in Tactical Nuclear Combat.* Alexandria, Va: George Washington University, Human Resources Research Office; 1965. HumRRO Technical Report 65–2.

27. Quarantelli EL. Images of withdrawal behavior in disasters: some basic misconceptions. *Soc Problems.* 1960;8:68–79.

28. Caldwell JM, Ranson SW, Sacks JG. Group panic and other mass disruptive reactions. *U S Armed Forces Med J.* 1951;2:541–567.

29. Smelser NJ. *Theory of Collective Behavior.* New York, NY: The Free Press; 1962.

30. Glass TA, Schoch-Spana M. Bioterrorism and the people: how to vaccinate a city against panic. *Clin Infect Dis.* 2002;34(2):217–223.

31. Quarantelli EL. The nature and conditions of panic. *Am J Sociology.* 1954;60:267–275.

32. Hammerman G. The psychological impact of chemical weapons on combat troops in World War I. In: Young RW, Drum BH, eds. *Proceedings of the Defense Nuclear Agency Symposium/Workshop on the Psychological Effects of Tactical Nuclear Warfare.* Washington, DC: Defense Nuclear Agency; 1987: 84–108.

33. Asukai N, Maekawa K. Psychological and physical health effects of the 1995 sarin attack in the Tokyo subway system. In: Havenaar JM, Cwikel JG, Bromet EJ, eds. *Toxic Turmoil: Psychological and Societal Consequences of Ecological Disasters.* New York, NY: Kluwer Academic/Plenum Publishers; 2002: 149–162.

34. Singer JE. Yes Virginia, there really is a mass psychogenic illness. In: Colligan MJ, Pennebaker JW, Murphy LR, eds. *Mass Psychogenic Illness.* Hillsdale, NJ: Lawrence Erlbaum Associates, Inc; 1982: 127–135.

35. Hulbert HS. Gas neurosis syndrome. *Am J Insanity.* 1920;77:213–216.

36. Salmon TW, Fenton N, eds. *Neuropsychiatry in the American Expeditionary Force.* In: *The Medical Department in the United States Army in the World War.* Vol 10. Washington, DC: Government Printing Office; 1929.

37. Struewing JP, Gray GC. An epidemic of respiratory complaints exacerbated by mass psychogenic illness in a military recruit population. *Am J Epidemiol.* 1990;132(6):1120–1129.

38. Petterson JS. Perception vs. reality of radiological impact: the Goiânia model. *Nuclear News.* 1988;31(14):84–90.

39. Ohbu S, Yamashina A, Takasu N, et al. Sarin poisoning on Tokyo subway. *South Med J.* 1997;90(6):587–593.

40. John TJ. Learning from plague in India. *Lancet.* 1994;344(8928):972.

41. Mavalankar DV. Plague in India. *Lancet.* 1994;344(8932):1298.

42. Madan TN. The plague in India, 1994. *Soc Sci Med.* 1995;40(9):1167–1168.

43. Kumar S. Plague in India. *Lancet.* 1994;344(8927):941–942.

44. Ramalingaswami V. Plague in India. *Nat Med.* 1995;1(12):1237–1239.

45. Ramalingaswami V. Psychosocial effects of the 1994 plague outbreak in Surat, India. *Mil Med.* 2001;166(suppl 12):29–30.

46. Centers for Disease Control and Prevention. Update: investigation of bioterrorism-related inhalational anthrax—Connecticut, 2001. *MMWR Morb Mortal Wkly Rep.* 2001;50(47):1049–1051.

47. Steinhauer J. Hysteria can be hazardous. *New York Times.* October 21, 2001. Available at: http://www.nytimes.com/2001/10/21/business/money-medicine-hysteria-can-be-hazardous.html. Accessed August 11, 2009.

48. Pomfret J. SARS inciting "mass panic" in Beijing. *Washington Post.* May 1, 2003:A11.

49. Eckholm E. Illness psychological impact in China exceeds its actual numbers. *New York Times.* April 24, 2003:A13.

50. McNeil DG. SARS fears shake Taiwan medical staffs. *New York Times.* May 21, 2003:A14.

51. Maunder R, Hunter J, Vincent L, et al. The immediate psychological and occupational impact of the 2003 SARS outbreak in a teaching hospital. *CMAJ.* 2003;168(10):1245–1251.

52. Avendano M, Derkach P, Swan S. Clinical course and management of SARS in health care workers in Toronto: a case series. *CMAJ.* 2003;168(13):1649–1660.

53. Nickell LA, Crighton EJ, Tracy CS, et al. Psychosocial effects of SARS on hospital staff: survey of a large tertiary care institution. *CMAJ.* 2004;170(5):793–798.

54. Kemeny JG, Babbitt B, Haggerty PE, et al. *The Need for Change, the Legacy of TMI: Report of the President's Commission on the Accident at Three Mile Island.* New York, NY: Pergamon Press; 1979.

55. Fabrikant JI. Health effects of the nuclear accident at Three Mile Island. *Health Phys.* 1981;40(2):151–161.

56. Organisation for Economic Co-operation and Development Nuclear Energy Agency. *Chernobyl: Assessment of Radiological and Health Impact. 2002 Update of Chernobyl: Ten Years On.* 3–155. Paris, France: OECD; 2002.

57. Gonzalez AJ. Chernobyl—ten years after. *IAEA Bull.* 1996;38:2–13.

58. Ginzburg HM. The psychological consequences of the Chernobyl accident—findings from the International Atomic Energy Agency Study. *Public Health Rep.* 1993;108(2):184–192.

59. International Atomic Energy Agency. *The Radiological Accident in Goiânia.* Vienna, Austria: International Atomic Energy Agency; 1988.

60. Lipsztein JL, Cunha PG, Oliveira CA. The Goiânia accident: behind the scenes. *Health Phys.* 1991;60(1):5–6.

61. Rosenthal JJ, de Almeida CE, Mendonca AH. The radiological accident in Goiânia: the initial remedial actions. *Health Phys.* 1991;60(1):7–15.

62. Hadden WA, Rutherford WH, Merrett JD. The injuries of terrorist bombing: a study of 1532 consecutive patients. *Br J Surg.* 1978;65(8):525–531.

63. Carley SD, Mackway-Jones K. The casualty profile from the Manchester bombing 1996: a proposal for the construction and dissemination of casualty profiles from major incidents. *J Accid Emerg Med.* 1997;4(2):76–80.

64. Brandao-Mello CE, Oliveira AR, de Carvalho AB. Psychological effects of the Goiânia radiation accident on the hospitalized victims. In: Ricks RC, Berger ME, O'Hara FM, eds. *Medical Basis for Radiation-Accident Preparedness III: The Psychological Perspective.* New York, NY: Elsevier, 1991: 121–129.

65. Janis IL. *Air War and Emotional Stress: Psychological Studies of Bombing and Civilian Defense.* New York, NY: McGraw-Hill; 1951.

66. Hersey J. *Hiroshima.* New York, NY: Knopf; 1946.

67. Showalter E. *Hystories: Hysterical Epidemics and Modern Culture.* New York, NY: Columbia University Press; 1997.

68. Gothe CJ, Molin C, Nilsson CG. The environmental somatization syndrome. *Psychosomatics.* 1995;36(1):1–11.

69. Rothman AL, Weintraub MI. The sick building syndrome and mass hysteria. *Neurol Clin.* 1995;13(2):405–412.

70. Weiss B. Neurobehavioral properties of chemical sensitivity syndromes. *Neurotoxicology.* 1998;19(2):259–268.

71. The Centers for Disease Control Vietnam Experience Study. Health status of Vietnam veterans. I. Psychosocial characteristics. *JAMA.* 1988;259(18):2701–2707.

72. The Centers for Disease Control Vietnam Experience Study. Health status of Vietnam veterans. II. Physical health. *JAMA.* 1988;259(18):2708–2714.

73. The Centers for Disease Control Vietnam Experience Study. Health status of Vietnam veterans. III. Reproductive outcomes and child health. *JAMA.* 1988;259(18):2715–2719.

74. Decoufle P, Holmgreen P, Boyle CA, Stroup NE. Self-reported health status of Vietnam veterans in relation to perceived exposure to herbicides and combat. *Am J Epidemiol.* 1992;135(3):312–323.

75. Johnson AA, Goetz JL, McRaney WK. *For the Record: A History of the Nuclear Test Personnel Review Program, 1978–1986.* Washington, DC: Defense Nuclear Agency; 1986. DNA 6041F.

76. Garcia B. Social-psychological dilemmas and coping of atomic veterans. *Am J Orthopsychiatry.* 1994;64(4):651–655.

77. Vyner HM. *Invisible Trauma. The Psychosocial Effects of Invisible Environmental Contaminants.* Lexington, Mass: Lexington Books; 1988.

78. White BW. *Desert Rock V: Reactions of Troop Participants and Forward Volunteer Officer Groups to Atomic Exercises.* Alexandria, Va: George Washington University, Human Resources Research Office; 1953.

79. Wachtel C. *Chemical Warfare.* Brooklyn, NY: Chemical Publishing Co, Inc; 1941.

80. Haldane JS. Lung-irritant gas poisoning and its sequelae. *J Roy Army Med Corps.* 1919;33:494–507.

81. Kawana N, Ishimatsu S, Kanda K. Psycho-physiological effects of the terrorist sarin attack on the Tokyo subway system. *Mil Med.* 2001;166(12 suppl):23–26.

82. Stolberg SG. For anthrax survivors, a halting, painful recovery. *New York Times.* May 7, 2002:F1.

83. Reissman DB, Whitney EA, Taylor TH Jr, et al. One-year health assessment of adult survivors of *Bacillus anthracis* infection. *JAMA.* 2004;291(16):1994–1998.

84. Parkinson DK, Bromet EJ. Correlates of mental health in nuclear and coal-fired power plant workers. *Scand J Work Environ Health.* 1983;9(4):341–345.

85. Baum A, Gatchel RJ, Schaeffer MA. Emotional, behavioral, and physiological effects of chronic stress at Three Mile Island. *J Consult Clin Psychol.* 1983;51(4):565–572.

86. Davidson LM, Fleming R, Baum A. Chronic stress, catecholamines, and sleep disturbance at Three Mile Island. *J Human Stress.* 1987;13(2):75–83.

87. McKinnon W, Weisse CS, Reynolds CP, Bowles CA, Baum A. Chronic stress, leukocyte subpopulations, and humoral response to latent viruses. *Health Psychol.* 1989;8(4):389–402.

88. Curado MP, Costa Neto SB, Helou S. Psychological aspects of the radiation accident in Goiânia: a general overview on victims and population. In: Ricks RC, Berger ME, O'Hara FM, eds. *Medical Basis for Radiation-Accident Preparedness III: The Psychological Perspective.* New York, NY: Elsevier; 1991: 143–154.

89. Collins DL, de Carvalho AB. Chronic stress from the Goiânia 137Cs radiation accident. *Behav Med.* 1993;18(4):149–157.

90. Novikov VS, Tsygan VN, Borisova ED, Rybina LA. Changes in cerebral bioelectric activity in the Chernobyl NPP accident liquidators. *Hum Physiol.* 1997;23(5):542–546.

91. Pastel RH. Radiophobia: long-term psychological consequences of Chernobyl. *Mil Med.* 2002;166(12 suppl):134–136.

92. Torubarov FS. Psychological consequences of the Chernobyl accident from the radiation neurology point of view. In: Ricks RC, Berger ME, O'Hara FM Jr, eds. *The Medical Basis for Radiation-Accident Preparedness III:. The Psychological Perspective.* New York, NY: Elsevier Science Publishing; 1991: 81–91.

93. Lifton R. *Death in Life: Survivors of Hiroshima.* New York, NY: Random House; 1967.

94. Nishikawa T, Tsuiki S. Psychiatric investigations of atomic bomb survivors. *Nagasaki Med J.* 1961;36:717–722.

95. Schnurr PP, Ford JD, Friedman MJ, Green BL, Dain BJ, Sengupta A. Predictors and outcomes of posttraumatic stress disorder in World War II veterans exposed to mustard gas. *J Consult Clin Psychol.* 2000;68(2):258–268.

96. American Psychiatric Association. *Diagnostic and Statistical Manual of Mental Disorders.* 4th ed. Washington, DC: APA; 1994.

97. Lettinga KD, Verbon A, Nieuwkerk PT, et al. Health-related quality of life and posttraumatic stress disorder among survivors of an outbreak of Legionnaires disease. *Clin Infect Dis.* 2002;35(1):11–17.

98. Schelling G, Stoll C, Haller M, et al. Health-related quality of life and posttraumatic stress disorder in survivors of the acute respiratory distress syndrome. *Crit Care Med.* 1998;26(4):651–659.

99. Weinert CR, Gross CR, Kangas JR, Bury CL, Marinelli WA. Health-related quality of life after acute lung injury. *Am J Respir Crit Care Med.* 1997;156(4 Pt 1):1120–1128.

100. Viel JF, Curbakova E, Dzerve B, Eglite M, Zvagule T, Vincent C. Risk factors for long-term mental and psychosomatic distress in Latvian Chernobyl liquidators. *Environ Health Perspect.* 1997;105(suppl 6):1539–1544.

101. World Health Organization. *International Statistical Classification of Diseases and Related Health Problems.* Vol 1. 9th rev. Geneva, Switzerland: WHO; 1977.

102. Cwikel J, Abdelgani A, Goldsmith JR, Quastel M, Yevelson II. Two-year follow-up study of stress-related disorders among immigrants to Israel from the Chernobyl area. *Environ Health Perspect.* 1997;105(6 suppl):1545–1550.

103. Tarabrina N, Lazebnaya E, Zelenova M, Lasko N. Chernobyl clean-up workers' perception of radiation threat. *Radiat Protection Dosimetry.* 1996;68:251–255.

104. Rahu M, Tekkel M, Veidebaum T, et al. The Estonian study of Chernobyl cleanup workers: II. Incidence of cancer and mortality. *Radiat Res.* 1997;147(5):653–657.

105. Bullman TA, Kang HK. Posttraumatic stress disorder and the risk of traumatic deaths among Vietnam veterans. In: Fullerton CS, Ursano RJ, eds. *Posttraumatic Stress Disorder: Acute and Long-Term Responses to Trauma and Disaster*. Washington, DC: American Psychiatric Press, Inc; 1997: 175–189.

106. North CS, Nixon SJ, Shariat S, et al. Psychiatric disorders among survivors of the Oklahoma City bombing. *JAMA.* 1999;282(8):755–762.

107. Curran PS, Bell P, Murray A, Loughrey G, Roddy R, Rocke LG. Psychological consequences of the Enniskillen bombing. *Br J Psychiatry.* 1990;156:479–482.

108. Abenhaim L, Dab W, Salmi LR. Study of civilian victims of terrorist attacks (France 1982–1987). *J Clin Epidemiol.* 1992;45(2):103–109.

Chapter 37

OPERATION IRAQI FREEDOM 05-07 MEDICAL CIVIL–MILITARY OPERATIONS: LESSONS LEARNED IN HUMANITARIAN ASSISTANCE

JEFFREY S. YARVIS, PhD*

*Lieutenant Colonel, Medical Service Corps, US Army; Chief, Behavioral Health, Department of Psychiatry, Borden Pavilion, Walter Reed Army Medical Center, 6900 Georgia Avenue NW, Washington, DC 20307; formerly, Director of Social Work, Uniformed Services University of the Health Sciences, Bethesda, Maryland

INTRODUCTION

The primary mandate of Task Force 30th Medical Brigade (TF 30) is force health protection. During Operation Iraqi Freedom (OIF) 05-07, TF 30 saved the lives of an unprecedented 96% of the wounded soldiers entering its facilities. Also historic was the way in which the task force commander employed behavioral health assets and their unique skills for the brigade's civil-military operations.

Medical brigades, with their organic clinical operations section and civil-military operations staff, represent a robust public health team capability unsurpassed by even the public health teams organic to a civil affairs brigade. Nearly half of the casualties seen in coalition hospitals were Iraqi; to transition these medical cases back to the Iraqis, Iraqi military and civilian medical capabilities must be enhanced.[1] TF 30 Medical Civil-Military Operations (CMO) joined together with the Department of State, Multi-National Force–Iraq (MNF–I), nongovernmental organizations (NGOs), private companies, and the Focused Stabilization Task Force of the Multi-National Corps–Iraq (MNC–I) to accomplish this goal. TF 30 also facilitated humanitarian assistance to vulnerable populations in Iraq.

In fiscal years 2005 and 2006, TF 30 assisted in securing more than $70 million to support humanitarian needs, including establishing emergency health services; enhancing water treatment and sewage plants, clinics, hospitals, and schools; and facilitating agricultural projects through effects-based planning with local and regional host-nation government officials. These efforts bolstered the legitimacy of the local medical officials, opened lines of communication between local individuals and local leaders with the Iraqi national government, created access to care, and promoted livelihoods. Due to the highly fluid nature of the internally displaced person (IDP) population in Iraq, TF 30 also supported ongoing preventive medicine operations for humanitarian assistance for IDPs. This chapter will discuss the medical civil-military lessons learned by TF 30 during OIF 05-07.

BACKGROUND

The US military routinely executes medical humanitarian missions. These missions encompass everything from medical support, to civic action, to capacity development or enhancement projects, to major theater wartime operations. The public affairs benefit of military medical forces providing support to another nation in conflict seems apparent. Assisting the injured, sick, and wounded, and providing access to care to displaced peoples seems beneficial. However, as Ritchie and Mott[2] point out, many pitfalls are associated with providing assistance. Past literature on the pitfalls of military humanitarian assistance was largely concerned with the ethical issues of providing care that cannot be sustained by the host nation, resulting in "doing more harm than good." This harm is often associated with the medical rules of engagement that are tied to the amount of resources the US military brings to support troops in a theater of operations. However, often overlooked are how the medical humanitarian assistance missions are tied to the strategic end state of an operation and how these missions may contribute to or detract from a mission.[3]

To frame military humanitarian assistance missions, it is necessary to go back to the purpose of all operations: to create a secure environment in which political and economic development can proceed. Therefore in Iraq, the end state of all missions, to include medical civil-military missions, is to create legitimate local and provincial Iraqi governments capable of continuing political and economic development. Furthermore, to stabilize the Iraqi government, the effect of the insurgency must be minimized. Insurgency is both a political and a military phenomenon. Insurgents will be frustrated if the government has a competent and capable administration that dispenses services and effectively coordinates a multitude of political, economic, and security policies. In Iraq, access to and delivery of medical care represents a tangible reminder that the government is functioning. These functions are also exploited by the insurgency. If the insurgency or those sponsoring it control service-oriented ministries, then the Iraqis will believe that it is the insurgency that is providing this care to them. In other words, healthcare is something that can be utilized by both the US military and the insurgency. The perceived Iraqi government response to the medical needs of its people is thus a key variable in achieving US political-military objectives.

President George W Bush recognized the importance of healthcare in achieving US political-military objectives when he said,

> America is now threatened less by conquering states than we are by failing ones....The United States should invest time and resources into building international relationships and institutions that can help

> manage local crises when they emerge....We will use our economic engagement with other countries to underscore the benefits of policies that generate higher productivity and sustained economic growth, including...investments in health and education that improve the well-being and skills of the labor force and population as a whole.[4]

Tommy G Thompson, the former US Secretary of Health and Human Services, noted that military missions must include medical strategies. He stated that the "[m]ost effective arsenal against terrorists [contains]: education, compassion, and medicine."[5] He also said that the "[b]est chance to defeat the terrorists [is] by enhancing our medical and humanitarian assistance."[5] History demonstrates the effectiveness of such strategies. During World War II, the US employed military humanitarian assistance in the Philippines. It has continued to do so in places such as Haiti and Bosnia because of a moral mandate in support and sustainment operations.[2]

The military operations other than war and peacetime engagement projects that represented the bulk of military humanitarian missions in the 1990s were inherently different than the missions occurring today in Iraq and Afghanistan. In Iraq, for example, the war began with kinetic fighting—attacking the enemy with weapons and destroying infrastructure along the way. As the United States approached the transition phase of operations during OIF 05-07, efforts were refocused on building projects. The various projects were undertaken to restore basic health services and address public health concerns to mitigate the health effects that were the result of the kinetic fight.

Now as the shift continues to the nonkinetic fight, the aim is to preserve existing structures, develop capacities, and target key structures critical to transitioning the health "battlespace." After three to four rotations in Iraq, medical civil-military operations were incorporated into all transition operations from the start and in all levels of planning—strategic, operational, and tactical. Waiting until the kinetic fight is over to plan and execute civil-military projects is not a workable concept.[6] Simultaneous integration of civil-military operations represents a shift in the operational effort following combat operations to a nonkinetic main effort. As the transition phase proceeded, the civil dimension became a part of the main effort. Following security gains, constructive engagement to repair damage and build on security success must begin in earnest. This is where longer-term success and true transition to civil control will become possible. The civil dimensions noted in Ritchie and Mott[2]—rule of law; facility / critical infrastructure assessment and repair; critical needs assessment (health, safety, and so forth); and local governance / leadership—all had to be focused. In addition, the TF 30 medical civil-military operations included nontraditional actors in the planning and execution process, such as NGOs and international organizations.

As mentioned earlier, medical civic action programs (MEDCAPs) and other medical military humanitarian assistance projects have apparent benefits such as "winning the hearts and minds." However, the contrary was true in Iraq; the apparent benefits of "tailgate" medicine were not realized because these missions were not tied to lines of operation and the strategic political-military objectives. Furthermore, the value to US medical personnel was not apparent. The need to transition patients back to an independent and capable host nation medical system was burdened by MEDCAPs. The medical civil-military end state defined by the XVIII Airborne Corps during OIF 04-06 was defined as: "To conduct coordinated cooperative medical engagements at the provincial level to strengthen governance and transition lines of operation in support of campaign plan and overall US objectives in Iraq."[7] No clear end state was identified in this mission statement. Past operational civil-military operations and plans did not effectively develop governance capacity in provinces. Furthermore, no standing organizations existed for coordination and support to medical civil-military operations at the national level. By OIF 05-07, it was clear that what was needed were fundamental changes in behavior, structure, and organization to address gaps in medical civil-military staffing and skill sets at the operational and strategic level. Inattention to these gaps led to inconsistent and "stovepiped" MEDCAPs that offered little long-term benefit and could not be quantified in terms of measures of effectiveness.

To implement the national strategy at the transition phase of operations in Iraq to achieve the political-military objectives set forth by the commander of the MNF–I, the following seven assumptions were made by the US medical civil-military operations team:

1. Increased governance capacity building and assistance is necessary to develop sustained capability of provincial governments.
2. Existing organic civil affairs public health teams will maintain current capability in provinces until their efforts are tied to the operational main effort, which when established will represent fully coordinated, joint

medical civil-military teams.

3. A need exists to develop a formalized mechanism for coordinating provincial activities and support at the Department of State and MNF–I.
4. Capability to provide enhanced health support to provincial governments must persist beyond elections.
5. The Iraqi national government will need to support increased medical outreach at the provincial and district levels.
6. Coalition resources necessary to support any new medical civil-military operations efforts will be available.
7. Medical civil-military efforts can be tailored to meet the needs and security situation existing in each province. Substantial capability of provincial governments will be developed in 2 years, allowing transition to more traditional US Agency for International Development (USAID), international organization, governmental organization, and NGO assistance delivery mechanisms to provincial and local governments for an additional 2 years.

Given these assumptions, the following mission statement for medical civil-military operations was developed:

- To assist Iraq's provincial director generals of health with developing a transparent and sustained capability to promote public health and provide provincial administration necessary to meet the basic health needs of the population.
- To provide timely and relevant assessments of health infrastructure and political developments in the Ministry of Health at the local level, and to promote Coalition governance and capacity development goals.

To implement the mission statement, the following eight tasks were identified:

1. Facilitate achievement of Coalition goals in Iraq by enhancing the capabilities of the Iraqi health sector from the district level within the Ministry of Health and the battalion level within the Ministry of Defense.
2. Promote health reform at the provincial level.
3. Assist local ministry representatives and Iraqi Army surgeons with developing a comprehensive strategy that results in a capable and accountable local government.
4. Assist provincial governments with identifying and prioritizing the needs of their citizens and with addressing those needs via the Iraqi government, Coalition, donor, and NGO resources.
5. Assess health capabilities of provincial governments and develop a joint plan of action to increase these capabilities, with emphasis on sustainability.
6. Assist provincial governments in developing short- and long-term goals for public health programs, and assist with their implementation.
7. Coordinate with other major subordinate commands to synchronize medical governance efforts with stability operations.
8. Coordinate with civil affairs assets to assess health sector developments at the local level, and to advocate Coalition goals and objectives.

These tasks were augmented with some of the peacetime concepts for civil-military operations noted in Ritchie and Mott[2]—train, coach, and mentor local government medical entities to develop their capacity to:

- develop core competencies and standards of care;
- establish effective linkages with ministries and central government;
- help Iraqi health officials plan and prioritize direction and activities;
- prepare critical needs lists, identify funding needs, and identify resources; and
- determine facility staffing requirements and assist medical officials to address these with their next higher minister or officer.

The G-5 (civil-military operations officer) of TF 30 also addressed systemic gaps through resource development activities for the MNC–I. Specifically, TF 30: (*a*) coordinated support by donors and NGOs; (*b*) communicated with stakeholders via effective public affairs and information operations activities; (*c*) provided and enhanced the delivery of provincial and municipal health services to include emergency medical services; (*d*) developed subordinate medical civil-military operations working groups; and (*e*) involved host-nation medical contacts in medical reconstruction activities to ensure the cultural relevance of all TF 30 projects. All of these efforts had to be observable in some meaningful way, therefore qualitative and quantitative measurements of success against established benchmarks were provided.

The involvement of Iraqi healthcare officials in TF 30's medical civil-military operations planning seems obvious, however, it had been routinely ignored by previous rotations. Upon implementation of the TF 30 medical civil-military engagement strategy, Iraqis were part of meetings at all levels of planning. This involvement was key to the paradigm shift from MEDCAP as the main thrust of medical humanitarian assistance to a more comprehensive process called "cooperative medical engagements." Cooperative medical engagements are specific humanitarian assistance opportunities led by Iraqi civilian or military medical personal for which US involvement is incidental to the overall engagement. Each cooperative medical engagement must focus on assisting the Iraqi medical system and the Iraqi Security Forces to provide for its civilian population. The projects must advance operational security goals; improve access (to regions and to the people); reinforce security and stability; and generate good will to enhance the US ability to shape the operating environment. Projects must be humanitarian in nature and must compliment the strategic goals and objectives of the Ministry of Health. Addressing the medical rules of engagement and misuse of MEDCAP, cooperative medical engagements do not allow for direct care to the Iraqi people unless it is a life, limb, or eyesight issue. The corps surgeon is the coordinating and approving authority for all cooperative medical engagements.

On August 18, 2005, then Secretary of Defense Winkenwerder stated that, "[t]he primary goal of the US Government in matters of world health is to build capability and capacity so that societies may address their healthcare needs." Cooperative medical engagements promote this concept. Initial reconstruction efforts had been designed to create entire healthcare systems for, and not with, the Iraqis. According to the Department of State,[7] $786 million from international and US sources was provided for health-sector development. However, few substantial gains were made in terms of transitioning healthcare back to the Iraqis or increasing access to care. TF 30's goals were more modest: building on existing platforms, identifying medical systems that could assist with the transition to the host nation through partnerships with the Iraqi Security Force and TF 30 facilities, or assisting medical systems key to stabilizing Iraq. Department of Defense Directive 3000.5 states, "Integrated civilian and military efforts are key to successful stability operations."[8] Executing this directive meant implementation at the local and regional levels, and allowing lower-level officials to communicate needs in a culturally acceptable way with the National Ministry of Health. Such open lines of communication and systemic cooperation across the country enhanced the legitimacy of all the health officials involved. Involving Iraqis through cooperative medical engagements addressed issues created by MEDCAPs. Ritchie and Mott[2] describe pitfalls of peacetime engagement projects. Some of the pitfalls that they identified—short-term focus, inadequate planning, disruption of local healthcare, and raising expectations for care—were all real problems that undermined long-term political-military objectives in Iraq. For instance, many medical civil affairs public health teams conducted "a MEDCAP a week," without any apparent reason. In addition to the problems discussed by Ritchie and Mott,[2] MEDCAPs also created parallel systems, vacuums of care when medical assets were moved around the battlefield, and resentment among Iraqi officials who often did not have an opportunity to vet these projects, determine if there was need for US interventions, or simply have the means to sustain US efforts once care was withdrawn. TF 30 and the corps surgeon's office were determined to achieve small, sustainable, and observable efforts.

Small sustainable humanitarian assistance projects created tangible results, increasing the legitimacy of Iraqi medical care and governance with potential for growth of Iraqi systems in a culturally relevant way. Using Natsios' "Nine Principles of Reconstruction and Development"[9] and considering the dimensions of nation building, TF 30 had highly successful cooperative humanitarian assistance operations, engaging Iraqis at the tactical, operational, and strategic levels (Exhibit 37-1).

These nine principles should guide medical planners in the targeting and execution of medical CMO and humanitarian assistance missions. Such planning is consistent with the effects-based planning conducted by military planners representing the full spectrum of battlefield operating systems and is not limited to medical planners. When employing these principles, the objectives of all CMO efforts should be to gain targeted effects that support the mission of the higher command, the commander's stated lines of operation, and the national strategy for the intervention for Iraq. It is also important, however, to understand that these concepts represent a departure from civil-military doctrine.[10]

EXHIBIT 37-1

NINE PRINCIPLES OF RECONSTRUCTION AND DEVELOPMENT

In 2005, Natsios[1] delineated nine principles that guide the US foreign assistance community, which includes the US military, in the provision of aid to a variety of war-torn countries:

> In a time of increasing collaboration between the two organizations [military and USAID], it is important that the military gain a better understanding of how USAID [US Agency for International Development] and development agencies generally approach their work, and how the two communities can beneficially build on this cooperation. . . .When a foreign assistance agency adheres to the Nine Principles, this greatly enhances the likelihood of success. Conversely, failure to take the Nine Principles into account when designing and managing a program increases the risk of program failure. . . . Just as a particularly skilled battlefield commander can violate one or two of the principles of war and still prevail, a development officer may violate one or two of the development principles and still succeed. But generally development agencies ignore these principles at great risk, particularly in countries like Iraq, Afghanistan, and Sudan, where major reconstruction efforts are under way.[1(p5)]

This table presents the nine principles for successful collaboration between the US military and other agencies, and the US military experience in Iraq with the utilization of the principles. The first two columns are from the Natsios article; the third column delineates how TF 30 interpreted and employed the "Nine Principles" in Iraq.

Principle	Description	Experience in Iraq
Principle 1: Ownership—*Build on the leadership, participation, and commitment of a country and its people.*	The first principle of development and perhaps the most important is ownership. It holds that a country must drive its own development needs and priorities.	Leadership, participation, commitment of host nation. Activities should enhance legitimacy of host nation.
Principle 2: Capacity Building—*Strengthen local institutions, transfer technical skills, and promote appropriate policies.*	Capacity building involves the transfer of technical knowledge and skills to individuals and institutions so that they acquire the long-term ability to establish effective policies and deliver competent public services.	Activities that enhance legitimacy of local professionals through accredited training models and certification programs. Activities that allow self-sustaining operational capability such as training in use of budgets and logistical systems. Activities that promote personal accountability and ownership of product and process.
Principle 3: Sustainability—*Design programs to ensure their impact endures.*	The core of the sustainability principle is that development agencies should design programs so that their impact endures beyond the end of the project.	Impact must endure, for example: TF 30 created the first self-sustaining Iraqi medical association in Iraq. Risk if ignored: alienation of local population.
Principle 4: Selectivity—*Allocate resources based on need, local commitment, and foreign policy interests.*	The selectivity principle directs US bilateral assistance organizations to invest scarce aid resources based on three notions: humanitarian need, the foreign policy interests of the United States, and the commitment of a country and its leadership to reform.	Needs assessment plus political-military objectives need not be expensive or time consuming.[2] Example: disease nonbattle injuries (DNBIs) at Iraq Security Force camps increased during the Ramadan holiday. Targeted Iraqi camps (nodes) were given handwashing campaign posters and water-testing strips for under $50/camp. In 2 months, DNBI from food- and water-borne sources went from approximately 300 Iraqi soldiers per month to zero. Lesson learned: did not have to create an entire preventive medicine program to address some immediate short- and potentially long-term problems.[3]

(**Exhibit 37-1** *continues*)

Exhibit 37-1 *continued*

Principle 5: Assessment—*Conduct careful research, adapt best practices, and design for local conditions.*	One of the most important tasks a development agency must undertake before designing and implementing a program is to conduct a comprehensive assessment of local conditions.	Research best practices, design for local conditions. Nongovernment orgnizations (NGOs) may already have this information. Example: International Medical Corps has been doing medical humanitarian assistance for nearly 30 years in Iraq.
Principle 6: Results—*Direct resources to achieve clearly defined, measurable, and strategically focused objectives.*	The principle of results is an outgrowth of the assessment principle. It means that before a donor agency even enters a particular country, it first determines its strategic objectives.	Results measured by standards, indicators, and effectiveness. Measures of standards; qualitative or quantitative. Example of qualitative standards: increased use of host-nation ambulances to clear battlefield and increased transportation of Iraqi casualties directly to host-nation facilities. Performance (process) indicators: decreased length of stay by Iraqi patients at targeted US facilities (nodes) by as much as 70% in one year's time. Impact indicators: increased host-nation care for burn patients through capacity enhancement projects with Iraqi hospitals. Measures of effectiveness: combination of key indicators, interdependent and multisectoral; more useful in longer missions; useful to determine transition criteria; need to partner with civilian agencies to do these right.
Principle 7: Partnership—*Collaborate closely with governments, communities, donors, nonprofit organizations, the private sector, international organizations, and universities.*	The partnership principle is a central element of USAID's business model and holds that donors should collaborate closely at all levels with partner entities, from local businesses and private voluntary organizations to government ministries.	Collaborate not only with the health attaché and host-nation minister of health, but also NGOs and international organizations.
Principle 8: Flexibility—*Adjust to changing conditions, take advantage of opportunities, and maximize efficiency.*	Development assistance is fraught with uncertainties and changing circumstances that require an agency to continuously assess current conditions and adjust its response appropriately.	Adjust to changing circumstances. Be aware of cultural, political environment.
Principle 9: Accountability—*Design accountability and transparency into systems and build effective checks and balances to guard against corruption.*	There are two important aspects to the accountability principle: donors should work to fight corruption in the countries where they operate, and donors must also ensure that the actual programs they implement are transparent and accountable.	Transparency (within security restrictions). Avoid corruption. Perception is everything.

(1) Natsios A. Nine principles of reconstruction and development. *Parameters*. 2005:5–20. (2) Bonventre G. Capacity-building in the health sector. Presentation to the Combatant Command Surgeons Conference. December 2005. Washington, DC. (3) Yarvis JS. Social workers as civil affairs officers: medical civil affairs in Iraq. In: Actionable strategies for caring for our warriors, veterans and our country. Presented at the 112th Annual Meeting of Association of Military Surgeons of the United States (AMSUS). San Antonio, Tex. November 2006.

PARTNERING WITH NONGOVERNMENTAL ORGANIZATIONS AND GOVERNMENTAL ORGANIZATIONS

TF 30 could not achieve optimal results without coordinating and synchronizing efforts with NGOs such as the International Medical Corps and Assisting Marsh Arabs and Refugees, and US governmental organizations such as USAID. These organizations are experienced in managing the second-order effects of combat and have substantive relationships in Iraq that often began well before OIF. Lacking a Commander's Emergency Response Program of its own, TF 30 relied on the resources of the MNC–I as well as the NGOs. In turn, the NGOs relied on the technical expertise, security capability, and networking ability of the military to effectively develop partnerships between the Iraqi military medical community, Iraqi civilian medical community, and the Coalition medical community to accomplish humanitarian assistance missions. For example, TF 30 facilitated the identification and movement of over $60 million in humanitarian assistance medical supplies for Iraqi hospitals and primary healthcare centers from Humanitarian Assistance-Kuwait and US donors (via the Denton Amendment[11]). TF 30 was the lead on medical issues for the MNC–I Humanitarian Assistance Working Group, working to match the needs of the Iraqi medical systems with available medical supplies and to focus the medical efforts being conducted by agencies working in the health sector. This coordination by the TF 30 CMO staff gave visibility to the "ground truth" from the tactical level of the health sector, thereby giving actionable intelligence to the health attaché for the US Department of State as it coordinated with the Iraqi National Ministry of Health.

The partnerships were not just focused on the delivery of tangible medical goods. Tangible goods, although extremely important in terms of demonstrating that Iraq can provide for its own people, are but one of many issues. Partnering with NGOs also involved sharing technical expertise and systems that enhance health promotion and delivery of services. Some of the enduring projects were the creation of three burn centers and a national trauma-training center, with an approximate cost of $2 million. These programs would allow Coalition hospitals to train and share expertise with their Iraqi counterparts while simultaneously developing the capacities of key Iraqi facilities. This will enable the Iraqis to gradually take over healthcare for critical neighborhoods and thus allow Coalition forces to transition out of caring for seriously ill and wounded Iraqi citizens and soldiers. An example of success in the area of Iraqi capacity was evidenced in their ability to "clear" or evacuate their own casualties from operational and civilian areas independent of Coalition evacuation assets. For example, during rotation 05-07, Iraqi medical facilities took over the health "battlespace," increasing the clearing rate from 41% to 81% and caring for casualties directly without the help of the Coalition medical assets, meaning the Iraqis were now clearing 81% of their casualties themselves. Another example of success was the decrease in the "length of stay" of Iraqi military and civilians in US medical facilities. Length of stay was defined as the number of days occupying a bed. In 7 months of capacity building, the length of stay in US beds decreased by an average of 6 days. This significant decrease occurred because Iraqi hospitals could now accept an increased number of patient transfers due to better Iraqi facilities, evacuation assets, and trained providers. Such capacity-building indicators were now being used by the MNC–I surgeon as measures of effect toward operational and strategic goals.

NGOs were well established in all 18 Iraqi provinces and therefore had relationships and credibility with the host nation. Because NGOs are neutral they can reach less approachable members of the health sector in the Iraqi Ministry of Health. NGOs must maintain the appearance of neutrality to be effective; military partnerships with them are less formal and not used as part of a military public affairs campaign. While humanitarian assistance activities make for good photo opportunities, the best public affairs stories come from programs that actually succeed. The worst example of health sector failures are structures that were built by the United States for Iraq, but sit empty or are used for other purposes by the enemy. Such failures can undermine US information operations. Typical focused humanitarian assistance partnership programs in the health sector are successful because the projects involve local contractors and workers, train local officials to staff programs and facilities, and are typically resourced at a degree that the community can maintain with its current level of financial, natural, and human resources. Furthermore, US medical CMO projects were linked to other civil-affairs projects to make them more comprehensive. TF 30's preventive and veterinary assets were heavily involved in sewer, water, electricity, and trash (SWET) projects. When SWET projects augment humanitarian efforts, the insurgency was diminished in those "Beladiyahs," or Iraqi districts. The key lesson learned from the NGO partners is that it takes much more than money and infrastructure development to be successful.

SUMMARY

TF 30 had highly successful civil-military operations and successfully transitioned its operations to the 3rd Medical Command for OIF 06-08. Recognizing the importance of CMO and humanitarian assistance in stability, security, transition, and reconstruction operations, the 3rd Medical Command deployed a more robust CMO capability to capitalize on the successes of TF 30. However, to date very few Army medics are trained in humanitarian assistance, and there is no proponent in the Army Medical Department for medical CMO or humanitarian assistance. The civil dimensions of war must be planned for. To facilitate medical planners' cognizance of the importance of CMO, doctrine and courses must be developed to meet needs of the operational commanders on today's battlefields.

REFERENCES

1. Swann S, Berry T. Task Force 30th medical brigade commander's overview: OIF 05-07. Presented at: The Medical Service Corps Conference; November 2006; Grassau, Germany.

2. Ritchie EC, Mott R. Military humanitarian assistance: the pitfalls of good intentions. In: Beam TE, Sparacino LR, eds. *Military Medical Ethics*. Vol 2. In: *Textbooks of Military Medicine*. Washington, DC: US Department of the Army, Office of The Surgeon General, Borden Institute; 2004: Chap 25.

3. Ritchie E, Mott R. Caring for civilians during peacekeeping missions: priorities and decisions. *Mil Med*. 2002;167(3 suppl):14.

4. Bush GW. *In the National Security Strategy of the United States of America*. September, 2002. Available at: http://georgewbush-whitehouse.archives.gov/nsc/nss/2002/index.html. Accessed July 28, 2010.

5. Thompson TG. The cure for tyranny. *The Boston Globe*. October 24, 2005. Available at: http://www.boston.com/news/globe/editorial_opinion/oped/articles/2005/10/24/the_cure_for_tyranny/. Accessed July 28, 2010.

6. Bonventre G. Capacity-building in the health sector. Presented at: The Combatant Command Surgeons Conference; December 2005; Washington, DC.

7. Bowersox J. Health sector update. Presented at: Task Force 30th Medical Brigade Commander's Conference; December 2005; Baghdad, Iraq.

8. Department of Defense. *Military Support for Stability, Security, Transition and Reconstruction (SSTR) Operations*. September 16, 2009. DoD Directive 3000.05. Available at: http://www.dtic.mil/whs/directives/corres/pdf/300005p.pdf. Accessed July 28, 2010.

9. Natsios A. Nine principles of reconstruction and development. *Parameters*. Autumn, 2005. Available at: http://www.carlisle.army.mil/usawc/parameters/Articles/05autumn/natsios.pdf. Accessed July 28, 2010.

10. Department of the Army. *Civil Affairs Operations*. Washington, DC: DA; 2000. Field Manual 41-10.

11. Information on the Denton Amendment is available at: http://www.usaid.gov/our_work/cross-cutting_programs/private_voluntary_cooperation/dentonguidelines.html. Accessed July 26, 2010.

Chapter 38

BEHAVIORAL HEALTH ISSUES IN HUMANITARIAN AND MILITARY RELIEF OPERATIONS: THE SPECIAL PROBLEM OF COMPLEX EMERGENCIES

THOMAS F. DITZLER, PhD*

*Director of Research, Department of Psychiatry, Tripler Army Medical Center, 1 Jarrett White Road, Honolulu, Hawaii 96859

INTRODUCTION

The provision of timely, effective, and culturally competent disaster behavioral health services is critical in all phases of a disaster response. Historically, disaster management and humanitarian assistance planners have divided events into three general categories: (1) natural, (2) technological, (3) and complex. Natural disasters include common geological and meteorological events such as floods, cyclonic storms, earthquakes, volcanic eruptions, and tsunamis. For those directly affected, these events can be catastrophic, but they do not constitute meaningful political threats for the public at large. The same may be said for most technological emergencies, such as the Bhopal, India, chemical accident of 1984, or for catastrophic infrastructure failure, such as the Chernobyl nuclear reactor meltdown in the Soviet Union in 1986. These disasters are often the result of human error, but they do not generally represent acts of political intention or willful malice. Local teams of trained personnel typically provide the response to these events, with regional or national assets deployed as required. However, in very large or regional natural disasters, such as the December 26, 2004, Indian Ocean tsunami, or in complex emergencies involving politically mediated security and logistical problems, such as the conflicts in Somalia or the former Yugoslavia, the operating environment may require an integrated multinational civil-military response.[1]

A number of recent events have provided opportunities to examine the capacities and limitations of civil-military collaboration in disaster response in general,[2] and in the provision of behavioral health support in particular.[3] Because of the organizational and logistical burden of large-scale and complex emergencies, civilian and military behavioral health providers must have a sound working knowledge of the shared operating space and the players who help shape the context of services. This chapter will consider (*a*) the humanitarian space and its players, (*b*) benefits and challenges to effective civil-military collaboration, (*c*) special behavioral health considerations in complex environments, and (*d*) principles with demonstrated utility in helping affected populations return to predisaster functioning.

OPERATIONAL BEHAVIORAL HEALTH IN CONTEXT: THE HUMANITARIAN SPACE AND ITS PLAYERS

Knowledge of the organizational and logistical aspects of integrated disaster response is critical to the efficacy of behavioral health services. The working environment is often referred to as the "humanitarian space"; it has been described in functional terms as an environment with the independence, flexibility, and freedom of action necessary to gain access and provide assistance to beneficiaries in a humanitarian emergency. For many civilian operators, including international and nongovernment organizations (NGOs), humanitarian space is achieved through acceptance of and adherence to the humanitarian principles of impartiality, neutrality, and independence as modeled by the International Committee of the Red Cross (ICRC).[4] Specifically, this means that aid is given regardless of race, creed, or nationality; aid is not used to further a particular political or religious position; and humanitarian and relief agencies do not act as tools of a state or policy.

Because military organizations responding to disasters are by definition not impartial, neutral, or independent, concern has arisen over the use of the term "humanitarian" in reference to military support in some contexts. The United Nations (UN) Inter-Agency Standing Committee provides useful guidance on this issue in a reference paper, *Civil-Military Relationship in Complex Emergencies*.[5] In part, the committee recommends that military efforts should be termed "relief" instead of "humanitarian." The difference in terminology is not just academic: the security and logistical support provided by the military can be critical to the success of the overall humanitarian effort; however, civilian humanitarians express concern that the perception of their affiliation with the military could negatively affect their security and ability to access vulnerable groups.

Well-orchestrated civil-military responses can offer great benefits, but such efforts take careful planning, a clear understanding of roles of civilian and military personnel, and effective communication between the two groups. This coordination is especially important in behavioral health services because of the profound effect of sociocultural issues in the acceptability of care. A central theme of disaster behavioral healthcare is the need for cultural competence in the delivery of services. Especially in large-scale disasters, it is critical for providers to know the context of services: what other agencies and activities are involved, how the range of services is coordinated, and what personnel and programs are available.

The first task for military personnel is to understand the types of organizations and personnel who share the environment—the "players." Personnel arriving on site should expect to find the humanitarian operating space shared by a range of "actors" (the acceptable generic reference in much of the literature in applied social and behavior science in political environments, such as terrorism, area studies, and complex disasters, especially when the mix includes a broad range of groups—in this case, active belligerents, military personnel, civilian agencies, and international organizations) presenting highly diverse organizational cultures and roles, as well as the affected population. In addition to various host nation assets, the key actors in a large-scale humanitarian response frequently include donor governments and agencies, UN operational agencies, NGOs, the International Red Cross and Red Crescent Movement, other international and regional organizations, and the media. Some of these organizations may provide acute behavioral health services, but the goal of many is the development of long-term, self-sustaining programs as an integrated part of capacity building and development. Successful behavioral health service is directly related to the physical, social, psychological, and spiritual support provided by these programs.

The International Community

Major donors in the international community include the European Community Humanitarian Office, Japanese International Cooperation Agency, Australian Council for International Aid, United Kingdom Department for International Development, US Agency for International Development, and Canadian International Development Agency. UN agencies, funds, and programs are also much in evidence. Although no agency has a primary behavioral health mandate, many UN activities make meaningful contributions to behavioral healthcare through pursuit of physical security, stability, sanitation, shelter, child development programs, and other essential support. Among these, the UN Development Program works in poverty reduction, development goals, democratic governance, crisis prevention, information and communication technology, human immunodeficiency virus/acquired immunodeficiency syndrome (HIV/AIDS) response, and landmine action in 166 countries. The UN High Commissioner for Refugees (UNHCR) has a mandate under international law to protect and assist refugees as specified in the 1951 Refugee Convention.[6] Focused on provision of food, shelter, and other basic necessities, this support is especially important in environments where the affected groups may include refugees, internally displaced persons, or migrants, a situation that can bring additional distress even in stable environments. UNHCR has approximately 5,000 staff in 120 countries with a current caseload of over 20 million people worldwide.

The World Food Program, the largest provider of food aid in the UN system, responds to both emergency needs and long-term economic and social development goals. In 2004, the program fed 113 million people in 80 countries. Operating in over 140 countries, the UN Children's Fund prioritizes girls' education, early childhood development, immunization, protection from violence and exploitation, HIV/AIDS services, health and nutrition programs for children and pregnant women, and children's rights. In recent years the program has also worked for the demobilization and reintegration of former child combatants through community-based efforts.[7]

The UN established the World Health Organization (WHO) in 1948; its constitutional objective is "the attainment by all peoples of the highest possible level of health." In disasters, WHO provides medical assessments and supplies and trains healthcare workers as part of building capacity. WHO is staffed by some 3,500 health experts, other experts, and support staff on fixed-term appointments, working at the Geneva, Switzerland, headquarters; in six regional offices; and in countries around the world. WHO actively pursues relations with NGOs to promote its policies, strategies, and activities.

A common feature of complex humanitarian emergencies (CHEs) is psychic trauma caused by the failure to maintain basic human rights. UNHCR, the secretariat for all UN human rights bodies, ensures that human rights are "mainstreamed" into all other UN activities. In addition to national capacity building, UNHCR maintains a field presence of human rights monitors and observers.

International organizations established by treaties also work closely with the UN and other actors. The International Organization for Migration, established in 1951 to assist with the movement of displaced persons in Europe, is the leading intergovernmental organization in the field of migration and now operates worldwide with 120 member states and offices in over 100 countries. This organization works closely with governmental, intergovernmental, and nongovernmental partners in managing the movement of migrants, resettling refugees to third countries or returning them to places of origin, and countering trafficking of people. The International Red Cross and Red Crescent Movement is the world's largest humanitarian network, with a presence and activities in almost every country. The Movement has three distinct entities: (1) the Geneva-based ICRC directs and coordinates international relief efforts in situations of conflict and promotes and strengthens humanitarian law (Geneva Conventions) and universal humanitarian principles; (2) the International Federation of Red Cross and Red Crescent Societies acts as the official representative of the member national societies and directs and coordinates the international assistance efforts of the individual member societies; and (3) the individual

National Red Cross and Red Crescent Societies provide a range of auxiliary disaster, development, and capacity-building services to the national authorities in their own countries. Although not officially a part of the UN, the Movement has observer status at UN headquarters in New York City.

Nongovernmental Organizations

The term "NGO" defines a very diverse group with respect to size, style of management, and type of operations. The World Bank defines NGOs as "private organizations that pursue activities to relieve suffering, promote the interests of the poor, protect the environment, provide basic social services, or undertake community development."[8] Tens of thousands of NGOs exist; many consult to governments and the UN, and some have a meaningful influence in world affairs. According to Hall-Jones,[9] the NGO sector now represents the eighth largest economy in the world. NGOs are generally funded by grants or private donations, although some receive large donations from governments. The groups may be national (indigenous) or international and are typically staffed by skilled professionals such as physicians, nurses, logisticians, engineers, and lawyers. NGOs are sometimes classified by their orientation (religious or secular); mission types (operational or advocacy); specific interests (medical care, child protection, food distribution); or operating area (community based, national, or international). Their size varies from small community-based groups to very large international organizations with equally large budgets.

Many NGOs have been working in particular locations for many years and have vast knowledge of the areas and access to the local population. InterAction is the largest alliance of US-based international development and humanitarian NGOs, with more than 160 member organizations.[10] The largest of these, in terms of financial assets, is currently the Bill and Melinda Gates Foundation, with an endowment of $28.8 billion.[9]

Military Support to Other Players

In recent years the military forces of many nations have deployed in response to humanitarian crises. These missions involve various forms of logistical and security support to protect civilian aid workers and ensure that relief reaches the populations in need. Types of military support can be conceptualized as belonging to five general service clusters, all of which have security as a central theme[11]:

1. Direct assistance: the face-to-face distribution of goods and services (these services often embrace a meaningful security component).
2. Indirect assistance: activities such as transporting relief goods or relief personnel (at least one step removed from the population).
3. Infrastructure support: general services such as road repair, airspace management, or power generation that facilitate relief but are not necessarily visible to or solely for the benefit of the affected population.
4. Peacetime missions: responses to large-scale natural disasters (eg, the Indian Ocean tsunami).
5. Training and exercises conducted in a region with no hostile intent.

The UN's *Guidelines on the Use of Military and Civil Defence Assets in Disaster Relief*,[1] originally released in 1994 and revised in December 2005, is the principal document specifying the obligations and limits of military support in humanitarian relief. Because the original document was developed at an international conference in Oslo, Norway, it is generally referred to as the "Oslo Guidelines." Under these guidelines, UN military and civil defense assets in humanitarian space are under UN control.

Other peace operations or support missions include a range of tasks undertaken by military forces that may not be under UN command, including peacekeeping, peace enforcement, peace building, and other operations with forces deployed under parameters that dictate a minimum necessary use of force. In some circumstances, the humanitarian mission may exist alongside traditional combat missions, including behavioral health services for detainees, as in Iraq and Afghanistan.

PRINCIPLES AND PRACTICE OF CIVIL-MILITARY COLLABORATION IN BEHAVIORAL HEALTH

The practice of civilian aid workers sharing the humanitarian space with the military is not new. Much of the recent interest in civil-military collaboration, however, may be traced to the success of Operation Provide Comfort in 1991, when NGOs and the military, working toward a common goal, achieved unprecedented success in providing humanitarian relief for the Kurds of northern Iraq.[12] Since that time, many senior military training institutions have developed curricula dedicated to civil-military issues. Civilian and military organizations differ greatly in their respective cultures, but each group possesses knowledge, skills, and assets that in collaboration create a synergy neither can achieve independently.

The coordination of these skills and assets, however, can be a critical challenge. Bessler and Seki[13] have provided a useful overview of common problems in the development of civil-military collaboration in the humanitarian space They point out, for example, that civilian humanitarians may express concern over the militarization of aid, especially in the area of military civil affairs projects designed to "win the hearts and minds" of the populace. These efforts are often a key part of the reconstruction process and have great pragmatic value; however, they can also create the perception that humanitarians might be used as de facto force multipliers or field operators of the local government. Humanitarians note that the perception of a military affiliation may compromise their principles of impartiality and neutrality, with a negative effect on the security of their staff or their ability to access affected populations. Given such problems, military and civilian workers must have a clear understanding of each other's needs to create a pragmatic and principled response.

Security Needs and Information Sharing

McHale[11] offers useful general guidance on security and informational requirements of civilian and military actors in the humanitarian space. Although specific needs of humanitarian actors vary widely, civilian humanitarians commonly seek military support for the following:

- security in the area to allow humanitarians to conduct operations, although usually not to the extent of one-on-one protection of their staff;
- reaction forces to assist personnel in danger, possibly requiring one-on-one security and evacuation of humanitarian staff;
- access to airfields, ports, and facilities if these are not readily open for humanitarian use;
- communication technology;
- logistical transport of materials and possibly personnel;
- emergency medical support and possible medical evacuation of personnel; and
- emergency infrastructure repairs.

McHale advises military operators in the humanitarian space to avoid classifying information unless necessary for security of operations or personnel. The military can often share with NGOs the following information:

- details on the security situation to inform humanitarian risk assessment, including areas of ongoing military action, banditry, or general instability;
- status of air and sea points of debarkation and lines of communication;
- checkpoint locations and pass-through procedures, which greatly reduces the chances of accidental injuries to humanitarian staff;
- location of unexploded ordnance, mines, and mine action activities;
- information on population movements, conditions, and activities;
- types of humanitarian (relief or support) projects planned by military; and
- poststrike information, including location of persons in need and unexploded ordnance.

Civilian humanitarian organizations are often hesitant to share information with the military, concerned over the perception of alignment with military intelligence. However, military personnel have suggested that security and efficacy is improved for both partners when NGOs offer the following information:

- location of humanitarian staff and operations, which lessens the chance of accidentally targeting areas with ongoing humanitarian operations or humanitarian staff;
- locations for possible evacuation of humanitarian staff if necessary; and
- a complete list of humanitarian projects, to avoid competition and duplication.

Practical Considerations

Because effective behavioral health services are an integral part of the overall disaster response, providers must be familiar with the coordination mechanisms and position themselves to be an ongoing and integrated part of the response. The most common administrative mechanism for coordination is the civil-military operations center (CMOC). The US Department of Defense defines a CMOC as

> an ad hoc organization, normally established by the geographic combatant commander or subordinate joint force commander, to assist in the coordination of activities of engaged military forces, and other United States Government agencies, nongovernmental organizations, private voluntary organizations, and regional and international organizations.

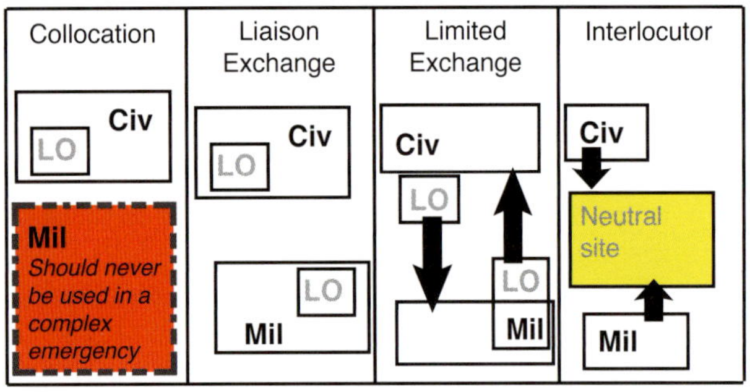

Figure 38-1. Civil-military coordination: four approaches to liaison arrangements. **Collocation:** humanitarian agencies and military units operate from within the same compound. The perception that civilian actors may be affiliated with the military can have negative security implications for the civilian humanitarian agency staff. For this reason, collocation is rarely used and should never be used in a complex emergency. **Liaison exchange:** liaison officers are assigned to and work in the offices of the other unit or agency. **Limited exchange:** liaison officers maintain an office in their own unit or agency but travel to the other actor's office to conduct business. **Interlocutor:** liaison officers maintain an office in their own unit or agency and travel to a neutral site to conduct business, such as a United Nations or local governmental office. This is often the most secure option for civilian humanitarian agency staff operating in an insecure environment.
Civ: civilian LO: liaison office Mil: military

> There is no established structure, and its size and composition are situation dependent.[14]

The Center for Excellence in Disaster Management and Humanitarian Assistance agrees that the physical structure of the CMOC and the liaison arrangement best suited for the mission are determined on a case-by-case basis, outlining four principal approaches to liaison placement (Figure 38-1).[11] Civil and military leaders benefit from a careful consideration of perceptions, accountability, the need for transparency, and how these issues may affect the security of civilian humanitarian staff and beneficiaries. The center also offers a number of operating principles obtained from successful CMOC endeavors (Exhibit 38-1).[11]

EXHIBIT 38-1

OPERATING PRINCIPLES LEARNED FROM SUCCESSFUL CIVIL-MILITARY OPERATIONS CENTERS

- Remember that coordination is personality and perception driven.
- Have respect for other actors and their operations; your personality and how you are perceived will dramatically affect whether coordination occurs.
- Have meetings chaired or co-chaired by civilian actors.
- Understand the roles, responsibilities, and constraints of the other humanitarian actors.
- Understand that nongovernmental organizations (NGOs) vary in their degree of comfort in working with the military; some NGOs will never be comfortable working with the military.
- When possible, work to establish areas of common responsibility.
- Establish open communications and sharing of information.
- Avoid classifying information unless necessary.
- Respond in a timely manner to requests for information or assistance.
- Understand that civilian actors may be hesitant to share information with you, especially in an open forum.
- Ensure that communications equipment (radio, mobile phones, e-mail) is compatible.
- Offer assistance when possible; understand that offers may be rejected.
- Know the market prices for local goods and services.
- Do not drive up prices by overbidding.
- Work with civilian actors to build consensus in operations.
- The collaborative process may benefit from a third party (eg, the US Office for the Coordination of Humanitarian Affairs) through which to share information.

Adapted from: McHale S. The International humanitarian community: overview and issues in civil-military coordination. Paper presented at: Combined Humanitarian Assistance Response Training; June 29, 2006; Marine Corps Bases Japan.

SPECIAL BEHAVIORAL HEALTH CONSIDERATIONS IN COMPLEX HUMANITARIAN ENVIRONMENTS

Equipped with an understanding of the players and a strategy for coordinating services, behavioral health providers can next consider important contextual issues that affect service delivery. Among the more important of these issues is how the psychic environment of CHEs differs from that of natural or technological emergencies. Although a CHE has several definitions, the UN Inter-Agency Standing Committee characterizes such a situation as

> a humanitarian crisis in a country, region or society where there is total or considerable breakdown of authority resulting from internal or external conflict and which requires an international response that goes beyond the mandate or capacity of any single agency and/or the ongoing United Nations country program.[15]

Many recent CHEs originated in the 1940s and 1950s, when the historical colonial powers began divesting themselves of overseas outposts. This trend accelerated at end of the Cold War, as the world experienced a dramatic rise in struggles for autonomy among newly liberated groups. These struggles often emerged along ethnic or religious lines, accompanied by a volatile mix of social, political, economic, and cultural variables that fueled internal conflicts. Humanitarian disasters that have emerged from these conflicts approximate civil wars and are labeled CHEs. CHEs are typically characterized by politically mediated excess mortality and morbidity; loss of civil police and judicial processes; massive displacement of people within the country (internally displaced persons) or across borders (refugees); destruction of critical infrastructure; and widespread damage to civil society and economies. The UN Office for Coordination of Humanitarian Affairs adds that

> [r]esponders typically face the need for a large-scale, multi-faceted humanitarian response in which delivery of assistance is hindered or prevented by political/military constraints, including significant security risks for humanitarian aid workers.[16]

Frequently, CHEs emerge from a weak or failed political infrastructure confronted by catastrophic economic distress or a natural disaster. The disaggregation of the former Yugoslavia and the Rwandan genocide of 1994 are illustrative of CHEs at the state level. The specific targeting of civilians to terrorize, displace, and create psychological distress is often a military goal. Garfield and Neugut note that World War I produced civilian casualty rates of approximately 14%; in World War II the rate had risen to 67%. By the 1990s the rate of casualties among noncombatants reached 90%.[17]

Factors Influencing Survivor Psychic Distress

Behavioral health providers should understand the ways in which the anarchic aspects of CHEs create psychic environments that differ greatly from those typically associated with natural or technological disasters. Any individual's subjective experience of psychic distress is a product of the complex interactions between the personal characteristics of the survivor and characteristics of the traumatizing event. Survivor characteristics may include a history of previous trauma, personality organization, physical health, availability of psychosocial support, and material resources.

The two principal characteristics of the traumatizing event itself are the gradient of exposure and the magnitude of personal loss and impact. The gradient of exposure defines how much trauma survivors were exposed to: how "close" it was and how many times they were exposed. The magnitude of personal loss and impact concerns the comprehensiveness of the event: Did the survivor hear about it, read about it, see it on electronic media, or witness it personally? Did it happen to someone they know? A loved one? Did they experience it personally? How many times? In general, the more directly and persistently an individual is affected, the higher the risk of meaningful behavioral health problems. In complex emergencies where losses result from intentional, human-mediated violence, the emotional proximity, comprehensiveness, and persistence of the trauma can be devastating to survivors and their greater communities.

Psychic Ground Effects

Measured by the gradient of effect and magnitude of personal loss, CHEs expose survivors to physical, emotional, and environmental sources of psychic trauma that are persistent and highly interrelated. Specific sources of distress may include persecution, oppression, marginalization, detention, incarceration, torture, witnessing atrocities, and separation from loved ones. In natural or technological disasters, emergency relief personnel and assets are limited largely by logistical constraints. In addition, the immediate cause of the threat is usually time-limited (eg, cyclonic storm, earthquake), so survivors can begin the response and recovery process in a fairly short time. CHEs, however, often involve an ongoing threat of armed aggression, including hostile resistance to both military humanitarian support and civilian aid workers.

Even following the official cessation of hostilities, threats in a CHE may extend into the "postconflict" environment for both survivors and responders. In the aftermath of a complex emergency, survivors may know not only victims, but also perpetrators. After the Rwandan genocide of 1994, aid workers frequently encountered Tutsi survivors who returned to their home areas only to encounter the very people who had killed members of their families.[18] Retributive violence can also persist long after the official "peace" has been declared.

In addition to ongoing physical and psychic threats to their safety and autonomy, survivors in CHEs often experience meaningful material deprivation, including loss of home, personal possessions, important records, economic and material resources, employment, social position, or authority. These problems are exacerbated by the loss of customary social, psychological, spiritual, and cultural institutions that could otherwise provide support.

Among the most distressing of behavioral health issues in CHEs is gender-based violence. Especially in CHEs involving ethnic conflict, sexual violence against women and girls is often a planned and systematic military weapon designed to humiliate, induce terror, and destabilize communities. Although reliable statistics are difficult to obtain, a large body of information obtained from NGO and international organization investigations documents the problem. Concerning the protracted conflict in Sudan, for example, the Watchlist Project notes that gender-related violence

> connected to conflict, including sexual slavery of women and children, rape by military forces, forced prostitution and forced marriage, is known to be a widespread problem in Sudan. No statistics are available. Children, especially girls from these areas, are victims of sexual exploitation, sexual slavery, forced marriage, rape and other forms of violence after abduction by . . . militias and opposition groups.[19]

Similarly, Roque reported,

> In Bosnia, for example, public rape of women and girls preceded the flight or expulsion of entire Muslim populations from their villages, and strategies of ethnic cleansing included forced impregnation In Rwanda, Hutu extremists encouraged mass rape and sexual mutilation of Tutsi women as an expression of contempt, which sometimes included intentional HIV transmission.[20]

In addition to the trauma of the violence itself, survivors of gender-based violence may also experience social rejection from their own group. In many traditional collectivist societies, family, tribe, or other group affiliation largely determines the sense of self and social role. Forcing women to bear the children of their enemies disrupts the social fabric of community organization. Gourevitch has described a Tutsi woman who had survived the Hutu massacre in Rwanda commenting on her relationship with the restored government:

> And they would say, "If they killed everyone and you survived, maybe you collaborated." To a woman who was raped 20 times a day, day after day, and now has a baby from that, they would say this.[18]

This circumstance might be thought of as an interethnic, multigenerational psychic insult A successful clinical response to such a problem would require an exceptionally well-resourced, culturally embedded, long-term commitment. UN-sponsored programs for the reintegration of former child combatants may provide a heuristic model for program development.

Environmental Threats

Environmental threats, both direct and indirect, negatively affect survivors' subjective sense of safety and security and are a major source of psychic distress. In addition to active armed conflict, direct threats may be represented by the loss of secure shelter or the presence of landmines and unexploded ordnance. Indirect threats often involve destroyed or degraded infrastructure, including utility and public health assets associated with transportation, power generation, water, sanitation, and basic health services. For many, living circumstances are austere and overcrowded. These problems often have the effect of forcing traumatized people to live in close proximity to others who are equally distressed, and with whom they may have to compete for scarce resources. The effects of this situation are especially deleterious for the most vulnerable people. Groups at high risk include children (especially unaccompanied minors), pregnant and lactating women, the elderly and infirm, the chronically and persistently mentally ill, displaced persons, and refugees.

During complex emergencies, the definition of "high-risk group" may evolve through the life span of the emergency. In general, anyone who is physically or psychologically vulnerable may be thought of as a high-risk individual, but because of the political nature of CHEs, high-risk groups may be determined by social, religious, educational, or political affiliation. For example, during many long-term CHEs such as the civil war in Mozambique (1975–1994), male adolescents became vulnerable to kidnapping and induction into irregular militias or paramilitary groups because of the depletion of older male soldiers lost in the fighting. Social and medical risks are often reflected in a high incidence of drug and alcohol abuse, domestic violence, and related pathology. These aspects of the psychic environment of CHEs have meaningful implications for behavioral health providers attending to the needs of both civilian survivors and military personnel operating in theater. Little doubt exists that the severity and persistence of human-mediated trauma in complex emergencies carries a much higher risk of long-term psychic distress than the trauma of natural or technological disasters.[21]

The most common behavioral health diagnoses among survivors of CHEs include anxiety disorders, especially acute or posttraumatic stress disorder, and mood disorders, especially depression. These conditions are often accompanied by a range of somatic complaints including body pains, sleep disturbances, and restlessness. Neglect of one's own health is common, as are substance use disorders. Apart from diagnosable disorders, however, the single greatest source of psychic distress is typically the problem of loss and grief. Loss and grief are axiomatic to human experience, but in CHEs the sheer magnitude of loss coupled with the absence of usual support structures can present a special clinical challenge for practitioners. The successful resolution of grief is an essential part of the recovery process; unresolved grief can be a rate-limiting factor in the successful return to predisaster functioning for both individuals and communities at large.

Although the response to acute grief is unique to each person, a number of descriptive models of bereavement and mourning have been advanced to describe common themes.[22–26] For a vast majority of survivors, the early grieving process includes preoccupation with persons or things lost and feelings of profound sadness, loneliness, fear, powerlessness, anger, anxiety, and despair. A central component of grief is the need to engage the mourning process to achieve appropriate levels of relief, resolution, reintegration, and return to functioning. In mourning, the reality of the pain is consciously identified and openly expressed with some degree of support seeking, psychological unburdening, and reestablishment of equilibrium. In unmourned loss, however, the reality of the pain is denied or suppressed, and the pain tends to remain fresh. The bereaved have a critical need for timely support to properly mourn their losses. Not grief itself, but grief that is unmourned, is associated with the development of more serious psychological problems; these may include pathological grief responses, depression, and posttraumatic stress disorder. These serious psychological problems are especially significant in complex emergencies, where the scale of destruction and social disorder creates cumulative risks at the same time that it precludes the ability of survivors to engage the normal mourning process in a timely way.

Despite the intensity of their experiences, some of the bereaved may initially fail to seek help because they are overwhelmed or immobilized by the shock and magnitude of their losses. Other survivors may actually decline help in an effort to preserve their sense of autonomy, competence, or dignity. Because social customs, religious practices, and traditional rituals exert great influence on the mourning process, behavioral health support should be integrated into other support and recovery activities provided by local providers and organizations. If possible, service providers should seek collaborative relationships with local traditional healers.

PRINCIPLES OF BEHAVIORAL HEALTHCARE IN HUMANITARIAN ENVIRONMENTS

Because of cultural and logistical problems, many traditional Western behavioral health interventions may be of limited use in disasters requiring a multinational response, especially complex emergencies. The most effective behavioral healthcare strategies pursue integration of sociocultural, medical, and psychological assets, ideally involving collaboration among relevant organizations. Practitioners are often less invested in direct clinical care for individuals and small groups and more focused on supportive and facilitative activities.

The WHO Department of Mental Health and Substance Dependence offers some general behavioral health service principles that have demonstrated utility across a range of disasters and cultures.[27] If circumstances permit, predisaster preparation should include a plan that identifies specific tasks, responsible personnel, and detailed communication and coordination strategies for key actors and agencies. If the key actors include international organizations, the leadership should be reminded that, to the degree possible, staff (including managers) should be hired from the local community. This practice increases the cultural competence of care and sets the stage for the development of long-term, self-sustaining programs.

Acute Phase

In the acute phase of a complex emergency, the crude mortality rate generally rises after loss of basic needs, including security, food, water and sanitation, and access to primary and public health services. Disaster behavioral health workers note that the reestablishment of these basic services is also essential in helping survivors recapture a sense of autonomy and efficacy in their environment. The process is enhanced by dissemination of information about relief efforts, including location of aid organizations and, when possible, information concerning the location of relatives. For survivors with behavioral disorders, whether disaster-induced or not, basic behavioral healthcare is best provided through general health services or through community-based primary healthcare resources within the health sector. In addition, providers should ensure the availability of essential medications for persons with acute psychiatric emergencies.

During complex emergencies, when the acute phase may be protracted, many survivors respond well to the principles of "psychological first aid."[28] Credentialed providers can also use psychological first aid materials to provide on-the-job training and supervision in core psychological care skills for existing healthcare providers, social service workers, and community leaders. This training expands the cadre of service providers available to the community while facilitating the integration of behavioral health into primary healthcare for the longer term. Also useful is the creation of community-based support and self-help groups to provide emotional support and enhance coping strategies, especially in grief management. Other helpful efforts, when possible, include encouraging the reestablishment of normal religious and cultural activities, specifically including orphans, those who have lost partners, and those without families.

One of the most practical behavioral health priorities is reopening schools. Schools normalize life for children and provide opportunities for them to interact with others in a familiar environment. Children in school are also much less likely to become involved in criminal or other high-risk behavior, and less likely to become victims of child exploitation, a tragically common occurrence following large-scale disasters. With children in a secure environment, other family members are freed to attend to pressing needs. Schools are also an accessible, low-visibility platform for disseminating behavioral health and social services information in an environment that is culturally confluent and preserves self-esteem. Uncomplicated, empathic information should focus on normal reactions, give practical advice, and provide specific information about availability and location of behavioral health and social service resources. These self-empowerment techniques provide immediate practical relief as they establish templates for self-sustaining, locally managed programs that can eventually serve the medium- and long-term needs of the community.

Reconsolidation Phase

In the reconsolidation phase, survivors often face a lengthy period of adjustment to the losses created by the disaster. Especially in response to very large-scale events, the enormity of the losses often predicts a rise in the most serious behavioral health problems, including posttraumatic stress disorder, depression, and suicidal thoughts. To meet the long-term needs of survivors, behavioral health services must be organized, sustained, and integrated into the local community.

The US Department of Veterans Affairs National Center for Posttraumatic Stress Disorder[29] recommends that following disasters, long-term tasks for behavioral health providers should include public education, screening, and where indicated, referral and treatment. Educational activities include programs on enhancing self-care and coping techniques, and providing information about social, financial, legal, and medical services. These activities help survivors normalize their reactions to trauma and develop healthy forms of coping. Screening seeks to identify those at increased risk for negative psychological outcomes. Survivors with a prior history of psychiatric illness, psychological trauma, or substance use disorders are particularly vulnerable, as are members of historically marginalized or disenfranchised groups. Survivors typically have a brief interview with a behavioral health provider and complete a risk-assessment questionnaire. Where appropriate, the screening process may rely on informal sources, including aid workers, friends, or family members. Based on screening assessments, survivors can be referred to counseling for specific problems, such as alcohol abuse or complicated bereavement, or to more medically or psychiatrically based interventions.

A principal behavioral health challenge of the reconsolidation phase is the establishment or reinvigoration of sustainable economic support programs to respond to the long-term consequences of the disaster's impact. Especially for survivors whose predisaster livelihoods depended on subsistence work, the ability to generate income is a critical link to emotional recovery. In disasters involving a multinational response, the success of these programs requires a high degree of collaboration among public and private programs from both the host nation and donor countries. Because of the sensitivities that invariably accompany humanitarian aid, the host government must be able to exercise maximum administrative influence over the community's return to predisaster functioning. Andrew Natsios, former director of the US Agency for International Development, describes the concepts of local ownership, capacity building, and sustainability as the "iron triad" of all successful reconstruction and development projects, an observation that generalizes well to behavioral healthcare.[30]

SUMMARY

Established principles and evolving research in the reconstruction and development fields inform the civilian and military humanitarian response communities, including behavioral health providers. In the humanitarian space, it is critical for behavioral health providers to know the key players, their respective roles, typical tasks, and relationships to each other. In part, this knowledge requires an understanding of the host culture, the challenges and opportunities of civil-military collaboration, and the best mechanisms to share resources and expertise among contributing groups. These knowledge sets permit practitioners to function as behavioral health force multipliers through their identification and support of community-based psychosocial and educational programs, the development of information networks, and collaboration with traditional healers and other local assets. The most effective practitioners also understand how the psychological ground effects in complex emergencies differ from those in natural and technological disasters, and how those differences affect the potential for psychological trauma and disability, especially in response to grief.

The greatest impetus and funding for behavioral health services typically occurs during the emergency phase of the response. However, evidence shows that the need for behavioral health services actually goes up over time, so that the most pressing needs often surface after the assets available in the acute period have diminished. The best strategy for responding to this problem is to ensure that local planners and other leadership are aware of the circumstance and that providers invest maximum effort in the establishment of culturally competent, indigenously managed programs. Behavioral health providers should initiate training and supervision of local personnel early in the response to ensure long-term behavioral health support.

Successful behavioral health service in the humanitarian space demands a high level of clinical expertise in an environment fraught with meaningful challenges. To meet these challenges, providers must develop skills in fields ranging from cultural anthropology to diplomacy, logistics, economics, and organizational behavior. The successful integration of these skills is rewarded with the development of timely, efficacious, and self-sustaining behavioral health services to help those in need.

REFERENCES

1. United Nations Office for the Coordination of Humanitarian Affairs. *Guidelines on Military and Civil Defence Assets in Disaster Relief—"Oslo Guidelines."* Rev 1. Geneva, Switzerland: UN; 2006.

2. March A. The Australian government's response to the Indian Ocean Tsunami. *Liaison*. 2006;3:50–54.

3. Perez JT, Coady J, De Jesus EL, McGuinness KM, Bondan S. Operation Unified Assistance: population-based programs of the US Public Health Service and international team. *Mil Med.* 2006;171:53–58.

4. International Committee of the Red Cross. *Proclamation of the Fundamental Principles of the Red Cross and Red Crescent*. ICRC Web site. Available at: http://www.icrc.org/web/eng/siteeng0.nsf/html/p0513. Accessed December 15, 2009.

5. United Nations Inter-Agency Standing Committee Working Group. *Civil-Military Relationship in Complex Emergencies*. Geneva, Switzerland: UN; 2004. Available at: http://ochaonline.un.org/mcdu/guidelines. Accessed December 15, 2009.

6. United Nations. Convention relating to the Status of Refugees; July 28, 1951. UN Office of the High Commissioner for Human Rights Web site. Available at: http://www2.ohchr.org/english/law/refugees.htm. December 15, 2009.

7. Ditzler T, Hubner M, Batzer W. Caring for former child combatants: evidence-based practices for reintegration. *Aust J Hum Security*. 2005;1:15–12

8. The World Bank. *Involving NGOs in Bank-Supported Activities*. Washington, DC: World Bank, USA; 1989. Operational Directive 14.70.

9. Hall-Jones P. The rise and rise of NGOs. Global Policy Forum Web site. May 2006. Available at: http://www.globalpolicy.org/component/content/article/176-general/31937.html. Accessed December 15, 2009.

10. InterAction: American Council on Voluntary International Action Web site. Available at: http://us.oneworld.net/member/interaction-american-council-voluntary-international-action. December 15, 2009.

11. McHale S. The International humanitarian community: overview and issues in civil-military coordination. Paper presented at: Combined Humanitarian Assistance Response Training; June 29, 2006. Marine Corps Bases Japan.

12. Successful aspects of the NGO-military interface. In: Davidson L, Daly-Hayes M, Landon J. *Humanitarian and Peace Operations: NGOs and the Military in the Interagency Process.* Washington, DC: National Defense University; 1996. Chapter 3. Available at: http://www.dodccrp.org/files/Davidson_Humanitarian.pdf. Accessed December 15, 2009.

13. Bessler M, Seki K. Civil-military relations in armed conflicts: a humanitarian perspective. *Liaison.* 2006;3:4–10.

14. US military glossary. About.com: US military Web site. Available at: http://usmilitary.about.com/od/theorderlyroom/l/blglossasry.htm. Accessed December 15, 2009.

15. United Nations Inter-Agency Standing Committee Web site. Available at: http://www.humanitarianinfo.org/iasc/content/default.asp. Accessed December 15, 2009.

16. US Office for the Coordination of Humanitarian Affairs. *OCHA Orientation Handbook of Complex Emergencies.* New York, NY: UN; 1999. Available at: http://www.reliefweb.int/library/documents/ocha__orientation__handbook_on__.htm. Accessed December 15, 2009.

17. Garfield RM, Neugut AI. The human consequences of war. In: Levy BS, Sidel VW. *War and Public Health.* New York, NY: Oxford University Press; 2000: 27–38.

18. Gourevitch P. *We Wish to Inform You That Tomorrow We Will Be Killed With Our Families.* New York, NY: Picador USA; 1998: 304–308.

19. Watchlist Project. *Watch List on Children and Armed Conflict.* New York, NY: Women's Commission for Refugee Women and Children; 2003. Available at: http://www.womenscommission.org/pdf/wl_sd.pdf. Accessed December 15, 2009.

20. Roque H. Addressing gender-based violence: if not now, when? *The United Nations Chronicle* [serial online]. 2002;39(3). Available at: http://www.un.org/Pubs/chronicle/2002/issue3/0302p77_gender_based_violence.html. Accessed December 15, 2009.

21. Ditzler TF. *Psychic Trauma in Complex Emergencies: Sources and Interventions. Health Emergencies in Large Populations 2005: A Training Course for the Management of Health Intervention in Armed Conflict* [CD-ROM]. Honolulu, Hawaii: DoD Center for Excellence in Disaster Management and Humanitarian Assistance and International Committee of the Red Cross; 2005.

22. Lindemann E. Symptomatology and management of acute grief. *Am J Psychiatry.* 1994;151(6 suppl):155–160.

23. Engel GL. Grief and grieving. *Am J Nurs.* 1964;64:93–98.

24. Kübler-Ross E. *On Death and Dying*. New York, NY: Macmillan; 1969.

25. Bowlby J. *Attachment and Loss.* Vols 1–3. New York, NY: Basic Books; 1979.

26. Westphal R. Dynamic grief model. Paper presented at: Shea-Arentzen Nursing Symposium; "Navigating New Frontiers of Nursing Practice: The Challenges of Health Care Reform," La Jolla, Calif. March 20–24, 1995; La Jolla, Calif.

27. World Health Organization, Department of Behavioral Health and Substance Dependence. *Behavioral Health in Emergencies: Mental and Social Aspects of Health of Populations Exposed to Extreme Stressors.* Geneva, Switzerland: WHO; 2003. Available at: www.who.int/whr/en. Accessed December 15,2009.

28. National Child Traumatic Stress Network, Department of Veterans Affairs National Center for Posttraumatic Stress Disorder. *Psychological First Aid: Field Operations Guide*. 2nd ed. Washington, DC: DVA; 2006. Available at: http://www.ncptsd.va.gov/. Accessed December 15, 2009.

29. Department of Veterans Affairs National Center for Posttraumatic Stress Disorder. Secondary behavioral health treatment following disasters. National Center for PTSD fact sheet. Available at: http://www.ncptsd.va.gov/. Accessed December 15, 2009.

30. Natsios AS. The nine principles of reconstruction and development. *Parameters*. 2005;Autumn:4–20.

Chapter 39

POPULATION-BASED PROGRAMS AND HEALTH DIPLOMACY APPROACHES OF THE US PUBLIC HEALTH SERVICE

JON T. PEREZ, PhD*; JEFFREY COADY, PsyD†; KEVIN McGUINNESS, PhD‡; and MERRITT SCHREIBER, PhD§

*Captain, Scientist Corps, US Public Health Service; Team Leader, US Public Health Service Disaster Mental Health Team II, Department of Health and Human Services, 801 Thompson Avenue, Suite 300, Rockville, Maryland 20852

†Commander, Scientist Corps, US Public Health Service; Deputy Team Leader, US Public Health Service Disaster Mental Health Team II, Department of Health and Human Services, 233 North Michigan Avenue, Suite 600, Chicago, Illinois 60601

‡Captain, Scientist Corps, US Public Health Service; Director and Medical Psychologist, HRSA/BCRS National Health Service Corps, Ready Responder Program, Department of Health and Human Services, c/o La Clinica de Familia, 510 East Lisa Drive, Chaparral, New Mexico 88081; formerly, Senior Clinical Scientist, Health and Human Services, US Department of Justice, Bureau of Prisons, Federal Correctional Institution La Tuna, New Mexico

§Captain, Scientist Corps, US Public Health Service (Inactive Reserve Corps); Senior Program Manager, Center for Public Health and Disasters, University of California at Los Angeles Center for the Health Sciences, 1145 Gayley Avenue, Suite 304, Los Angeles, California 90024; Operations Lead, USPHS Mental Health Team II

Go to the people
Live with them
Learn from them
Care about them

Start with what they know
Build with what they have
But with the best leaders
When the work is done
The task accomplished
The people will say
"We have done this ourselves"

—Lao Tzu (700 BC)[1]

INTRODUCTION

The Commissioned Corps (Corps) of the US Public Health Service (USPHS) is an all-officer corps of approximately 6,000 members.[2] The Corps is capable of providing highly trained and mobile healthcare professionals to carry out programs that promote the health of the nation and, when needed, furnish health services and expertise in times of war or other national or international emergencies.

As demonstrated in its healthcare relief response to the Indian Ocean tsunami of December 26, 2004, the Corps provided distinct leadership approaches and methodologies that proved useful to that extraordinary international effort. Several of the key leadership precepts and approaches are now known as the "*Mercy* model" and constitute an important guide for USPHS health diplomacy efforts worldwide.[3]

THE INDIAN OCEAN TSUNAMI AND RELIEF EFFORTS

The Indian Ocean tsunami, also known as the "Sumatra tsunami," was the result of a massive earthquake, with a magnitude of at least 9.0 on the Richter scale, that occurred when the India tectonic plate subducted beneath the Burma plate.[4] Waves reached a height of 35.5 feet, and killed an estimated 230,000 people, 168,000 in Indonesia alone. (When earthquakes occur in landmasses above sea level, their initial effects are felt immediately and precautions can be taken in anticipation of follow-on tremors and structural collapse. Attachment 1 to this chapter provides a description of land-based earthquake disaster relief.)

Operation Unified Assistance (OUA) was an unprecedented undertaking to support victims of a massive natural disaster. The USNS *Mercy* sailed from San Diego on January 5, 2005, less than 3 days after being ordered to assist, and arrived in Banda Aceh, Indonesia, on February 6, 2005. From that point through to its departure on April 29, 2005, the ship and crew treated over 17,500 patients in the region. It brought together an untested capability (the USNS *Mercy* as a humanitarian service platform) and an untested mix of uniformed and civilian personnel to accomplish an overarching humanitarian mission that was not clearly defined until well into its eventual execution.

The OUA teams were sent into an area of extraordinary human devastation where there was active military conflict, devastated healthcare infrastructure, and an uncoordinated mix of governmental and nongovernmental organization (NGO) programs with widely divergent approaches and capabilities. Logistics of ship-to-shore lift, security, unknown length of time on station, limited understanding of and commitment to population-based programs by key leadership personnel, and initial relief agency reticence to accept US help, limited preliminary activities and very nearly stopped them completely. Ashore, the *Mercy* team was met with suspicion by many who questioned the sincerity of the overall US commitment to tsunami relief and, in particular, the team's commitment. It was in this environment that the eventual collaborations, programs, and successes were achieved, and it was the *Mercy* leadership approach that helped build them.

Although not especially unique or groundbreaking in many of its individual specifics, the overall intervention approach developed and implemented by the USPHS behavioral healthcare team was seen as a marked advance for behavioral health programming in multinational relief efforts. The people and agencies of Aceh Province embraced this approach, as well as the larger international relief community supporting them. It significantly altered the view of the United States' ability to work in an integrated, international behavioral health relief effort.

At its most basic level, the *Mercy* model represents a public health leadership approach, not a program or a product. That approach is composed of specific knowledge, attitude, and collaboration precepts that guide efforts to create teams and programs. Relief personnel face operational environments that vary in nature, severity, and complexity. The basic *Mercy* approaches have proven themselves to help relief leadership maximize what resources are available, and mobilize systems far larger than the coordinating team itself to create large-scale, population-based recovery programs.

The precepts are highly adaptable to international and domestic systems. In its tsunami relief form, the *Mercy* model was composed of 21 general precepts that fostered collaborative interaction among diverse organizations and stakeholders (detailed in Attachment 2 to this chapter). Most recently, virtually the same precept set was used with substantial success in the Hurricanes Katrina/Rita (in 2005) response where it was shared with the Louisiana Department of Education and ultimately directly contributed to the successful development of a psychosocial recovery program for over 200,000 displaced schoolchildren.[5]

The *Mercy* model precepts have been applied most effectively to facilitate delivery of population-based behavioral health interventions. However, they have also been adapted for use across an array of disciplines from biomedical engineering to primary care medicine. Given the scope of hazards that the United States faces in the world as a nation, in which very large numbers of the population may develop enduring mental health consequences as a result of disaster exposure,[6] *Mercy* model percepts are particularly needed.

THE *MERCY* MODEL: "LEADERSHIP OF THE OPEN HAND"

The *Mercy* model is designed to effect large-scale, coordinated change in damaged or fragmented systems following major disasters by providing collaborative leadership to help the system regain operational status. The model is called "Leadership of the Open Hand," in deference to the Lao Tzu quotation that opened this chapter. It details the means and methods to work in a response environment where US agencies are neither completely in control nor have the resources to effect unilateral action or mission accomplishment. Instead, the strategy in such cases is to increase response impact through effectively harnessing collaborations with other agencies, forces, NGOs, international organizations, and even nations.

This is accomplished by

- addressing, first and foremost, public health and system-level interventions;
- providing essential health system leadership support for damaged systems during highly chaotic and difficult times;
- seeking and promoting collaborative approaches, not unilateral action;
- assessing system needs rapidly and determining the best placement of limited resources to maximize system effects;
- partnering with the most promising and resourceful agencies;
- providing partner agencies with capacity-building tools;
- working with partner agencies from program conception through implementation; and
- accomplishing it all in time frames measured in days, not weeks or months.

In Indonesia, the model was utilized to help coordinate relief agencies and the Indonesian government's disaster relief effort to provide specific infrastructure and program support for children's services. Through this effort an array of population-based services was created in the posttsunami relief environment that was eventually delivered to all 200,000 school-aged children in Aceh Province. Equally important, the approach taught local agencies methods to independently develop and deliver their own programs without any outside support.

In the post-Katrina recovery efforts, the *Mercy* model was used to help the Louisiana Department of Education regain its operational footing and create a statewide system of behavioral health interventions for students affected by the hurricane. In Indonesia, the process, from initial conception to implementation, was completed in just 9 days. In Louisiana, it took 12 days. There were seven officers directly assigned to population-based operations in Indonesia; there were four officers assigned to the Louisiana Department of Education. This chapter will focus more specifically on the Indonesian mission, but the reader should understand it represents many missions with similar leadership challenges.

Far from a closed fist, "my-way-or-the-highway" leadership approach, the *Mercy* approach is open-handed leadership, designed to help pull people and systems back up and forward following major catastrophic disruption. It utilizes the leadership approaches described in the WICS ("wisdom, intelligence, and creativity, synthesized") model by Robert Sternberg,[7] to achieve this collaborative partnership for the common good. Future relief situations will have many of the associated leadership challenges present in the OUA response, as well as others not even imagined here. Thus, understanding the transitions from chaos to clarity, and suspicion to collaboration are critical to understanding the ultimate mission successes. In particular, decisions were made and approaches were adopted at several key junctures that, if carried out differently, would have resulted in mission failure. For future planning, it is important to fully appreciate how fragile the situations were and how easily the missions could have failed. It is the team's belief that the leadership approach embodied in the open-handed *Mercy* model precepts contributed to these significant transitions and was critical to the ultimate successes of the international team missions.

Another important aspect of the leadership approach involved the OUA team aboard the USNS *Mercy* and around the world working to support novel programming outside of their traditional operating spectrum. International relief organizations, many of which had never worked with or were suspicious of US uniformed services support, were also of critical importance because these organizations provided many of the resources that were crucial to successful program implementation. Also, research and program institutes from around the world provided significant amounts of information, often in real-time, via email and other digital technologies in support of the team's training efforts, despite the significant time zone differences.[8]

In a related Department of Health and Human Services effort, a team at the Centers for Disease Control and Prevention Emergency Operations Center facilitated the use of the novel, rapid mental health triage platform—PsySTART (psychological simple triage and rapid treatment)—that enabled use of a population-based rapid triage platform in an affected area. This work began empirical validation of this non–symptom-based approach to rapidly determine levels of risk in mass casualty events. When the results of the PsySTART triage "tags" are aggregated to form population estimates, they can be used as a common metric for *Mercy* model population approaches using evidence-based risk indicators.[9,10] The *Mercy* model and the PsySTART rapid mental health triage system are now key competencies of a training initiative for new federal disaster response assets—the USPHS Disaster Response Teams—created after Hurricane Katrina.

The *Mercy* model approach did not begin with all of these pieces in place. How the people and processes were assessed, understood, and guided forward is the real leadership success story of the *Mercy* effort by the USPHS team; this effort continues to evolve.

THE USPHS *MERCY* MISSION: "GO WEST AND DO GOOD THINGS"

The overall mission order was to "go west and do good things." It meant that actual operations would be developed and based, in no small measure, upon what was encountered when the USNS *Mercy* arrived on station. Mission definition depended to a large degree upon the resources already in place in the region, the priority needs of the local Indonesian people, and resources that the USNS *Mercy* and her crew could bring to bear in the relief effort. Mission clarity was only that which could be conjured or inferred, not what was provided, nor even what could be seen or verified until arrival in the area of operations.

The USPHS team took the mission order as a mandate to develop its own mission contingencies and integrate them with the larger Navy mission as it developed, sometimes minute by minute. To meet its own developing mission demands, the USPHS team prepared several operational capabilities. Contingency planning included direct clinical services for the ship's personnel and those patients who would be received on station; environmental health missions; biomedical engineering missions; and population-based behavioral health missions. The first three mission capabilities were immediately discernible and clearly understood. The last was not. Among the USPHS team there developed a desire to take services "beyond the boat," meaning going to shore-based operations and moving beyond direct-service provision to include large-scale, population-based public health missions.[11]

While the USPHS team brought direct clinical service capability, it also brought unique expertise to help local agencies create service programs in relief environments, methods to work collaboratively with a wide range of relief operations, and the ability to integrate seamlessly with operating relief systems and structures already in place. However, these capabilities were seen as novel by much of the leadership, and even useless by some of them. Indispensable support for these capabilities came from Rear Admiral William C Vanderwagen, commander of the USPHS team and the Secretary of Health and Human Services representative on station, and Captain DM Llewellyn, the medical treatment facility (MTF) commander. Early on, they communicated their support for the population-based approaches[12] recommended by the USPHS behavioral health team. Trusting the team's expertise and advice, they enabled the mission to go forward despite the fact that such methods were outside the normal operating spectrum of the MTF and untested in previous deployments. Rear Admiral Vanderwagen, in particular, saw the approach as critical to any large-scale response, directed the team to develop it, and advocated for it across the leadership lanes from Washington, DC, to the MTF itself.

Initial Assessments and Collaboration

USPHS personnel were on the first helicopter in to Banda Aceh from USNS *Mercy* and began assessment and collaboration efforts at that time. The operational assessment and initial collaboration efforts for population-based services lasted 5 days. During that time, individual meetings were scheduled with over a dozen NGO and governmental agencies engaged in psychosocial recovery activities, local schools were visited to determine the needs as expressed directly by local school teachers and head masters, and USPHS team members participated in various meetings with representatives of over 50 NGOs and agencies that provided behavioral health services in the province.

Very quickly the assessment indicated:

1. The needs were beyond anything any of the team members had ever seen before.
2. There were over 200 agencies/forces/NGOs operating in the theater with widely varying capabilities, only limited coordination, and very divergent approaches to relief efforts.
3. The USPHS team would be in this immediate area of operation for an unknown, but presumably very short, length of time, possibly only days.
4. Of 17 USPHS officers initially available for shore-based operations, only seven officers were available for population-based behavioral health services; the remaining personnel were needed for other healthcare missions and to provide direct services on the ship.

The behavioral health personnel, unlike other capabilities shipboard, faced an ambiguous situation and three key initial decision points, only the first two of which were under their direct control:

1. What can reasonably be done in days, not weeks, given the enormity of need?
2. What should be offered and to whom?
3. Will anyone want what the behavioral health personnel have to offer?

The behavioral health climate was sensitive, particularly for the USPHS team members from the *Mercy*. The prevailing feeling among the NGOs in Banda Aceh was that the USNS *Mercy* was late to the response, would be there only long enough to take part in a public relations event, and would probably look to "take over" as opposed to "work with" programs already in place. It was also expected that western psychological/psychiatric interventions would be used with little regard for deeply held spiritual and traditional belief systems that may not be congruent with them. This was not an open or initially welcoming operational environment, but one that viewed *Mercy* personnel and their offers with cool distance.

It was also a situation that began to change with a critical exchange that has since become known by international colleagues of the US team as "the diplomatic pants incident." In this particular incident, the open-hand leadership approach was demonstrated, with particular attention paid to mission success, not personal success.

The United Nations Children's Fund (UNICEF) and the Australian Agency for International Development (AusAID) were the organizations with which the *Mercy* personnel saw the most potential for collaboration and at-scale impact for programs. Highly professional, experienced, and respected throughout the relief area, they had resources, infrastructure, and personnel, and were there for the long haul. Three meetings were held with various personnel from those agencies over the course of the first few days after arrival. The first two meetings appeared to be very encouraging, with many ideas shared and possibilities for collaborations discussed. At the third meeting, however, there was a distinctly disquieting change, particularly with respect to UNICEF response to the USPHS personnel.

The USPHS team was confronted with an impromptu, but mission-critical, decision point. It proved to be a moment of leadership awareness that substantially changed the overall behavioral health mission outcome. In retrospect, the US team's recognition of the potentially course-changing implications of subtle changes in vocal tone, physical posture, and interpersonal distance proved to be as important to mission success as the actual words exchanged between team members and their international partners. The following case study demonstrates the importance of follow-up conversations in these circumstances.

Case Study 39-1: After the formal meeting completed,

when just a couple of the *Mercy* USPHS team members were together, the obvious question that hung in the air was asked:

Did the USPHS team do something to offend?

The UNICEF colleagues politely replied, "Why are you wearing uniforms today?"

It was explained that the team members were uniformed officers of the United States Public Health Service. The behavioral health team leader went on to explain that although the team had worn civilian attire to previous meetings, they were wearing uniforms on this particular day because the team leader's only pair of civilian pants had been permanently stained with helicopter hydraulic fluid the day before and, not wanting to be disrespectful, he opted to wear a clean uniform instead of the soiled civilian pants. The rest of the team had followed suit. The answer to the question that followed was a bit more complicated, however.

"Are you military?"

It was explained that, although the team was assigned to the US Navy for this humanitarian mission, as USPHS officers, they were part of the US Department of Health and Human Services and generally prefer to fight disease, not people.

The UNICEF partners responded with smiles of relief.

"We would much prefer the dirty pants," they commented, "as it is against our [UNICEF] charter to work with military forces unless it is absolutely necessary."

"Then dirty pants it shall be."

After this exchange, the tension evaporated. Assurances were made, collaborations sealed, and operations began in earnest. Understanding that they had become a symbol of the collaboration, the USPHS team leader wore the "diplomatic" (ie, dirty) pants ashore for the remainder of the mission.

Good-natured humor and self-effacement were embodied in such behaviors and approaches, and, although seemingly secondary to specific program delivery, it was exactly these processes that created the interpersonal environment that allowed the programs to be delivered at all. For the US personnel to be seen by the international relief community, and the Achenese in particular with the fears they associated with US involvement, as approachable and capable of personal humility and self-effacement was critical to their accepting US content and programmatic support. The importance of these approaches and processes cannot be overstated. The United States was seen with human faces and supportive, helping hands through these approaches, which spanned the breadth of services provided by the entire MTF. Those friends with expertise, in the case of the population-based programs, were readily welcomed when expertise absent such personal connection was not.

Program Development and Delivery

The next critical leadership decision was to *integrate* the USPHS behavioral health team of seven into the initial UNICEF and AusAID planning team of five, to create a single management team. That team, in turn, chose to develop programs and train a cadre of individuals to deliver psychosocial interventions for school-aged children in every school in the province.

The collective plan called for the USPHS team, within 1 week's time to:

- develop a training curriculum;
- train the UNICEF/AusAID staff in its delivery;
- prepare and distribute associated documentation; and
- administer to 45 governmental and NGO staff the final training program of 40 contact hours covering 43 content areas.

The Indonesian colleagues were unsure whether the USPHS team was capable of developing and delivering such a program within such a short time frame, especially with Indonesian interpreters. The team provided assurances that it could do so. The program would create a network of trainers to carry on long after the *Mercy* mission was completed, and it could be delivered in a short period of time, although some thought privately that it was an impossibly short period of time.

The first critical step in the development of the program involved collecting, evaluating, and preparing the necessary materials. Using e-mail, the Internet, and a large international virtual team from academic and NGO organizations, the US team relied almost completely on the information provided to it electronically from these sources around the world. That information was received within 24 hours of the first request and amounted to over 500 pages of training and intervention documentation.

The next critical decision point came during a planning meeting when the USPHS/UNICEF/AusAID/Aceh team was evaluating training information. Originally, the mission concept called for USPHS personnel to provide the training with Indonesian translation. The Indonesian members of the planning team, however, included professors of psychology and other human-service subject-matter experts. Most of these personnel had advanced degrees, were residents in the province, and were highly capable trainers and facilitators. The conversation during the meeting suggested that the quantity of training information might need to be cut by half to provide adequate time for translation during the presentations. The specter of such a loss of information yielded a substantial change in approach: what if the collective international team gave the Indonesian members all the information, partnered with them as they created their own training program, and mentored them as they delivered it in Indonesian to Indonesians?

This was perhaps the most important and powerful shift in approach throughout the entire mission. The "Black Wave" devastated the people of Aceh. Lives, property, infrastructure, and ways of life were destroyed. Following the physical destruction, community confidence was also damaged as armies of personnel and foreign assistance descended upon the province and began "doing things for" the victims rather than "doing things with" the community. Until members of the US team took an important second look at their own approach, they were engaged in the very same damaging process.

With this new strategy, the long-term power of the program began to grow and the US team members were accepted as colleagues, not outside "experts." The new approach provided a vehicle for the Indonesian people to take charge of their own and their province's psychosocial recovery, beginning with their children. The shift put the Indonesians on the team in charge of everything. The international team—meaning everyone else—became their support team. The US team members were now seen as trustworthy, and thus transitioned from intruders to welcome advisors and collaborators.

Two days were added to the preparation time to allow for this change in approach. Two more Indonesian facilitators were contracted by UNICEF to assist. This international group then began developing what eventually became known as the "assembly line" for choosing program content and having it immediately translated and packaged for delivery. The entire training program content was developed in this manner in less than 5 days.

The most important aspect of the health diplomacy model that emerged from this mission was that the model facilitated a diverse group of people, from all over the world, to become an integrated team. It was promoted, in no small measure, as a direct result of this change in approach. Consensus became the standard for program development—roles were created and people filled them based on program needs, not necessarily professional credentials, and those team members who would soon leave stepped back and supported those who would remain.

Final Preparations and One Last Hurdle

When the second *Mercy* precept was formulated ("We are not 'the pros from Dover'"),[13] it was with the USPHS team members in mind. It was modified to include "We are not the pros from Djakarta" after the final Indonesian members of the team arrived from the capital and the whole training curriculum came close to unraveling 2 days before it was to be delivered. One of the new members wanted to try a very different approach to several aspects of training. The Indonesian members met with the international team for advice about how to proceed. They then met as a team to address the concerns, educate the new members about why the program was as it was, and welcomed them into the process. It worked; consensus was achieved, only minor and very beneficial adjustments were made, and the program was finalized for delivery with everyone's roles clearly delineated and agreed upon. Most importantly, the team integrated new membership, incorporated new ideas without losing the overall approach, and did it without altering the consensus approach that was the hallmark of the entire process.

The trainings themselves were the culmination of a short but intense period of development filled with deep emotion and renewed spirit of hope for the training staff and the approximately 90 people from throughout Aceh Province who would themselves become trainers. The training brought together a wide range of both governmental and NGO personnel from across northern Sumatra, gave them detailed content and a network of people upon whom they could rely to help them, and instilled confidence that they could deliver this training themselves upon their return home. As of this writing, the programs are still operating and the Abidin University Hospital in Banda Aceh has dedicated space for the programs there to support their ongoing operation.

SUMMARY

The program described in this chapter developed from a USPHS leadership approach. It was then modified into an international collaboration among several agencies in the middle of the chaos of the relief effort, and transitioned from a program given by outside "experts" to one ultimately formulated and delivered by the people of Indonesia themselves. The development team included many who were directly affected and suffered significant personal losses, while others knew only what they saw reported via news media prior to their arrival. Several team members had no previous relief experience, although others had years of experience in such efforts. Several of the relief agencies represented had never before worked together, nor worked directly with the US Navy or USPHS; the initial levels of suspicion about motives and capabilities in the response were high. That they all ultimately came together in a spirit of common cause is a testament to the best of what is possible in times of great human need, and when personal interests are subsumed to support the greater good and provide large-scale successes for others.

The success of this program also demonstrates the significant benefits that can result when quiet, but informed leadership principles are understood and acted upon. Absent the open-handed leadership approach, there would have been no collaboration and no subsequent program. Future missions and their commanders will face similar chaos and unknowns, but some of the precepts developed in the *Mercy* model may prove useful in developing the clarity and collaborations necessary to effect change at-scale in health systems following major conflagration or catastrophic emergencies. Attachment 2 to this chapter contains these precepts, exactly as they were written by the USPHS team during relief efforts and as reported in their after-action report. Emerging operational approaches such as the PsySTART rapid mental health triage platform can also be used as tools to further these aims. They are particularly effective when the relief and response lanes are shared among agencies and forces, rather than wholly "owned" by a particular command structure. Because these cases make up the vast majority of international relief efforts, the *Mercy* approaches appear to maximize effectiveness via better collaboration where command and control would be either counterproductive or rejected outright by the other agencies involved in the response.

REFERENCES

1. Tzu L, Wieger L, Bryce D. *Tao-Te-Ching: The Classic Chinese Work in English Translation.* New York, NY: Random House; 2005.
2. US Department of Health and Human Services. What is the commissioned corps? United States Public Health Service Web site. Available at: http://www.usphs.gov/aboutus/questions.aspx#whatis. Accessed August 18, 2010.
3. Perez J, Coady J, DeJesus E, McGuinness K, Bondan, S. Operation Unified Assistance population-based programs: US Public Health Service and international team. *Mil Med.* 2006;1:S53–S58.
4. Magnitude 9.1–off the west coast of northern Sumatra 2004 December 26 00:58:53: UTC. US Geological Survey Web site. Available at: http://earthquake.usgs.gov/earthquakes/eqinthenews/2004/usslav/#summary. Accessed September 30, 2010.
5. McGuinness KM, Coady JA, Perez JT, Williams NC, Mcintyre DJ, Schreiber MD. Public mental health: the role of population-based and macrosystems interventions in the wake of Hurricane Katrina. *J Prof Psychol: Res Pract.* 2008;39(1):58–65.
6. Norris F, Murphy A, Baker C, Perilla J. Severity, timing, and duration of reactions to trauma in the population: an example from Mexico. *Biol Psychiatry.* 2003;53(9):769–778.
7. Sternberg R. A systems model of leadership: WICS. *Am Psychol.* 2007:62(1):34–42.
8. Reissman D, Schreiber M, Klomp R, et al. The virtual network supporting the front lines: addressing emerging behavioral health problems following the tsunami of 2004. *Mil Med.* 2006;1:S40–S43.
9. Thienkrua W, Cardozo BL, Chakkrab M, et al. Thailand Post-Tsunami Mental Health Study Group. Symptoms of posttraumatic stress disorder and depression among children in tsunami-affected areas in southern Thailand. *JAMA.* 2006;296:549–559.
10. Schreiber M. Learning from 9/11: toward a national model for children and families in mass casualty terrorism. In: Daneli Y, Dingman R, eds. *On the Ground After September 11: Mental Health Responses and Practical Knowledge Gained.* New York, NY: Haworth Press; 2005: 605–614.
11. Coady J, Perez J, Schreiber M. The way forward: innovations in disaster mental health. *Calif Psychol.* 2007;40(2):41–44.
12. Schreiber M, Gurwitch R, Coady J, Perez J, Wong, M. *Toward a National Model for Children and Families in Mass Casualty Events.* New York, NY: Springer Publishing; in press.
13. Hooker R. *M*A*S*H.* New York, NY: Simon & Schuster; 1969.

ATTACHMENT 1: EARTHQUAKE DISASTER RELIEF

Major earthquakes have the potential to be one of the most catastrophic natural disasters affecting humanity, as evidenced by the recent earthquakes in Bam, Iran, Pakistan, and Peru. Earthquakes of significant size set off a chain of events that significantly affects the public health and medical infrastructures of the region. Accelerated urbanization in seismically active parts of the world dramatically increases the vulnerability of these regions. Worldwide, more than a million earthquakes occur each year, with nine countries accounting for 80% of earthquake fatalities (China, Japan, Pakistan, Chile, Russia, Turkey, Peru, Iran, and Italy[1–6]). In the United States, the state experiencing the most earthquakes is Alaska.[1,2]

Numerous factors influence earthquake mortality and morbidity, including natural factors, structural factors, and individual factors. Aftershocks are a particular concern and may occur for a prolonged period of time. For example, during the Northridge, California, earthquake more than 14,000 aftershocks occurred in the region over the next 5 years.[3] Landslides and mudflows after earthquakes account for significant morbidity and mortality. Hazardous materials (chemical, biological, radioactive) are an increasing risk after earthquakes due to accelerated urbanization. Following the Loma Prieta earthquake in California in 1989, toxic materials were responsible for about 20% of after-earthquake injuries. Flooding from dams with structural damage and fires continue to be additional causes of mortality and morbidity after earthquakes.[7–9]

Structural factors affecting injury or death rates include trauma caused by building collapse. In fact, approximately 75% of earthquake fatalities are caused by collapse of buildings that were poorly constructed or not earthquake resistant.[10–12] Individual risk factors include age, health, and emotional stability. Demographic factors associated with increased risk for death and injury are persons over the age of 60, children between 5 and 9 years of age, and chronically ill persons.[12] The increased vulnerability of these groups is because of lack of mobility, exacerbation of underlying diseases, and inability to withstand major traumatic injury. Entrapment, the occupants' locations within a building, their behavior during the earthquake, and time until rescue, constitute the factors affecting mortality and morbidity.

Logistical support is an essential element of disaster relief and an area in which the military excels. The mass casualty response to earthquakes includes four essential elements of disaster medical response: (1) search and rescue, (2) triage and initial stabilization, (3) definitive medical care, and (4) evacuation.[13] The requirements for search and rescue and definitive care, and the need for outside assistance from military and civilian teams, are significantly increased in earthquake disasters compared to other natural disasters because of the severity of wide-spread damage and the complexity of injuries.

Psychological trauma and other adverse psychological sequelae are frequently the side effects of earthquake disasters for a number of reasons. Earthquakes occur with little or no warning compared to hurricanes (several days of storm tracking) or even tornadoes (often with several hours of meteorological information). This lack of warning deprives victims of time to take psychological and physical protective action, and exacerbates a sense of loss of control over the destructive event. Earthquakes expose victims to serious threats to personal safety, increasing their vulnerability to future psychological symptoms. One of the important lessons learned in disaster medical response is the necessity to configure teams based on functional capacities, not professional titles. A capacity for mental health interventions is critical, and mental healthcare teams are now incorporated into most civilian and military disaster response teams in the United States.

Earthquakes are a major cause of the full spectrum of traumatic injuries, both physical and psychological, and frequently require outside medical and public health disaster assistance. Ultimately, disaster mitigation will be the most significant factor in decreasing mortality and morbidity from earthquakes.

Acknowledgment

This attachment was prepared by Susan Miller Briggs, MD, MPH, Associate Professor of Surgery, Harvard Medical School; Director, International Trauma and Disaster Institute, Massachusetts General Hospital, Boston, Massachusetts.

REFERENCES

1. Noji EK, ed. *The Public Health Consequences of Disasters*. New York, NY: Oxford University Press; 1997.

2. Hays WW. Perspectives on the international decade for natural education. *Earthquake Spectra*. 1990;6:125–143.

3. Prager EJ. *Furious Earth: The Science and Nature of Earthquakes, Volcanoes, and Tsunamis*. New York, NY: McGraw-Hill; 1999.

4. Perez E, Thompson P. Natural hazards: causes and effects. Lesson 2–earthquakes. *Prehosp Disaster Med*. 1994;9:260–271.

5. US Geological Survey. *Scenarios of Possible Earthquakes Affecting Major California Population Centers, With Estimates of Intensity and Ground Shaking*. Menlo Park, Calif: USGS; 1981. Open-File Report 81-115.

6. Blake P. *Peru Earthquake, May 31, 1970. Report of the CDC Epidemiologic Team*. Atlanta, Ga: Centers for Disease Control and Prevention; 1970.

7. Showalter PS, Myers MF. Natural disasters in the United States as release agents of oil, chemicals, or radiological materials between 1980–1989: analysis and recommendations. *Risk Anal*. 1994;14:169–182.

8. Durkin ME, Thiel CC, Schneider JE, et al. Injuries and the emergency medical response in the Loma Prieta earthquake. *Bull Seismological Soc Am*. 1991;81:2143–2166.

9. Hayes BE, Freeman C, Rubin JL, et al. Medical response to catastrophic events: California's planning and the Loma Prieta earthquake. *Ann Emeg Med*. 1992;21:368–474.

10. Colburn AW, Murakami HO, Ohta Y. *Factors Affecting Fatalities and Injury in Earthquakes. Engineering Seismology and Earthquake Disaster Prevention Planning*. Hokkaido, Japan: Hokkaido University; 1987. Internal Report.

11. EQE Engineering. *The October 17, 1989 Loma Prieta Earthquake: A Quick Look Report*. San Francisco, Calif: EQE Engineering; 1989.

12. Coburn AW, Spence RJS, Pomonis A. *Factors Determining Human Casualty Levels in Earthquakes: Mortality Prediction in Building Collapse*. Reston, Va: US Geological Survey; 1992.

13. Briggs SM, ed. *Advanced Disaster Medical Response Manual for Providers*. Boston, Mass: Harvard Medical International; 2003.

ATTACHMENT 2: THE *MERCY* MODEL

The *Mercy* (ship and concept) was an untested capability arriving at the site of an unprecedented event. Extraordinary devastation, great chaos, much need, little information about overall response, and, of equal importance, little information on the ground and among agencies there about us, who we were, and what we might do. We did not know ourselves what we might be capable of doing. There was fear, particularly among the international mental health community, that we were going to interfere or otherwise act unilaterally without cooperation or coordination. The international relief community, including our own US organizations, viewed us with suspicion. Western psychological methods were not widely understood, or greatly accepted, and our reputation—real or conjured—was that we would come in for a few days, see a limited number of patients (more to use as props for media opportunities than genuine assistance), get our pictures taken, congratulate ourselves, and then leave. As a team, we assumed this going in and swore we would do nothing of the sort. The *Mercy* model began with that promise. The precepts as they were formulated were:

1. "Go West and Do Good Things…" This was essentially the mission order until the ship arrived on station: our overarching precept was to promote the greater good, not our particular role in the effort.
2. We are not "the pros from Dover"—borrowing the line from the book M*A*S*H.[1] The principle here is collaboration, not independent action. Egos and personal ownership of information and approaches are checked at the helicopter door.
3. We are here as students of the people and culture we are here to assist, because the better we understand, the better we can serve.
4. We work for and with agencies ashore, not the other way around. We do not work independently, unless we have capabilities that are useful, support those that are already in place, or are desired by the agencies with whom we work.
5. For behavioral health, given limited time, personnel, and resources, we will focus on public health and population-based approaches to maximize program development, penetration, and effects. Responding to the area's behavioral health relief systems and infrastructure needs is our primary concern, not direct service. We are responding to a disaster of unprecedented proportions. We could limit our overall impact by only delivering direct services, or we could take our limited personnel resources and seek to maximize potential impact by working with systems programmatically. Somewhat novel, but not at all unprecedented.
6. Initial work will be assessing the mental health infrastructure, programming, agencies, and services, then developing relationships with agencies, not developing programs independent of them. The building of the relationships with other agencies is the most critical step in the entire process; without the relationship, there is no program. New relationships with agencies may be met with suspicion; we should approach this as an opportunity, not a threat.
7. Collaborative leadership, consensus approach: coordination not control, development not ownership, shine spotlight on others not ourselves, and collaboration among the team and the teams with whom we work. Seek consensus wherever possible and defer to others when conflict arises or differences threaten the process. Adopt local approach when such exists. Simple concepts, though extremely difficult to execute and should neither be overlooked nor undervalued.
8. We will not promise anything that we can't deliver, period.
9. Team members do what needs to be done regardless of position or professional background.
10. Promote respect for divergent people, professions, worldviews, and spiritual beliefs.
11. "Wisdomkeepers" must be sought and welcomed—language and cultural guidance are essential. We will learn as much as we teach.
12. International team formation is critical; positive interpersonal relationships, group formation, promotion, and collaboration are primary goals.
13. Focus on facilitation for program development, not instruction, so the process of program development is taught by doing. Through this process new leaders are developed and the people are empowered.
14. Create tools for program development and show how to use them: don't just provide the programs themselves.
15. Focus on approach for paraprofessionals and nonprofessionals, not professionals…because there aren't any, or at least not enough to make any substantive difference. The "paraprofessionals" are both the

experts of the culture and the facilitators of the programs. They bring valuable and essential skills to the trainings and must be empowered to implement programs.

16. We are an international team with a local presence. We are, in a very real sense, a local presence for an international team and knowledge trust, including many of the finest disaster recovery people around the world. Utilizing digital and other technologies, we are in this together and will work together as a worldwide virtual team.
17. Programs will need to be formulated with great speed, will be discrete and time limited—we do not know how long we will be on station in any given place and we will not start something we can't finish. Thus, we will work as quickly as possible to provide stand-alone programming.
18. Mobilize local expertise and capability, wherever possible, then support it with programming and disseminate the overall process widely, particularly where there has not been such an approach before. This was particularly true in Aceh, where there was limited infrastructure, and what infrastructure was there developed posttsunami. This offered an opportunity to support the new network and capability in ways that might not otherwise have been possible.
19. Use a program assembly line approach to maximize collaboration and speed of program production. It is during this process that the relationships and trust developed between organizations and people. We did what we said we would do and we promoted active collaboration, not passive acceptance, for the program's development:
    a. Team consensus on program specifics; we began by asking the question: "If we could do anything, what would the program look like?" Taking that ideal, we then asked, "How can we do this?" and mobilized the network, both in Aceh and internationally, to try to get as close to the ideal as possible. This we learned from AusAID [Australian Agency for International Development] and UNICEF [United Nations Children's Fund].
    b. Content gathering: gathering as much information as possible as quickly as possible in the areas requested, then reduce that information to a usable set of reference materials from which to choose final products.
    c. Logistical and resource support: where, how, who, funding, mechanisms of support, travel, security, local transportation and housing, etc. Completely UNICEF and AusAID managed.
    d. Editorial/programmatic: consensus collaboration on what content, from all that was received, would finally be used in the presentations.
    e. Media preparation: taking the selected information and putting it into the proper format, PowerPoint, reference documents, etc, for participants.
    f. Translation: taking the final training products and translating them, primarily from English into Indonesian, and placing them into the day's presentation curriculum and reference documentation.
    g. Trainer preparation: review materials with trainer and promote input on feasibility of content and method.
    h. Presentation: as much as possible, use local trainers and program people. We will support and supervise as needed, but this is their show, not ours. We helped produce, but they star.
20. Evaluation: current evaluations are being completed by members of UNICEF, AusAID, Karinivasu, and Women's Crisis Counseling. The evaluation will cover other international agencies' experiences in working with the behavioral health team and its role in the collaboration.
21. Ongoing collaboration: while the programs might be time limited, the relationships are not and the potential for ongoing support and collaboration is very real, particularly with technology and digital capabilities to maintain and support it. Plan for and promote it.

REFERENCE

1. Hooker R. *M*A*S*H*. New York, NY: Simon & Schuster; 1969.

Chapter 40

BEHAVIORAL HEALTH ISSUES AND DETAINED INDIVIDUALS

RICHARD TOYE, PhD,* and MARSHALL SMITH, MD†

*Lieutenant Colonel, Medical Service Corps, US Army Reserve; Company Commander, 883rd Medical Company (Combat Stress Control), 495 Summer Street, Boston, Massachusetts 02210; formerly, Brigade Behavioral Health Consultant, 804th Medical Brigade, Fort Devens, Massachusetts

†Lieutenant Colonel, Medical Corps, US Army; Chief, Behavioral Health, Landstuhl Regional Medical Center, CMR 402, Box 1357, APO AE 09180; formerly, Chief, Outpatient Behavioral Health, Landstuhl Regional Medical Center

INTRODUCTION

The US military provides appropriate healthcare services for enemy prisoners of war and other individuals detained during operations. Doctrine and international treaties require that detainees be provided "equivalent care" to prevent deterioration of their condition. The scope of detention healthcare operations is dictated variously by the magnitude of the detention activities in theater, the typical duration of an individual's detention, cultural norms and situational factors affecting the problems presented by detainees, and the availability of resources in theater.

In Operation Iraqi Freedom, behavioral health services to detainees first emerged as a critical operation in 2003, when it was discovered that local psychiatric inpatients had been released into the streets by retreating enemy forces, and that Coalition troops had captured and detained many of them in facilities at Umm Qasr. The emergent need to distinguish between distressed psychotic individuals and acting-out enemy combatants required immediate diversion of combat and operational stress control assets to the detention mission. At that time, noncombatant detainees who were seriously mentally ill were discharged to community care. In 2004, as detainee operations stabilized, nongovernmental organization surveyors expressed concern that seriously mentally ill individuals retained in detention were receiving care from providers other than licensed behavioral healthcare practitioners and that the standard of equivalence of care was not being met. At the time of this text's preparation, three separate medical task forces with augmented behavioral health teams have rotated through theater detainee healthcare operations in Iraq. This chapter provides a basic framework of operations in detainee behavioral healthcare, reflecting the lessons learned by the first two contingents, Task Force Medical (TF MED) 115 and TF MED 344. To help the units tasked with this challenging job apply these lessons, the chapter will discuss critical mission activities and common problems in the process of preparing and executing the detention behavioral healthcare mission.

TRAINING THE TEAM

Predeployment Preparation

Predeployment is a stressful time for all involved. The unit mission focus is on common training tasks; the command emphasis is on facilitating service members' transition from the home environment to the combat environment. Nevertheless, every effort should be made for personnel to receive appropriate mission-specific training prior to deployment to a detention mission. Predeployment preparation should include, at a minimum, four essential components: (1) reviewing current Department of Defense (DoD) and federal and state corrections healthcare policy and procedures, (2) establishing communication with unit personnel currently on site in theater, (3) reviewing cultural information specific to the host nation, and (4) gaining familiarization with the detention care setting.

Most DoD behavioral health providers have never worked in the corrections environment, much less the detention healthcare environment; a review of current corrections policy and procedures is a must. Detention healthcare is similar to healthcare given to patients overseen by the Federal Bureau of Prisons, an agency of the US Department of Justice. Bureau of Prisons standard operating procedures (SOPs) provide the model used to develop military protocols for detention care. These various SOPs[1,2] address essential topics including suicide prevention, medication distribution, and screening procedures, all key elements in the detainee care mission. If time permits, personnel should consider visiting a local corrections establishment to talk with the medical personnel about providing care in a corrections environment.

Perhaps the most important step in preparing to deploy is establishing communication with the personnel being replaced. This point cannot be stressed enough. The current active unit has implemented SOPs that will be suitable for most purposes, and deploying staff should obtain and review them to become familiar with current operations and capitalize on lessons learned before arriving in country. The currently deployed unit can also provide information on particulars of the environment such as billeting information, recreational facilities, supplies to bring, and available resources. Communication may be difficult because of time zone differences, but multiple channels exist: e-mail, telephone, or even videoconference, if available. Exchanging contact information benefits everyone; for the outgoing unit, the process of training the incoming unit has its own value. Most units have tremendous pride in their organization and appreciate others' interest and willingness to accept their feedback and experiences. Changes in existing protocols will undoubtedly be needed, but current SOPs provide a good place to start.

If no behavioral health unit was previously in country and the mission is to establish the first detention behavioral healthcare program in the area occupied, it is especially important to understand the standards by which behavioral healthcare will be evaluated, as well as learning what assets will be available to support the mission. Although the program is mandated to provide detainees with equivalent care, the perception of what "equivalent" means can vary widely, so it is important to establish as soon as possible what services and level of care are intended. DoD doctrine, US Bureau of Prison standards, and community standards within the area of operations (AO) can help inform this decision.[1–5]

In most cases, detainees are from a different culture than the typical service member patient. Cultural differences can be an obstacle to establishing rapport and to patient care delivery. Misunderstandings between patient and clinician can be frustrating in an already tense environment, so it is important for providers to be familiar with common local customs and courtesies. This information can be found on the Internet, in textbooks, and in other historical sources. If possible, a briefing by someone from the particular culture will be very helpful. Prior to deployment in 2005, TF MED 344 enjoyed extensive cultural briefings from Iraqi expatriates, which made the transition into that environment much smoother than it might otherwise have been.

Additionally, briefing by a medical provider from the culture is invaluable. Names of medications and the social significance of different forms of treatment may differ. It is essential to know some of the cultural differences in the way medicine is practiced; for instance, the perception of mental illness can vary tremendously among cultures. Understanding some of the basic differences and perceptions increases the effectiveness of even basic treatments; however, it is important to assess the quality of source information. For example, TF MED 344 was repeatedly informed that rural Iraqis considered behavioral health issues to be signs of malign influence, and that the indigenous personnel were unsophisticated and wary of behavioral health issues. In fact, the population appeared to have a good knowledge of behavioral health issues and protocols. One illiterate farmer, detained during a sweep of his community, thanked providers for their interest in his mental state and acknowledged that he was depressed, but stated his preference to work with his local cleric about his feelings of loss over the death of his sons in the conflict.

Cultural issues and phenomena are limitless, and there is no way to be totally prepared for the situation in theater. For example, it is common knowledge that psychosis often presents differently in different cultures. When TF MED 344 staff encountered a detainee who reported concerns about his visions of a talking chicken, the question arose as to whether this was a psychosis or malingering. Certainly in a US population, malingering was more likely. Discussion with translators and other detainees provided no indication that chickens had any particular significance in this culture, and other psychotic individuals in camp tended to have auditory hallucinations without visual manifestations. While it was not possible to be sure, the subsequent presentation of several other patients with exactly the same hallucinations suggested to staff that the "talking chicken" phenomenon was malingering behavior. In stark contrast, the extremely high incidence of self-injurious behavior turned out to have several cultural antecedents, including both an acceptance of excoriation as a religious ritual and a history of self-mutilation among prisoners during the Saddam Hussein regime to avoid being brutalized even more by their guards.

While cultural issues are legion, it also is important to recognize the universal nature of mental illness. For example, one patient managed by TF 344 reported that God spoke directly to him and told him that all infidels would die. This presentation could certainly have reflected the social-political context of the conflict; however, other camp residents repudiated the patient's statements and were concerned for his welfare and safety. The individual was truly psychotic and responded well to antipsychotic medications. Another detainee presented with a long history of self-injurious behavior, and swallowed any sharp object he could find. His behaviors increased as attention to them increased. He was diagnosed as a self-destructive borderline personality and required extremes of behavioral management.

The context of care in a detention camp differs significantly from deployment to any other forward operating base or operations center. In a detention camp, the enemy is not only outside the perimeter, but has a large presence within the perimeter as well. This has two main effects. First, security protocols assume a significant place in day-to-day operations. Second, coalition personnel are confronted with a uniquely stressful task of interacting on a daily basis with the enemy, creating a number of behavioral health issues that can affect operations.

Security issues are always legion during deployment to a hostile AO. In detention care, security is doubly important. Access to the patient routinely requires special clearance and passes, and time must be planned to allow for multiple security checks. Patients are not seen privately. "Outpatient" interactions may be through a security barrier. Armed guards accompany hospitalized patients or those seen in a clinic. Clinical schedules must be coordinated with the guards' transportation schedules for these custodial staff. Daily operations are likely to be interrupted by head counts, missing person checks, or crowd control operations. In the Iraq AO, detainees were assigned numbers rather than being referred to by name, making it difficult to track cases, especially because detainees were routinely shifted from camp to camp as a security precaution.

Medical and custodial staffs are patently affected by having to interact with the enemy on a daily basis. They cannot treat the enemy aggressively, and must provide compassionate care even when threatened or disparaged by the detainee. They cannot establish friendships or trusting relationships with the individuals they see most often each day. The stress of detainee care causes irritability, anger, and dissatisfaction rarely seen in other healthcare or operations centers. Management of this distress is an important part of the behavioral healthcare mission.

The Clinical Process in Detainee Care

The clinical process in detention care also differs markedly from that in other clinic-based operations. Staff may or may not need a refresher in basic clinical assessment and brief counseling techniques, but the team invariably requires training in detention operations. Training should address screening, assessment, intervention expectations, crisis response, and coordination of care.

Every new detainee is screened for behavioral health risk factors as part of their initial medical evaluation. A brief questionnaire covering previous behavioral health treatment and current behavioral health concerns is administered through an interpreter. Familiarity with the screening process and with typical detainee reactions to the behavioral health interview is a must. Intake screening is a volume business: screening must proceed at the pace of internment operations. This can range from 50 screenings a week to 150 a day, with little advance notice, depending on the pace of operations in theater. It will be tempting to assign one or two individuals to the screening process, because it is inherently different from other clinical operations and can be accomplished best by personnel who are experienced with the procedure. Even when this is done, however, every member of the team must be able to complete the screening interview both to provide surge capacity and because this is a must-do procedure that if not completed delays the movement of the detainee into the camp.

The intake screen identifies new detainees who need follow-up evaluation. Detainees may also be referred for evaluation by military police, by the medical team, by other detainees, or through self-referral. At Abu Ghraib in 2004 and 2005, after systematic improvements in the detention facility were established, it was typical for providers to see a dozen individuals for new assessment and disposition each week. Personnel must be comfortable with conducting a functional assessment leading to initial diagnosis and disposition in sparse conditions, using an interpreter for the interview portion of the assessment. Clear criteria for assessment and disposition should be established and practiced prior to deployment. Mobilization site training will most likely provide "typical" cases that are florid in their presentation, a training model that is unrealistic and not useful. Instead, training should focus on assessment of anxiety disorders in an anxiety-provoking situation, identification of malingering, and differential diagnosis of adjustment disorder and major depression. The patient cannot be expected to be a reliable informant; the information received will be distorted by translation; and the setting will create ambiguities that make a typical assessment model untenable. The behavioral health clinician must rely on behavioral signs and reports of functional impairment from collateral sources at least as much as on the patient's own report.

Ongoing review of the active caseload is more complex in detention care than in the clinic or in the corrections setting. Patients do not have regular appointments; they are scattered across a barbed wire encampment and are moved frequently for security reasons. A concerted effort must be made to develop and sustain a patient tracking system. Once continued care is established, clear outcome criteria should be established and monitored for each case. Establishing outcome criteria will probably be the part of this process most reminiscent of normal clinical practice.

One of the most frequent questions asked by providers outside of this setting is whether the military really "does therapy with those guys." Odds are that most intervention will involve medication management, behavioral intervention, and education or brief supportive counseling rather than psychotherapy per se. Among the many factors mitigating against the establishment of therapeutic trust are the likely brevity of care, as well as cultural and privacy issues preventing in-depth treatment in most cases. However, as in any setting, treatment approaches should be adjusted to meet the needs of the individual.

Detention care can be volatile, and is a 24-hour operation. The clinical team is on call at all times. Although the facility includes physical safeguards to keep aggressive and suicidal detainees secure, custodial staff values the reassurance and direction that on-call behavioral health consultants provide when detainees have problems off-shift. Clinicians must respond to every call, even if the situation is under control. A common problem is threats of self-harm to obtain camp privileges. In Iraq, where many historical factors facilitated self-excoriation, it was not uncommon to be called to attend to a detainee who had cut himself shallowly across the chest and threatened further self-harm if his demands were not met. In the United States, this behavior would be an indication of serious underlying pathology, but in this setting the behavior was more often than not an extreme example of manipulative or coercive behavior on the part of a detained individual.

Finally, the behavioral health team will not operate in isolation. Detainees receiving behavioral health services are also under care of the medical team. Some primary healthcare providers will prefer to prescribe their own psychotropics, and some will use medicines from the behavioral health formulary for other purposes, such as pain management. Nongovernmental organizations are often involved in coordinating social services for the detainee. It is necessary to establish protocols for coordinating medication procurement as well as coordinating care with the healthcare team, including medication procurement, record keeping, and social service contact management. The behavioral health team should train on and practice these protocols before entering the operational area.

Unit Transition

Several things can be done to optimize the transition from one unit to its replacement at the detention center. The outgoing unit will probably know their replacements at least a month or two before the transition. If the incoming unit has not contacted the outgoing unit in that period, the outgoing unit should work through their leadership to contact and establish a working relationship with their replacements. In addition to preparing for a successful handoff, preparing the detainees over a period of about a month is useful in minimizing disruption. Replacements should arrive early enough that outgoing staff can demonstrate current procedures for at least a week.

This staffing overlap is commonly referred to as the "left seat/right seat ride." To set up the new unit for success, it is strongly recommended that staff with similar roles be paired with outgoing staff during duties for several days, allowing newcomers to adjust to the environment, see the day-to-day operation, and ask questions. A date should be designated for the takeover of duties by the new staff, accompanied the first time by outgoing staff. Optimally, the oncoming unit should have at least a day or two to function independently prior to the departure of the outgoing unit, although this schedule can run into problems. In both TF MED 115 and TF MED 344 some medical teams were ready to relinquish their duties the day replacements arrived. Others, feeling pride of ownership, did not feel comfortable standing by while the replacement staff took over and learned the job.

Tours are generally for 1 year and invariably rapport will be established between staff and detainees. Detainees talk among themselves and with other medical and nonmedical staff, and often have some idea when units are scheduled to depart, knowing that units usually change somewhere around the 11- or 12-month point. Detainees have an active interest in the transition and may ask detailed questions. They will understand the transition process and probably try to find out exactly when the new unit will take over. Some appreciate the care they received and will feel anxiety about the upcoming transition and termination. However, operational security should be kept in mind: detainees should not be given specific dates or any other information that may be used to threaten security. Personnel should be vague and ensure detainees that their care will continue; no information about troop movements should be divulged.

Units preparing for departure often shift focus to the task of reintegration and manage ongoing tasks with less interest and enthusiasm. Personnel should maintain operational focus: the outgoing unit has the responsibility to prepare both the detainees and the gaining unit for a successful, seamless transition. A modified termination process and a well-planned and executed left seat/right seat ride will give the outgoing unit closure, knowing that the mission they conducted and improved upon will be handed over to people they were able to train. The gaining unit will build upon and modify procedures to optimize the care they deliver over the course of their tour.

EFFECTIVE USE OF TRANSLATORS

Communication with detainees is essential to effectively assess and treat them. Most detainees will not speak English, and unless the medical staff speaks the detainee's language, the use of a translator is vital in obtaining a good history. In some settings, translators are intentionally rotated among sites and services as a security measure, making it impossible to thoroughly train a few select individuals. This may be a source of contention. Frequently, as a medical team becomes familiar with a translator, they feel confident in them and request sole access to them. This is not good practice. During TF MED 344's tenure, no fewer than three proficient and apparently friendly translators were removed from service: two were found to have passed information to hostile elements, and one was removed for continually asking for cast-off uniforms. Incessant questions about vacation plans or other personal information, which might be normal in other settings, are not a sign of a reliable interpreter.

It is unlikely that many translators will have expertise in behavioral health or behavioral health terminology. Some cultures may have different understanding of terms such as "hallucinations" or "delusions," so questions about these symptoms may get lost in translation and render the assessment ineffective. Other concepts may be uncommon in a particular culture, and some questions might be seen as offensive or disrespectful. Translators may have their own opinions about the patient's problems, and may not make the effort to translate the questions exactly. Furthermore, personnel must be aware that hired translators may be traditional enemies of the detained population: they may come from neighboring countries in conflict with that of the detainee, or they may have opposing politics.

Personnel should take time up front to get to know the translators and ascertain their understanding of behavioral health terminology, as well as their ability to convey information to a detainee. Translators should understand the importance of asking the patient every question posed, rather than providing answers themselves. Hired translators should be used when possible, but the unavailability of hired translators should not impede the successful execution of the mission. In the absence of a hired translator, detainees who are fluent in English may be required to serve as translators. Custodial staff may be able to recommend a detainee who has proven to be effective and may have assisted them on other occasions. Although clinicians might initially be reluctant to use a detainee as a translator, having a trusted detainee assist can be both extremely effective and enlightening. Detainees may feel more comfortable opening up to a fellow detainee who they respect and admire than to a hired translator they may not trust. Establishing a rapport with the detainees is important for successful treatment, and sometimes having a working relationship with one of their peers who speaks English can facilitate an effective therapeutic relationship.

DEVELOPING A TREATMENT PLAN

It is important to bear in mind, in this setting more than most, that diagnosis is functional: the goal is not necessarily to determine the etiology and nature of the disorder but to develop effective treatment. International standards for care in this setting specify treatment of mental disorders that result in incapacity to care for oneself or in increased risk of deterioration of function or health; the emphasis on functional impairment must be highlighted. Functional impairment is a critical ingredient in deciding to provide care, especially if resources are limited. To that end, personnel must

- diagnose only to the level of the available data;
- develop treatments using rubrics that maximize functional outcome as simply and as safely as possible; and
- rely on outcome monitoring to adjust and eventually to titrate treatment.

Diagnosis and treatment in detention care is vulnerable to many problems not experienced in other settings: language and cultural barriers to establishing good communication, subtle cultural factors associated with the meaning of mental illness for the detainee, pressure in detention to acquire marketable drugs or to garner attention or respite from the compound, and group dynamics affecting the individual's behavior. The absence of good collateral information and the biases of the interpreter and custodial staff toward mental illness and toward the detainee complicate matters immeasurably. Available information includes the self-report of the detainee, third-party reports from camp mates and custodial staff, records from medical services provided during detention, observation, and functional assessment. Because the translation may be unreliable, the clinical interview should rely more heavily on behavioral observation than most clinicians are accustomed to.

Behavioral Management Considerations

Establishing a program for managing behavioral problems, or providing consultation, is an essential part of a successful detainee behavioral healthcare mission. Military police deal with behavioral challenges daily and often turn to the behavioral health team for advice and support. Some detainees test the limits of acceptable behavior, which must be handled effectively to prevent others from acting in similar fashion. Often, unacceptable behavior occurs to achieve secondary gain, and the behavioral health team can educate the corrections staff on appropriate means to address the behavior without rewarding the detainee (which reinforces the behavior and causes others to engage in the same or similar behavior). The behavioral management program can empower the corrections staff and significantly curtail inappropriate detainee behavior.

Detainee custodial staff members have one of the most challenging jobs in the military. Staff members may have a corrections background, and these personnel can utilize their prior experience and training to effectively manage inappropriate behavior. Others have no prior corrections experience and may be operating in a detainee environment for the first time with very limited training. Faced daily with hostile and belligerent detainees, most custodial staff do an exceptional job maintaining order and discipline. When detainees engage in behavior that poses a threat to themselves or others, custodial staff will call on the behavioral health team for assistance. To facilitate teamwork, behavioral health personnel should establish a working relationship with custodial staff early in deployment. Behavioral health personnel should introduce custodial staff to the most common behaviors associated with mental illness and encourage them to get the behavioral health team involved early if they have concerns or are unsure of how to handle a particular situation. Custodial staff will appreciate knowing they can call on behavioral health professionals if they need assistance. Often, the behavior can be controlled by simply removing the detainee from the environment or by giving the detainee some time alone away from other detainees. Furthermore, the behavioral health team is responsible for training the custodial staff to recognize when a detainee may be psychotic, experiencing another Axis I disorder, or having a primary Axis II problem so they can contact the team to make an assessment. A good clinical assessment will aid in determining what the primary problem is and help in making the appropriate decision to resolve the situation.

Primary Axis II problems, common in any corrections population, can be expected in the detainee population as well. Common reasons for acting-out behavior involve secondary gain such as wanting more cigarettes, wanting to get out of the heat and into an air-conditioned building, and a host of other reasons primarily viewed by the detainee as obtaining pleasure and reducing suffering. Inappropriate behavior may include self-injurious behavior such as cutting, eating barbed wire, making suicidal statements, making suicidal gestures, and faking seizure-like activity or other medical conditions that commonly require removal from confinement and evaluation in the hospital setting. This behavior can be significantly reduced by having a medical or behavioral health team evaluate detainees in their living space and by transporting them only if medically indicated. However, contact with the behavioral health team on site can itself become a detainee's goal.

Despite some similarities to corrections setting, the detention care setting is unique, and common clinical assumptions about the etiology of acting-out behavior must be suspect. Although some detainees cut themselves or threaten suicide for reasons such as trying to leverage a move to a better tent, other acting-out behavior may have a more malign purpose: creating a distraction so that another detainee may be threatened or killed, distracting custodial staff from efforts by detainees to build a tunnel, or signaling a plan for a riot. At times there may be no apparent reason for such behavior. On one occasion in 2005, detainees were received at Abu Ghraib from an Iraqi prison. All were screened for health and behavioral health needs, and most were found to be in poor condition because of harsh conditions at the Iraqi prison. Somewhat to the surprise of providers, most expressed pleasure at being returned to Abu Ghraib, where they had initially been triaged months earlier before being turned over to the Iraqis. One such individual, who was extremely vocal in his pleasure at returning to the relative comfort of American detention, nevertheless faked a seizure within an hour of being returned to the camp.

Having a designated observation area located in the detainee compound allows medical staff to bring the care to the detainee and limits the need for transport outside of the compound. In addition to observation, basic first aid, including suturing, bandaging, checking vital signs, administering medications, and other necessary interventions that do not require transport to the hospital can be done in the detainee compound. The designated area should be near the corrections staff command post or another area where detainees can be watched constantly but within their compound and as close to their living area as possible, so even direct contact with the behavioral health team can be limited if malingering to obtain such contact is suspected. TF MED 115 dealt with the increasingly self-injurious behavior of one detainee by strictly limiting the patient's access to the hospital, a treatment plan that required constant reassurance to the emergency medical teams that were called on to dress moderately severe self-inflicted injuries in the camp's field setting. This strict restriction on access to the hospital eventually reduced the frequency of self-injurious behavior by the detainee, proving its value.

Medication Management and Distribution

Although some detainees with mental illness will not require medications, others will, and should be offered the appropriate medication to effectively treat their respective illness. Mental illnesses among detainees reflect those in the general population and include mood disorders, anxiety disorders, psychotic disorders, substance use disorders, personality disorders, and others listed in the *Diagnostic and Statistical*

Manual of Psychiatric Disorders. Many medications commonly used and available in the United States are not available throughout the world, so cultural awareness can play an important role in prescribing appropriate medications. A given detainee may have been effectively treated on a psychotropic medication prior to being detained and should remain on that medication. Additionally, if the treatment is going to be necessary and continued after the detainee is released, selection of a medication that is available in the local economy should be strongly considered to facilitate accessibility and ongoing treatment. Otherwise, the indications, contraindications, side effects, and prescribing guidelines for a particular class of medications remain the same as in other settings.

Depending on the size of the detainee population and the number of detainees on medication, distribution can be a complicated and time-consuming process. Care must be given to prevent hoarding; consideration should be given to potential lethality or medical complications; and if possible selection of medications that can be taken daily, rather than more often, will increase compliance and decrease the demand on the staff distributing each medication.

Each staff member responsible for distributing medication should be trained on the proper distribution technique. The technique is essentially the same as what is practiced in many US prisons: distributing each dose separately and watching closely to prevent deception and hoarding. A sequence of actions needs to take place to ensure that the right patient receives the medication, and actually swallows it (Exhibit 40-1).

EXHIBIT 40-1

MEDICATION DISTRIBUTION PROCESS FOR DETAINEES

- Confirm the patient's identity by comparing the detainee's identity card or armband to the person presenting for treatment (trading armbands for favors is not unknown); do not administer the medication if identification is not positive.
- Administer each medication as a single dose; do not give a detainee requiring medication twice a day both doses in the morning.
- Ask the detainees to hold out their hand, and then place the medication in their hand.
- Ensure they have water to help with swallowing the medication.
- Watch them carefully as they put the medication into their mouth and swallow.
- After they swallow, have them open their mouth and stick out their tongue to check for "cheeking" the medication. Have them open their hands with their fingers spread apart to ensure they don't have the medication still in their hands.
- After making sure they have actually swallowed the medication, the detainees can be excused from the area.

This is required for each medication, and each detainee must be required to follow the procedure. Hoarding medications can be a serious problem, and abuse of psychotropics is endemic in this population. Medical staff, including behavioral health personnel, must be trained in this process, and leadership should make spot checks to ensure the process is being adhered to. Mental health personnel should take the lead in this process. Detainees may protest initially, but with continued practice most comply without hesitation. Furthermore, the process of interacting with detainees twice a day improves the therapeutic alliance: some detainees view the interaction as extremely supportive and benefit clinically from the interaction, although this process can be time consuming and very demanding on the medical staff member. Staff members can rotate administering medications. This also helps prevent burnout and helps the staff get to know the detainees.

Some detainees may be on other medications prescribed by different providers. It should be routine to review the medical record or to check with the pharmacy to get a list of all prescribed medications for each detainee to ensure there are no contraindications or overlaps in medication. Medical providers should discuss potential side effects for each medication with detainees and ensure each detainee has given informed consent prior to starting a medication. A medication education program is useful to prepare detainees for eventual release, when they will probably be provided a several-day supply of medication.

Communicating With Other Sites

Interacting with behavioral health staff at other detention sites should be facilitated early in the deployment. Detainees often are transferred from one site to another depending on the legal issues associated with their case. Communication between detention camps allows the effective transfer of detainees with behavioral health problems and enhances the continuation of treatment without interruption. The gaining facility should prepare by reviewing pertinent medical records, obtaining appropriate medications, and discussing any concerns with the staff members who have been treating the detainee. Without a working relationship between staff, detainees will be transferred and the gaining team can potentially be caught off guard and this may impact patient care. Communication between staff at different sites should occur on a regular basis, because moves often are sudden and unanticipated. The frequency can be determined based on patient acuity and need. Sometimes the gaining team receives information about transfers before the losing staff. Problems arise when detainees arrive at the new location and say they were taking psychiatric medications or receiving psychiatric treatment, and there is no record of the treatment. Often the detainee does not know what medications are being administered. Without the knowledge of current diagnosis and treatment, an effective treatment plan may be interrupted and the detainee will have to start the assessment and treatment process from the beginning, a frustration for both the detainee and the behavioral healthcare staff.

SPECIAL CLINICAL ISSUES

Common syndromes in detention care include situational reactions to capture and adjudication, fear of other detainees, distress related to being separated from family, and reactions to the inevitable inactivity associated with detention. Detainees often present with acute anxiety immediately after transfer to the facility or before trial. They often complain of insomnia, fatigue, or depressed mood, symptoms that on inquiry are related to poor sleep habits and inactivity. Awareness of these situational factors can reduce overdiagnosis and overuse of medication with this population.

Individuals in detention often attempt to assert control, gain special privileges, or reduce boredom in ways that bring them to the attention of the behavioral health team. Aggression toward others, unusual behavior such as bathing in sewage, and suicidal statements or parasuicidal behavior may be typical signs of mental illness, but in this context often are manipulative or testing behaviors. Hunger strikes, another behavior of significance seen in the detention population, are discussed in detail below because of their unusual political nature. Differential functional diagnosis and training of custodial staff in behavioral management are important tools in managing these potentially disruptive concerns.

Cognitive disorders present a special challenge in military detainee care. Primary disorders that may present include the entire gamut of these illnesses: developmental disorders including mental retardation; acquired traumatic brain injury, acute or chronic; metabolic, vascular, or other invasive lesions from a medical cause; or age-related dementia. All represent special circumstances affecting the detainee's ability to function and therefore trigger a special obligation on the part of the military caretaker. Unfortunately, most instruments designed to detect cognitive impairment are insensitive to cultural factors and to educational deprivation, making them unsuitable in this setting, even when effective, nonbiased translation services are available.

Privacy and confidentiality are recurring issues in behavioral health service systems. Although it is benevolent to argue that the detained individual has a right to confidentiality, in this setting even the right to refuse treatment may be arguable if detainees' behavior causes substantial risk to themselves or others. Command has a legitimate interest in the mental state of detainees with serious emotional or cognitive issues, as do custodial staff responsible for the compound. It is likely that other residents of the compound will be aware of the patient's behavioral health issues, especially if the behavior is disturbed. Interviews must be conducted in the public view, or at least with a guard present. Reasonable respect for human dignity and privacy is always indicated, but in this setting confidentiality in its strictest interpretation is unlikely and should not be promised.

Medical record management is another special clinical issue in the military detention setting. International standards require a single portable medical record that follows the patient and that can be accessed by the patient, his or her representative, or oversight agencies such as the International Red Cross. This apparently simple requirement is complicated by the typically dispersed nature of forward base detention settings: the record-keeping facility is likely to be in the hospital, not the camp, necessitating maintenance of a local working record in many instances. In the current conflict, detainees are identified by number, rather than by name, because of ambiguities in establishing identities and also to protect the individual. This makes matching the patient to the record difficult as well. Frequent movement of detainees for security or legal reasons further complicates compliance with medical record standards.

HUNGER STRIKES: A UNIQUE CLINICAL ISSUE

Behavioral health consultation to hunger strikes constitutes a special or command-directed assessment and as such requires the involvement of a doctoral-level behavioral health provider to meet the criterion of equivalent care to detainees. The military psychologist, psychiatrist, or doctoral social worker involved must be aware of international standards for the treatment of hunger strikers and the theater policy on hunger strikes; must be cognizant of cultural factors impinging on the detainee's decision to fast; and if at all possible must consult with the facility commander, with Judge Advocate General staff, and with the detainee's primary care provider to determine relevant contextual and situational issues before engaging with the detainee or making recommendations to command.

There is strong international sentiment in favor of hunger strikers, based on a history of their use to protest repressive political regimes. The international medical community supports self-determination by the detainee and proscribes forced feeding.[6,7] Nevertheless, not all hunger strikes have the same degree of legitimacy.[8] Reactive food refusers, much more common than political hunger strikers, are much more likely to rapidly terminate their fast without adverse consequences.

A typical hunger strike protocol[9] requires the behavioral health provider to assess the competence of the fasting detainee at the outset of the hunger strike and daily thereafter. In addition to the complications created by the adversarial nature of a detention setting, the crosscultural aspects of assessment in a military context make this a challenging task. Because assessment will be ongoing throughout the hunger strike, the provider must be aware of the typical course of a hunger strike and of the impact of starvation on an individual's emotional and cognitive status.

Assessment

The detainee engaging in a hunger strike is not allowed to refuse reasonable evaluations. The situation is analogous to evaluating a reluctant person suspected of dementia: the assessment is in the patient's best interest. However, it is important to attempt to obtain informed consent for this and subsequent assessments, if only to establish a reasonable working relationship with the patient. The purpose, extent and limitations of evaluation, boundaries of the relationship with the provider, role conflicts that may develop, and issues of medical record confidentiality should be described. If the detainee refuses to be interviewed, observation and information from collateral sources become critical in establishing the person's competence. In one such instance in theater, the attending physician was given a fixed interview protocol to follow that allowed assessment of immediate, delayed, and procedural memory, and was primed with specific questions to ask. The psychologist observed the interaction on closed-circuit television to allow clinical assessment of the patient's cognitive status.

Relevant factors in determining initial competence to fast include the presence of a mental disorder affecting judgment and decision making; problems with impulse control leading to importune behavior; a cognitive disorder including mental retardation, brain injury, or dementia; coercion by or influence of others; and inaccurate situational information. Personal history, facility records, and clinical observation during the interview are essential tools in the assessment. Standard cognitive instruments are unlikely to be available, making psychometric evaluation of dementia or cognitive disorder difficult. The last two factors listed, coercion or influence by others and inaccurate situational information, are less accessible to historical review or direct assessment, but are important areas of concern. One incipient hunger strike during the TF MED 344 experience was avoided by clarifying the process of judicial review for the detainee.

The initial interview should clarify that the detainee does intend to engage in a hunger strike. Language problems and confusion on the battlefield can create inaccurate perceptions: one detainee transferred from a division internment facility to the tertiary internment facility or theater internment facility for a hunger strike protocol in early 2006 immediately denied intent to fast when interviewed in the emergency room and ate as soon as his gastrointestinal distress and nausea were treated. As part of clarifying intent, the behavioral health provider discusses with each detainee whether he plans to fast to death, or if he will accept medical advice and limit his hunger strike when his health is imperiled.

The behavioral health provider is mandated to clarify the detainee's reason for entering into a hunger strike. The provider does not, however, become engaged in negotiating with the detainee concerning demands, for a variety of reasons: maintaining a useful neutrality with the detainee separates the issue of refusal to eat from the issue that the detainee wishes to bring to public attention, an important strategy in managing the hunger strike situation. In one typical hunger strike situation, the detainee began every conversation with a request to see the combatant commander; each request was met with a response that the commander was aware of the request and the psychologist could do nothing to facilitate this matter.

Daily reassessment of the detainee's emotional and cognitive status is required. A routine should be established with the primary care provider that allows the behavioral health provider to review any medical factors that may be affecting the detainee and to interview the primary care provider about his or her interactions with the detainee. Initial reassessments are usually not fruitful except to help establish a pattern and a relationship, as cognitive and emotional changes are unlikely in the first week of the hunger strike.

Follow-up assessments include evaluation of subtle cognitive changes caused by altered nutritional status, such as a tendency to make more risky decisions, become irritable, and be increasingly oppositional, especially in situations involving confrontation.[10] Minor memory or concentration problems that may signal the onset of delirium resulting from reduced metabolism, medications, altered nutrition, or organ dysfunction must be recognized early to avoid rapid cognitive deterioration. Hunger strikers with suicidal or morbid ideation, alteration in future orientation, or reduced interest in pleasurable activity, may be depressed—a condition for which they may allow treatment. The assessment also evaluates the detainee's confidence in his physician, his understanding of the medical information he is provided, and his intent to persist in the hunger strike.

Cognitive measures are sensitive to educational and cultural factors (few instruments have been normed for use in different cultures) and are vulnerable to practice effects; repeated administration on a daily basis will invalidate their use just as the information they can provide becomes more critical. The behavioral health provider should design an observational protocol using routine interactions in the detention setting to assess memory, concentration, verbal fluency, and motor coordination rather than relying on tests.

Documentation of findings is critical. There are three possible outcomes of a hunger strike: the detainee ends the hunger strike voluntarily, the detainee is fed forcibly, or the detainee dies from complications related to not eating. Especially in the event of forced feeding or death, the basis for medical and subsequent administrative decisions about care must be clearly documented and communicated.

Intervention

The behavioral health provider cannot collaborate with coercive or deceptive strategies, nor agree to strategies that might be perceived as maltreatment of the detainee. Although it is reasonable to withdraw privileges or hold the detainee in isolation to prevent contagion or coercion, for example, it is not reasonable to restrict access to hygiene facilities or exercise. Exposing the patient to pleasant aromas and pleasing presentations of meals may be useful; deliberate exposure to others eating, taunting with food, or excessive exposure to food may constitute abuse and is likely to be counterproductive. Threats of forced feeding are counterproductive, create an adversarial atmosphere, and are considered coercive by the international community.

Psychological management of the hunger strike should focus on limiting unwarranted attention to the detainee during the hunger strike to reduce unintended reinforcement of the unwanted behavior. Medical management and administrative negotiations should be matter-of-fact and without emotional overlay. Effort should be made to separate treatment of the hunger strike and treatment of the concerns raised by the detainee: the decision-maker for the demands should be distinct from the medical and custodial personnel who work with the detainee. These two issues should never be linked during discussions with the detainee.

Consultation

The military behavioral health provider consults to the attending physician and to command regarding various aspects of the hunger strike situation, often in ways not anticipated by the command authority. It was the senior author's experience that command expectations may exceed the role of the consultant: there may be an expectation that the behavioral health provider has greater insight into the hunger striker's motivations than is possible, or that the provider may in some way be able to intervene and somehow induce the hunger striker to end the fast. Clear delineation of roles and capabilities is essential.

Healthcare providers do have a valuable role in protecting both the patient and the military command from the adverse consequences of the hunger strike. The careful balance between consulting to the care of the hunger striker, balancing competing ethical issues often associated with this situation, acknowledging international standards of care, and advising command regarding effective actions requires a thoughtful approach to this type of situation.

The behavioral health provider discusses with the treating physician the available literature on hunger strikes, the ethics associated with managing both hunger strikers with a terminal goal and those willing to accede to medical advice, and the importance of avoiding an adversarial relationship with the patient. The physician should be encouraged to establish benchmarks for various decisions, including informing the patient of critical medical milestones and what findings to use to signal command that medical incapacity may be imminent.

Command is likely to consider forced feeding very early in the hunger strike, in part because the consequences of allowing the detainee to die in custody are extreme and in part because of limited knowledge about the likely time frame of the hunger strike. Keeping the detainee alive through forced feeding, however, may simply prolong the hunger strike, carries its own medical risks, and is not likely to be necessary for health reasons in the first weeks of the strike. Good medical advice is critical to limiting the commander's reactive responses, and effective consultation on approaches to the hunger striker will give command options other than coercive methods.

SUMMARY

Providing psychiatric care in a battle zone to an enemy combatant poses unique professional and personal challenges. There is no true civilian analogue to this situation. Because the mission is unique, it is important to develop a clear understanding of the clinical mission and its inherent systemic issues before entering the area of operations. It is vital to understand the full political and humanitarian impact of the behavioral healthcare provider's role in this setting to appreciate the importance of the mission and to reconcile the accompanying complex and often contradictory emotions and reactions.

REFERENCES

1. US Department of Justice, Federal Bureau of Prisons. Program statements for medical, dental, and health policies (6000 series). Available at: http://www.bop.gov/DataSource/execute/dsPolicyLoc. Accessed July 8, 2010.

2. American Public Health Association. *Standards for Mental Health Services in Correctional Institutions*. 3rd ed. Washington DC: APHA; 2003.

3. US Department of the Army. *Enemy Prisoners of War, Retained Personnel, Civilian Internees and Other Detainees*. Washington, DC: DA; 1997. Army Regulation 190-8.

4. US Department of the Army. *Medical Support to Detainee Operations*. Washington, DC: DA; 2006. Field Manual 4-02.46.

5. US Department of the Army. *The Law of Land Warfare*. Washington, DC: DA; 1956. Field Manual 27-10.

6. World Medical Association. WMA Declaration of Malta on Hunger Strikers. Available at: http://www.wma.net/en/30publications/10policies/h31/index.html. Accessed July 8, 2010.

7. English V, Gardner J, Romano-Critchley G, Sommerville A. Management of prisoners on hunger strikes. *J Med Ethics*. 2001;27:203–204.

8. Reyes H. Medical and ethical aspects of hunger strikes in custody and the issue of torture. International Committee of the Red Cross Web site. 1998. Available at: http://www.icrc.org/web/eng/siteeng0.nsf/htmlall/health-article-010198?opendocument. Accessed July 8, 2010.

9. Oklahoma Department of Corrections. Hunger strikes. Operations Memorandum 140122. Available at: www.doc.state.ok.us/Offtech/op140122.pdf. Accessed July 8, 2010.

10. Fessler DMT. The implications of starvation induced psychological changes for the ethical treatment of hunger strikers. *J Med Ethics*. 2003;23:243–247.

Chapter 41

MENTAL HEALTHCARE IN THE UNITED KINGDOM ARMED FORCES

NEIL GREENBERG, MD*; JAMIE HACKER HUGHES, PsychD†; MARK EARNSHAW, BA(Hons), MSc‡; and SIMON WESSELY, MD§

*Commander, Medical Corps, United Kingdom Armed Forces; Defence Professor of Mental Health, King's College, London, Weston Education Centre, Cutcombe Road, London SE5 9RJ; formerly, Senior Lecturer in Military Psychiatry, Academic Center for Defence Mental Health, King's College, London

†Head of Defence Clinical Psychology, Ministry of Defence, Joint Medical Command, Coltman House, Whittington Barracks, Lichfield, United Kingdom WS14 9PY; formerly, Senior Lecturer in Military Psychology, Academic Center for Defence Mental Health, London, United Kingdom

‡Lieutenant Colonel QARANC, Ministry of Defence, St Georges Court, Bloomsbury Way, London, WC1A 2SH, United Kingdom; formerly, Research Fellow, Academic Centre for Defence Mental Health, London, United Kingdom

§Department Head, Department of Psychological Medicine, King's Centre for Military Health Research, King's College, Weston Education Centre, 10 Cutcombe Road, London SE5 9RJ United Kingdom; formerly, Honorary Lecturer in Forensic Psychiatry, Institute of Psychiatry, London, United Kingdom

INTRODUCTION

Defense mental health services (DMHS) in the United Kingdom (UK) are primarily community based and provide both operational and homeland services to all 200,000 of the personnel in the UK armed forces. This chapter will examine the history of military mental health in the UK and bring readers up to date on important procedural and operational aspects of the DMHS today.

HISTORY

In keeping with its tradition as the senior military service in the UK, the Royal Navy first established formal services to manage and treat service personnel who suffered from psychological problems. In August, 1818, a lunatic asylum was opened at the Royal Naval Hospital Haslar[1]; today a Royal Navy Department of Community Mental Health (DCMH) remains at Haslar Hospital. With the outbreak of World War I, British Army psychologists and neurologists deployed to France in 1914 in support of British troops. Operating from field hospitals, casualty clearing stations, and, later, "NYDN" (not yet diagnosed neurological) hospitals, these practitioners saw large numbers of personnel suffering from "shell shock," "disordered action of the heart," and related syndromes. Personnel deemed unfit for further combat, at least in the immediate future, were evacuated to rear areas or to the UK.[2] A large number of hospitals were established in Britain, including Craiglockhart[3]; Seale Hayne, a converted agricultural college; and Sir Edward Mapother's No. 2 General Hospital in Stockport.[4] These institutions provided treatment for shell shock and other disorders, aiming, if possible, to return individuals to the front to continue fighting. Specialist training courses in military psychiatry were also established at the Maudsley Hospital in London and, by Gordon Mott, at Maghull Hospital in Liverpool. Specialist centers for the treatment of disordered action of the heart were also established at Mount Vernon in Hampstead and Sobraon House in Colchester.

Although the British Psychological Society had been founded at University College London in the 1890s, psychology was a largely experimental science in World War I; it was some years before psychotherapy and clinical psychology became disciplines in their own right. The first military psychological practitioners, such as Charles S Myers and William H Rivers, were mostly medical doctors. Myers later became consultant psychologist to the British Expeditionary Force, and Gordon Holmes was consultant neurologist. Myers established four forward NYDN centers modeled on the French system,[5] and, later, five forward "disordered action of the heart" centers in France, in addition to the hospitals in Britain. These facilities were established well before Thomas Salmon, the American psychiatrist, visited France in 1917 and influenced what has since become known as "forward psychiatry."[6]

Following World War I, the UK built up a network of special civilian treatment centers and hospitals to treat the ongoing casualties generated by the war, peaking in 1921. (At that time nearly 15,000 inpatients and 3,000 outpatients were still suffering with war-related psychological disorders.) Although the vast majority of those who worked throughout the war for the British military mental health services returned to civilian employment, some remained in the services, forming a core of psychological practitioners during the build up to World War II. For the additional practitioners necessary for the Royal Navy, Army, and new Royal Air Force (RAF), formed between the wars from the Royal Flying Corps (originally part of the Army), neurologists and psychiatrists were recruited from four main sources (all in London): the Tavistock Clinic (Army), the Maudsley Hospital (Royal Navy), Saint George's Hospital (Royal Navy), and Guy's Hospital (RAF).[7]

For the first time psychologists were also recruited to work in personnel selection. Otherwise, the pattern of British Army military mental health service provision in World War II nearly mirrored that in the earlier war. In addition to a number of forward hospitals, treatment facilities also operated in the UK, including No. 41 Neuropathic Hospital in Bishop's Lydeard (where the Tavistock Clinic psychoanalyst JA Hadfield, one of the first to use collective hypnosis and abreaction, was based) and the better-known centers at Northfield (where Wilfred Bion, John Rickman, and Michael Foulkes, the founders of group psychotherapy, worked). In addition, forward psychiatry began to be practiced, often by accident or through necessity, but increasingly by design, in North Africa, Italy, and northwest Europe.

Support for the psychiatrists was far from unanimous, however; many saw them as fifth columnists (a clandestine group seeking to undermine the government), and Winston Churchill referred to psychiatrists as "gentlemen asking odd questions."[8] Stigma was still attached to patients with mental illness. The RAF Neurological Hospital at Matlock was established as the final treatment center for the growing number of "lack of moral fiber" (LMF) cases, an administrative category rather than a diagnosis. This category was begun after 250 "breakdown" cases occurred after the Battle of Britain in 1940; by the end of the war the LMF category included nearly 3,000 cases of breakdown per year.[9] It is believed that fear of being labelled as LMF was essential to keeping RAF pilots motivated to fly despite the high risk of being shot down (mission attrition rates of 50% were common, especially during the early days of the war).[10] Sergeants labeled as LMF were reduced to the lowest rank and put to work shovelling coal, peeling potatoes, or even mining coal. LMF officers were asked to resign or transferred to desk jobs in administration. Many of those categorized as LMF had already completed a dozen or more operational raids, but the designation was deemed useful for encouraging continuous operational flying in the face of extreme risk.

By the end of 1943, the number of psychiatrists totalled 227 in the British Army, 43 in the RAF, and 35 in the Royal Navy.[11–13] The majority of the 35 military psychologists[14] worked with selection panels and designed aptitude tests to ensure that officers were up to standard. These World War II selection tests included the "leaderless group," a method by which a group of potential officer candidates are encouraged to come up with a plan to deal with a mock incident without a leader being assigned in order to see what transpires (ie, does a "natural" leader emerge?). It remains the basis for selecting the officers' cadre today. Unlike in the United States during World War II, mental health professionals were rarely used in screening for vulnerability to future breakdown. This aptitude testing policy represented a major "democratization" of officer selection, in keeping with the social transformations the war brought about across society. At the end of the war, however, all the psychologists were demobilized, leaving only the psychiatrists in the service.

In the late 1960s, the UK began deploying large numbers of forces to contain the increasingly unstable situation in Northern Ireland. The particular demands of this counterinsurgency operation—effectively asymmetric warfare with an unknown and unseen enemy—began to take its toll on the mental health of troops. The Northern Ireland "troubles" continued until the late 1990s. Although no concrete evidence suggests that the conflict was more traumatogenic than other military operations, many of its veterans suffered from posttraumatic stress disorder (PTSD) and other psychological injuries.

In 1982, Britain again went to war, this time thousands of miles away across the Atlantic,[15] to recapture the Falkland Islands invaded by Argentina weeks before. Although the Royal Navy deployed psychiatrists to the conflict, the overall mental health burden was thought to be small. However, some current anecdotal evidence indicates that marines who sailed back to the UK after the war fared better in mental health outcomes than their airborne colleagues and other infantry units that were air-trooped home. These stories suggest that the marines settled back into their day-to-day lives after talking through their experiences during the sea voyage, as there was no formal mental health support made available for the troops during the voyage home. The airborne paratroopers, in contrast, displayed violent and aggressive behavior at home because they missed the necessary time to "decompress."[16] However, no research has been carried out to support or refute these claims.

At the end of the 20th century, UK forces were deployed on a number of fronts. Operation Banner, the name given to the Northern Ireland deployment, continued, with troops rotated at regular intervals for 3-month "emergency" tours, 6-month tours, and 2-year "permanent" tours. In addition, British troops were deployed on United Nations and North Atlantic Treaty Organization peace and stabilization missions to Bosnia-Herzegovina, Kosovo, and Macedonia. Army field mental health teams (FMHTs) deployed in the majority of these operations, often led by psychiatrists in the initial "surge" phases, but increasingly relying on a pool of well-trained, highly skilled, and relatively autonomous mental health nurses drawn from the hospitals and community clinics to operational roles.[17] At the same time, however, defense cuts and downsizing led to the closure of all but three military hospitals; these have since shut. Today, there is no dedicated military hospital in the UK, and military medical care is provided in military wings of civilian hospitals called "military district hospital units."

In addition to these and other peacekeeping operations (eg, in Lebanon, Rwanda, and Sierra Leone),[18] the UK was involved in two major, if short-lived, wars, followed by ongoing and increasingly intense operations in the hostile theaters of Iraq and Afghanistan. Saddam Hussein's invasion of Kuwait in 1991 led to a rapid British military deployment—Operation Granby—as part of a multinational coalition led by the United States to reclaim the country from the Iraqi forces. British Army psychiatrists and mental health nurses deployed with the Army field hospitals as field psychiatric teams but, where possible, adopted a freestanding roving role providing mental health briefings, psychological debriefings, and mental health assessments as required throughout theater. A Royal Navy mental health team deployed with a hospital ship, offshore in the Mediterranean Sea, and RAF mental health teams supervised the aeromedical evacuation and repatriation of mental health casualties. This role continues outside times of major conflict, with RAF mental health nurses on standby to escort service personnel with mental health and other problems back to the UK from anywhere in the world.

When British and American forces invaded Iraq in 2003 (the British component of the invasion and occupation is known as Operation Telic), FMHTs composed of psychiatrists and Army mental health nurses again deployed with the UK's air assault and armored brigades, and were part of two military field hospitals. Again, the Royal Navy supplied a mental health capability on the primary casualty-receiving facility—Royal Fleet Auxiliary Argus—and the RAF continued to operate as before. All mental health aeromedical evacuations and repatriations went to Duchess of Kent's Psychiatric Hospital (since closed) for assessment, treatment, and, if necessary, admission. Those requiring outpatient treatment, including mobilized reservists (who made up a large percentage of some Operation Telic units, especially medical units), were referred to the network of DCMH.

CONTEMPORARY DEFENSE MENTAL HEALTH SERVICES

The goal of DMHS is to provide military personnel with speedy access to skilled, effective, flexible treatment based on individual needs.[19] The DMHS approach aims to foster recovery and rehabilitation, ensuring that personnel are rapidly returned to duty whenever possible, or supported and enabled to make a smooth, seamless, and effective transition back into civilian life. Treatment, care, and rehabilitation are provided in close proximity to the person's work environment to maximize occupational recovery and in close partnership with primary and secondary care facilities. A clear understanding of the unique nature of military ethos, composition, and task underpins the effective delivery of mental healthcare to service populations. Delivery of this care is multidisciplinary, provided by a variety of skilled professionals, depending on individual needs.

The UK armed forces emphasize that stress management and day-to-day mental health hygiene are functions of the chain of command rather than medical or support services. The same principles apply for physical and psychological disorders; for instance, the management of hydration is directed by unit leaders in the same way as stress management. Both may need a subject matter expert to provide appropriate information and training; however, the subject matter expert does not assume responsibility for the process.[19,20]

When the chain of command is unable to continue to support personnel, three levels of mental healthcare provision exist: (1) primary care, (2) community mental healthcare, and (3) inpatient care. Provision of mental healthcare has moved from a hospital-based to a community-based service, mirroring changes in the UK's civilian National Health Service. Care in the community, as the process is termed in the National Health Service, has been a key element of UK government health planning over the last 2 decades and is considered well-suited to both military and civilian mental healthcare delivery. A report by an independent team of experts led to the closure of the last military inpatient facility in early 2004. Currently all inpatient care is provided by an independent service provider (a private psychiatric hospital) on a pay-per-patient basis. Military protocols advocate using inpatient care for the minimum amount of time possible because community management is seen as the key to effective occupational rehabilitation.

The "workhorse" of the system is the DCMH, which carries out all specialist mental health functions within the DMHS. There are 15 DCMHs in the UK, with additional units in Germany, Cyprus, and Gibraltar. The departments are tasked with treating service personnel, providing a range of mental health educational programs, liaising with the independent service provider, and facilitating medical discharges when appropriate. The current cadre of some 200 military mental health professionals across the services are primarily uniformed members of the Royal Navy, Army, or Air Force. However, social work and psychology services are provided by civil servants. Most of the service members (75%) are nurses, with the remainder composed of psychiatrists, clinical psychologists, and social workers. Presently occupational psychologists and occupational therapists do not form part of the uniformed cadre.

Policy and strategy for the DMHS comes from the surgeon general's department through executive and professional advisory committees. In the UK, the military surgeon general, who may be a member of any service, is the head medical officer of all three services. The head of DMHS is the defense consultant advisor, and each service has a consultant advisor and a senior nursing officer. Although DMHS care is delivered on a triservice basis (ie, mental health professionals from each service routinely provide care to personnel of all three services), each service is responsible for career development and personnel management of its members.

Operational Organization

The deployable uniformed mental health assets are composed of registered mental health nurses (also called community psychiatric nurses), and consultant psychiatrists. The consultant psychiatrists traditionally have deployed only during the initial surge phase of operational deployments; at later stages, community psychiatric nurses form FMHTs with telephone supervision and a visiting service from a consultant psychiatrist. Experience has shown that the most effective FMHTs comprise one officer at captain-to-major level (or equivalent) and one senior noncommissioned officer. This structure helps remove barriers across the military rank structure and destigmatize military mental health.

Operational planning includes a casualty estimate, which, in conjunction with the size of the deploying force, dictates which mental health assets are deployed. In the majority of traditional war fighting scenarios, an FMHT consisting of a psychiatrist and two or three community psychiatric nurses is deployed at role 2 (role 2 is usually collocated with the dressing station in the region of 1-hour travel by road from the fighting troops). Traditionally based at role 3 (3–4 hours traveling time by road from the front line) and collocated with the field hospital is a further complement of mental health personnel including a consultant psychiatrist and community psychiatric nurses.

Predeployment

Before deployments, the DCMH and FMHT assess medically downgraded personnel or those undergoing mental health treatment to give a clear indication to commanders about whether these personnel might be fit to deploy, and if so, whether there are employability restrictions. Ideally, the deploying FMHT also assists with preoperational stress management presentations[5] and meets the commanders of units they will support in the operational theater to clarify arrangements (mental health personnel are often logistically prevented from deploying with units they supported in peacetime locations). The provision of formal briefings to all deploying personnel is mandated by policy. Such briefings are intended not only to provide factual information on stress reactions but also to detail the mental health provision (and how to access it) during the forthcoming operation. Specific briefings on subjects such as body handling or dealing with prisoners of war may be given, depending on the nature of the forthcoming deployment.

During Deployment

Teams aim to travel to all units in theater seeing patients as required (usually referred from medical services) and undertake a command liaison role within the unit lines. Operational travel restrictions sometimes prevent this mode of operations, and mental health professionals can then find themselves stuck in one location, unable to respond to other needs. In these instances patients may travel to the FMHT, but they will consequentially lose proximity support from their units.

Assessment of potential patients in theater loosely follows the flowchart in Figure 41-1, which explains the referral pathway according to the seminal work undertaken by Goldberg and Huxley concerning the pathways to care followed by psychiatric patients in the community.[21] Mental health nurses work with unit commanders and medical staffs to provide occupationally relevant advice aiming to maintain the fighting force whenever possible. However, unit commanders hold the ultimate responsibility in assigning operational duties. These decisions are based on a number of factors including the operational situation, the unit support available, and the location of medical and psychiatric assets.

Postdeployment

In line with postdeployment operational stress management policy,[20] DMHS professionals assist with any decompression process. The level of decompression package is left to the brigade commander to decide in consultation with medical or psychiatric advisors. The surgeon general's policy dictates that some form of homecoming brief will be delivered to returning troops, which should be tailored to suit the intensity of the operation once the unit has returned to the decompression area (a low-threat location in theater or another base such as Cyprus) or peacetime location.

Ministry of Defence Posttraumatic Stress Disorder Legal Case

In 2002, a number of former military personnel sued the Ministry of Defence (MOD) over claims of psychological injury related to their operational service.[22] The claimants did not dispute their assignment of operational duties but claimed that the MOD was negligent in failing to provide appropriate predeployment screening and training as well as appropriate postoperational care that might have prevented, or at least detected and treated, their disorders prior to discharge from the services. Judgment in the PTSD group action was handed down by Lord Justice Owen on May 21, 2003. The judge found for the MOD on almost all of the generic issues, despite criticizing the ministry in several areas. The judge found against the MOD in 4 of the 16 lead cases, but these cases turned on their individual facts and did not represent institutional failure.

During subsequent examination of the case, the judge made clear that the MOD has a duty to provide a safe system of work for its personnel where reasonable

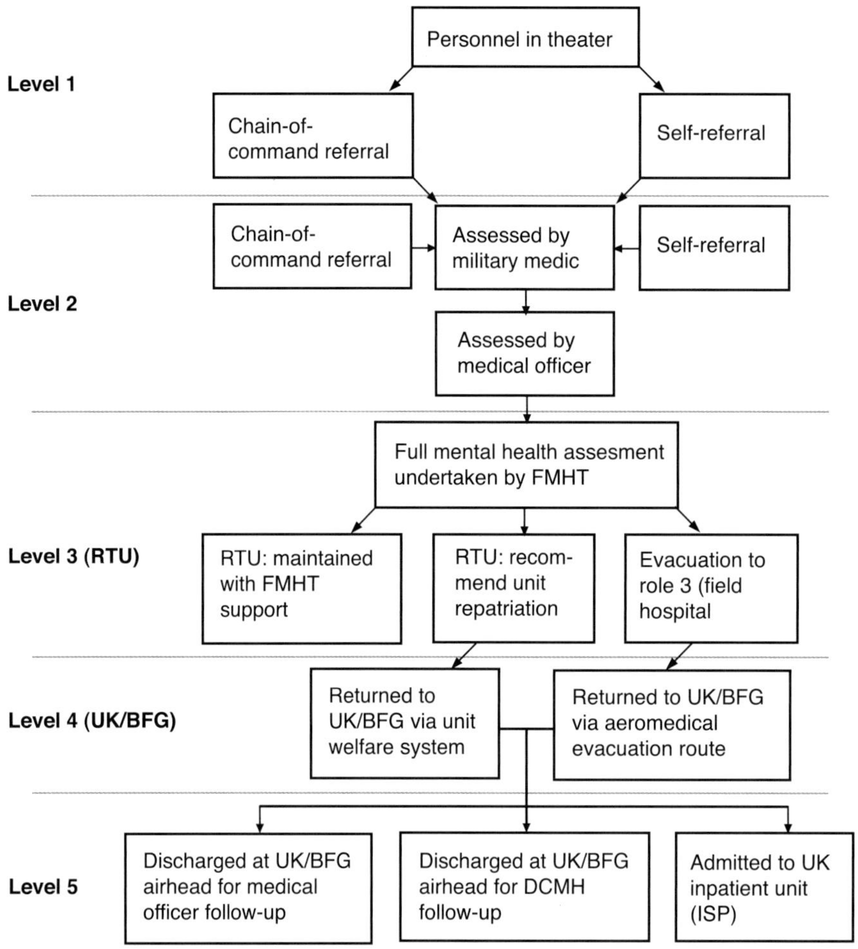

Figure 41-1. Operational mental health referral flowchart.
BFG: British Forces Germany
DCMH: Department of Community Mental Health
FMHT: Field Mental Health Team
ISP: inpatient service provider
RTU: return to unit
UK: United Kingdom

and practical. It does not, however, have a duty to do so in the course of combat, where the interests of personnel are subordinate to the military objective; this is known as "combat immunity." The judge defined combat so that the immunity was not restricted to troops in the presence of the enemy but also all active operations against the enemy when personnel are exposed to the threat of attack, including attack and resistance, advance and retreat, pursuit and avoidance, and reconnaissance and engagement. Immunity extends to the planning of and preparation for operations in which there is the possibility of attack or resistance, including peacekeeping or policing operations in which personnel are exposed to the threat of attack.

The case was heated, and 16 subject matter experts from the UK, United States, Israel, and Australia gave evidence at the trial. Subjects discussed included screening before recruitment and before and after deployment, the potential use of critical incident psychological debriefings, preventative stress inoculation, and decompression or postdeployment briefings. None of these measures were found to be robustly effective in the prevention or treatment of psychological injury.[22] An MOD internal report,[23] providing guidance for the future management of operational mental health issues, called for initiating a robust research program, training the chain of command to identify the signs of stress and assist anyone likely to "break down," and instituting a stress awareness strategy to destigmatize mental health problems and encourage those who need help to request it.[6]

Trauma Risk Management

In the late 1990s, the brigadier in charge of the Royal Marines Commandos, an elite group of military maritime personnel who often form the UK's rapid reaction force, tasked a staff officer to investigate ways to improve his troops' mental health in response to operational stress. An initial critical incident psychological debriefing program was rejected within the robust culture of the marines. Staff subsequently developed a more successful peer support/psychological risk assessment program called Trauma Risk Management (TRiM), which has since been adopted by a number of UK organizations, including some of the emergency services and the diplomatic service.

The program, now fully integrated into the Royal Marines and many parts of the Royal Navy and Army, aims to equip nonmedical personnel with the skills to detect service members who might be suffering from traumatic stress problems. TRiM practitioners are trained to provide relevant mentoring and support in the aftermath of potentially traumatic events and deployments and, when necessary, to encourage persistently distressed personnel to seek referral from professional sources of mental health support.[24,25] The program has been embedded within the existing personnel management systems. For example, during initial training young marines are instructed in field craft, shooting skills, and using TRiM support. Potential TRiM practitioners are selected for their interpersonal skills, experience, and common sense. Once trained, they provide basic psychoeducational packages to their units. Furthermore, all promotion courses within the Royal Marines Command provide some detail on TRiM, ensuring that all marines, and especially those in leadership positions, are aware of TRiM and able to use the system. The training program has gained external certification and has also been considered by the US military[26] (preliminary training courses for US personnel were held in Washington, DC, in 2003, and San Diego, California, in 2005). The TRiM system is also to form part of the new US Army Psychological First Aid package designed for use by Army medical staff.

Among the TRiM program's strategic aims is to be a vehicle for organizational culture change. The course aims to destigmatize mental health issues and provide a pool of informed peers or mentors who are likely to be more acceptable than mental health professionals as sources of support. Research on UK military peacekeepers showed that more than 90% of personnel talked to peers about their deployments, whereas only 8% talked to medical or welfare staff.[27]

A cluster randomized controlled trial is underway in the Royal Navy to ensure that TRiM does not suffer the same fate as the critical incident psychological debriefing program. The trial will attempt to identify any potential for TRiM to do harm, as well as any positive or negative cultural changes that occur on warships that have received TRiM training. A possible positive result of the trial would be an increase in referrals with no increase in mental health problems.

CURRENT RESEARCH AND FUTURE DIRECTIONS

The King's Centre for Military Health Research (KCMHR) is the primary UK military mental health research institution. Although numerous other academic centers conduct relevant research into both serving and retired UK military service personnel, none has a solely military orientation. The center boasts close links with an internationally acclaimed war studies department at King's College London and offers a master of science degree in war and psychiatry.

KCMHR has just completed a 3-year study on the health of about 12,000 randomly sampled UK military personnel, examining the recurrence of "Gulf War syndrome" problems and the rates of psychiatric injury following Operation Telic. Results so far show no rise in multisymptom conditions.[28,29] Furthermore, regular military personnel have not been especially affected by service in Iraq in terms of posttraumatic stress or general psychological or physical symptoms. Veterans of Iraq deployments drink more alcohol and display more risky behaviors than those who did not deploy, but the absolute risk increase has been small. This result does not appear to be true for reservists, who are displaying significant changes in both psychological and physical health. The absolute risk increase is still small (a doubling of PTSD symptoms from about 3% to 6%); however, the research has prompted MOD attempts to mitigate the problem (made more acute because veteran and reservist mental healthcare is not provided by the military).

With predeployment data on a subset of those deployed in Operation Telic, KCMHR was able to model the effects of predeployment mental health screening (when it had been conducted). The results showed that predeployment screening would not have reduced postoperational psychiatric illness, but would have had a significant deleterious effect on the numbers of personnel deployed.[30]

Other work underway is investigating the impact of military service on family life, the usefulness of medical countermeasures to mental illness, and the effects of potential exposure to depleted uranium. KCMHR intends to follow the cohort for many years to gain relevant insights into the health of the UK service member in the 21st century. Preliminary results that have influenced strategic MOD policy include the finding that providing too much informed choice can adversely influence vaccine compliance[31] and that predeployment mental health screening is likely ineffective.[30]

The recently established Academic Centre for Defence Mental Health is a small cadre of MOD mental health staff attempting to stimulate DMHS research. The center also provides the defense consultant advisor in psychiatry, an advisor to the surgeon general, with regular reports on emergent research findings into potentially useful MOD policy actions. The MOD is increasingly realizing the need to use relevant research findings to inform future policy making.

SUMMARY

UK military psychiatry has a rich historical basis. Modern mental health provision is heavily community based, with operational provision being delivered by rendering appropriate support to the chain of command, which, in UK military doctrine, is primarily responsible for the psychological welfare of troops. The DMHS cadre of single-service uniformed and civilian staff provide triservice care, with a recently increased emphasis on research that is already providing a plethora of useful data informing and influencing MOD policy. Having weathered a protracted legal case and the shrinkage of the armed forces, the DMHS will continue to focus on supporting the sailors, soldiers, and airmen of the UK armed forces, as well as personnel and operational commanders in their missions, while ensuring the use of the ever-increasing body of research evidence to inform future practice.

REFERENCES

1. Jones E, Greenberg N. Royal Naval psychiatry: organisation, methods and outcomes 1900–1945. *Mariner's Mirror.* 2006;92:190–203.
2. Johnson W, Rows RG. Neurasthenia and the war neuroses. In: McPherson WG, Herrringham WP, Elliott TR, eds. *History of the Great War, Diseases of the War.* Vol 2. London, England: HMSO; 1923.
3. Salmon TW. The care and treatment of mental diseases and war neuroses ('shell shock') in the British Army. *Ment Hyg.* 1917;1:509–547.
4. Jones E, Wessely S. *Shell Shock to PTSD: Military Psychiatry from 1900 to the Gulf War.* Hove, UK: Psychology Press; 2005.
5. Myers CS. *Shell Shock in France, Based on a War Diary.* Cambridge, England: Cambridge University Press; 1940.
6. Salmon TW. Care and treatment of mental diseases and war neurosis ("shell shock") in the British army. In: Salmon TW, Fenton N, eds. *Neuropsychiatry.* Vol X. The Medical Department of the United States Army in the World War. Washington, DC: GPO; 1929: 497–547.
7. Shepard B. *A War of Nerves: Soldiers and Psychiatrists 1914–1994.* London, England: Jonathan Cape; 2000.
8. Churchill WS. War cabinet minutes (TNA PREM4/15/2. December 1942). In: Jones E, Wessely S. *Shell Shock to PTSD: Military Psychiatry from 1900 to the Gulf War.* Hove, UK: Psychology Press; 2005.
9. McCarthy J. Aircrew and "lack of moral fibre" in the Second World War. *War Soc.* 1995;18:87–101.
10. Jones E. "LMF": The use of psychiatric stigma in the Royal Air Force during the Second World War. *J Milit Hist.* 2006;70:439–458.
11. O'Connor R. Work of Psychologists and Psychiatrists in the Services. TNA/WO32/11974, 5 December 1946. UK National Archives (Kew, Richmond, Surrey).
12. Rees JR. *The Shaping of Psychiatry by War.* London, England: Chapman and Hall; 1945.
13. Sandiford HA. Army Psychiatry Advisory Committee Minutes (TNA, WO32/13462, 5 July 1945). In: Jones E, Wessely S. *Shell Shock to PTSD: Military Psychiatry From 1900 to the Gulf War.* Hove, UK: Psychology Press; 2005.

14. Hacker Hughes JGH. Unpublished MSc Dissertation. *British Naval Psychology 1937–1947: Round Pegs Into Square Holes?*: University of London. 2007.

15. Freedman L. *The Official History of the Falklands Campaign.* Vol II. *War and Diplomacy*. London, England: Frank Cass; 2005.

16. Hughes JG, Earnshaw NM, Greenberg N, et al. Use of psychological decompression in military operational environments. *Mil Med*. 2008;173(6):534–538.

17. Deahl MP, Gilham AB, Thomas J, Searle NM, Srinivasan M. Psychological sequelae following the Gulf War: factors associated with subsequent morbidity and the effectiveness of psychological debriefing. *Br J Psychiatry.* 1994;165:60–65.

18. Hacker Hughes JGH, Campion BC, Cameron F, Devon M. Results of a survey on psychological health of British peacekeepers deployed during 2002. *European Psychother* [special edition]. 2003: 204.

19. Greenberg N, Temple M, Neal L, Palmer I. Military psychiatry: a unique national resource. *Psychiatr Bull.* 2002;26:227–229.

20. Surgeon General's Policy Letter 03/06. The Prevention and Management of Traumatic Stress Related Disorders in AFs Personnel on Operations. Ministry of Defence: London, England; 2006

21. Goldberg D, Huxley P. *Mental Illness in the Community*. London, England: Tavistock Publications; 1980.

22. McGeorge T, Hacker Hughes J, Wessely S. The MOD PTSD class action—a psychiatric perspective. *Occup Health Rev.* 2006;122:21–28.

23. Applegate D. Lessons learnt from the PTSD group actions. Service Personnel Board: a paper by the stress project leader. Ministry of Defence: London, England; 2003.

24. Jones N, Roberts P, Greenberg N. Peer-group risk assessment: a post-traumatic management strategy for hierarchical organizations. *Occup Med (Lond).* 2003;53:469–475.

25. Greenberg N, Cawkill P, Sharpley J. How to TRiM away at posttraumatic stress reactions: traumatic risk management—now and the future. *J R Nav Med Serv*. 2005;91:26–31.

26. Keller RT, Greenberg N, Bobo WV, Roberts P, Jones N, Orman DT. Soldier peer mentoring care and support: bringing psychological awareness to the front. *Mil Med.* 2005;170:355–361.

27. Greenberg N, Thomas S, Iversen A, Unwin C, Hull L, Wessely S. Do military peacekeepers want to talk about their experiences? Perceived psychological support of UK military peacekeepers on return from deployment. *J Ment Health.* 2003;12:6:561–569.

28. Hotopf M, Hull L, Fear NT, et al. The health of UK military personnel who deployed to the 2003 Iraq war: a cohort study. *Lancet.* 2006;367:1731–1741.

29. Horn O, Hull L, Jones M, et al. Is there an Iraq war syndrome? Comparison of the health of UK service personnel after the Gulf and Iraq wars. *Lancet.* 2006;367:1742–1746.

30. Rona R, Jones M, Hull L, et al. Would mental health screening of the UK armed forces before the Iraq War have prevented subsequent psychological morbidity? *BMJ.* 2006;333:983–984.

31. Murphy D, Hooper R, French C, Jones M, Rona R, Wessely S. Is increased reporting of symptomatic ill health in Gulf War veterans related to how one asks the question? *J Psychosom Res.* 2006;61:181–186.

COMBAT AND OPERATIONAL BEHAVIORAL HEALTH

Section VIII: Other Military Issues

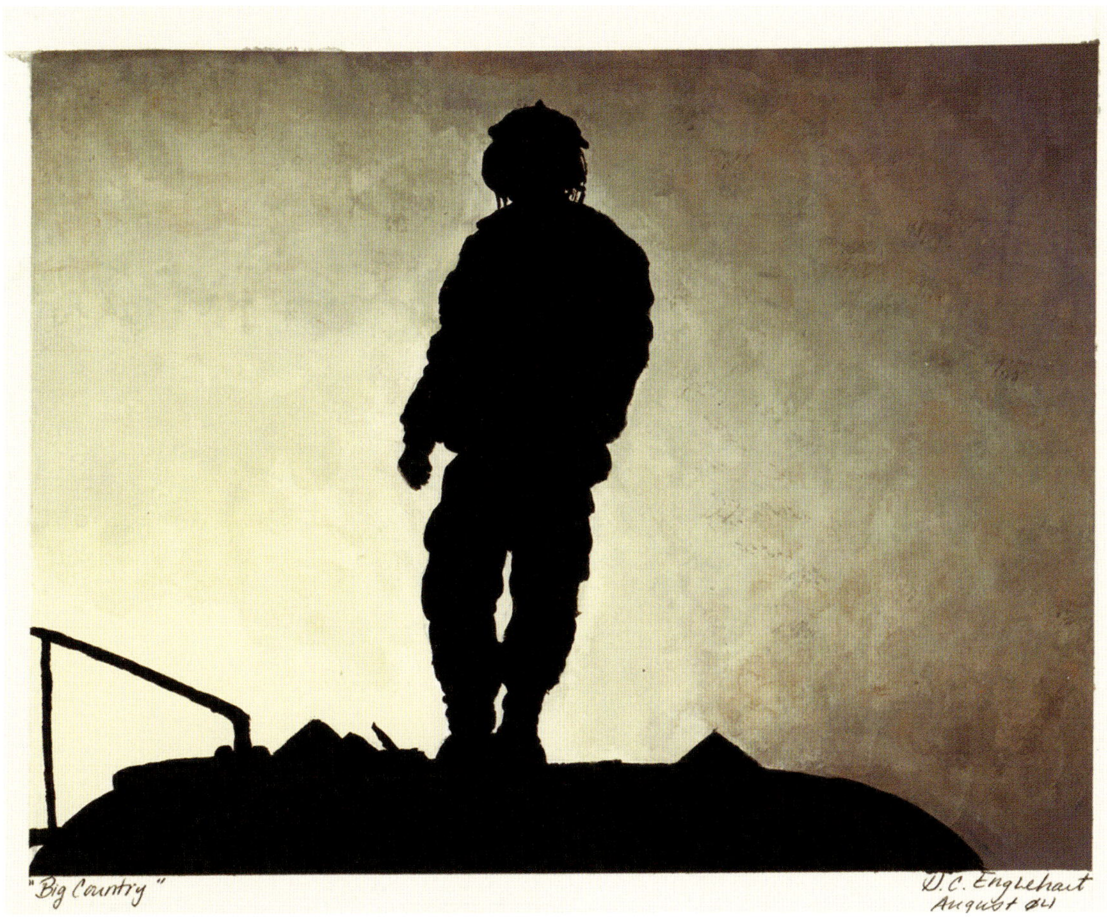

Big Country, by Heather Englehart, watercolor on paper, 2004.

Art: Courtesy of the Army Art Collection, US Army Center of Military History.

Chapter 42

MILITARY PSYCHIATRY GRADUATE MEDICAL EDUCATION

CARROLL J. DIEBOLD, MD*; WENDI M. WAITS, MD†; MILLARD D. BROWN, MD‡; AND DAVID M. BENEDEK, MD§

*Colonel, Medical Corps, US Army; Chief, Department of Psychiatry, Tripler Army Medical Center, 1 Jarrett White Road, Honolulu, Hawaii 96859-5001

†Lieutenant Colonel, Medical Corps, US Army; Chief, Inpatient Psychiatry Service, Department of Psychiatry, Tripler Army Medical Center, 1 Jarrett White Road, Honolulu, Hawaii 96859-5001; formerly, Child and Adolescent Psychiatry Fellow, Tripler Army Medical Center, Honolulu, Hawaii

‡Major, Medical Corps, US Army; Psychiatry Residency Director, Tripler Army Medical Center, 1 Jarrett White Road, Honolulu, Hawaii 96859-5001

§Colonel, Medical Corps, US Army; Professor and Deputy Chair, Department of Psychiatry, Uniformed Services University of the Health Sciences, 4301 Jones Bridge Road, Bethesda, Maryland 20814

INTRODUCTION

Graduate medical education (GME) is an essential aspect of military medicine. To maintain a healthy and productive operational force primed for success in varied environments and scenarios, medical personnel must possess adequate training and experience to provide appropriate and timely healthcare to service members. The unique skills required for a military healthcare provider to thrive in both operational and garrison environments necessitate comprehensive training and education. General lessons learned from past conflicts revealed that healthcare providers acquired knowledge and experience treating casualties on the battlefield rather than relying on training received from civilian medical institutions. From the advent of military GME in the early 20th century, the primary mission has been to prepare medical personnel to function in all types of operations.

As military graduate medical education evolved, military-specific proficiencies were introduced early in the training process. Before beginning the first year of GME, most trainees complete the Basic Officer Leadership Course, in which rudimentary knowledge such as extending military courtesies, proper wear of the uniform, elementary leadership skills, and basic soldier proficiencies are taught.[1] Students who do not have the opportunity to complete the basic course prior to entering GME will complete this training shortly after graduation. Consistent with training given to all assigned soldiers, a military treatment facility (MTF) with a GME program may require trainees to participate in annual common task training to maintain proficiency in basic military skills such as nuclear, biological, chemical response; weapons familiarization and maintenance; and military communication procedures.

Psychiatry is the medical specialty with the greatest number of military-unique tasks. Like a civilian psychiatrist practicing in a public institutional setting such as a prison or forensic healthcare facility, the military psychiatrist is consistently confronted with dual-agency issues, necessitating consideration of the needs of the organization versus those of the patient.[2] However, unlike civilian behavioral healthcare providers, who can decide their degree of involvement in forensic and administrative psychiatric issues, military psychiatrists do not have a choice in participating in such cases, thereby requiring extensive training in military-unique behavioral health topics such as command-directed mental health evaluations, Rule for Courts-Martial 706 evaluations, security clearance assessments, and medical evaluation boards.[3–6] Each of these military-unique administrative evaluations requires specific training and experience to perform competently. In addition to unique administrative tasks, the military psychiatrist must develop diverse skills such as consulting with commands, briefing nonmedical military leaders, providing psychoeducation to soldiers and leaders, and constructing realistic treatment plans while taking into account a service member's duties.

This chapter will present the evolution of psychiatry GME in the military healthcare system from its origins in the early 20th century to the current process of training military psychiatrists. The US Army, Navy, and Air Force all participate in psychiatry GME, maintaining a pipeline of well-trained graduates who are frequently deployed to combat zones shortly after completion of training. Training programs vary in size and structure, including service-specific programs, programs sponsored by one service that accept trainees from other services, partnerships with civilian and Veterans Administration programs, and a joint service program in Washington, DC. All programs are accredited by the American Council of Graduate Medical Education (ACGME), fulfilling the same academic requirements observed by civilian programs, in addition to providing education in unique military psychiatric skills.[7] In addition to residency training in adult psychiatry, military psychiatry GME programs can offer subspecialty fellowship training in child and adolescent, forensic, addiction, and geriatric psychiatry.

Areas addressed in the chapter will include leadership of a GME program, role of the program director, faculty development and recruitment, curriculum, contribution of undergraduate medical education to psychiatry GME, and research opportunities within training programs. The relevance of military psychiatric training will be presented, in addition to recommendations on how this unique specialty education can be enhanced in the future.

HISTORY

Formal psychiatric GME in the US military is a relatively new entity, the development of which has mirrored civilian psychiatric training in the United States in many ways. In other ways, however, it has developed independently, establishing a unique legacy and creating for its alumni a broader clinical skill set than that acquired by most graduates of civilian training programs. Colonel (Retired) Michael

G Wise authored an excellent summary of military GME through the mid 1980s, the highlights of which are summarized below.[8]

The first psychiatric "residents" in the Department of Defense (DoD) appear to have been four servicemen—two from the Navy and two from the Army—assigned to work at Saint Elizabeths Hospital in Washington, DC, for a period of 2 years beginning in 1909[9] (the same year that Sigmund Freud first lectured at an American university, introducing the psychoanalytic movement to the United States and increasing American interest in psychiatry[10]). At the beginning of World War I, psychiatrists in the Army numbered only 50,[11] an amount drastically insufficient to treat the 4 million US soldiers who would eventually serve in the war.[12] In an effort to address this issue, the Army commissioned many psychiatrists from state hospitals, and nonpsychiatric Army physicians were enrolled in civilian neuropsychiatric training programs that lasted an average of 6 weeks.[11] By the time of the 1918 armistice, nearly 700 psychiatrists were serving in the Army.[11]

Following World War I, psychiatrists gradually left the military, to such an extent that by 1940 uniformed psychiatrists on active duty numbered less than 100.[13,14] One year after the attack on Pearl Harbor, an improved and standardized neuropsychiatry course for nonpsychiatric military physicians was established and offered at a handful of civilian institutions.[14] During the remainder of World War II, this 12-week course produced 1,300 graduates, referred to as "90-day wonders."[15]

In 1946, Congress passed the National Mental Health Act, which provided federal funds for a number of mental health initiatives, including training for mental health professionals.[10] Over the course of the next decade, eight military psychiatry residency programs opened and received accreditation from ACGME (Table 42-1).[8] The "90-day wonder" program remained active at Fort Sam Houston, Texas, from 1946 to 1950, while physicians in the new psychiatric residencies completed their training.[16]

The field of psychiatry was also gaining a foothold in the civilian sector. During this same decade, the first Institute on Psychiatric Services meeting was held, the *Psychiatric Services* journal was established, the American Psychiatric Association authorized the creation of district branches, the first meeting of the American Psychiatric Association Assembly was held, the first *Diagnostic and Statistical Manual of Mental Disorders* was published, and psychoactive drugs were introduced in the United States.[9]

Perhaps as a result of psychotropic medications being introduced and the subsequent decreased number of psychiatric hospital admissions, three of the US military's first psychiatric residencies closed shortly after opening: the Navy's Great Lakes, Illinois, program in 1948; the Navy's San Diego, California, program in 1954; and the Army's Fitzsimons, Colorado, program in 1958.[8] However, the remainder of the programs stayed open for many years (Figure 42-1).

TABLE 42-1

AMERICAN COUNCIL OF GRADUATE MEDICAL EDUCATION ACCREDITATION HISTORY OF US MILITARY PSYCHIATRY RESIDENCIES

Year	Programs Accredited or Discontinued
1946	Bethesda (Md), Great Lakes (Ill), and Philadelphia (Penn) Navy programs accredited
1948	Walter Reed (Washington, DC) and Letterman (Calif) Army programs accredited; Great Lakes program discontinued
1950	Fitzsimons (Colo) Army program accredited
1951	San Diego (Calif) and Oakland (Calif) Navy programs accredited
1954	San Diego program discontinued
1958	Fitzsimons program discontinued
1965	Wilford Hall (Tex) Air Force program accredited
1976	Dwight D Eisenhower (Ga) Army program accredited; Philadelphia program moved to Portsmouth (Va) and accreditation continued
1977	Wright-Patterson (Ohio) Air Force program accredited
1978	Tripler (Hawaii) Army program accredited
1981	San Diego program reaccredited
1983	Oakland program discontinued
1993	Letterman program discontinued
1999	Dwight D Eisenhower program discontinued

Data source (through 1987): Wise MG. The past, present, and future of psychiatric training in the US armed services. *Mil Med*.1987;152:550–553.

During the 1980s, as memories of the Vietnam War were fading and a Cold War conflict seemed increasingly less likely to materialize, pressure from the federal government to consolidate US military installations increased.[17] After a preliminary round of DoD-initiated closures in 1988, Congress passed the US Department of Defense Base Realignment and Closure Act of 1990 (also known as the "BRAC law" or Public Law 101-510),[18] which established a non-DoD committee and a schedule for the evaluation of military bases for closure. As a result of this legislation, additional BRAC rounds occurred in 1991, 1993, and 1995.

Closure of military psychiatry residency programs took varied paths. The Presidio in San Francisco, California, home of Letterman Army Medical Center,

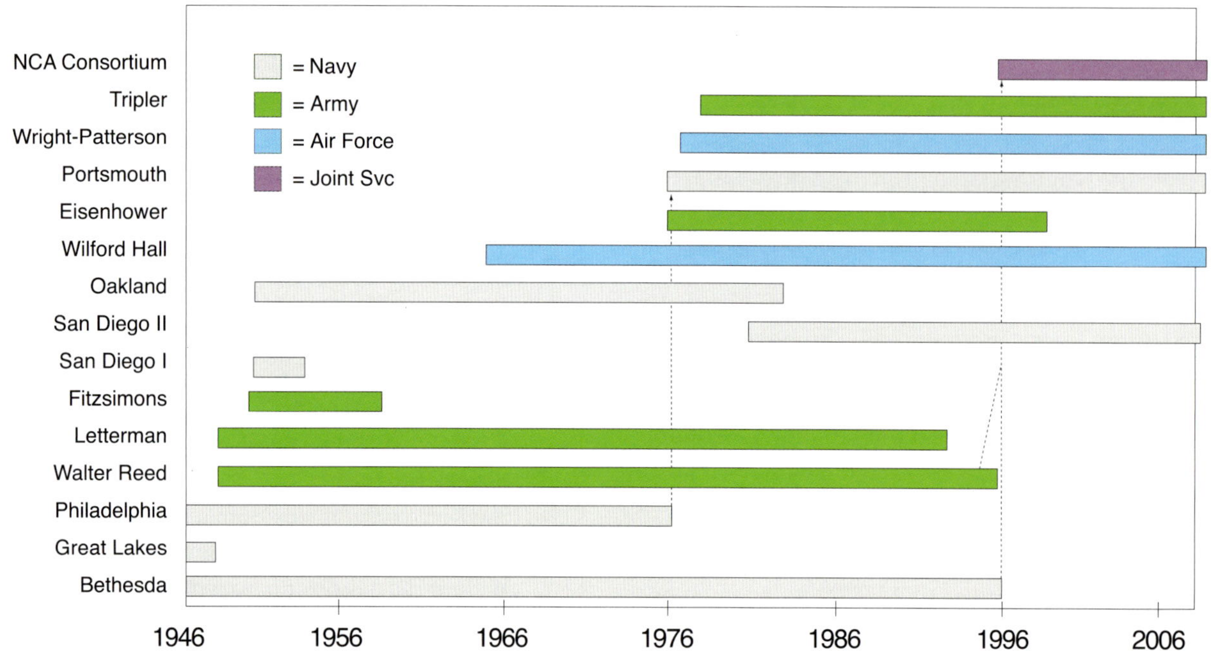

Figure 42-1. A graphic timeline of accredited US military psychiatry programs. The dotted lines represent when programs were either transferred to another location or merged.
NCA: National Capital Area; Svc: Service

was identified for closure in 1988.[19] Its final cohort of psychiatry residents graduated in 1993, and the hospital closed 1 year later.[20] The training program at Eisenhower Army Medical Center in Augusta, Georgia, although not an official casualty of the BRAC, was closed preemptively by the Army in 1999 because of a dwindling pool of applicants.[21] Similarly, although Oak Knoll Naval Hospital in Oakland, California, was not identified for closure until the 1993 BRAC, the Navy had already relocated the psychiatry training program from Oakland to San Diego in the mid-1980s.

In 1995, in an effort to fortify their programs against the threat of closure, the three DoD hospitals in the national capital area—Walter Reed Army Medical Center in Washington, DC; the National Naval Medical Center in Bethesda, Maryland; and Malcolm Grow Air Force Hospital in Prince George's County, Maryland—combined forces, creating the National Capital Area Consortium. Affiliated with the Uniformed Services University of the Health Sciences (USUHS), in Bethesda, Maryland, the consortium program is currently the largest active military psychiatry training program.

A new BRAC initiative in 2005 has called for the closure of Walter Reed by 2011,[22] but the consortium psychiatry residency program is expected to remain intact and headquartered at what is currently the National Naval Medical Center. The 2005 BRAC initiative also called for the consolidation of Wilford Hall Air Force Medical Center with Brooke Army Medical Center in San Antonio, Texas. By 2011, only a San Antonio Military Medical Center is expected to exist, with the north campus (Brooke) being primarily an inpatient facility and the south campus (Wilford Hall) having only outpatient services.[23] As in Washington, DC, the Air Force psychiatry residency program in San Antonio is expected to remain intact.

The global war on terror (GWOT) has contributed to an increase in behavioral health problems among active duty personnel and their families, as well as among veterans and civilians in the United States. Interest in psychiatry as a career field also appears to be on the rise, perhaps as a direct result of this GWOT-influenced increased demand.[24] The future of military psychiatry GME will likely continue to parallel the need for services during times of war, as has been the case for the past century.

PROGRAM LEADERSHIP

The military stresses competent leadership as an essential factor in successful completion of the mission. Much of an officer's military education is composed of development and utilization of proper leadership techniques.[25] Although the majority of military medical officers will never serve in command positions, many will become service, section, or department chiefs, directly responsible for delivering high-quality medical care in addition to promoting the professional development of subordinates. A fortunate few will be appointed to lead GME programs, taking on the responsibility of training future military clinicians to excel in varied environments.

The department chairperson performs diverse roles in a military psychiatry GME program. Besides the requirements established by ACGME, the chairperson must also meet the standards expected of a military leader.[7] Essential attributes include articulating a clear vision, prioritizing the mission, managing personnel, and overseeing the budget, all while supporting the goals of the MTF commander. As the military healthcare system evolves into a managed care model emphasizing clinical productivity as a measurement of fiscal success, GME leaders are challenged with demonstrating financial success while maintaining a quality training program. GME-related activities such as clinical supervision, didactics, trainee performance assessments, medical education committees, psychiatric clinical report reviews, and research-related activities do not produce workload credit, resulting in a lower productivity standing compared with other MTFs that do not have GME programs.

Success of a military psychiatry program is predicated on the department leadership being able to incorporate GME into four essential tasks: (1) direct patient care delivery, (2) deployment cycle support, (3) operational readiness of personnel, and (4) research activities. Until the mid-1990s, military psychiatry GME programs were relatively insulated from external influences such as managed care and operational taskings. Programs readily focused on psychiatric education, utilizing direct patient care, clinical supervision, didactics, and research, augmented by a military psychiatry curriculum, to prepare trainees for success as clinicians in an MTF practice or as a garrison-based division psychiatrist. GME leaders were not pressured by the requirement to formulate intricate business plans to predict and subsequently demonstrate clinical productivity. Specific military psychiatric curriculum consisted of several didactic courses and focused on familiarization with basic military organization structure and function, dual-agency issues, performing military-unique administrative mental health evaluations, interacting with operational leadership, and operational military mental health doctrine, much of which was from the Vietnam era and in the process of being updated. The operational experience for trainees was limited to a rotation during the final year of residency to a post with a large troop population, and in many instances such rotations lacked formal structure or stated goals and objectives.

As the evolution of managed care within the military healthcare system of the late 1990s coincided with the changes in defense strategy after September 11, 2001, conducting military GME became much more complex and challenging. Leaders of GME programs wer no longer able to dedicate resources exclusively to the training mission but were forced to balance multiple requirements while devising methods to maximize the learning experience of trainees. GME programs became directly affected by the GWOT through deployment of faculty and taskings to participate in deployment cycle support at locations serving as deployment platforms. Advantageously, trainees were given the opportunity to participate directly in many deployment cycle support activities, as well as to provide treatment for casualties evacuated from the theater of operations. A challenge for the GME leadership was to ensure that adequate supervision and training occurred during the provision of such services.[26]

With the extended GWOT-related campaigns of Operation Iraqi Freedom and Operation Enduring Freedom in the first decade of the 21st century, most graduates from Army psychiatry GME programs deployed to a combat zone within 2 years of completing training, requiring the programs to provide comprehensive instruction and practical experience in operational psychiatry. Faculty at the two Army GME programs became part of the psychiatry deployment pool and served in diverse assignments throughout both theaters of operations, directly enhancing the quality of the operational psychiatry curriculum. Prior deployment experience became a determining factor for prospective faculty, and by the end of 2006, over 75% of the active duty staff psychiatrists at the two Army psychiatry programs had deployed to a combat theater.[27]

Role of the Program Director

A residency program's existence and viability critically depends on a program director who is fully engaged and active in the program's daily activities. In the field of psychiatry, such active participation is even more paramount in running a successful residency program. The field of psychiatry requires that residency graduates not only be skilled in diagnostic assessments and treatment modalities, but that they also be capable of engaging patients and systems to construct realistic individualized treatment plans. Such capabilities can be utilized effectively only if the psychiatrists are fully aware and in control of their own personal mental health. Therefore, a quality psychiatry residency program encourages trainees to develop an awareness of how their own histories can potentially affect their ability to engage patients in clinical service delivery and program faculty in their educational pursuits. The psychiatry residency program director must therefore possess skills as an effective parent, colleague, arbitrator, visionary, and leader when interacting with residents and faculty.

When groups are formed in which some have power and control over other members, acting out behaviors will inevitably follow. In a residency program, the program director must anticipate these behaviors and develop methods of preventing them when possible, in addition to maintaining proper boundaries when challenged. The faculty and program director are expected to avoid leveraging their power differential while guiding the trainees through a process of personal growth and learning. The program director must learn to respond appropriately to acting out behaviors with the requisite amount of action, while redirecting residents with such behaviors toward more constructive use of their energies.

Psychiatry residency training evolves along a developmental continuum. The beginning section usually involves encouraging residents to apply newly learned knowledge in patient care and to develop clinical instincts in evaluation and treatment procedures. During the middle phase, the program director helps residents consolidate basic skills and begin developing more advanced skills in therapeutics through treatment of challenging and treatment-resistant cases. Finally, during the end stage of training, the program director develops situations for the resident to become a leader of junior colleagues and begin taking on independent responsibilities as a credentialed provider.

The visionary program director must be aware of the future of psychiatry as an evolving medical specialty while remaining cognizant of how the military plans to address its future behavioral health challenges. The latter requires the program director to maintain connections with military behavioral health leaders so the needs of the military system can quickly be built into the training of future military psychiatrists. These changing needs force the program director to continually refine the vision and mission of the program, articulating these refinements clearly and concisely to the faculty and residents. Program directors must also stay current with the latest developments and research in psychiatry, which is rapidly developing from a field of general syndromes to a complex specialty containing significant advances in neuroscience and therapeutics.

Leaders of organizations are tasked with many responsibilities that can quickly become overwhelming and burdensome, and those whom they lead look to them for mentorship and guidance. Leaders' behaviors set the tone for the entire organization and are naturally scrutinized by subordinates. Program directors must therefore be aware of the significance an action can have across the residency training program. The fundamental operating principles of a residency must be repeatedly articulated so that residents and faculty can understand the rationale and potential outcomes of certain decisions. Faculty and trainees may not agree with a decision, but they need to be made aware of how decisions are consistent with the stated principles of the program. With so many ongoing issues to incorporate into a residency program, the program director must balance being open to feedback at all levels with making decisive and timely decisions to keep the program current with psychiatry as a specialty and also with the needs of the military.

Faculty Development

In addition to capable GME leadership, recruitment and selection of appropriate faculty is a critical element to program success. Besides uniformed clinicians, the teaching staff is composed of civilian faculty employed by the federal government, clinicians on personal service contracts, and possibly faculty members from local civilian psychiatry GME programs.

As with any enterprise, the recruitment and retention of bright, experienced, and energetic supervisors directly affects program success. A psychiatry GME faculty member should possess the inner drive for personal growth, passion to promote learning in trainees, and professional experience to provide capable supervision and guidance.[7] The composition of a military psychiatry GME faculty should be a mix of established clinicians with significant experience in academic settings and midcareer psychiatrists with an interest in further development of teaching and mentoring skills. In many instances, the more professionally mature members of the faculty are retired military clinicians who possess a wealth of practical military psychiatric experience.

Retention of military physicians beyond completion of initial active duty service obligation has been a challenge since the conclusion of Operation Desert Storm. The potential of prolonged operational deployments combined with dwindling resources and the evolution of managed care within the military healthcare system has produced a less attractive environment for prolonged service. However, one extremely favorable aspect of military medicine is the wide scope of career tracks available.[28] Within several tours of duty post-training, active duty psychiatrists are in a position to mold their careers in a single area, such as a clinical, operational, command, academic, or research-based concentration, with the flexibility to shift between these tracks. For the academically oriented military psychiatrist, the potential to become faculty at one of the military GME programs is a tremendous incentive to continue practicing medicine on active duty.

Potential faculty members are identified throughout the entire career path of the military psychiatrist. Occasionally, an outstanding trainee demonstrating a talent for academic psychiatry may be recruited to remain on staff as a junior faculty member while further refining teaching and mentoring skills under the guidance of senior faculty. More likely, promising graduates with an interest in teaching and academics will serve at least one tour as an MTF or operationally based psychiatrist to gain practical clinical and administrative experience as an independent healthcare provider. Another group consists of clinicians who initially were not recognized as future faculty members, but through a combination of experience, reassessment of career aspirations, and possibly attaining specialized skills such as forensic or addictions psychiatry training, may be deemed faculty material at midcareer or later.

No codified requisite criteria exists for consideration for faculty appointment to a military psychiatry GME program, but the candidate should demonstrate superior clinical, leadership, management, scholarship, and military skills with an underlying passion to develop future military psychiatrists. A search committee composed of current faculty members should be formed to identify and interview candidates. One method to screen potential faculty is using ACGME competencies to predict a resident's level of performance as an independent practitioner.[7] The potential faculty member should markedly exceed the baseline standard for each of the competency areas, with focus on the ability to provide mentorship and guidance (Exhibit 42-1). Additional data to be assessed are performance during GME training, scope of assignments post-GME, input from supervisors and colleagues, and unique skills to enhance the training program.

Recruitment of a dedicated and multitalented faculty is essential for the success of a military psychiatry training program. The increased frequency of operational deployments since September 11, 2001, has necessitated frequent shifting and restructuring of faculty duties. To provide future military psychiatrists with the necessary skills to thrive in multiple complex environments, the GME faculty must be dedicated to the mission of being teachers, mentors, and role models.

EXHIBIT 42-1

AMERICAN COUNCIL OF GRADUATE MEDICAL EDUCATION COMPETENCIES

1. Patient care that is compassionate, appropriate, and effective for the treatment of health problems and the promotion of health.
2. Medical knowledge about established and evolving biomedical, clinical, and cognate sciences, as well as the application of this knowledge to patient care.
3. Practice-based learning and improvement that involves the investigation and evaluation of care for their patients, the appraisal and assimilation of scientific evidence, and improvements in patient care.
4. Interpersonal and communication skills that result in the effective exchange of information and collaboration with patients, their families, and other health professionals.
5. Professionalism, as manifested through a commitment to carrying out professional responsibilities, adherence to ethical principles, and sensitivity to patients of diverse backgrounds.
6. Systems-based practice, as manifested by actions that demonstrate an awareness of and responsiveness to the larger context and system of healthcare, as well as the ability to call effectively on other resources in the system to provide optimal healthcare.

Data source: Accreditation Counsel for Graduate Medical Education. Psychiatry program requirements. ACGME Web site. Available at: http://www.acgme.org/acWebsite/RRC_400/400_prIndex.asp. Accessed October 28, 2009.

CURRICULUM

During the last 2 decades, the establishment of the core competencies and the psychotherapy competencies as the basic evaluation tools has brought significant changes to psychiatry GME. Training requirements are gradually shifting to an outpatient-centered treatment model as the inpatient rotation standard has been steadily reduced. Specific didactic requirements have also been expanded with the evolution of psychiatric subspecialties such as forensic, geriatric, and psychosomatic medicine, as well as with advancements in psychopharmacology. Training programs must also provide residents with adequate exposure to the challenges of managed care, because most psychiatrists-in-training will not have a practice composed exclusively of direct-payment patients. In addition to the elements unique to psychiatry training, military programs have unique training requirements pertinent to the diverse role of the uniformed psychiatrist.

Core Competencies

The core competency movement within ACGME began with the "outcomes movement" by the US Department of Education in the 1980s and accelerated in Canada in 1996 through the publishing of the Canadian Medical Education Directions for Specialists (CanMEDS) 2000 Project report.[29] This movement grew out of a recognition that the role of the physician has changed from a paternalistic medical expert model to a model in which the medical expert is part of a medical decision-making team that includes the patient. Also, the rapid pace of advancement of medical knowledge has repeatedly emphasized the need for physicians to be avid life-long learners and for residency training programs to teach new physicians how to develop life-long learning skills. In response to the change in the mechanism of healthcare delivery, ACGME and the American Board of Medical Specialties launched the core competencies program for all American residencies in 1999.[30] In 2001, the psychiatry residency review committee (RRC) became the first RRC to change its official program requirements. The following year, site reviewers began assessing whether or not programs had begun to implement the core competencies. Similar to the overall emphasis in healthcare on the ability to assess quality in medicine by such certifying organizations as the Joint Commission, ACGME mandated outcome measures to assess competency in the core areas.[31]

The core competencies consist of six main elements: (1) medical knowledge, (2) patient care, (3) interpersonal and communication skills, (4) practice-based learning and improvement, (5) professionalism, and (6) systems-based practice.[7] Medical knowledge and patient care emphasize the traditional elements of physician medical education over the past century. Medical school and clinical experiences in residency form the foundation of medical knowledge that physicians use to perform competent, safe patient care. The patient care competency focuses on interactions with patients, including the psychiatry-specific psychotherapy core competencies. Interpersonal and communication skills have become increasingly more important as fully informed consent and a focus on patient choice have steadily increased throughout the past 60 years, since the passage of the Nuremburg Code in 1947.[32] Practice-based learning and improvement emphasizes the ability to understand and grow from clinical experiences in addition to keeping current on recent advances. The goal is to instill such abilities during training so that practitioners continue the process throughout their entire medical careers.

Professionalism is an essential aspect of any occupation, encompassing the requisite skills and sense of commitment needed to function in a competent and safe manner. No amount of medical expertise can overcome the requirement for strict standards of behavior that define professionalism and serve as the backbone for a strong physician-patient relationship. In addition to acting professionally with patients and healthcare colleagues, the military clinician has an additional obligation to maintain the high standards of a military officer.[33] Finally, advances in medical practice have resulted in effective management and control of many chronic illnesses in the outpatient setting, which in turn has created a need for increasing collaboration with many different organizations to maximize the well-being of patients. The systems-based training competency emphasizes this ability to operate within systems of care, in coordination with many types of healthcare professionals, thereby maximizing quality of life for patients. By training within a systems-based environment, the military psychiatry resident gains an appreciation for the importance of utilizing primary, secondary, and tertiary prevention.[34]

Implied in the competency model is the idea that length of time in training alone is insufficient to establish competence. Rather, a consistent ability to use a specific set of knowledge, skills, and attitudes must be demonstrated by the trainee prior to clearance for graduation. Further development will produce a longitudinal assessment tool for competence as opposed to completion of a set of timed requirements. However, little evidence exists on what outcome measures can reliably assess the psychiatric core competencies. Currently, many programs use some form of standardized assessment tool in conjunction with subjective input from multiple sources such as supervisors, instructors, and mentors to assess overall competency of trainees.[35]

Medical Students and Core Competencies

The core competencies of interpersonal and communication skills, professionalism, and systems-based practice in particular require trainees to demonstrate the ability to interact effectively with persons other than patients. Because they are so crucial to successful medical practice, development of these competencies begins very early in the medical education process. At the heart of these competencies is the theme of working cooperatively within multidisciplinary teams of other medical professionals in a manner that synergizes efforts to provide the best care for patients. With nurses, occupational therapists, medical technicians, and administrative staff, medical students are often members of these multidisciplinary teams.

At USUHS, the only US federal medical school and the principle source of future military physicians, military medical students are introduced to the concepts of team learning, practice, and interpersonal communication through a variety of small-group laboratory exercises based on clinical vignettes. Students also participate in Introduction to Clinical Medicine small-group courses, where they learn and practice medical interviewing and physical examination skills with patients from the treatment facilities in the national capital area.

Psychiatry residents from the National Capital Consortium's psychiatry GME training program are actively recruited and encouraged to participate as co-instructors with full-time university faculty members in these exercises and courses. In this manner, residents are afforded opportunities to demonstrate their medical knowledge, to discuss principles of systems-based medicine, and to role model professional relationships with junior medical officer students and senior co-faculty.

Third-year USUHS medical students currently participate in clinical clerkship rotations on psychiatry wards and clinics at the three medical centers within the National Capital Consortium; at Tripler Army Medical Center, Hawaii; and at Wilford Hall Air Force Medical Center (soon to be known as the San Antonio Military Medical Center–South). Additionally, 3rd- and 4th-year students from USUHS and other medical schools may also rotate at civilian treatment facilities and other military medical centers. At these sites, residents (under the appropriate guidance of military GME faculty) also hone their skills as mentors, teachers, supervisors, role models, and team leaders.

GME program faculty members appointed by the USUHS Department of Psychiatry as clinical site directors at each of these sites assure that residents contribute to the core knowledge and competency requirements of the Liaison Committee on Medical Education for psychiatry clerkship students. Students are responsible for learning the fundamentals of psychiatric assessment, differential diagnosis and treatment, mental status examination, safety assessment, treatment planning, and case presentation to multidisciplinary teams during these rotations. In providing both didactic and "hands-on" training for medical students, GME residents also develop and demonstrate the RRC-required core competencies, as well as honing the professional and leadership skills necessary for the practice of psychiatry in military medical settings.

Psychotherapy Competencies

Psychiatry residency programs have had to restructure their training strategy to meet the competency requirements for various psychotherapies, including supportive therapy, psychodynamic therapy, brief therapies, cognitive-behavioral therapy, and combined medication and psychotherapy. The evolution of managed healthcare converging with marked advancement in psychopharmacology shifted the emphasis of psychiatry GME away from long-term psychotherapeutic treatment and toward a crisis intervention model. In response, many psychiatry residency programs experienced a shift in culture away from emphasis on psychotherapy skills toward a more neurobiology-based approach that led to increased reliance on safer, less burdensome medications for treating mental illnesses. By the end of the 1990s, numerous programs around the country were struggling to find the financial resources necessary for robust psychotherapy training.[36] In contrast, military residency programs faced less financial pressure to demonstrate productivity and thus were able to maintain a strong emphasis on psychotherapy skills development.

In 2001, the psychiatry RRC mandated not only that residencies must start implementing the six core competencies, but additionally that they must develop assessment tools to certify that their graduates are trained and competent in all five psychotherapies.[37] No directives have been written on how to teach, develop, or assess each of these psychotherapies, and development of competencies was left to individual programs to design and implement.

General Psychiatry Residency Curriculum

An accredited psychiatry residency program must be 48 months in length, including the postgraduate year 1, also known as internship. Graduation from medical or osteopathic school is a prerequisite to enter such a program. The psychiatry internship usually consists of approximately 6 months of basic medical training in primary medicine areas, such as internal medicine, family medicine, or pediatrics, and about 6 months of neurology and psychiatry training. Postgraduate year 2 typically involves mostly inpatient psychiatry rotations, as well as rotations in addictions, consultation-liaison, geriatric psychiatry, and other clinical experiences. The majority of outpatient psychotherapy and medication management training occurs during postgraduate year 3. Finally, postgraduate year 4 involves consolidating medication management and psychotherapy skills, mentoring junior trainees, and learning administrative skills necessary for interacting in the larger system of medical care.[7]

Requirements for completion of GME training in psychiatry have evolved over time. During the past 2 decades, focus has shifted from inpatient psychiatric experience to outpatient rotations, mirroring the medical industry's evolution of an outpatient-based treatment model. For example, the required time for inpatient psychiatry rotations in 1984 was 12 months, compared to a minimum of 6 months in 2007.[7,38] ACGME mandates specific time requirements for certain rotations, and others are left to the discretion of the training program (Exhibit 42-2).

Three other aspects to psychiatry residency training are unique and increase the complexity and cost of executing a training program. First, much of psychiatric care occurs in one-on-one sessions with a patient. The duration of a typical appointment can be from 30 to 90 minutes, with a low reimbursement rate compared to other medical specialties. Because of the very sensitive nature of topics discussed and the structure of psychotherapy sessions, there are significant barriers to having a supervisor directly observe a trainee's interactions with patients. Some programs in the military are beginning direct observations via video links to offices with consent by the patient as a means to observe but not intrude on the patient-physician interaction.

Secondly, as mandated by ACGME, psychiatry trainees must meet with supervisors individually at designated times to review clinical encounters that have already occurred.[7] Each trainee must have 2 hours a week of individual time with faculty supervisors to discuss recent evaluations and therapy cases. Therefore, if a program has 25 residents, faculty must spend 50 hours a week of nonclinical time reviewing cases with the trainees, leading to a large amount of fiscally nonproductive time for both residents and supervisors.

Third, much of psychiatry training involves trying to understand the enormously complex field of human behavior. Residents need to understand human development across the lifespan and how it manifests differently at various points in development. For example, a 5-year-old girl might be displaying normal developmental behavior when she states that she sees an invisible friend standing next to her, whereas such behavior would be abnormal for a 13-year-old child. In addition to learning through clinical experiences and case supervision, psychiatry GME training requires a greater amount of didactic learning than any other medical specialty. The total time spent participating in didactics does not include advanced preparation or individual reading and research pertinent to the resident's cases. Learning how to distinguish normal behaviors from mental disorders, understanding various medication and therapy treatment modalities, and learning how to develop realistic treatment plans necessitate a large reading and didactic program.[7] To satisfy all of the academic requirements, most psychiatry GME programs have developed didactics schedules of about 3 to 5 hours per week per year level, resulting in an overall didactic schedule of approximately 13 to 15 hours per week for the entire program, all of which is nonbillable time for faculty and resident participants.

EXHIBIT 42-2

SUMMARY OF AMERICAN COUNCIL OF GRADUATE MEDICAL EDUCATION RESIDENCY REVIEW COMMITTEE REQUIREMENTS FOR PSYCHIATRY RESIDENTS, AS OF 2007

Timed Experiences

- Primary Care Medicine: 4 months in internship year
- Inpatient Psychiatry: minimum of 6 months
- Outpatient Psychiatry: 12 consecutive months
- Neurology: 2 months
- Consult-Liaison Psychiatry: 2 months
- Child and Adolescent Psychiatry: 2 months
- Addiction Psychiatry: 1 month
- Geriatric Psychiatry: 1 month

Untimed Experiences

- Forensic Psychiatry
- Community Psychiatry
- Family/Couples Therapy
- Group Therapy
- Electroconvulsive Treatment
- Psychological Testing

Research and Scholarly Activity

Although not specifically mentioned as a GME core competency, the ACGME RRC requires that involvement in scholarly activity or research be incorporated into residency training.[7] All military psychiatry GME programs require participation in a research project or scholarly endeavor as a requirement for graduation.

Historically, such scholarly endeavors have included literature reviews presented at department-wide or hospital grand rounds. Increasingly, however, general psychiatry residents have been paired with research mentors—GME faculty members with specific skills and interest in research. As a result, many GME residents graduate with a sophisticated understanding of study design, institutional review board procedures, and research report writing skills. In addition to numerous book chapters, military residents have authored or coauthored publications accepted in the *American Journal of Psychiatry, Journal of the American Academy of Psychiatry and the Law, Jefferson Journal of Psychiatry, Psychosomatic Medicine, Military Medicine,* and *American Journal of Disaster Medicine,* among others. These efforts have not only advanced the practice of psychiatry within the military, but have also expanded the knowledge and understanding of specific military psychiatric issues within the larger civilian community.

Military Psychiatry Curriculum

In addition to satisfying all of the standard ACGME requirements for a psychiatry residency program, military GME programs must prepare trainees to function as capable leaders immediately upon completion of training. New graduates can be placed into various leadership positions, such as chief of a division mental health clinic or officer-in-charge of a brigade combat team mental health section.[39] The staff of a mental health clinic or section may include other officers, several enlisted personnel, and possibly civilian employees. New graduates can also be assigned to combat stress control units or to other medical units in a deployment setting, where they will be expected to serve in leadership roles.

A well-executed military psychiatry curriculum spans the entire 4-year training cycle. Issues emphasized in the military psychiatry curriculum include dual-agency issues, utilizing the military structure to support soldiers in need, and ways to reduce stigma and perform primary prevention efforts. Dual-agency issues arise more often in military psychiatry because Army psychiatrists serve simultaneously as physicians and Army officers.[40] Most of the time these two roles do not conflict, but in some situations duty to the mission may be of higher priority than the immediate best interest of the soldier. Especially during combat operations, the needs of the group and the mission may sometimes trump the needs of the individual, potentially creating a dilemma for physicians trained and sworn to act in the best interests of the patient.[41] This dual-agency issue is addressed frequently in the training of military psychiatrists.

One benefit of the military structure is the ability to develop and execute a comprehensive biopsychosocial formulation and treatment plan for a service member. Military psychiatry GME programs provide trainees with practical experience in performing clinical psychiatry while addressing pertinent military issues. Applying an occupational health model by working closely with the service member's chain of command, the military psychiatrist has influence in structuring a soldier's work environment via the scope of work, physical setting of work, and even duty hours.[6] An in-depth understanding of the challenges and constraints faced by military units is essential for the military psychiatrist when consulting with service members' chains of command to develop realistic treatment plans. To promote familiarity with the practice of psychiatry in a military environment, trainees participate in rotations at posts and bases with large cohorts of operational units. Through such interactions, the psychiatrist-in-training gains practical experience in military group dynamics and learns to develop realistic treatment plans within the constraints posed by the unit's mission.

Many military psychiatry GME graduates deploy to an operational environment shortly after completion of training, so familiarity with unit structure and dynamics is tremendously important to the psychiatrist aspiring to be of optimal service to both active duty patients and unit leaders. Learning about the critical role of mental health in the entire deployment cycle support process prior to completion of residency training will greatly aid the military psychiatrist in the initial assignment.[42]

Unlike most civilian occupations, military service does not impact solely upon the service member, but affects the entire family unit. The high percentage of married service members makes adequate knowledge and experience in managing family dynamics, particularly in the face of deployment, necessary for military psychiatry trainees. The mental health needs of military children have been recognized through research and practical experience.[43] Military psychiatry trainees should have experience with programs that address such needs outside of the traditional office setting, such as in school-based mental health programs.[44]

Over the last 5 to 10 years, increasing emphasis has been placed on early identification of mental health problems through education and primary prevention efforts. After the September 11, 2001, terrorist attacks, the Army instituted Operation Solace to offer assistance to Pentagon employees. Military psychiatry trainees played a prominent role as members of the assistance team.[45] Boundaries of traditional methods of patient care had to be crossed to allow survivors easy access to mental healthcare providers while simultaneously decreasing the stigma to seeking help. For example, mental health teams of various types of providers were assembled to bring outreach efforts directly to employees in work areas, creating the term "therapy by walking around." Outcome data suggest that such efforts may have resulted in a smaller-than-expected incidence of mental illness at the Pentagon following the attack.[46]

Combat operations since then have provided multiple opportunities for mental healthcare providers to further improve educational activities, to refine screening of service members during the entire deployment cycle, and to minimize the traumatic effects of the combat experience. Further advances in military psychiatry curricula will result in graduates being better prepared for the complex military mental health treatment mission.

Postresidency Fellowship Training

Postresidency psychiatric subspecialty education and training (fellowship programs) are currently offered at several military medical centers.[47] These programs provide the Army and Navy Medical Corps with the majority of their military psychiatric subspecialists. Historically, the Air Force has opted to permit relatively few of their psychiatrists to complete fellowship training (and these primarily through civilian channels), but Air Force physicians have also participated in the training programs described below. The opportunity to apply for and, if selected, receive subspecialty training in child and adolescent psychiatry, forensic psychiatry, geriatric psychiatry, and addictions psychiatry serves as a retention incentive for physicians who might otherwise terminate their active duty service. Military psychiatrists with subspecialty training continue to primarily practice adult general psychiatry in most operational billets. However, those assigned to tertiary care facilities and teaching hospitals are often assigned duties specifically related to their subspecialty skills (eg, working several days a week at the child psychiatry service, or as a medical review officer for the base substance abuse program). Those assigned to smaller clinics or medical detachments are given duties that utilize their expertise. For example, although military regulations do not require a forensic psychiatrist for the evaluation of competency and criminal responsibility,[4] forensically trained psychiatrists are called upon to conduct these assessments by commanders or medical service chiefs whenever possible. Thus, the opportunity to practice specialized psychiatric skills also serves as a retention incentive for specialty-trained psychiatrists.

Fellowship programs in child and adolescent psychiatry accredited by the ACGME RRC are presently offered at Tripler Army Medical Center and Walter Reed Army Medical Center (as part of the National Capital Consortium). Walter Reed also offers RRC-accredited fellowship training in forensic and geriatric psychiatry, and Tripler offers addictions psychiatry fellowship training. Army GME plans currently permit two Army psychiatrists to enter forensic training each year, five psychiatrists to enter child and adolescent training, and one to enter geriatric or addictions training in alternate years. The programs also offer training to Navy and Air Force psychiatrists on a space-available basis, provided their parent service agrees to permit their matriculation. In this way, the training programs generate a pool of psychiatric subspecialists sufficient to fulfill forecasted needs and to justify continued program accreditation.

The US Army, Navy, and Air Force have also recently established annual training billets for the National Capital Consortium's Disaster Psychiatry Fellowship at USUHS. This military-unique training opportunity combines a competitive master's in public health program with research and clinical mentorship in military operational response to disasters, war, and terrorism, as well as rotating internships at various federal agencies involved in disaster response. Disaster psychiatry subspecialty training, though not formally recognized by the ACGME through an accreditation process, has emerged to fill a need within the military for psychiatrists specifically trained in public health interventions, health surveillance, and principles of disaster mental health research and practice. Because the military is uniquely positioned and often tasked to provide medical and mental healthcare in natural and human-caused disasters, military psychiatrists with subspecialty training in this arena can augment the response of general psychiatrists and behavioral health specialists.

The opportunity to apply subspecialty skill sets in military operational environments—whether addressing the mental health needs of child victims of the southeast Asian tsunami or the medico-legal issues surrounding the mental health of service members accused of war crimes—often encourages specialty-trained psychiatrists to remain on active duty beyond their contractual obligations.

RELEVANCE IN MISSION PERFORMANCE

The delivery of mental health services in a military environment differs in multiple ways from civilian mental healthcare. Just as an attorney who relocates to a new state must learn the laws and culture of that state before establishing a practice, military mental health providers must thoroughly understand their service branch's laws and culture to be effective caregivers. Military GME provides trainees with necessary exposure to the knowledge, skills, and attitudes required of military mental healthcare providers. Additionally, trainees in military programs receive guidance and supervision from experienced military supervisors while providing healthcare directly to service members and their dependents. Instruction and training in military-unique mental health issues is not available in civilian training, and being comfortable practicing in a military environment may be a major determinant of the length of time a military psychiatrist will ultimately remain in the service.[8] As the Society of Medical Consultants to the Armed Forces emphasized in a 1987 white paper, "[Military] graduate medical education is the chief guarantor of quality medical care and an unmatched incentive for the recruitment and retention of active duty medical officers. It is the essential prop supporting the entire voluntary military medical structure."[48]

The material presented in this section focuses on Army psychiatry GME training. Although the other mental health disciplines such as psychology, social work, psychiatric nursing, and occupational therapy may also offer graduate training programs in military healthcare facilities, psychiatry training is the longest and the most comprehensive. The authors of this chapter, all Army psychiatrists, are most familiar with Army standards and procedures. However, all branches of the US armed forces currently endorse a similar approach to evaluating, treating, and managing service members with psychiatric conditions. Additionally, each service recognizes the importance of addressing the issues of the entire military family when developing a mental healthcare delivery strategy. Each service also follows the same regulatory guidance, albeit with different nomenclature. Most of the information presented in this section is applicable to all mental health disciplines and all branches of the armed forces. Regardless of specialty or uniform, exposure to military systems as a trainee greatly contributes to the development of confidence and competence in caring for service members and their families during peacetime and war.

The military mental health field is unique, with many inherent challenges that are not addressed in civilian residency training programs. Besides simply offering cultural immersion, military residencies include both didactic and experiential training opportunities that appropriately prepare trainees for the jobs they will enter following graduation. These programs are a crucial component of military medicine and have been identified as the largest guarantor of provider longevity in the military. Additionally, appropriate implementation of the aforementioned knowledge, skills, and attitudes by well-trained military mental health providers will enhance overall unit readiness and improve mission performance by the units they support.

Military psychiatry is distinguishable from civilian adult psychiatry by two major constructs, both requiring years of experience to master. The first is the aforementioned dual-agency role, referring to the psychiatrist's constant but necessary struggle to balance the best interest of the patient with the best interest of the patient's unit, which includes overall unit health and successful completion of the military mission.[45] The second construct is the extensive amount of technical, military-specific knowledge required to practice successfully within the military culture (Table 42-2).

As mentioned above, all US military psychiatry programs are accredited by ACGME. Like psychiatrists trained in civilian programs, military psychiatrists are expected to demonstrate competence through successful development of specific knowledge, skills, and attitudes.[7] Thriving as a military mental health provider requires the nurturing of career-specific knowledge, skills, and attitudes that can be gained only by repeated clinical encounters within military systems under the direction of an experienced supervisor. This section will introduce and explain these elements of competence as they relate to military psychiatry, accompanied by case examples pertinent to each.

Knowledge

Knowledge begins with a basic understanding of the military culture, such as appropriate wear of the uniform, rank recognition, salutations, customs, and courtesies.[49] It also involves an appreciation of the mindset of military leaders, who are responsible for the safety of hundreds of service members and millions of dollars worth of equipment, and whose success depends on their ability to motivate their troops to accomplish potentially life-threatening tasks under adverse conditions for minimal pay. Leaders often have neither the time nor the incentive to make special accommodations for service members who are not mentally fit for the mission at hand. Additionally, knowledge consists of understanding military occupations in terms of education, content, scope, typical duty environment, and inherent stressors. For example, the military psychiatrist should know that cooks and infantry soldiers require one of the lowest entrance examination scores,[50] that recruiters have one of the most stressful jobs,[51] and that aviation crew members are prohibited from taking certain types of medications.[6]

TABLE 42-2

OFFICIAL DOCUMENTS WITH WHICH US ARMY PSYCHIATRISTS SHOULD BE FAMILIAR

Number	Title
Army Regulations and Pamphlets	
AR 40-1	*Composition, Mission, and Functions of the Army Medical Department*
AR 40-66	*Medical Record Administration and Documentation*
AR 40-400	*Patient Administration*
AR 40-501	*Standards of Medical Fitness*
AR 380-67	*Personnel Security Program*
AR 600-8-4	*Line of Duty Investigations*
AR 600-8-22	*Military Awards*
AR 600-8-24	*Officer Transfers and Discharges*
AR 600-85	*Army Substance Abuse Program*
AR 608-18	*The Army Family Advocacy Program*
AR 623-3	*Evaluation Reporting System*
AR 635-40	*Physical Evaluation for Retention, Retirement, or Separation*
AR 635-200	*Active Duty Enlisted Administrative Separations*
AR 670-1	*Wear and Appearance of Army Uniforms and Insignia*
DA Pamphlet 600-24	*Suicide Prevention and Psychological Autopsy*
Department of Defense Directives and Instructions	
DoD Directive 1332.14	*Enlisted Administrative Separations*
DoD Directive 1332.30	*Separation of Regular and Reserve Commissioned Officers*
DoD Directive 6490.1	*Mental Health Evaluations of Members of the Armed Forces*
DoD Instruction 6490.4	*Requirements for Mental Health Evaluations of Members of the Armed Forces*
Army Field Manuals	
FM 4-02.51 (formerly FM 8-51)	*Combat and Operational Stress Control*
FM 6-22.5	*Combat Stress*
Other Documents	
DoDSER	*Department of Defense Suicide Event Report*
Air Force Instruction 41-307	*Aeromedical Evacuation Patient Considerations and Standards of Care*

Furthermore, knowledge includes familiarity with community resources and programs available to assist troubled service members and their families. Each branch of the armed forces has its own service-specific support agencies, several of which psychiatrists are required by regulation to contact under specific circumstances, and others that are simply available for anyone who needs them. The first category includes substance abuse education and treatment programs,[52] child and family welfare programs,[53] patient administration offices,[54] physical evaluation board liaison offices,[55] other mental health treatment programs in the community, and law enforcement agencies. The second category includes organizations such as the command chaplain group, local community service agencies (eg, Army Community Service, Fleet and Family Services, Airman and Family Readiness Centers), the staff judge advocate (legal), the inspector general, Military OneSource, and the Veterans Administration.[56,57]

Another aspect of knowledge is the military psychiatrist's ability to predict the effect of clinical decisions and administrative recommendations on service members, their command, and the military as a whole. For example, military psychiatrists must have an idea of realistic alternative duties available to a service member who is given a mental health profile or is prescribed sedating medications. They must proactively liaison with unit leaders to minimize stress on the service member, to help the unit accommodate the service member's duty limitations, and to limit adverse effect upon the unit's mission. Military psychiatrists must have an appreciation for how long it takes an individual to be administratively or medically separated from the service and how peers are likely to treat that individual during the separation process. An additional concern for commanders is that a recommendation for an administrative separation may trigger a flurry of requests for separation from other service members. This is especially concerning during times of high operational tempo, when a unit's attrition rate is a critical factor that can degrade the unit's ability to accomplish its mission. Additionally, the psychiatrist should know something about financial compensation and other benefits available to veterans upon leaving active duty service.

Finally, and perhaps most importantly, knowledge refers to being intimately familiar with a host of military regulations and instructional manuals.[2] Because of their obligation to protect units as well as individual service members, military psychiatrists must know the medical conditions that disqualify recruits from entering military service, as well as those conditions that require a recommendation for medical discharge.[6] They must be familiar with the regulation that addresses the medical disability program and know how to conduct a separation history and physical examination.[55] In addition to knowing which mental health conditions warrant medical separation, military psychiatrists must be familiar with regulations pertaining to administrative (nonmedical) separations, which differ for officer and enlisted personnel, and some of which require an evaluation and recommendation for discharge by a doctoral-level mental health professional. During these separations, knowledge of the psychiatrist's role as either a patient advocate or a neutral evaluator is essential.[58,59]

As part of a safeguard to prevent coerced mental health referral of service members, military psychiatrists must be very familiar with the tenets of the DoD policy on command-directed mental health evaluations, including service members' rights in such proceedings, the limits of confidentiality, the psychiatrists' obligations, the personnel involved, specific time limits, and required documentation.[3] This policy was implemented in 1993 in response to congressional-level concern that service members were being inappropriately referred for mental evaluations after blowing the whistle on suspicious activities within their commands.[60] Deviation from the prescribed process could result in significant administrative sanctions against the military psychiatrist.

Additional administrative duties that do not have a correlate in civilian mental healthcare include security clearance evaluations,[5] participation in suicide investigations and appropriate documentation of suicide attempts,[61–64] and transportation of patients via the military aeromedical evacuation system.[65] Regulations pertaining to basic charting standards, maintenance of military medical and mental health records, and dispositioning of retired records are other duties required of a military psychiatrist.[54,66] Since September 11, 2001, having an understanding of service-specific medical and mental health units, their placement on the battlefield, and the behavioral health officer's specific roles and obligations during wartime has become even more critical for the military psychiatrist.[67–69] Such knowledge could conceivably be acquired through a concentrated training period shortly after entering active duty,[8] but the depth and scope of such training would not remotely approach the training and experience gained from a 4-year military training program. The following case studies, as well as the others in the chapter (all from the clinical experience of one of the authors [WW]), demonstrate the benefits of such a program.

Case Study 42-1: A deployed Army psychiatrist identifies a number of immature and maladaptive coping skills in many of the soldiers she evaluated. Concerned about their ability to successfully complete the deployment, she recommends most of them for personality disorder separations under Chapter 5-13, Army Regulation 635-200.[59] Even though some of these soldiers are aggressive and unpredictable, the majority of them are not separated. The frequency with which the psychiatrist recommended separation reduced her credibility with the unit's commander, who ultimately stops following through on any of the psychiatrist's recommendations whatsoever.

Case Study 42-2: A 25-year-old deployed Army aviation soldier comes to the mental health clinic requesting treatment for insomnia. The soldier describes initial insomnia related to worries about upcoming missions that involved flying into hostile territory. In addition to clarifying the soldier's psychiatric symptoms, the psychiatrist asks him about his job and work schedule. Knowing that aviation personnel are grounded while using psychotropic medications, as well as realizing that the soldier's job could require him to wake up in the middle of the night and quickly perform an equipment check prior to flying, the psychiatrist does not feel comfortable prescribing a sleep medication for the soldier. Instead, she provides him with instructions in deep breathing and progressive muscle relaxation and schedules him to attend a sleep hygiene class offered by the clinic.

Case Study 42-3: A soldier walks into the mental health clinic with a memorandum stating that he needs a psychological evaluation to get his security clearance renewed. Having just graduated from a civilian residency program, the psychiatrist is unaware that he should have received additional documents pertaining to the soldier's background prior to the appointment and that the memorandum's questions must be answered in a very specific fashion. He conducts a one-on-one assessment of the soldier and types up a letter stating that he thinks the soldier should be granted a security clearance. His letter is rejected by the requesting security agency because it does not address a key question raised during the background check and was not submitted in the proper format.

Skills

Many of the skills required of military psychiatrists, including assessment, formulation, crisis management, consultation, and various psychotherapies, are taught in civilian training programs. Other skills, however, are required uniquely by military psychiatrists, and can only be learned by working within a military environment. Such skills are mastered through successful completion of a military psychiatry GME program followed by experience at the initial duty assignment. Military-related skills include the specific interpersonal skills required for interacting with individual patients as well as their patients' commanders and military support personnel. Additionally, numerous technical and administrative skills related to both patient care and career management are required of military psychiatrists. Even unique clinical skills are required, particularly during times of overseas deployment (Exhibit 42-3).

EXHIBIT 42-3

UNIQUE SKILLS REQUIRED OF MILITARY PSYCHIATRISTS

Military psychiatrists must possess the ability to

- connect with service members who are patients;
- connect with service members who are not patients;
- connect with unit leaders;
- be a "salesperson" and an ambassador for the field of mental health;
- provide appropriate interventions following traumatic events;
- interact within and among various military agencies;
- access pertinent regulations;
- format and write military memoranda;
- prepare official reports;
- provide quality care in austere environments;
- counsel subordinates; and
- prepare counseling statements, award recommendations, and performance reviews.

Military psychiatry is not unique in requiring good interpersonal skills. However, the specific interpersonal skills required of a military psychiatrist are unique and vary depending upon the setting. For example, because some service members feel uncomfortable interacting with providers who do not maintain the decorum they expect of a military officer, the psychiatrist must maintain appropriate military bearing, yet not be so formal and rigid as to negatively influence the formation of a therapeutic alliance. Like patients in the civilian sector, service members will open up in a supportive, somewhat relaxed environment. A military psychiatrist who is too authoritative may have difficulty connecting with a service member who is having trouble with one or more supervisors, and thus may inadvertently create a barrier to care. Conversely, a style that is too casual may give service member patients permission to behave unprofessionally or spend excessive amounts of time at the mental health clinic—behaviors that will inevitably lead to or worsen preexisting occupational difficulties.

Working with unit commanders requires an entirely different interpersonal skill set, consisting of a business-like attitude, a focus on data and regulations, emphasis on mission success, and a willingness to accept that the commander will not always seem appreciative of the psychiatrist's efforts to help the unit or the soldier. Commanders often have preconceived negative opinions of mental health providers secondary to prior personal or family contacts with mental healthcare professionals, a perceived adversarial role, and a skewed opinion of the ability of mental health to enhance mission readiness.

As clinicians, psychiatrists are expected to maintain their clinical skills and to keep up with current medical literature. As military officers, they are expected to maintain their physical fitness and be familiar with current military tactics, procedures, and regulations. Often, the most challenging interpersonal skill required of a military psychiatrist is expert marketing to a population that may be resistant to receiving psychiatric assistance. Unlike their civilian counterparts, military mental health professionals must actively participate in primary prevention activities through education and outreach efforts for the units they support. By proactively getting to know their post's units and commanders, they can reduce stigma associated with mental health interventions, an identified barrier to care.[70] The ability of military psychiatrists to establish themselves as viable members of a unit's healthcare team will enhance access to mental healthcare for soldiers. Enhanced access to care is vital in an era of repeated combat operations when a large percentage of service members self-report operational mental health issues.[71]

Military psychiatry also requires a number of unique technical skills, many of which include researching and writing official correspondence and reports of various types (Exhibit 42-4).[2] Failure to take the appropriate course of action or failure to document recommendations or actions in the correct manner could reduce the psychiatrist's credibility, negatively impact the effectiveness of the unit, and potentially have lifelong consequences for uniformed patients. The military psychiatrist must be familiar with pertinent regulations, how to access the regulations, and how to apply them while providing high-quality mental healthcare for service members and commands. In the US Army, regulations dictate how a medical chart is prepared,[54] what elements of the physical examination are required for a disability evaluation,[55] how to schedule a command-directed mental health evaluation,[3] what information must be provided to commanders after a command-directed evaluation,[72] how to communicate recommended duty limitations to soldiers and their commanders,[6] how to dispose of closed behavioral health charts,[54] and even how to write in the "military style."[73] Significant failure to practice in accordance with these regulations could adversely affect a provider's reputation, credentials, and medical license.

EXHIBIT 42-4

DOCUMENTS AND REPORTS PREPARED BY MILITARY PSYCHIATRISTS

- Clinical notes
- "Sick slips"
- Extended sick slips (eg, physical profile, limited duty board)
- Safety precaution recommendations to commanders
- Security clearance evaluations
- Medical review officer findings
- Medical board narrative summaries
- Suicide line-of-duty statements
- Sanity boards
- Psychological autopsies*
- Military memoranda
- Standard operating procedures
- Counseling statements
- Officer evaluation report support forms
- Officer evaluation reports
- Award recommendations
- Line-of-duty investigations

*In the US Army, as of 2001, these are completed only by forensically trained psychiatrists.

Technical skills required of military psychiatrists also include those relevant to their career progression and to that of their subordinates. If conducted appropriately, the military's performance evaluation system ensures that service members are provided with timely feedback and ample opportunities to improve upon their deficits.[74] Similarly, the military's award system recognizes exceptional performance, providing incentives for exceeding the standard.[75] Both mechanisms to recognize performance are complex and can be quite confusing, even to individuals with years of experience. Promotions and accompanying pay raises depend upon the ability to successfully navigate these two systems. All military leaders, including most military psychiatrists, are responsible for counseling and rating their subordinates, as well as for submitting award requests months before they will be presented. The psychiatrist must be familiar with subordinates' accomplishments, know what level of award such accomplishments warrant, and what language to use to ensure the requested award is approved. Procedure and language is of equal, if not greater, importance when preparing performance reports, and information on these elements is not available in any official document. It is available primarily through mentoring and guidance by senior officers and supervisors.

Military psychiatry GME programs provide trainees the opportunity to learn about the military performance rating system because trainees, like all military officers, require an annual evaluation report. Through formal instruction and individual guidance by a supervisor, trainees learn how to document personal goals and accomplishments.[74] They also become familiar with the process of mentoring and evaluating subordinates, which they will most likely have to perform at their initial postresidency duty station. Trainees in civilian psychiatry GME programs do not have the same opportunity to experience the military rating system and thus are at a great disadvantage when evaluating other mental health professionals upon completion of residency training.

Military psychiatry also requires unique clinical skills during deployment or other duty in austere environments. The practice of "combat psychiatry" requires the ability to conduct problem-focused interviews in suboptimal clinical settings with little privacy, loud ambient noise, extremes of temperature, and unreliable computer and telephonic support. Interventions must be brief (two to four sessions) and solution-focused. Long-term psychotherapy is not an option. The military psychiatrist must learn to trust the clinical capabilities of staff members, which often include enlisted mental health specialists with less than a year of training. Laboratory services are often very limited, commonly consisting of basic serology and urine screens only. The results of liver and thyroid function tests, drug levels, and advanced drug screens may take weeks to return, if they are available at all. Stocked medications are sometimes limited to one or two selective serotonin reuptake inhibitors (SSRIs), bupropion, one sleep agent, one benzodiazepine, and a first-generation antipsychotic such as haloperidol. Mood stabilizers, atypical antipsychotics, non-SSRI antidepressants, and stimulants may not be available at all. Subspecialty consultants are also difficult to access, and at times a military psychiatrist may be the only actual physician at the location. Such topics are integrated into the curriculum of military residencies to prepare trainees for successful practice in diverse and challenging environments. The following vignettes, as well as those elsewhere in the chapter, are illustrative of materials prepared for military physicians in training.

Vignette 42-1: A psychiatrist is treating a soldier who is extremely angry with his chain of command. He claims that his commander "plays favorites" and fails to take care of his subordinates' basic needs. The soldier mentions several unsafe practices allegedly occurring in the unit and gives the psychiatrist permission to investigate. The psychiatrist discovers that an unusually high number of individuals within the soldier's company are being seen at the mental health clinic, their charts all documenting similar complaints. He requests a meeting with the company commander to discuss the allegations. At the scheduled appointment time, the psychiatrist arrives in a pressed uniform, prepared with a briefing that includes specific data about recent behavioral trends in the unit, evidence-based information about how unsafe and unfair practices could contribute to reduced unit readiness, and very specific recommendations on how to improve the situation. The company commander states that he's interested in trying to implement the recommendations.

Vignette 42-2: A new military psychiatrist was active in his residency's psychotherapy interest group and authored several publications on dialectical behavioral therapy. One of his first patients as a division psychiatrist is a young woman with a very troubled past whom he diagnoses with borderline personality disorder. Intrigued by the case, the psychiatrist begins to see the patient for 50 minutes twice a week. Enlisted mental health specialists in the clinic complain to their noncommissioned officer in charge that the psychiatrist is always in session and is never able to staff cases. The patient herself seems to be getting worse and insists that she needs a sick slip excusing her from her upcoming field training exercise. At the end of the 4th week, the patient's first sergeant accompanies her to the appointment and angrily asks the psychiatrist whether or not he understands the impact that her absence from the training exercise will have on the rest of the unit, and whom he expects to look after her while the unit is in the field.

Vignette 42-3: A deployed Army psychiatrist is working at a small base at a hostile location in Iraq. Late one night, he is sleeping in his cot at the back of his clinic tent when he is awakened by a weary-appearing soldier requesting help. The soldier is dirty, malodorous, and exhausted. Earlier in the day, he returned from a long convoy during which his platoon was attacked with small-arms fire and rocket-propelled grenades. He claims to be tense and worried about his wife, whom he has been unable to call in 2 weeks. He tearfully tells the psychiatrist that he is scheduled to go out again the next morning, but that he doesn't feel like his "head is in the game," and that he questions his ability to defend his comrades. The psychiatrist conducts a brief assessment and contacts the soldier's commander to recommend he be removed from convoy duty for a couple of days and be allowed to participate in a "restoration" program offered by the clinic.

Attitudes

The development of appropriate attitudes may seem less essential than the acquisition of sufficient knowledge and skills in the field of military psychiatry. However, psychiatrists who approach clinical and administrative tasks in the military with the wrong attitudes may inadvertently make their lives more stressful and find it difficult to achieve job satisfaction. They must adopt an attitude of selflessness and advocacy for patients while maintaining a skeptical eye for malingering. They may have to treat a patient while simultaneously providing support for the patient's unit. They must adopt an attitude of flexibility and humility, including a willingness to take on challenging tasks for minimal recognition. Finally, they must excel in their role as a leader to ensure their subordinates receive the recognition and promotions they deserve.

The dual-agency role discussed earlier perfectly demonstrates the importance of having the right attitude for the job. Military psychiatrists must be willing to adopt a utilitarian viewpoint.[76] They must regard the entire population of service members as their "patient" and endeavor to protect that "patient" from harm, even at the cost of violating the confidentiality of individual service members. Unforeseen violations of doctor-patient confidentiality are rare, but are necessary and appropriate if the identified patient is experiencing symptoms that could compromise the safety of the unit. Depending on the patient's job, such symptoms might include poor concentration, sleep deprivation, errors in judgment, severe anxiety, profound depression, delusions, hallucinations, cognitive deficits, impaired impulse control, and of course, suicidal and homicidal fantasies.

Military psychiatrists must be flexible and creative, satisfied with limited available resources and treatment capabilities, and moderately comfortable as the sole psychiatrist serving troop populations as large as 15,000.[77,78] They must accept the inability to help everyone, a difficult concept to acknowledge for many psychiatrists, who presumably entered the field to help their patients live happier, more productive lives. Because of the high service-member-to-psychiatrist ratio, military psychiatrists must also believe in the power of primary prevention and commit themselves to the concept that psychiatric care begins in the foxhole, where troops help one another overcome adversity.

Psychiatrists in the military should maintain an air of humility and understand that a caring friend, a chaplain, or a commander may be more effective and therapeutic than a mental health professional in certain situations. They must also accept that the title of "captain" or "major" is sometimes preferable to "doctor" in military units, because the former more clearly identifies them as a part of the military team. Additionally, they will come to realize that most of the troops they serve have no idea what the difference is between a psychiatrist, a psychologist, and a social worker.

The military psychiatrist must be willing to work under and alongside other mental health professionals, such as psychiatric nurses, social workers, and occupational therapists. They must also be willing to place a great deal of trust in the clinical abilities of their enlisted mental health specialists, who are often the first providers to make contact with service members seeking treatment. These personnel serve a crucial role in triaging patients, performing and documenting initial assessments, conducting educational groups, providing supportive counseling, and managing acute crises, often with fewer than 12 months of mental health training.[79] Mental health specialists in the Reserves and the National Guard may have completely unrelated civilian jobs, requiring an extensive amount of training prior to providing patient care. Military psychiatry training programs incorporate into the curriculum specific experience working with other mental health professionals and paraprofessionals.

Operating in a military environment under close scrutiny also creates a number of unique challenges. Military psychiatrists must always remember they are representatives of the US armed forces. Many military bases are relatively small, and psychiatrists commonly encounter patients and their families at various locations on post and in the surrounding communities. Many military psychiatrists have had the experience of sharing a lunch table, a medical waiting room, and even a shower area with their patients. Such situations, while essentially unheard of in a civilian setting, are commonplace in today's military environment, and uniformed psychiatrists must be capable of maintaining good military bearing and a professional demeanor at all times.

Case Study 42-4: A military psychiatrist is seeing an intelligence analyst who has had difficulty sleeping since she was switched to the night shift 4 weeks ago, and has had a limited response to sleep medications. Her energy and concentration have reached dangerously low levels and she has already made a couple of mistakes on the job. While recognizing the soldier's right to seek treatment confidentially, the psychiatrist has valid concerns that his patient's ability to accurately report important intelligence data may be compromised. He contacts the soldier's commander to recommend that she be given a day shift job because of her compromised ability to perform her duties, knowing that her security clearance may be suspended as a result.

Vignette 42-4: A military psychiatrist graduated with honors from an esteemed medical school on the East Coast and completed a civilian residency before joining the Army. She was used to wearing a white coat to work and having a large administrative staff to assist her. She was also accustomed to calling her staff by their first names and to joining them regularly at educational dinners sponsored by pharmaceutical companies. She has a very difficult time adjusting to the Army and feels disrespected by the other members of her department, whom she regards with an air of contempt. Her department chief, a psychologist, counsels her multiple times on the importance of being a team player and interacting regularly with the local commands. She ultimately deploys to Iraq, and as soon as possible following her miserable 15 months in the desert, elects to resign from the Army.

Vignette 42-5: A young soldier in Afghanistan walks into the combat stress control clinic in the middle of a chaotic afternoon. The psychiatrist, who is finishing up with one patient and has two more waiting to see him, just learned that a patrol from the base was attacked and that a unit is requesting a critical event debriefing. He missed lunch and has three phone calls to return, plus a tobacco cessation class to teach in 30 minutes. Noticing the new soldier standing in the entryway, he snarls at her and tells her she'll have to come back unless it's an emergency. The next morning the psychiatrist goes to the motor pool to catch a convoy to a neighboring base, and discovers that this soldier will be his driver.

FUTURE OF GRADUATE MEDICAL EDUCATION

Military psychiatry GME faces numerous pressures on different fronts. As emphasis on efficiency in the direct care side of the military healthcare system increases, a decision on whether GME should be financed within the system or contracted out to the civilian side may become necessary. Because the field of military psychiatry is distinctly different than its civilian counterpart, the training of psychiatrists outside the Army is less tenable than in other medical specialties. The large shift into the core competency movement will directly affect the structure and content of all training programs. The current conflicts in the Middle East and the GWOT will have direct effects on the future of GME in psychiatry as issues involving behavioral health gain even more national attention.

The viability of GME within the military, because of its high costs, has always been debated. As medical services inside and outside the military strive for optimal efficiency, medical education is placed under increasing pressure because of the costly general apprenticeship model of medical education, which emphasizes personal experiences with teachers, mentors, and patients. Only through personal relationships with teachers and mentors and plentiful patient care experiences can a clinician develop sophisticated synthesizing capabilities. Traditionally, military GME was not affected as much as civilian training programs by the managed care model, but MTF commanders are now assessed by workload productivity via the relative value unit. GME-related tasks do not produce relative value units and therefore have no workload credit, a critical factor in whether the military decides to continue supporting GME with military and civil service faculty or contract the mission to nongovernment organizations.

The competency movement carries some promise for transition from time-based experiences toward a competency standard independent of time. Although more applicable to procedure-dominant medical specialties, the development of treatment portfolios of medication and psychotherapy cases will benefit psychiatry, allowing more longitudinal, rather than cross-sectional, evaluations. The competency movement will also leverage psychiatry to develop more relevant clinical outcome measurements, enabling programs to start objectively measuring their trainees' patient care skills.

The current conflicts in the Middle East and the ongoing GWOT will necessitate an elevated operational tempo for years to come and require that the mental wellness of all service members receive attention from the military. Added emphasis on treatment of posttraumatic stress disorder and traumatic brain injury must be incorporated into training programs. As proximity, immediacy, expectancy, and simplicity (PIES) principles and force sustainment and resetting efforts take on increasing importance in behavioral health force-shaping in all environments, further emphasis on military psychiatry doctrine in GME programs will become paramount. Because the overall number of matriculates from USUHS and the Health Professions Scholarship Program has decreased in recent years, increased recruitment efforts will be necessary to ensure adequate numbers of future psychiatrists.

SUMMARY

GME is an essential aspect of ensuring safe, high-quality healthcare in the United States. Training programs for each medical specialty must abide by a specific set of requirements and guidelines and maintain available faculty to provide adequate physician-in-training supervision and mentoring. Psychiatry GME has very extensive didactic, clinical, and supervision requirements, resulting in the development of a comprehensive skill set over the course of the training period. Military psychiatry GME programs observe all of these requirements, in addition to providing education in military-specific behavioral health skills, which are essential for psychiatrists to function adequately in both garrison and operational environments.

Lessons learned from military conflicts over the last 40 years indicate that psychiatric trauma from war is a significant medical issue; this issue has become a prominent concern for American society. Service members returning from combat deployments can carry psychological scars that make reintegration into society challenging and stressful, affecting both veterans and their families. Military psychiatry GME programs have enhanced training in all aspects of the deployment cycle support process to ensure that military psychiatrists are prepared to address the varied needs of the military family during the deployment cycle. With behavioral health issues secondary to military service receiving extensive scrutiny in the media and by government agencies, military psychiatrists must be comfortable practicing in potentially high-profile environments, necessitating a comprehensive training experience.

With the anticipated long-term duration of the GWOT, military psychiatry GME will continue to be an essential aspect of military readiness. Ongoing refinement of behavioral health screening throughout the deployment cycle, treatment of psychiatric conditions related to combat stress, and deployment-related interventions for military families will require military psychiatry GME programs to be flexible in modifying military-specific training while complying with the standard requirements mandated by ACGME. Retention of qualified military GME program faculty as mentors, role models, and subject matter experts will ensure the continued development of competent military psychiatrists prepared to support US service members and their families.

REFERENCES

1. US Department of the Army. *Commissioned Officer Professional Development and Career Management*. Washington, DC: DA; 2007. DA Pamphlet 600-3.

2. Diebold CJ. Military administrative psychiatry. In: Lande G, Armitage D, eds. *Principles and Practice of Military Forensic Psychiatry*. Springfield, Ill: Charles C Thomas; 1997.

3. US Department of Defense. *Mental Health Evaluations of the Members of the Armed Forces*. Washington, DC: DoD; 1997. DoD Directive 6490.1.

4. Joint Service Committee on Military Justice. *Manual for Courts Martial United States*. Washington, DC: US Government Printing Office; 2005.

5. US Department of the Army. *Personnel Security Program*. Washington, DC: DA; 1988. Army Regulation 380-67.

6. US Department of the Army. *Standards of Medical Fitness*. Washington, DC: DA; 2007. Army Regulation 40-501.

7. Accreditation Counsel for Graduate Medical Education. Psychiatry program requirements. ACGME Web site. Available at: http://www.acgme.org/acWebsite/RRC_400/400_prIndex.asp. Accessed November 23, 2007.

8. Wise MG. The past, present, and future of psychiatric training in the US armed services. *Mil Med*.1987;152:550–553.

9. Heaton LD, Anderson RS, Glass AJ, Bernucci R, eds. *Zone of Interior*. Vol 1. In: *Neuropsychiatry in World War II*. Washington, DC: Department of the Army, Office of The Surgeon General; 1966.

10. Ozarin LO, McMillan G. The American Psychiatric Association: historical highlights. American Psychiatric Association Web site. Available at: http://www.psych.org/public_info/libr_publ/apahighlights.cfm. Accessed November 23, 2007.

11. Bailey P, Williams FE, Komora PO. *Neuropsychiatry*. Vol X. In: *The Medical Department of the United States Army in the World War*. Washington, DC: US Government Printing Office; 1929.

12. US Army Center of Military History. Number of Army personnel who served during each major war, and the number of casualties incurred. US Army Center of Military History Web site. Available at: http://www.army.mil/cmh-pg/faq/FAQ-C&C.htm. Accessed November 23, 2007.

13. Steyn RW. Retrospections: a sketch of nautical psychiatry through World War II. *Mil Med*. 1980:145:407–412.

14. Taylor RR, Mullins WS, Parks RJ. *Medical Training in World War II*. Washington, DC: Department of the Army, Office of The Surgeon General; 1974.

15. Menninger WC. Psychiatric experience in the war, 1941–1946. *Am J Psychiatry*. 1947:104:577–586.

16. Forrer GR, Grisell JL. US Army psychiatric training program. *AMA Arch Neurol Psychiatry*. 1957:77:218–277.

17. Department of the Army. *Department of Defense Report to the Defense Base Closure and Realignment Commission*. Vol III. Washington, DC: DA; 1995. Available at: http://www.defenselink.mil/brac/army.htm. Accessed November 23, 2007.

18. Defense Base Closure and Realignment Act of 1990. Pub L No. 101-510 (1990).

19. The Defense Secretary's Commission on Base Realignment and Closures. *Report of the Defense Secretary's Commission*. Washington, DC: DoD; 1988. Available at: http://www.defenselink.mil/brac/army.htm. Accessed November 23, 2007.

20. Pincus SH, Staff Psychiatrist, Madigan Army Medical Center, Fort Lewis, Washington. Personal communication, February 2007.

21. Orman DT, Director, PTSD-TBI/BH Integration Office, USAMEDCOM, Fort Sam Houston, Texas. Personal communication, April 2007.

22. Defense Base Closure and Realignment Act of 1990 (as amended in 2004). Pub L No. 101-510 (2004).

23. Department of Defense, San Antonio Military Medical Center. San Antonio medical BRAC. SAMMC Web site. Available at: http://www.sambio.amedd.army.mil/About.htm. Accessed November 23, 2007.

24. Moran M. Medical school grads' interest in psychiatry holds steady. *Psychiatry News*. 2007;42(8):1.

25. US Department of the Army. The leader, leadership, and human dimensions. In: *Army Leadership Be, Know, Do.* Washington, DC: DA; 1999. Army Field Manual 22-100. Part 1.

26. Accreditation Counsel for Graduate Medical Education. Duty hours language. ACGME Web site. Available at: http://www.acgme.org/acWebsite/dutyHours/dh_Lang703.pdf. Accessed November 23, 2007.

27. Ritchie EC. Colonel, Medical Corps, US Army; Psychiatry Consultant to the Army Surgeon General. Personal communication, February 2007.

28. Barthel HJ. US Army Medical Corps Chief's Briefing, presented at Tripler Army Medical Center, Hawaii, August 2006.

29. Canadian Medical Education Directions for Specialists (CanMEDS) 2000 Project. *Skills of the New Millennium: Report of the Societal Needs Working Group*. Ottawa, Ontario, Canada: Royal College of Physicians and Surgeons of Canada; 1996.

30. American Board of Medical Specialties Task Force on Competence. *Proceedings From the 1999 Professional Competence and Board Certification Conference, Chicago, Illinois, 18–19 March, 1999*. ABMS Web site. Available at: http://www.abms.org/About_ABMS/ABMS_History/Extended_History/Competency_Movement.aspx. Accessed February 28, 2011.

31. Joint Commission on the Accreditation of Healthcare Organizations. *Comprehensive Accreditation Manual for Hospitals*. Oakbrook Terrace, Ill: Joint Commission; 2007.

32. National Cancer Institute. A guide to understanding informed consent. NCI Web site. Available at: http://www.cancer.gov/clinicaltrials/conducting/informed-consent-guide/allpages. Accessed November 23, 2007

33. US Department of the Army. *Oath of Office—Military Personnel*. Washington, DC: DA; 1999. Department of the Army Form 71.

34. Sadock BJ, Sadock VA. Public and hospital psychiatry. In: *Kaplan and Sadock's Synopsis of Psychiatry*. 9th ed. Philadelphia, Penn; Lippincott, Williams & Wilkins; 2003: 1376–1377.

35. My Evaluations Web site. Available at: https://www.myevaluations.com/Logon.asp. Accessed November 23, 2007.

36. Bender E. New residency requirements divide training directors. *Psychiatric News*. 2003;38(7):14.

37. Accreditation Counsel for Graduate Medical Education. ACGME Outcome Project. ACGME Web site. Available at: http://www.acgme.org/outcome. Accessed November 23, 2007.

38. Accreditation Council for Graduate Medical Education. Essentials of accredited residencies. In: *Directory of Graduate Medical Education Programs*. Chicago, Ill: American Medical Association; 1984: 81.

39. US Department of the Army. *Heavy Brigade Combat Team Combined Arms Battalion*. Washington, DC: DA; 2005. Field Manual 3-90.5.

40. Howe EC. Special problem for military psychiatrists. In: Simon RI, ed. *Review of Clinical Psychiatry and the Law*. Washington, DC: American Psychiatric Association Press; 1992: 305–307.

41. American Medical Association. Principles of medical ethics. AMA Web site. Available at: http://www.ama-assn.org/ama/pub/category/2512.html. Accessed November 23, 2007.

42. US Department of the Army. *Deployment Cycle Support (DCS) Directive*. Washington, DC: DA; 2007. Army Directive 2007-02. Appendix A-6.

43. Jensen PS, Martin D, Watanabe H. Children's response to parental separation during Operation Desert Storm. *J Am Acad Child Adolesc Psychiatry*. 1996;35:433–441.

44. Faran ME, Weist MD, Saito AY, Yoshikami L, Weiser JW, Kaer B. School-based mental health on a United States Army installation. In: Weist MD, Evans SW, Lever NA, eds. *Handbook of School Mental Health: Advancing Practice and Research*. New York, NY: Kluwer Academic/Plenum Publishers; 2003: Chap 14.

45. Waits WM, Waldrep D. Application of Army combat stress control doctrine in work with Pentagon survivors. *Mil Med*. 2002;167(9 suppl):39–43.

46. Milliken CS, Leavitt WT, Murdock P, Orman DT, Ritchie EC, Hoge CW. Principles guiding implementation of the Operation Solace plan: "Pieces of PIES," therapy by walking around, and care management. *Mil Med*. 2002;167(9 suppl):48–57.

47. Accreditation Counsel for Graduate Medical Education. Reports—list of programs by specialty. ACGME Web site. Available at: http://www.acgme.org/adspublic/. Accessed November 25, 2007.

48. Society of Medical Consultants to the Armed Forces. *Military Graduate Medical Education Under Stress: A White Paper*. Fredericksburg, Va: SMCAF; 1987. Available at: http://www.smcaf.org/Military%20GME%20Under%20Stress%201987.pdf. Accessed November 25, 2007.

49. Bonn KE. *Army Officers Guide*. 50th ed. Mechanicsburg, Penn: Stackpole Press; 2005.

50. Powers R. Army enlisted job descriptions and qualification factors. About.com: US Military Web site. Available at: http://usmilitary.about.com/od/enlistedjobs/a/92g.htm. Accessed October 27, 2009.

51. Cave D. For Army recruiters, a hard toll from a hard sell. *New York Times*. March 27, 2005. Available at: http://www.nytimes.com/2005/03/27/nyregion/27recruit.html. Accessed October 26, 2009.

52. US Department of the Army. *Army Substance Abuse Program*. Washington, DC: DA; 2006. Army Regulation 600-85.

53. US Department of the Army. *The Army Family Advocacy Program*. Washington, DC: DA; 2006. Army Regulation 608-18.

54. US Department of the Army. *Medical Record Administration and Health Care Documentation*. Washington, DC: DA; 2006. Army Regulation 40-66.

55. US Department of the Army. *Physical Evaluation for Retention, Retirement, or Separation*. Washington, DC: DA; 2006. Army Regulation 635-40.

56. US Department of the Army. *Army Community Service Center*. Washington, DC: DA; 2006. Army Regulation 608-1.

57. Military OneSource Web site. 2007. Available at: http://www.militaryonesource.com/skins/MOS/home.aspx. Accessed November 25, 2007.

58. US Department of the Army. *Officer Transfers and Discharges*. Washington, DC: DA; 2006. Army Regulation 600-8-24.

59. US Department of the Army. *Active Duty Administrative Separations*. Washington, DC: DA; 2005. Army Regulation 635-200.

60. Military Whistleblower Protection Act of 1988, 10 USC § 1034 (1988).

61. US Department of the Army. *Suicide Prevention and Psychological Autopsy*. Washington, DC: DA; 1988. DA Pamphlet 600-24.

62. US Department of the Army. *Line of Duty Policy, Procedures, and Investigations*. Washington, DC: DA; 2004. Army Regulation 600-8-4.

63. Department of Defense. Psychological autopsies. TRICARE Web site. Available at: http://mhs.osd.mil/pdfs/policies/2001/01-016.pdf. Accessed November 25, 2007.

64. US Army Suicide Risk Management and Surveillance Office. Army Suicide Event Report. ASER Web site. Available at: https://aser.amedd.army.mil/aser. Accessed November 25, 2007.

65. US Department of the Air Force. *Aeromedical Evacuation Patient Considerations and Standards of Care*. Washington, DC: US Government Printing Office; 2003. Air Force Instruction 41-307, Attachment 6.

66. US Department of the Army. *Patient Administration*. Washington, DC: DA; 2006. Army Regulation 40-40.

67. US Department of the Army. *Composition, Mission, and Functions of the Army Medical Department*. Washington, DC: DA; 1983. Army Regulation 40-1.

68. US Department of the Army. *Combat and Operational Stress Control*. Washington, DC: DA; 2006. Field Manual 4-02.51 (formerly Field Manual 8-51).

69. US Department of the Army. *Combat Stress*. Washington, DC: DA; 2000. Field Manual 6-22.5.

70. Office of the Surgeon, Multinational Force–Iraq. *Mental Health Assessment Team (MHAT-III) Operation Iraqi Freedom Report*. Washington, DC: Department of the Army; 2006. Available at: http://www.behavioralhealth.army.mil/research/index.html. Accessed November 25, 2007.

71. Hoge CW, Castro CA, Messer SC, McGurk D, Cotting DI, Koffman RL. Combat duty in Iraq and Afghanistan, mental health problems, and barriers to care. *N Engl J Med*. 2004;351:13–22.

72. US Department of Defense. *Requirements for Mental Health Evaluations of the Members of the Armed Forces*. Washington, DC: DoD; 1997. DoD Instruction 6490.4.

73. US Department of the Army. *Preparing and Managing Correspondence*. Washington, DC: DA; 2002. Army Regulation 25-50.

74. US Department of the Army. *Evaluation Reporting System*. Washington, DC: DA; 2007. Army Regulation 623-3.

75. US Department of the Army. *Military Awards*. Washington, DC: DA; 2006. Army Regulation 600-8-22.

76. Beauchamp TL, Childress JF. *Principles of Biomedical Ethics*. 4th ed. New York, NY: Oxford University Press; 1994.

77. Ritchie EC, White R. Becoming a successful division psychiatrist: guidelines for preparation and duties of the assignment. *Mil Med*. 1993;158(10):644–648.

78. Hill JV, Lange C, Bacon B. Becoming a successful division psychiatrist: the sequel. *Mil Med*. 2007;172(4):364–369.

79. US Army Recruiting Command. Careers & jobs: mental health specialist (68X). GoArmy.com Web site. Available at: http://www.goarmy.com/JobDetail.do?id=160#training. Accessed November 25, 2007.

Chapter 43

MILITARY FORENSIC MENTAL HEALTH

ELSPETH CAMERON RITCHIE, MD, MPH*

*Colonel, US Army (Retired); formerly, Psychiatry Consultant to The Surgeon General, US Army, and Director, Behavioral Health Proponency, Office of The Surgeon General, Falls Church, Virginia; currently, Chief Clinical Officer, District of Columbia Department of Mental Health, 64 New York Avenue NE, 4th Floor, Washington, DC 20002

A portion of this chapter appeared as: Ritchie EC, Benedek D, Malone R, Carr-Malone R. Psychiatry and the military: an update. *Psychiatr Clin North Am*. 2006;29(3):695–707.

INTRODUCTION

As the wars in Iraq and Afghanistan continue, the US military medical system is required to address many issues at the interface of psychiatry and the law. Service members with mental health consequences from war impact not just the healthcare system, but also the military justice and disability systems. This chapter highlights some of the most topical forensic issues facing military providers, attorneys, and the courts.

The extent to which violent and aggressive behavior in the aftermath of deployment can be attributed to combat experience remains an area of debate and ongoing investigation.[1–3] However, of the hundreds of thousands of veterans deployed in these wars, only a small subgroup has been involved in violent crimes. For this group, military forensic psychiatrists will be called upon to make determinations of competency and criminal responsibility and to inform the courts about the potential contributions of war-related distress or disorder to criminal behavior.

Complicating the widespread occurrence of war-related psychological disorders is the "signature wound" of these wars: traumatic brain injury (TBI). The numerous causes of head trauma include blast exposure, gunshot wounds, motor vehicle injuries, and other accidents. The severely wounded are routinely screened for head trauma; however, some soldiers who experience periods of unconsciousness may not present for treatment. They may later develop difficulty concentrating or irritability but be misdiagnosed or receive no medical treatment. More recently, updates in screening for TBI have been widely implemented. Now all deployed soldiers receive screening for TBI, as well as posttraumatic stress disorder (PTSD), upon their return from an overseas deployment. PTSD, although a well-recognized and validated psychiatric disorder, has also long been associated with malingering, allegedly for the purposes of both avoiding prosecution or punishment, and/or obtaining disability compensation.

Forensic psychiatry, psychology, and social work focus on the intersection of mental health issues and the law. Core topics include competency, criminal responsibility, sexual trauma, and disability. This chapter focuses on forensic psychiatry, rather than the other disciplines, as that is the best-developed discipline in the military; however, the concepts will apply across the disciplines.

Military forensic psychiatrists currently serve in the US Army, Navy, and Air Force. Forensic psychiatry in the military has many similarities to forensic psychiatry as practiced in the civilian world, but some key differences exist. This chapter will accentuate some of the differences. It opens with a description of military law, determination of competency and criminal responsibility, and the role of expert witnesses in the courts-martial system. The next sections discuss malingering and psychological autopsies. Numerous forensic issues also relate to detainees. Although the care of detainees is presented in another chapter in this volume, this chapter will briefly discuss sanity boards on detainees and the behavioral science consultation team policies. A full discussion of the military forensic psychiatry issues and the military legal system is beyond the chapter's scope but may be found in other sources.[4–8] Several case examples, which are composites, are presented and are meant to illustrate principles.

Case Study 43-1: A soldier was returned from Afghanistan in the early years of the global war on terror (GWOT). After serving a hard 6 months there, he received an e-mail from a neighbor, saying: "I have seen a red pick-up truck in your driveway overnight the last few nights. What's up?" The soldier applied for emergency leave, saying his mother was dying. The day after he returned home, he and his wife had a fight over his perceptions that she had a lover. He pulled his personal gun out of the nightstand and shot and killed her. He then turned the gun on himself.

THE PSYCHIATRIST AND THE CRIMINAL JUSTICE SYSTEM

Military Law

The birth of American military law can be traced to the first American Articles of War, which consisted of 69 separate articles enacted by the Continental Congress on June 30, 1775, governing the conduct of the Continental Army.[5,6] Congress enacted today's Uniform Code of Military Justice (UCMJ) in 1950.[8–10] The UCMJ combined the laws formerly governing the US Army, Navy, and Air Force into one uniform code. As a result, the US military has its own system of criminal justice with hierarchical sources of rights. In addition to the UCMJ, military law is based on the US Constitution, federal statutes, executive orders containing the Military Rules of Evidence (MRE), Department of Defense (DoD) directives, service directives, and federal common law. The US Constitution applies to service members unless superseded by military or operational necessity.[9,10]

The UCMJ established several levels of courts-martial. General courts-martial are analogous to felony trials, and special courts-martial are analogous to misdemeanor trials. The summary courts-martial, comparable to a justice-of-the-peace court, is a single-officer court with significantly limited authority.[9] The Fifth Amendment of the Constitution specifically denies the right to grand jury indictment to service members.[9] In place of the grand jury, the military states that no case may be referred to a general court-martial unless there has been a UCMJ Article 32 investigation.[9]

An Article 32 investigation is an open hearing designed to inquire into the facts of the case surrounding the charges. Although similar to both civilian preliminary and grand jury hearings, an Article 32 investigation is a more protective procedure because it affords the opportunity for discovery, to confront adverse witnesses, and to present evidence. Additionally, the recommendation of the Article 32 investigating officer is advisory only and not a final decision.[9]

Forensic Evaluations or "Sanity Boards"

The issue of criminal responsibility is addressed in many military settings, typically during Article 32 hearings and special and general courts-martial. In accordance with Rule for Courts-Martial 706, if it appears to any commander who considers the disposition of charges, or to any investigating officer, trial or defense counsel, military judge, or court member, that there is reason to believe that the accused (or defendant in civilian legal proceedings) lacked mental responsibility for any offense, the fact and basis of the belief is transmitted ultimately to the officer authorized to order such an inquiry.[10]

Determinations of mental or criminal responsibility are referred to a board, commonly referred to as a "706 board" or "sanity board." Sanity boards determine the capacity of the accused to stand trial and address any other questions requested by the convening authorities, usually related to the clinical diagnosis and criminal responsibility. The board officially consists of one or more persons who must be either a physician or a clinical psychologist. Normally, at least one board member is either a psychiatrist or a clinical psychologist.[10]

Although not specifically required by the rule, a military forensic psychiatrist or psychologist is in many cases best qualified to serve as a member of the board.[7,10] This is especially true for cases with complicated mental health issues or those involving very serious crimes, when the potential for appellate scrutiny of the sanity board findings is high. Military lawyers usually acknowledge the specialized training and experience that a military forensic psychiatrist or psychologist brings to sanity boards, frequently asking convening authorities and military judges to request such specialists to participate during assessments of criminal responsibility.[7]

According to Article 50a of the UCMJ,

> [i]t is an affirmative defense in a trial by court-martial that, at the time of the commission of the acts constituting the offense, the accused, as a result of a severe mental disease or defect, was unable to appreciate the nature and quality or wrongfulness of the acts.[11]

The above is often called the cognitive prong of the insanity defense (ie, that the accused knows the difference between right and wrong). This military standard, like the federal standard since the Insanity Defense Reform Act of 1984, does not include a volitional prong (eg, the capacity of the accused to conform his conduct to the requirements of the law). The burden of proving lack of mental responsibility falls on the accused, who must prove the defense by clear and convincing evidence. The court can then find the accused guilty, not guilty, or not guilty by reason of lack of mental responsibility.[11]

Because the accused is obligated to participate in the sanity board process, protections afforded to the defense limit discovery of the findings. Two reports are prepared: (1) a full report that includes all of the board's findings and the basis for its opinions, and (2) an abbreviated report containing only the board's ultimate conclusions on all questions specified in the order. The full report is furnished only to the defense counsel and, upon request, to the commanding officer of the accused. The full report may be released by the board (or other medical personnel) only to other medical personnel for medical purposes. Release of the full report to any person not authorized to receive it is allowed only pursuant to an order by the military judge. The abbreviated report is provided to the officer ordering the examination, the commanding officer of the accused, the investigating officer (if any) appointed pursuant to Article 32, and to all counsel in the case.[8] If the accused chooses to raise a mental health defense, the full report (redacted to exclude direct statements made by the accused) may become discoverable.

Case Study 43-1 (continued): The gunshots were heard by the neighbor who had previously sent the soldier the e-mail about his wife. The soldier survived, although with severe brain damage and hearing loss. The defense requested a sanity board, on the basis that the soldier had PTSD and traumatic brain injury, and therefore was neither competent to stand trial nor criminally responsible because of his PTSD.

Sanity Boards on Detainees

In July 2008, requests for "706 Boards" or sanity boards began to be made for the detainees at Guantanamo Bay. This author did four sanity boards that fall, until the trials ceased. While no individual issues are discussed here, a few thorny questions will be reviewed. Issues of culture and coercion are central. If a detainee discusses "djin" or spirits, is that psychosis or cultural belief? If he says that Allah made him do it, is that religiosity or terrorism? If he goes on a hunger strike, is that depression or coercion from other detainees? If it seems he cannot understand the questions, is that poor education, language difficulties, or deliberate refusal to cooperate with the examiners?

Courts-Martial Expert Consultants and Expert Witnesses

In accordance with MRE 706, "[t]he trial counsel, the defense counsel, and the court-martial have equal opportunity to obtain expert witnesses under Article 46 [of the UCMJ]."[10(p275)] MRE 706 also allows for accused individuals to select expert witnesses at their own expense. MRE 702 states that

> [i]f scientific, technical, or other specialized knowledge will assist the trier of fact to understand the evidence or to determine a fact in issue, a witness qualified as an expert by knowledge, skill, experience, training, or education, may testify thereto in the form of an opinion or otherwise . . .[10(p275)]

MRE 703 addresses the bases of opinion testimony by experts. It states that

> [t]he facts or data in the particular case upon which an expert bases an opinion or inference may be those perceived by or made known to the expert, at or before the hearing. If of a type reasonably relied upon by experts in the particular field in forming opinions or inferences upon the subject, the facts or data need not be admissible in evidence in order for the opinion or inference to be admitted.[10(p275)]

Sources for these facts and data include stipulations of fact, investigative and police reports, medical and service records, testimony heard during a court-martial, and personal and professional knowledge.[10] However, MRE 403 states that an expert's reliable and relevant testimony

> may be excluded if its probative value is substantially outweighed by the danger of unfair prejudice, confusion of the issues, or misleading the members, or by considerations of undue delay, waste of time, or needless presentation of cumulative evidence.[10(p255)]

MRE 704 allows experts to testify on the ultimate issue, stating that the expert's "opinion or inference otherwise admissible is not objectionable because it embraces an ultimate issue to be decided by the trier of fact."[10(p275)] MRE 705 allows the expert to testify

> in terms of opinion or inference and give the expert's reasons therefore without prior disclosure of the underlying facts or data, unless the military judge requires otherwise. The expert may in any event be required to disclose the underlying facts or data on cross-examination.[10(p275)]

The defense may request an expert consultant if a sanity board's opinions are deemed favorable to the prosecution, if mitigating factors might affect sentencing, or in both cases.[6] The expert may be either civilian or military. In accordance with a seminal military case, *United States v Toledo*, the defense must specifically request appointment of a confidential expert consultant for the consultant to be protected by the attorney–client privilege. Such requests are often subject to intense scrutiny during pretrial motions.[7] If the appointment is not granted, the military forensic psychiatrist may still function as an expert within the limitations of rules of discovery.

The defense may request a military forensic psychiatrist or psychologist to testify during the merits phase (or "guilt phase") or after conviction during the sentencing phase. For example, the expert witness may be asked to provide expert testimony during the merits or sentencing phases about the impact of combat-related PTSD, "Gulf War syndrome," or the "Vietnam syndrome" on the mental state or behavior of the accused.[12] In addition, the expert witness may be specifically asked to provide testimony on mitigating factors during the sentencing phase. For example, issues addressed by military forensic psychiatrists include the cumulative effects of sleep deprivation (secondary to combat stress or combat-related PTSD) and operational tempo on judgment and decision-making capacity.

Either defense or trial counsel may request expert consultation if a sanity board reaches a conclusion that is not favorable to its side. In addition, sanity boards have been successfully challenged on the basis of thoroughness, accuracy, and misapplication of the proper military standard for criminal responsibility.

The military forensic psychiatrist may also be asked to provide expert testimony for the prosecution during the merits phase on counterintuitive behaviors of an alleged victim, such as "rape trauma syndrome" or "battered spouse syndrome."[13] Because the accused may not be compelled to submit to any psychiatric evaluation beyond that of a sanity board, any testimony on aggravating factors at sentencing is often limited to a review of collateral documents and observation of the accused during the court-martial, which requires the military forensic psychiatrist to testify to this limitation.

Case Study 43-1 (continued): The sanity board did an extensive evaluation, including reviewing interviews of numerous witnesses, and a week-long assessment of the accused, including psychological testing. Although they agreed that he had PTSD, they did not think it rendered him not criminally responsible. The damage from the head wound did interfere with some of his activities of daily living. However, he knew the functions of the judge and jury and the basic elements of the case. He was able to cooperate with the defense attorney and to behave in the courtroom. Therefore he was found both competent and criminally responsible. Perhaps because of his diagnoses of PTSD and organic brain syndrome, he received a sentence of only 10 years.

Board certification in the subspecialty of forensic psychiatry now requires completion of an accredited 1-year fellowship program, and then a board examination in forensic psychiatry. Currently only one forensic psychiatry program exists in the DoD—the National Capital Consortium's Military Forensic Psychiatry Fellowship Program (in existence since 1992), located in Washington, DC. Recently a forensic psychology program was started there as well. In addition to the training requirements specified by the Accreditation Council for Graduate Medical Education, fellows receive training to serve as consultants and expert witnesses in courts-martial involving military-specific offenses.

MALINGERING

Case Study 43-2: A soldier presented to the combat stress control unit in Balad, Iraq. He had been in an improvised explosive device attack the day before. Two of his buddies had been severely wounded. He had hit his head against the hatch in the explosion, but was otherwise unhurt. His chief complaint was, "I just want to go home." He said he might shoot himself if he could not. The brief screen for traumatic brain injury and for PTSD was negative. He also said he could not stop shaking. The junior psychologist thought he might have a factitious disorder (tremor).

Malingering has always presented a challenge for forensic psychiatrists, especially in the armed forces, where it can be a specific criminal offense under the UCMJ. Healthcare professionals are reluctant to label patients as malingerers for many reasons, including the perception that it is tantamount to accusing the individual of fraud and deceit. Clinicians, accustomed to using their skills to diagnose and treat those who seek help for problems, often feel uncomfortable when confronted with patients who seek not therapeutic assistance to improve their well-being, but rather "official" corroboration of an attempted deception. However, reluctance to diagnose an obvious case of malingering or, even worse, treating patients as if they had the feigned illness (perhaps seen as the path of least resistance), may actually violate the maxim of "*primum non nocere*" (first do no harm). Insulating the patient from the consequences of malingering might be tempting, with the shortsighted view that either the benefits accrued by a successful deception or avoiding the penalties associated with fraud would be in the patient's best interest. This action may promote a dysfunctional psychosocial developmental process and foster longer-term negative effects. Military healthcare practitioners must find ways to make their ethical and fiduciary responsibility to act in the patient's best interest coincide with the needs of the system. Such dual responsibilities, of course, are not limited to the military; therapeutic practice often requires balancing the individual needs of the patient with broader social obligations.

Malingering has a longstanding history of recognition in the military, as highlighted by "avoidance of military duty" topping the list of external incentives in its description in the *Diagnostic and Statistical Manual of Mental Disorders*.[14] This text describes malingering as

> the intentional production of false or grossly exaggerated physical or psychological problems, motivated by external incentives such as avoiding military duty, avoiding work, obtaining financial compensation, evading criminal prosecution, or obtaining drugs.[14]

Malingering may be viewed as adaptive behavior under extreme circumstances, for example, when a prisoner of war feigns illness to escape maltreatment. This issue has predictably come to the forefront of clinical practice during wartime. Malingering might increase in the attempt to avoid combat duty by service members who otherwise lack the antisocial tendencies usually associated with this behavior. In this context, malingering can also be seen as a maladaptive response in an extremely stressful situation.[15,16] However, because military service in the United States is now voluntary, recruits know they are going to a theater of operations. In the author's experience, soldiers are more likely to deny symptoms than to exaggerate them, a phenomenon known as "negative malingering."

The treatment of the malingering patient in combat is complicated by dual agency and ethical considerations. Although the motivation may appear as no more than a superficial attempt to return home, it is often predicated by a primal fear for personal safety. In either sense, individual malingering creates a concern for an "epidemic" of malingering within the unit. Furthermore, malingerers' actions create a danger to the lives of their fellow soldiers, which creates a need for discipline and a duty to third parties when such deception has been detected. Military psychiatrists are challenged with balancing these considerations and the employment of limited therapeutic resources, including their own time and energies. Often the adage of "greatest good for the greatest number" dictates the type of treatment that can be offered in the combat zone, with substantial pressures to treat "bona fide" combat stress reactions, rather than "misconduct stress behavior."

A "diagnosis" of malingering does not necessarily equate to the crime of malingering. Article 115 of the UCMJ describes the criminal offense of malingering as follows:

> Any person subject to this chapter who for the purpose of avoiding work, duty, or service (1) feigns illness, physical disablement, mental lapse or derangement; or (2) intentionally inflicts self-injury; shall be punished as a court may direct.[10(p344)]

Military law recognizes the two distinct forms of malingering—feigning illness and intentional self-injury—with different punishments for each (greater for self-injury than for feigning illness). If the offense was committed in time of war or in a hostile-fire pay zone, the more serious offense of malingering to avoid combat duty brings even stronger penalties. Maximum prison sentences may range from 1 year for feigning illness in a noncombat situation to a maximum of 10 years for intentional infliction of self-injury to avoid combat duty.

Again, although there is a perception that malingering is common, in today's all-volunteer military malingering is probably much less common than believed. In actuality, it is the author's belief that soldiers are far more likely to conceal psychiatric symptoms than to embellish.

Case Study 43-2 (continued): The combat stress team treating soldiers in Balad was presented with a common dilemma. Should the team send him home, and therefore potentially have an epidemic of soldiers who had the same complaint of "I just want to go home"? The team members consulted with the division psychiatrist, who diagnosed a conversion disorder, rather than a factitious disorder. They elected to try the classic principles of combat psychiatry (eg, immediate treatment with the expectation of recovery and return to his unit). Unfortunately, the soldier did not respond and eventually had to be evacuated to Landstuhl. He was then evacuated to Water Reed Army Medical Center in Washington, DC, where he received numerous diagnoses. When he learned that he was going to be discharged from the Army, he ended his life by jumping off a bridge in Washington, DC.

PSYCHOLOGICAL AUTOPSIES

Before 2001, a report known as a "psychological autopsy" was required on every suicide in the US Army. After completion, it was submitted to the Army Surgeon General and the Walter Reed Army Institute of Research. These retrospective suicide investigations were designed to gather information from the soldier's unit and family to provide lessons learned that might prevent future suicides. However, many of these postmortem investigations were performed by mental health officers who may not have had any specific training in this particular task. Investigators generated long narrative reports that seldom produced any feedback or change to the system. Furthermore, the report format made data extraction and analysis difficult. Another major issue of the psychological autopsies was who had access to their information. Before 2001, psychological autopsies were accessible under the Freedom of Information Act, which resulted in violation of patient privacy. For example, a reporter from the Raleigh *News and Observer* published salacious and intimate details obtained from over 50 psychological autopsies from Fort Bragg, North Carolina.[17]

DoD changed the requirements for psychological autopsies first in a Health Affairs policy letter in 2001 and later in a DoD directive in 2003.[1,18] The policy requires a formal psychological autopsy only if the death were equivocal, that is, it was not known whether the death was a suicide, homicide, or accident. All suicides still must be evaluated. A DoD suicide event report is now generated for both attempted and completed suicides. If mental health personnel had been following the soldier, a quality assurance review—known as a root cause analysis—should be conducted. As part of the new requirement, practitioners must receive additional training in conducting psychological autopsies. The additional training should cover basics of crime scene investigation, physical autopsy procedures, toxicology, and understanding of suicidal behavior and determinants. Forensically trained psychiatrists have usually already received this training.[19]

Cases that require psychological autopsies tend to cluster in the following categories:

- an accidental or deliberate drug overdose;

- an accidental or deliberate motor vehicle accident;
- a gunshot wound, which may have been self-inflicted, accidental, or a homicide; or
- a hanging, which may have resulted accidentally from autoerotic asphyxia or intentionally from suicide.

Case Study 43-3: A soldier in the Warrior Transition Unit was found deceased. In his room were found numerous pill bottles and an empty bottle of whisky, but no suicide note. The investigation found that he had recently gotten a divorce, but had seemed upbeat in the past several days. He had told his therapist that he was glad the divorce was finalized and was excited about the future. His command did not think it was a suicide. His family thought it might be a homicide, with his ex-wife giving him the pills for an overdose. The medical examiner agreed to a psychological autopsy. The results eventually supported an accidental overdose, although suicidal intent was suspected.

BEHAVIORAL SCIENCE CONSULTATION TEAMS

Although psychologists have supported detention operations and interrogations for many years, the events of September 11, 2001 and the ongoing GWOT have required the unprecedented and sustained involvement of behavioral science consultants (BSCs) in support of both detention operations and intelligence interrogations/detainee debriefing operations. Prior to GWOT, support for these missions was provided by personnel organic to the intelligence and special operations communities. However, the expanded demand for BSCs to support these missions has required assignment of psychologists and forensic psychiatrists from other mission areas within the DoD.

The Army is the executive agent for the administration of DoD detainee policy. The GWOT has resulted in the detention of large numbers of detainees by US forces. The intelligence interrogation and debriefing of detainees is a vital and effective part of the GWOT. It is designed to obtain accurate and timely intelligence in a manner consistent with applicable US and international laws, regulations, and DoD policy. Behavioral science personnel provide expertise and consultation to commanders to directly support the detention and interrogation/debriefing operations.

BSCs are psychologists and forensic psychiatrists, not assigned to clinical practice functions, but to provide consultative services to support authorized law enforcement or intelligence activities, including detention and related intelligence, interrogation, and detainee debriefing operations. Because BSCs are not engaged exclusively in the provision of medical care, they may not qualify for special status accorded retained medical personnel or carry DoD-issued identification cards identifying themselves as engaged in the provision of healthcare services. Analogous to behavioral science unit personnel of a law enforcement organization or forensic psychiatry or psychology personnel supporting the criminal justice, parole, or corrections systems, BSCs employ their professional training not in a provider-patient relationship but in relation to a person who is the subject of a lawful governmental inquiry, assessment, investigation, adjudication, or other proper action.

BSCs function as special staff to the commander in charge of both detention and interrogation operations (ie, the Commander, Detainee Operations). BSCs should be aligned to report directly to this commander, not to one charged solely with command of the detention facility or Joint Interrogation Debriefing Center. This arrangement enhances the BSC's ability to provide comprehensive consultation regarding all subjects within the BSC's area of expertise on combined aspects of detention operations, intelligence interrogations, and detainee debriefings. Often behavioral science consultation to detention operations, intelligence interrogations, and detainee debriefings is conducted by individual BSCs working alone.

"Behavioral drift"—the continual reestablishment of new, often unstated, and unofficial standards in an unintended direction—is commonly observed in detention and other settings in which individuals have relative control or power over others' activities of daily living or their general functioning. It often occurs when established official standards of behavior are not enforced. Ambiguous guidance, poor supervision, and lack of training and oversight contribute to this change in observed standards. Certain psychological and social pressures can greatly increase the likelihood of behavioral drift. Drift is detrimental to the mission and may occur very quickly without careful oversight mechanisms and training

The mission of a BSC is to provide psychological expertise and consultation to assist the command in conducting safe, legal, ethical, and effective detention facility operations, intelligence interrogations, and detainee debriefing operations. This mission is composed of two complementary objectives:

1. To provide psychological expertise in monitoring, consultation, and feedback regarding

the whole of the detention environment to assist the command in ensuring the humane treatment of detainees, prevention of abuse, and safety of US personnel.

2. To provide psychological expertise to assess individual detainees and their environment and provide recommendations to improve the effectiveness of intelligence interrogations, detainee debriefings, and detention facility operations.

SUMMARY

The United States has historically been concerned about the successful adjustment of its military members returning from war. Although the greater population of war veterans will not be involved in criminal proceedings, a substantial minority will develop career-ending disabilities as a result of mental illness. In rare instances, these will be life-ending events. For a very small yet highly visible minority of returning veterans, questions about the cause, precipitants, and manner of death will necessitate psychological autopsies. This chapter highlighted recent updates in military forensic psychiatry and the mechanisms through which answers to questions of competency, criminal culpability, and motivation underpinning self-injurious behavior are determined within the US military. As the GWOT progresses, so, too, will the experience and study of combat-related mental health. Military judicial processes and the policies and procedures governing psychological autopsies must continue to evolve to meet increasing demands.

REFERENCES

1. Fontana A, Rosenheck R. The role of war-zone trauma and PTSD in the etiology of antisocial behavior. *J Nerv Ment Dis*. 2005;193:203–209.

2. McCarroll JE, Ursano RJ, Liu X, et al. Deployment and the probability of spousal aggression by US Army soldiers. *Mil Med*. 2000;165(1):41–44.

3. Epidemiological Consultation NO. 14-hk-ob 1 U 0-9. Investigation of homicides at Fort Carson, Colorado, November 2008–May 2009, July 2009.

4. Lande RG, Armitage DT, eds. *Principles and Practice of Military Forensic Psychiatry*. Springfield, Ill: Charles C Thomas Publishers, Ltd; 1997.

5. Lande RG. The history of forensic psychiatry in the US military. In: Lande RG, Armitage DT, eds. *Principles and Practice of Military Forensic Psychiatry*. Springfield, Ill: Charles C Thomas Publishers, Ltd; 1997: 3–27.

6. Lande RG, Benedek DM. Forensic psychiatry in the United States military. *J Am Acad Psychiatry Law*. 1998;26(2):295–304.

7. Ritchie EC, Benedek D, Malone R, Carr-Malone R. Psychiatry and the military: an update. *Psychiatr Clin North Am*. 2006;29(3):695–707.

8. Zonana HV. Legal regulations of psychiatric practice in the military. In: Lande RG, Armitage DT, eds. *Principles and Practice of Military Forensic Psychiatry*. Springfield, Ill: Charles C Thomas Publishers, Ltd; 1997: 452–468.

9. Gilligan FA. Military law. In: Lande RG, Armitage DT, eds. *Principles and Practice of Military Forensic Psychiatry*. Springfield, Ill: Charles C Thomas Publishers, Ltd; 1997: 28–56.

10. US Department of Defense. *Manual for Courts-Martial, United States*. Washington, DC: DoD, Joint Service Committee on Military Justice, 2008. Available at: www.usapa.army.mil / pdffiles / mcm.pdf. Accessed December 4, 2009.

11. Uniform Code of Military Justice, 10 USC § 801–946 (2005).

12. Filbert BG. Disorder and syndrome evidence. In: Lande RG, Armitage DT, eds. *Principles and Practice of Military Forensic Psychiatry*. Springfield, Ill: Charles C Thomas, Ltd; 1997: 187–198.

13. Ritchie EC. Reactions to rape: a military forensic psychiatrist's perspective. *Mil Med.* 1998;163(8):505–509.

14. American Psychiatric Association. *Diagnostic and Statistical Manual of Mental Disorders: DSM-IV-TR.* 4th ed, text revision. Washington, DC: APA; 2000.

15. Ritchie EC: Malingering and the United States military. In: Lande RG, Armitage DA, eds. *Principles and Practice of Military Forensic Psychiatry.* Springfield, Ill: Charles C Thomas, Ltd: 1997.

16. Malone RD, Lange CL. A clinical approach to malingering. *J Am Acad Psychoanal Dyn Psychiatry.* 2007;35:1,13–21.

17. Richissin T. When "tough it out" backfires. *News and Observer.* October 26, 1997:A1.

18. US Department of Defense. *Armed Forces Institute of Pathology Operations.* Washington, DC: DoD; 2003. DoD Instruction 5154.30.

19. Ritchie EC, Gelles MG. Psychological autopsies: the current Department of Defense effort to standardize training and quality assurance. *J Forensic Sci.* 2002;47(6):1370–1372.

Chapter 44

WOMEN, MENTAL HEALTH, AND THE MILITARY

DEBORAH CROWLEY, MD*; TRISHA BENDER, MD†; ASHLEY CHATIGNY, DO‡; TINA TRUDEL, PhD§; AND ELSPETH CAMERON RITCHIE, MD, MPH¥

*Captain, Medical Corps, US Army; Child and Adolescent Psychiatry Fellow, Department of Psychiatry, Tripler Army Medical Center, 1 Jarrett White Road, Honolulu, Hawaii 96859

†Major, Medical Corps, US Army; Division Psychiatrist, 25th Infantry Division Headquarters, Building 580, DIVSURG CELL, Schofield Barracks, Hawaii 95857-6000; formerly, Child and Adolescent Fellow, Tripler Army Medical Center, Honolulu, Hawaii

‡Captain, Medical Corps, US Army; Fellow, Department of Child and Adolescent Psychiatry, Tripler Army Medical Center, 1 Jarrett White Road, Honolulu, Hawaii 96859-5000

§Site Director, Defense and Veterans Brain Injury Center at Virginia NeuroCare, 1101-B East High Street, Charlottesville, Virginia 22902; Assistant Clinical Professor of Psychiatry and Behavioral Neurobehavioral Sciences, University of Virginia Medical School, Charlottesville, Virginia 22902; formerly, Executive Director, Lakeview NeuroRehabilitation Center, Effingham Falls, New Hampshire

¥Colonel, US Army (Retired); formerly, Psychiatry Consultant to The Surgeon General, US Army, and Director, Behavioral Health Proponency, Office of The Surgeon General, Falls Church, Virginia; currently, Chief Clinical Officer, District of Columbia Department of Mental Health, 64 New York Avenue NE, 4th Floor, Washington, DC 20002

INTRODUCTION

Before the military operations in Afghanistan (Operation Enduring Freedom [OEF]) and Iraq (Operation Iraqi Freedom [OIF]), reproductive and gynecological issues dominated the medical concerns of most women in uniform. What was important to female soldiers was how to juggle family and career, with the occasional deployment to Korea, Somalia, or Kosovo, for a period of 6 to 12 months. "How do I manage with a baby? How do I figure out breastfeeding when I go to the field? How do I keep clean when the porta potties are all stinky and I'm having my period in the field? How do I deal with that?"

Since the terrorist attacks of September 11, 2001, the world for female soldiers has changed. Women still constitute about 15% of the military. In the US Army, women are not still assigned in technical combat units, such as infantry and artillery. However, they are definitely and clearly in combat. Women are military police and truck drivers, as well as involved in a wide range of other fields where they have to be prepared to defend themselves. In the other military services, they do have technically combat roles. Because there are no safe lines anymore and no rear areas, women are increasingly being wounded and killed, although clearly not as frequently as men.

PSYCHOSOCIAL STRESSORS FOR WOMEN IN MILITARY SERVICE

It is no surprise that life in the military brings a unique set of psychosocial stressors to women who serve. A multitude of expectations need to be met to succeed in the military, including a high level of physical fitness, extended work hours, a far-reaching network of rules and regulations, and 24-hour availability for duty. Service members can also be deployed at short notice, for varying lengths of time, and to almost any continent around the globe. Many potential benefits to military service also exist, such as employment stability, financial incentives for higher education, a unique camaraderie, and family support. The following section addresses unique challenges that can affect female service members and can have a significant impact on their mental health.

Physical Fitness

All service members are expected to maintain physical fitness to perform their jobs. Although each service has its own particular standards of fitness, there are more similarities than differences. Physical aptitude is measured in an annual or semiannual formal fitness test that evaluates muscular endurance and aerobic capacity.

Each service also has standards established for varying categories of height and weight of each member.[1] This is also based on age and gender. If service members exceed the maximum allowable weight, they must meet a standard body fat percentage. Soldiers, both male and female, will frequently use various methods to meet the weight standards. Some of these methods involve physician-approved diet and exercise regimens. However, various other methods are used, to include crash diets, extreme exercise regimens, and alternative approaches, such as body wraps and wearing sauna suits. In some cases, this can result in development of an eating disorder, which is addressed in more detail in other chapters.

Physical fitness is an obvious requirement for successful military service, with different jobs requiring different levels of physical strength and endurance. Generally speaking, male soldiers are expected to run faster and have greater muscular strength than female soldiers. This is based on the physical differences in muscle mass and distribution between the sexes. However, male and female soldiers are often required to complete the same physical tasks. For example, soldiers on jump status are expected to bear a certain load when they exit an aircraft, and that load is the same whether the parachutist is male or female. During deployments, female soldiers are required to wear the same load of combat gear as male soldiers. Completing these tasks is generally more difficult for female soldiers than for male soldiers, again because of the differences in body composition, muscle mass, and average size of each gender. This often becomes an added stressor for female soldiers, expected to meet the same standards as their male counterparts, but beginning with a different physiological makeup.

If service members exceed the maximum allowance for body fat percentage, they are enrolled in a weight control program, which can include monthly weigh-ins, mandatory classes and meetings with a nutritionist, and a specialized physical fitness regimen. If they fail to meet the standards for the physical training test, they can be enrolled in specialized physical training regimens. For physical training failure, soldiers can be barred from favorable actions, which can prevent them from being promoted, going on leave, or receiving awards. Soldiers can also be administratively separated from the service if they consistently fail to meet physical fitness standards.[2]

However, compared to their civilian counterparts, female soldiers may actually have an advantage by being expected to be physically fit. Studies have shown that regular exercise regimens decrease the incidence or severity of symptoms of depression and anxiety.[3,4] Exercise can be a very valuable coping skill to deal with the other stresses that the military imposes, both in and of itself, as well as in its role in improving sleep.

Job Assignment

For enlisted service members, military job opportunities are often assigned based on a test score resulting from the Armed Services Vocational Aptitude Battery (ASVAB).[5] Many enlistees enter the service with an idea of the type of job they would like to have, but there is no guarantee the service will offer them the specific job they desire. Many soldiers are offered a limited number of jobs, and it can be quite upsetting when it is not something they are interested in. This often sets the stage for how soldiers will either look forward to, or dread, the time for which they have committed to serve. This is in contrast to employment in the civilian world, where most people are able to turn down the job they do not want or simply interview with a different employer.

These same job assignment constraints also apply to commissioned officers. Officer candidates are given the opportunity to submit a preference list for their branch assignment. These assignments, however, are first and foremost based on the needs of the military; officer preferences are secondary. It can be a significant long-term stressor for someone who, for example, wants to be an aviator but is instead assigned to the Quartermaster Corps. Female soldiers are restricted to the noncombat arms branches with a few exceptions—such as aviation and field artillery. For some women this is frustrating because they believe that if they can meet the same physical and technical standards of the job as men, they should be given the opportunity to perform that job. For other women who do not desire these jobs, the restrictions are a relief because they, unlike their male counterparts, do not run the risk of being assigned to them.

Location and Social Support

The military is a culture in which its people are expected to adapt to change. This change appears in many different ways—living environment, daily routine, job assignments, command as well as peer composition, and structure. For some individuals, the change is welcomed, and for others the change is dreaded. For all, it poses a significant stressor.

Many people join the military as an opportunity to travel the world. Frequent moves are often experienced, whether desired or not. Soldiers can voice a preference in assignment location, but ultimately service members are distributed according to the needs of the military. For young enlisted service members, basic training is often the first time away from home for an extended period of time. This removes them from everything that is familiar to them—families, friends, homes, daily routines, jobs, and ways of life. They are limited in their contact with their main social support network, and placed in an environment where they are told how to dress, how to walk, how to behave, and what to value. Most of these soldiers are relatively young, without a firm idea of who they are or their plan for their lives. This is a stressful time for all service members, male or female.

The nature of the military requires soldiers to be mentally and physically strong, bold, and aggressive. Society has traditionally reserved these characteristics for men, but recently women in the military have assumed an increased presence in customarily male roles, both as a result of changes in the country's social values and the needs of the military.[6] In these surroundings, young female soldiers away from home for the first time all too often succumb to the temptation to engage in unhealthy behavior to fit in and be viewed as part of the team. This is their attempt to develop a new social support network in this stressful environment, as well as to be accepted by male colleagues.

Deployments

Deployments are another major source of change unique to military service. At short notice, soldiers can be taken from the daily routine they have been accustomed to and transported halfway around the world for months at a time. This usually includes time away from loved ones, although the military has greatly improved deployed soldiers' opportunities to communicate with loved ones back home.

Deployments can also mean harsh field conditions or climates to which the soldier is not accustomed. These austere conditions have an impact on personal privacy on a daily basis. Most significantly, deployments can place soldiers in situations of unpredictable or even certain danger with a threat to their lives. Any field situation, whether a training exercise at their home station or a deployment abroad, poses significant difficulties in the area of personal hygiene for female soldiers, who have to be prepared to deal with daily hygiene associated with menstruation even while in the field. Facilities for changing and disposing of hygiene products are not always available in the field, and time availability to take care of hygiene is often an issue as well. In addition to menstruation, urination is another stressor for female soldiers. During a field exercise, this becomes a matter of both privacy and convenience. However, during a deployment it can be a significant safety issue as proper wear of protective gear and avoidance of hostile fire become considerations.[7]

Deployments have become more common and more frequent for military service members over the last few decades. Recent studies estimate that soldiers entering the service today will have an average of 14 deployments over a 20-year career.[8] These include both combat deployments and peacekeeping missions. Studies have shown that service members generally want the opportunity to do what they have been trained to do, and most will find meaning in serving on a deployment.[9] However, over time, the stressors of a deployment will begin to take their toll on the physical and mental well-being of soldiers.

Deployment length appears to be a factor in the development of mental health problems for service members. Several studies have indicated that the longer a deployment lasts, the more psychological stress soldiers will experience, which, in turn, leads to development of symptoms such as depressed mood, sleep disturbances, increase in anxiety, and impairment in concentration.[10] Most of these studies, however, focused on male soldiers. A study done by Adler and colleagues demonstrated that this relationship between length of deployment and stress may not be true for female soldiers. This may be related to a physiologic difference in stress response between men and women, a topic that in itself needs further research.[10]

Pregnancy

Pregnancy is a major stressor to military and nonmilitary women alike. There are physical changes, potential health problems, hormonal variations, and the adjustment to becoming a mother. In accordance with service-specific regulations, pregnant service members are given a medical profile, excluding them from regular unit physical training.[11] This makes them exempt from formal physical fitness testing during pregnancy and for 180 days after delivery of the baby.

Restrictions are placed not only on physical fitness requirements, but also on duty hours and tasks. This is to prevent potential complications in the pregnancy, for which the rate is already higher for women in the military than for their civilian counterparts.[12] For example, after the 28th week of pregnancy the Army limits female soldiers to 8 hours of work at one time and 40 hours of work in a week.[12] There are also restrictions that prevent working in motor pool areas, rifle ranges, from heights, or on aircraft. This can have varying effects on service members, depending on their assigned job and unit. For instance, for a female military physician, although this will reduce work hours and prevent being on call overnight, otherwise there may be little change to the daily routine. For a mechanic, however, a temporary job reassignment may be needed. Not only would this require a service member to learn a new job and adjust to a new work schedule, but her work as a mechanic would still need to be done by someone else in the unit.

The scenario with the mechanic poses yet another stressor for pregnant service members—potential social conflicts with her unit mates. As service members can be overtasked and overworked at baseline, extra work left by a pregnant service member is rarely welcomed. This can lead to resentment of the pregnant soldier by the other soldiers in the unit. In some units, however, just the opposite can happen. In cohesive units, soldiers rally around teammates who are facing challenges, and the resulting support can be much greater than what is found in civilian workplaces.

The combination of a pregnancy and a pending deployment presents unique challenges. Because pregnancy precludes female service members from deploying,[12] there is sometimes a perception that the service member intentionally became pregnant to avoid deploying. Not only can this prevent deployment, but the military also offers administrative separation for enlisted members who become pregnant.[13] This can be seen by other soldiers as an abandonment of duty and obligation, regardless of the true intent of the pregnancy.

After the baby arrives, if the pregnancy is without complications, the service member is allotted 6 weeks of maternity leave. After these 6 weeks, the service member is expected to return to regular duty hours with her assigned job, although she is still exempt from physical fitness testing for 180 days postpartum. If the delivery required a Caesarean section, she may have difficulties with sit-ups. Women may have additional challenges meeting the military's weight standards following pregnancy, even when given this 180-day recovery period.[14]

The US Army Center for Health Promotion and Preventive Medicine has now developed and disseminated a pregnancy physical training program for female soldiers. The "long-range goal of this program is to reduce the impact of pregnancy on individual soldier fitness and unit readiness by mitigating losses from attrition and reduced fitness."[15] Service members also continue to be nondeployable for 6 months following delivery, after which time they are expected to deploy like any other service member. Soldiers can choose to waive this 6-month "bonding period" and deploy shortly after delivery.[16]

One psychiatrist related his experience of deploying with a unit that contained several female soldiers who had chosen to waive their option to remain behind during their allowed bonding period.[17] These female soldiers cited various reasons for their decisions, including not wanting to let their fellow soldiers down and wanting to perform the jobs they were trained to do. However, once deployed these women had significant problems, both mentally and physically. They experienced the expected emotional issues associated with being separated from their newborns. Physically they had not yet recovered from 9 months of pregnancy and subsequent childbirth. Many of these soldiers developed depression, and for some this led to suicidality. Not only did this scenario have a significant impact on the individual soldiers, but in turn it became an additional stress to their units in the deployed environment.[17]

This section addressed some of the psychosocial stressors unique to women in the military; however, it is not comprehensive. Some female service members are readily able to adapt and cope with these stressors, but for others they can lead to development of a mental illness. The rest of this chapter will address specific diagnoses in further detail.

MENTAL HEALTH DISORDERS IN WOMEN

Although women are affected by the same major mental illnesses as men, there have been key differences noted in studies and a review of the literature of women's mental health. These differences, such as history of presentation and course of illness, have an important impact on diagnostic and treatment considerations for the female patient. Furthermore, pregnancy, breastfeeding, perimenopause, and menopause can complicate mental well-being. This section will first consider each major mental illness separately.

Schizophrenia

Even though the ratio does not differ between genders, the onset of the disorder occurs later in women than in men (20–29 vs 15–24). A small percentage of women have their first psychotic episode in their forties.[18] Women are more likely to have a good premorbid functioning history prior to their illness and during the course of their illness, display more positive symptoms with affective signs, and experience fewer negative symptoms than men.

Treatment of schizophrenia in the female patient does not differ from the standard practice guidelines, but a few gender-specific situations do occur. Some antipsychotic medications (risperidone, haloperidol) can induce hyperprolactinemia (normal prolactin 5–25 ng/ml), thus causing menstrual irregularities or amenorrhea (prolactin over 60 ng/ml). In cases in which the medication cannot be switched or lowered, the hyperprolactinemia could be managed by adding the dopamine agonist bromocriptine (2.5–7.5 mg twice daily) or cabergoline (0.5 mg/week).[19] Alternatively, oral contraceptives could be used to restore the menstrual regularity disrupted by the hyperprolactinemia, in addition to providing contraception.

Women with schizophrenia are at high risk for unplanned pregnancy because of ineffective use of contraception and high rates of sexual assault. Prevention should include counseling about preferred choice of birth control, sex education, and psychosocial support. Patients with schizophrenia who do become pregnant require frequent monitoring. Reemergence of psychotic symptoms can lead to failure to obtain prenatal care, paranoid delusions about the medical team that prevent cooperation, poor self-care, and adverse pregnancy outcomes (ie, low birthweight, low Apgar scores, prematurity). These factors, in addition to previous functioning, must be considered when deciding treatment during pregnancy.

There are limited data on the effects of antipsychotic medications on the fetus. Some data showed no increased risk of congenital malformation with high-potency agents (haloperidol and trifluoperazine), although low-potency phenothiazines appear to have a higher incidence of nonspecific congenital anomalies and neonatal jaundice.[20] The newer atypical antipsychotics have only a few case reports. These do not indicate adverse effects; however, with their small numbers, these reports give the clinician little guidance. With either the decision to treat with medication or to watch symptoms, the patient will need close follow-up and involvement of any psychosocial supports that the patient has enlisted.

Depression

The prevalence of unipolar depression for women is statistically higher (10%–25%) compared to men (12%).[21] Dysthymia is twice as prevalent in women as in men.[22] Similarly, seasonal affective disorder is also more prevalent in women than men.[23] Although the symptoms of depression do not differ significantly between the sexes, women are at risk for depressive episodes during reproductive transitions such as premenstruation, pregnancy, postpartum, periomenopause, and menopause.

Premenstrual dysphoric disorder (PMDD) is listed as a mood disorder not otherwise specified in the fourth edition of the *Diagnostic and Statistical Manual* (DSM-IV-TR) of the American Psychiatric Association, which describes the severe spectrum of recurrent physical and emotional symptoms associated with the late luteal phase of the menstrual cycle, which resolve with the onset of menstruation. The physical symptoms include headaches, cramping, breast tenderness, and bloating, while the emotional symptoms include depression, irritability, anxiety, and insomnia. After ruling out other causes of symptoms (including other medical and psychiatric disorders such as unipolar depression, dysthymia, and anxiety), PMDD can be monitored with daily symptom charting over a 2-month period. Treatment is based on the severity of symptoms and ranges from nonpharmcological approaches, such as sleep hygiene, relaxation therapy, and cognitive-behavioral therapy, to the addition of selective serotonin reuptake inhibitors (SSRIs) for the more severe cases.

Maternal depression during pregnancy creates risks for both the woman and her children, such as alcohol abuse, poor nutrition, failure to obtain adequate prenatal care, and suicidal behaviors. Obstetrical complications have also been studied and have shown increased risk for slow fetal growth,[24] small infant head circumference,[25] and increased risk of preterm delivery.[26]

The US Food and Drug Administration (FDA) uses a pregnancy rating system[27] to guide clinicians on potential safety of a medication during pregnancy or lactation (Exhibit 44-1). However, the rating system does not always reflect the available data. Also, there can be some lag time before new data are incorporated into the system. It is important to note that to date, in the absence of controlled trials, the FDA has not approved any medications for use during pregnancy or lactation. Thus, it is important to obtain informed consent with each patient about the risk-to-benefit ratio when using a psychotropic.

When medications are used in pregnancy, the

EXHIBIT 44-1

US FOOD AND DRUG ADMINISTRATION CATEGORIES AND LABELING REQUIREMENTS FOR DRUG USE IN PREGNANCY

Pregnancy Category:

A Studies in pregnant women have not shown that (*name of drug*) increases the risk of fetal abnormalities if administered during the first (*second, third, or all*) trimester(s) of pregnancy. If this drug is used during pregnancy, the possibility of fetal harm appears remote. Because studies cannot rule out the possibility of harm, however, (*name of drug*) should be used during pregnancy only if clearly needed.

B Reproduction studies have been performed in (*kind(s) of animal(s)*) at doses up to (x) times the human dose and have revealed no evidence of impaired fertility or harm to the fetus due to (*name of drug*). There are, however, no adequate and well-controlled studies in pregnant women. Because animal reproduction studies are not always predictive of human response, this drug should be used during pregnancy only if clearly needed.

C (*Name of drug*) has been shown to be teratogenic (or to have an embryocidal effect or other adverse effect) in (*name(s) of species*) when given in doses (x) times the human dose. There are no adequate and well-controlled studies in pregnant women. (*Name of drug*) should be used during pregnancy only if the potential benefit justifies the potential risk to the fetus.

D (*Name of drug*) can cause fetal harm when administered to a pregnant woman. (*Describe the human data and any pertinent animal data.*) If this drug is used during pregnancy, or if the patient becomes pregnant while taking this drug, the patient should be apprised of the potential hazard to a fetus.

X (*Name of drug*) may (*can*) cause fetal harm when administered to a pregnant woman. (*Describe the human data and any pertinent animal data.*) (*Name of drug*) is contraindicated in women who are or may become pregnant. If this drug is used during pregnancy, or if the patient becomes pregnant while taking this drug, the patient should be apprised of the potential hazard to a fetus.

Data source: Code of Federal Regulations,Title 21, Volume 4, Revised as of April 1, 2008 (21CFR201.57). Available at: https://www.accessdata.fda.gov/scripts/cdrh/cfdocs/cfCFR/CFRSearch.cfm?fr=201.57. Accessed September 2, 2009.

minimal effective dose should be administered. That is, the dose that effectively treats a patient's symptoms without unduly exposing the fetus to higher than necessary doses. To date, the SSRIs, in particular fluoxetine, have the most extensive published data about their use during pregnancy. One study on the long-term neurobehavioral effects of SSRIs during pregnancy compared children exposed to fluoxetine, or a tricyclic antidepressant, or no antidepressant. No significant differences between the three groups were noted.[28] All SSRIs have FDA risk category of "C," with the exception of paroxetine, which has a risk category of "D" and is not recommended for use during pregnancy. In the United States, physicians have increasingly prescribed bupropion during pregnancy to treat depression, apparently as a consequence of its FDA "B" risk category. However, there are currently no published data regarding its safety or tolerability during gestation.

The postpartum period can be a particularly vulnerable period for a woman, with up to 85% of women experiencing postpartum "blues" within the first 2 weeks after giving birth. This condition usually remits spontaneously, and thus treatment is not required. However, psychoeducation of physician and patients to distinguish postpartum blues from a more serious condition, postpartum depression, is warranted. The prevalence of postpartum depression is about 10%. Any previous history of depression significantly increases the woman's risk dramatically. A history of PMDD prior to conception increases her risk for developing postpartum depression to 24%. An episode of depression endured during pregnancy increases the risk of postpartum depression to 35%. Any woman with a prior history of postpartum depression has a 50% to 60% risk of developing postpartum depression during subsequent pregnancies.[29] Treatment is multimodal and includes psychoeducation, individual and group psychotherapy, support (community resources), and pharmacotherapy. Breastfeeding should be discussed thoroughly as all psychotropic medications pass through breast milk and there are limited data establishing the effects on the infant. For the patient whose depression is complicated by psychosis or suicidality, hospitalization is generally required until the patient is no longer dangerous to self or others. Postpartum psychosis is considered an acute emergency and reason for acute admission, as it carries a risk of infanticide (1/1,000) if left untreated, in addition to the risks to the mother associated with psychosis.

Bipolar Disorder

Bipolar disorder occurs in 1% of the population and is equally prevalent in men and women. Women tend to experience more depressive and mixed episodes than men, with fewer manic episodes. This may lead to diagnosis of unipolar depression and treatment with antidepressants, which then exacerbates the condition and results in rapid cycling—a condition seen more often in women than in men.[30] Another precipitation of rapid cycling is thyroid dysfunction, which can be caused by lithium-induced hypothyroidism. Women are at greater risk for thyroid dysfunction than men, thus levels of thyroid stimulating hormone should be checked every 6 months for any woman receiving lithium.

Management of bipolar disorder can be particularly challenging during the perinatal period because the current first-line agents either have known teratogenicities, are associated with congenital malformations, or have little data to support their safety during pregnancy or lactation. In particular, lithium has been demonstrated to increase the risk for Ebstein's anomaly (also called Ebstein's malformation, in which the tricuspid valve is abnormally formed) from 1 in 20,000 to 1 in 1,000 when the fetus is exposed during organogenesis.[31] Exposure later in gestation can lead to fetal or neonatal cardiac arrhythmias, fetal hypoglycemia, nephrogenic diabetes insipidus, polyhydramnios, or premature delivery.[32,33] The American Academy of Pediatrics discourages the use of lithium during lactation. This recommendation is based on a study that revealed that infant serum levels are double maternal serum levels postbreastfeeding. Lithium use during lactation is also correlated with adverse events such as lethargy, hypotonia, hypothermia, and electrocardiogram changes.[34]

Prenatal exposure to valproate is associated with neural tube defects and craniofacial, cardiovascular, and limb anomalies.[35] A metaanalysis revealed the risk for neural tube defect during valproate exposure to be 3.8%—38 times greater than prevalence in the general population.[36] There is a paucity of data regarding the use of the atypical antipsychotics during pregnancy and lactaction.

Anxiety Disorders

Overall, anxiety disorders are more prevalent in women than in men (with the exception of obsessive-compulsive disorder, which has equal prevalence). Compared to men, women are twice as likely to suffer from posttraumatic stress disorder (PTSD), three times as likely to experience panic disorder with agoraphobia, and four times as likely to have social phobia.[37,38]

Although other comorbid psychiatric disorders occur in 91% of patients with panic disorder, and 84% of patients with panic disorder and agoraphobia, panic disorder with agoraphobia is more common in alcoholic women than alcoholic men.[39] The treatment for panic disorder does not differ between the genders, with the most effective treatments consisting of cognitive behavioral-therapy and pharmacotherapy.

Comprehensive evaluation to rule out disorders that mimic anxiety, to include thyroid disorders, lupus, iron deficiency anemia, cardiovascular disease, and periomenopause, should be included in the work up. Other causes of anxiety—such as alcohol use, nicotine, caffeine, nonsteroidal decongestants, herbal supplements, and appetite suppressants—should also be ruled out.

TRAUMATIC BRAIN INJURY IN WOMEN

Background

Traumatic brain injury (TBI) is one of the most complex conditions of high risk to military personnel, affecting physical, cognitive, and behavioral health. Rates of TBI in the general population and military are high, making this condition a major public and military health problem. In the current war on terror, brain injury has become a predominant injury for military men and women in a wide variety of roles. The focus on TBI has increased with the occurrence of such injuries in OIF and OEF. With regard to OIF, the Office of The Surgeon General of the Army notes that 64% of wounded-in-action injuries have occurred as a result of blast from improvised explosive devices, rocket-propelled grenades, land mines, and mortar or artillery shells.[40] Improvements in helmet design and body armor have resulted in reductions in penetrating injuries, including penetrating head trauma. As a direct result of the improved survivability of blast injuries, closed-head trauma has become the signature injury of these military operations.

The detailed review of military TBI—from moment of injury through medical and rehabilitation setting and finally to vocational and family outcome—has been addressed in a prior volume of the *Textbooks of Military Medicine*.[41] Therefore, this section will only focus on familiarizing the reader with research findings regarding gender differences and their implications for women. Even though male TBI outnumbers female TBI approximately 2:1 in the general population, and men in the military population far outnumber women, the rates of female TBI and female service members have both increased over the past decade. Understanding the implication of female gender in all aspects of TBI has developed during this time, although it is still in its infancy.

Traumatic Brain Injury, Gender, and Outcome

The analysis of gender as a variable in neurotrauma is a fairly recent phenomenon, with discrepant results across a number of studies. Animal models suggest positive effects of hormone treatment (progesterone, estrogen) on outcome, and potential differential risk/benefit for women who are either pre- or postmenopausal. Progesterone modulates gamma-amino butyric acid and inhibits apoptosis, gliosis, and production of inflammatory agents, thereby reducing brain edema. Estrogen is known as a powerful antioxidant with vasoprotective action. However, in animal models, although exogenous administration of estrogen was beneficial to males, administration to females was detrimental, and increased rates of injury-related mortality.[42–44]

Hormonal issues may also play a significant role in mild TBI diagnosis among periomenopausal, menopausal, and postmenopausal women, due to symptom overlap. For example, in examining population base rates, in excess of 20% of these women report concentration difficulties, sleep disturbance, anxiety, depression, and irritability, all symptoms common to mild TBI. In excess of 30% of these women also report fatigue and nervousness.[45]

A metaanalysis on gender differences in TBI outcome identified only nine studies where data were reported based on gender. In analyzing these available studies, women were observed to have worse outcome on 85% (17 of 20) of the variables discussed.[46] Other individual studies, often with relatively small samples of women, present conflicting results wherein women demonstrated greater response to coma stimulation,[47] gains in postacute rehabilitation,[48] maintenance of cognitive level relative to age norms,[49] and lower risk for dementia.[50]

Among those with moderate to severe TBI, female survivors were noted to have a 1.28 times higher mortality rate and a 1.57 times higher poor-outcome rate than male survivors.[51] Research regarding the much more common concussion/mild spectrum of TBI demonstrates that female gender is associated with a greater likelihood of subjective cognitive complaints.[52] Women were also noted to have significantly higher rates of postconcussive syndrome at 1-month postinjury, with continued trends in this direction at 3 and 6 months postinjury.[53] Women sustaining sports-related concussions demonstrated significantly greater decline in simple and complex reaction time and reported more postconcussion symptoms than male peers. In this sports-related concussion study, female subjects were cognitively impaired roughly 1.7 times more often than comparison male subjects. They also experienced more subjective and objective adverse effects from concussion, even with adjusting for helmet use (such as comparison male football players).[54] Thus, especially in mild TBI, it is critical that women have thorough evaluation and follow-up to reduce risk of complications, avoid repeat injury, and ensure optimal recovery.

Psychological Sequelae of Traumatic Brain Injury in Women

Results related to gender, overall outcome, and quality of life are also mixed, because few of the many TBI studies present results by gender. A recent larger sample study contradicts early findings of higher perceived quality of life among females post-TBI.[55] A number of studies specifically examining depression post-TBI demonstrate a significant association between female gender and post-TBI depression.[56–58] The finding of higher rates of post-TBI depression among women is not unexpected given the higher rates of depression among them in the general population. Thus, detailed depression screening is strongly recommended.

TBI with concomitant PTSD is a particular concern in military settings. When experiencing the same trauma, women have higher rates of PTSD than men in the general population. This finding appears to hold true for PTSD post-TBI. A number of studies report that women manifest higher rates of post-TBI PTSD.[59–61] One study noted that symptoms increased over time, and that both the severity of the TBI and memory for the event were not associated with the PTSD diagnosis, which involved predominant intrusion and avoidance symptoms.[62] Complicating factors associated with PTSD and female TBI survivors include a premorbid history of sexual trauma and abuse, which occurs at a significantly higher rate for women in population studies.

In some instances, the experience of TBI is noted to trigger reemergence of intrusive recollections and symptoms associated with abuse, at times after years of nonoccurrence. This PTSD-related complication can disrupt the rehabilitation process through flashbacks, behavioral and affective disturbance, nightmares, and hypervigilance. Issues related to prior sexual trauma and abuse should be proactively addressed in the history and treatment planning process.[62] Also related to post-TBI psychological status and PTSD risk is the high rate of TBI from domestic violence, wherein women are more frequently the victims. Studies of battered women indicate extremely high frequency of blows to the head (92%) and loss of consciousness (40%), with a significant correlation between frequency of blows to the head and severity of cognitive symptoms.[63] Along with blows to the head, battered women also may experience anoxic injuries from choking, and are very likely to suffer from multiple brain injuries. Women sustaining brain injuries in the context of domestic violence often present both cognitive impairment as well as psychological symptoms, including generalized distress, depression, anhedonia, worry, anxious arousal, and PTSD.[64] Screening for TBI following domestic violence, and for domestic violence risk among those women presenting with TBI, is advised.

Family and Vocational Issues for Women Following Traumatic Brain Injury

Examination of the burden of TBI on family members indicates spouses and primary caregivers typically experience the most stress. Divorce and family dysfunction are extremely common occurrences post-TBI. Research indicates that male caregivers of female relatives with TBI displayed more distress on clinical inventories than any other gender combination. Time since injury and days in coma (a measure of severity of injury) did not affect family caregiver distress ratings.[65] Thus, family treatment and support should be initiated as early and as intensely as possible, especially in those circumstances where the woman with TBI will likely be dependent to some degree on a family caregiver.

Women with TBI additionally may have difficulty functioning in their spousal role, as the injury may affect satisfaction with gender role, body image, self-esteem, and sexuality. Gender-role satisfaction relates to a woman's ability to engage in preinjury activities that defined and supported her sense of femininity and womanhood. It is particularly beneficial for women to reconnect with rites of passage and developmental life-stage transitions, such as partnership with another or parenting children, or both, as a means of expressing the ability to participate.[66] In moderate to severe TBI, rehabilitation may be extended and involve stays in various settings, all of which may separate the female service member from military, family, and gender roles—an experience associated with diminished personal satisfaction and self-esteem. Nontraditional rehabilitation and therapeutic activities may be needed to enhance ability to function in the multitasking role as mother for those service women with children at home and parenting responsibilities.

Body-image concerns and sexual dysfunction also adversely affect self-esteem and may contribute to depression. Following TBI, body image difficulties may influence feelings of attractiveness and comfort being seen by a partner; physical difficulties may impact sexuality through body positioning, sensation, and movement; and physiological problems may reduce energy for sex, sex drive, ability to initiate sex, and ability to achieve orgasm. Predictors of women's sexual dysfunction post-TBI include degree of depression and evidence of endocrine disorders. Significant problems reported by women with TBI include difficulties with sexual arousal; pain with sexual activity; decreased ability to masturbate; diminished vaginal lubrication; and altered, delayed, or lack of orgasm.[67] Rehabilitation and psychotherapy professionals must be able and willing to engage in frank discussion of sexuality post-TBI. They must also have some familiarity with treatment approaches and resources, because problems in this area are associated with depression, loss of self-esteem, and increased family strain.

Successful recovery from TBI results in return to work for military personnel with TBI. Some soldiers are even able to return to active duty. Others may no longer be able to serve in such roles and may require vocational rehabilitation to achieve community reintegration. Studies have demonstrated worse vocational outcome for women post-TBI than for men. At times data suggesting good outcome for women are deceiving, in that successful vocational outcomes have included the category of "homemaker," often with minimal definition or analysis of tasks and function. Significantly fewer women return to work full-time post-TBI.[68] A review of state vocational rehabilitation services was conducted comparing men and women with similar injuries, neuropsychological test results, and demographics. Women were noted to have vocational rehabilitation services terminated after being accepted, but before successfully initiating active services, almost 50% more often than men; women received vocational rehabilitation maintenance services half as often as men; and only 4.4% of women (vs 23.6% of men) were employed successfully through vocational rehabilitation.[69] The return-to-work outlook is challenging for anyone post-TBI. However, the vocational outlook for women is particularly disconcerting, and may necessitate extra efforts on the part of vocational rehabilitation counselors and advocates.

Thus, the sequelae of TBI are complex and may involve rehabilitation of cognitive, physical, and behavioral impairments. Women with TBI are especially vulnerable to cognitive complaints and problems such as depression and PTSD. It may be difficult for women post-TBI to return to family and vocational roles. The clinician is advised to be aware of, and proactive regarding, women's unique issues post-TBI, because early intervention may improve outcome and reduce risks of long-term disability and the emergence of comorbidities.

SUMMARY

This chapter has discussed the unique and challenging situation that women face in today's military. From childbirth to specific disease pathology, women's mental health needs are constantly changing with their ever-diversifying roles as service members. This is a new era for women, in both medicine and the military. Women are a significant part of the fighting force. However, for their true potential to be reached, the military must adapt to those needs that are gender specific. The ability of the military to be sensitive to these mental health issues will maximize the fighting force. It will also encourage more women to join, knowing that the services are "female friendly."

Although women are prohibited from joining certain branches of the military, there continue to be new and exciting opportunities. Importantly, it must be remembered that with new opportunities come new risks. This chapter has presented an overview of the different risk factors, presentations, and treatments of mental health issues unique to female service members. In this wartime era, it is important to be cognizant of the diverse pathological mental health illnesses and the unique differences among the sexes. With the help of providers and military leadership, utilization of these data should improve outcomes for female service members.

REFERENCES

1. US Department of the Army. *The Army Weight Control Program*. Washington, DC: DA; 2006. Army Regulation 600-9.

2. US Department of the Army. *Active Duty Enlisted Administrative Separations*. Washington, DC: DA; 2005. Army Regulation 635-200. Chap 18.

3. Harris AH, Cronkite R, Moos R. Physical activity, exercise coping, and depression in a 10-year cohort study of depressed patients. *J Affect Disord*. 2006;93:79–85.

4. De Moor MH, Beem AL, Stubbe JH, Boomsma DI, De Geus EJ. Regular exercise, anxiety, depression and personality: a population-based study. *Prev Med*. 2006;42(4):273–279.

5. US Department of the Army. *Enlist: Ace the Placement Test (ASVAB)*. Available at: http://www.army.com/enlist/ace-the-placement-test.html. Accessed on January 8, 2007.

6. Lindstrom KE, Smith TC, Wells TS, et al. The mental health of US military women in combat support occupations. *J Women's Health*. 2006;15:162–172.

7. Ritchie EC. Issues for military women in deployment: an overview. *Mil Med*. 2001;166(12):1033–1037.

8. Castro CA, Adler AB. The impact of operations tempo on soldier and unit readiness. *Parameters*. 1999;86–95.

9. Britt TW, Adler AB, Bartone PT. Deriving benefits from stressful events: the role of engagement in meaningful work and hardiness. *J Occup Health Psychol*. 2001;6:53–63.

10. Adler AB, Huffman AH, Bliese PD, Castro CA. The impact of deployment length and experience on the well-being of male and female soldiers. *J Occup Health Psychol*. 2005;10:121–137.

11. US Department of the Army. *Standards of Medical Fitness*. Washington, DC: DA; 2006. Army Regulation 40-501. Chap 7-9.

12. Tam LW. Psychological aspects of pregnancy in the military: a review. *Women's Health Issues*. 1995;5:237–237.

13. US Department of the Army. *Active Duty Enlisted Administrative Separations*. Washington, DC: DA; 2005. Army Regulation 635-200. Chap 8.

14. Weina SU. Effects of pregnancy on the Army Physical Fitness Test. *Mil Med*. 2006;171(6):534–537.

15. US Army Center for Health Promotion and Preventive Medicine. *Pregnancy/Postpartum Physical Training (PPPT), Program Overview*. Available at http://chppm-www.apgea.army.mil/dhpw/Readiness/PPPT.aspx. Accessed February 12, 2007.

16. US Department of the Army. *Overseas Service*. Washington, DC: DA; 2008. Army Regulation 614-30. Chap 3: 6–17.

17. Drouillard G. Major, Medical Corps, US Army. Interview, January 3, 2007.

18. Goldstein JM, Link BG. Gender and the expression of schizophrenia. *J Psychiatr Res*. 1988;22:141–155.

19. Hales RE, Yudofsky SC, eds. *Textbook of Clinical Psychiatry*. Washington, DC: American Psychiatric Publishing; 2003: 1527.

20. Edlund MJ, Craig TJ. Antipsychotic drug use and birth defects: an epidemiologic reassessment. *Compr Psychiatry*. 1984;25:32–37.

21. American Psychiatric Association. *Diagnostic and Statistical Manual of Mental Disorders*. 4th ed, text revision. Washington, DC: American Psychiatric Association; 2000.

22. Kessler RC, McGonagle KA, Zhao S, et al. Lifetime and 12-month prevalence of DSM-III-R psychiatric disorders in the United States. Results from the National Comorbidity Survey. *Arch Gen Psychiatry*. 1994;51:8–19.

23. Rosenthal NE, Sack DA, Gillin JC, et al. Seasonal affective disorder: a description of the syndrome and preliminary findings with light therapy. *Arch Gen Psychiatr*. 1992;53:289–292.

24. Hedegaard M, Henriksen T, Sabroe S, Secher NJ. The relationship between psychological distress during pregnancy and birth weight for gestational age. *Acta Obstet Gynecol Scand*. 1996;75:32–39.

25. Lou HC, Hansen D, Nordentoft M, et al. Prenatal stressors of human life affect fetal brain development. *Develop Med Child Neurology*. 1994;36:826–832.

26. Korebrits C, Ramirez MM, Watson L, Brinkman E, Bocking AD, Challis JR. Maternal corticotrophin-releasing hormone is increased with impending preterm birth. *J Clin Endocrinol Metab*. 1998;83:1585–1591.

27. Schatzberg A, Nemeroff C, eds. *Textbook of Psychopharmacology*. 3rd ed. Washington, DC: American Psychiatric Publishing; 2004.

28. Nulman I, Rovet J, Stewart DE, et al. Neurodevelopment of children exposed in utero to antidepressant drugs. *N Engl J Med*. 1997;336:258–262.

29. O'Hara MW, ed. *Postpartum Depression: Causes and Consequences*. New York, NY: Springer-Verlag; 1995.

30. Tondo L, Baldessarini RJ. Rapid cycling in women and men with bipolar manic-depressive disorders. *Am J Psychiatry*. 1998;155:1434–1436.

31. Altshuler LL, Cohen L, Szuba MP, Burt VK, Gitlin M, Mintz J. Pharmacologic management of psychiatric illness in pregnancy: dilemmas and guidelines. *Am J Psychiatry*. 1996;153:592–606.

32. Wilson N, Forfar JC, Godman MJ. Atrial flutter in the newborn resulting from maternal lithium ingestion. *Archives Dis Child*. 1983;58:538–549.

33. Mizrahi EM, Hobbs JF, Goldsmith DI. Nephrogenic diabetes insipidus in transplacental lithium intoxication. *J Pediatr*. 1979;94:493–495.

34. American Academy of Pediatrics–Committee on Drugs. The transfer of drugs and other chemicals into human milk. *Pediatr*. 2001;108:776–789.

35. Centers for Disease Control and Prevention. Spina bifida incidence at birth—United States, 1983–1990. *MMWR Morb Mortal Wkly Rep*. 1992;41:497–500.

36. Samrén E, van Duijn C, Koch S, et al. Maternal use of antiepileptic drugs and the risk of major congenital malformations: a joint European prospective study of human teratogenesis associated with maternal epilepsy. *Epilepsia*. 1997;38:981–990.

37. Kessler RC, Sonnega A, Bromet E, Hughes M, Nelson CB. Posttraumatic stress disorder in the National Comorbidity Survey. *Arch Gen Psychiatry*. 1995;52:1048–1060.

38. Schneier FR, Johnson J, Hornig CD, Liebowitz MR, Weissman MM. Social phobia: comorbidity and morbidity in an epidemiologic sample. *Arch Gen Psychiatry*. 1992;49:282–288.

39. Task Force on Panic Anxiety and Its Treatments. Panic anxiety and panic disorder. In: Klerman GL, Hirschfield RMA, Weisman MM, et al, eds. *Panic Anxiety and Its Treatments*. Washington, DC: American Psychiatric Press; 1993: 3–38.

40. Defense and Veterans Brain Injury Center. Providing care for soldiers with traumatic brain injury. Washington, DC: The Henry M. Jackson Foundation for the Advancement of Military Medicine, Inc; 2006. Available at: http://www.hjf.org/research/featureDVBIC.html. Accessed November 13, 2008.

41. Zasler ND, Devaney Serio C. Traumatic brain injury. In: Dillingham TR, Belandres PV, eds. *Rehabilitation of the Injured Combatant*. Vol 1. In: Zajkchuk R, Bellamy RF, eds. *Textbook of Military Medicine*. Washington, DC: Department of the Army, Office of The Surgeon General, Borden Institute; 1998: 207–269.

42. Bramlett HM. Is there a role for hormonal therapy after traumatic brain injury? *Restor Neurol Neurosci*. 2005;23:165–166.

43. Melton L. What can sex hormones do for the damaged brain? *Lancet*. 2001;358:818.

44. Rogers E, Wagner AK. Gender, sex steroids and neuroprotection following traumatic brain injury. *J Head Trauma Rehab*. 2006;21:279–281.

45. O'Bryant SE, Palav A, McCaffrey RJ. A review of symptoms commonly associated with menopause: implications for clinical neuropsychologists and other healthcare providers. *Neuropsychol Rev.* 2003;13:145–152.

46. Farace E, Alves WM. Do women fare worse: a meta-analysis of gender differences in traumatic brain injury outcome. *J Neurosurg.* 2000;93:539–545.

47. Wilson SL, Powell GE, Brock D, Thwaites H. Vegetative state and responses to sensory stimulation: an analysis of 24 cases. *Brain Inj.* 1996;10:807–818.

48. Goranson TE, Graves RE, Allison D, La Freniere R. Community integration following multidisciplinary rehabilitation for traumatic brain injury. *Brain Inj.* 2003;17:759–774.

49. Himanen L, Portin R, Isoniemi H, Helenius H, Kurki T, Tenovuo O. Longitudinal cognitive changes in traumatic brain injury: a 30-year follow-up study. *Neurol.* 2006;66:187–192.

50. Starkstein SE, Jorge R. Dementia after traumatic brain injury. *Int Psychogeriatr.* 2005;17(suppl 1):S93–S107.

51. Kraus JF, Peek-Asa C, McArthur D. The independent effect of gender on outcomes following traumatic brain injury: a preliminary investigation. *Neurosurg Focus.* 2000;8:e5.

52. Chamelian L, Feinstein A. The effect of major depression on subjective and objective cognitive deficits in mild to moderate traumatic brain injury. *J Neuopsychiatry Clin Neurosci.* 2006;18:33–38.

53. Bazarian JJ, Wong T, Harris M, Leahey N, Mookerjee S, Dombovy M. Epidemiology and predictors of postconcussive syndrome after minor head injury in an emergency population. *Brain Inj.* 1999;13:173–189.

54. Broshek DK, Kaushik T, Freeman JR, Erlanger D, Webbe F, Barth JT. Sex differences in outcome following sports-related concussion. *J Neurosurg.* 2005;102:856–863.

55. Steadman-Pare D, Colantonio A, Ratcliff G, Chase S, Vernich L. Factors associated with perceived quality of life many years after traumatic brain injury. *J Head Trauma Rehab.* 2001;16:330–342.

56. Ruddle JA, Coetzer BR, Vaughan FL. Grief after brain injury: a validation of the Brain Injury Grief Inventory (BIGI). *Illness Crisis Loss.* 2005;13:235–247.

57. Glenn MB, O'Neil-Pirozzi T, Goldstein R, Burke D, Jacob L. Depression amongst outpatients with traumatic brain injury. *Brain Inj.* 2001;15:811–818.

58. Levin HS, Goldstein FC, MacKenzie EJ. Depression as a secondary condition following mild and moderate traumatic brain injury. *Semin Clin Neuropsychiatry.* 1997;2:207–215.

59. Greenspan AI, Stringer AY, Phillips VL, Hammond FM, Goldstein FC. Symptoms of post-traumatic stress: intrusion and avoidance 6 and 12 months after TBI. *Brain Inj.* 2006;20:733–742.

60. Levin HS, Brown SA, Song JX, et al. Depression and posttraumatic stress disorder at three months after mild to moderate traumatic brain injury. *J Clin Exp Neuropsychol.* 2001;23:754–769.

61. Ohry A, Rattock J, Solomon Z. Posttraumatic stress disorder in brain injury patients. *Brain Inj.* 1996;10:687–695.

62. Reeves RH, Beltzman D, Killu K. Implications of traumatic brain injury for survivors of sexual abuse: a preliminary report of findings. *Rehab Psychology.* 2000;45:205–211. Available at: http://www.nhchc.org/TBIandsexualabuse.pdf. Accessed November 13, 2008.

63. Jackson H, Philp E, Nuttall RL, Diller L. Traumatic brain injury: a hidden consequence for battered women. *Prof Psychol Res Pract.* 2002;33:39–45. Available at: http://www.lscny.org/TBIMaterials/TbiDVConsequence.pdf. Accessed November 13, 2008.

64. Valera EM, Berenbaum H. Brain injury in battered women. *J Consult Clin Psychol.* 2003;71:797–804.

65. Gervasio AH, Kreutzer JS. Kinship and family members' psychological distress after brain injury: a large sample study. *J Head Trauma Rehab.* 1997;12:14–26.

66. Gutman SA, Napier-Klemic J. The experience of head injury on the impairment of gender identity and gender role. *Am J Occup Ther*. 1996;50:535–544.

67. Hibbard MR, Gordon WA, Flanagan S, Haddad L, Labinsky E. Sexual dysfunction after traumatic brain injury. *NeuroRehabilitation*. 2000;15:107–120.

68. Klonoff PS, Lamb DG, Henderson SW. Outcomes from milieu-based neurorehabilitation at up to 11 years post-discharge. *Brain Inj*. 2001;15:413–428.

69. Bounds TA, Schopp L, Johnstone B, Unger C, Goldman H. Gender differences in a sample of vocational rehabilitation clients with TBI. *NeuroRehabilitation.* 2003;18:189–196.

Chapter 45

MENTAL HEALTH SUPPORT TO OPERATIONS INVOLVING DEATH AND THE DEAD

JAMES E. MCCARROLL, PhD, MPH*, AND ROBERT J. URSANO, MD†

*Colonel, US Army (Retired); Psychologist, Center for the Study of Traumatic Stress and Department of Psychiatry, Room B3068, Uniformed Services University of the Health Sciences, 4301 Jones Bridge Road, Bethesda, Maryland 20814; formerly, Psychologist, Walter Reed Army Institute of Research, Silver Spring, Maryland

†Colonel, US Air Force (Retired); Director, Center for the Study of Traumatic Stress, and Chair, Department of Psychiatry, Room B3068, Uniformed Services University of the Health Sciences, 4301 Jones Bridge Road, Bethesda, Maryland 20814

INTRODUCTION

Exposure to the dead and death is common in military and civil conflict, disaster, crime, and other violent events such as transportation accidents. "Exposure to the dead" means the viewing and handling of human remains. "Exposure to death," on the other hand, refers to connotations associated with the deceased that bring forth cognitive and emotional reminders of the individual to the family and to other groups such as military units, communities, and even nations.

Many publications have addressed the effects of traumatic death on posttraumatic symptoms,[1] but none has focused on the role of the mental health provider in assisting soldiers and commanders with adjusting to the stress of caring for deceased soldiers on the battlefield or at a site of mass casualties. Mental health personnel should be familiar with this topic for three major reasons: (1) to understand the nature of distress in personnel exposed to the dead; (2) to recommend policies to medical and line commanders to reduce soldier distress; and (3) to understand their own vulnerability to these same stresses.

In the medical field, mental health personnel are probably among the most insulated from death. Psychiatrists dissect cadavers as medical students and attend medical school lectures about confronting the deaths of patients, but are unlikely to be exposed to traumatic death or even surgical or medical deaths on a routine basis. Psychologists and social workers may never have seen the dead outside of funerals. As a result, many, if not most, mental health personnel are largely unprepared to understand the nature of contact with the dead from mass disasters or war. These situations often involve large numbers of casualties, and most of the remains will not appear like those prepared for viewing in funeral homes. In the US Army mortuary affairs community, the term "remains" is used to refer to the dead; other terminology is often considered disrespectful. The term "bodies" is frequently used in the medical field and is occasionally used here to avoid repetition, but no disrespect is intended.

The purposes of this chapter are to (*a*) explain the stresses of handling remains, (*b*) describe common feelings and responses of persons who have handled or seen the dead, (*c*) provide procedures to help mental health workers support personnel exposed to the dead, and (*d*) prepare mental health workers to effectively communicate the situation of those caring for the dead to higher authorities, who may fail to understand the nature of the services of both the remains' handlers and mental health professionals.

Persons who encounter remains may themselves have had a variety of previous experiences with the dead or no experience at all. Some gain experience through their professions. Among these are medical personnel such as pathologists, nurses, and some technicians; police, firefighters, and emergency service workers; and professionals who attend the dead such as military personnel who recover bodies from the battlefield, morticians, funeral directors and their staffs, and forensic investigators. Professional groups, for the most part, are protected from distress by their roles and identities. For example, pathologists are still serving a patient and achieve professional satisfaction in solving a mystery; they routinely provide the final medical procedures for their patients. The major goal of public service workers is to save lives, but over time their professionalism and frequent exposure to the dead generally protects them from the adverse consequences of such encounters.

A second group has encountered the dead episodically. Among these are people who have lived in a violent community, those involved in a natural or community disaster such as a building explosion or fire, victims of violent crime or violent civil disturbance, and military personnel whose regular job is handling the dead. A third group is composed of people who have rarely or never encountered the dead except at funerals or, secondarily, through the media. Members of these groups anticipate and experience exposure to the dead in a different manner.[2] Because of their relative lack of experience, the two latter groups usually need more preparation before exposure and more assistance afterward.

MILITARY CARE-OF-THE-DEAD POLICY AND TRAINING

The history and documentation of wartime care for the dead is very limited, although some official records of these services are publicly available.[3] A recent history, prompted by the invasion of Iraq in 2003, has updated the record with personal stories and photographs.[4]

When a service member dies, the remains are no longer the responsibility of the Army Medical Department, but are handled through the military logistics system. Enlisted Army soldiers whose military profession is to collect, process, and return remains to the families are in the military occupational specialty of mortuary affairs and belong to the Army Quartermaster Corps. Following their basic training, they attend a 7-week course at the Mortuary Affairs Center and School at Fort Lee, Virginia. The course curriculum consists of familiarization with the physical and psychological aspects of dying and death, search and recovery operations, tentative identification, decontamination, and accountability for the personal effects of the deceased. Students receive classroom and field experience at a morgue or mortuary where they are exposed to remains. They are also trained in the numerous Army procedures for the care of the dead, which helps ensure that the dead are handled in a dignified, reverent, and respectful manner, principles that are continually emphasized in the training. Following their initial training, mortuary affairs personnel can obtain additional experience in a variety of military and civilian mortuaries where they observe and sometimes assist in autopsies. Unfortunately, however, mortuary affairs operations are not usually included in Army training exercises, which limits the ability of commanders to understand mortuary affairs functions and operations in wartime.

Quartermaster Corps officers receive familiarization training in mortuary affairs and may command a mortuary affairs company, but this command is only one of a variety of positions these officers are expected to assume. Of the other US military services, only the Navy has a dedicated career field for persons who handle remains. The Navy requires that personnel at sea who handle remains be licensed embalmers to care for bodies that cannot be returned quickly to the United States.

STRESSES OF EXPOSURE TO REMAINS

Research on groups of experienced (mortuary affairs soldiers) and inexperienced (those whose military profession did not require exposure to the dead) soldiers found three main concerns about working with remains[5]: (1) physical characteristics of the remains, (2) personal safety, and (3) emotional involvement associated with the remains.

Physical Characteristics of Remains

Senses seem to serve different cognitive and emotional processes. Each sense has special qualities that may produce distress in an individual.

Smell

The odor sensation has many special qualities[6]; aside from being immediately unpleasant, the smell of remains has additional effects. Smell is the most likely of the senses to trigger reminders at a later time. Odor memory is highly resistant to extinction, that is, there is long-term recognition of odors. A smell cannot be conjured up from the past, but can be recognized almost instantly (although a lemon's smell cannot be mentally conceptualized, its appearance can be visualized). Also, the strength of the memory varies with the involvement a person has with the odor.

People working with remains often try to mask odors by some means, such as wearing a mask laced with a strong fragrance. However, this strategy can be problematic for several reasons. Fragrances may not always be available, and the use of an additional olfactory stimulus adds another scent to the mix already present, which may also bring back unpleasant associations later. Breathing through the mouth is an effective way of avoiding unpleasant odors.

Sight

The sight of grotesque remains (burned, mutilated, dismembered, decomposed) may be the most dramatic aspect of casualties. Scenes of death are likely to be remembered and form the basis of conscious or intrusive memories. However, the most grotesque remains may not be the most bothersome to all observers. A body that looks natural with no or few visible signs of wounds may cause more distress than damaged remains. In addition, bodies that are badly burned or otherwise grossly distorted may not look human, which may make it easier for the handler to gain cognitive and emotional distance.

Touch

Tactile qualities of remains are disturbing to some workers, even when wearing gloves. For example, the skin of decomposing bodies will easily slip off the underlying tissue. Some tactile sensations are familiar, some are unfamiliar, and each has the capacity for disturbance.

Sounds

Dropping a body on a floor, truck bed, or table may remind the remains handler of sounds that would be painful to a living person. An example of such a sound is that of a head making a cracking noise against a hard surface. Autopsy equipment also produces potentially distressing sounds.

Taste

Sensations of taste are usually associated with

smell. Some remains handlers have an aversion to grilled meats after handling burned remains, but this reaction is not universal. People react individually to foods following exposure to remains, just as they have individual food references in other circumstances.

Types of Remains

What will bother individuals, or what will relieve their distress, is not completely predictable. However, with varying degrees of certainty, the categories that bother almost everyone can be enumerated and described, providing a framework for understanding situations and reactions peculiar to one person or another. Almost without exception, caring for the bodies of children is the most distressing type of exposure to the dead. Also distressing to most people are the remains of torture victims, innocent persons (such as casualties of friendly fire in the military), women who died in combat, and persons killed in a grotesque manner, as well as body parts and large numbers of remains. On the other hand, some types of remains, or some scenes or situations, are bothersome to some people but not others. In one case, remains wrapped in gauze in preparation for casketing reminded an experienced handler of a rag doll.

Each military conflict is likely to involve a unique type of death or types of remains and situations. Examples from the current wars in Iraq and Afghanistan are torture victims, fragmented remains from bombings, mass graves, and civilian casualties including children. Additionally, cultural differences in procedures for handling remains are often poorly understood by Americans.

Personal Safety

Remains handlers must protect themselves against battlefield dangers, disease, contamination, and occupational hazards. Battlefield recovery of remains can be hazardous. For example, remains can be booby-trapped with explosives. Local populations can be hostile, and the possibility of combat cannot always be ruled out. Physical contact with remains requires the same personal protective measures as are routinely taken by doctors and dentists to protect themselves from blood products and other sources of contamination. In addition to naturally occurring contamination, the enemy can contaminate remains with toxins such as chemical, biological, or radiological substances. Decontamination of remains and of the handler pose similar hazards.

In areas where certain diseases are endemic, remains handlers should be aware of necessary protective measures. Persons who die due to combat or disasters rarely have medical conditions that cause epidemics. Remains (including animal remains) do not cause disease except under certain circumstances. This point is especially important for commanders, supervisors, and medical personnel to understand because misconceptions can cause errors in the handling and processing of remains.[7] For example, if commanders or public officials incorrectly believe that remains can cause disease, a rush to bury or cremate them can occur, preventing the bodies from being returned to families or investigated for cause and manner of death.

Remains *can* cause disease when diseases are present in the area—microorganisms causing disease can survive in remains after death, and environmental conditions can facilitate the microorganisms' growth. Examples of such conditions are overcrowding, contaminated water, poor sanitation, and endemic disease. Some diseases that can be spread by remains are blood-borne diseases such as hepatitis B and C, human immunodeficiency virus, gastrointestinal diseases such as hepatitis A, *Escherichia coli*, cholera, and respiratory diseases such as tuberculosis. However, the most common risks to the remains handler are occupational hazards such as cuts, spills, sprains and strains, fatigue, and dehydration.

Emotional Involvement

Emotional involvement refers to the feeling of distress by the remains handlers when some quality of the remains creates a sense of shared humanity, weakening or destroying the handlers' psychological distance. The remains lose some of their inanimate quality, and the handler feels some sense of the loss of the life of another person. Emotional involvement often occurs when the handler is of similar age as the remains or has a child the same age. Other circumstances that can create a sense of emotional involvement are obtaining or preparing personal documents for deceased, media reports on the individual or situation that caused the death, contact with unit members in which more is learned about the history of the deceased, and contact with the family. These situations make the remains "like me." Emotional involvement is sometimes referred to as identification with the deceased.[8]

The personal effects of the deceased are highly likely to create a sense of emotional involvement with the deceased and, often, with the survivors of the deceased.[9] Pictures, letters, and personal possessions and mementoes all help contribute to building a picture of the life of the deceased and a sense of loss or even threat for the handler ("it could have been me"). In the military, personal effects are given the same degree of care and concern as the remains. Personal effects are sent to a personal effects depot where they are sorted, catalogued, inventoried, cleaned, and shipped to the next of kin. Mortuary affairs personnel staff these depots and are exposed in detail to the lives of the deceased. Policy requires that mortuary affairs staff read letters before they can be returned to the family to ensure that the material is returned to the correct recipient and to remove material that might be sensitive or embarrassing to the family. Government property and morbid material (such as blood-soaked clothing) are not returned to the next of kin. A summary court officer is appointed to review all personal effects and to assure that all legal matters are observed.

PSYCHOLOGICAL EFFECTS OF CARING FOR REMAINS

Reactions to death and the dead are varied and difficult to catalogue or predict. Some reactions are immediate, and others may not appear until later. Typical immediate reactions are surprise and shock, withdrawal, nervousness, and shame at one's own reactions. Overworking is also common and leads to fatigue and errors. Other reactions are intrusive thoughts, avoidance of reminders of the situation, feeling "keyed up," and problems with daily functioning. These reactions are normal and expected unless prolonged. More extreme reactions can impact negatively on health, including substance abuse, excessive smoking, failure to seek needed medical care, and other behaviors that indicate a lack of self-care.

Additional behaviors can be expressed, and people respond differently and at different times. A longitudinal study of posttraumatic responses over a 13-month period in a group of mortuary workers found that intrusive and avoidance symptoms were elevated at 1, 4, and 13 months, but decreased over time. The level of probable posttraumatic stress disorder symptoms was 11% at 1 month, 10% at 4 months, and 2% at 13 months. Depression was not increased. Marital status was a factor in response: single remains handlers reported more avoidance and somatization than married remains handlers.[10]

Anticipation of exposure to traumatic death is stressful. In any remains-handling situation, anticipation of one's own reaction must be considered,[2] especially for inexperienced people. Training and experience can reduce anticipated stress and result in improved performance, decrease fatigue, and decrease the risk of adverse psychological effects. For example, inexperienced forensic dentists working with the remains of the badly burned victims of a fire reported more distress from handling decomposed, burned, and fragmented remains than the experienced dentists.[11] However, both experienced and inexperienced dentists reported distress from handling the remains of children. These findings challenge the common belief that highly trained professionals are immune to distress.

In most circumstances, the groups with the most exposure have the most distress. For example, the distress for forensic dentists who handled burned remains was related to the hours of exposure to the remains.[11] In another study, the responses of mortuary workers were measured before and after exposure to the remains of service members killed in war.[12] When age, sex, volunteer status, and experience were controlled, intrusion symptoms increased significantly for all groups exposed to the dead, and avoidance symptoms increased in the two groups with the most exposure. Even after controlling for symptoms expressed in anticipation of exposure to the dead, exposure itself increased posttraumatic symptoms.

ROLE OF THE MENTAL HEALTHCARE PROVIDER IN MASS DEATH SITUATIONS

To be maximally effective in assisting soldiers, the mental health provider must be knowledgeable about the stresses of operations and their likely effects on exposed personnel; be available, known, and trusted; and coordinate efforts with the local chaplain or other first lines of support outside the military unit or civilian organization.

Recognizing Signs of Stress

No particular reactions or signs of distress shown by remains handlers differ from reactions of other persons. Experienced supervisors have reported witnessing or hearing about many common stress-related behaviors and feelings (Exhibit 45-1). It cannot be overemphasized that these reactions are usually normal signs of understandable distress about a difficult situation. Only when these reactions are prolonged should mental health workers seek to intervene. For day-to-day distress reactions, first-line supervisors and colleagues should offer understanding and allow respite for a reasonable period of time. Mission demands rarely prevent such temporary respite. Mental health workers can assist in preparing supervisors to

EXHIBIT 45-1

SIGNS OF STRESS IN MORTUARY OPERATIONS AND COPING WITH THE WORK

Behavioral signs of stress

- Fatigue, agitation, withdrawal, sleeplessness
- Loss of, or gain in, appetite
- Quitting (not reporting for work)
- Extreme agitation or crying

Psychological signs of stress

- Depression, sadness, apathy
- Major change of personality
- Other feelings
  - Anxiety
  - Frustration
  - Anger
  - Feeling sick and nervous
  - Fear
  - Loneliness

recognize the normal stresses of working in a mass casualty environment and provide temporary relief. Exhibit 45-2 provides examples of ways mortuary affairs soldiers deal with stress.

Assisting Soldiers With Exposure to Mass Death

The plan recommended here for mental health professionals to assist soldiers, commanders, and other medical personnel after a mass death is based on a three-stage model: (1) preparation, (2) on-site actions, and (3) follow-up (Exhibit 45-3). Commanders should be visible and available to soldiers for at least part of

EXHIBIT 45-2

HOW DO MORTUARY AFFAIRS SOLDIERS SAY THEY DEAL WITH STRESS?

- "Stay focused" (concentrate on doing their job)
- Exercise or engage in sports
- Keep busy
- Read and write letters
- Talk to others
- Listen to music
- Get away from the mass death scene
- Communicate with family back home

EXHIBIT 45-3

GUIDELINES FOR ASSISTING SOLDIERS AND COMMANDERS IN CARING FOR THE DEAD

Before: Anticipate operational procedures and train for them

- Obtain and share information
- Brief plans up (command) and down (soldiers) the chain of command
- Expose inexperienced personnel gradually
- Practice
- Anticipate reactions and prepare for them

During: Limit exposure to the remains and scene and support the soldier

- Avoid or decrease exposure to strong stimuli
- Provide respite: breaks, food, sleep
- Provide supervision
- Pair inexperienced with experienced person
- Encourage talk among workers and supervisors
- Recognize signs of stress and act
- Provide respectful and visible command or authority
- Emphasize job and role of remains handlers

After: Inform, talk, and listen

- Provide operational debriefing and education on the facts of the event
- Acknowledge the existence of intense personal feelings
- Encourage family and organizational support systems
- Reinforce the positive aspects of the work accomplished

Long-term: Follow-up guidelines for soldiers and commanders

- Posttraumatic symptoms are usually not lasting—most people "move on"
- Time is the most effective treatment for most people
- Watch for problems that do not go away
- Problems that persist should not be neglected

the operation and ensure that all necessary logistic support has been provided. In the follow-up phase, they should speak to soldiers as a group about their work, reinforcing the soldiers' role and the importance of their work. The question usually arises as to when soldiers should be ready to go back to work. Although there is no firm answer to this, it is recommended that soldiers be given some time off after the operation to rest and attend to personal matters. Several days of respite is common following a difficult mission. Sending soldiers back to work immediately, unless absolutely necessary, is likely to be detrimental to their functioning and may be interpreted as a lack of appreciation for them and their work. Support of soldiers in mass death operations involves three domains: (1) personal, (2) organizational, and (3) logistical.

Personal Support

In addition to normal social support, the supervisor and the mental health worker should attempt to reinforce in the soldier a pride of accomplishment whether the individual is distressed or not. Exhibit 45-4 lists many points that can be made by the mental health worker, the supervisor, and the commander. The exhibit includes unique military aspects of caring for remains with which the individual, particularly the lower ranking soldier, should be aware. Immediately obvious are the services to the deceased and the family of the deceased. Less obvious are the honor of upholding military service traditions and fulfilling the nation's cultural expectations. It is also vital that persons outside the mortuary affairs field understand the importance of recognizing these principles.

Personal support of soldiers also includes access to mental health and spiritual care. Because of the broad dispersion of mortuary affairs collection points and interruptions in transportation capabilities, mental health teams in the current Middle East conflicts often have difficulty establishing relationships with soldiers. Also, contact between soldiers and mental health personnel can be a touchy issue. In spite of the competency, good will, and attempts of mental health workers to be helpful, soldiers will not often engage with them if they are not known and trusted. Being credible requires frequent contact. Chaplains are often the primary resource for personal assistance, and mortuary affairs personnel report that chaplains from all the services are available and often spend time with them eating meals and staying overnight. Chaplains, medics, and mental health workers must be known as regular visitors to achieve credible status with soldiers. Regardless of these relationships, however, the commander or other supervisor who has the authority to refer a soldier to mental health personnel should do so when the situation warrants.

EXHIBIT 45-4

REINFORCE THE POSITIVE

Common individual reasons for care of the dead in war

- Upholding American military service traditions
- "Everybody comes back home"
- "If I do it for them, somebody will do it for me"

Personal pride in care of the dead in war

- Doing something important for the deceased soldier
- Doing something important for the families
- Doing a job that others cannot do
- Personal mastery of a difficult job

Practical considerations of families in having remains returned

- Document place and cause of death
- Assist with grieving
- Resolve legal and personal issues
    - Wills and inheritance
    - Remarriage
    - Government compensation
    - Insurance

Effects on society

- Respect for and care of the dead as an American tradition
- Social identity of the dead
- Funerals, memorials, and monuments
- National pride or shame

Organizational Support

For mortuary affairs soldiers, the presence of commanders and their respectful attitude are extremely important when remains are being cared for. It is considered highly disrespectful for commanders and other visitors not to remove headgear or wipe their feet before entering the processing area when remains are present. Commanders and mental health personnel can assist the soldiers by adhering to these practices and preparing visitors to do the same.

Other forms of organizational support are related less to the stress of handling remains and more to occupational functioning. In widely dispersed conflicts such as Iraq and Afghanistan, soldiers operate many collection points, often with minimal personnel. Soldiers may be required to recover remains from distant locations and are always on duty. Processing remains requires physical work in lifting and moving the deceased as well as the transfer cases in which they are shipped. A large number of remains can require several hours to process. As a result, opportunities for rest, recreation, and personal time are limited. Commanders must ensure that soldiers have time for sleep and recuperation. Finally, collection points and mortuaries are often located at air fields away from Army support or are isolated to prevent unnecessary troop exposure. This isolation can have a positive effect in the freedom to accomplish the work without interference, but isolation can sometimes result in the mortuary affairs soldiers being shunned by others. Such situations require a great deal of command support for the soldier.

Logistical Support

The psychological stress of mortuary affairs work can be greatly reduced if soldiers have the necessary supplies and equipment, adequate transportation, and good area or unit support. Mortuary affairs soldiers often do not operate at an organic organizational level (platoon or company) in war. In the current Middle East conflicts, soldiers who staff collection points in the field are usually assigned to other Army organizations, such as a division, or even to other military services. Soldiers returning from Iraq and Afghanistan have reported excellent support from the US Air Force and Marine Corps. However, occasionally collection points lacked some logistic support, including refrigeration equipment and vehicles for transporting personnel and remains. Army command authorities may have limited control over mortuary affairs personnel when those personnel are attached to another Army unit or military service. However, they can take steps to ensure that the organizations to which the mortuary affairs soldiers are attached provide them proper support.

Social Effects of Proper Care of the Dead

The effects on society are far from the battlefield but should be impressed on mortuary affairs soldiers to reinforce the positive aspects of their work. The requirement for dignified care of remains is not only doctrine, but becomes a creed for these soldiers. Members of American society must have faith that this tradition is carried on and that mortuary affairs soldiers accomplish this mission.

The social identity of the dead has meaning for the survivors of the deceased.[4] Social identity refers to the place that the deceased will have in the minds of survivors such as fellow soldiers, the family, and others who may or may not have known the individual. After death, an identity can be broader than the identity the individual had in life. This identity includes, but is not limited to, knowledge of the place and manner of death, the place of burial, and how the individual is remembered. The return of the remains and personal effects contribute greatly to the formation of this identity.

Wartime funerals and memorials are legion. Whether humble or grand, funerals and memorials are less than complete without remains to memorialize. Families, without exception, want a remembrance of the deceased; if the remains are unrecoverable, then a memento is required. The memento can be a personal effect, soil from the area of death, or a symbol of the individual's life or death.

SUMMARY

The mortuary affairs soldier has an important role in the long chain of events that support the recovery and return of the dead from war. The soldiers who perform this role obtain support primarily from each other, but also from their organization and those above them. The job stresses are largely compensated for by the soldiers' own sense of accomplishment in performing an honorable but difficult task. Support from mental health workers, chaplains, or commanders, comes from (*a*) recognition of the work, including an understanding of the duties; (*b*) respect for the remains-handling process; (*c*) spending time with personnel to decrease any possible isolation caused by the nature or location of the work; and (*d*) understanding how the stress of this particular job interacts with those stresses that affect all soldiers in a deployed environment.

The way a country cares for the remains of its war dead contributes to national pride or shame. This is reinforced in the soldier by the credo, "no one left behind." The commander, the mortuary affairs soldier, and the mental health provider all play important roles in ensuring the endurance of this tradition.

Acknowledgment

Thanks to Mr Tommy D Bourlier and Mr Douglas L Howard, Director and Deputy Director, respectively, of the US Army Mortuary Affairs Center and School, Fort Lee, Virginia, for their reading and comments on the manuscript. Thanks also to Jodi McKibben, PhD, Center for the Study of Traumatic Stress, Department of Psychiatry, Uniformed Services University of the Health Sciences, Bethesda, MD, for her reading and commentary on the manuscript. And, finally, a special thanks to the many soldiers who shared their time and stories with the authors.

REFERENCES

1. Ursano RJ, McCarroll JE, Fullerton CS. Traumatic death in terrorism and disasters: the effects on posttraumatic stress and behavior. In: Ursano RJ, Fullerton CS, Norwood AE, eds. *Terrorism and Disaster*. New York, NY: Cambridge University Press; 2003: 308–332.

2. McCarroll JE, Ursano RJ, Ventis WL, et al. Anticipation of handling the dead: effects of gender and experience. *Br J Clin Psychol*. 1993;32:466–468.

3. Risch E, Kieffer CL. Care of the dead. In: *United States Army in World War II. The Technical Services. The Quartermaster Corps: Organization, Supply, and Services.* Washington, DC: US Government Printing Office; 1955: 361–494.

4. Sledge M. *Soldier Dead.* New York, NY: Columbia University Press; 2005.

5. McCarroll JE, Ursano RJ, Fullerton CS, et al. Gruesomeness, emotional attachment, and personal threat: dimensions of anticipated stress of body recovery. *J Trauma Stress*. 1995;8:343–347.

6. Engen T. Remembering odors and their names. *Am Scientist*. 1987;75:497–503.

7. Pan American Health Organization and World Health Organization. *Management of Dead Bodies in Disaster Situations.* Disaster Manuals and Guidelines Series, No 5. Washington, DC: PAHO and WHO; 2004: 71–83. Available at: http://www.paho.org/english/dd/ped/DeadBodiesBook.pdf. Accessed November 18, 2008.

8. Ursano, RJ, Fullerton CS, Vance K, Kao TC. Posttraumatic stress disorder and identification in disaster workers. *Am J Psychiatry*. 2003;156:353–359.

9. McCarroll JE, Blank AS, Hill K. Working with traumatic material: effects on Holocaust Memorial Museum Staff. *Am J Orthopsychiatry*. 1995;65:66–75.

10. Ursano RJ, Fullerton CS. Vance K, Kao TC, Bhartiya VR. Longitudinal assessment of posttraumatic stress disorder and depression after exposure to traumatic death. *J Nerv Ment Dis*. 1995;183:36–42.

11. McCarroll JE, Fullerton CS, Ursano RJ, Hermsen JM. Posttraumatic stress symptoms following forensic dental identification: Mt. Carmel, Waco, Texas. *Am J Psychiatry*. 1996;153:778–782.

12. McCarroll JE, Ursano RJ, Fullerton CS, Liu X, Lundy A. Effect of exposure to death in a war mortuary on posttraumatic stress symptoms. *J Nerv Ment Dis*. 2001;189:44–48.

Chapter 46

ETHICS AND MILITARY MEDICINE: CORE CONTEMPORARY QUESTIONS

EDMUND G. HOWE, MD, JD*; ROBERT C. McKENZIE, DO†; AND CHAD BRADFORD, MD‡

*Professor of Psychiatry, Associate Professor of Medicine, and Director, Programs in Medical Ethics, Uniformed Services University of the Health Sciences, 4301 Jones Bridge Road, Bethesda, Maryland 20814; and Senior Scientist, Center for the Study of Traumatic Stress, Bethesda, Maryland; formerly, Major, Medical Corps, United States Army

†Lieutenant Colonel, Medical Corps, US Army; Department of Behavioral Health, US Army Health Clinic-Vicenza, Caserma Ederle, Italy, Unit 31401, Box 13, APO AE 09042

‡Commander, Medical Corps, US Navy; Division Psychiatrist, 2nd Marine Division, Division Surgeon's Office, Attn: Division Psychiatry, HQBN 2MAR DIV, Camp Lejeune, North Carolina 28547; formerly, Forensic Psychiatry Fellow, National Capital Consortium, Washington, DC

INTRODUCTION

Numerous new ethical issues have arisen in the past few decades as a result of developments in biology and technology. Others have arisen as a result of different kinds of warfare, as manifested by the terrorist attacks of September 11, 2001.[1] These changes have resulted in a need for reevaluation of traditional military medical ethics and some unprecedented paradigm shifts.[2–6]

The need for military behavioral healthcare providers to have a sound, basic understanding of these issues has also increased and is much wider in scope. Military physicians must now, more than ever, be aware of ethical considerations that may affect their clinical practices. They must also be cognizant of how ethical considerations can bear on policies the military is developing, whether these are behavioral or medical in intent. Furthermore, because military behavioral healthcare providers may be involved as ethics consultants or on ethics committees, they must understand core ethical arguments that have to be taken into account in these relatively new practices.

Consequently, this chapter will seek to address those major issues in which it can reasonably be expected that military behavioral healthcare providers might be involved. When appropriate, this discussion will describe specifically how these military behavioral healthcare providers might become involved in the topic areas discussed. This chapter also will highlight areas in which the need for *de novo* analysis has been posed. It will do this in the same order as the sections presented in this book—prior to, during, and after deployment.

ISSUES ARISING PRIOR TO DEPLOYMENT

Recruitment Issues

During the initial years of the ongoing war on terror, with mounting casualties, sustaining the needed flow of volunteers to enter the military became problematic. The need to meet recruiting goals led to a relaxation of enlistment standards. Changes included increasing the number of waivers being given for individuals with legal difficulties, lowering the Armed Services Vocational Aptitude Battery (ASVAB) scores, and becoming more permissive concerning tattoos that have specific pejorative connotations for some target groups. It is unclear what the effects will be on individuals recruited under the new conditions and how these precedents will affect short-term and more long-term military standards. However, since the overall economy worsened in 2008 recruits have been plentiful, and standards for waivers have again tightened.

One ethical dilemma here involves the competing factors of individuals' right or wish to serve their country, the mission's requirements, and the military's need to maintain standards among soldiers who enlist. A second dilemma concerns how much recruits should be screened prior to being accepted. Individuals with lower ASVAB scores or criminal histories may become more of a burden on units as limitations are reached or antisocial behaviors recur. These outcomes may lead to situations in which unit efficacy is compromised or atrocities are committed. However, it might be an ethical error to exclude 100 individuals with previous legal difficulties if only one would reoffend. Furthermore, recent data have shown that individuals who have waivers are actually less likely to commit violent crimes. They also have a higher retention and promotion rate than the majority of soldiers, perhaps because these cases are scrutinized much more closely.[7] Individuals with prior misdemeanor convictions, a lower ASVAB score, or a previous gang or racist group affiliation may want to serve their country or better their own financial or educational standing through military service. Allowing these individuals to serve may be in their best interests, but they may encounter continued difficulties within the services, possibly ending up with a shortened enlistment or a less than favorable discharge.

In addition, a military unit's morale and readiness can suffer directly when standards are lowered. Having an individual with extreme racist views or a gang affiliation can divide and undermine the cohesion in a military unit, in which every member must be willing to save or assist every other member. Individuals with racist views may only be willing to pull individuals they like out of harm's way, while allowing those of a "different persuasion" to remain exposed. Anything short of a completely integrated team may not operate effectively in high-stress combat environments. The potential complications that may occur as these individuals rise in the ranks and take over positions of leadership could also increase. In these positions, their choices could be based on affiliations or ethnicities, rather than abilities, which would erode the principles of equality and fairness. One possible solution: an additional probationary period for these special populations. This is already done for recruits who are obese or do not fit fitness standards so that they can meet fitness standards prior to basic training.

The questions of what level of screening needs to be implemented and whether there should be a special "probational" track to allow these individuals into full service may need to be addressed. As there is no current empirical data to use to assess these arguments, this may remain an ongoing dilemma.

Treatment Concerns

Suicidal Depression During Basic or Preliminary Combat Training

An ethical problem of an entirely different sort, but which also may occur before deployment, is what military behavioral health providers should do when soldiers state that they feel suicidal during basic or early training. Providers may believe that sometimes this is because these soldiers don't want to be in the military, and not because they are truly suicidal. Well-known procedures are in place for soldiers to request discharge. Soldiers may, however, not elect to take these, for various reasons, such as to save face. Indeed, sometimes soldiers may try to get out of the military by presenting with suicidal ideation; however, this is less common in today's all-volunteer Army.

Military psychiatrists or other mental health workers to whom these soldiers present may over time: (*a*) initiate measures to give them an administrative separation to release them from service, because they see their depression as a preexising condition not responsive to treatment, (*b*) judge them to have a personality disorder, or (*c*) discharge them back to duty. Customarily, providers respond by giving the soldier a trial of psychotherapy and/or antidepressants.

The ethical problem primarily posed to providers stems from the fact that soldiers presenting during basic or advanced indivitual training, and before deployment, may (as at any other time) be genuinely depressed and suicidal.[8,9] Thus, if military care providers don't take all the precautions they could, this may increase the likelihood that some, even if only a few, of these soldiers will commit suicide. To the degree that providers take all possible precautions, they are acting in support of military needs as well as those of the soldiers.

The possibility of other soldiers temporarily or permanently feeling they want out of the military, and thus pursuing this same psychiatric out, may lead to military physicians treating soldiers with combat fatigue as they now do; that is, they treat most such soldiers with the expectation that they will return to their units in combat. If providers instead released these soldiers from their units and from further combat duty, inordinate numbers of soldiers could follow suit.

A reason often given as an ethical justification for treating soldiers with the expectation of return to duty is that if soldiers return to their unit, they will be less vulnerable to having permanent psychiatric symptoms later because of survivor guilt, should the unit eventually lose members in combat. Factually this may be true, but as an ethical argument, this reasoning is fallacious. Respecting soldiers' autonomy would in other contexts prevail over the value of doing what is best for these soldiers' later symptoms. Respecting their autonomy "normally," or in civilian contexts, would require military physicians to give soldiers the choice of risking these symptoms or risking death.

The justification for military physicians to treat soldiers with combat fatigue with the expectation that they will return to their unit is both for the sake of the mission and the individual soldier in one sense, though not in another. That is, soldiers may do better in both the short and longer run if they can return to their unit. They may, for example, feel better being back among those they have known and be less prone to later psychiatric symptoms that would be due, most likely, to their previously having left their unit and never having returned.

Soldiers who are evacuated out of the theater usually do not stay in the Army, and they often do not remain in contact with the "buddies" they left behind. The loss of their social networks, the structure of the military, and associated healthcare may lead to a downward spiral into joblessness and even homelessness. Still, their being treated with this return-to-duty expectation is to some extent coercive and, thus, differs from what civilians seeking psychiatric treatment after trauma will encounter; indeed, this expectation deprives them of a source of additional autonomy.

A similar rationale supports military care providers treating soldiers in basic training who present with suicidal depression. Treating them with psychotherapy and medications, when there is a possibility that they are genuinely depressed, has a good likelihood of keeping these soldiers from leaving the Army and/or possibly ending their lives, even if at the time this does not seem the best that providers could do for patients who say they feel suicidal. In civilian settings, providers might try more to eliminate or reduce the source of ongoing stress. Military physicians treating these patients as they do now, in any case, reduces the possibility that too many other soldiers in basic training or other predeployment settings will present with suicidal depression, again for unconscious or conscious reasons, as a means for seeking a way out.

A final, additional ethical dilemma here is whether military behavioral healthcare providers should inform soldiers presenting in this manner of the "ground rules" of seeking discharge by this means. They could tell soldiers that to be discharged for depression, they must generally first undergo a trial of psychotherapy and medication for approximately 6 months. However, in the current climate of increasing suicides during the last 6 years, this option is unlikely to be politically palatable. Nonetheless, there is an ethical obligation to disclose such facts, as opposed to allowing outcomes to be determined or significantly affected by keeping some information unknown. The question then becomes: Should providers regard soldiers reporting suicidal depression in this same category and not inform them of the ground rules or should they inform them?

The optimal compromise between military physicians meeting the needs of the mission and those of these soldiers may be somewhat contradictory and paradoxical. It may be that optimally they should insist on treating and even giving these patients medication for 6 or more months while at the same time giving them full information concerning how these ground rules work. Providing this information may, in addition, be the only way in which they can treat these patients most successfully by gaining their trust. If this practice stems the potential flood of soldiers gaining discharge by this means (as it appears it would), treatment with disclosure in this manner should suffice to support the mission needs.

Predeployment Distress

The policy of deploying soldiers who are not emotionally prepared, or who have certain home-front issues to resolve, may cause undue distress to these soldiers and their families. A more liberal deployment policy may be in the best interests of soldiers and their units. The ethical dilemma of weighing the readiness needs of military units against the individual needs of such soldiers and/or their families can be problematic. Certainly, military units need to be at maximal strength, but having several soldiers "whose heads aren't in the game" will be counterproductive. Individual soldiers may themselves be at risk or, because of distraction, they may put their team members at risk, and they may ultimately compromise a mission.

During the current war on terror, enlisting soldiers, all voluntary, know the potential risks of pending deployments. In the current situation it is just a matter of time until a soldier deploys; whether a soldier will deploy is not in question. Despite this knowledge, some individuals are less prepared to deploy than others. These individuals may be struggling with short-term adjustment issues, or they may have a family circumstance that could be resolved if they were just given a short period of time. Perhaps as little as 30 days would be required to get them emotionally prepared to deploy, or to get their family circumstances resolved. Examples of the latter would be moving a wife stateside from Germany or making sure all financial matters are in order.

The risk to military units from such a "lenient" approach is 2-fold. First, allowing exceptions to, or delaying, individual deployments may violate the fundamental premise of fairness, in that the rest of their team is expected to be ready to deploy and to deploy on orders. Presumably, many other members of their unit would also prefer to delay, or even avoid, the deployment. Second, a military unit is only as good as its members, and if they aren't present, the unit suffers. If some members are allowed to delay their deployment, this may be critical to the mission, as when the soldier not deployed is a generator mechanic, or the most competent communications specialist.

It may be ethically optimal to develop a way to deal with each individual circumstance on a case-by-case basis, with the general presumption that all units would deploy in entirety, as much as possible. A multitracked system to evaluate and clear deploying soldiers, with one track for those who require a short period of reconstitution or to accomplish family-related issues, another track for those soldiers who should not be deployed, and a third track for those ready to deploy may be the best of all options. By keeping commands informed about the process and the status of their soldiers, the needs of individuals and the needs of military units may jointly be best met. Current policy is to only deploy service members who have been stable for at least 3 months; otherwise they must get a waiver from the combatant surgeon, who is usually the Central Command surgeon.

Further Treatment Issues

Military behavioral healthcare providers must consider how social and emotional distance from members of their unit may affect treatment of potential unit member patients. Both at work and outside of work, military behavioral healthcare providers are likely to interact with their future patients on a regular basis. Maintaining too much distance from their units may give the impression of their being aloof and unapproachable, decreasing the likelihood of future referrals. Maintaining too close a relationship may establish a friendly, rather than a therapeutic, relationship. Close relationships may also hinder military behavioral healthcare providers' ability to make an accurate diagnosis.

Military behavioral healthcare providers and their future patients are likely to be stationed on the same base, in the same unit, and may frequent common work areas. Military bases tend to be insular, with those on the base frequently coming into contact with each other. They may share similar collateral duties such as command committees or other work projects. They may frequently cross paths and interact with each other at military functions such as awards ceremonies, formations, and command education and training. Outside of work they may frequent the same stores or use the same daycare.

Vignette 47-1: A military psychiatrist maintained a distinct social and emotional distance from those in his unit. It was not his practice to socialize with staff or interact at command functions. When not in session with a patient, he would remain in his office with the door shut. When approached about this behavior the psychiatrist explained that he was indeed not socially phobic, but was rather purposefully maintaining his social and emotional distance from others in the command in case one day they should become his patients. He explained that if he were to get too close, he might be expected to be a "friend" to his patients; they might expect him to do the things that a friend might, such as to socialize together and share personal details of his life. Both of these, he reasoned, could be harmful to treatment. He also reasoned that if he became too close to his unit, he may have more difficulty recommending that they go to combat should the need arise. He also reasoned that this might hinder his ability to make an accurate diagnosis; that his pretreatment conceptions of the person might cloud his ability to perceive mental illness; and that this might lead him to diagnose mental illness that is not there.

Is this psychiatrist's social behavior ideal or does it go too far? Or is it altogether inappropriate and unnecessary? Why?

Although it is important to maintain the appropriate social and emotional distance, it is also important for military behavioral healthcare providers to be approachable and to facilitate referrals. It is difficult for military behavioral healthcare providers to help if no one is willing to make appointments with them. Military behavioral healthcare providers interacting with the unit while maintaining their professional bearing may be ideal. Keeping a "finger on the pulse" of unit morale is important to maintaining the fighting ability of the unit, and often is one of the jobs of military behavioral healthcare providers. Military behavioral healthcare providers should be educated about how their relationship to their unit may affect their treatment should such soldiers become their patients. The goal for these providers should be to offer appropriate treatment to their patients while maintaining maximum unit combat effectiveness. In order to achieve these goals military behavioral healthcare providers must maintain objectivity despite their social and emotional relationships with their unit.

ISSUES ARISING DURING DEPLOYMENT

One of the most important medical considerations that has arisen is how military physicians should treat prisoners of war (POWs). Under the Geneva Conventions, it is clear that military physicians should treat POWs equally to allied soldiers, but it is unclear how this equal treatment should be carried out. Suppose, hypothetically, that US soldiers and POWs have identical injuries. Military physicians could treat each on an alternating or random basis, or they could treat all US soldiers with identical injuries first. Or, military physicians using this second approach could use broad categories of injuries so that they could treat more US soldiers first and still, in a technical sense, treat both US soldiers and POWs equally.[2]

An ethical question arising in regard to detainees is whether military physicians should also treat detainees equally, even though from a legal standpoint, detainees may not meet criteria to be POWs, and the Geneva Conventions may not apply. Leaving aside the practical difficulty of determining who is a POW and who is a detainee, a key question regarding the treatment of detainees is the extent to which military physicians' obligations as medical professionals should take precedence over their duties as military officers.

At a seminar on military medical ethics, a group of military physicians who recently served in Iraq were asked what they thought they should do if an enemy were brought in injured, they knew that US soldiers with "identical injuries" were on the way, and their commanding officer ordered them to withhold treatment until their own soldiers arrived and then to treat them first. All the military physicians present felt that they should refuse the commanding officer's order. They thought that they should treat first whoever was before them because this was what, as physicians, they should do.

Legally and ethically, the military holds that all service persons should disobey an illegal or unethical order. Difficulties may exist, however, in determining what constitutes "illegal" or "unethical." The integrity of the military system would require that military physicians, like other service persons, defer to orders when ambiguity exists in urgent situations. Afterwards, they should have these decisions reviewed as widely and quickly as possible.

Ethically, however, it may be possible to establish in advance when an order would conflict with a priority that military physicians hold as medical professionals and to decide then which priority should prevail. This endeavor could favor two outcomes. First, the military's mission might undergo less risk of being significantly compromised. Second, it might help ensure that the highest medical standards were upheld.

Since the disclosure of abuses of detainees at Abu Ghraib, numerous concerns regarding detainees have been raised.[10,11] The US government has invited experts on human rights from the United Nations and others to visit the detainee facility at Guantanamo Bay, Cuba, to inspect the activities there and confirm that present policies meet appropriate ethical standards. The results of these visits can become more conclusive, of course, only if all aspects of all operations there can be fully examined.

One core concern that has received particular public scrutiny and attention is the way in which military health professionals, especially psychiatrists, psychologists, and other medical care providers, have interacted with, and should interact with, detainees. The underlying presupposition is that care providers, being devoted to healing, should set the highest ethical standards in this as in all military contexts.[12] Some healthcare professionals, however, question even this presupposition. Michael Gross, who wrote a recent text on military medical ethics, believes that military care personnel owe a higher duty to their country than to their profession.[4] The converse of this position is that if there is a moral value that care providers should hold, presumably this value is important enough that it should also be held by all.

This second section of this chapter will examine core ethical questions that military care providers' involvements with detainees pose. It will do this in three parts. The first part will consider basic questions regarding detainees, such as what approaches should be permitted during interrogations, whether a mechanism should be provided to allow exceptions to practices proscribed during interrogations, whether the permissible approaches should be enumerated specifically beforehand, whether detainees' conditions should be made better over time, and who should decide all of these issues. These basic questions must be considered first because those that follow and involve care providers are to some extent contingent on these initial answers.

The second part of this section of the chapter will involve questions specifically related to military medical personnel. These will include healthcare provider involvement in interrogations, if they should be involved at all, and confidentiality when treating detainees as patients. The third part will concern what is now the most difficult ethical problem faced by military healthcare providers treating detainees: what to do when detainees refuse to eat. This section will include a brief discussion of whether military care providers should have more opportunity to express their views and the nature of any special duties as military physicians during combat.

The ethical issues military psychiatrists may face in regard to detainees' care are numerous. Military psychiatrists may be asked to serve as consultants during interrogations under the present Department of Defense (DoD) regulations (though psychologists, usually, will take on this role); they must, however, treat detainees solely and exclusively as clinicians would.

This discussion will not attempt to provide the "right" answers to these ethical questions. Rather, it will presume that ethical analysis can't provide these answers, because the values that should warrant highest priority may reasonably differ. It will, however, attempt to provide useful frameworks for considering the more difficult questions these situations pose. It will also present key considerations that those making these determinations should consider. It will finally suggest values that the ethical solutions eventually reached should take into account, regardless of what these solutions will be.

General Questions Regarding the Nonmedical Treatment of Detainees

The core question involving detainees is the extent to which they should be regarded and, accordingly, treated primarily as persons who could have information that could save many lives, or as persons who no longer pose an immediate threat, and thus, like POWs, should be warranted optimal respect and care as persons who are no longer combatants. When detainees are first incarcerated, the ethical justification for treating them primarily as persons who may have information that could save others' lives is greatest. Over time, increasingly, the strength of this justification will probably decrease.

Three more specific key questions raised by nonmedical treatment of detainees concern (1) what approaches should interrogators be permitted to use during interrogations, (2) should the conditions under which detainees are incarcerated change over time, and (3) who should decide both of these questions.

What Approaches Should Interrogators Be Permitted to Use?

Widespread agreement exists that, ethically and legally, the United States should be prohibited from engaging in cruel, inhumane, or degrading treatment of detainees. Specifically, the question involves the concrete concern as to whether any harm—permanent or transient, physical or psychological—should be permitted at all. A starting point for addressing all these questions is to ask what approaches law enforcement personnel now take in the United States with US citizens when they suspect that these individuals have already committed or may commit heinous crimes. Some believe that what the general public currently permits in these situations goes too far. Still, assuming that what is now legally permitted is at least ethically acceptable, if not ideal, brings into focus the key questions that should now be asked regarding limits to interrogators' actions: should interrogators be permitted to cause detainees greater harm than what is allowable with citizens, and, if so, how much greater, and why?

The main argument in favor of allowing interrogators to inflict greater harm to detainees by using more harmful techniques is to further the possibility of saving more lives. As a starting point in this discussion, a suspected serial killer is a paradigmatic example of a US citizen wanting to kill others now or in the future. Such persons, if released, may continue to kill. A second paradigmatic example that can be used for the purpose of conducting this analysis is a person such as Timothy McVeigh, when it was suspected that he blew up the Murrah Federal Building in Oklahoma City in 1995.

In cases such as these, law enforcement personnel in the United States are limited in spite of the fact that if they used more harmful techniques, they might potentially save greater numbers of lives in future terrorism cases. Detainees may differ in several ways from "ordinary" criminals. Chief among these are three: First, they may have information that could save many more lives, even more than individuals like McVeigh. The number of lives saved could be in the tens, hundreds, thousands, or even more. If a terrorist planned to release a lethal biological agent in New York City and a detainee could identify a plot and potential perpetrators before this took place, it could save the lives of perhaps millions.

The likelihood of this occurring may be remote. It may, also, be uncertain whether a detainee has this information and if so, whether duress during an interrogation will elicit the information in time for it to be of value. Research indicates that most information obtained by coercive measures is unreliable[13]; still, some of this information may be of value. The ethical conflict then is between respecting detainees optimally, such as treating them as one would US citizens suspected of being serial killers or mass murderers, like McVeigh, versus possibly gaining information through severe treatment that could save countless lives.

Second, the present threat is different from what it was during even World War II when the Nazis committed genocide. Now, terrorists can live alone, out of communication with each other for years or decades, only then to emerge and possibly endanger an entire city. The only means of finding these terrorists and preventing such harm may be to learn their identities from detainees.

Third, many contemporary terrorists may be motivated to kill others for a variety of reasons, including religious ones. Terrorists motivated by religious reasons, however, may not care whether they live or die in the course of killing others. Indeed, they may actively seek to die as they carry out their attacks. This "new" motivation may escalate the means they are willing to take, such as killing themselves or even their children, thus adding another reason that interrogators might be more ethically justified in using interrogation techniques harsher than US civilian law enforcement personnel use.

The indignity and harm that using more "vigorous" techniques would cause detainees are the main ethical arguments against using these techniques. What should be further said regarding these arguments? First, even if tens of thousands of persons could be saved as a result of detainees having specific and valuable information, it doesn't follow that any and all means possible to produce this outcome are ethically justifiable. Interrogation approaches, at the extreme, include torture, threats of torture, and torture or threats of torture to detainees' families. At some point, especially in ancient times, these approaches were used, in large part for their deterrent effect. Now, these approaches are generally deemed unconscionable choices that might destroy the values initially worth fighting for.

Second, in other contexts in the United States, absolute priority is given to respecting *all* persons' dignity regardless of the numbers of lives that could be saved by not doing this. The best example and paradigm here is the present practice in the conduct of research. Regardless of the possible gain, no participants can be used against their will.

Some, such as Michael Gross, the author of the previously mentioned military medical ethics text, question whether traditional value priorities should continue to prevail at this time.[4] Gross cites the question of what to do if terrorists infiltrate themselves among civilians so that they will not be caught. He argues that there are only two options: (1) doing nothing and becoming defenseless, or (2) departing from previous values and accepting a greater loss of "innocent" civilian lives in the effort to rout out the terrorists who have infiltrated them.

Should limits be proscribed and, if so, should these

be explicitly and specifically publicized? The first question to be answered here is where the line should be drawn between permissible and impermissible interrogation approaches. The second question that must be answered is the extent to which this line should be established by enunciating and publishing concrete, specific limits. If these limits are too vague, interrogators may more easily stretch them. Interrogators may do this for a worthy reason—hoping to save the greatest number of lives. Thus, due to the merit underlying this aim, many interrogators may seek to do this to the extent that they legally can.

Specific limits help prevent this stretching. An example is the abuses that occurred at the prison in Abu Ghraib, Iraq. All military service persons know that they are legally required to refuse unethical or illegal orders. If it is unclear whether an order is unethical or illegal, a service person given such an order may be less clear on what to do. The cost of disobeying is potentially a court-martial. Thus, this is a strong, prima facie argument for establishing prior, specific, and concrete limits.

Too much specificity, however, that is too well publicized also carries a price when persons such as detainees may have information that could save lives. If limits are spelled out in too much detail and detainees come to know what these specific limits are, they may find it easier to "steel themselves" during interrogations so that they do not give information before these limits are reached. Consequently, they may give out less information and as a result fewer lives may be saved.

Should Detainees' Conditions Be Improved Over Time?

A similar price potentially exists in regard to giving detainees greatly improved conditions over time, such as to be able to communicate again with their families. Knowing that they can look forward to such privileges also may help them "hold out." On the other hand, it is most humane to improve detainees' conditions and give them the fullest access to their families after they have been interrogated and after the predominant likelihood of their giving information has passed.

Once interrogation efforts have most likely exhausted the degree to which interrogators can "succeed," logically the argument for giving detainees greater privileges, such as regaining contact with their families, should be greater. From this perspective, detainees should be regarded more and more over time as persons warranting greater respect and care, as opposed to their continuing to be regarded more as potential sources of life-saving information. If detainees know that in time this opportunity will occur, it may likewise make it easier for them to steel themselves during interrogations so that they don't give out information that they otherwise would. Some might suggest that seeing their families could be used as a "carrot," or incentive to give information. This approach would more extensively exploit detainees' vulnerability and may be more ethically problematic and, in the view of some, even unconscionable for this reason.

As a possible alternative and a moral compromise between these conflicting values, greater opportunities could be given to some detainees but not all. Then, all wouldn't know with certainty that they would ever gain these opportunities. It may be that, empirically, detainees' knowledge of better futures will have no effect on their capacity or decision to withhold information during interrogations. Their knowing that they could see their families could, on the other hand, possibly increase their positive regard for the United States, and thus their willingness to give out more information.

In general, detainees who are treated humanely may become more willing to give information over time. Even this possibility is ethically problematic, however, because it involves viewing detainees primarily not as ends in themselves, because they are humans, but as means to an end. Alternatively, it may be that detainees should only be ultimately regarded as ends in themselves. In this case, their captors should treat them humanely even at the expense of other losses, even including loss of other lives.

Remaining questions to be answered are whether, in extreme cases, there should be exceptions and a mechanism to implement the exceptions. Exceptional interrogation techniques might be permissible, in rare circumstances, when extremely extenuating criteria exist. These criteria might include many lives being endangered, the danger being imminent, and it being highly likely that a detainee has information that could save lives. In these situations there could also be a mechanism for outside review before exceptional interrogation approaches are used, as well as observation during the interrogation. The major argument in favor of permitting such a mechanism for exceptions is that it could save more lives.

There are two ethical questions involved in interrogating detainees and having mechanisms for making exceptions to limits. First, what is the highest moral road? And second, what, if any, criteria would justify the United States not taking this usual "highest" moral road? In making these decisions, it may that a high price would be paid to maintain moral standards that most people can accept. This price would involve allowing persons' lives to be lost and accepting this loss in advance.

Who Should Decide These Questions?

Who should decide what the limits for interrogators should be, notwithstanding the potential loss of lives? If established, should these limits then be made public and explicit?[14(pp89–90)] International codes may be one source of answers. Yet, ethically, using international codes alone to determine policy is problematic for many reasons. First, if the codes were enacted before the terrorist attacks of September 11, 2001, they could not have taken into consideration newer circumstances and possibly greater risks terrorists now pose. Codes enacted since this time, on the other hand, could. Second, codes by their nature are limited. Likewise, the ethical soundness of the tenets in all codes may be less sound in exceptional circumstances, such as when a detainee has information that could save thousands of lives.

These limitations inherent in codes may justifiably result in supporting interrogations that are harsh, or in allowing military medical personnel to treat POWs in ways that are unequal, as delineated in the discussion above. Military medical personnel may, consistently with international requirements, categorize all service persons and all POWs with abdominal wounds in the same group, notwithstanding these wounds' seriousness and urgency. The code says that care providers must treat service persons and POWs equally. However, because it doesn't specify whether both groups of patients must be treated alternately or on a random basis, military care providers could treat all their own soldiers in the same category of medical illness first, followed by treatment of POWs.[2]

Analogously, if a code prohibits interrogators from using cruel or inhumane approaches, it could, by its obverse implication, condone interrogators using harsh approaches that don't quite meet the standard of cruel or inhuman, but nonetheless go beyond those permitted to US law enforcement personnel interrogating US citizens. It may be that these standards should be the same or, perhaps, that even the present policies for US citizens go too far—or not far enough—in allowing the use of harsh interrogation techniques.

Third, the risk of codes not being specific enough and not going far enough is especially possible because codes often represent a compromise. They may reflect political pressures and may, like laws, express the least demanding, but still permissible ethical action that persons should take, rather than expressing the highest ethical standards to which they can and should adhere. Because international codes represent a compromise that requires finding areas in which all can agree, codes may represent a "bottom line" acceptable to all participants.

This situation currently poses a problem for the United States. Codes may proscribe certain practices with detainees, such as forced-feeding if the detainee is on a hunger strike. What may be optimal for countries in general may not be optimal or even acceptable for specific countries, such as those most targeted by terrorists for attack. Thus, the losses to these latter countries—such as the United States—for following the code may be greater and the benefits less than for other countries. Ethical analysis often can't provide the right answers to these questions, any more than it can give an answer that is self-evidently valid.

Achieving the best ethical outcome may be attempted by submitting what is at question to the optimal process of consideration. In the United States, this may mean submitting ethical questions such as these to legislators, who are the persons the greater society chooses to decide these questions, checked and countered, from time to time, by the courts. The decisions made at any one time may be overturned. Still, allowing legislation to determine ethical codes may be the best process possible.[15,16(pp37–40)] The "best antidote to bounded rationality—as manifested by cognitive biases and resulting errors in judgment—may be to deploy the law as a debiasing tool."[16(p37)]

How Should Military Medical Care Providers Be Involved With Detainees, If At All?

The military's general policies in regard to detainees, as just considered, are critical to the contingent question of how military care providers should interact with detainees.[17] A first, core ethical issue in regard to military medical care providers' involvement with detainees is the extent, if any, to which military care providers should isolate themselves from other military endeavors on the basis that they, as care providers, have a medical, profession-based, patient-oriented ethical standard to uphold, as opposed to a mission-oriented moral standard. Key subquestions include the following: (*a*) how much should providers be involved in nonmedical actions, such as interrogations, and (*b*) what should providers do when they give detainees medical care. Should they, for instance, participate in force-feeding them?

In What Ways, If Any, Should Care Providers Be Involved in Nonmedical Acts?

There are many ways in which military care providers could be nonmedically involved with detainees.[18]

Psychiatrists and psychologists could work with interrogators during interrogations to try to find and probe areas in which detainees are most vulnerable in the hope of obtaining more information that could ultimately save lives. During interrogations, military care providers could also serve an opposite function: they could watch interrogations through a one-way mirror to attempt to ensure that the techniques interrogators use stay within their permissible limits and thus better protect detainees from harm.

What some view as the most overriding ethical concern here is that care providers have separate duties as care providers to detainees that may interfere or conflict with their obligations as military personnel or clash with military goals. The classical example in principle here is physicians' obligation as physicians to do no harm, as proscribed under their Hippocratic Oath. Some view such care providers as having a higher moral standard regarding detainees' well-being than interrogators, who are expected to at least be coercive if not harmful to detainees in seeking information. Thus, questions have been raised as to whether physicians should provide a safeguarding function for detainees by viewing them during interrogations through one-way mirrors.

Ethically, the assumption that military care providers have, or should have, a higher standard, as characterized above, may be more problematic than some have assumed. Persons in the military knowingly and willingly risk and often give their lives for their country. This is especially true when there is no draft. If there is a highest road in terms of behavior, it may be soldiers' being willing to give their lives and carrying out other behaviors that also further the highest moral standards possible. Military noncare providers, such as interrogators, may be viewed as within this group in that they, like those willing to die during combat, give ultimate priority to trying to save others' lives.

However, it is not self-evident that care providers should serve some oversight function of interrogators merely because they and many others believe that they uphold a higher moral standard. What this suggests is that there may be, and perhaps should be, ethical conduct that both care providers and noncare providers would support equally. The military could adopt practices for interrogating detainees that most physicians, military or not, and most soldiers and most citizens would agree with. The military could decide also what actions, if any, it would need to take to enforce these standards. It would make sense, were this to occur, to view military personnel and military care providers as having moral values of equal status and to not see care providers as being the right group to serve an oversight function, practically or theoretically, because they serve higher moral values.[4]

A second, related area of current controversy is whether physicians and particularly psychiatrists should not participate in the same ways as other care providers, specifically psychologists. The American Psychiatric Association (APA) has passed guidelines that forbid psychiatrists from being directly involved in interrogations, whereas the American Psychological Association has allowed participation to a greater extent. Inasmuch as both psychiatrists and psychologists may have clinical training, some psychologists question the basis on which psychiatrists—or physicians—should be excluded from participating in military actions carried out to further the needs of the greater society, when psychologists aren't, and possibly should not be, excluded.[19–21] Nurses have raised this same question; however, their situation remains theoretical because nurses haven't been asked to assist in interrogations. The same concern also applies to other mental healthcare providers, such as social workers. A possible overarching ethical question underlying these debates is whether it is possible for all military personnel, including interrogators and various care providers, to see themselves as pursuing the same ethical standards in serving the needs of the greater society.

A further source of values that warrant moral weight and may conflict with those of care providers or those of the military is the greater society. A primary ground for society's views warranting moral weight in regard to what physicians should do is that the public makes certain sacrifices so that medical students can learn to be physicians. Society funds medical schools and, more importantly, allows these students special privileges, such as to "practice" on bodies, whether cadavers or live patients, so they can learn the skills they will need later to be able to "cure." This is also true in regard to other professionals such as nurses, clinical psychologists, and social workers.

Physicians, in return, at least implicitly promise to use their skills for good. This "good" may include conducting practices that society by inaction has implicitly condoned. Thus, in that society has allowed exceptions on this basis, exceptions justifiably exist. Physicians serve in some roles that serve society's needs more than patients' needs. An example is forensic psychiatry. Society, presumably, wants and accepts this.

One core ethical question regarding military care providers being involved in interrogations and other nonmedical military actions is whether society expects and accepts this, because if not, care providers may be violating their implicit promise to society to not harm but to "cure." This question may be uniquely complicated, because the greater society might want physicians—psychiatrists in particular—to participate in interrogations so that society may have greater protection. What the greater society wants and expects is, in theory, an empirical question. Society's view may be expressed over time in how persons vote. The question remains, regardless of legislative outcomes, what moral weight should society's view of the appropriate roles of care providers in the military have? Society may, on one hand, not want care providers to violate their implicit promise to cure, but on the other hand, society may want psychiatrists and other care providers to help protect society as much as possible.

The above question is of added importance because professional organizations may believe they, too, have a stake that warrants significant or even overriding weight in deciding what those within their profession should do. They may believe that their view should be decisive. Physicians have been told by the American Medical Association that they should not take on certain roles during criminal executions and psychiatrists, by the APA, that they shouldn't evaluate criminal offenders and deem them sane to meet legislative criteria for execution. Organizations may take this same view in regard to psychiatrists or other care providers participating directly or indirectly in interrogations.

Thus, care providers within the military may fear that if the military asks them to serve in certain roles that depart from what their professional organizations have proscribed, they may jeopardize their good standing within these organizations or even lose their licenses to practice. This is again an instance in which, if possible, the military and these organizations becoming united and working toward adopting a shared, highest ethical value would be ideal.

Both the military and the APA may have grounds on which they could agree. Psychiatrists could, for instance, participate in formulating policy. Their agreeing on the level of participation in interrogations might make sense to both groups because behavioral healthcare providers offering suggestions in this capacity may help both the military and detainees. They may be able to suggest interrogation approaches that (*a*) are as effective but pose less of a risk of potential harm and (*b*) pose no more risk of potential harm but are more effective in eliciting information. These two possibilities illustrate an important general consideration regarding ethics that should always apply in cases such as this. That is, it is generally not difficult to recognize negative ethical aspects of a situation. What is more difficult ethically is to go one step beyond this and then find a better solution.

An important question regarding whether psychiatrists and other care providers should participate either indirectly or directly in interrogations is, therefore, what the relative gains and losses of each approach would be. One core consideration here is what would occur if psychiatrists, and other care providers, were not included in interrogations. The focus of controversy in regard to interrogations is, however, on military care providers being involved directly. Many care providers wince in response to the idea that they, themselves, as well as others, could rightfully perceive them as caring for patients on one day and stopping just short of inhumane treatment when working with detainees on the next.

It is not ethically clear that the solution of having mixed roles from one day to the next, sometimes in a forensic setting, which is generally accepted by forensic psychiatrists and psychologists, is sufficiently analogous to the interrogation issue to allow the justifications for one to apply to the other. When care providers evaluate suspected criminal offenders for insanity, they inform them that anything they say may be used against them. This warning helps respect these interviewees' autonomy and helps behavioral healthcare providers in this role avoid engaging in implicit deceit.

Some believe that if care providers do the same thing with detainees, this may suffice, or at least reduce the extent to which the role of care providers, such as psychiatrists, is objectionable, so that they can, from an ethical standpoint, be justifiably involved in interrogations. This argument, however, may miss this point. The ethical presupposition made when forensic psychiatrists give this warning is that their conducting the evaluation is ethically justifiable even if psychiatrists find the interviewees to be sane as opposed to insane—though the judge or jury will ultimately make this determination. This is because if psychiatrists don't interview defendants to try to discern whether or not they were severely emotionally impaired when they committed their crime, the judge or jury will then have to make this determination. Without the psychiatry opinion, the judge or jury may be much more likely to infer that the defendants were sane. This could in some instances result in execution.

In the interrogation of detainees, these same presuppositions don't exist. The detainee is being pressured, purposefully, in the hope of affecting him or her sufficiently adversely to give up information. If the psychiatrist adds to this pressure, the psychiatrist is also doing harm. The psychiatrist could, however, also serve only as an ally to the detainee. For example, US military physicians have helped detainees greatly, some military care providers report, by developing their trust. This will be discussed in greater detail in the next section, which deals with detainees who refuse to eat.

A final question that should be asked is how could psychiatrists and other care providers help interrogators? It may be that the experience of interrogating detainees has no harmful effect on interrogators. Alternatively, however, it may. This especially may be the case if detainees are from a different ethnic group. This also may be truer if the approaches interrogators can use are harsher. Military care providers being present can help confirm for interrogators that while in the process of the interrogation, detainees remain persons not inherently different from the interrogators. Psychiatrists and others participating in this way could then be allies who might benefit interrogators as well as detainees.

How Should Military Care Providers Treat Detainees?

Ethical treatment of detainees by military care providers is complex. A potential scenario could involve a detainee with diabetes. Here, clinicians informing interrogators of this condition may be essential so that interrogators respond in ways that will maximally meet detainees' medical need for drugs such as insulin. Interrogators with this knowledge may require medical providers to monitor food intake so that the detainee is unlikely to become hypoglycemic. Yet, at the same time, if clinicians provide clinical information, interrogators could misuse it. Interrogators could threaten to allow detainees' blood sugar level to dangerously fluctuate (whether or not they could or would, in actuality, do this) to try to get detainees to provide the information they want.

It may be wholly implausible that this would happen. Rather, if clear specific limits are in place, interrogators are obligated to stay within the rules previously proscribed by the DoD, even if these rules are to some extent vague and thus allow "loopholes."[22] Furthermore, the military could develop mechanisms to ensure that if care providers give interrogators information like this to help detainees, interrogators don't misuse it. Such mechanisms could include outside review, ensuring greater transparency, as indicated above. In other contexts, care providers couldn't be reasonably expected to be able to treat detainees optimally unless they could wholly respect detainees' confidentiality. If detainees were depressed, they might share their feelings, honestly, only if they felt that they had trustworthy care providers.

Military physicians, in innumerable cases, have reportedly shown extraordinary compassion to detainees and, as a result, gained their trust. In these cases compassion was shown not to gain trust in hopes of improved information gathering, but to treat detainees with respect, simply as persons, regardless of whether it would affect provision of information or not. To attain and maintain this confidentially may require additional resources. An example here is the need for sufficient numbers of interpreters. If the interpreters for clinicians and interrogators are different, it could be expected, both theoretically and practically, that detainees would have greater trust in their care providers. Otherwise, they might fear that information interpreters hear during the "clinical hour" could then be passed on to interrogators, who could use the information against them.

More money spent by the military, and by extension the greater society, to provide the necessary conditions for optimal medical care should be a high priority. Treating detainees with optimal respect should, perhaps, generally take priority over other, competing ethical values. Plausibly, the military's doing this would serve to enhance detainees' trust. The military at Guantanamo now may provide first-class medical care to detainees. For example, medical care previously offered to detainees of a certain age includes evaluation of elevated prostate-specific antigen blood levels to possibly detect early prostate cancer and endoscopic examinations of their lower bowels to assess for possible early colon cancer. Does the military do everything for detainees that care providers would for prisoners in the United States or civilians in the best US hospitals? Should it?

The answers to these questions are analogous to many others considered above. Some of these decisions may rightfully be those for the greater society. However, the greater society may be unjust. What is clear is that what should be done can be known with greater certainty only as what is being done now becomes increasingly transparent. Then, wherever the lines are drawn now can be subjected to greater scrutiny, and society, through legislation or the courts, can decide whether or not what is done now is what should be done.

The main reason for the military's acting on behalf of the greater society to maximize detainees' trust may not be to "win them over" in the hope that they would then give information that could save lives. Rather, the reason may be to regard detainees as primarily ends in and of themselves. The idea that humans should never be used unduly as means to others' ends, as opposed to ends in themselves, is a common principle accepted in ethics and put forth by Kant. It is based on what respect for humans and human dignity requires. If, for example, interrogators pretend they are friends of detainees to get information, these interrogators are deceiving detainees and using them as primarily means to US ends. Ethically this is problematic, though it may be justifiable if one can argue for other reasons, such as saving millions of lives.

Optimal care may then be warranted merely because detainees should, as fellow humans, have care providers they can trust regardless of what they have done or may have done. As persons and captives, they still warrant utmost respect. This value, and this value alone, generally is presumed to be overriding unless a compelling case against it can be made. Similarly, this principle should be adhered to in all instances in which detainees are involved unless some other, convincing case can be made. Thus, providing detainees with the utmost respect can be a core, initial ethical position on which all persons—interrogators and physicians alike—could agree, at least initially.

In regard to specific approaches permitted during interrogations, it may be that a resolution acceptable to most concerned parties is achievable. All parties should seek ethical unity, if possible. A next strategy to resolving the many potential conflicts between care providers and other military personnel is to seek out and find value priorities on which most parties, both military and civilian, can agree.

The value in regard to which pursuing this stragey may be most plausible may occur after detainees have been incarcerated and later, during every moment of their interrogations. This value is that detainees should be respected as persons. This fundamental concept is paramount not only in this country's ethics, but also internationally. Thus, it may be that greater ethical agreement both nationally and internationally may be possible. With this agreement it may be that applications shared to a greater extent by all can be brought about.

How Should Military Care Providers Respond When Detainees Refuse To Eat?

Substantial numbers of detainees may refuse to eat. The core ethical conflict this brings about is whether military care providers should force-feed detainees against their protests and thus maintain their lives, or if providers should respect detainees' autonomy by going along with what they request.[23,24] The key question here is what care providers should do and why.

Should Care Providers Force-Feed Detainees or Respect Their Autonomy?

In this situation, the context is most important ethically. Generally it is considered a first ethical priority to respect persons by allowing them autonomy. The one value that may most reasonably override this is another deontological value—that is, respecting detainees in another way by maintaining their lives. Detainees may have uncertain futures and be denied physical contact with their families. Thus, respecting their autonomy by allowing them to choose to die is especially problematic. This is because showing respect for detainees as persons may better be accomplished by improving the conditions under which they live. Respecting their autonomy warrants more moral weight if the context in which they live maximizes their welfare and if, as a result of this, their capacity to make choices is unfettered by pressing personal or emotional needs.

If the detainees' situations are improved as much as possible, it may be that it is justifiable to still force-feed them against their will because this maintains their lives. Thus, it may be more effectively determined at a later time whether this same refusal to eat, if they still are refusing food, should be respected. This rationale may lose moral weight over time because it will be increasingly implausible to believe that detainees will decide they really want to live at some point if they have continued to refuse to eat.

This principle, attending to persons' greater context as opposed to their most immediate needs, is exemplified most notoriously by an example involving research in Willowbrook, New York. Here, several thousand children who were "retarded" were institutionalized and lived in poor hygienic conditions. Many, if not most, of the children contracted hepatitis. Researchers wanted to study hepatitis by intentionally giving the disease to a group of these children. They justified this because the children participating in this research would be better off in two ways: (1) they would live under better conditions, and (2) the hepatitis they acquired would be less severe in the research setting than if naturally acquired from the general population at the institution.

The study began in the 1950s and continued into the 1960s. After the study was completed, it was criticized on the basis that it had exploited the children's poor condition and in doing so treated them primarily as means to others' ends. To treat them as ends in themselves would have meant to change their surroundings and make their surroundings better. Since then, this has been done. These children, now adults, were placed in small group homes; Willowbrook Institution no longer exists.

The analogy here is that respecting detainees' autonomy by allowing them to die in their present context may be problematic because efforts could be taken to improve their situation. Respecting them more may require establishing rigorous criteria to determine when detainees are much more likely to give useful information, and once this "window" had passed, creating for them better living conditions (according to their views of what these should be). Otherwise, care providers granting detainees autonomy under conditions that offer them little to no present source of meaningfulness in their lives would respect their autonomy literally and, in this one sense, also further the likelihood of their wanting to die.

Ethically, the practice of allowing detainees who wanted to starve to death to do so could risk military care providers meeting the requirement of international law but violating its spirit, just as they could when treating US soldiers and POWs "equally," as described earlier in this chapter.[2] Care providers could literally respect detainees' autonomy while knowing that their environment is impoverished and intentionally leaving it that way. Thus, detainees could live and be allowed to remain in an environment unnecessarily conducive to increasing the likelihood that they would want to die.

In the case of care providers granting detainees autonomy to starve themselves to death, a similar question of intent may be involved. Suppose that detainees remain living under conditions in which they can find little or no meaning and that the likelihood of them providing useful information has become remote. If they are then allowed to die, allegedly to respect their autonomy, this could be done due to an underlying intent to further the likelihood that they would choose to die, as opposed to an overt intent to respect their autonomy. It would be unclear what the genuine underlying intent of those allowing the detainees to die really is.

In like manner, care providers respecting detainees' autonomy in a context that they find meaningless, when this context could be changed, may not be ethically justifiable. Care providers may be implicitly accepting and supporting the circumstances that may contribute to these detainees' deaths. It may be, on the other hand, that improvements in detainees' lives aren't possible for reasons related to security. If so, significant harms that could result from making these changes might preclude these changes from being made.

Military care providers, even knowing all this, may have limited choices. Regardless, if they act in ways that accept and support a suboptimal environment, they may be ethically guilty of moral complicity. Still, if they do respect the prisoners' autonomy by allowing them to not eat—whether this is the providers' choice or that of others higher in their chain of command—they may then have an ethical duty to offer detainees sedation so that as they starve to death, they don't suffer. By giving this sedation, these care providers would be facilitating these detainees' deaths, because sedation would most likely shorten their lives. Providing sedation might be viewed for this reason as ethically unjustifiable. Yet, the military care providers' intent would be to relieve the suffering of the detainees. Giving sedation might ethically be not only justifiable but also mandatory because it is more humane.

A second choice of military care providers under these conditions would be to refuse to participate, even in giving sedation. Care providers are outside the combat setting and thus they should have greater opportunity to express and adhere to personal values that they hold within their moral conscience. Their refusing to participate could violate the principle of military necessity if detainees' starving was viewed as likely to rally persons throughout the globe to carry on their fight. Then, and only then, might military care providers have a higher, overriding ethical military duty to do what they must to further the military mission of protecting society.

The possibility of rallying other countries or organizations against the United States could be the ethical justifification to require physicians to force-feed detainees. If important military needs are not at stake, however, military care providers should be able to adhere to their own moral values and views to the same extent as their civilian colleagues.

What this should require in practice is itself an ethical question. Assuming military necessity isn't present, should a recruiter of physicians who will care for detainees on a hospital ward only ask them whether they have moral scruples or, if they say that they do have moral scruples, then ask them further what these are? Asking them only whether they have scruples most respects physicians as persons by not requiring them to come up with "valid" reasons. Asking them the specifics of their scruples, in comparison, in effect disrespects them, because their moral values are respected to a lesser extent. In other words, in the latter case, their values and moral conscience would be respected only if they give "acceptable" reasons.

Furthermore, recruiters' asking military care providers for the reasons for their scruples presupposes that logical reasons underlie all valid emotional "qualms." However, this isn't the case. Many times, what persons experience as a violation of their moral conscience is a felt emotion, and persons may or may not be able to articulate why they feel this way. Likewise, in its effect, this question also would discriminate between those physicians who report "good reasons" and those who do not. This may violate a morally important aspect of care providers being treated with equality and, as an unwanted consequence, it might divide them as a group.

The highest road for physicians to take with most

patients who want to refuse treatment and die by this means may be for these care providers to take measures to try to ensure that dying is what these patients really most want. Then, if and when providers have taken these measures, their highest moral road may be to accept the detainees' wishes. For example, if patients have just undergone trauma and acquired quadriplegia, hours later they may request that their respirator be shut off. These patients' care providers might well ask them whether they might be willing to take a bit more time because there are many persons in this situation who respond like the late Christopher Reeve, who lived for 9 years after suffering a catastrophic cervical vertebrae fracture in 1995. They may in time also find meaning in this wholly altered state. Military physicians may see their optimal ethical task as to take an analogous route with detainees.

The ethical idea at stake here is to try to enable such patients to be more truly autonomous and not unduly driven by overriding needs when these needs can be better met. This is especially important when one choice patients can make, namely death by starvation, is irreversible. The longer these patients persist in making this same request, the stronger the argument becomes for granting it, despite the fact that these patients may seem, from an objective perspective, to have unchanged needs. Subjectively, of course, even though their external environment hasn't changed, detainees may be quite different "inside."

Applying these ethical guidelines to detainees would suggest that an optimal ethical course might be to maximize the immediate benefits detainees could enjoy once reasonable time had been given to attempt to obtain information from them. After giving them maximal possible benefits, time should be allowed to help ensure that not eating was what a detainee really wanted to do. Detainees might change their minds over time and subsequently want to live without being aware beforehand that this might occur. Many patients with terminal illness want to die at one time only to feel later that they want to live on as long as they can. For this reason, even in the two states in the United States in which patients can have assistance in dying, their request generally must be repeated and sustained over a significant intervening period of time before care providers can go along with their request.

It might be claimed that because detainees' external conditions are in so many respects impoverished, such as their not being able to have physical contact with their families, it is likely that many are genuinely depressed and thus their depression could deprive them of sufficient mental capacity to be competent to then choose to die. This concern, though ethically reasonable, would in principle be inconsistent with the possibility in civilian contexts in the United States that persons depressed or significantly emotionally impaired can still determine their outcomes. Thus, in this country, even if patients are severely depressed, this generally does not preclude them from making even life-ending decisions regarding themselves.

A question implicit throughout the above discussion is, however, whether patients who are ill or even have a terminal illness are the most appropriate subjects to use as an ethical analogy. It may be that no group will suffice as an analogy. Other analogies, such as prisoners incarcerated with life sentences, may be as, or more, valid, although not sufficient. This prisoner analogy could be cut in different ways. It might suggest that detainees should have much greater rights, such as to be able to meet physically with their families. But it might also imply (unlike the use of the medical analogy) that they should not have the option of choosing to die by starvation. The present policy of not allowing detainees to refuse to eat and thus to die by this means is based on US law regarding prisoners.

The prisoner analogy may be flawed, depending on whether allowing prisoners to refuse to eat, even when they will be executed, is or isn't ethically justifiable. The underlying rationale for not allowing the refusal to eat may be one of punishment. If so, the rationale of punishing detainees by this same means wouldn't suffice. A second possible rationale some might offer for not allowing persons on death row to refuse to eat is that persons on death row may be depressed and for this reason incompetent to choose whether they want to die by starvation. This, too, wouldn't suffice because even if patients are depressed, they still may be deemed sufficiently competent to refuse life-saving treatment.

In this instance there may be no adequately analogous situations. Military care providers not participating directly in interrogations may not be sufficiently like forensic psychiatrists, nor like physicians giving lethal injections to effect criminals' deaths, nor like psychiatrists determining that persons are incurable sociopaths such that death should or should not be imposed. Likewise, a detainee wanting to starve to death may not be sufficiently like a patient with terminal illness wanting to refuse a respirator (or food and water) so that death is hastened.

None of these examples may be a close enough replica of the detainee situation to serve as an ethically adequate model. If these analogies are insufficient, the answers to the above questions may thus be more difficult. Ethics may at best only shed light on the key factors to be considered. This analysis has considered both the importance and the limitations of codes. These codes emphasize the importance of respecting prisoners' autonomy. Allowing detainees to die under suboptimal conditions may, however, be qualitatively different from what those enacting these codes, which require respect for autonomy, had in mind. Thus, this different context should be considered.

The sanctity of persons' lives is an important deontological value, as is respecting persons' dignity in other ways, such as respecting their autonomy. In some situations it is considered ethically justifiable for physicians to override patients' autonomy and to exercise therapeutic privilege. This is allowed by law in all states and recently has been reaffirmed by the Council on Ethical and Judicial Affairs, a body within the AMA.[25] Physicians can exercise this privilege only when not doing so would, in their view, harm patients unduly. Whether overriding detainees' refusals to eat would meet these same criteria is open to challenge. However, furthering detainees' interests, such as in the use of therapeutic privilege, may be the only basis on which overriding detainees' autonomy could be justifiable.

Soldiers' Opportunity to "Speak Up"

Military care providers may have markedly different, even heart-felt, views on whether or not detainees should be force-fed. This raises a question in regard to not only this situation, but to all areas concerning the extent to which soldiers should be free to express their views and more specifically whether or not they should have more freedom than they have now. During combat operations, it is imperative that every soldier follows orders and works together with other soldiers to accomplish the mission, as directed. There is little room to question commands, unless the orders are in violation of the Uniform Code of Military Justice or the rules of engagement. Soldiers having a dissenting opinion may be vulnerable to highly significant sanctions if they speak out.

There are also clear guidelines that limit a soldier's first amendment right to free speech. But are the present limitations ethically optimal, or could the creation of an environment with more free flow of communication serve both soldiers and their commands better? Might the military be stronger if soldiers are allowed to verbally dissent?

If soldiers could do this, they would need to be aware of the appropriate method to make their disagreements known, and a more "liberal" process would need to be set in place. This change might create a better system by instilling a pressure valve to allow soldiers an outlet for expressing themselves. This might work to increase morale by allowing even the lowest ranking individual an avenue to be heard. Many improvements may even be identified by this same method.

POSTDEPLOYMENT PROBLEMS

Three recently occurring postdeployment problems particularly warrant ethical discussion. These are (1) whether soldiers with posttraumatic stress disorder (PTSD) should be redeployed, (2) what should be done when soldiers have or may have head injuries due to blasts, and (3) when, if ever, military physicians should make decisions on behalf of their soldiers' interests and "against" rules and regulations, and "outside the box." The appropriate role for military behavioral healthcare providers in these ethical issues is particularly evident. PTSD is among the most important of the disorders they must treat.

Posttraumatic Stress Disorder

The first of these problems focuses on whether soldiers who have deployed, and then been diagnosed with an acute stress disorder or PTSD, should be deployed again into a combat environment. This ethical dilemma revolves around the competing needs of the individual and the needs of the military. The needs of the individual may be best served by allowing them to delay deployment to allow treatment and healing or by avoiding another deployment altogether.

This could, however, have a negative effect on soldiers by decreasing their expectancy that they will improve and may lead to a fixation of their symptoms and subsequent disability. This may also cause soldiers to experience increased guilt over not being with their buddies and unit during future operations. Some soldiers, especially those suffering from more mild degrees of PTSD, might not only want to return to the theater, but may do better if they do.

Allowing these individuals to avoid a deployment can also have a significant effect on their unit's readiness. Many individuals may begin to mimic these illnesses intentionally to avoid deployment. This "copycat" scenario is seen throughout military units. This phenomenon isn't exclusive to deployments. There have been many accounts of one individual in a unit being administratively separated, or avoiding an agreed-upon military service commitment, and then this being followed by several other unit members claiming the same level of distress. Suicidality is an example, as well as soldiers alleging that continued military service would keep them at risk. They may then request to be administratively separated. This can affect a unit's readiness and decrease the available number of trained troops. A competing concern is the potential negative consequences for units that may have these individuals with them in theater. These individuals, in addition, may be more vulnerable to recurrent or progressive impairments, can consume a disproportionate amount of human resources, and may compromise security.

Allowing this means of exclusion, especially for those more mildly affected, may also have effects on recruiting. Indicating to potential recruits that soldiers in distress will be taken care of, even to the extent that continued deployments may not be required, may facilitate recruiting. The extent of this effect, if any, is open to speculation. In the present state of uncertainty, three key variables should be weighed and considered. Two are in favor of deploying these soldiers, and one opposes deployment. Suppose that deploying the soldiers, overall, does help their healing process. This may benefit these individuals and their families. Military units may also benefit by allowing them to maintain their needed unit strengths, and therefore having the needed numbers of trained soldiers to complete their missions.

Recruiting, which currently faces many challenges, may be enhanced by going the "other" way, namely, by allowing affected individuals to delay deployment to receive treatment, or to avoid another deployment altogether. Empirical data will indicate more clearly over time how soldiers with PTSD respond overall to being redeployed. Until this information is better known, the best ethical solution to this question may remain more open to debate.

Head Injuries

The second postdeployment ethical issue involves soldiers who return with head injuries caused by blast injuries, primarily in Iraq. Here what has been found is that these soldiers' impairment may differ from that caused by other head injuries, such as those sustained in a car accident.[26,27] These soldiers may remain literally competent or able to acknowledge accurately the pluses and minuses of accepting or declining treatment or of participating in research, but, at the same time, they may still have extensive underlying difficulties. These difficulties may become apparent only through formal cognitive testing. Most importantly, these difficulties may profoundly affect their judgment. The question has arisen whether the usual methods of assessing competency prior to allowing these soldiers to consent to treatment or to participate in research should suffice, or whether a special new category should be established in both treatment and research contexts to better take into account the recently discovered, unique cognitive impairments and needs of soldiers with head injuries.

Respect for these persons might require that a higher, stricter standard for determining competency be established. This would be, however, the first time that a special category of this type has been developed for such a specific group. Establishing such a standard could have the adverse effect of stigmatizing these individuals. It could also result in some soldiers becoming fearful or angry by limiting their autonomy or by alerting them for the first time that they had deficiencies of which they were unaware. This abrupt overwhelming of their denial could do exceptional harm.

The best approach in both these instances—treatment and research—might be to provide greater procedural safeguards, individualized according to the harms potentially at stake. Depending on these harms, review of each soldier's competency could be evaluated in detail by a specially constituted board with varied and exceptional expertise. This board could apply a graded standard, which would require a higher threshold for competency only when the treatment or research proposed posed a significantly greater risk. This approach might be roughly analogous to the greater protections provided now in regard to both treatment and research involving children. Requirements are established concerning children in research that don't exist for adults and that vary according to the extent of children's personal risks. DoD research regulations provide exceptional requirements for doing research that involves children, especially when the research involves more than minimal risk.

These additional innovative measures might be required on the basis of compensatory justice. Because these soldiers have taken extra risks on behalf of their country, safeguards that would help ensure that they make the best choices, even when they don't know that they can't make them, may be not only ethically optimal, but from the perspective of compensatory justice, may be ethically mandatory.

Decisions "Outside the Box"

The third postdeployment ethical issue to be discussed here involves whether it is ever justifiable for military physicians to make treatment decisions that are inconsistent with official policy. Should the military behavioral healthcare provider, for instance, always make decisions that are consistent with official policy, even if that policy may have a negative impact on patients' treatment?

Official policy dictates that those active duty service members not physically or mentally capable of deploying should be placed on limited duty. Limited duty status is temporary, often removes the member from the current job, and serves several purposes. It allows the service member's parent command the opportunity to obtain a deployable replacement. It also allows the nondeployable service member's condition to improve so that return to full duty can occur. Without this limited duty option, this return may not be possible. Limited duty can, however, negatively impact treatment by reinforcing the patient role and delaying recovery.

There may be instances, however, when a patient who is not mentally capable of deployment should not be placed on limited duty. For example, patients recently returned from war and diagnosed with PTSD from trauma that occurred during the war may not be mentally fit just yet to return to the war. It is often possible to continue to treat such patients clinically but not to place them on a limited duty status because they would not be deployed for some time. This can be highly advantageous and desired by such soldiers because it may prevent unwanted consequences from being placed for any length of time on limited duty status.

Is it ethical for the military behavioral healthcare provider in such a case to not follow official policy and to not place the patient on limited duty in order to provide or facilitate additional treatment? What is the best ethical choice in these instances? All rules tend by their nature to create some "bad results." Military physicians making off-the-record exceptions may prevent some bad results. If, on the other hand, all such physicians commonly use their individual discretion, this would undermine the rules and possibly cause greater harm. In this case, it may be that military physicians would be ethically justified in making exceptions if the cases in which they would do so occur but rarely. In such instances, they should also establish and specify criteria that should be met. One such criterion might be that both the spirit and purpose for which the rule was made in the first place are not fundamentally violated.

What the relevant criteria warranting moral weight should be may vary depending on the type of case. Military physicians may vary on the criteria they choose and the moral weight they place on each if they use their discretion. Still, using discretion, and the foreseeable harms this may bring about, may ethically outweigh the harms that will occur if they followed the rules so absolutely that no exceptions would occur.

SUMMARY

This last example of military physicians making exceptions is, perhaps, paradigmatic of all the problems examined in this chapter and thus an ideal one with which to end this discussion. Most ethical questions involve a determination not so much of what the decision or decisions should be "across the board," but rather where along the spectrum of real and imagined circumstances one should "draw the line," why, and who should draw it.

In this chapter, the authors have attempted to highlight many of the existing ethical questions as well as new and emerging ones that have arisen. There generally are no self-evident answers to these questions that all reasonable persons will agree on. Still, the principles and most relevant facts should always be considered by those having the responsibility to make these decisions. This is what, more than anything else, ethics and ethical analysis has to offer. This analysis may enable decision makers to more maximally consider "both sides."

In some cases, "ethics" can clearly show something is wrong. The rationales for genocide used by the Nazis during World War II are an obvious and unequivocal example. In most, more difficult ethical problems, however, the questions that arise are and must remain open to debate. In these situations, the debate is not, however, so much over what is right and what is wrong, but as just discussed, what should be the general rule; when, if ever, one should make exceptions; and who should decide.

REFERENCES

1. Grönvall GK. A new role for scientists in the Biological Weapons Convention. *Nat Biotechnol.* 2005;23(10):1213–1216.

2. Howe EG. Dilemmas in military medical ethics since 9/11. *Kennedy Inst Ethics J.* 2003;13(2):175–188.

3. Beam TE, Sparacino LR, eds. *Military Medical Ethics.* In: Zajtchuk R, Bellamy RF, eds. *Textbooks of Military Medicine.* Washington, DC: Department of the Army, Office of The Surgeon General, Borden Institute; 2003.

4. Gross ML. *Bioethics and Armed Conflict: Moral Dilemmas of Medicine and War.* Cambridge, Mass: MIT Press; 2006.

5. Howe EG. Ethical issues in military medicine: mixed agency. In: Lande RG, Armitage DT, eds. *Principles and Practice of Military Forensic Psychiatry*. Springfield, Ill: Charles C Thomas; 1997.

6. Howe EG. Ethical issues regarding mixed agency of military physicians. *Soc Sci Med*. 1986;23(8):803-815.

7. Tan M. Study: waiver troops OK, but need discipline. *Army Times*. May 12, 2008. Available at: http://www.armytimes.com/news/2008/05/army_waivers_051008w/. Accessed July 22, 2010.

8. Martin PD, Williamson DA, Alfonso AJ, Ryan DH. Psychological adjustment during Army basic training. *Mil Med*. 2006;171(2):157–160.

9. Mahon MJ, Tobin JP, Cusack DA, Kelleher C, Malone KM. Suicide among regular-duty military personnel: a retrospective case-control study of occupation-specific risk factors for workplace suicide. *Am J Psychiatry*. 2005;162(9):1688–1696.

10. Bloche MG, Marks JH. Doctors and interrogators at Guantanamo Bay. *N Engl J Med*. 2005;353(1):6–8.

11. Rubenstein L, Pross C, Davidoff F, Iacopino V. Coercive US interrogation policies: a challenge to medical ethics. *JAMA*. 2005;294:1544–1549.

12. Johnson WB, Bacho R, Helm M, Ralph J. Multiple-role dilemmas for military health care providers. *Mil Med*. 2006;171(4):311–315.

13. Intelligence Science Board. *Educing Information: Interrogation: Science and Art*. Washington, DC; National Defense Intelligence College Press; 2006.

14. Howe E. Further considerations regarding interrogations and forced feedings. In: Goodman R, Roseman MJ, eds. *Interrogations, Forced Feedings, and the Role of Health Professionals: New Perspectives on International Human Rights, Humanitarian Law, and Ethics*. Cambridge, Massachusetts: Harvard University Press; 2009: 75–102.

15. US Army Medical Command. MEDCOM policy on US Army Behavioral Science Consultation to detention operations, intelligence interrogations, detainee debriefing, and tactical questioning (unpublished policy, 2009).

16. Marks JH. Looking back, thinking ahead: the complicity of health professionals in detainee abuse. In: Goodman R, Roseman MJ, eds. *Interrogations, Forced Feedings, and the Role of Health Professionals: New Perspectives on International Human Rights, Humanitarian Law, and Ethics*. Cambridge, Massachusetts: Harvard University Press; 2009: 21–47.

17. US Department of Defense. *Medical Support Program for Detainee Operations*. Washington, DC: DoD; June 6, 2006. DoD Instruction 2310.08E.

18. Lewis NA. Interrogators cite doctors' aid at Guantanamo. *N Y Times*. June 24, 2005:A1, A19.

19. American Psychiatric Association. Psychiatric participation in interrogation of detainees. Position statement, approved by the Board of Trustees May 2006, and the Assembly of District Branches, May 2006 #200601. Available at: http://www.psych.org/Departments/EDU/Library/APAOfficialDocumentsandRelated/PositionStatements/200601.aspx. Accessed July 16, 2010.

20. O'Reilly KB. AMA adopts policy on interrogations. *Am Med News*. July 3, 2006. Available at: http://www.ama-assn.org/amednews/2006/07/03/prse0703.htm. Accessed July 22, 2010.

21. Behnke S. Ethics and interrogations: comparing and contrasting the American Psychological, American Medical and American Psychiatric Association positions. *Monitor Psychol*. 2006;37(7):1–5. Available at: http://www.apa.org/monitor/julaug06/interrogations.html. Accessed July 22, 2010.

22. US Department of the Army. *Human Intelligence Collector Operations*. Washington, DC: DA; September 2006. Field Manual 2-22.3.

23. Annas GJ. Hunger strikes at Guantanamo—medical ethics and human rights in a "legal black hole." *N Engl J Med*. 2006;355(13):1377–1382.

24. Nicholl DJ, Atkinson HG, Kaik J, et al. Forcefeeding and restraint of Guantanamo Bay hunger strikers. *Lancet.* 2006;367(9513):811.

25. American Medical Association. Withholding information from patients (therapeutic privilege). AMA House of Delegates, policy adopted June 2006. Available at: http://www.ama-assn.org/go/cejareports. Accessed July 22, 2010.

26. Warden DL. Military TBI during the Iraq and Afghanhanistan wars. *J Head Trauma Rehabil.* 2006;21(5):398–402.

27. Tauber KH, Warden DL, Hurley RA. Blast-related traumatic brain injury: what is known? *J Neuropsychiatry Clin Neurosci.* 2006;18:141–145.

Chapter 47

COMBAT AND OPERATIONAL BEHAVIORAL HEALTH: FINAL THOUGHTS AND NEXT STEPS

ELSPETH CAMERON RITCHIE, MD, MPH,* AND MICHAEL DOYLE, MD†

*Colonel, US Army (Retired); formerly, Psychiatry Consultant to the Army Surgeon General, and Director, Behavioral Health Proponency, Office of The Surgeon General, Falls Church, Virginia; currently, Chief Clinical Officer, District of Columbia Department of Mental Health, 64 New York Avenue NE, 4th Floor, Washington, DC 20002

†Colonel, Medical Corps, US Army; Deputy Chief of Clinical Services, US Army Medical Activity, US Military Academy, 900 Washington Road, West Point, New York 10996; formerly, Commander, US Army Health Clinic, Wiesbaden, Germany

INTRODUCTION

While this book has been in production, Department of Defense (DoD) behavioral healthcare delivery has improved dramatically. From the beginning of the conflicts in Afghanistan and Iraq, a robust combat stress control presence has been operating in theater. Much of the initial improvement was in the management of patients in theater and as they redeploy (return home) to the United States. Many chapters, such as those focused on patient care at Landstuhl Regional Medical Center in Germany and Walter Reed Army Medical Center in Washington, DC, have highlighted these improvements. Back in the United States, improving the reintegration of soldiers and their families is a continuous priority for leaders at all levels and for the nation.

RECENT BEHAVIORAL HEALTH INITIATIVES

Multiple new organizations and initiatives emerged in the last few years, such as: (*a*) the Behavioral Health Proponency; (*b*) the Defense Center of Excellence; (*c*) the Comprehensive Soldier Fitness Program; and (*d*) the Behavioral and Social Health Outcomes Program at the former Center for Health Promotion and Preventive Medicine (CHPPM), now the Public Health Command (Provisional). The Army Campaign Plan for Health Promotion, Risk Reduction, and Suicide Prevention was formed in the spring of 2009. In 2010, the Army's Comprehensive Behavioral Health System of Care was implemented. The November 5, 2009, shootings at Fort Hood, Texas, spurred numerous recommendations for both the DoD and the military services. Finally, there is a new DoD–Department of Veterans Affairs Integrated Mental Health Strategy. All of these new programs and organizations have sought improved approaches to the emerging challenges facing military behavioral health.

Behavioral Health Proponency

The Army Medical Department (AMEDD) Behavioral Health Proponency, the first of these new initiatives, was established in 2007 to coordinate all the different behavioral health functions in the AMEDD. Modeled after AMEDD's Proponency of Preventive Medicine, this organization is a multidisciplinary group, with its director located at the Office of The Surgeon General (this volume's senior editor was the first director of the Behavioral Health Proponency). A Suicide Prevention Program Office was also established in 2007 to help centralize the diverse AMEDD elements that assist with education, training, and tracking of suicide prevention efforts. However, this latter office became redundant with the Behavioral Health and Social Outcomes Program and the Army Campaign Plan for Health Promotion, Risk Reduction, and Suicide Prevention and is not currently active.

Defense Centers of Excellence

The congressionally mandated Defense Centers of Excellence (DCoE) also started in 2007 and grew with congressional support due to a recommendation from the DoD Mental Health Task Force. The Department of Veterans Affairs and all of the military services are represented at DCoE, including the Public Health Service. The mission statement of the DCoE (available at: http://www.dcoe.health.mil/) is:

> **Mission:** The DCoE assesses, validates, oversees and facilitates prevention, resilience, identification, treatment, outreach, rehabilitation, and reintegration programs for psychological health (PH) and traumatic brain injury (TBI) to ensure the Department of Defense meets the needs of the nation's military communities, warriors and families.

Comprehensive Soldier Fitness

The Army's chief of staff, General George W Casey, Jr, requested the establishment of the Comprehensive Soldier Fitness (CSF) program, which was begun in 2008. Under the umbrella of the G-3 (ie, the training directorate), the Army developed a comprehensive behavioral health strategy—"whole-life fitness"—that includes multiple categories of wellness (physical, emotional, social, family, and spiritual). This strategy recognizes the need to incorporate enhancement of current health (of the soldier and family), prevention of future problems, and treatment when problems arise. The strategy also emphasizes the use of standardized metrics to determine success, standardized screening and treatment modalities, and the use of evidence-based clinical guidelines. Ultimately the strategy recognizes that the Army team is successful when leadership and behavioral health professionals partner to remove any stigma associated with identifying the need for help and receiving behavioral health intervention. This strategy encompasses a holistic approach to behavioral health issues.

The "Army Strong" campaign has been a success. But mental, emotional, and spiritual strength, like physical strength, do not just "happen"—these attributes can and must be taught, practiced, and perfected. As with physical capability, everyone enters the Army with a variable amount of strength in each of these domains, everyone has the potential to improve, and both the rate of improvement and ultimate achievement will be different for every soldier and family. At 9 years into the global war on terror, with its unrelenting operational tempo, a focus on comprehensive fitness has become an operational mandate.

The vision and mission statements of whole-life fitness (available online at: http://www.army.mil/csf/about.html) are:

> **Vision:** An Army of balanced, healthy, self-confident Soldiers, families and Army civilians whose resilience and total fitness enables them to thrive in an era of high operational tempo and persistent conflict.
>
> **Mission:** Develop and institute a holistic fitness program for Soldiers, families, and Army civilians in order to enhance performance and build resilience.

The CSF program ensures that all soldiers undergo appropriate assessment of their total fitness, encompassing all the "Army Strong" components. The results of the assessment will direct further training, intervention, or treatment as needed. This begins at accession and, like physical fitness, includes reassessment at appropriate intervals. Furthermore, the CSF office makes certain that all training, interventions, and treatments utilized have demonstrated effectiveness, applying accepted methodology and scientific rigor. They are also chartered to ensure timely reassessment, to demonstrate value added to both the soldier and the leadership.

The CSF office also ensures that the training programs, services, and interventions offered complement one another, are not duplicative, are resourced based on objective outcomes, and are standardized across the Army, including the Reserve components. Lastly, CSF is dedicated to making sure that all stakeholders, both internal (soldiers, families, leaders, and Army commands) and external (members of Congress and staff, media, and veterans' groups) understand the absolute necessity of a comprehensive, coordinated effort to enhance the fitness and resiliency of the Army, which is particularly important during this era of persistent conflict and for the foreseeable future.

Behavioral and Social Health Outcomes Program

A new focus on surveillance of behavioral health emerged at the former CHPPM, now the Public Health Command (Provisional). Great demand exists for such capacity, as evidenced by increasing requests from Army leadership for actionable data from population health indicators in this area. Recent Mental Health Advisory Team surveys and epidemiological consultation investigations have clearly demonstrated that no single data source is sufficient for acquiring the information necessary to perform analysis of individual, community, or military health system factors that are associated with suicides and related adverse behavioral outcomes. Timely and effective intervention requires data to be collected and reviewed in a way that allows a comprehensive understanding of both individual suicide cases and the broader community context (psychological and physical health, installation and unit factors, social ties, and other applicable factors). The former CHPPM received funding from the US Army Medical Command for the establishment of this capability, as well as funding from the Army G-1 to establish a separate "strategic analysis cell" to collect and follow data for the specific purpose of generating actionable data in the effort to mitigate suicides in the Army.

CHPPM's Behavioral and Social Health Outcomes Program (BSHOP) is a comprehensive behavioral health epidemiology and surveillance program formed to evaluate the full spectrum of psychological health and social wellness in Army communities. BSHOP's mission is to establish and operate a central behavioral health and social health outcomes epidemiologic resource for the Army and to bolster ongoing behavioral health program development and evaluation capability at CHPPM. The program is structured to analyze, interpret, and disseminate information on the status, trends, and determinants of the behavioral health and fitness of America's Army. The end objective is to provide a ready means to identify and evaluate impediments to medical readiness and establish a basis for preventive action.

In the spring of 2009, the Army's vice chief of staff established the Army Suicide Prevention Task Force (ASPTF) in response to the Army's increasing suicide rate. The ASPTF's effort has resulted in roughly 250 initiatives throughout the Army that are currently being executed, in addition to the development of the Army Campaign Plan for Health Promotion, Risk Reduction, and Suicide Prevention.

Efforts to mitigate the psychological effects of war continue. The shootings at Fort Hood led to both DoD and service-specific recommendations. The recommendations relevant to behavioral health, published in "Protecting the Force" (available at: http://www.army.mil/-news/2010/01/15/33006-protecting-the-force-lessons-learned-from-fort-hood/), emphasized caring for medical personnel and screening for violence. It is unclear at this point how well these recommendations will be implemented.

The Army's Comprehensive Behavioral Health System of Care, begun in 2010, seeks to implement best practices in optimal integration across the Army.

Begun in the Western and Pacific regions, under the leadership of Brigadier General Patricia Horoho and Brigadier General Steve Jones, it seeks to improve the reintegration process using lessons learned throughout the Army. The new DoD–Veterans Affairs Integrated Mental Health Strategy incorporates 28 strategic actions aimed at aligning the two healthcare systems. Although many of the recommendations are similar to others already made, the new program focuses on transitions from military to civilian life.

The shootings at Fort Hood have led to three major health-related efforts for the Army and DoD: (1) to seek to uncover violent tendencies in individuals; (2) to build upon the comprehensive behavioral response to the shooting; and (3) to expand provider resiliency training. There have also been concerted efforts to improve access to care by increasing the number and availability of providers and decreasing stigma. In the Army, the number of behavioral healthcare providers has increased almost 70% between 2007 and 2010.

When this chapter was written, the Army had 2,579 behavioral health providers available, with a conservative need estimate of 3,072 military, civilian, and contract behavioral healthcare providers. This represented an 84% fill, or a shortage of 493 providers. The Army is currently attempting to hire or contract the additional providers (87 psychiatrists, 146 psychologists, 222 social workers, and 38 psychiatric nurses). However, these numbers continually change, as providers are hired or leave and as new requirements are developed.

Provider hiring difficulties are not due to lack of funding; rather, the difficulties stem from a lack of civilian providers willing to practice in remote locations, compensation limitations inherent to government employment, and a national shortage of qualified providers. To address these limitations, the Army has employed selected behavioral health recruitment and retention incentives. These include

- implementing a critical skills retention bonus for master's level clinical psychologists;
- including social work officers (captains) in the critical skills retention bonus program instituted by the Army;
- establishing incentive special pay for psychiatric nurse practitioners;
- providing increases in multiyear special pay for psychiatrists
- utilizing the active duty health professions loan repayment program for both accession and retention of behavioral healthcare providers;
- making health professions scholarship program allocations available as a tool for the US Army Recruiting Command to recruit psychiatric nurse practitioners; and
- increasing the number of health professions scholarship allocations dedicated to clinical psychology and increased the seats available in the clinical psychology internship program.

SUMMARY

This volume began with a brief look at the history of behavioral healthcare in the US military, especially the genesis of the two volumes on military psychiatry in the *Textbooks of Military Medicine* series that were published over 15 years ago. Many of the "lessons learned" described in those two volumes were based on military experiences during Vietnam. Both the military and civilian society have dramatically changed since Vietnam, but one point that remains constant is that the human ability to adapt to the horrors of combat is finite. It is through the evolution of both proactive measures to help soldiers "steel" themselves against their experiences and therapeutic interventions by the behavioral healthcare system that the best possible outcomes can be achieved for military personnel. This project has summarized the experiences of more than 150 behavioral healthcare providers, in all fields and specialties, who have given their time and words to capture these latest battlefield conditions and lessons learned.

The system of behavioral healthcare in the US military is always in flux, with numerous individuals and organizations attempting to improve it via various innovative programs. One constant theme, as demonstrated in the discussion in this chapter, is that the many attempts at both quick and comprehensive solutions only demonstrate the complexity and difficulties of the mission. Clearly the effects of the conflicts in Operation Enduring Freedom and Operation Iraqi Freedom, as well as tsunamis and other natural and manmade disasters, will continue to take their toll on US military members, their families, and the nation. It is thus a national duty to continue providing our service members the best behavioral healthcare available.

Appendix 1

PROVISION OF BEHAVIORAL HEALTH SERVICES DURING OPERATION IRAQI FREEDOM ONE

ROBERT D. FORSTEN, DO*; BRETT J. SCHNEIDER, MD†; SHARETTE KIRSTEN GRAY, MD‡; COLIN DANIELS, MD§; AND GARY J. DROUILLARD, MD¥

*Lieutenant Colonel (P), Medical Corps, US Army; Command Psychiatrist, US Army Special Operations Command (AOMD), 2929 Desert Storm Drive (Stop A), Fort Bragg, North Carolina 28310-9110; formerly, Staff Psychiatrist, Department of Psychiatry, Walter Reed Army Medical Center, Washington, DC

†Lieutenant Colonel, Medical Corps, US Army; Deputy Chief, Department of Psychiatry, Building 61, Child and Adolescent Psychiatry Clinic, Walter Reed Army Medical Center, 6900 Georgia Avenue NW, Washington, DC 20307

‡Lieutenant Colonel, Medical Corps, US Army; Chief, Hospital and Administrative Psychiatry Services, Department of Behavioral Health, Building 36000, Darnall Loop, Carl R. Darnall Army Medical Center, Fort Hood, Texas 76544; formerly, Division Psychiatrist, 4th Infantry Division, Fort Hood, Texas

§Lieutenant Colonel, Medical Corps, US Army; Psychiatrist, Department of Psychiatry, Madigan Army Medical Center, 9040 Fitzsimmons Drive, 7BLM, Tacoma, Washington 98431; formerly, Chief, Behavioral Health Services, 28th Combat Support Hospital, Operation Iraqi Freedom 2003

¥Lieutenant Colonel, Medical Corps, US Army; Chief, Chemical Addiction Treatment Service, Department of Psychiatry, 1 Jarrett White Road, Tripler Army Medical Center, Honolulu, Hawaii 96859; formerly, Chief, Consultation Liaison Psychiatry, Tripler Army Medical Center, Honolulu, Hawaii

INTRODUCTION

In 2003, the US Army deployed four different medical units with behavioral health assets during Operation Iraqi Freedom One (OIF I). Each of these units provided varying levels or echelons of healthcare throughout the war zone. A review of care echelons and each behavioral health unit is discussed later in this appendix. The primary mission of these behavioral health units was to provide evaluation and treatment for all behavioral health disorders and operational stress issues, in addition to administrative psychiatric support services. The structure of each unit and how it delivered its services varied markedly, depending on numerous factors, including the unit supported, location, command, logistic support, and assigned personnel. Behavioral health assets were located throughout Iraq at the combat stress control (CSC) detachment or company, division mental health section (DMHS), combat support hospital (CSH), and area support medical battalion/company. Of these different types of behavioral health assets, two are medical units (CSH and area support medical battalion), and two are assigned directly to the combat units (DMHS and CSC). The area support medical battalion/company's behavioral health capability was phased out in 2007 and will not be discussed in this appendix; also, the forward support medical company (FSMC), as part of the forward support medical battalion (FSMB), may have had behavioral health assets assigned to it but this organizational structure will be phased out. Only the CSC company and detachment, DMHS, and CSH will be discussed.

Although many other resources on medical topics and military operations exist, this appendix focuses on helping behavioral health providers understand the challenges identified during the conventional ground phase of OIF I (2003), amid highly uncertain conditions characteristic of the early stages of combat operations, as well as potential differences between behavioral health operations during future deployments or campaigns.

During peacetime, US Army physicians, nurses, medical administrators, and enlisted medical personnel primarily work in post hospitals and clinics. The aforementioned behavioral health units have key personnel assigned to them at all times to operate the unit in garrison. During war or contingency operations, these personnel may receive activation orders to augment medical units through the Army's Professional Officer Filler Information System (PROFIS). PROFIS assigns personnel working in hospitals and clinics to deploying Forces Command (FORSCOM) units.

The Army attempts to assign behavioral health officers (psychiatrists, psychologists, social workers, psychiatric nurses, occupational therapists, and behavioral health specialists [formerly military occupational specialty 91X, now 68X]) who are geographically located close to their PROFIS unit (in many cases the personnel are located on the same base as the unit), so these personnel can train or coordinate with the unit in garrison. However, some personnel assigned to units as PROFIS providers have duty stations hundreds (and in some cases thousands) of miles away from their FORSCOM unit's home station or garrison. In addition, Reserve component medical and behavioral health units also participated in OIF I, with some active duty PROFIS personnel augmentees filling Reserve vacancies.

Most PROFIS personnel who met the deployment challenge—coming together to comprise the treatment aspect of the medical and behavioral health units—had never met prior to deployment, in contrast to FORSCOM units (combat arms, combat support, and combat service support branches) that train for wartime missions continuously in garrison, and US Army medical branches that perform "real life" missions on a daily basis. However, moving into a battlefield setting to treat medical and behavioral health casualties presents different challenges, such as the logistics of patient care in the austere or hazardous environment, compared to the more complex and heavier case loads typically managed in garrison medical organizations. Despite the challenges, most professional personnel adapted to their new environment and completed the medical mission admirably.

ECHELONS OF TREATMENT IN THE COMBAT THEATER

Every behavioral health unit in a theater of combat operations provides different treatment options, increasing with the treatment echelon (level) of care. There are five echelons of care, with echelon 5 possessing the most comprehensive or definitive options (similar to a medical center in the continental United States [CONUS]) and echelon 1 composed of self-aid, aid from other unit members (buddy aid), and care from combat medics. As the echelon increases, so does the evaluation capability and medical care provided. In terms of behavioral health assets, each unit at the battalion level—echelon 1—was assigned an enlisted behavioral health specialist whose activities were coordinated by the DMHS.

Each behavioral health specialist is an enlisted soldier or noncommissioned officer (NCO) with varying degrees of experience in the diagnosis, treatment, and management of behavioral disorders. Starting at the brigade level—echelon 2—a CSC detachment (also assigned at corps or echelons-above-brigade [EAB] level) focuses on interventions to prevent combat operational stress response casualties through critical incident debriefings, stress management classes, "walk-about" marketing contacts, and some restoration/fitness programs resembling brief day-treatment programs, as well as providing conventional clinic-based behavioral health evaluation and treatment. Each brigade also has an organically assigned behavioral health officer—usually a psychologist or social worker—who may conduct evaluations of brigade soldiers or facilitate command liaisons with area CSC/CSH elements. Echelon 3 consists of CSC companies providing fitness or restoration units, the CSH (which is typically assigned at corps-level EAB), and the DMHS, if the theater organization utilizes conventional division structure instead of modular independent brigades. On a linear battlefield, echelons of care also show predictable positions relative to the forward line of troops, but a nonlinear battlefield obscures this relationship, with many behavioral health resources (units or detached slices/elements) located across large areas, such as a forward operating bases (FOBs) or logistic support areas (LSAs). However, some behavioral health resources may support small camps or outposts with small elements positioned locally or rotating out from FOBs, depending on local needs, resources, distances, transportation/logistics, and expected travel-related hazards.

Prior to wartime deployment, all units (augmented with their PROFIS personnel) complete tasks such as medical screening; legal documents (wills, powers of attorney); weapons qualification; training in unexploded ordinance; CBRNE (chemical, biological, radiological, nuclear, and explosive) hazards; and all other training required by unit readiness training matrices. PROFIS personnel join the unit for this specified "train-up" period to ensure they are familiar with the standard operating procedures, mission essential task list, and internal workings of the host unit. Many PROFIS personnel may lack prior experience with the specific unit or its chain of command and may never have met face-to-face with any of the unit's members. The exception is DMHS, which operates in garrison with most of the personnel required during deployment, but may be augmented with PROFIS personnel depending on wartime mission requirements.

Garrison division mental health personnel will need to train all the personnel within the behavioral health section with whom they will be deploying. At a minimum, this training should consist of setting up standard operating procedures related to evaluation, diagnosis, treatment, clinic management, and prevention techniques. The training also gives the unit leaders an assessment of each team member's technical proficiency and experience, and the extent to which that provider is able to function independently. Supervision may be required depending on training, licensure, and credentialing levels.

ARRIVING IN KUWAIT

Prior to entering Iraq, most units from OIF I landed in Kuwait at the SPOD/APOD (sea [for equipment]/aerial [for personnel] point of embarkation/debarkation). Many units had expected to arrive at another SPOD/APOD in Turkey and approach from the north but received last-minute redirection to the overcrowded Kuwait staging area due to diplomatic issues. From the APOD, most units moved to a "cabal," or tactical assembly area, where they reassembled their operating capability and prepositioned while awaiting movement north into Iraq. These cabals were small base camps with minimal infrastructure located in the remote Kuwaiti desert. The majority of OIF I soldiers then convoyed into Iraq from Kuwait, loaded into high mobility multipurpose wheeled vehicles (HMMWVs or Humvees), family of medium tactical vehicles (FMTVs) or the older M939 series 2.5 ("deuce-and-a-half") vehicles, and 5-ton trucks. These convoys often took up to 3 days to complete because anytime a vehicle broke down, the entire convoy waited until the vehicle was remobilized or recovered. Furthermore, early-phase convoys also contended with nearby combat or threatened engagement by Iraqi Army forces. Additionally, the early unit convoys faced challenges related to unlabeled and undeveloped routes through an unmapped country with minimal signage and many roads that were inadequate for large and heavy military vehicles. While some units possessed global-positioning-satellite capability, many navigated with uncertain means in a landscape with few reliable visual landmarks during a season where large dust storms could completely obstruct visibility and stifle breathing for extended periods (soldiers deploying to OIF now fly directly into Iraq via the nearest air strip to where they will assume mission responsibility).

Units typically resided in tents, although some moved into dirty, decrepit, abandoned masonry structures. Tent space became very limited in both Kuwait and Iraq during OIF I; many personnel were fortunate to have 2 linear feet of space on either side of the cot on which they slept and stored all their gear. Many less-fortunate soldiers, especially in combat arms units, did not have either a cot or a tent and slept on the ground or on their vehicles, in extremely variable stifling heat or bitter cold. Overcrowded tents, stress, and close living proximity accelerated viral spread and increased the frequency of infectious illnesses. Anecdotally, the average weight loss per soldier during the first month was 5 to 10 lb; many infantry soldiers lost 20 to 40 lb during the conventional ground combat phase due to limited food consumption, along with irregular and continuous combat operations. However, most soldiers within these units adjusted physically and behaviorally, bonding into a cohesive team and unit. During this period, officers had to avoid complaining, especially around the enlisted soldiers, who tended to lose respect for officers they heard complaining. However, among some officers, complaining, mostly through humor, was a helpful way to vent frustration, improving overall officer morale, mood, and bonding.

The largest stressor in Kuwait was not the Scud missile alerts and subsequent donning of the mission-oriented protective posture (MOPP) 4 suits (thick, carbon-based chemical weapons protection suits), or joint-service lightweight integrated suit technology (JSLIST) equipment, but boredom coupled with overcrowding and the austere environment, which tended to fuel gossip behaviors and interpersonal conflicts. Additionally, soldiers experienced emotional stress from a perceived conspicuous absence of information on each unit's specific mission, leading to speculation on justifications for deployment, chain-of-command motives, and when each unit would actually move forward to begin operations in Iraq. In most cases, unit equipment arrived in port (SPOD) after unit personnel had been flown into the APOD, causing personnel to wait in the cabals for their equipment while residing in overcrowded tents with minimal infrastructure or recreational opportunities.

Units with responsive and competent commanders who fostered group cohesiveness and subordinate communication, keeping their soldiers busy with mission-focused operational training, appeared to have less disruptive drama and stress-related behavioral health issues or conduct problems. These leaders effectively implemented the primary preventive actions to control and reduce the stressors known to increase combat and operational stress reactions, validating the basic precepts of combat psychiatry, as per Field Manual (FM) 4-02.51 (formerly FM 8-51), *Combat and Operational Stress Control.*

Most soldiers seen by medical personnel on the cabals were not "emergent," but rather had interpersonal problems with supervisors, were homesick or had home-front problems, or did not adjust well to the high operation tempo the deployment could demand. The first two stressors (unit/command problems and home-front worries) emerged as the top two most common stressors of deployed service members, as shown in the first and subsequent Mental Health Advisory Team (MHAT) reports. Each cabal had a small clinic set up for seeing medical emergencies and sick call, but these battalion aid station equivalents did not have behavioral health assets unless augmented individually by providers in units temporarily assembling at a particular base.

Privacy became an issue while evaluating patients on the cabals because no structures approximating "clinical space" had been set up, nor was there a mechanism for medical recordkeeping. Despite this, commanders knew where the medical units were located on the cabals and sent their personnel to "walk in" for evaluations. Soldiers were often evaluated by medical personnel who sat down with them on the sand, in the shade of a vehicle or tent. Documentation remained an unresolved issue without any means of copying files, and no soldier had a medical record to review or document care. Most of the medical notes completed during OIF I were handwritten on SF600 forms, and soldiers typically lost these notes. Records kept at facilities would not follow soldiers through their care at different locations. The Armed Forces Health Longitudinal Technology Application (AHLTA) or the Composite Healthcare System (CHCS) electronic medical records did not become operational until later rotations (approximately 2006–2007). The role of the behavioral health professional on the cabal during OIF I was primarily evaluation to determine which soldiers were safe and could move north to Iraq and which soldiers needed to be evacuated from theater for further evaluation, treatment, or administrative separation. Some soldiers had unexpected panic responses to the MOPP-4 protective mask. This required either prompt successful desensitization (sometimes with benzodiazepine-induced relaxation) to learn to tolerate the mask or evacuation from theater. Behavioral health emergency patients had to join a convoy to the hospital in Kuwait, which was staffed by one psychiatrist.

COMBAT SUPPORT HOSPITALS

Two combat support hospitals—the 21st and 28th CSHs—were at cabals in Kuwait by March 2003, preparing to deploy their hospitals north to Iraq after initiation of the ground invasion. Because the 21st CSH was an early Medical Reengineering Initiative (MRI) CSH, it did not have a neuropsychiatric group as the 28th CSH had. The primary mission of the new MRI CSH was to perform split operations in two locations, separating into two smaller hospitals, both capable of operating independently but with the same chain of command. Campaign evolution soon demonstrated the need for smaller hospital organizations that maintained similar capability levels but provided more geographically dispersed support, prompting the 28th CSH to perform a split operation as well, as did all subsequent CSH units. The lack of a neuropsychiatric group meant that the behavioral health section of the 21st CSH brought no equipment such as bedding, tentage, or cots, and only a limited number of behavioral health personnel: a psychiatrist, a psychiatric nurse, and two behavioral health specialists. In contrast, the 28th CSH had a psychiatrist, a social work officer, three psychiatric nurses, and approximately six enlisted behavioral health specialists. The 28th CSH did not operate a separate neuropsychiatric ward and planned to use only one or two beds from the medical–surgical ward to house psychiatric patients. They also did not plan to operate an outpatient clinic or behavioral health holding capability (resembling a fitness program at a CSC).

Once operations commenced, the number of psychiatrically hospitalized patients exceeded the number of medical patients on the ward. Additionally, units often packed a ground evacuation vehicle with soldiers requiring behavioral health evaluations. These convoys would go directly to the CSH, bypassing other echelons and flooding the CSH with outpatient evaluations. Some units also sought to "medicalize" the behavioral problems within their unit and send misconduct cases to the CSH for presumed evacuation instead of administering disciplinary action and initiating administrative returns. These numerous outpatient evaluations resulted in many soldiers who did not require hospitalization or evacuation but needed several days of observation before returning to duty. Furthermore, delays in transportation also increased needs for a holding requirement and some supervision by behavioral health staff.

Once the 21st CSH split, a professional provider and a behavioral health specialist went with each hospital slice. As an MRI CSH, the 21st was composed of three companies: A Company (CO), B CO, and Headquarters CO. As stated above, the primary mission of the new MRI CSH was to perform split operations so that one slice could set up and operate independently of the other. B CO left approximately 5 days before A CO in mid-April and was located in Mosul, Iraq, approximately 160 miles north of A CO, which was located on a large airfield in Balad, Iraq, about 40 miles north of Baghdad. The 28th CSH set up its main unit initially in Camp Dogwood, a patch of desert near Baghdad, and subsequently packed up the tent hospital to move into a fixed facility (Ibn Sina) in Baghdad, maintaining a smaller slice in Tikrit.

One of the earliest goals of the CSH was to set up the emergency room (ER) and operating rooms (ORs) within 48 hours or less to be ready to accept patients. Once this "main line" is set up, the remainder of the CSH is then built adjoining it. There is no set procedure on how or where to put clinics, wards, and so forth, so the hospital is usually arranged by the experience within the command. For example, the 21st CSH in Balad had a section of tents between the ER and the OR that acted as an "exchange," so patients could overflow if needed into this area. The exchange made coordination of patients easier for mass casualty events, air evacuation, and movement to and from the ER, OR, and radiology. The 21st CSH set up an outpatient clinic in addition to inpatient services. In this case, the psychiatrist worked in both settings seeing routine outpatients as well as inpatients usually admitted through the emergency room. The outpatient service was located in the "specialty clinic" area of the hospital in an "office" consisting of half of one of the sections in the eight-section tent, with a field desk and two chairs. The 28th CSH had a similar arrangement, except that the behavioral health "clinic" was located at the other end of the hospital tent complex, away from any other clinics and next to the chaplain's "office." The clinic space also consisted of a small tent section, with patient interviews often conducted in hallways during busy periods.

As soon as the 21st CSH arrived at Balad, behavioral health consultations began. Because the 21st was the first medical treatment facility on the base, the psychiatrist and behavioral health specialist quickly started seeing patients. Initially, behavioral health patients were seen on an outpatient basis because the hospital ran sick call for the base from the specialty clinic. Three fourths of the behavioral health referrals at sick call were sent by the chain of command to rule out danger to self or others. These were soldiers who had threatened to hurt themselves or others. The other 25% needed medication refills because they did not deploy with enough medication or were close to running out after being in Kuwait for several months before moving forward into Iraq. The 28th CSH saw a similar preponderance of danger evaluations and medication refills. Units also sent numerous evaluations for chapter separation, conscientious objection, or other administrative issues. Army Reserve and Army National Guard units seemed to have a disproportionate number of chapter evaluations, as the active duty deployment gave these Reserve units an unanticipated opportunity to evaluate actual duty performance and separate those incapable of meeting mission requirements. However, the main active duty unit supported by the 28th CSH, the 3rd Infantry Division (ID), appeared to supply most of the malingering and misconduct cases seen at this CSH.

The 21st CSH pharmacy section deployed with a small supply of paroxetine and fluoxetine, but these drugs were quickly depleted within the first week after the hospital was set up. However, the CSH was collocated next to a medical logistics battalion that was able to coordinate future medication supplies. After 6 to 8 weeks, the pharmacy stocked up on oral medications, including several selective serotonin reuptake inhibitors, second-generation antidepressants, stimulants, atypical antipsychotics, benzodiazapines, and sleep medications. The 28th CSH pharmacy also deployed with a minimal supply of medications, forcing providers to dispense medications in 1-week increments to delay or minimize stock-outs, which still occurred. In contrast to the 21st CSH, the 28th CSH did not have logistics support and sustained operations with the limited drug supplies the psychiatrists personally carried into theater. In addition, behavioral health specialists from the 28th CSH who went to Landstuhl Regional Medical Center (LRMC) in Germany on medevac escort missions requested and obtained medication resupply from the psychiatrists there to bring back into theater. For future reference, any psychiatrist deploying to an immature theater should have a lockbox (or several) of medications and coordinate as soon as possible with the medical logistics battalion and pharmacist for resupply.

The dynamics of a deployed CSH were such that it took a physician with a great deal of military experience as well as an approachable, healthy personality to function as the deputy commander for clinical services (DCCS). The DCCS is particularly helpful in organizing the physicians into a tight-knit team. The DCCS acts as a buffer between providers and along the chain of command, engaging in the medical administrative battles to allow other physicians to focus on their medical mission, and to ensure that their junior rank did not result in others ignoring or overruling their expert recommendations based on rank alone. The DCCS also mentors junior medical officers by arranging training—military and nonmilitary—as well as normalizing the deployment experience.

Many referrals to the CSHs were soldiers requiring dispositions from outlying behavioral health units. Early in OIF I, if a soldier was evacuated to a hospital remote from the referring unit, that soldier usually ended up being evacuated out of theater to Kuwait and then to Germany. Discussing cases with commanders and behavioral health teams during the early phases of OIF I was often difficult due to limitations in communication lines, which were down at least half the time. It was also not uncommon for all convoys to be halted for several days at a time secondary to increased fighting. This frequent lack of any communication abilities with commands, via either telephone line or in person, discouraged providers, overburdened holding capabilities, and led to medical evacuation of soldiers who might otherwise have returned to duty. The division psychiatrist had multiple examples of soldiers being dropped off at the DMHS clinic for an evaluation, and the unit then convoyed for hours back to their assigned FOB prior to contacting the DMHS. Although most of these soldiers received fit-for-duty dispositions, they remained at the DMHS for several weeks because no one could contact their command, and it could take 2 weeks or so for the referring unit to convoy back and pick up the soldier. At the 21st CSH, providers usually admitted soldiers for observation and safety to the medical–surgical intermediate care ward (and later, the five-bed neuropsychiatric unit of the 28th CSH). However, a theater policy to admit patients to a CSH for no more than 7 days resulted in evacuations to a higher level of care where return to duty (RTD) became even more difficult and improbable. Most unit commanders supported providers who recommended patient evacuation, but on some occasions they objected to evacuation and wanted their soldiers returned to them. A chain-of-command representative (the commander, first sergeant, or senior NCO) then came to the CSH or CSC to pick up the soldier in person.

The 21st CSH did not have neuropsychiatry assets to establish an inpatient milieu; behavioral health patients admitted to this CSH did not have the benefit of a psychiatric ward setting with groups, confidentiality, or a multidisciplinary approach to treatment. However, the milieu remained very limited and public at the 28th CSH as well. Patients had a few groups run by psychiatric nurses but shared the ward with medical and surgical patients. Nursing care was generally delivered to these patients by a psychiatric nurse; however, medical and surgical nurses also contributed to nursing care of psychiatric patients due to staffing necessities. While some staff sought to increase privacy by hanging blankets as dividers around a psychiatric patient's bed, this effectively identified them as a psychiatric patients and increased interest in them when they stepped out from behind the hanging blanket. Open space anonymity provided better confidentiality because other patients would not know why another patient had been hospitalized.

Very few psychiatric cases evacuated from Iraq

returned to Iraq. Once soldiers were evacuated to the 47th CSH in Kuwait, the psychiatrist assigned to the 47th noted that:

> most soldiers sent to Kuwait markedly improve as they "move Westward" and most of what is sent here for air evacuation to Germany (Landstuhl Regional Medical Center) is not battle fatigue and not severe behavioral illness but rather a failure to adapt to the deployment due to occupational stress and problems back home. Because of this, more soldiers were sent back to their commands with recommendations for administrative separation. However, many were transported out of the theater on a medical evacuation because they were "conditionally suicidal" but we still recommend for a chapter separation.

Some behavioral health providers were unwilling to make the recommendation for a chapter separation. One of the psychologists in a reserve CSC unit stated, "I'm just not comfortable making a decision like that that will have such an impact on someone's life," meaning that this provider thought a separation would affect a soldier's career in civilian life. However, these administrative duties remain an integral part of the job for military behavioral health providers, either in garrison or on deployment. During OIF I, the chief of psychiatry at LRMC stated that, "it helps Landstuhl tremendously to have recommendations like these because these soldiers look fine when they get there and we don't get to see them when they are in Iraq, when they have mentally decompensated." Such was the case in the CSHs in Iraq when soldiers were sent for evaluation from smaller behavioral health units (DMHS, CSC, chaplain, behavioral health technicians) or battalion surgeons embedded within combat units. These soldiers usually improved quickly but also decompensated quickly when told they were being sent back to their unit. Providers at the CSH would then spend extensive time trying to reach the unit at a distant location for collateral information via primitive telephonic infrastructure to make the necessary determinations. Without collateral information providers would often not know the relevant conditions and observed behaviors of the soldier. However, some units became more available for discussion when they received notification from the patient administrative section or the CSH patient administrative section that their soldier was in RTD status and needed pick-up for transportation back to the unit.

As stated, the policy of the CSH was to evacuate any soldier admitted for more than 7 days. Usually, units off the base could not be reached in this period of time and these soldiers were sent to Germany via the 47th CSH in Kuwait. However, the 28th CSH accumulated a large holding population awaiting RTD, sometimes exceeding the 7-day hospitalization policy if RTD appeared probable. Extensive holding populations entailed some risk and caused some concern to the hospital command, but the command then used its resources and influence to achieve contact with the original unit and arrange transportation. Some of the psychiatric patients at 28th CSH needed evacuation and went to LRMC, which facilitated pharmacy resupply, as already discussed. However, these evacuations presented another issue as it typically took 2 to 3 weeks for a behavioral health specialist who escorted the patient to return to the CSH for routine duties. Sometimes the CSH sent other nursing personnel on these missions, but that depleted other sections of their nursing or enlisted medical personnel. The poor lines of communication to units and limited treatment options presented challenges that the CSH units handled differently; the 21st CSH usually evacuated these soldiers from theater, whereas the 28th CSH held them for RTD to prevent personnel depletion (at the CSH and sending unit). Early in OIF I, when commanders were able to locate their soldiers and call or visit the CSH to see how they were doing, the commanders were occasionally angry that they had "lost" their soldiers to the medical evacuation system. Getting soldiers to agree to commit themselves to maintaining personal safety and return to their units was sometimes very difficult with only supportive therapy and "three hots and a cot," especially if the soldier had the expectation of release from theater.

Soldiers' mood and affect usually brightened when they were away from the stress of their unit; had some rest, a shower, and three meals; and were in an air-conditioned hospital. Many soldiers evaluated in this setting stated they had joined the Army for "college money" and "never thought [they] would deploy"; they often acted out when told they were going back to their units. This situation became an ethical dilemma for psychiatrists sending soldiers back to combat knowing they might be killed, injured, or deteriorate behaviorally, but these issues applied to any soldier ordered into a combat environment.

After the end of the major combat offensive, roughly the end of April 2003, it was not considered very dangerous for units to convoy to hospitals or clinics, although sporadic attacks with small arms and rocket-propelled grenades continued. However, after the insurgency became more organized, these ground convoys decreased in frequency as improvised explosive devices (IEDs) hidden around roadways became the primary weapon against coalition forces. Camps received regular mortar (indirect) fire after early July 2003, and the roadside IEDs and rocket indirect fire attacks also increased dramatically. For example, the Balad (Arabic for "in the country or countryside") airfield (aka Camp Anaconda), a huge, sprawling airbase of many square miles, received multiple mortar attacks from July 3 to September 26, 2003. Most of these mortar attacks occurred in the quadrant of the base containing the CSH.

Commanders reported difficulty in referring soldiers to DMHS or CSC units where they would normally have been seen for evaluation and treatment. Because CSHs were located on large LSAs, units brought their soldiers to the CSHs when they convoyed to the LSA to pick up supplies. A very small percentage of cases seen involved florid psychosis or mania; most referrals were lower-ranking enlisted personnel with adjustment disorders. However, the behavioral, logistical, and combat stressors of OIF I affected all ranks and branches. For example the psychiatrist of the 21st CSH evacuated two aviators due to panic attacks and anxiety that affected their flying, caused in each case by "brown out" situations (caused by sand and dust from the rotor wash during landings). This resulted in such significant anxiety about future recurrences that it impaired overall mission capability. Other cases were more serious and involved stress confronted by higher level commanders.

Case Study A1-1: A 40-year-old combat arms battalion commander with 19 years active duty presented as a self-referral for worsening depressed mood with suicidal thoughts to shoot himself in the head with his 9-mm pistol. His brigade commander described him as "the strongest and most reliable battalion commander in the brigade." His depression centered on the lack of control he felt over the lives of his troopers and the lack of training his men had been given for "extra duties" such as security and patrols. While on a patrol two of his soldiers had been killed by insurgents. After admission to the hospital for 5 days followed by 3 weeks of outpatient treatment consisting of counseling and medication, his mood and suicidal thoughts continued to worsen. He was evacuated from theater for more intensive treatment. In follow-up, he was noted to be doing well and still on active duty.

Another factor that led to referrals to behavioral health was the guilt associated with killing enemy combatants or the sheer terror of seeing friends killed by insurgent attacks. Many soldiers did not confront these stressors until seen by a behavioral health provider. Many would break into tears when asked the simple question of whether or not they had killed anyone in combat. Another common source of guilt came (correctly or incorrectly) from whether one's actions or inactions led to a negative outcome for a friend, civilian noncombatant, or fellow soldier.

Case Study A1-2: A 22-year-old enlisted soldier presented to the CSH, referred by his unit for depressed and psychotic symptoms. He blamed himself for the death of his commander. His commander had reached up to catch a line that was falling on top of the Bradley fighting vehicle that the commander was on top of. It electrocuted the commander. The presenting soldier had been the gunner but was inside the vehicle at the time of the electrocution. He felt guilty and demonstrated severe depression with psychotic features, hearing voices telling him he was a "poor soldier" and that he "should have done something to help his commander," with whom he had a good working relationship. In reality, there was nothing he could have done to save his commander, yet he believed it was his fault that his commander died. Traumatic event management with the soldier and unit proved helpful in this case, and his psychotic symptoms improved significantly with an antidepressant and low-dose atypical antipsychotic medication, allowing him to return to duty.

One behavioral health unit referred a soldier to the CSH for medevac to LRMC for a "sleep study to rule out sleepwalking." While conceptually it was easy to send this soldier back to the unit for observation, the increase in mortar and rocket attacks made his return more complicated and potentially hazardous. The provider admitted this soldier instead, observing him at the CSH before sending him back to his unit. In most cases, sleepwalking referrals were returned to the unit after brief medical work-up to avoid an epidemic of sleepwalking "evacuation syndrome" in these units.

During the period in late 2003 when insurgent attacks increased, word began to spread that most units would remain deployed for a year rather than the 6 months many had expected. From May to June 2003, there were six suspected cases of self-inflicted gunshot wounds to the foot seen at the 21st CSH in Balad and several at the 28th CSH at Camp Dogwood. The psychiatrist at the 21st consulted for the surgical team to evaluate one of these cases that appeared suspicious.

Case Study A1-3: An orthopaedic surgeon consulted psychiatry to evaluate an enlisted soldier in his mid-20s to determine whether the soldier's injury was accidental or self-inflicted, and to assess the soldier's risk of self-harm. The soldier stated that he shot his foot by accident. During the initial evaluation he reported depressed mood "ever since I've been deployed," and noted that he wanted to go home. He also complained of having interpersonal problems with his chain of command. He reported poor sleep, guilt about the deployment, anergia, and poor concentration since being deployed. He denied having these symptoms prior to deployment and felt they would "go away if he were home." He expressed surprise that the orthopaedic surgeon would send him back to duty, even though his foot had a clean injury without any fractures. He commented that, "I might as well shoot myself intentionally in order to leave if I have go back there." The provider also noted that during the initial evaluation the soldier stated that his first concern was where he would be "sent from here," expecting "that it would be Germany."

Initial psychiatric evaluation recommended that after sufficient orthopaedic recovery, he follow up with a CSC unit near his unit duty location with a stress management group. In the following days, his unit started a line-of-duty investigation, which contributed to his stress. The hospital chaplain then consulted psychiatry 3 days later when the soldier hinted that he would display violent behavior if he returned to the unit. When questioned about suicide or homicide, he stated, "I don't know what will happen if I go back to my unit." He still insisted that the initial incident was an accident. He denied pulling the trigger and could not come up with a reason for the weapon discharging. Ten days after the second evaluation, his chain of command contacted the hospital and informed the medical team that they wanted to court-martial the soldier. However, the line-of-duty investigation remained incomplete and would take 2 to 3 more weeks to complete. The CSH informed the unit that the soldier's foot had healed sufficiently for discharge from the hospital, but because of the unit's remote location and lack of medical facilities to change his foot dressings, he would need air evacuation to LRMC in Germany. When the soldier learned of this decision, his affect and mood brightened to euthymic and he reported, "I expected that." He appeared happy that he would be getting out of the Army, stating, "Any way is good." He reported feeling "glad that I'm not going back to my unit with a loaded weapon."

After the soldier had been at the CSH for approximately 6 weeks, due to the nature of his injury, the line-of-duty investigation, and the poor communication with his unit, he was sent to Kuwait for evacuation to Germany. However, his unit intercepted him in Kuwait and told him he was returning to Iraq for a court-martial, at which point it required several personnel to restrain him. He was nonetheless eventually evacuated from Kuwait to an Army hospital in Germany due to his combative behavior.

From June to July 2003, a suicide cluster occurred, with each case likely having had multiple contributing factors, but ultimately leading each individual to feel hopelessness and intolerable depression. These soldiers may have felt trapped in a situation with no clear departure or end date (unprecedented in this generation of deployed soldiers). Additionally, all soldiers carried their weapons and ammunition at all times. Added deployment stressors were the following: separation from family and loved ones; receiving "dear John/Jane" letters ending relationships; no lines of communication home; threat of being killed or injured; high temperatures; perceived harassment from chain of command; and poor sleep, latrines, hygiene, and food. Behavioral health planners and commanders discussed relocating the 113th CSC fitness teams from Mosul and Baghdad to the 21st CSH in Balad to start a neuropsychiatric unit after these suicides. This collocation never occurred, but a CSC fitness or restoration unit should collocate with an MRI CSH to share resources, treatment, and evaluation of soldiers, since the post-MRI CSH has limited behavioral health assets. (This arrangement worked very well during subsequent deployment rotations observed in the authors' subsequent deployments, including the 1908th CSC and 10th CSH in 2006 in Baghdad, and the 47th CSH and the 528th CSC at COB Speicher, in 2009.) Such collocation could improve RTD rates, as well as reduce evacuations from theater. At the 21st CSH in Mosul, the 98th CSC ran an outpatient clinic next to the hospital with two CSC psychiatrists (who admitted patients to the hospital if needed), a social worker, and five behavioral health specialists.

COMBAT STRESS CONTROL UNITS

The US Army's behavioral health community has long recognized the impact of acute and chronic stressors, as well as traumatic events, on the functioning of individual soldiers and military units. The Army currently maintains two types of CSC units: (1) CSC companies and (2) CSC detachments. The former are primarily staffed by reservists and contain 80 personnel of various disciplines, including psychiatrists, psychologists, psychiatric social workers, psychiatric advanced practice nurses, general psychiatric nurses, a medical-surgical nurse, numerous psychiatric technicians, and administrative support staff (eg, a cook, mechanics, and so forth), so they can function as self-sustaining units in a deployed environment. The active duty component CSC detachments grew 50% larger after the introduction of MRI units and are approximately half the size of a CSC company, but with fewer psychiatrists. Also, they do not contain the same mix of personnel as pre-MRI units or CSC companies.

CSC units are designated primarily as units tasked to perform preventative activities. As such, personnel in a CSC usually are configured into teams, known as prevention teams, consisting of one professional and two paraprofessionals (behavioral health specialists). These teams are usually assigned to specific units for which they provide primary and secondary prevention for combat-stress–related issues. Specifically, these teams present psychoeducational briefings focusing on suicide prevention, stress management, identification of combat fatigue or depression, and briefings preparing soldiers to reconnect with their families near the end of their deployment. At the beginning of OIF, military doctrine recommended critical event debriefing as the preferred intervention for traumatic events experienced by groups of soldiers. However, concurrent studies, both in the military and in civilian settings, questioned the efficacy of these critical event debriefings.

Even more important to the practitioner, some studies reported that critical event debriefings had the potential to actually harm some participants, possibly through reexperiencing the trauma or by overwhelming the psychological defense mechanisms that had otherwise been allowing the soldier to manage the trauma without intervention. Furthermore, many providers had not attended courses certifying proficiency in conducting critical event debriefings. These factors contributed to a wide variation in the utilization of the debriefings and the consistency of responses to potentially traumatizing events. The military behavioral health community had previously promoted the utility of critical event debriefing to Army leaders during the years leading up to OIF, which resulted in commanders requesting a debriefing for their soldiers anytime any adverse event happened. The following case study describes some of the issues involved in this process.

Case Study A1-4: A military chaplain phoned a local CSC unit after a fire had broken out in a hangar that served as the "barracks" for a military unit. The chaplain said that the unit's commander had requested a critical event debriefing. The chaplain asked for the assistance of the CSC unit inasmuch as the chaplain was inexperienced in performing such a debriefing and because the large unit would require multiple group debriefings (debriefings are usually limited to 20 people).

The consulted behavioral health officer evaluated the situation and determined that no one's life had been threatened by the fire, only property was lost, and that finding new housing was the unit's most immediate concern. The CSC staff discussed the situation with the chain of command and decided that instead of critical event debriefings (where everyone participated in groups discussing their experience, both factual and emotional), they would take a different approach with this particular event. This approach consisted of a meeting with the whole unit at once. The unit's commander spoke first to reassure his unit that new housing was in process and expected imminently. Furthermore, the Army would help the soldiers replace items lost in the fire. The behavioral health staff then gave an educational briefing about stress management and coping skills to the assembled soldiers along with specific contact information if any soldier wanted individual meetings.

Adaptive doctrine allows these CSC teams more flexibility to evaluate and treat soldiers with combat fatigue and behavioral health disorders. The teams also engage in traumatic event management and critical event debriefings, providing evaluation and appropriate intervention for involved units. The teams provide consultation to military commanders, both in ways to help the whole unit prevent combat-stress–related dysfunction and also by performing command-directed behavioral health evaluations on individuals when commanders are concerned about their safety and reliability. Finally, the teams provide assessment and treatment for soldiers who self-refer for evaluation of their own distress.

These functions require that the prevention teams live with units and travel within the operational area of the units for which they provide support services. Due to the travel hazards in the evolving Iraqi theater and in any nonlinear battlefield, routine travel plans decreased somewhat during OIF I. These prevention teams are "assigned" to cover the unit, but are not actually organic to the unit, so living and integrating with the host unit becomes imperative to develop trust from the unit's leaders and soldiers. Without developing these strong relationships, including being perceived as available and "useful" to the commander and soldiers, a prevention team would not accomplish its defined mission; not due to lack of skill or personnel, but due to an inability to earn credibility and trust with their customers. Without the credibility, barriers inevitably arise and limit the prevention team's access to the soldiers who need their care.

Despite the task of prevention and the doctrinal mission of psychoeducation classes, this pivotal underlying mission of relationship-building conveys a similarity with marketing functions. Although philosophically debatable, a unit's referral rate from the first sergeant or sergeant major provides a useful practical indirect metric of a prevention team's effectiveness, as these NCO leaders keep their fingers on the metaphorical pulse of the unit and will only refer when their skeptical trust has been earned. Some CSC units sought to justify their existence by optimistically counting social and coincidental contacts as "prevention" (marketing) contacts to report as statistics, but these contacts provide minimal actual care. Genuine individual or small-group sessions, usually with credentialed providers, not initiated by CSC staff, constitute substantive care and adverse outcome prevention.

In contrast to the established doctrine promoting team travel, some observations provide insights requiring diligent consideration to optimally balance benefits with costs. Travel tended to increase breadth of contact, but greatly decreased the depth of intervention. Soldiers needing behavioral health services tend to get directed to nearby behavioral health components perceived as helpful and competent, and whose personnel accumulate into provider panels. These panels quickly evaporate when disrupted by travel, as soldiers move on instead of establishing a perceived new relationship with another provider. Command elements directing behavioral health activities often do not appreciate the differences inherent in behavioral health relationships and expect a comparable portability from behavioral health as they might expect from other medical providers, such as sick call or dental or surgical services. New locations established after travel rarely yield a client/patient panel to match the size of the panel at the previous location.

Professional providers practicing in the best interest of beneficiaries maintain some degree of skepticism towards disruptive relocations that do not appear warranted or logical on clinical grounds. Directed activities may serve as perceived requirements or even a beneficial bullet in someone's reports or evaluations that actually detracts from collective soldier care. For example, an author questioned an ill-advised tasking that appeared more politically motivated than care-driven because the decision makers did not permit any merit discussion or consult actual subject matter experts. This particular tasking decimated a robust panel at a large base with ten to twelve substantive appointments per day while yielding two to three appointments per day after relocation. After returning in 8 weeks, the panel required another 8 to 12 weeks of rebuilding before approaching its previous productivity level.

CSC units also had a second type of function—restoration—with the restoration (formerly known as fitness) team. This team had more personnel assigned and usually operated from a stationary location, unlike the prevention teams. In addition to providing marketing activities similar to those provided by prevention teams, the restoration team also served as a treatment alternative for the prevention teams, commanders, or other nonbehavioral health providers, for soldiers who needed an evaluation and may have benefited from a spectrum of intervention activities ranging from prescriptions with interval aftercare to an intensive outpatient/partial hospitalization program equivalent to daytime groups and self-care quarters. By doctrine (specifically FM 4-02.51), restoration teams were meant to provide a stable place, somewhat removed from the front lines, where a soldier could be "restored" through the basic principles of the acronym BICEPS (brevity, immediacy, contact, expectancy, proximity, and simplicity). (PIES—proximity, immediacy, expectancy, and simplicity—was the previous acronym, used in FM 8-51.) Nonetheless, these treatment concepts led to the practice of "three hots and a cot," with the belief that the majority of combat stress casualties could be reconstituted in a short time, usually 1 to 3 days with close attention, to avoid accumulating large numbers or permitting extended care (> 3–4 day), which decreased the soldier's expectation of RTD, possibly prompting symptom sustainment to delay RTD and maximize reprieve at the relatively comfortable CSC. In concept, referrals managed with BICEPS would adapt better in the long run if returned to their units than if "medicalized" and evacuated. Doctrine also discourages labeling these soldiers as "patients," since labels also shape expectations (this appendix uses the term "patient" in the CSC context for consistency to denote a beneficiary receiving services, without intending to imply any particular treatment/intervention model or outcome expectation). In practical settings, care often transitioned fluidly across environments dictated by external circumstances (eg, care could occur at the CSC for one encounter, then a dining facility table, and then a CSH clinic office, with various combinations of pharmacological, psychological, educational, and behavioral interventions).

During OIF I, most restoration teams were based in camps that also housed a soldier's unit headquarters and that sometimes took frequent indirect fire. Thus, providers observed little difference between, or benefit from, quartering soldiers in the CSC versus leaving them with their host unit. While providing a respite from the immediate unit environment and command interactions may provide some benefit for certain cases, it may also adversely affect soldiers' perceived proximity to their unit and expectation for prompt RTD. Typically, documentation given to unit commanders recommended environmental and behavioral modifications as part of the treatment/restoration program, including the expected CSC aftercare. Anecdotally, by not keeping soldiers separated from their peers, commanders reduced the general unit perception that the soldier was "mental" or "crazy," thus reducing the stigma of care within these units. As discussed, restoration teams often functioned like community behavioral health clinics, providing psychiatric evaluation and treatment of ambulatory patients. This function also provided a referral resource for nonpsychiatric clinicians and the prevention teams.

The most common complaint from soldiers presenting to the CSC, consistent with the CSH, was for evaluation of "home-front issues," such as difficulties with significant others or family members at the home station or elsewhere in the United States or Germany. Depressed mood, insomnia, and anxiety, most commonly in the form of panic attacks, hypervigilance, or "jumpiness," remained prevalent symptom complaints, but frank posttraumatic stress disorder (PTSD) was very rarely diagnosed among soldiers during their deployment.

With the chief complaints listed above, most practicing psychiatrists would recognize that targeted psychopharmacologic interventions would have an important role in helping to alleviate symptoms. As previously mentioned, military doctrine for CSC was written to support a linear Cold-War–style combat campaign. Linear battlefields with conventional mobility warfare feature a rapidly moving, fluid battlefield requiring more prevention and triage than formal diagnoses, treatment, and aftercare plans. Doctrine writers appeared to conceive definitive psychiatric care (permitting RTD) as a separate activity to occur in rear areas after CSC doctrinal interventions failed to achieve prompt RTD, or after the rapidly moving campaign concluded. Thus, no provisions in FM 8-51, the doctrine at the beginning of OIF I, detailed how a CSC should obtain or store medications or a recommended formulary. Since the beginning of OIF I, the Army recognized this change in underlying assumptions and the consequent need to revise CSC doctrine in OIF II (2004). Of note, treatments with potentially sedating medications, especially atypical antipsychotics for insomnia or anxiety and benzodiazepines for anxiety, received increasing scrutiny. Media coverage of the issue and command concern understandably arose about ensuring that soldiers remain alert during missions. Providers must use these options responsibly to alleviate symptoms while recognizing that soldiers may display less optimal performance or alertness if their symptoms remain unaddressed. Benzodiazepines demonstrated good efficacy in overcoming or desensitizing acute stressors, but these drugs require vigilance, responsible prescribing, and commensurate psychological interventions. Without this attention, escalating use occurred frequently, leading to habituation and perpetuation of anxiety symptoms after return to CONUS.

DIVISION MENTAL HEALTH SECTIONS

During OIF I, combat forces deployed as entire divisions, under the organizational structure of the "Operational Force" (all divisions except the 4th and 25th IDs) or "Force XXI" (the 4th and 25th IDs had changed to Force XXI by the beginning of OIF I). This organization differed from the new "modular" organizational structure now in place due to the Army's transformation after OIF I. This appendix relates specifically to the DMHS assets during OIF I, prior to the Army's transformation to the current modular organizational structure and operation.

The organically assigned DMHS assets belong specifically to the division, as permanent and integral parts of the division in peacetime and wartime. During a deployment, the DMHS can occasionally receive supplemental behavioral health PROFIS personnel if there is a shortage of assigned but needed personnel. In contrast to the DMHS, CSH and CSC-type units have few organic medical assets and receive most of their medical personnel from PROFIS. DMHS personnel operate within the division, both in garrison and in a deployed environment, as the primary behavioral health resources for the division. They evaluate and treat division soldiers, liaison with chain of command, and provide command consultation services for the various units within the division.

In garrison, the DMHS usually operates from one location as a full behavioral health section, generally located near other division medical assets. If division brigades are located in different geographical areas, such as Germany or Korea, then the DMHS will have more than one operating clinic. DMHS staff provide the full range of behavioral health services, including

- evaluation for all behavioral health disorders (whether self-referrals, command referrals, or medical referrals);
- treatment, including individual therapy, group therapy, and medication management; and
- prevention services (usually via command consultation and liaison).

In divisions structured in either the Operational or Force XXI structure, the DMHS generally has one division psychiatrist, one division psychologist, one division social worker, and six to eight behavioral health specialists (military occupational specialty 68Xs, previously designated as 91Xs). Depending on the organizational structure of the division (ie, Operational vs Force XXI), DMHS personnel were either all assigned to the main support battalion (as part of the division support command brigade) or to a specific support battalion within the division.

In an Operational structured division (eg, the 101st Airborne [Air Assault] Division), all DMHS personnel were assigned to the main support battalion. However, in a Force XXI structured division (eg, the 4th ID), the DMHS operated together in garrison but were actually assigned to the various support battalions. In these divisions, the division psychiatrist and noncommissioned officer-in-charge (NCOIC) were assigned to the division support battalion. The other DMHS personnel were assigned to the FSMCs, part of the forward support battalions, designated to support a specific brigade combat team during deployment. Under this structure, usually one behavioral health officer (either the division social worker or division psychologist) along with one or two behavioral health specialists were assigned to each of the FSMCs. However, with three FSMCs but only two available behavioral health officers (ie, a social worker and a psychologist), one FSMC would have a team of only behavioral health specialists assigned to it, with no assigned officer.

According to linear battlefield doctrine, the division psychiatrist provided behavioral health service support to division personnel evacuated from the maneuver brigades, as well as to personnel assigned or attached to units collocated with the division support units and division headquarters. However, as stated previously in this appendix, OIF I did not develop according to a "linear" battlefield model, particularly with the various maneuver brigades and brigade combat teams located on different FOBs throughout Iraq, with nonlinear patterns of enemy engagements or orientation of combat forces. Therefore, patients from the various maneuver brigades could be routed directly to the division or main support battalion according to doctrine, or directly to a nearby higher echelon of care (eg, CSC or CSH). Proximity became more important as travel hazards increased and soldiers understandably presented to the closest asset with the capability to adequately evaluate the problem and minimize overall risk.

Once receiving deployment orders, the DMHS shifted operations from the garrison mission to the deployment or operational mission. This included screening for and identifying division soldiers whose behavioral health conditions made them unsuitable for deployment, transferring their care to the garrison hospital behavioral health assets, and processing recommendations for medical separations (via Medical Evaluation Board) or administrative separations (ie, AR 635-200, Chapter 5-13/5-17), as indicated. Reserve component units frequently referred soldiers for evaluation prior to deploying, but sometimes these referrals occurred after arrival in theater when medical screening revealed that the soldier was taking mood stabilizers or antipsychotic medications for the treatment of bipolar disorder or psychotic disorders that the Reserve unit did not fully recognize. Subsequent screening processes became more comprehensive and prevented deployment of these vulnerable soldiers in later rotations. As expected, other routine referrals to behavioral health included cases of existing depression, anxiety disorders, or substance-use disorders.

Case Study A1-5: A 44-year-old E-8 reservist with over 25 years in service was referred for anxiety and alcohol dependence. He had been drinking one half of a fifth of whiskey in Kuwait every other day. Prior to deployment he drank a case of beer from Friday night to Sunday night, with an occasional beer on the weekdays. The soldier initially presented prior to deployment, secondary to increasing anxiety and depression related to recent activation to active duty and occupational difficulties. He minimized his alcohol use at this time. He was assigned as his unit's first sergeant but did not feel he could handle the position's responsibility. In addition to symptoms of anxiety, he also reported uncontrollable crying spells, poor concentration, fatigue, and decreased appetite. The initial CONUS provider diagnosed him with an adjustment disorder with anxious and depressed mood, starting him on citalopram, clonazepam, and zolpidem. He was found fit to deploy but directed to seek behavioral health services once he arrived in theater. He returned for aftercare 2 weeks later while still in CONUS and reported that his symptoms had improved and that he had stopped the prescribed medications.

After deploying to theater, his symptoms of anxiety returned and he sought help at the CSH in Kuwait. His provider restarted him on his previous medications but he stopped these again after 4 weeks. He subsequently presented again in relation to pending Uniform Code of Military Justice charges due to his alcohol consumption while deployed, a violation of General Order Number 1. He did not feel that he could go on with his job and was evacuated from theater for treatment of his alcohol dependence and anxiety.

As preparations for deployment continued, all garrison DMHS operations were shut down and the care of soldiers remaining behind transferred to the garrison hospital behavioral health assets, while the DMHS focused on equipment readiness, packing, and training for the upcoming deployment missions. Packing followed existing up-to-date load plans and focused on identifying what supplies and equipment would be needed in theater. Packing included inventory, assessment, and loading the equipment already "owned" by the DMHS, per the Table of Organization and Equipment (tents, light sets, field desks, chairs, cots, and vehicles). It also included assessing the need for and acquiring other anticipated useful supplies necessary to conduct the mission (eg, supplies for writing patient notes, maintaining charts, performing command referrals, writing mental status evaluations, useful templates, prescription pads, and any important resources such as textbooks or field manuals).

Of note, supplies of psychotropic medications were not obtained prior to leaving the garrison environment. Once deployed and OIF I began, the absence of pharmaceutical supplies quickly became apparent, with poor availability in theater and lengthy delays to establish dependable supply chains. By approximately midsummer 2003, a dependable supply chain had developed and medications became readily accessible through the division's own supply chains or at the various CSH units.

Maneuver brigades and their supporting units convoyed from Kuwait into Iraq during the initial assault that began OIF I. Some combat units, such as the 101st Airborne (Air Assault) Division, that were directly involved in the initial assault "jumped" from one location to the next. This occurred from the beginning of formal combat operations until approximately May 2003, as units repositioned with a northerly movement direction and support units completed their convoys afterwards. As the mission evolved, permanent FOBs became established, with designated units operating out of a given location. During the previous "jumping" phase, conducting behavioral health and support operations had the unique challenge of operating in temporary environments without the stability, infrastructure, or luxuries of an established base. Prior to arriving and setting up at their permanent FOBs, the various maneuver brigades and supporting units (main and forward support battalions) remained in one location for only a few days to weeks, conducting operations from tents and makeshift buildings. Conditions remained austere for all units during this time, and did not provide ideal conditions for conducting sustainable operations. Fortunately the behavioral health mission did not have significant equipment requirements, and the DMHS teams experienced limited adverse effects because they required only a pen and paper to document encounters and a location to see patients. Providers could see patients in any safe, convenient, and relatively comfortable place. Providers utilized their ingenuity to create clinical spaces, for instance, in the small DMHS tent, in the back of a HMMWV, or in any "field-expedient" location providing a minimal amount of privacy for soldiers. Once established in the permanent FOBs, units dedicated more time and resources to setting up tents for permanent operations or occupying and improving old, abandoned Iraqi buildings on the FOB premises, converting them for living and working accommodations.

As previously mentioned, in a deployed environment, the DMHS section was divided into small two- to three-person teams (usually composed of a behavioral health officer—psychiatrist, psychologist, or social worker—and one or two behavioral health specialists) integrally located with the support battalion. Therefore, these were small operations, usually working out of a small tent or other accommodations, available 24 hours a day to accommodate soldiers who could present at any time (because soldiers presented unexpectedly day or night after convoying several hours from another FOB that lacked behavioral health assets). These DMHS teams were able to provide a range of behavioral health services and support to all the soldiers in the supported brigade and in their vicinity or catchment area. They were responsible for direct behavioral health patient care, as in garrison, with services that included

- evaluation of acute behavioral health issues whether presented via self-referral or command referral;
- command consultation; and
- treatment, including brief supportive therapy and medication management, if required.

In terms of the types of cases presenting for treatment to DMHS, the whole spectrum of behavioral health concerns was represented, from significant Axis I disorders to subthreshold symptoms consistent with adjustment disorders related to situational stressors (occupational, home-front, or other operational stressors, classified, per Army doctrine, as "combat and operational stress reactions") to misconduct stress behaviors. The most common cases presenting were those not meeting the threshold for actual significant Axis I disorders but rather were more consistent with misconduct stress behaviors (eg, substance abuse, fighting) or combat and operational stress reactions—problems that might formerly have been diagnosed, per the *Diagnostic and Statistical Manual of Mental Disorders*, 4th edition, terminology, as occupational problems, adjustment disorders, or even partner-relational problems. Soldiers were presenting with symptoms of stress related to the "operational" stress of functioning in an austere environment with extreme temperatures, extended separation from home and family, lack of privacy, and increased behavioral and physical demands. There was significant occupational stress from difficulties with peers or superiors; home-front stress from family, partner-relational, or financial concerns; or just frustration with the environment and the cumulative effect of the various stressors.

Soldiers also presented with symptoms of actual Axis I depressive disorders, anxiety disorders, bipolar illness, psychosis, and attention deficit hyperactivity disorder (ADHD), either newly presenting or with diagnoses present prior to deployment (the latter cases needing continued treatment and routine medication management, particularly for depression, ADHD, or anxiety). A significant number of soldiers also presented with substance use issues, usually related to alcohol or other drugs (such as "Iraqi valium," which they acquired illegally from Iraqis). The presentation of soldiers with acute stress disorder (ASD) or PTSD-type symptoms related to traumatic combat experiences was rarer at the beginning of OIF I prior to the maturation of the insurgency. However, by approximately August 2003, after the increase in insurgent attacks (eg, IEDs, rocket-propelled grenades, mortar attacks), the number of soldiers presenting with ASD/PTSD symptoms notably increased. Overall, the ratio was approximately 6 to 4 for soldiers presenting with either "misconduct stress behaviors" (eg, substance abuse, assault on other soldiers) or subthreshold symptoms classified in Army parlance as "combat and operational stress reactions" to those presenting with significant Axis I disorders.

The number of patients presenting to DMHS usually ranged from eight to twelve soldiers per day. Soldiers generally presented as walk-ins (either as self-referrals or as command referrals). Most presentations were patients with an acute crisis; those who presented for routine treatment (ie, medication refills or follow-up) usually came whenever their operational mission would allow or, if located on another base, whenever they could "hop" a ride on a convoy that was traveling to the FOB where DMHS was located. Command referrals were usually acute (ie, for soldiers with imminent risk issues) but were also occasionally for routine, nonacute concerns.

In addition to evaluation and treatment of both acute and routine issues, DMHS teams accomplished other associated behavioral health activities, similar to those in a garrison-type environment. These included behavioral health evaluations, as required, for administrative separations (Chapters 13 and 14 separations) and recommendations to command for Chapter 5-13 or 5-17 administrative separation for soldiers whose conditions clearly indicated unsuitability for continued service. Sanity boards were also conducted for soldiers undergoing court-martial. In addition, evaluations were done occasionally for soldiers planning to attend drill sergeant or recruiting school upon redeployment. The DMHS staff also provided consultation on a regular basis to commanders, first sergeants, chaplains, other medical personnel, and Judge Advocate General personnel, to ensure the safest, most appropriate, and most efficient dispositions for soldiers.

Examples of cases that presented to DMHS included the following:

- soldiers who "locked and loaded" their weapon against their unit members; there were several cases a month of significant soldier versus soldier violence.
- soldiers in acute suicidal crises, including soldiers of all ranks, who had locked and loaded their weapon and held it to their head;
- a soldier with a past history of clinical depression who had been barred from convoys/patrols by his unit because he had been taking "pot shots" at local Iraqis;
- a soldier involved in "horseplay" with two other soldiers that "got out of hand" when the soldier pulled out his bayonet, which caused the threatened soldier to pull out his 9-mm pistol;
- single or married soldiers presenting in recurrent suicidal crises after learning that soldiers with whom they were sexually involved were, simultaneously, sexually involved with other soldiers in the unit;
- cases of soldiers who consumed alcohol and became belligerent, suicidal, and/or homicidal, and occasionally assaulted other soldiers, or held their squad at gunpoint while intoxicated (two cases occurred on one FOB);
- soldiers who made suicide attempts by overdose or who had unintentionally overdosed on "Iraqi valium" obtained from local Iraqis (with prolonged sedated, amnestic periods);
- multiple soldiers who "head-butted" brick or concrete walls (or fractured hands from punching walls) due to anger involving NCOs, coworkers, or home-front issues;
- a sergeant major with anxiety, panic attacks, and nightmares of death after being accidentally electrocuted by another soldier;
- soldiers with acute manic or psychotic presentations (although rarer); and
- soldiers with notable ASD- and PTSD-type anxiety symptoms resulting from involvement in combat operations.

The 4th ID DMHS psychiatrist/NCOIC team was collocated with a CSC restoration team on the same FOB, which was very helpful for soldiers who presented acutely and who could benefit from a brief period of restoration away from their acute stressors. Soldiers who required evacuation to higher echelons of care, including out of theater, were evacuated to the closest CSH.

From April 2003 to November 2003, the 4th ID psychiatrist and DMHS NCOIC at the 4th ID DSB, located at FOB Speicher in Tikrit, Iraq, evaluated over 600 soldiers. Of this number, 22 were referred to the CSC restoration program (due to operational stress reactions that made them temporarily nonmission capable), and 12 were evacuated to higher echelons of medical care (including some out of theater), resulting in an RTD rate of a minimum of 94.4%. This rate improved later in the year when the same team (although with a new division psychiatrist) saw an additional 480 soldiers from mid-November 2003 until March 2004, when the 4th ID redeployed stateside, with only three soldiers requiring evacuation out of theater.

SUMMARY

Over the past 8 years, behavioral health issues in the Army and the Department of Defense have changed greatly and continue to do so. This appendix is historical in nature. It may be used as a training tool for military residents and fellows (for example, in a military psychiatry seminar) or to assist in preparation of future providers deploying to an immature theater. The case studies may be used for discussions about varying stressors and other conditions that might be encountered during deployments. Regardless of the use of this material, the discussion of each major unit during OIF I and the challenges faced should be considered in future operations.

RECOMMENDED READING

American Psychiatric Association. *Diagnostic and Statistical Manual of Mental Disorders, 4th edition, Text Revision (DSM IV-TR).* Arlington, Va: APA; 2008.

US Department of the Army. Mental Health Advisory Team (MHAT) Reports I-VI. Available at: http://www.behavioralhealth.army.mil/research/index.html. Accessed November 23, 2010.

US Department of the Army. *Combat Stress Control in a Theater of Operations.* Washington, DC: DA; 29 September 1994. Field Manual 8-51.

US Department of the Army. *Combat and Operational Stress Control.* Washington, DC: DA; July 2006. Field Manual 4-02.51.

US Department of the Army. *Active Duty Enlisted Administrative Separations.* Washington, DC: DA; April 27, 2010. AR 635-200.

Jones FD, Sparacino LR, Wilcox VL, Rothberg JM, Stokes JW, eds. *War Psychiatry.* In: Zajtchuk R, Bellamy RF, eds. *Textbooks of Military Medicine.* Washington, DC: DA, Office of The Surgeon General, Borden Institute; 1995.

Appendix 2

OPERATIONAL PSYCHIATRY IN OPERATION ENDURING FREEDOM

BRYAN L. BACON, DO*; MATTHEW J. BARRY, DO†; AND JAMES DEMER, MD‡

*Major, Medical Corps, US Army; Disaster Psychiatry Fellow, Department of Psychiatry, Uniformed Services University of the Health Sciences, 4301 Jones Bridge Road, Bethesda, Maryland 20814; formerly, Chief, Behavioral Health, Bavaria Medical Department, Vilseck, Germany

†Major, Medical Corps, US Army Reserves; Staff Psychiatrist, Department of Behavioral Health, Rochester Veterans Affairs Outpatient Clinic, 465 Westfall Road, Rochester, New York 14620; formerly, Major, Medical Corps, US Army; Chief of Psychiatric Service USA MEDDAC and 10th Mountain Division Psychiatrist, Fort Drum, New York

‡Attending Child Psychiatrist, Inpatient Child Psychiatry Service, Hutchings Psychiatric Center, 7682 Warrior's Path, Baldwinsville, New York 13027; formerly, Major, Medical Corps, US Army; Division Psychiatrist, 10th Mountain Division, Fort Drum, New York

INTRODUCTION

The mental health mission in support of Operation Enduring Freedom (OEF) possesses numerous challenges unique to the region and history of the nation. To best understand the complexities associated with mental health operations in this theater, a logical starting point is a brief history of Afghanistan itself and the United States military involvement in support of OEF. This will provide the basic construct as to the evolution of the mission and its inherent obstacles.

The appendix will then cover deployment-related mental health issues and an overview of the mental health mission in OEF. Five clinical cases are presented at the end of the appendix to facilitate learning by emphasizing the wide array of subject matter that will test the skills of the deployed mental health clinician.

A BRIEF HISTORY OF AFGHANISTAN

The Islamic Republic of Afghanistan has a turbulent history dating back to 2000 BCE and has endured countless warring factions and oppressive regimes. From the Aryans to Alexander the Great, from Genghis Khan to the Soviet Union, and most recently, the Taliban, Afghanistan has known little stability and peace.

Afghanistan, or "Land of the Afghans," emerged from the Iranian state of Khorasan and won its independence from Britain in 1919. Failing economic and social reforms in the 1960s and 1970s led to public discontent and invigorated the Marxist People's Democratic Party of Afghanistan (PDPA). In 1978, the PDPA overthrew the government and established the Democratic Republic of Afghanistan. Unfortunately, political infighting and Marxist-based reforms imposed upon the overwhelmingly Muslim population fueled a rebellion and ultimately a civil war. To bolster the communist influence, the Soviet Union deployed the 40th Army in December 1979. The Soviet war in Afghanistan, aimed at crushing the antigovernment Mujahideen insurgency and empowering the PDPA, ended in failure 9 years later.

The social, economic, and cultural void that ensued provided fertile ground for the rise of the Taliban, a politico-religious force that oppressively imposed a strict interpretation of Sharia law. By the mid-1990s, the Taliban had seized control of the majority of the country. Their tenure was relatively short, however, as the Taliban's support and harboring of international terrorists led to its demise in 2001. Significant steps toward achieving national self-sufficiency and stability have occurred recently. A ratified constitution, free elections, emphasis on education, and enhancement of a national infrastructure are all prominent examples of this progress.

Although the recent discovery of vast mineral stores, valued at approximately 1 trillion US dollars, may translate to economic security and prosperity for the nation, the realization may take decades. Currently Afghanistan remains one of poorest nations outside of Africa, and one that relies on an agriculturally based economy. Unfortunately, only 1% of its land is suitable for agroindustry, and only one-tenth of that used for farming. Cash crops are in demand and poppy production fills that void. Poppy production accounts for 57% of Afghanistan's gross domestic product. Aside from Afghanistan's reliance on the poppy industry, the ongoing insurgency, susceptibility to corruption, high rates of illiteracy and unemployment, oppression of the female population, rugged terrain, and rich history of tribalism present formidable challenges to the nation and its people.

US MILITARY INVOLVEMENT IN AFGHANISTAN

In response to the terrorist attacks of September 11th, President George W Bush demanded on October 7th, 2001, that the Taliban "close terrorist training camps; hand over leaders of the al Qaeda network; and return all foreign nationals, including American citizens, unjustly detained in your country." This ultimatum was rejected. On October 20th, 15 land-based bombers, 25 Navy strike aircraft, and Tomahawk missiles from US and British ships launched the first strikes of Operation Enduring Freedom. The initial aerial assault targeted terrorist strongholds in Kandahar, Jalalabad, and Kabul, and was soon followed by the deployment of ground forces.

The theater of operations in Afghanistan has matured significantly since the onset of military action. A multinational coalitional force, dominated by US personnel, is now directed by the International Security Assistance Force (ISAF). The North Atlantic Treaty Organization (NATO) took command and coordination of the ISAF in August 2003; it represents NATO's first mission outside the Euro-Atlantic area. ISAF's role is to assist the government of Afghanistan and the international community in maintaining security within its area of operation. ISAF supports the government of

Afghanistan in expanding its authority to the rest of the country, and in providing a safe and secure environment conducive to free and fair elections, the spread of the rule of law, and the reconstruction of the country.

US ARMY MENTAL HEALTH OPERATIONS IN DEPLOYMENT

The primary mission for US Army psychiatry and the mental health team derives from the US Army Medical Department's mission to "conserve the fighting strength." In the combat theater, mental health providers accomplish this mission through an array of services that assist the chain of command in controlling mental illness and combat and operational stress through sound prevention programs and effective treatment modalities that establish the expectation of recovery.

Mental health providers deploy immediately with a combat force and may include psychiatrists, psychologists, psychiatric nurse practitioners, social workers, or mental health technicians. Typically, the total number and type of providers vary from one rotation to the next. Assets are often in the form of combat and operational stress control (COSC) teams, division mental health providers, brigade behavioral science officers, and technicians or activated reservists, and may incorporate all branches of the military at any given time. Such a convoluted arrangement demands a well-delineated command structure and working agreements between all parties to greatly improve mission effectiveness and quality of care. To successfully execute the mission in any combat endeavor, providers must employ sound preparation, outreach, prevention, education, and consultative and clinical practices.

Preparation

Predeployment planning is often limited in its scope or absent altogether. However, when the opportunity avails itself, the behavioral health professional should identify the mission, its requirements, and available assets. Familiarizing oneself with the theater prior to deployment is crucial and can be accomplished in myriad ways, ranging from participation in the predeployment site survey to a simple call or email to the team that will be replaced. Reviewing after-action reports and speaking with providers from previous deployments may be beneficial as well. Collecting pertinent and accurate information will greatly assist with the determination of staffing needs. Once staff members are identified, it becomes possible to know the team prior to departure. Furthermore, establishing relationships with commands, chaplains, and medical providers and screening deploying troops before departure will serve the mission well.

Outreach

Recent combat operations have engaged the enemy in a low-intensity, nontraditional battlefield. Such conflicts are characterized by an insidious sense of randomness and loculated pockets of activity within a large geographical space, using conventional weapons typically combined with asymmetrical tactics ("terrorism") and applied use of intelligence.

In accommodating this type of mission, troops are often strategically scattered across the area of operations and reside in rustic installations called firebases or forward operating bases (FOBs). Based on mission necessity, the troop population, capability, and firepower, these outposts are in a nearly constant state of fluidity. Accordingly, it is critical that a relationship develops between key personnel at the smaller forward posts and mental health providers in theater. Meeting the senior leadership, medical assets, and chaplaincy will be essential, as they will serve as liaisons between individual and unit needs, and the mental health assets. Assigning specific providers (who periodically visit their catchment) to particular FOBs and firebases will further this dynamic by advocating for basic needs to improve morale. These behavioral health personnel provide a sense of familiarity to both the local troop population and leadership, and a commitment to

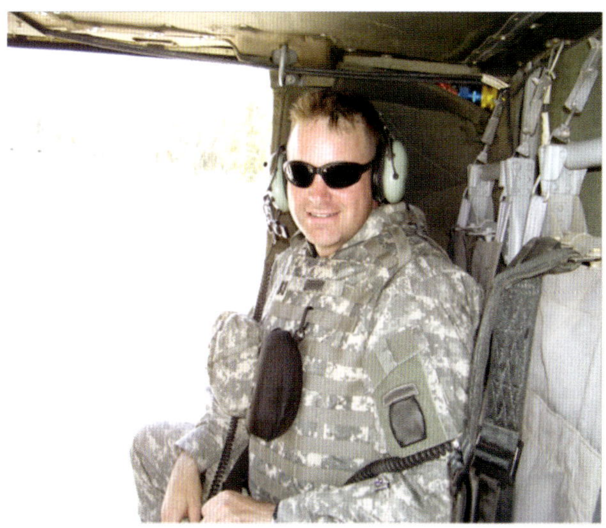

Figure A2-1. The mental health mission in OEF demands mobility from its providers.

a

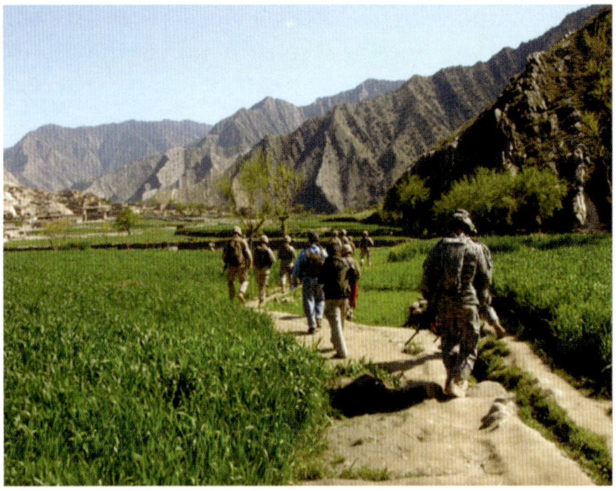

b

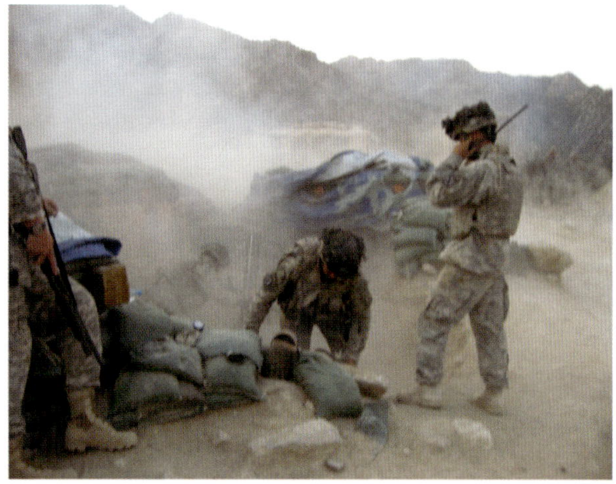

c

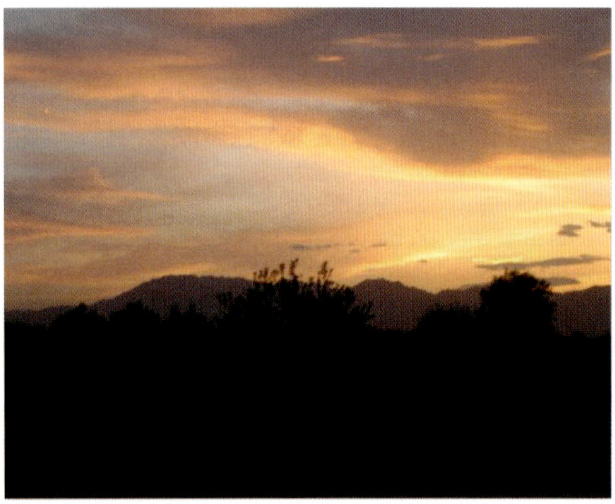

Figure A2-2. Credibility is gained not only with clinical knowledge but also by sharing soldiers' experiences, such as foot patrols (**a**); sharing in their daily activities in remote locations (**b**); or just enjoying an Asian sunset with them (**c**).

continuity of care for those relying on their services (Figure A2-1 and Figure A2-2).

Prevention

From a classic medical model, prevention is any activity by which an individual avoids the development of a disease or condition (primary prevention), diagnoses a disease in an early stage or prevents its recurrence (secondary prevention), or avoids a disease's worsening and restores oneself to an optimal level of functioning (tertiary prevention). The importance of prevention efforts cannot be understated in the theater; they can play a pivotal role in troop readiness and mission effectiveness.

Most often, deploying service members receive an array of predeployment training that typically includes psychoeducational briefs on broad mental health topics, such as the emotional cycle of deployment or general psychiatric symptomatology. However, this training is not guaranteed, and the content and quality may vary; primary prevention must be augmented in theater. An excellent means of accomplishing this is securing a platform at the theater-wide inprocessing brief that all arriving US personnel attend. Another option is meeting with local chaplains and medical providers to provide information on common symptoms and issues, and how to engage mental health services.

As in any wartime period, there will be certain military occupational specialties (MOSs) with greater exposure and risk for emotional issues. These groups should be identified early and visited regularly utilizing the "therapy by walking around" concepts described by Milliken with the goal of providing a means of decompression, assessment, and formal mental health services if needed. Typically, mortuary affairs, combat medics, medical evacuation (medevac) crews, physicians (surgeons and trauma doctors in particular), nurses, chaplains, vehicle drivers, and senior leadership, among others, would benefit from secondary prevention.

Following a discrete, often traumatic event, tertiary prevention may be implemented. Currently, there is much debate as to the value and efficacy of critical incident stress management or debriefings, the seven-step Mitchell model in particular. Army mental health now supports the concept of traumatic event management (TEM), which enables the clinician to develop a program tailored to the specific needs of the unit considering the actual event, theater tempo, unit history, and response.

Regardless of the model employed, tertiary prevention will be a high-profile item in theater. Clinicians will be responsible to intervene at their discretion, while assessing, supporting, and educating various command elements that may still be fluent in the "antiquated" critical incident stress management (CISM) dialect.

Education

Developing a modified, yet aggressive, education plan will enhance quality of care while blunting the workload burden. A well-trained mental health technician can effectively serve as an intake coordinator, supportive or skills-based therapist, group facilitator, prevention specialist, liaison to the enlisted ranks, and representative to forward installations. Investing time in supervision and basic instruction will greatly improve the efficiency of the deployed team.

Besides enhancing intrinsic resources, educational efforts intended for medics, physician assistants, physicians, and chaplains can improve care throughout the area of operations. Broad topics such as terminology, diagnostic assessments, basic psychopharmacology, relaxation training, and sleep hygiene instruction can effectively accelerate initiation of treatment plans and reinforce their efficacy, reduce the need for unnecessary evacuations, and filter legitimate mental health cases from administrative or occupational issues of discord.

Consultation

Deployed mental health providers serve as the subject matter experts for mental health and combat and operational stress. Commanders will often seek the expertise and recommendations of the behavioral health professional concerning individual or unit issues in the forms of a command-directed mental health evaluation or unit climate assessment, respectively. Furthermore, input will be requested for larger policy issues affecting the deployed force, such as suicide prevention, sexual assault programs, and redeployment planning. The behavioral health provider will also serve as a theater-wide consultant to medical providers from all branches of the US military, as well as those employed by civilian contracting agencies and coalition nations.

Clinical Operations

Although much of the mission will be firmly rooted in the principles and practices of COSC, placing a provider at each site in theater is impossible because of the numerous forward locations and limited mental health staffing resources. Thus, the mental health assets are typically divided into smaller teams and placed at several mature locations that have sizeable troop populations, access to intratheater transportation, and appropriate medical, intelligence, and command support services.

The pace of routine clinical work in the deployed setting is usually less demanding than one might experience while in garrison. It is recommended that set hours of operation are established and an on-call schedule is developed to preserve boundaries and protect against burnout while maintaining availability for those in need. The scope of practices in the clinic depends on the vision, resources, and staffing of the unit but ordinarily consists of individual counseling and brief therapy, time-limited skills and cognitive behaviorally based groups, medication management, mental status evaluations (for special schools/duties or administrative separation), command-directed evaluations, and seminars on topics such as anger management, stress reduction, smoking cessation, and relationship issues.

As with all clinical operations, standard operating procedures should be developed and followed. Roles, responsibilities, command structure, documentation, record storage, admission, evacuation, on-call coverage, and policies for various programs (such as suicide prevention, command-directed evaluations, TEM, and so forth) are topics that should be formally outlined in a standard operating procedure that is clear, concise, and understood by all members of the mental health team.

MENTAL HEALTH OPERATIONS IN AFGHANISTAN

In late 2001, mental health assets sparsely populated the Afghanistan theater of operations. A pair of mental health technicians supported Kandahar, and a team of four (social worker, occupational therapist, and two technicians) were in Uzbekistan before relocating to Bagram Airfield in early 2002. A psychiatrist and social worker in Kuwait provided consultative services. Each rotation since then has witnessed an improved presence.

Common presentations include occupational discord, partner-relational problems, sleep problems, and stress. Psychosomatic, anxiety, and depression conditions represent a modest number of overall cases, while psychotic disorders and purely combat-related presentations are fairly rare. One can expect a robust stream of requests for command-directed evaluations and other administrative psychiatry tasks, and providers must maintain a healthy skepticism for secondary gain issues.

Effective screening and prevention programs, access to care in theater, and an underlying expectation of recovery has led to a return-to-duty rate in excess of 98% in recent years. Despite the success, Afghanistan presents an array of unique obstacles that may compromise satisfactory execution of the mental health mission. These obstacles must be addressed to ensure mission effectiveness.

Chain of Command

Serving under ISAF, there are many layers of command intricacies that are often magnified by joint-service endeavors and the modularity of the Army. Providers should anticipate working closely with other branches of service and learn to negotiate across command structures. Further, roles and responsibilities, and the chain of command, should be promptly established so that all stakeholders understand mission specifics.

Logistics

Clinical operational sites are selected based upon activities in theater, troop populations, and the availability of infrastructure, intelligence, command support, resources, and travel opportunities. Considering these variables, recent clinical sites in Afghanistan have included Bagram, Kandahar, Orgun-E, Jalalabad, Kabul, and Salerno. With troops spread across the theater, and highly mobile in response to mission evolution, clinical sites may have to change during the course of a rotation. Additionally, temporary prepositioning of mental health assets at selected FOBs and firebases based on tactical operational intelligence can be a valuable tool. Ultimately, COSC forward activities must possess flexibility to accommodate the fluid battlefield.

Communication

Although the theater has evolved significantly, telephone and Internet access remain unreliable. Developing contingency plans and creative problem solving must suffice until communication systems fully mature.

Travel

Movement throughout the area of operations is critical to mission success but remains profoundly inefficient. COSC teams tasked to forward locations routinely wait multiple days for travel on both sides of the mission. Flights are often cancelled due to combat operations, maintenance issues, or weather conditions. Ground convoys present many of the same limitations, along with the risk for attack from improvised explosive devices (IEDs) and vehicle-borne improvised explosive devices (VBIEDs). To ameliorate this situation, establish a good rapport with the local air and ground movement request officers, learn all the potential means of travel to particular areas (scheduled "ring" helicopter flights, special rotary flights, C-130 and STOAL [short take off and landing] flights, and ground convoys), and prepare for delays.

Documentation

OEF has introduced the electronic theater medical information (TMIP) program. This will ultimately help with patient care, but not all locations will possess the same technology or maintenance capabilities. Establish documentation standard operating procedures and rely on "FOB logs" to create a patient list and foster seamless transitions of care at each site.

Data Collection

Historically speaking, there has never been a consistent outcome measure or statistical collection system that has passed between rotations. Hence, it is nearly impossible to compare relevant statistical rates with previous deployments. TMIP will assist with some of the demographic and diagnostic data collection, but the development of a comprehensive program that provides meaningful outcome measures has yet to be implemented.

CONCLUSION

Providers face an array of challenges in delivering quality mental health services in the deployed setting. Further, OEF introduces unique obstacles that synergistically complicate the already challenging mission. However, relying on sound strategies firmly rooted in conceptual military psychiatry will foster a comprehensive system of care for soldiers on the ground and will be effective in conserving the fighting force.

CASE STUDIES

Case Study A2-1: Importance of History of Present Illness (HPI)

Situation: A married active duty Army E4 white male with no past psychiatric history self-presented to the mental health clinic in Bagram complaining of suicidal ideation and poor sleep for the past 5 days. The soldier explained that his wife was possibly cheating on him and the only way to salvage the marriage was getting home. If he could not get home, "life is not worth living." A detailed interview and suicide assessment revealed low risk for self-harm, with no plan. He had just returned from midtour rest and recuperation (R&R) leave 3 days prior to presentation and was waiting in transient status at Bagram for a flight back to his FOB.

Assessment: marital discord, occupational problem with conditional suicidality.

Treatment: supportive therapy daily while awaiting flight, symptom relief with Ambien, return to FOB as soon as possible.

Teaching points:

1. Expect to see a bump in self-referrals during the midtour R&R leave window.
2. Conduct a thorough evaluation of every soldier.
3. Target tangible symptoms such as sleep; educate and support.
4. Firmly set expectation that service members will return to their unit.
5. Identify funneling points for R&R and establish a clinical presence at those locations. When soldiers return to theater, they often have to wait days for travel back to their FOB. During that time they are in transient status with no significant accountability. Work with unit liaisons at such sites to assign daily tasks for these personnel and expedite their return to the FOB and unit.

Case Study A2-2: Traumatic Event Management Gone Wrong

Situation: A tragic helicopter crash occurred in theater resulting in several deaths. Approximately 1 week later, the clinic was asked by the chaplain and flight surgeon to assist with a "debriefing." Eager to help with this high-profile incident, mental health resources were pledged in support.

Process: The accident was detailed by the flight surgeon; the chaplain provided the unit history. A suitable place of meeting familiar to the unit was selected. Due to the number of individuals, it was decided to have two sessions—one for officers and another for enlisted. The sessions began with the commander providing a review of the accident and an update on the investigation. He then entertained questions. Troops were then allowed to depart or continue with the voluntary group debriefing. All stayed, many of them reluctantly. Unknown to the mental health providers, members of the command stayed in the room, taking notes. The chaplain assumed a role as a co-facilitator, yet would leave the group, interrupt, and make off-target statements. The resentment among the soldiers was palpable and the provider was clearly seen as an agent of the command.

Teaching points:

1. Obtain a thorough unit history; an inadequate report was provided in this situation because there was long-standing animosity, stemming from myriad issues, between the soldiers and command.
2. If your TEM includes a group modality, make sessions truly voluntary, with no command influence and no note taking.
3. Determine who is facilitating before proceeding.
4. Be sensitive: don't patronize or insult the dynamics by splitting up teams that may include both officers and enlisted.

Case Study A2-3: Use Skills and Get Creative

Situation: A unit was involved in a noncombat motor vehicle accident in an area densely populated with civilians. Despite their best efforts, civilian casualties and deaths resulted. As the soldiers began to aid the injured, the crowd swelled in number and voracity. Many soldiers likened the masses and situation to the film *Blackhawk Down.* All feared for their safety as the atmosphere soon became confrontational; rocks and other debris rained down on the soldiers. Upon return to their FOB, the unit commander requested assistance for his soldiers. A psychiatrist visited the FOB, spending a few days helping soldiers normalize their reactions and consolidate their feelings. He suggested, if at all possible, a graduated return to activities outside the wire. Accordingly, a humanitarian mission was arranged at a nearby village. The psychiatrist accompanied the unit on the convoy, serving as a primary care physician for the medical component of the humanitarian mission. He was also present for the soldiers, many of whom were ambivalent about departing the confines of the FOB.

Teaching point:

1. Credibility is achieved through clinical competence, effective communication, honesty, and relating with soldiers. Creative approaches in developing rapport will augment this process.

Case Study A2-4: The Barber From Russia

Situation: The division psychiatrist was walking across the post and came upon a suspicious young man squatting alone by the roadside. Efforts to negotiate the language barrier were fruitless, so the psychiatrist went for help. The man followed and lunged for the officer's sidearm. The psychiatrist swatted the hand away; the man then retreated to seclusion. Shortly thereafter, the military police brought the man to the combat support hospital; they had found him scaling a fence to a minefield. A Russian interpreter translated a psychiatric diagnostic interview. The young man had a history of depression that was treated successfully in Russia. He was hired by a contractor to work at the installation barbershop. Since his arrival in Afghanistan, he became increasingly depressed with ruminations, hallucinations, and suicidal ideation. He was maintained at the combat support hospital (CSH) with a company escort and improved slightly with olanzapine. He was evacuated from theater 48 hours later and returned to Russia for definitive treatment.

Teaching points:

1. Although there are rigorous screening procedures for US service members, the same cannot be said for the large numbers of contractors working in support of OEF.
2. As one of only a few behavioral health subject matter experts in the country, you will find that skills in cultural psychiatry—from local Afghan nationals to civilian contract employees and Coalition forces—will be tested.
3. There are no inpatient psychiatric units in the CSH system. If individuals need admission, they can usually board in the CSH with an escort until they are evacuated.

Case Study A2-5: Keep the End State in Mind

Situation: Medical providers in southeastern Afghanistan became increasingly frustrated with the medical rules of engagement (ROE) of perserving "life, limb, or eyesight" as they pertained to the hundreds of local nationals who came to the front gate begging for medical care. The physicians organized and contacted the Minister of Health as well as the dominant nongovernmental organizations that were providing medical assistance in Kandahar. In the process, the former dean of the then-defunct medical school was found, a medical library was created through donations from the deployed physician's home departments, and classes were taught. The US physicians instructed the medical students in their specialties and arranged for logistical medical support for the local hospital. By the end of the 12-month rotation, the local hospital could handle treating mild and moderate wounds from an IED mass casualty event in the city.

Teaching points:

1. Counterinsurgency conflicts are partially won with robust humanitarian efforts.
2. If frustrated by the challenges offered by deployment, do something productive to change the situation.

Appendix 3

GOOD OR BAD NEWS? MEDIA COVERAGE OF SOLDIERS: FOCUS ON BEHAVIORAL HEALTH IN IRAQ DURING OPERATION IRAQI FREEDOM 05-07

JEFFREY S. YARVIS, PhD,* AND ELSPETH CAMERON RITCHIE, MD, MPH†

*Lieutenant Colonel, Medical Service Corps, US Army; Chief, Behavioral Health, Department of Psychiatry, Borden Pavilion, Walter Reed Army Medical Center, 6900 Georgia Avenue NW, Washington, DC 20307; formerly, Director of Social Work, Uniformed Services University of the Health Sciences, Bethesda, Maryland

†Colonel, US Army (Retired); formerly, Psychiatry Consultant to the Army Surgeon General, and Director, Behavioral Health Proponency, Office of The Surgeon General, Falls Church, Virginia; currently, Chief Clinical Officer, District of Columbia Department of Mental Health, 64 New York Avenue NE, 4th Floor, Washington, DC 20002

INTRODUCTION

The mental health of soldiers during the wars in Iraq and Afghanistan has generated ongoing media interest, focusing on major issues such as suicide, administrative discharges, psychiatric medications, fitness to deploy, care of wounded soldiers, and traumatic brain injury. This appendix provides some basic guidance for interacting with the media, followed by a discussion of media coverage during a specific period of time. Questions raised include: Does the media's portrayal of soldiers with mental illnesses present the public with an accurate picture? How does the representation of the behavioral health of soldiers affect behavioral health operations?

This appendix explores the possible operational impact of negative portrayals of soldiers with mental illnesses, using examples from Operation Iraqi Freedom (OIF) 05-07, through discussions of sensitive behavioral health issues such as suicide, portrayals of the combat environment to the public via documentaries such as *Baghdad ER*, and controversial events such as the killings in Haditha. In some cases media reporting can magnify the stigma experienced by soldiers with behavioral health problems, in addition to affecting the practices of military behavioral health. In other cases, the media can shed light on problems that need to be, and indeed are, addressed by military behavioral healthcare providers and policy makers.

BASICS OF INTERATING WITH THE MEDIA

Members of the media often approach military behavioral healthcare providers. If approached by a journalist, the first rule for the provider is to contact the public affairs office (PAO). PAO staff will handle negotiations with the media, and decide if it is an appropriate interaction. If an interview is approved, the interviewee should be prepared for surprise questions and always remember that quotations can be taken out of context. If giving a lecture, the speaker should keep in mind that media are often in the audience. Again, PAO staff should provide guidance for any public speaking or media interactions by military practitioners.

ISSUES AND CONCERNS WITH BEHAVIORAL HEALTH REPORTING ON IRAQ

During OIF 05-07, the war in Iraq entered its fourth year. Like all wars, the Iraq War is an extremely complex set of ever-changing dynamics. The battlefield has evolved considerably since US forces first invaded Iraq in 2003, changing from largely combat operations during the first months into civil-military endeavors since then. During this time the enemy had also evolved from organized Iraqi forces into varying militias, including some foreign fighters. Over 1,100 tribes live in the country; tribal territories often extend beyond Iraq's national boundaries. Other nation states also put external pressure on Iraq. Various religious and ethnic groups compete for scarce resources in the Bedouin cultural tradition. Privateers and black-marketeers make a living in chaotic social and economic circumstances. Iraqi politicians maintain different views about the best way to govern. Despite this complex and evolving environment, media reports have sometimes given a simplified impression that the ongoing conflict results from sectarian violence between the Sunni, Shia, and Kurdish groups.

Combat stress or behavioral health assets were positioned throughout Iraq to help soldiers negotiate their way through these complex operational and emotional terrains. During OIF 05-07, the ongoing war in Iraq affected behavioral healthcare in two important ways. First, enough time had elapsed by then for military leaders to be aware of outcomes and problems that had arisen from OIF I (the first rotation) and OIF II (the second rotation). Consequently, new policies involving the behavioral health community were initiated (ie, suicide prevention, use of psychiatric medications; see Chapter 25, Suicide Prevention, and Chapter 10, Psychiatric Medications in Military Operations, respectively, for further discussion of these topics). Secondly, the length of the conflict and the number of casualties had generated increasing media interest in the war and in behavioral health services available to soldiers. Although it is impossible to determine to what extent the media influenced the day-to-day operations of behavioral health providers, the increased scrutiny did concern military leadership. This translated into greater cognizance of behavioral health activities.

The media has covered wars since the advent of print journalism. With the introduction of motion pictures, war coverage reached larger audiences throughout World War II. During this period, as well as during the Korean War, most of the video reporting of the war was seen in movie theaters. It was not until Vietnam that images of war were televised into the homes of the US populace. This footage, however, was generally edited at a network before it was aired because the media lacked the capability of a live feed from the battlefield. Beginning with the Persian Gulf War (1990–1991), however, journalists were able to send live feeds from their embedded positions directly to television broadcasts. Commanders and politicians had virtually no time to review what might be broadcast, and in many cases heard of issues raised by the media only after they had been aired.

The following three issues—suicide, *Baghdad ER*, and Haditha—all of which involved situations during OIF 05-07, will be examined as they were reported by the media and acted upon by the military. Neither the nature of recent advances in media technology nor the media's effect on public opinion has been fully measured. However, it is not difficult to imagine that media coverage of behavioral health could have operational impacts and affect the behavior of soldiers. Mention Abu Ghraib or Haditha and one will elicit a wide range of reactions, from well informed to hearsay, from those responding. It is then that one can sense the true power and influence the media can have. The positive impact of this phenomenon is that the military often gains the attention and the political support it needs to address important psychological health needs of soldiers, for example, suicides in the Army.

Suicide Rates in the Army

Various media sources began reporting in 2003 that Army suicide rates were on the rise and that those soldiers deployed to Iraq and Kuwait experienced the greatest increase.[1] Although Army suicide statistics remained lower than for comparable age groups in the civilian population, the Army surgeon general, Lieutenant General James Peake, said that "any suicide is something we worry about and want to stop."[2] Despite the trend data being consistent with the civilian sector, recommendations were immediately implemented, including augmenting the Army's suicide prevention program and making behavioral healthcare more accessible to soldiers in combat and other high-stress environments. However, media reports, such as the articles on suicide, may alter mission focus and influence military behavioral health resources by diverting limited assets to respond to the reporting.

The Army's first mental health survey ever conducted in a combat zone took place in 2003 (see Chapter 5, Walter Reed Army Institute of Research Contributions During Operations Iraqi Freedom and Enduring Freedom, in this volume, for a more detailed discussion of the survey process). At the request of the commanding general, Combined Joint Task Force-7 of the US Central Command established and dispatched the first Mental Health Advisory Team (MHAT) to survey and provide recommendations on OIF-related behavioral health services. A team of 12 military and civilian psychiatrists, psychologists, social workers, and combat-stress experts surveyed 756 soldiers in Iraq between late August and early October 2003. They also surveyed behavioral health and medical care providers, unit leaders, and unit ministry staffs. The survey was conducted when conditions were at a low point: at the end of a very hot summer, before much of the infrastructure that created more comfortable living conditions had been put in place, and before most soldiers knew when they would redeploy to their home stations. The team leader of this first MHAT, Colonel Virgil Patterson, said one in four soldiers surveyed reported moderate or severe emotional, alcohol, or family problems. More than half reported low or very low morale.

After media reports on suicide began appearing, military behavioral health experts found themselves adding one additional task to their already significant duties: to maintain current and accurate data on suicide in theater and remain prepared to respond to media reports. For example, in 2003 the *Baltimore Sun* ran an article with the title "Army's Suicide Rate Has Outside Experts Alarmed," and the follow-on subtitle of "Most died serving in Iraq after major combat phase."[3] Similar reports were carried by most of the major news networks and papers. Later articles used language similar to that used by the *Baltimore Sun* in 2003. For example, the *Hartford Current* noted in 2007 that the "Army continues to struggle with suicides," and the "2006 Rate Of Self-Inflicted Deaths In Iraq Could Exceed Record Set In 2005."[4] Since OIF 05-07, an upward trend in suicide rates in active duty military has occurred, as discussed further in Chapter 25, Suicide Prevention, in this volume.

Baghdad ER

The 2006 HBO (Home Box Office) documentary *Baghdad ER* was a graphic and emotional account of the realities of war through the emergency room experiences of a combat support hospital. At the very outset of *Baghdad ER*, the producers pointed out that 90% of soldiers wounded in Iraq survive—the highest survival rate in American military history. (During OIF 05-07, survival rates exceeded 96%.[5])

Visual documentaries can serve as powerful reminders or "triggers" for soldiers who have been exposed to the sights, sounds, and smells of combat injuries; *Baghdad ER* was such a harsh reminder of the brutal realities of war. Military officials were allowed to preview the documentary and proactively prepare for its impact. The Army surgeon general at the time,

Lieutenant General Kevin Kiley, recommended that Army medicine plan for the effect that *Baghdad ER* might have on those who saw it. Said Kiley, "This film will have a strong impact on viewers and may cause anxiety for some soldiers and family members."[6] He noted that, "some may have strong reactions to the medical [surgical] procedures such as the amputation of a limb."[6] Kiley said military medical treatment facilities should be ready to assist troops and family members who might be upset after watching the film. He suggested that behavioral health facilities should extend their treatment hours and reach out to the troops proactively.[6] Kiley recognized that families and soldiers with ongoing psychological difficulties might have additional behavioral healthcare needs after the program aired. There were no known negative effects from viewing the program, although this was not systematically studied. From conversations with viewers, one of the authors (ECR) reported positive response to the program.

Haditha

Additional media interest in the military in Iraq came in the wake of the killing of 23 Iraqis on November 19, 2005, in Haditha, a city in the western Iraq province of Al Anbar. It was alleged that the killings were retribution for the attack on a convoy of US Marines with an improvised explosive device that killed Lance Corporal Miguel Terrazas.[7] A Marine Corps communiqué initially reported that 15 civilians were killed by the bomb's blast and 8 insurgents were subsequently killed when the Marines returned fire against those attacking the convoy. However, evidence provided by the media contradicted the Marines' account.[7] According to these media reports, at least 15, and allegedly all, of those killed were noncombatant civilians and were killed by the Marines.

Discussing the events in Haditha, psychiatrist Robert Jay Lifton explains that, "atrocity is a group activity."[8] Therefore, he wrote, "[t]o attribute the likely massacre at Haditha to 'a few bad apples' or to 'individual failures' is poor psychology and self-serving moralism."[8] Lifton says that the Haditha incident can be understood as what he calls "an atrocity-producing situation"—which he defines as

> one so structured, psychologically and militarily, that ordinary people, men or women no better or worse than you or I, can commit atrocities....Recognizing that atrocity is a group activity, one must ask how individual soldiers can so readily join in. I believe they undergo a type of dissociation that I call doubling—the formation of a second self. The individual psyche can adapt to an atrocity-producing environment by means of a sub-self that behaves as if it is autonomous and thereby joins in activities that would otherwise seem repugnant.[8]

In environments where sanctioned brutality becomes the norm, homicidal ideation and homicidal impulses, dormant in most individuals, are likely to be expressed.[9] The violent energy of the group becomes such that an individual soldier who questions it could by turned against by his or her peers. (For example, a Vietnam veteran who had been at My Lai told this author [JY] that he had refused to fire and pointedly lowered the barrel of his gun to the ground.) To resist intense group pressure requires a combination of conscience and moral courage, the very qualities that the military seeks to instill in soldiers as "core values."

Previously, Lifton explained his concept of atrocity-producing situations during a lecture about the possible torture of prisoners at Abu Ghraib.[8] In such situations, Lifton explained, although individuals are responsible for their own actions, when attempting to assign blame for atrocities it is perhaps more instructive to examine the conditions and examples set by higher commanders. When the rules of engagement do not appear to apply, or when ambiguities exist about what means may be used to achieve a "worthy" end, soldiers are less likely to adhere to the values that the military has sought to instill within them. Likewise, stress results from not knowing who the enemy is, not feeling safe, and witnessing evil. Cumulatively, these situations can contribute to behaviors that at times might exceed the rules of engagement. Additionally, the rules are sometimes difficult for a soldier to apply in the heat of battle or under circumstances outside normal soldier experiences or training. This explanation does not purport to dismiss the notion of accountability; however, it speaks to the process of "pathologizing" a new generation of soldiers.

Politics, social control, and mental health have long been tied together. For instance, diagnostic terms can reflect the bias of people and the times, such as "hysteria"—a term inherently biased against women. "Mental health" has been used both to limit civil rights and to advocate for civil rights. The former was discussed in the writings of the psychiatrist Thomas Szasz,[10] who suggested in 1961 that "mental illness" and the threat of being institutionalized were the means by which societies controlled those who strayed from the common morality. He advocated for the rights of those who had been institutionalized, setting in motion a movement that resulted in the release of many previously confined patients.[10]

SUMMARY

Behavioral healthcare in the military differs from the civilian practice in one distinct way: military behavioral health providers are tasked to conserve the fighting strength of the military. Thus, although they treat individuals, their focus is on the overall institution. Military providers accomplish their mission by caring for both US military personnel and their families. These providers, however, can be distracted by the situations that inevitably arise when complex mental health issues are reported in a simplified manner. The media can bring attention to areas indeed needing corrective action; however, the media can also sensationalize stories, as evidenced by titles like "Potent Mixture: Zoloft & a Rifle."[11]

The accurate presentation of behavioral health data is essential to combat and operational stress policy and doctrine; however, when data are misunderstood or reported out of context, they can undermine popular support for soldiers and potentially impact soldiers' mental health. Possible areas of operational consequences due to media coverage include changing policies on evacuation of behavioral health casualties, limiting use of psychotropic medication in theater, and lessening the trust in clinician "instincts." This operational impact has been termed the "CNN [Cable News Network] effect" and is seen as a double-edged sword—a "strategic enabler" and a potential operational risk.[12]

It is difficult to quantify the operational impact or strategic effect the media can have on behavioral health planning and execution. However, it is clear that the media are powerful forces shaping the environment in which behavioral health practitioners can work. Therefore, clinicians must be proactive as scientist-practitioners to demonstrate the efficacy of their practices, to plan effective battlefield interventions and operations for combat and operational stress control, and to assist with screening and surveillance of the service members within the scope of their responsibility. The media can also play a crucial role in drawing needed attention to situations in the military affecting soldiers in both garrison and operational settings. This unique convergence of two professional communities can contribute to conserving the fighting strength, which is, of course, the mission of all members of the military medical community.

REFERENCES

1. Miles D. 2003 Suicide rates elevated among [Operation] Iraqi Freedom troops; 2004 rates dip. *American Forces Press Service*. March 25, 2004. Available at: http://www.defenselink.mil/news/newsarticle.aspx?id=27000. Accessed August 4, 2010.

2. Miles D. Army suicide rate in combat zones elevated. *American Forces Press Service*. March 26, 2004. Available at: http://usmilitary.about.com/cs/terrorism/a/arsuicide.htm. Accessed August 4, 2010.

3. Martinez M. Army's suicide rate has outside experts alarmed: most died serving in Iraq after major combat phase. *Baltimore Sun*. December 30, 2003. Available at: http://www.commondreams.org/headlines03/1230-01.htm. Accessed August 4, 2010.

4. Chedekel L, Kauffman M. Army's suicide struggles continue: 2006 rate of self-inflicted deaths in Iraq could exceed record set in 2005. *Hartford Courant*. January 31, 2007. Available at: http://www.courant.com/news/specials/hc-unfit-strugglescont-jan31-2007,0,4648693.story. Accessed August 4, 2010.

5. Swann S, Berry T. Task Force 30th Medical Brigade Commander's Overview: OIF 05-07. ERMC Medical Service Corps Conference, Grassau, Germany, November, 2006.

6. Starr B. Army: HBO documentary could trigger stress disorder. *CNN*. May 15, 2006. Available at: http://www.cnn.com/2006/SHOWBIZ/TV/05/15/baghdad.ER/index.html. Accessed August 4, 2010.

7. McGirk T. Collateral damage or civilian massacre in Haditha? *Time*. March 19, 2006. Available at: http://www.time.com/time/world/article/0,8599,1174649,00.html. Accessed August 4, 2010.

8. Lifton RJ. The psychology of atrocity. *Editor and Publisher*. 2006. Available at: www.editorandpublisher.com/.

9. Kirkland FA. Honor, combat ethics, and military culture. In: Beam TE, Sparacino LR, eds. *Military Medical Ethics.* Vol 1. In: Lounsburg DE, Bellamy RF, eds. *Textbooks of Military Medicine.* Washington, DC: Department of the Army, Office of The Surgeon General, Borden Institute; 2003: 157–198.

10. Szasz TS. *The Myth of Mental Illness: Foundations of a Theory of Personal Conduct.* New York, NY: Hoeber-Harper; 1961.

11. Kauffman M, Chedekel L. Potent mixture: Zoloft & a Rifle. *Hartford Courant.* May 16, 2006. Available at: http://www.courant.com/news/specials/hc-unfitzoloft0516.artmay16,0,3148380.story. Accessed August 4, 2010.

12. Belknap MH. *The CNN Effect: Strategic Enabler or Operational Risk?* Carlisle Barracks, Penn: US Army War College; 2001. Available at: www.au.af.mil/au/awc/awcgate/army-usawc/cnn-belknap.pdf. Accessed August 4, 2010.

ABBREVIATIONS AND ACRONYMS

25th ID: 25th Infantry Division Light
5-HT1a: serotonin

A

AA 77: American Airlines Flight 77
AAA: animal-assisted activity
AAR: after-action review
AAS: American Association of Suicidology
AAT: animal-assisted therapy
ACE: Ask, Care, and Escort
ACGME: American Council of Graduate Medical Education
ACPHP: Army Campaign Plan for Health Promotion, Risk Reduction and Suicide Prevention
ACR: Army Central Registry
ACRM: American Congress of Rehabilitative Medicine
ACS: Army Community Service
ACU: Army combat uniform
ADAPT: Alcohol and other Drug Abuse Prevention Training
ADCO: Alcohol and Drug Control Officer
ADHD: attention deficit hyperactivity disorder
AFB: Air Force Base
AFHSC: Armed Forces Health Surveillance Center
AFIP: Armed Forces Institute of Pathology
AFMAC: Adult Family Member Assistance Center
AFME: Armed Forces Medical Examiner's Office
AHEC: Area Health Education Center
AIT: advanced individual training
AKO: Army Knowledge Online
AMEDD: Army Medical Department
AMEDDC&S: Army Medical Department Center and School
AN: anorexia nervosa
AO: area of operations
AOC: alteration of consciousness
APA: American Psychiatric Association
APA: American Psychological Association
APOE/APOD: aerial point of embarkation/debarkation
AR: Army Regulation
ARNG: Army National Guard
ARS: acute radiation sickness
ARVN: Army of the Republic of Vietnam
ASAM: American Society of Addiction Medicine
ASAP: Army Substance Abuse Program
ASD: acute stress disorder
ASER: Army Suicide Event Report
ASF: aeromedical staging facility
ASIST: Applied Suicide Intervention Skills Training
ASMB: area support medical battalion
ASMC: area support medical company
ASPP: Army Suicide Prevention Program
ASPTF: Army Suicide Prevention Task Force
AST: aspartate aminotransferase
ASVAB: Armed Services Vocational Aptitude Battery
ATM: automated teller machine
AusAID: Australian Agency for International Development
AW2: Army Wounded Warrior
AWOL: absent without leave

B

BAC: blood alcohol concentration
BAMC: Brooke Army Medical Center
BCT: brigade combat team
BDE: brigade
BDU: battle dress uniform
BED: binge-eating disorder
BFG: British Forces Germany
BH: behavioral health
BHL: behavioral health liaison
BHO: behavioral health officer
BICEPS: brevity, immediacy, centrality, expectancy, proximity, and simplicity
BKA: below-the-knee amputation
BMI: body mass index
BN: bulimia nervosa
BRAC: Base Realignment and Closure
BSC: behavioral science consultants
BSHOP: Behavioral and Social Health Outcomes Program

C

CAAC: Child and Adolescent Assistance Center
CACO: casualty assistance call officer
CanMEDS: Canadian Medical Education Directions for Specialists
CAO: casualty assistance officer
CAPS: Child and Adolescent Psychiatry Service
CASF: contingency aeromedical staging facility
CAST: Chaplain Annual Sustainment Training
CBRN: chemical, biological, radiological, and nuclear
CBRNE: chemical, biological, radiological, nuclear, and explosive
CBT: cognitive-behavioral therapy
CDC: Centers for Disease Control and Prevention
CDT: carbohydrate deficient transferrin
CED: critical event debriefing
CENTCOM: Central Command
CG/USARV: Commanding General, United States Army Republic of Vietnam
CHCS: Composite Health Care System
CHCS-ITT: Composite Health Care System–Interactive Training Tool
CHE: complex humanitarian emergency
CHPC: Community Health Promotion Council
CHPPM: Center for Health Promotion and Preventive Medicine
CID: Criminal Investigation Division
CIP: command interest profile
CIR: critical incident report
CISD: critical incident stress debriefing
CISM: critical incident stress management
Civ: civilian
CMAOC: Casualty and Mortuary Affairs Operation Center
CMO: civil-military operations
CMOC: civil-military operations center
CNN: Cable News Network
CO: Company
COMT: catechol-o-methyltransferase
COMUSMACV: Commander US Military Assistance Command, Vietnam
CONUS: continental United States
COSB: combat and operational stress behavior
COSC: combat and operational stress control
COSC-WARS: Combat/Operational Stress Control Workload Activity Reporting System
COSFA: combat and operational stress first aid
COSR: combat and operational stress reaction
COSR/SR: combat and operational stress/staff resiliency
COTA: certified occupational therapy assistant
COX-2: cyclooxygenase-2
CPIP: Clinical Psychology Internship Program
CPT: cognitive processing therapy
CQ: charge of quarters
CRH: corticotropin-releasing hormone

CSC: combat stress control
CSC: combat stress casualty
CSCT: combat stress control team
CSF: cerebrospinal fluid
CSF: Comprehensive Soldier Fitness
CSH: combat support hospital
CSR: combat stress reaction
CT: cognitive therapy
CT: computed tomography
CY: calendar year
CYP2D6: cytochrome p450 enzyme

D

DA: Department of the Army
DAI: diffuse axonal injury
DAMIS: Drug and Alcohol Management Information System
DCCS: deputy chief of clinical services
DCMH: Department of Community Mental Health
DCOE: Defense Centers of Excellence
DCS: Deployment Cycle Support
DCSP: Deployment Cycle Support Program
DEROS: date of expected return from overseas
DHC: Deployment Health Clinic
DHEA: dehydroepiandrosterone
DHHS: Department of Health and Human Services
DIF: division internment facility
DISCOM: Division Support Command
DMH: division mental health
DMHA: division mental health activity
DMHS: defense mental health services
DMHS: division mental health section
DNA: deoxyribonucleic acid
DNBI: disease nonbattle injury
DoD: Department of Defense
DoDSER: Department of Defense Suicide Event Report
DoE: Department of Education
DRRI: Deployment Risk and Resilience Inventory
DSB: division support battalion
DSCOT: doctorate of science in occupational therapy
DSM: *Diagnostic and Statistical Manual of Mental Disorders*
DSM-III: *Diagnostic and Statistical Manual of Mental Disorders*, 3rd edition
DSM-III-R: *Diagnostic and Statistical Manual of Mental Disorders*, 3rd edition, revised
DSM-IV: *Diagnostic and Statistical Manual of Mental Disorders*, 4th edition
DSM-IV-TR: *Diagnostic and Statistical Manual of Mental Disorders*, 4th edition, text revision
DSN: Defense Satellite Network
DTI: diffusion tensor imaging
DUI: driving under the influence
DVA: Department of Veterans Affairs
DVBIC: Defense and Veterans Brain Injury Center
DWI: driving while intoxicated
DWMMC: Deployed Warrior Medical Management Center

E

ECT: electroconvulsant therapy
EDNOS: eating disorder not otherwise specified
EEG: electroencephalography
EFMP: Exceptional Family Member Program
EMDR: eye movement desensitization and reprocessing
EMF: expeditionary medical facility
EPA: Environmental Protection Agency
EPICON: epidemiological consultation
EPS: extrapyramidal symptom
ER: emergency room
EtG: ethyl glucuronide
ETOh: ethanol

F

FAP: Family Advocacy Program
FDA: Food and Drug Administration
FEMA: Federal Emergency Management Agency
FLAIR: fluid attenuated inversion recovery
FM: Field Manual
FMHT: field mental health team
FOB: forward operating base
FORSCOM: Forces Command
FRAGO: fragmentary order
FRG: family readiness group
FSB: forward support battalion
FSMC: forward support medical company

G

G-3: operations
G-5: civil-military operations officer
GABA: gamma-amino butyric acid
GAO: Government Accountability Office
GCS: Glasgow Coma Scale
GDP: gross domestic product
GE: gradient echo
GERD: gastroesophageal reflux disease
GGT: gamma glutamyl transferase
GI: government issue
GKO: Guard Knowledge Online
GME: graduate medical education
GOAT: Galveston Orientation and Amnesia Test
GPMRC: Global Patient Movement Requirements Center
GSA: GWOT Support Assignment
GTA: graphic training aid
GTO: girls' time out
GTP: guanine triphosphate
GWOT: global war on terror

H

HA: humanitarian assistance
hemcon: hemorrhage control
HI: homicidal ideation
HIPAA: Health Insurance Portability and Accountability Act
HIV/AIDS: human immunodeficiency virus/acquired immunodeficiency syndrome
HMMWV: high mobility multipurpose wheeled vehicle
HOPE: Health Opportunities for People Everywhere
HOSP: hospital
HPA: hypothalamic-pituitary-adrenocortical
HPI: history of present illness
HRA: Health Risk Appraisal
HS: hour of sleep (at bedtime)

I

IA: individual augmentation
IBTC: installation biochemical testing coordinator
ICD-10: *International Classification of Diseases*, 10th edition
ICD-9: *International Classification of Diseases*, 9th edition
ICD-9-CM: *International Classification of Diseases*, 9th edition, clinical modification
ICP: intracranial pressure
ICRC: International Committee of the Red Cross
ICU: intensive care unit
ICW: intermediate care ward

ID: Infantry Division
IDF: Israeli Defence Forces
IDP: internally displaced person
IED: improvised explosive device
IMA: installation management activity
IMCOM: Installation Management Command
IOM: Institute of Medicine
IPT: interpersonal therapy
IRT: imagery rehearsal therapy
ISAF: International Security Assistance Force
ISP: inpatient service provider
ITO: in the theater of operations

J

JAG: Judge Advocate General
JFHQ: Joint Forces Headquarters
JIDC: Joint Interrogation Debriefing Center
JLIST: Joint Service Integrated Suit Technology
JPTA: Joint Patient Tracking Application

K

KCMHR: King's Centre for Military Health Research
KIA: killed in action
KO teams: hospital augmentation detachments

L

LINN: Living in the New Normal
LMF: lack of moral fiber
LO: liaison office
LOC: loss of consciousness
LOD: line-of-duty
LRMC: Landstuhl Regional Medical Center
LSA: logistic support area
LSD: lysergic acid diethylamide

M

MACE: Military Acute Concussion Evaluation
MATC: Military Advanced Training Center
MCEC: Military Child Education Coalition
MCE: mass casualty event
MCV: mean corpuscular volume
MDNOS: mood disorder not otherwise specified
MEB: medical evaluation board
MED: medical
MEDCAP: medical civic action program
MEDCMO: medical civil-military operations
MEDCOM: Medical Command
MEDDAC: Medical Department Activity
MEDEVAC: medical evacuation
MEF: marine expeditionary force
MEPS: Military Entrance Processing Station
METT-TC: mission, enemy, terrain and weather, troops and support available, time available, and civil considerations
MFLC: Military Family Life Consultant
MHAT: Mental Health Advisory Team
MHCS: Mental Health Consultation Service
MHCTO: Mental Health Casualty Tracker for OIF
Mil: military
MIRECC: Mental Illness Research, Education, and Clinic Center
MMB: multifunctional medical brigade
MNC-I: Multi-National Corps–Iraq
MNF-I: Multi-National Force–Iraq
MOA: memorandum of agreement
MOD: Ministry of Defence
MOPP: mission-oriented protective posture
MOS: military occupational specialty
MP: military police
MRE: meal, ready-to-eat
MRE: military rules of evidence
MRI: medical reengineering initiative
MRI: magnetic resonance imaging
MRO: medical review officer
MS: multiple sclerosis
MSB: main support battalion
MSE: mental status evaluation
mTBI: mild traumatic brain injury
MTD: Medical Transient Detachment
MTF: medical treatment facility
MTOE: modified Table of Organization and Equipment
MUPS: medically unexplained physical symptoms
MWR: Morale, Welfare and Recreation

N

NATO: North Atlantic Treaty Organization
NBC: nuclear, biological, and chemical
NBCOT: National Board for Certification in Occupational Therapy
NCA: National Capital Area
NCO: noncommissioned officer
NCOER: noncommissioned officer evaluation report
NCOIC: noncommissioned officer in charge
NCPTSD: National Center for PTSD
NE: norepinephrine
NES: night-eating syndrome
NGB: National Guard Bureau
NGF : nerve growth factor
NGO: nongovernmental organization
NMDA: *N*-methyl-D-aspartic acid
NNMC: National Naval Medical Center
NPDB: National Practitioner Data Bank
NPSP: New Parent Support Program
NPY: neuropeptide Y
NSAID: nonsteroidal antiinflammatory drug
NVA: North Vietnamese Army
NVVRS: National Vietnam Veterans Readjustment Study
NYDN: not yet diagnosed neurological

O

OCCH: Office of the Chief of Chaplains
OCD: obsessive-compulsive disorder
OCONUS: outside the continental United States
ODS/S: Operation Desert Shield/Storm
OEF: Operation Enduring Freedom
OER: officer evaluation report
OIF: Operation Iraqi Freedom
OIF 05-07: Operation Iraqi Freedom 05-07
OIF I: Operation Iraqi Freedom One
OIF-II: Operation Iraqi Freedom Two
OIH: opioid-induced hyperalgesia
OMUS: outbreak of multiple unexplained symptoms
ONE: Operation Noble Eagle
OPNAVIST: Operational Navy Instruction
OPTEMPO: operations tempo
OR: operating room
OSCAR: Operational Stress Control and Readiness
OT: occupational therapy
OTA: occupational therapy assistant
OTSG: Office of The Surgeon General
OUA: Operation Unified Assistance

P

P-U-L-H-E-S: profile serial system

PAM: Pamphlet
PAO: public affairs office/officer
PA: physician assistant
PASBA: Patient Administration Systems and Biostatistics Activity
PC: psychological casualty
PCA: patient-controlled analgesia
PCLS: Psychiatry Consultation Liaison Service
PCM: primary care management
PCOS: postcombat and operational stress
PDHA: Post-Deployment Health Assessment
PDHA: predeployment health assessment
PDHRA: Post-Deployment Health Re-Assessment
PDPA: People's Democratic Party of Afghanistan
PE: prolonged exposure
PET: positron emission tomography
PFA: psychological first aid
PFA: personal fitness assessment
PGA-CI: Parent Guidance Assessment–Combat Injured
PGD: prolonged grief disorder
PH: psychological health
PHC(P): Public Health Command (Provisional)
PHI : protected health information
PICK: Premarital Interpersonal Choices and Knowledge
PKC: protein kinase C
PMCS: Preventative Maintenance Checks and Services
PMD: psychiatric mental disorder
PMDD: premenstrual dysphoric disorder
PMP: Preventive Medical Psychiatry
PMR: Patient Movement Record, Patient Movement Requirement, or Patient Movement Request
po: per os (by mouth, orally)
POC: point of contact
POPM: Proponency of Preventive Medicine
POW: prisoner of war
PROFIS: Professional Officer Filler Information System
ProQOL: Professional Quality of Life Scale
PRT: provider resiliency training
PSA: prostate-specific antigen
PSP: patient support pallet
PsySTART: psychological simple triage and rapid treatment
PT: physical training
PTA: posttraumatic amnesia
PTE: potentially traumatic event
PTG: posttraumatic growth
PTSD: posttraumatic stress disorder
PTSS: posttraumatic stress symptoms

Q

q: quodque (every)
QPR: Question, Persuade, Refer

R

R&R: rest and recuperation
RAF: Royal Air Force
RANKL: receptor activator of nuclear factor-κB ligand
RASS: Richmond Agitation-Sedation Score
RCS: Readjustment Counseling Service
RCT: randomized controlled trial
REM: rapid eye movement
RFO: request for orders
RGA: retrograde amnesia
RMC: regional medical center
RNAi: antisense ribonucleic acid
ROE: rules of engagement
RRC: Regional Readiness Command
RRC: residency review committee
RTD: return to duty
RTU: return to unit

S

S-3: operations officer
SA: substance abuse
SAC: Soldier Assistance Center
SAC: Standardized Assessment of Concussion
SAFAC: Soldier and Family Assistance Center
SAMHSA: Substance Abuse and Mental Health Services Administration
SARS: severe acute respiratory syndrome
SAV: staff assistance visit
SDH: subdural hemorrhage
SDQ: Strengths and Difficulties Questionnaire
SERE: Survival, Evasion, Resistance, and Escape
SeRV-MH: Services for Returning Veterans-Mental Health
SFLC: Soldier and Family Life Consultants
SI: suicidal ideation
SIC: stress injury continuum
SIR: serious incident report
SIT: stress inoculation training
SITREP: situation report
SME: subject matter expert
SM: service member
SNP: single-nucleotide polymorphism
SNRI: serotonin-norepinephrine reuptake inhibitor
SNS: sympathetic nervous system
SOP: standard operating procedure
SPPM: suicide prevention program manager
SPRINT: Special Psychiatric Rapid Intervention Team
SPSS: Statistical Package for the Social Sciences (version 16, SPSS Inc, Chicago, IL)
SRMSO: Suicide Risk Management and Surveillance Office
sRNA: small ribonucleic acid molecules
SRP: Soldier Readiness Program
SSRI: selective serotonin reuptake inhibitor
STOAL: short take off and landing
SWAPP: Soldier Wellness Assessment Pilot Program
SWEP: Solomon Wellness Educational Program
SWET: sewer, water, electricity, and trash

T

TAI: traumatic axonal injury
TAMC: Tripler Army Medical Center
TAPS: Tragedy Assistance Program for Survivors
TBI: traumatic brain injury
TCA: tricyclic antidepressant
TEM: traumatic event management
TF 30 Med: Task Force 30th Medical Brigade
THR: target heart rate
TIF: tertiary internment facility or theater internment facility
TIPPS: Therapeutic Intervention for the Prevention of Psychiatric Stress
TMD: temporomandibular dysfunction
TMI: Three Mile Island
TMIP: theater medical information program
TOE: Table of Organization and Equipment
TRAC2ES: TRANSCOM Regulating and Command and Control Evacuation System
TRANSCOM: Transportation Command
TRiM: Trauma Risk Management
TSG: The Surgeon General
TSH: thyroid-stimulating hormone
TTY: text telephone
TWA: Trans World Airlines

U

UBHNA: Unit Behavioral Health Needs Assessment
UCMJ: Uniform Code of Military Justice
UK: United Kingdom
UMT: unit ministry team
UN: United Nations
UNHCR: UN High Commissioner for Refugees
UNICEF: United Nations Children's Fund
USAID: US Agency for International Development
USAMEDCOMV: US Army Medical Command Vietnam
USAR: US Army Reserves
USAREUR: US Army, Europe
USARV: US Army Republic of Vietnam
USDOT: US Department of Transportation
USMACV: United States Military Assistance Command, Vietnam
USPHS: US Public Health Service
USUHS: Uniformed Services University of the Health Sciences

V

VA: Veterans Affairs
VA: Veterans' Administration (pre-1980 name)
VAS: verbal or visual (or both) analogue scales
VBA: Veterans Benefits Administration
VBIED: vehicle-borne improvised explosive device
VCSA: vice chief of staff for the Army
VHA: Veterans Health Administration
VTC: video teleconference

W

w/: with
w/o: without
WHO: World Health Organization
WHO-EURO: World Health Organization Regional Office for Europe
WIA: wounded in action
WICS: wisdom, intelligence, and creativity, synthesized
WRAIR: Walter Reed Army Institute of Research
WRAMC: Walter Reed Army Medical Center
WTC: World Trade Center
WTP: Warrior Transition Program
WTRP: Warrior Training and Rehabilitation Program
WTU: warrior transition unit

INDEX

A

B

D

F

G

H

M

N

O

P

Q

R

S

U

V

W

Y

Z

ISBN 978-0-16-088756-7

90000

9 780160 887567